Nursing the Critically Ill Adult

THIRD EDITION

Brief Contents

UNIT 1: INTRODUCTION 1

CHAPTER 1: Introduction 3
CHAPTER 2: Dimensions in Critical Care Practice 15

UNIT 2: COMMUNICATION 29

CHAPTER 3: Communication: Patient and Family 31

UNIT 3: STIMULATION 49

CHAPTER 4: Stimulation Assessment 51
CHAPTER 5: Stimulation Disorders 80
CHAPTER 6: Stimulation Treatment Techniques and Pain Management 117

UNIT 4: AERATION 133

CHAPTER 7: Aeration Assessment 135
CHAPTER 8: Aeration Disorders 160
CHAPTER 9: Aeration Treatment Techniques 185

UNIT 5: FLUID BALANCE 213

CHAPTER 10: Cardiovascular Physical Assessment 215
CHAPTER 11: Cardiovascular Diagnostic Procedures 237

CHAPTER 12: Dysrhythmias and Conduction Defects 259
CHAPTER 13: Cardiovascular Disorders 304
CHAPTER 14: Cardiovascular Interventions 345
CHAPTER 15: Renal Assessment and Acute Renal Failure 368
CHAPTER 16: Fluid, Electrolyte, and Acid-Base Imbalances 395
CHAPTER 17: Endocrine/Metabolic Disorders and Treatment 426
CHAPTER 18: Hematologic/Immunologic Disorders 445

UNIT 6: NUTRITION 461

CHAPTER 19: Nutrition 461

UNIT 7: ACTIVITY 496

CHAPTER 20: Activity 496
CHAPTER 21: Trauma 519

APPENDIX 1 FANCAS 572
APPENDIX 2 Pharmacology 592
Index 617

Contents

UNIT 1: INTRODUCTION   1

CHAPTER I: INTRODUCTION   3

NURSING MODEL   4
NURSING PROCESS   4
Assessment 6
Diagnosis 8
Planning and Intervention 11

Evaluation 13
CORE CONCEPTS AND SKILLS   13
CONCLUSIONS   13
References 13
Supplemental Reading 14

CHAPTER 2: DIMENSIONS IN CRITICAL CARE PRACTICE   15

THE CRITICAL-CARE ENVIRONMENT   16
ADVANCES IN TECHNOLOGY   17
CHANGES IN THE NURSING ROLE   17
Satisfactions of Critical-Care Nursing 17
Stresses of Critical-Care Nursing 17
STRESS-REDUCTION MECHANISMS   19
ETHICS: PRINCIPLES AND DILEMMAS   20
Types of Ethical Dilemmas 21
LEGAL ISSUES   23
Reasons for Lawsuits 23

Protection Against Lawsuits 24
Special Legal Problems 24
What to Do if You Are Sued 24
EXAMPLE: THE CASE OF ORGAN
DONATION   25
Stress of Organ Donation 25
Ethical Aspects of Organ Donation 26
Legal Aspects of Organ Donation 26
References 27
Supplemental Reading 28

UNIT 2: COMMUNICATION 29

CHAPTER 3: COMMUNICATION: PATIENT AND FAMILY 31

ASSESSMENT 32
Process: History and Physical Examination 32
Content 35
PLANNING AND IMPLEMENTATION OF CARE 38
Impaired Verbal Communication Related to Vision Deficit, Hearing Deficit or Loss of Speech 38
Sensory-Perceptual Alterations Related to Excessive and/or Meaningless Stimuli, Chemical Imbalances, or Drugs 39

Ineffective Individual Coping Related to Crisis 41
Ineffective Family Coping (Compromised or Disabling) Related to Crisis 43
OUTCOME EVALUATION 47
References 47
Supplemental Reading 48

UNIT 3: STIMULATION 49

CHAPTER 4: STIMULATION ASSESSMENT 51

HISTORY 52
PHYSICAL EXAMINATION 52
Assessment of the Level of Consciousness 52
Assessment of Mentation 56
Examination of the Head and Neck 56
Assessment of the Cranial Nerves 57
Assessment of the Sensorimotor Function 62
Examination of the Vital Signs 70

DIAGNOSTIC PROCEDURES 74
Cerebrospinal Fluid Sampling 74
Electroencephalography 75
Computerized Tomography (CT) 75
Cerebral Arteriography 76
Magnetic Resonance Imaging (MRI) 77
References 79
Supplemental Reading 79

CHAPTER 5: STIMULATION DISORDERS 80

INCREASED INTRACRANIAL PRESSURE 81
Assessment 81
Planning and Implementation of Care 86
Outcome Evaluation 89
HERNIATION SYNDROMES 89
Assessment 89
Planning and Implementation of Care 93
Outcome Evaluation 93
STATUS EPILEPTICUS 93
Assessment 94
Planning and Implementation of Care 95
Outcome Evaluation 97

VASCULAR DISORDERS 97
Arterial Syndromes 97
Stroke Classification 97
Diagnosis of Stroke 99
Management of Stroke 100
Planning and Implementation of Care 101
Outcome Evaluation 103
▪ AUTOIMMUNE DISORDERS 103
GUILLAIN-BARRÉ SYNDROME 103
Assessment 103
Planning and Implementation of Care 105
Outcome Evaluation 107

MYASTHENIA GRAVIS 108
Assessment 108
Planning and Implementation of Care 111

Outcome Evaluation 114
References 114
Supplemental Reading 116

CHAPTER 6: STIMULATION TREATMENT TECHNIQUES AND PAIN MANAGEMENT 117

CRANIOTOMY 118
Assessment 118
Preoperative Planning and Implementation 119
Postoperative Planning and Implementation 119
Outcome Evaluation 121
VENTRICULAR SHUNTS 121
Assessment 121

Planning and Implementation of Care 125
Outcome Evaluation 126
PAIN 126
Assessment 126
Planning and Implementation of Care 128
Outcome Evaluation 130
References 130

UNIT 4: AERATION 133

CHAPTER 7: AERATION ASSESSMENT 135

HISTORY AND PHYSICAL EXAMINATION 136
The Lungs and Thorax 137
Inspection 138
Palpation, Percussion, Auscultation 140
PULMONARY FUNCTION TESTS 142
Lung Volumes and Capacities 142
Airway Resistance 145
Compliance 145
Deadspace 146
V_D/V_T Ratio 146
BLOOD GAS VALUES 146
Interpreting Blood Gas Values 146

DIAGNOSTIC PROCEDURES 154
Chest X-ray 154
Lung Scans 157
Bronchoscopy 157
Pulmonary Angiography 158
Thoracentesis 158
Open Lung Biopsy 159
References 159
Supplemental Reading 159

CHAPTER 8: AERATION DISORDERS 160

PULMONARY EDEMA 161
Assessment 161
Planning and Implementation of Care 162
Outcome Evaluation 162
ADULT RESPIRATORY DISTRESS
SYNDROME (ARDS) 163
Assessment 163
Planning and Implementation of Care 165
Outcome Evaluation 166

ATELECTASIS 166
Assessment 168
Planning and Implementation of Care 169
Outcome Evaluation 169
PNEUMONIA 170
Assessment 170
Planning and Implementation of Care 171
Outcome Evaluation 171

PNEUMOTHORAX 171
Assessment 171
Planning and Implementation of Care 172
Outcome Evaluation 173
PLEURAL EFFUSION 173
Assessment 173
Outcome Evaluation 174
PULMONARY EMBOLUS 174
Assessment 174
Planning and Implementation of Care 176
Outcome Evaluation 177

▪ CHRONIC RESPIRATORY FAILURE 177
BRONCHITIS AND EMPHYSEMA 177
Assessment 177
Planning and Implementation of Care 178
Outcome Evaluation 179
STATUS ASTHMATICUS 179
Assessment 180
Planning and Implementation of Care 180
Outcome Evaluation 183
References 183
Supplemental Reading 183

CHAPTER 9: AERATION TREATMENT TECHNIQUES 185

OXYGEN THERAPY 186
Guidelines for Initiation F_1O_2 Selection 186
Methods of Oxygen Therapy 186
Complications 188
Outcome Evaluation 189
CHEST PHYSIOTHERAPY 189
Techniques of Chest PT 189
Outcome Evaluation 192
ARTIFICIAL AIRWAYS 192
Types of Artificial Airways 192
Prevention of Complications 194
Treatment of Complications 196
Removal of Artificial Airways 197
Outcome Evaluation 197
TRACHEAL SUCTIONING 197
Prevention of Complications 198
Treatment of Complications 200
Outcome Evaluation 200

MECHANICAL VENTILATION 201
Procedure for Mechanical Ventilation 201
Prevention of Complications 203
Treatment of Complications 205
Discontinuation of Mechanical Ventilation 206
Outcome Evaluation 207
CHEST DRAINAGE 207
Techniques of Chest Drainage 207
Maintenance of Chest Drainage 208
Prevention of Complications 209
Removal of Chest Tubes 210
Outcome Evaluation 210
THORACIC SURGERY 210
Preoperation Assessment 210
Operative Procedures 210
Postoperative Complications 211
References 211
Supplemental Reading 212

UNIT 5: FLUID BALANCE 213

CHAPTER 10: CARDIOVASCULAR PHYSICAL ASSESSMENT 215

HISTORY 216
PHYSICAL EXAMINATION 218
General Inspection 218
Examination of the Skin 219
Evaluation of Peripheral Arterial Pulses 220

Blood Pressure Auscultation 220
Examination of Neck Veins 226
Examination of the Heart 227
References 236
Supplemental Reading 236

CHAPTER 11: CARDIOVASCULAR DIAGNOSTIC PROCEDURES 237

LABORATORY TESTS 238
Evaluation of Serum Enzymes 238
DIAGNOSTIC PROCEDURES 239
Chest Roentgenology 240
Echocardiography 240
Doppler Ultrasonography 241
Radionuclide Studies 242
Electrophysiologic Studies 244
Cardiac Catheterization 244
Arteriography 247

HEMODYNAMIC MONITORING 247
The Cardiac Cycle and Pressure Waves 247
Uses of Hemodynamic Lines 247
Pressure Measurements 247
Central Venous Pressure (CVP) Lines 249
Pulmonary Arterial (PA) Lines 252
Arterial Lines 257
References 258
Supplemental Reading 258

CHAPTER 12: DYSRHYTHMIAS AND CONDUCTION DEFECTS 259

DYSRHYTHMIA DIAGNOSIS 260
ECG Recording 260
ECG Analysis 264
Common Dysrhythmias 275
Conduction Defects 276
Funny-Looking Beats 292
Differentiation of General ECG Patterns 294
NURSING CARE RELATED TO DYSRHYTHMIA 294
Assessment 294

Risk Conditions 295
Planning and Implementation of Care 301
Intervention 302
Outcome Evaluation 303
References 303
Supplemental Reading 303

CHAPTER 13: CARDIOVASCULAR DISORDERS 304

▪ ACUTE CHEST PAIN 305
▪ ACUTE MYOCARDIAL INFARCTION 307
ASSESSMENT 308
Risk Conditions 308
Signs and Symptoms 308
Diagnostic Procedures 308
PLANNING AND IMPLEMENTATION OF CARE 314
OUTCOME EVALUATION 314
▪ CARDIAC FAILURE 322
ASSESSMENT 323
Risk Conditions 323
Signs and Symptoms 324
PLANNING AND IMPLEMENTATION OF CARE 325
Pharmacologic Therapy 328
OUTCOME EVALUATION 331

▪ ACUTE CARDIAC TAMPONADE 331
ASSESSMENT 331
Risk Conditions 331
Signs and Symptoms 332
PLANNING AND IMPLEMENTATION OF CARE 332
Assisting with Pericardiocentesis 333
OUTCOME EVALUATION 333
▪ SHOCK 333
ASSESSMENT 333
Risk Conditions 333
Pathophysiologic Changes 334
Signs and Symptoms 336
Laboratory Data 337
Prevention 337

PLANNING AND IMPLEMENTATION OF
CARE 339

Alteration in Tissue Perfusion Related to Loss of
Circulating Blood Volume 339

Alteration in Tissue Perfusion Related to Diminished Myocardial Contractility 341

Alteration in Tissue Perfusion Related to Excessive Vasoconstriction 343

Impaired Gas Exchange Related to Ventilation-Perfusion Imbalance 343

Altered Urinary Elimination Related to Decreased
Renal Perfusion 343

Altered Nutrition (Less Than Body Requirements)
Related to Diminished GI Perfusion 343

Definitive Care 344

OUTCOME EVALUATION 344

References 344

Supplemental Reading 344

CHAPTER 14: CARDIOVASCULAR INTERVENTIONS 345

EMERGENCY CARDIAC DRUG THERAPY 346

Sudden Death 346

Emergency Cardiac Drugs 346

Defibrillation and Cardioversion 349

PACEMAKERS 350

Indications 350

Approaches 350

Modes of Pacing 351

Pacing Catheters 352

Bedside Insertion 352

Postinsertion Nursing Care 354

PERCUTANEOUS TRANSLUMINAL
CORONARY ANGIOPLASTY (PTCA) 356

Candidates for PTCA 356

Patient Preparation for PTCA 357

PTCA Procedure 357

Mechanism of Dilatation 358

Care Following PTCA 358

CARDIOPULMONARY BYPASS 359

Principles of Cardiopulmonary Bypass 359

Postoperative Implications of CPB 360

INTRA-AORTIC BALLOON
COUNTERPULSATION 361

Physiologic Effects 362

Indications 362

Equipment 362

Insertion 362

Nursing Care 363

Weaning 364

Conclusions 365

OUTCOME EVALUATION 365

References 366

Supplemental Reading 366

CHAPTER 15: RENAL ASSESSMENT AND ACUTE RENAL FAILURE 368

▪ **ASSESSMENT** 369

HISTORY AND PHYSICAL EXAMINATION 370

LABORATORY TESTS 370

Related Anatomy and Physiology 370

Tests of Renal Function 374

▪ **ACUTE RENAL FAILURE** 376

ASSESSMENT 376

Risk Conditions 376

Signs and Symptoms 377

Phases 378

PLANNING AND IMPLEMENTATION OF
CARE: OLIGURIC PHASE 380

Excess Fluid Volume Related to Inability to Excrete Water and Waste Products 380

Potential for Injury Related to Hyperkalemia-Induced Dysrhythmias 381

Activity Intolerance Related to Anemia 381

Potential for Infection Related to Decreased Immunologic Defenses 381

Potential for Injury Related to Diminished Drug
Excretion 381

Altered Nutrition (Less Than Body Requirements)
Related to GI Distress and Decreased Mental
Alertness 381

Potential Pain Related to Uremic Pericarditis
381

Potential Pain Related to Bone Disease 382

Fear Related to Seriousness of Illness 382

PLANNING AND IMPLEMENTATION OF
CARE: DIURETIC PHASE   382

Potential Fluid Volume Deficit Related to Excessive Diuresis 382

Potential Injury Related to Hypokalemia 382

DIALYSIS   382

Hemodialysis 382

Peritoneal Dialysis 388

Continuous Ultrafiltration/Hemofiltration 390

RENAL TRANSPLANTATION   392

Potential Fluid Volume Deficit 392

Alteration in Tissue Perfusion Related to Graft Rejection 392

Potential for Infection 393

OUTCOME EVALUATION   393

References 393

Supplemental Reading 393

CHAPTER 16: FLUID, ELECTROLYTE, AND ACID-BASE IMBALANCES   395

▪ FLUID AND ELECTROLYTE
  IMBALANCES   396

ASSESSMENT   396

Serial Body Weights 396

Fluid Intake and Output 397

Body Fluid Osmolality 398

Electrolytes 398

FLUID IMBALANCES   399

Fluid Volume Deficit 399

Fluid Volume Excess 400

Outcome Evaluation 400

SODIUM IMBALANCES   401

Roles of Sodium 401

Hyponatremia 401

Hypernatremia 402

Outcome Evaluation 403

POTASSIUM IMBALANCES   404

Roles of Potassium 404

Hypokalemia 404

Hyperkalemia 407

Outcome Evaluation 407

CALCIUM IMBALANCES   408

Roles of Calcium 408

Hypocalcemia 409

Hypercalcemia 410

Outcome Evaluation 411

MAGNESIUM IMBALANCES   411

Roles of Magnesium 411

Hypomagnesemia and Hypermagnesemia 411

Outcome Evaluation 412

▪ ACID-BASE IMBALANCES   413

ASSESSMENT   413

Key Physiologic Concepts 413

Classification of Acid-Base Imbalances 414

Overview of Imbalances 414

Signs and Symptoms 417

Arterial Blood Gas Analysis 418

Electrolyte Imbalances 421

Other Laboratory Data 423

PLANNING AND IMPLEMENTATION OF
CARE   423

Respiratory Acidosis 423

Respiratory Alkalosis 424

Metabolic Alkalosis 424

Mixed Disorders 424

General Nursing Care Measures 424

OUTCOME EVALUATION   424

References 424

Supplemental Reading 425

CHAPTER 17: ENDOCRINE/METABOLIC DISORDERS AND TREATMENT   426

▪ DIABETIC KETOACIDOSIS   427

ASSESSMENT   427

Pathophysiology 427

Risk Conditions 427

Signs and Symptoms 428

Laboratory Tests 428

PLANNING AND IMPLEMENTATION OF
CARE   428

Fluid Volume Deficit Related to Urinary Losses Secondary to Osmotic Diuresis 428

Chemical Imbalance Related to Electrolyte Losses and Lack of Insulin 429

Acid-Base Imbalance Related to Abundance of Metabolic Acids Secondary to Insulin Deficiency 430

Sensory-Perceptual Alteration Related to Changes in Level of Consciousness Secondary to Cellular Dehydration 430

Altered Gas Exchange Related to Respiratory Pattern Changes Secondary to Acidosis and Decreased Level of Consciousness 430

Knowledge Deficit Related to Mechanisms of DKA 430

OUTCOME EVALUATION 430

▪ HYPERGLYCEMIC HYPEROSMOLAR NONKETOTIC COMA 431

ASSESSMENT 431

Risk Conditions 431

Signs and Symptoms 431

PLANNING AND IMPLEMENTATION OF CARE 432

Fluid Volume Deficit Related to Decreased Volume Secondary to Osmotic Diuresis 432

Chemical Imbalance Related to Changes in Serum Levels Secondary to Relative Lack of Insulin 432

Sensory-Perceptual Alteration Related to Decreased Level of Consciousness Secondary to Cellular Dehydration 433

Alteration in Tissue Perfusion Related to Decreased Plasma Volume Secondary to Osmotic Diuresis 433

Altered Respiratory Function Related to a Disturbance in Respiratory Center Functioning 433

Knowledge Deficit Related to Insufficient Information Regarding Mechanisms of HHNK and Prevention 433

OUTCOME EVALUATION 433

▪ HYPOGLYCEMIA 434

ASSESSMENT 434

Risk Conditions 434

Signs and Symptoms 434

Chemical Imbalance Related to Low Serum Glucose Level 434

Sensory-Perceptual Alteration Related to Decreased Cerebral Cellular Metabolism Secondary to Hypoglycemia 435

Knowledge Deficit Related to Mechanisms of Hypoglycemia 435

OUTCOME EVALUATION 435

▪ THYROID CRISIS 435

ASSESSMENT 435

Risk Conditions 435

PLANNING AND IMPLEMENTATION OF CARE 436

Fluid Volume Deficit Related to Increased Metabolic Activity Secondary to Increased Circulating Thyroid Hormone 436

Potential Alteration in Body Temperature Related to Increased Metabolic Activity Secondary to Increased Thyroid Hormone 436

Potential Decreased Cardiac Output Related to Increased Cardiac Workload Secondary to Increased Adrenergic Activity 436

Potential for Impaired Gas Exchange Related to Decreased Muscle Strength Secondary to Protein and Muscle Catabolism 437

Alteration in Nutrition: Less Than Body Requirements Related to Increased Nutrient Requirements Secondary to Increased Metabolic Activity 437

OUTCOME EVALUATION 437

▪ THERAPEUTIC HYPOTHERMIA 437

ASSESSMENT 437

Candidates 437

Signs and Symptoms 438

PLANNING AND IMPLEMENTATION OF CARE 438

Introduction of Therapeutic Hypothermia 438

Expected and Potential Effects 439

REWARMING 442

Possible Complications 443

OUTCOME EVALUATION 444

References 444

Supplemental Reading 444

CHAPTER 18: HEMATOLOGIC/IMMUNOLOGIC DISORDERS 445

LABORATORY TESTS 446

Complete Blood Count (CBC) and Reticulocyte Count 446

Blood Coagulation 448

▪ DISSEMINATED INTRAVASCULAR COAGULATION (DIC) 450

ASSESSMENT 450

Risk Conditions 450

Signs and Symptoms 451

PLANNING AND IMPLEMENTATION OF CARE 451

Fluid Volume Deficit Related to Bleeding 451

Potential Fluid Volume Excess Related to Frequent Infusions 453

Pain Related to Tissue Ischemia 453

Impaired Skin Integrity Related to Ischemia 453

Altered Tissue Perfusion Related to Peripheral Microthrombi 453

Altered Urinary Elimination Related to Renal Microthrombi 453

Impaired Gas Exchange Related to Pulmonary Microthrombi 454

Altered Level of Consciousness Related to Neurological Microthrombi 454

Altered Oral Mucous Membrane Related to Ischemia 454

Fear Related to the Unknown and to Death 454

Disturbed Self-Concept Related to Loss of Ability to Care for Self and Unattractive Appearance 454

OUTCOME EVALUATION 454

▪ ACQUIRED IMMUNE DEFICIENCY SYNDROME 454

ASSESSMENT 454

Pathophysiology 454

Risk Conditions 455

Signs and Symptoms 455

PLANNING AND IMPLEMENTATION OF CARE 456

Altered Gas Exchange Related to Diffuse Consolidative Process 456

Sensory-Perceptual Alteration Related to Viral Invasion of the CNS 456

Potential for Additional Infection Related to Decreased Immune Function 457

Altered Nutrition: Less Than Body Requirements, Related to Anxiety, Diarrhea, and Increased Metabolic Need 457

Impaired Tissue Integrity Related to Bedrest and Deficient Immune System 457

Altered Comfort: Pain Related to Damaged Nerves, Edema, and Immobility 457

Self-Care Deficit Related to Progressive Weakness 458

Anxiety Related to Life-Threatening Illness 458

Fluid Deficit 458

OUTCOME EVALUATION 458

CURRENT INVESTIGATIONAL AREAS 458

CURRENT GUIDELINES FOR PREVENTING TRANSMISSION OF HIV 459

References 459

Supplemental Reading 460

UNIT 6: NUTRITION 461

CHAPTER 19: NUTRITION 461

▪ GASTROINTESTINAL SYSTEM (GI) 462

GI ASSESSMENT 462

History 462

Physical Examination 462

UPPER GI HEMORRHAGE 465

Assessment 465

Planning and Implementation of Care 466

Outcome Evaluation 473

ACUTE PANCREATITIS 473

Assessment 473

Planning and Implementation of Care 474

Outcome Evaluation 475

HEPATITIS 475

Assessment 475

Diagnosis 476

Planning and Implementation of Care 477

Guidelines for Prophylaxis 477

Outcome Evaluation 478

LIVER FAILURE 478

Liver Functions 478

Assessment 478

Planning and Implementation of Care 480

Outcome Evaluation 482

▪ NOURISHMENT OF THE CRITICALLY ILL 482

NUTRITIONAL ASSESSMENT 482

History 482

Physical Examination 483

Laboratory Data 484
MALNUTRITION   485
Physiology of Starvation 485
Planning and Implementation of Care 486

Outcome Evaluation 494
References 494
Supplemental Reading 495

UNIT 7: ACTIVITY   496

CHAPTER 20: ACTIVITY   496

ASSESSMENT   497
History 497
Physical Examination 498
Diagnostic Procedures and Laboratory Tests
    498
PLANNING AND IMPLEMENTATION OF
CARE   498
Fluid Balance 498
Aeration 501

Nutrition 502
Communication 502
Activity 503
Stimulation 508
OUTCOME EVALUATION   514
References 516
Supplemental Reading 518

CHAPTER 21: TRAUMA   519

▪ INTRODUCTION   520
NURSING ROLES   521
▪ MULTIPLE TRAUMA   522
KEY CONCEPTS   522
Principles of Injury in Blunt Trauma 523
Principles of Injury in Penetrating Trauma 524
ASSESSMENT   525
Risk Conditions 525
History 525
Physical Examination 526
Cardinal Rules in Major Multiple Trauma 527
PLANNING AND IMPLEMENTATION OF
CARE, EMERGENT PERIOD   527
Ineffective Airway Clearance Related to Ob-
    structed Airway 528
Ineffective Breathing Patterns 529
Impaired Gas Exchange 529
Alteration in Cardiac Output: Decreased 529
Decreased Tissue Perfusion Related to Acute
    Loss of Circulating Blood Volume 530
Fluid Volume Deficit Related to Acute Loss of
    Circulating Blood Volume 530
Altered Tissue Perfusion: Cerebral 530

Impaired Physical Mobility Related to Spinal Cord
    Injury 531
OUTCOME EVALUATION, EMERGENT
PERIOD   531
PLANNING AND IMPLEMENTATION OF
CARE, ACUTE PERIOD   532
Potential for Infection 532
Impaired Tissue Integrity 532
Ineffective Individual/Family Coping Related to
    Traumatic Experience 532
OUTCOME EVALUATION, ACUTE PERIOD   533
SUMMARY   533
▪ HEAD INJURY   533
ASSESSMENT   533
Mechanism of Injury 533
PLANNING AND IMPLEMENTATION OF
CARE   536
Maintaining a Patent Airway with Adequate Re-
    spiratory Exchange 536
Monitoring and Assessing Neurologic Status 537
Preventing/Controlling IICP 537
Maintaining Normal Body Functions 537
Preventing/Controlling Seizure Activity 538

Preventing/Controlling Infection 538

OUTCOME EVALUATION   538

▪ **SPINAL CORD TRAUMA**   **539**

KEY CONCEPTS   539

Mechanisms of Injury 539

Classification of Spinal Cord Injury 539

ASSESSMENT IN THE EMERGENCY
DEPARTMENT   541

PLANNING AND IMPLEMENTATION OF
CARE   541

Potential Ineffective Breathing Pattern Related to
  Spinal Cord Injury 542

Potential Altered Tissue Perfusion Related to
  Spinal Cord Shock 542

Potential Ineffective Thermoregulation Related to
  Spinal Cord Shock 542

Impaired Physical Mobility Related to Spinal Cord
  Injury 542

Altered Urinary Elimination Pattern Related to
  Spinal Cord Injury 542

Altered Bowel Elimination Related to Spinal Cord
  Injury 542

Alteration in Comfort: Pain Related to Injury or
  Surgical Intervention 542

Potential for Infection 543

Altered Tissue Perfusion Related to Autonomic
  Dysreflexia 543

Disturbance in Self-Concept: Body Image, Self-
  Esteem, Role Performance, Personal Identity
  Related to Spinal Cord Injury 543

OUTCOME EVALUATION   544

▪ **CHEST TRAUMA**   **545**

KEY CONCEPTS   545

Etiology 545

Mechanism of Injury 545

Pathophysiology 546

ASSESSMENT   546

Signs and Symptoms 546

Diagnostic Considerations 546

PLANNING AND IMPLEMENTATION OF
CARE   548

Resuscitation and Stabilization 548

Impaired Gas Exchange 548

Ineffective Breathing Patterns 548

Fluid Volume Deficit Related to Blood Loss 548

Alteration in Comfort: Pain Related to Disruption
  of Nerves and Tissues 548

OUTCOME EVALUATION   549

▪ **ABDOMINAL TRAUMA**   **549**

ASSESSMENT   549

Signs and Symptoms 549

Diagnostic Considerations 550

PLANNING AND IMPLEMENTATION OF
CARE   551

Fluid Volume Deficit Related to Blood Loss 551

Potential for Infection Related to Ruptured Hollow
  Viscus 551

OUTCOME EVALUATION   552

▪ **ORTHOPEDIC TRAUMA**   **552**

ASSESSMENT   552

Risk Conditions 552

Pathophysiologic Changes 552

Signs and Symptoms 553

Diagnostic Considerations 554

PLANNING AND IMPLEMENTATION OF
CARE   554

Alteration in Comfort: Pain 555

Impaired Skin Integrity 555

Selected Orthopedic Injuries 555

Selected Complications 556

Definitive Care 557

OUTCOME EVALUATION   557

▪ **BURNS**   **557**

KEY CONCEPTS   557

ASSESSMENT   557

Signs and Symptoms 558

PLANNING AND IMPLEMENTATION OF
CARE   561

Pain Related to Continued Burning or Exposure of
  Sensory Receptors 561

Impaired Gas Exchange Related to Upper and
  Lower Airway Injury 561

Decreased Cardiac Output Related to Burn Shock
  and Other Factors 562

Potential Decreased Cardiac Output Related to
  Potassium Imbalances 563

Decreased Tissue Perfusion Related to Progressive Thrombosis 563

Altered Urinary Elimination Pattern Related to
  Volume Changes 564

Altered Bowel Elimination Related to Paralytic
  Ileus and Gastric Hemorrhage 564

Potential Altered Level of Consciousness 564

Potential for Injury Related to Anemia 564

Ineffective Thermoregulation Related to Heat
  Loss 564

Altered Nutrition Related to Stress Response 564

Potential for Infection Related to Broken Skin, Traumatized Tissue, and Suppressed Inflammatory Response 565

Potential Impaired Gas Exchange Related to Shock, Trauma, and Infection 565

Potential Activity Intolerance Related to Contractures 566

Potential Poor Wound Healing Related to Inadequate Wound Care 566

Potential Ineffective Individual and/or Family Coping Related to Psychotraumatic Experience 568

OUTCOME EVALUATION   569

APPENDIX 1 FANCAS   572

APPENDIX 2 Pharmacology   592

Index   617

Preface

Clinical insight—that intuitive "knowing" or grasp of a situation that enables you to be intimately involved in a patient's care and yet "there" for the patient on an emotional level—is an amalgam of perceptual awareness, practical knowledge, expertise, and clinical experience. But just how important is insight in the high-technology world of the critical-care unit?

Nursing diagnosis is a concept that fires the imagination. But given the day-to-day reality of a busy critical-care unit, can you translate the concept into practice? And more importantly, does nursing diagnosis actually improve the quality of patient care?

This text is founded on three key beliefs: that clinical insight distinguishes the nurse who is merely technically competent from the one who is an expert clinician; that nursing diagnosis is *central* to the provision of professional nursing care; and that nursing diagnosis is the link between technology and humanism in the critical-care environment.

Continuing Features

The third edition continues the tradition of excellence established by the first edition, winner of an *American Journal of Nursing* Book of the Year award, and the second edition, the first critical-care book to use nursing diagnosis as an organizing theme. The book retains many popular features, including:

- Anatomy and physiology *integrated* into all the steps of the nursing process

- The emphasis on nursing diagnosis, utilizing the diagnoses approved by the North American Nursing Diagnosis Association's (NANDA) Seventh Conference (1986). The text is specially designed to develop confidence and competence in applying nursing diagnosis in day-to-day critical-care nursing practice. Easy-to-find screened boxes emphasize the most appropriate nursing diagnoses for each disorder discussed. The diagnoses also provide structure for the presentation of related nursing interventions.

- An emphasis on practical applications of clinically relevant information

- Specific outcome criteria for evaluating the effectiveness of nursing care

- Critical-care pharmacology in an easy-to-use format that emphasizes anticipated effects and nursing responsibilities

- FANCAS, the conceptual framework developed by a nurse that focuses on patient needs for Fluid balance, Aeration, Nutrition, Communication, Activity, and Stimulation

New Features

Several distinguishing new features have been added to the third edition. They include:

- Clinical Insights opening each chapter, described in the next section.

- Nursing Research Boxes, that concisely report nursing research findings on topics of importance to critical-care nurses.

- Nursing Care Plans on shock, cardiac failure, renal failure, adult respiratory distress syndrome (ARDS), gastrointestinal bleeding, and cerebral aneurysm.

- *New content* on neurovascular disorders, acquired autoimmune deficiency syndrome (AIDS), percutaneous transluminal coronary angioplasty (PTCA), continuous arteriovenous hemofiltration (CAVH), neurologic, cardiac, and pulmonary surgery, and other topics.

- A new chapter, "Dimensions in Critical Care Practice," that explores the intricacies of the intensive care unit: technological advances, nursing role changes, stress, ethical dilemmas, legal issues, and organ donation.

- An entirely new chapter on trauma.

Clinical Insights

These insights, unique among critical-care books, are paradigms that illuminate the day-to-day practice of critical-care nursing. (A paradigm case is a clinical experience that forever alters the nurse's way of perceiving and interpreting clinical situations.) Although the paradigms describe the utilization of a skill or care of a person with a disorder described in the chapter, they also are designed to be appreciated on their own. Taken together, the paradigms poignantly present the issues important to critical-care nurses and illuminate with crystalline clarity the individual acts of grace and mercy that form the tapestry of expert nursing practice in critical care.

The paradigms draw on the research of Benner, Diekelmann, Crabtree, Jorgenson, and Tanner.[1] In her groundbreaking work, Benner (1984) provided a description of expert nursing care within the context of everyday practice. Her journey of exploration, intended to uncover the knowledge embedded in clinical nursing practice, asked nurses to describe critical incidents, as well as typical and atypical days at work. Analysis of their responses revealed 31 expert competencies derived from actual nursing practice. As Benner emphasizes, these competencies, not intended to be a complete description of nursing expertise, can only be understood within the context of a situation; and that is why these insights are brought to you in the nurse's own words.

The Crabtree and Jorgenson study, a part of Diekelmann's research, extended Benner's work by focusing exclusively on critical-care nurses and asking them to compare their practice to Benner's competencies. Their research provided further insight into the values and behaviors of expert nurses. Benner and Tanner honed in on how expert nurses use intuition.

Paradigms uncovered in these studies are exemplars—positive examples, to be used as models. Together, they represent a wide variety of the 31 competencies, and a stimulus for thoughtful reflection on your own practice.

Overview

Chapter 1 introduces the concepts central to the book, particularly nursing diagnosis, the development of excellence in critical-care nursing, and the competencies of expert nurses. Chapter 2 discusses professional issues in critical care. Chapter 3 examines the emotional experience of critical illness, focusing on crisis stage, family needs, and communication techniques. Chapters 4–21 present clinical information, grouped into units that progress from patient assessment techniques through diagnostic techniques, clinical disorders, and related interventions. Appendix 1 describes the FANCAS model and presents a patient assessment and care plan based on it. Appendix 2 presents critical-care pharmacology you'll want to have at your fingertips.

[1]Benner, Patricia (1984): *From Novice to Expert: Excellence and Power in Clinical Nursing Practice.* Menlo Park: Addison-Wesley Publishing.
Benner, Patricia and Christine Tanner (1987): "Clinical judgment: how expert nurses use intuition." *Am J Nurs* 87:23–31.

Crabtree, Anne and Marcy Jorgenson (1986): "Exploring the practical knowledge in expert critical-care nursing practice." Unpublished master's thesis, University of Wisconsin, Madison.
Diekelmann, Nancy, Anne Crabtree and Marcy Jorgenson (1987): "Preserving personhood in the ICU—a Heideggerian hermeneutical analysis of the paradigm cases of expert critical-care nurses." Unpublished research manuscript, University of Wisconsin, Madison.

The Audience

This book is for you:

- The nursing student wanting a solid foundation on which to base your clinical experience
- The graduate nurse beginning your career in critical care
- The experienced critical-care nurse wanting to update and strengthen your knowledge base
- The critical-care educator wanting to convey both the art and science of critical-care nursing

Instructor's Guide

An instructor's guide is available to accompany this text. The guide contains learning objectives, teaching strategies, a testbank of sample questions, and transparency masters.

Acknowledgements

An editor is but one member of the team necessary to publish a book. Although a book flows from the editor's vision, it takes many talented, committed people to produce it. Special recognition is paid to the contributors (acknowledged by name on a separate page), who gave so generously of their expertise; the talented publishing team at Addison-Wesley, including Nancy Evans, Jamie Spencer, Glenda Epting, and Wendy Earl; the production team, including Wendy Calmenson, Elliot Simon, and Kathy Lee, and the artists, especially Richmond Jones. To each, I extend my gratitude and appreciation. I am particularly indebted to Patricia Benner, Christine Tanner, Anne Crabtree, Marcy Jorgenson, and Nancy Diekelmann for their generosity in sharing paradigms.

A special thank you to our reviewers:

Susan Bennett, RN, MSN, CCRN
Ball State University
Muncie, Indiana

Vicki Buchda, RN, MS, CCRN
Good Samaritan Medical Center
Phoenix, Arizona

Randy Caine, RN, MS, CCRN
California State University, Long Beach
Long Beach, California

Sandra Carden, RD, BS
Health Care Plan
Buffalo, New York

Diane Dressler, RN, MSN, CCRN
Midwest Heart Surgery Institute
Milwaukee, Wisconsin

Diana Field, RN, MSN
Memorial Medical Center
Long Beach, California

Lorraine Fitzsimmons, RN, DNS
San Diego State University
San Diego, California

Linda Haggerty, RN, MS
Rush-Presbyterian-St. Luke's Medical Center
Chicago, Illinois

Jeanette Hartshorn, RN, PhD, CCRN
Medical University of South Carolina
Charleston, South Carolina

Linda Land, RN, MS
California State University, Chico
Chico, California

Sandi Martin, RN, BSN, CCRN
Abbott Northwestern Hospital
Minneapolis, Minnesota

Linda Miers, RN, MSN
University of Alabama, Birmingham
Birmingham, Alabama

Nancy Ginkus-O'Connor, MSN, MBA
Lehigh Valley Hospital Center
Allentown, Pennsylvania

Marlene Reimer, RN, MN
University of Calgary
Calgary, Alberta (Canada)

Margaret Slota, RN, MN
Pediatric Critical-Care Nursing Consultant

Barbara Tueller, RN, MS, CEN, CCRN
Samuel Merritt Hospital College of Nursing
Oakland, California

Judith A. West
Clinical Nurse Specialist and Wound Care Consultant
San Francisco, California

Elizabeth Hahn Winslow, RN, PhD
Methodist Medical Center
Dallas, Texas

On a personal level, I continue to be nourished by the love and support of my family. My husband, Mike, kept me centered and upbeat even during the "tough times." My son, Jason, shared his wonder and excitement in the ever-expanding world around him, diverting me and reminding me of the primacy of love in a meaningful life.

Enjoy yourself, have fun with this book, and never forget that your human caring is the most valuable gift you have to offer the critically ill.

Nancy Meyer Holloway

Contributors

Patricia E. Benner, RN, PhD, FAAN
Associate Professor, Department of Physiological
  Nursing
University of California San Francisco
San Francisco, California
Clinical Insights

Barbara A. Bires, RN, MSN, CCRN, CEN
Educator and Consultant in Trauma Care
Donald Cook and Associates
Los Angeles, California
Chapter 21, Trauma

Anne S. Crabtree, RN, MS
Nurse Education Coordinator
Saint Joseph's Hospital
Marshfield, Wisconsin
Clinical Insights

Nancy L. Diekelmann, RN, PhD, FAAN
Professor
University of Wisconsin
Madison, Wisconsin
Clinical Insights

Claire A. Dyer, RN
Nursing Education Coordinator
Saint Francis Memorial Hospital
San Francisco, California
Chapter 21, Trauma

Madeline E. Fassler, RN, BSN, CEN
President, Creative Education Resources, Inc.
San Leandro, California
Chapter 12, Dysrythmias and Conduction Defects

Loretta Forlaw, RN, MSN, CNSN, LTC, AN
Clinical Nurse Specialist Nutrition Support
Walter Reed Medical Center
Bethesda, Maryland
Doctoral Student (Nursing)
The Catholic University of America
Chapter 19, Nutrition

Anna Gawlinski, RN, MSN, CCRN
Cardiovascular Clinical Nurse Specialist
UCLA Medical Center
Los Angeles, California
Chapter 10, Cardiovascular Physical Assessment
Chapter 11, Cardiovascular Diagnostic Procedures

Edward J. Glogowski, RN, MS, CRRN
Neurological Clinical Nurse Specialist
Alta Bates-Herrick Hospitals
Berkeley, California
Chapter 3, Communication: Patient and Family

Catherine R. Gregory, RN, CCRN
Nurse Educator and Staff Nurse Critical Care Unit
Goleta Valley Community Hospital
Santa Barbara, California
Santa Ynez Valley Hospital
Solvang, California
Chapter 5, Stimulation Disorders
Chapter 6, Stimulation Treatment Techniques and Pain
  Management

Susan Pfettscher-Hopper, RN, MSN
Clinical Specialist, Doctoral Student
University of California
San Francisco, California
Chapter 2, Dimensions in Critical Care Practice

Susan S. Jacobs, RN, MS
Cardiopulmonary Nurse Specialist
Menlo Park, California
Chapter 7, Aeration Assessment
Chapter 8, Aeration Disorders
Chapter 9, Aeration Treatment Techniques

Marcille J. Jorgenson, RN, MS
Education Specialist
University of Wisconsin Hospital and Clinics
Madison, Wisconsin
Clinical Insights

Leslie S. Kern, RN, MN, CCRN
Cardiothoracic Surgery Clinical Nurse Specialist
UCLA Medical Center
Los Angeles, California
Chapter 13, Cardiovascular Disorders

Julie A. Shinn, RN, MA, CCRN
Educational Coordinator—Critical Care Region
Stanford University Medical Center
Stanford, California
Chapter 14, Cardiovascular Interventions

Gary Sparger, RN, MSN, CEN, MICN
Associate Professor
California State University
Long Beach, California
Chapter 21, Trauma

Charleen A. Strebel, RN, CCRN, CNRN
Critical Care Educator
Santa Barbara Cottage Hospital
Santa Barbara, California
Chapter 4, Stimulation Assessment
Chapter 5, Stimulation Disorders
Chapter 6, Stimulation Treatment Techniques and Pain
  Management
Chapter 21, Trauma

Betsy Todd, RN, BSN
Staff Nurse, The Presbyterian Hospital
New York, New York
Drug Columnist, *Geriatric Nursing*
Appendix 2, Pharmacology

Barbara L. Tueller, RN, MS, CEN, CCRN
Faculty, Department of Medical-Surgical Nursing
Samuel Merritt College of Nursing
Oakland, California
Chapter 16, Fluid, Electrolyte, and Acid-Base
  Imbalances
Chapter 17, Endocrine/Metabolic Disorders and
  Treatment
Chapter 18, Hematologic/Immunologic Disorders
Chapter 19, Nutrition

Alice A. Whittaker, RN, MS, CCRN
Director of Clinical Nursing
University Medical Center
Tucson, Arizona
Chapter 15, Renal Assessment and Acute Renal Failure

Unit 1

INTRODUCTION

1

Introduction

CLINICAL INSIGHT

Domain: The helping role

Competency: Providing comfort measures and preserving personhood in the face of pain and extreme breakdown

In the emotionally treacherous atmosphere of the intensive care unit, acts of simple human kindness take on special poignancy. In this excerpt, from Crabtree and Jorgenson (1986, pp. 96–99), Kim, a nurse, describes the bond that she developed with Jack, a gravely ill cardiac surgical patient dying after numerous surgeries, and his wife Kate, who has resisted the painful realization that her husband will not survive much longer. Shortly after Jack survives a code, his 40th birthday occurs:

It was the night of Jack's 40th birthday, and I was working nights, and another nurse and I went nuts; we decorated his room; we had balloons all over. We got him a corsage, and we got Kate a corsage, too. We decorated the whole room. And, when Kate came in the next morning, she just went nuts! She was so touched that somebody would do this. I don't think she knew that we knew that it was his birthday, except for the fact that it's on the admission sheet. And,

we had gone to the hilt. We had a birthday party to behold! . . . Kate was so touched that I think it made all the difference in the world. She was a different lady after that; she was even to the point where she was saying things like, I know that this is probably going to be Jack's last birthday. Because, I've seen how he does better, and then how he's gotten worse.

Later, Kim shares her reflections on the bond that developed among them and her gratitude for their gifts of love to each other:

That's the kind of situation that I think it's so important to become emotionally involved. You can have all the book knowledge in the world, and I think it's important. Maybe it's important not to get too involved, but maybe we need to be slapped in the face sometimes with reality. That's the kind of situation where I knew what the full picture was; I knew the man was dying, and I got so emotionally involved, but it felt so good. It felt so good to feel like I touched that lady and her family . . . and Jack; even if she didn't admit that he was dying, at least she could feel good, you know. She didn't have to say to me, I know my husband has a dying heart, and he's not going to live very long but, for even just one day, to make them feel good. They had a nice day. And, to a certain degree, I think that is very important in nursing. . . .

Not only do I think that we need to represent patients and their families, and be their advocates, but who else is going to make them feel good? And, I, maybe for that reason . . . maybe I should thank them for that. We had just had a horrendous stretch, and it was kind of like he and his wife slapped me in the face, you know; like, don't forget about us poor souls here who, even though you might not be able to give him this drug and make him better, or you might not be able to put me on this drip and I'll be all better. . . . You know, don't forget about us and feel good about the fact that you can cry and feel bad, but you're still human, and you haven't lost that. And, you know, after that time it was like—yes, I do want to be a nurse, and, yes, I do want to keep doing what I'm doing. I don't want a new job, and I want to stay here and keep doing what I'm doing because I feel good about it. And, they gave that back to me, and I think that's really important. So . . . he's my favorite patient. I'll never forget him as long as I live.

Critical-care nursing is the nursing of people undergoing life-threatening physiologic crises. As a critical-care nurse, you offer your patients and their families something very special: direct assistance with life-and-death crises. This assistance can be both an awesome responsibility and a tremendously exciting challenge. The Clinical Insight nearby eloquently describes a further special contribution of the critical-care nurse: preserving personhood in the face of such crises.

The scope of critical-care nursing has been defined by the American Association of Critical Care Nurses (AACN) as encompassing three components: the critically ill patient, the critical-care nurse, and the critical-care environment (Table 1-1). As implied in the AACN Scope of Practice, the very essence of critical-care nursing is anticipation and early intervention in problems besetting the critically ill. Prediction of patient problems must be based on a sound understanding of anatomy and physiology and astute patient assessment. For this reason, significant portions of this book are devoted to helping you acquire this understanding and skill. Critical-care nursing also requires adeptness at nursing care planning, intervention, and evaluation. These subjects also are discussed in depth in this book.

Three unifying concepts guided the selection and organization of the material in this book:

- The importance of a nursing model in guiding practice.

- The nursing process, incorporating nursing diagnosis.

- The concept of core knowledge and skills.

Nursing Model

Nursing education long has been patterned upon the traditional "body systems" approach. That approach reflects the biomedical model, which is based on the Cartesian view that distinguishes between the body and the mind or soul (Feild and Winslow 1985). Although a biomedical model is appropriate for use in fulfilling the responsibilities that nurses share with physicians (nursing's interdependent role), a nursing model is needed to focus attention on nursing's core concerns (its independent role). Feild and Winslow point out that a nursing model is used *with*—not in place of—a medical model. By adding a nursing model to the biomedical model, this book promotes a holistic approach to patient care, one that integrates nursing's independent functions with its collaborative ones. The model used is FANCAS, a conceptual approach developed by Dr. June C. Abbey. Appendix 1 contains a description of its components and an example of a patient assessment and care plan based on this approach. This model is compatible with most nursing models that are based on a framework of problem solving, basic needs, general systems, or adaptation (Abbey 1980).

Nursing Process

In a short time of clinical practice, you can learn the mechanics of critical care—the application of electrocardiogram (ECG) electrodes, manipulation of hemodynamic monitoring lines, and so on. You can become adept at these technical skills, however, without truly comprehending the principles on which they are based. Without understanding the underlying principles, you may find yourself depending upon physicians' orders and the habitual behavior of other nurses for guidance; crises seem to occur with alarming frequency, and you may become increasingly anxious about your ability to cope with them. Your patients suffer, too, because you are unable to spot problems early and prevent them from reaching crisis proportions. Tired and tense, you may also find you cannot give patients and families the emotional support they desperately need. Slowly, the satisfaction and pride you initially felt as a critical-care nurse evaporates and your nursing becomes just a crisis-oriented, highly stressful job beset with staff shortages, "assembly line" patient care, and too many dying

TABLE 1-1 SCOPE OF CRITICAL-CARE NURSING PRACTICE

Introduction

AACN builds on the ANA definition of nursing[2] and defines critical-care nursing as that specialty within nursing which deals with human responses to life-threatening problems.[1] The scope of critical-care nursing is defined by the dynamic interaction of the critically ill patient, the critical-care nurse, and the critical-care environment.

The goal of critical-care nursing is to ensure effective interaction of these three requisite elements to effect competent nursing practice and optimal patient outcomes within an environment supportive of both. The framework within which critical-care nursing is practiced is based on a scientific body of knowledge, the nursing process, and multidisciplinary collaboration in the care of patients.

Although a distinct specialty, critical-care nursing is inseparable from the profession of nursing as a whole. As members of the profession, critical-care nurses hold the same commitment to protect, maintain, and restore health as well as to embrace the *Code for Nurses.*[3]

The Critically Ill Patient

Central to the scope of critical-care nursing is the critically ill patient, who is characterized by the presence of, or being at high risk for developing, life-threatening problems. The critically ill patient requires constant intensive, multidisciplinary assessment and intervention in order to restore stability, prevent complications, and achieve and maintain optimal responses.

In recognition of the critically ill patients' primary need for restoration of physiologic stability, the critical-care nurse coordinates interventions directed at resolving life-threatening problems. Nursing activities also focus on support of patient adaptation, restoration of health, and preservation of patient rights, including the right to refuse treatment or to die. Inherent in the patients' response to critical illness is the need to maintain psychological, emotional, and social integrity. The familiarity, comfort, and support provided by social relationships can enhance effective coping. Therefore, the concept of the critically ill patient includes the interaction and impact of the patient's family and/or significant other(s).

The Critical-Care Nurse

The critical-care nurse is a licensed professional who is responsible for ensuring that all critically ill patients receive optimal care. Basic to accomplishment of this goal is individual professional accountability through adherence to standards of nursing care of the critically ill and through a commitment to act in accordance with ethical principles.

Critical-care nursing practice encompasses the diagnosis and treatment of patient responses to life-threatening health problems. The critical-care nurse is the one constant in the critical-care environment. As such, coordination of the care delivered by various health care providers is an intrinsic responsibility of the critical-care nurse. With the nursing process as a framework, the critical-care nurse uses independent, dependent, and interdependent interventions to restore stability, prevent complications, and achieve and maintain optimal patient responses. Independent nursing interventions are those actions which are in the unique realm of nursing and include manipulation of the environment, teaching, counseling, and initiating referrals. Dependent nursing interventions are those actions prescribed by medicine. Interdependent nursing interventions are actions determined through multidisciplinary collaboration. Underlying the application of these interventions is a holistic approach that expresses human warmth and caring. This art, in conjunction with the science of critical-care nursing, is essential to the interaction between the critical-care nurse and critically ill patient in attaining optimal outcomes.

The critical-care environment is constantly changing. The critical-care nurse must respond effectively to the demands created by this environment for the broad application of knowledge. Realization of this goal is accomplished through entry preparation into professional nursing practice at a baccalaureate level and a commitment to maintaining competency in critical care nursing through ongoing education concurrent with an expanding base of experience.

The Critical-Care Environment

The critical-care environment can be viewed from three perspectives. On one level the critical-care environment is defined by those conditions and circumstances surrounding the direct interaction between the critical-care nurse and the critically ill patient. The immediate environment must constantly support this interaction in order to effect desired patient outcomes. Adequate resources, in the form of readily available emergency equipment, needed supplies, effective support systems for managing emergent patient situations, and measures for ensuring patient safety are requisites. The framework for nursing practice in this setting is provided by standards of nursing care of the critically ill.

The institution or setting within which critically ill patients receive care represents another perspective of the critical-care environment. At this level, the critical care management and administrative structure ensures effective care delivery systems for various populations of critically ill patients through provision of adequate human, material, and financial resources, through required quality systems, and through maintenance of standards of nursing care of the critically ill.

Additional elements contributing to effective care delivery include:

- Participatory decision-making which ensures that the critical-care nurse provides input into decisions affecting the nurse-patient interaction.
- A collaborative practice model that facilitates multidisciplinary problem-solving and ethical decision-making.
- Education of critical-care nurses consistent with standards for critical-care nursing education and practice.

The broadest perspective of the environment encompasses a global view of those factors that impact the provision of care to the critically ill patient. Monitoring of legal, regulatory, social, economic, and political trends is necessary to promote early recognition of the potential implications for critical-care nursing and to provide a basis for a timely response.

(Adopted by AACN Board of Directors, November 1986)
[1]AACN, "Definition of Critical Care Nursing" AACN Position Statement, February, 1984.
[2]ANA, Nursing: A Social Policy Statement, ANA, Kansas City, Missouri, 1980.
[3]ANA, Code for Nurses, ANA, Kansas City, Missouri, 1985.

From Thierer J. et al: *Standards for nursing care of the critically ill.* 1981. By permission of the American Association of Critical-Care Nurses, Newport Beach, Ca.

patients. Eventually, "burnt out," you decide critical-care nursing really is not for you and leave the field.

This scenario, replayed many times in critical-care nursing, is one reason for rapid turnover of nursing staff in many critical-care units. It is tragic: the nurse feels she somehow has failed to "measure up," and patients are deprived of an experienced critical-care nurse. Worse, it is a tragedy that could be prevented.

The critical-care nurse must be assisted in evolving a nursing style that both nurtures her and enables her to provide optimum patient care. The keys to such a nursing style—anticipation, judgment, and creativity—depend on skillful application of the nursing process in critical-care situations.

The nursing process is so important in critical care that the American Association of Critical Care Nurses (AACN) has formally incorporated standards for use of the nursing process into its *Standards for Nursing Care of the Critically Ill* (1981). This document recognizes five steps in the nursing process: (1) continuous data collection; (2) problem/need identification and prioritizing; (3) formulation of a plan of nursing care; (4) care plan implementation according to the priority of problems/needs; and (5) continuous evaluation of the results of nursing care. For each of these steps, AACN has identified pertinent standards of critical-care nursing practice.

Although the labels for the phases of the nursing process may differ among authors, the concepts are similar. *Nursing the Critically Ill Adult* recognizes five phases of the nursing process: (1) assessment; (2) diagnosis; (3) planning; (4) intervention; and (5) evaluation (Figure 1-1). Although separated in this book for analysis, the phases of the nursing process interact synergistically in practice.

Assessment

Any professional process starts with data collection and analysis. What distinguishes medical from nursing assessment is the goal of each professional.

The nurse's goal in the assessment phase is the acquisition of a nursing database, that is, information from which the patient's nursing care needs can be identified. Comprehensive nursing assessment thus necessitates collection of data from many sources: the health record, your own physical assessment of the patient, interviews with the patient and family, monitoring devices, diagnostic studies, and laboratory tests. When gathering data from these sources, remember that your focus is on the patient's current condition and that you want information with nursing implications. The sections of this book addressing patient assessment present one way to examine these data systematically. By following a logical sequence in assessment, you avoid accidentally overlooking an important source of information about your patient.

In contrast, the physician's goal in the assessment phase is the acquisition of a medical database. To this end, the physician will perform a comprehensive history and physical examination to the extent appropriate to the patient's current status. The health history usually consists of the patient's chief complaint, profile, family history, past health history, history of the present problem, and a review of systems. To perform the review, the physician questions the patient about the presence and characteristics of symptoms. A detailed physical examination follows.

There is no one "right" way to assess a patient; many assessment formats have been developed. Those most commonly used are head-to-toe and body systems. Because these are medically derived databases, this book offers a third option: the FANCAS database for use in critical care, adapted from the original (see Appendix 1). Close comparison of the three formats reveals that each includes the same items for assessment; what varies is their organization. You may choose to use one of these formats or you may develop one appropriate to your own patients and practice setting. Other nursing conceptual models you might wish to explore and from which you might want to use assessment tools are Roy's adaptation model (1976), Orem's self-care competency model (1980), Rogers' unitary-man model (1969), King's systems model (1971), and Gordon's model of eleven functional health patterns (1987).

Obviously, it is neither expedient nor appropriate to collect all the data presented via any assessment tool for every patient. Within the first 5–10 minutes of admission, you should obtain a brief nursing history and perform a rapid examination guided by the patient's symptomatology. In this rapid assessment, you should seek to identify the patient's major problems, the rapidity with which they are developing, and how well he or she is compensating for them. You then will be able to determine priorities and initiate any urgent care. More complete assessment can be undertaken once care for the patient's immediate life threats has been instituted.

By developing knowledge and skill in patient assessment, you can enhance your ability to deliver comprehensive, high-quality patient care. You will be better able to detect significant changes early, institute care, and evaluate the results of your actions. You also will be better able to understand the detailed examinations performed by physicians and appreciate the significance of their findings. Finally, you will be able to demonstrate

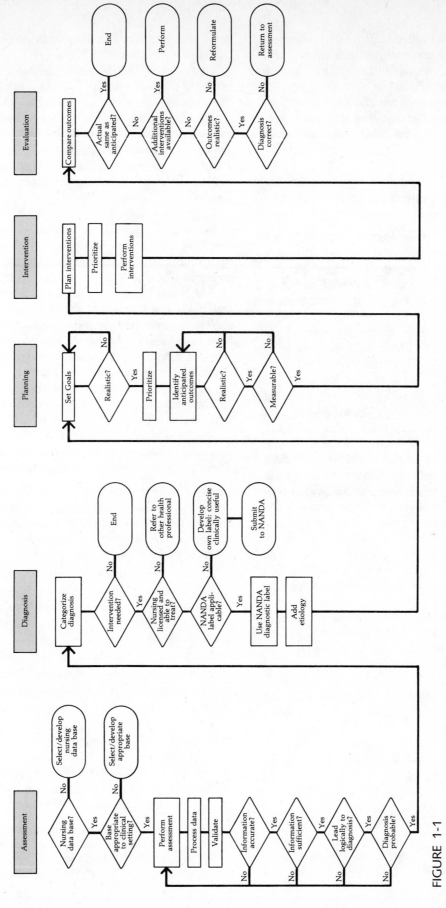

FIGURE 1-1

Nursing process flowchart.

to patients, visitors, and other staff the increasing responsibility nurses are assuming for anticipation, prevention, and early intervention in the myriad disorders that can plague the critically ill.

Whatever assessment tool you choose, it should be practical, flexible, and systematic, and should lead naturally into the next phase of the nursing process—*nursing diagnosis.*

Diagnosis

Several definitions of nursing diagnosis have been developed. The most widely accepted, and the most practical from an operational viewpoint, is Gordon's (1976), which defines nursing diagnosis as "A concise term representing a cluster of signs and symptoms and describing an actual or potential health problem . . . which nurses, by virtue of their education and experience, are licensed and able to treat." This definition clearly delineates the crucial difference between medical and nursing diagnosis: if you as a nurse are not licensed to or able to identify and treat a problem, it is not a nursing diagnosis. For example, coronary artery disease is a medical diagnosis because nurses are neither educated to nor legally authorized to diagnose or treat disease processes. Related problems that might be appropriate nursing diagnoses for a patient with coronary artery disease, however, could include ineffective individual coping, spiritual distress, or altered tissue perfusion. If you question whether a problem you have recognized is a nursing diagnosis, ask yourself these two crucial questions: Am I *licensed* to identify and treat this problem? Am I *able* to identify and treat it? If the answers to both questions are yes, you have made a *nursing diagnosis.*

Historical Background Although the term *nursing diagnosis* is new, the process itself is not. Nurses have been diagnosing for years, but the accepted labels for their decisions have been "patient problems" or "needs." Nurses' diagnostic efforts often have been intuitive, haphazard, not shared explicitly with colleagues or patients, and in some cases poorly differentiated from medical diagnoses.

Nursing diagnosis was formally recognized as a professional nursing function in 1973 when it was included in the American Nurses' Association (ANA) *Standards of Nursing Practice.* A major contribution to the profession has been the systematic definition and classification of diagnoses by the National Group for the Classification of Nursing Diagnoses. This pioneering group has met biannually in St. Louis, Missouri, since 1973. At the Fifth National Conference in 1982, the group was formalized as the North American Nursing Diagnosis Association (NANDA).

The goals of NANDA include formal acceptance and testing of diagnostic labels. NANDA maintains a national clearinghouse to serve as a central information exchange. Clearinghouse activities include storing materials on nursing diagnosis, providing bibliographies on diagnostic categories, disseminating information about activities of nurses using nursing diagnosis, publishing a newsletter, and coordinating arrangements for national conferences.

Nursing Diagnosis in Critical Care To enrich the development and utilization of nursing diagnosis from a critical-care perspective, National Conferences on Nursing Diagnosis in Critical Care, jointly sponsored by AACN and Marquette University, were held in 1983 and 1987. The purpose of the first conference was to explore the evolution of nursing diagnosis and issues related to its use in critical care. The issues receiving the greatest debate were the appropriateness of including physiologic diagnoses and the nature and degree of autonomy in critical-care nursing practice.

The purpose of the second conference was to move beyond conceptual controversy to address clinical use of nursing diagnosis in critical care. Critical care poses a unique challenge in the use of nursing diagnosis. There are several reasons for this challenge:

1. The very nature of the problems with which critical-care nurses deal. As noted at the start of the chapter, critical-care nursing involves the care of people undergoing life-threatening physiologic crises. As such, the prominence of physiologic problems is undeniable.

2. The inseparability of physiologic and psychologic factors underlying patient problems, for example, postcardiotomy delirium, which can result from postoperative chemical imbalances as well as anxiety, powerlessness, and so on.

3. The close collaboration between nursing and other disciplines. This collaboration exists both in assessing patients and in making and carrying out therapeutic decisions.

4. The theoretical and practical confusion regarding the dependent, interdependent, and independent roles of the nurse. These roles have been the source of major philosophic disagreements and controversy in nursing. Nowhere is this more apparent than in the field of critical-care nursing. Guzzetta and Dossey (1983) assert:

One of the major problems with using nursing diagnosis in critical care is related to the so-called "dependent" role vs. the interdependent and independent roles of the critical-care nurse. . . . Although the "dependent" and independent roles of the nurse can be *theoretically* defined, the lines that separate these roles in practice become fuzzy. Perhaps it is time to rethink these concepts and reexamine the premises on which they are based. . . . Perhaps the reason that the nurse's "dependent" and independent roles cannot be clearly defined in critical care is that *in practice* these roles do not exist. Perhaps we should stop wasting our time trying to delineate these roles and realize that the *critical-care nurse's role is one of interdependence* and co-participation with the patient, the family, the physician, and other members of the health team.

5. The nature of the NANDA list of diagnoses. The levels of conceptualization vary from very concrete to very abstract. Some of the diagnoses appear to rename medical problems, for example, *decreased cardiac output* and *altered tissue perfusion.*

Nursing diagnosis in critical care is in an evolutionary phase. The issues of the appropriateness of including physiologic diagnoses in patient care plans and the type and degree of nursing autonomy necessary to treat nursing diagnoses will remain an area of exciting, stimulating debate. Until these issues are resolved, there are some guidelines that are appropriate for those of us engaged in clinical practice who want to use nursing diagnosis.

1. *The plan of patient care should reflect all the problems with which the critical-care nurse must deal.* Whether the medical and nursing diagnoses and interventions are listed in separate areas of the care plan, or whether the list of nursing diagnoses includes all problems encountered by the critical-care nurse, is less important than having accessible to the nurse all the data he or she needs to get a clear picture of the patient and his or her problems.

2. *A physiologic diagnosis is not synonymous with a medical diagnosis.* Many physiologic terms are used by both physicians and nurses, for example, *diarrhea.* Furthermore, a physiologic diagnosis may require nursing interventions *as well as* medical interventions. For example, the patient with diarrhea could require special skin care (a physiologic nursing intervention), interpersonal acceptance by the nurse despite the distasteful body excretions (a psychologic nursing intervention), and administration of anti-infective drugs to kill the causative organism (a medical intervention).

3. Use the diagnoses that have meaning for you.

Benefits of Nursing Diagnosis   Considerable confusion has surrounded "nursing diagnosis" in the minds of nurses, physicians, and the public. By custom, "diagnosis" has been so long and so strongly associated with medicine that many people think the use of this term automatically implies that the nurse is trying to

practice medicine. In actuality, diagnosis simply is the generic term for the intellectual process by which a person makes judgments from data gleaned during the assessment phase. What are the benefits of using nursing diagnosis? There are two major ones: the impact on day-to-day nursing practice, and the influence on the nursing profession. Patient benefits from nursing diagnosis include (1) clear identification of the problem, which directs specific planning, implementation, and evaluation of care, and (2) clear identification of the nurse's accountability. Nursing diagnosis provides a clinical language that facilitates reporting, team conferences, charting, computerization, teaching, research, and publishing. Even more important, nursing diagnosis facilitates accountability, in the nurses' own eyes, their colleagues' eyes, and the public's eyes. As Diers (1981) has written:

> Nursing is exceedingly complicated work since it involves technical skill, a great deal of formal knowledge, communication ability, use of self, timing, emotional investment, and any number of other qualities. What it also involves, and what is hidden from the public, is the process of thinking that leads from the knowledge to the skill, from the perception to the action, from the investment to the touch, from the observation to the diagnosis. Yet it is the process of nursing care that is at the center of nursing's work and is so little attended to, so little described, that no wonder people think nurses are just nice people with a minimum of training, dumbly following doctors' orders.

Nursing diagnosis represents an important way for us to document nursing thinking and thus to differentiate ourselves from other professions and to validate ourselves as autonomous professionals.

Nursing vs Medical Diagnosis   Many nurses have trouble articulating the distinctions between medical diagnosis and nursing diagnosis. This difficulty is particularly serious in critical care, where nurses may be called upon in emergencies to make medical diagnoses and to treat them under standing orders or protocols. A delineation of the most distinct differences follows.

1. The physician focuses on the diagnosis of a specific disease process. In contrast, the nurse focuses on the diagnosis of human responses, both those resulting from the disease and those unrelated to it. The nursing diagnosis considers the medical diagnosis and treatment but zeroes in on the patient's physical, emotional, and social responses to disease, treatment, surroundings, other people, and him or herself (Shoemaker 1979). As every experienced nurse knows, two patients with the same disease label may have widely varying problems, depending on their personal differences and on their progress along the health–illness continuum.

2. The intent of medical diagnosis is to prescribe treatment to cure the disease process. Medical treatment typically consists of diet, medication, surgery, and physical therapy. The intent of nursing diagnosis is to prescribe treatment to relieve patient problems falling within nursing's independent area of practice. Nursing treatment typically consists of physiologic interventions, health education, crisis intervention, counseling, therapeutic use of self, and referral to other professionals.

3. Medical diagnoses usually are limited and static during the course of an illness. In contrast, nursing diagnoses are numerous and flexible, reflecting dynamic alterations in the patient's status during illness and recovery.

4. Medical diagnoses are short, commonly accepted phrases. Nursing diagnoses are not—yet. Nursing diagnoses are not yet ordered in a universally accepted taxonomy. As a result, nurses may use different phrases to describe the same problem, further contributing to confusion in the development and use of nursing diagnoses. NANDA is working to develop a universally acceptable taxonomy. As it struggles with the balance between conciseness and comprehensiveness in terminology, it sometimes adopts phrases that appear long and somewhat awkward to use. In the interest of supporting this important attempt toward nursing unity, this text uses the diagnoses approved by NANDA for clinical testing, in spite of any difficulties with length or awkward phrasing. The order of words in accepted diagnoses has been revised to reflect the order used in ordinary conversation, for example, the accepted diagnosis of "coping, ineffective, individual" appears in this book as "ineffective individual coping." In situations where NANDA has not yet identified or accepted specific diagnoses, new ones have been created. These are identified clearly as such, by an asterisk (*) following the diagnosis.

Process of Nursing Diagnosis The two essential components of a nursing diagnosis are the problem and the etiology. The *problem* is a statement of an undesirable health response. It reflects a nursing judgment that this condition is one that nurses are capable and licensed to treat. The *etiology* is a statement of the most probable cause of the problem.

Because many nurses are uncertain about how actually to identify nursing diagnoses in their day-to-day practice, the following section includes some clear, use-

*Information about the procedure for submitting new diagnoses for evaluation is available from North American Nursing Diagnosis Association, St. Louis University Dept. of Nursing, 3525 Caroline St., St. Louis, MO 63104.

ful guidelines drawn from the works of Shoemaker (1979), Dossey and Guzzetta (1981).

Step 1. Assess Your Patient Do a baseline physical and emotional assessment as early as possible in your care of the patient. Use a nursing database, as it is difficult to derive nursing diagnoses from a medical database. Many nursing databases are available in the literature, including the ones in this book, or you can develop your own to assess the nursing data you consider important.

Step 2. Process the Information intellectually. Shoemaker (1979) suggests you use three general steps: cognitive processing, pattern recognition, and validation. *Cognitive processing* means comparing the data you have assessed against your knowledge base of normal versus abnormal findings. *Pattern recognition* is the clustering of related findings and the identification of possible causes. For instance, the signs of restlessness, tachycardia, sweating, and dilated pupils can be clustered together in a pattern that may be associated with pain, shock, or anxiety. Pattern recognition enables you to form tentative diagnoses and then gather further data to rule out inappropriate diagnoses. Pattern recognition thus is essentially the same step as the identification of the signs and symptoms that define the problem and the identification of a tentative diagnosis. *Validation* involves careful review of each step to be certain that you have sufficient, accurate information, that the information leads logically to the diagnosis, and that the chosen diagnosis is reasonably probable. It is validation that differentiates nursing diagnosis from nursing intuition.

Step 3. Diagnose the Problem For each pattern recognized in Step 2, decide whether you are able and licensed to identify and treat it. If not, consult a physician about it. If the problem does fall within the nursing realm, try to label it using an accepted diagnosis. The NANDA list is alphabetical, making it somewhat impractical to use for quick location of an appropriate label. It is easier to use a categorized list, which groups related diagnoses together. Such lists include this book's grouping of diagnoses under the FANCAS model of patient needs (Appendix 1), Bockrath's (1982) grouping of diagnoses under 10 common responses to illness, and Gordon's (1982) grouping of diagnoses under 11 functional health patterns. Whatever list you choose, carry a copy of it with you for easy reference when you are on duty.

Step 4. Add the Etiology The etiology should be a concise, clinically useful description of the factor(s) maintaining the problem. Use the words "related to" to join the problem and the etiology, for example: "Ineffective individual coping related to lack of support system."

For most nursing diagnoses, the problem–etiology

linkage is an inference based on clinical judgment (Gordon 1987). In this book, the editor and contributors take the position that is unnecessary to limit etiologies only to factors within the area of independent nursing practice. Based on the criterion of clinical usefulness, they believe that acceptable etiologies may be pathophysiologic factors (e.g., anemia) or medical or surgical disorders or interventions (e.g., thoracotomy). Limiting etiologies to factors amenable only to independent nursing interventions, as has been advocated by some nursing diagnosis proponents, can lead to convoluted attempts to "force-fit" phraseology, e.g., "potential wound infection related to impaired skin integrity secondary to surgical incision resulting from thoracotomy" rather than concise, easily understood "potential wound infection related to thoracotomy."

Step 5. Write Your Own Diagnosis If Necessary If there is no accepted diagnosis that fits the problem you have identified, *write your own.* You may wish to consult the nursing literature or simply to state the problem clearly. Remember to use concise, clinically useful terms that describe problems nurses can treat. Avoid jargon and terms with legal implications, such as "pain related to fall from bed when siderails left down." If you do develop your own diagnosis, consider sending it to NANDA—you just may have made an important contribution to the development of nursing practice!

Don't be afraid of physiologic diagnoses. Try them out and see how they work for you. Do they make your practice clearer? easier to explain to others? more satisfying? Keep notes on your experiences—and be sure to share them with NANDA.

Planning and Intervention

An analogy can be made between a neophyte cook and a neophyte critical-care nurse. When you are learning to cook, a cookbook guides you into selecting the proper ingredients in the proper proportions and informs you what others have found to be the most effective ways to prepare the dish so that it ends up a delight instead of a disaster. As you develop skill in cooking, you begin to experiment, adapting the ingredients and techniques to fit what you have on hand. Eventually, for familiar dishes you may not need the cookbook at all, consulting it only when you prepare a dish you serve infrequently. You may even become a gourmet cook, inventing your own recipes. Although this book describes concepts and techniques used in critical-care nursing, just as you cannot become a great cook by blind adherence to recipes, you cannot become an excellent critical-care nurse by rote application of con-

cepts; nor can you learn motor skills from written descriptions only. Benner's (1984) groundbreaking study of clinically expert nurses illuminates some of the competencies that contribute to their excellence. These competencies, derived from actual practice, are presented in Table 1-2.

Based on the Dreyfuss model of skill acquisition, Benner discusses five levels of skill acquisition in nursing: novice, advanced beginner, competent, professional, and expert. Briefly, these stages can be characterized as follows:

- *Novice.* Because the person has no experience in the situation, he or she must use previously taught rules to guide action. Behavior is inflexible and limited.
- *Advanced beginner.* The person has coped with enough situations to begin to recognize recurring meaningful aspects of a situation. Performance is barely acceptable. He or she can't yet sort out what's most important.
- *Competent.* The person feels a growing ability to cope with nursing's demands. Plans are conscious and deliberate, so the person is organized and efficient. Actions are beginning to be based on long-term goals.
- *Proficient.* The person understands the situation as a whole. Having learned from experience what typical events to expect, he or she recognizes when something unusual is happening. He or she is able to quickly zero in on the most important aspects of a situation.
- *Expert.* The person intuitively grasps a situation, no longer relying on rules and guidelines. The meaning of events and actions depend on the context of the situation.

These levels of skill reflect changes in three characteristics of skilled performance:

- Transformation from relying on abstract principles to using prior concrete experience to predict and project events.
- Growing recognition of salience, that is, a change in perception from seeing all parts of a situation as equally important to viewing the situation as a complete whole in which only some parts are important.
- Transformation from a detached observer to an involved participant.

Benner points out that experience is required for developing expertise, and that a sound educational base is necessary for acquiring advanced skills because it forms

TABLE 1-2 COMPETENCIES OF THE EXPERT NURSE

DOMAIN	COMPETENCIES
Helping role	The healing relationship: creating a climate for and establishing a commitment to healing Providing comfort measures and preserving personhood in the face of pain and extreme breakdown Presencing: being with a patient Maximizing the patient's participation and control in his or her own recovery Interpreting kinds of pain and selecting appropriate strategies for pain management and control Providing comfort and communication through touch Providing emotional and informational support to patients' families Guiding a patient through emotional and developmental change by providing new options and closing off old ones through channeling, teaching, mediating Acting as a psychologic and cultural mediator Using goals therapeutically Working to build and maintain a therapeutic community
Teaching-coaching function	Timing: capturing a patient's readiness to learn Assisting patients to integrate the implications of illness and recovery into their lifestyles Eliciting and understanding the patient's interpretation of his or her illness Providing an interpretation of the patient's condition and giving a rationale for procedures The coaching function: making culturally avoided aspects of an illness approachable and understandable
Diagnostic and monitoring function	Detection and documentation of significant changes in a patient's condition Providing an early warning signal: anticipating breakdown and deterioration prior to explicit confirming diagnostic signs Anticipating problems: future-think Understanding the particular demands and experiences of an illness: anticipating patient care needs Assessing the patient's potential for wellness and for responding to various treatment strategies
Effective management of rapidly changing situations	Skilled performance in extreme life-threatening emergencies: rapid grasp of a problem Contingency management: rapid matching of demands and resources in emergency situations Identifying and managing a patient crisis until physician assistance is available
Administering and monitoring therapeutic interventions and regimens	Starting and maintaining intravenous therapy with minimal risks and complications Administering medications accurately and safely: monitoring untoward effects, reactions, therapeutic responses, toxicity, and incompatibilities Combating the hazards of immobility: preventing and intervening with skin breakdown, ambulating and exercising patients to maximize mobility and rehabilitation, preventing respiratory complications Creating a wound management strategy that fosters healing, comfort, and appropriate drainage
Monitoring and ensuring the quality of health care	Providing a backup system to ensure safe medical and nursing care Assessing what can be safely omitted from or added to medical orders Getting appropriate and timely responses from physicians
Organizational and work-role competencies	Coordinating, ordering, and meeting multiple patient needs and requests: setting priorities Building and maintaining a therapeutic team to provide optimum therapy Coping with staff shortages and high turnover: contingency planning Anticipating and preventing periods of extreme work overload within a shift Using and maintaining team spirit; gaining social support from other nurses Maintaining a caring attitude toward patients even in the absence of close and frequent contact Maintaining a flexible stance toward patients, technology, and bureaucracy

Adapted from Benner P: *From novice to expert* (compiled from individual boxed tables in Benner). 1984. Menlo Park, Ca: Addison-Wesley Publishing Company, Inc.

the best position for developing salience. *Nursing the Critically Ill Adult* is intended to help provide the basis on which you can safely enter practice. Accordingly, the experts who have contributed to the book focus on the salient aspects of various types of patient care situations, indicate nursing priorities, and offer guidelines for action.

To become an expert, you must care for patients under the guidance of an experienced practitioner who can help you develop your ability to sort through concepts and facts, select the ones pertinent to your patient and practice setting, and synthesize them into a plan of action. Even in seemingly routine situations, you must be alert to special circumstances and adapt your care accordingly. With practice, you may discover that you no longer need this book's guidelines in familiar situations. Instead, you will return to them from time to time to refresh your memory and to guide your care in unfamiliar circumstances.

Evaluation

Evaluation is a crucial phase of the nursing process because it enables you to judge the accuracy of your decisions and actions during the earlier phases. To help you evaluate your assessments, plans, and interventions, each chapter of this book contains a list of patient outcome criteria, that is, the desirable outcomes toward which your care is oriented. These are *ideal* outcome criteria, and you must use your judgment about their applicability in a given situation.

Core Concepts and Skills

The concept of core knowledge and skills implies that there are common principles and techniques in the care of critically ill patients. These standard elements provide a fruitful approach to mastering the general principles and skills of critical-care nursing, which can be applied to a wide variety of patients. Appendix 1 lists the core concepts and skills discussed in this book.

Conclusions

In the past nursing has functioned largely on a perceptual basis; that is, the nurse perceived a problem and then acted upon it. Her behavior often was prescribed by common sense or ritualistic practice. In recent years, the profession increasingly has emphasized an intellectual approach to patient care. Such an approach is crucial for developing the body of nursing knowledge, but it must be tempered by an awareness of the realities of day-to-day practice in the clinical setting. According to Doona (1976), the dynamic interaction of perceptual and conceptual data is the key to ideal judgment. Tempering your scientific knowledge with judgment will enable you to become a wise critical-care nurse. Add imagination to the mix, and you also will become a creative one.

REFERENCES

Abbey J: FANCAP: What is it? Pages 107–118 in *Conceptual models for nursing practice,* 2d ed. Riehl J, Roy C Sr (eds). New York: Appleton-Century-Crofts, 1980.

American Nurses' Association: *Standards of nursing practice.* Kansas City, MO: The Association, 1973.

Benner P: *From novice to expert.* Addison-Wesley, 1984.

Bockrath M: Your patient needs two diagnoses—medical and nursing. *Nurs Life* (Mar/Apr) 1982; 29–32.

Crabtree A, and Jorgenson M: Exploring the practical knowledge in expert critical-care nursing practice (unpublished Master's thesis, University of Wisconsin, Madison, 1986).

Diers D: Why write? Why publish? *Image* 1981; 13:1–7.

Doona M: The judgment process in nursing. *Image* 1976; 8:27–29.

Dossey B, Guzzetta C: Nursing diagnosis. *Nursing 81* (Jun) 1981; 34–38.

Feild L, Winslow EH: Moving to a nursing model. *Am J Nurs* (Oct) 1985; 1100–1101.

Gordon M: Nursing diagnosis and the diagnostic process. *Am J Nurs* 1976; 76:1298–1300.

Gordon M: Historical perspective: the national conference group for classification of nursing diagnosis. Pages 2–8 in *Classification of nursing diagnosis: Proceedings of the third and fourth national conferences.* Kim M, Moritz D (eds). New York: McGraw-Hill, 1982.

Gordon M: *Nursing diagnosis; Process and application,* 2d ed. New York: McGraw-Hill, 1987.

Guzzetta C, Dossey B: Nursing diagnosis: Framework-process-problems. *Heart Lung* 1983; 12:281–291.

Hurley M (ed): *Classification of nursing diagnoses: Proceedings of the sixth conference.* St Louis: Mosby, 1986.

King I: *Toward a theory of nursing.* New York: Wiley, 1971.

Orem D: *Nursing: Concepts of practice,* 2d ed. New York: McGraw-Hill, 1980.

Rogers M: *Introduction to the theoretical basis of nursing.* Philadelphia: FA Davis, 1969.

Roy C Sr: *Introduction to nursing: An adaptation model.* Englewood Cliffs, NJ: Prentice-Hall, 1976.

Shoemaker J: How nursing diagnosis helps focus your care. *RN* (August) 1979; 57–61.

Theirer J et al. (eds): *Standards for nursing care of the critically ill.* Reston, VA: Reston Publishing Co., 1981.

SUPPLEMENTAL READING

Campbell C: *Nursing Diagnosis and intervention in nursing practice,* 2d ed. New York: Wiley, 1984.

Carnevali D: *Nursing care planning: Diagnosis and management,* 3d ed. Lippincott, 1983.

Carpenito L: *Handbook of nursing diagnosis.* Philadelphia: Lippincott, 1985.

De Gasperis M: Implementing nursing diagnosis in the critical care setting. *Dimen Crit Care Nurs* 1983; 2:44–49.

Grady RM: Comprehensive management of nursing care delivery. *Nurs Manag* 1985; 16(5):47–49.

Kim M: Nursing diagnosis in critical care. *Dimen Crit Care Nurs* 1983; 2:5–6.

Thompson J et al.: *Clinical nursing.* St Louis: Mosby, 1986.

Ziegler S et al.: *Nursing process, nursing diagnosis, and nursing knowledge.* Norwalk, CT: Appleton-Century-Crofts, 1986.

2

Dimensions in Critical Care

CLINICAL INSIGHT

Domain: The helping role

Competency: Presencing: being with a patient

Ethical dilemmas, especially those related to impending death, are a poignant part of critical-care nursing. Although ICU nurses are committed to making the culturally avoided subject of death approachable, the ethical dilemmas surrounding death in the ICU can be wrenching. In the following paradigm, from Crabtree and Jorgenson (1986), pp 110–111), Chris, a nurse, reflects on a situation in which a family is paralyzed over whether to discontinue ventilatory support. The patient, a male, has had respiratory disease for over 30 years and multiple hospitalizations. After being transferred out of the unit, he suffers a cardiac arrest and is returned to the unit brain-dead.

When I finally took him as a primary nurse, because I knew this man needed to be allowed to die, and there was an impasse between the family and the physician, the family was angry at the physicians and wouldn't speak to them. I didn't know much more about it than that. I looked in the chart, and it was plainly evident why the family was unwilling to speak

with the physicians that day he arrested; when the family came back and said, "Why did you move him out? Why did you do this?", the resident told the family, and recorded a note in the chart, that this family was totally unrealistic. They should have understood from the day he was admitted to this hospital that there was very little we could offer him. And that . . . and this was what the resident said . . . that he was unable to help himself in any way; he was too weak to feed himself, too weak to breathe on his own, and this family should have known from the start that he was terminal.

Fighting to honor the patient's previously expressed wish to die naturally, Chris makes concerted efforts to improve communication between the family and the medical staff. One daughter strongly resists discontinuing ventilatory support—and after lengthy discussion with her, Chris discovers why.

She said, look, the reason why I can't stop this ventilator, why I can't say, go ahead and do this, is because my father's suffered for 30 years with a disease where he couldn't breathe. His father was hanged, and he talked many times with me about how he couldn't bear the thought of dying for lack of air, because that's the way his father died. She said, I am not going to agree to stop a ventilator. So that was the basic issue. That was why this woman was holding out. I had no idea. I had no idea about any of this. And, everybody else just thought she was being unreasonable. Because they had been, at a certain time, unreasonable in the past. But, nobody had any idea that there was some promise between father and daughter.

Chris's attempts to draw out this daughter reveal a powerful reason for the daughter's resistance. This insight provokes considerable soul-searching for Chris, following which she is able to use compassion and wisdom to resolve the impasse:

So, then I had to rethink my whole position on this thing, because I was arguing that it's unethical to prolong the death and suffering of a dying person. Which is a reasonable argument. But, on the other hand, there's a very good chance that this man wasn't suffering; this patient wasn't suffering. And, yet, stopping the ventilator would cause an enormous amount of suffering for the daughter. Well, in that case, it seems much less reasonable to stop the ventilator on the patient when we could do all sorts of other things, like stopping all labs and all other kinds of treatment, and put the patient on at least morhine and Valium or some combination like that, so we were certain he wasn't suffering, and let him go.

In the ICU, advanced technology gives us the power to view death as a symptom—to be treated and reversed when possible—rather than as a life event (Crabtree and Jorgenson, p. 189). But with this power comes terrible knowledge, for we have seen the consequences of defying death. Assisting patients and families to experience death in a way meaningful to them is an act of grace and mercy.

This chapter examines many of the threads that make up the tapestry of life and death in the intensive care unit: the critical-care environment, changing technology, the changing role of the nurse, ethical issues, and legal issues. All of these threads are integrated and illuminated in the concluding section on organ donation.

The explosion of biomedical technology in the second half of the twentieth century has created the environment of the critical-care unit, a specialized unit viewed as the ultimate site for delivery of the "best" in acute and life-saving medical care. For such an environment to be effective, however, an expert nursing staff is crucial.

The Critical-Care Environment

The physical structure and specific functions of a critical-care unit are as variable as the general United States hospital system. Ranging from the smallest of units in a primary community hospital to the large, multiple units in a major tertiary-care facility, these units and their nursing staffs share the responsibility for care of the critically ill patient who requires both constant surveillance and multiple technically sophisticated interventions.

What kind of patients are admitted to the critical-care unit? The many criteria for admission include: the patient's diagnosis and age, individual physician practices, community standards, formal criteria of hospital committees, bed availability, and nursing staff availability (both within the critical care unit and elsewhere in the hospital). Thus, patients may be admitted for observation and surveillance of their primary medical condition or its complications, for care and treatment of an acute illness or injury, postoperative care (routine or for complications), or for delivery of specialized technological monitoring or treatment.

The location of the individual hospital also determines who becomes a patient in the critical-care unit. For instance, is the hospital service area one of young adults? Or is the community one of elderly individuals? Age also is related to the nature of the critical-care patient's illness. Younger patients may suffer from an acute illness or injury, whereas older patients are more likely to be hospitalized with a combination of acute and chronic illness or complications of a chronic illness.

The aging of the American population necessarily affects the patient population being admitted to critical-care units for acute illness; changes in the American population must be considered in identifying the types of patients to be served by the critical-care unit in the individual hospital.

The extension of life of patients suffering from chronic illnesses may also affect the patient population admitted to the critical-care unit. As medical knowledge has been employed to maintain the life of these individuals, acute episodes of a disease or illness or its complications may bring these patients to the critical-care unit repeatedly.

The organization of health care delivery also affects

the type of patients receiving care in the critical-care unit. The current emphasis on hospital competition is creating services that affect the use of the critical-care unit—for example, emergency medical services and provision of high-technology services (cardiac procedures, organ transplantation, research therapies and procedures). Other hospitals and their critical-care units are feeling the impact of economic shifts in health care, particularly those that provide critical care for the uninsured—the indigent, those covered by various local and state welfare (Medicaid) programs.

Critical-care nurses should understand the population served by the hospital facility and its critical-care unit and be aware of the goals and objectives of the hospital to best meet the needs of their patients.

Advances in Technology

Critical-care nurses work on the cutting edge of the technologic developments in acute medical care. The development and implementation of life-saving equipment and procedures occur routinely in the critical-care setting. These technologic advances and changes require that critical-care nurses be flexible in their practice and able to quickly integrate such advances into their knowledge base and skills. Because our technologies are so diverse, we have witnessed the subspecialization of critical-care nurses, who develop special expertise in one area of patient care (one disease process) and the technologies associated with it. Subspecialization in areas such as coronary care, open heart surgery, burn care, and trauma has allowed critical-care nurses to become and remain expert practitioners.

Critical-care patients share the common need for highly competent and expert technologic nursing care to save or maintain their lives. To maintain expertise and skills in the face of rapidly changing technology of the critical-care unit, nurses find it essential to participate in continuing education courses, read the various journals specifically directed to critical-care nursing practice, and maintain membership in professional organizations. In addition, many hospitals provide a clinical/ education specialist for its critical-care nursing staff. Nurses who have chosen critical-care nursing as their specialty have available many opportunities and resources to maintain their expertise and skills in providing patient care in the rapidly changing technological environment.

Changes in the Nursing Role

Along with the changes in biomedical technology have come new challenges for critical-care nurses.

Satisfactions of Critical-Care Nursing

Critical-care nursing today is intellectually and emotionally demanding. To successfully provide care to desperately ill, unstable patients, the nurse must have a more extensive base of scientific knowledge and be more technologically astute than at any previous time. The opportunity to exercise intellectual skills and receive recognition for them is satisfying. In addition, many nurses thrive in the fast-paced atmosphere of the critical-care unit. The very intensity of the experience is thrilling, and the opportunity to affect people emotionally during a highly charged time in their lives is profoundly satisfying.

Stresses of Critical-Care Nursing

The practice of critical care nursing may exact a price, however. The sources and impact of stress on the critical-care nurse have been the subject of increasing interest for over a decade. In spite of much study and attention, nurses continue to feel stress and suffer from "burn-out" leading to multiple job changes and even to leaving the field of nursing. Discussions of stress and methods to resolve stress felt by critical-care nurses have been popular subjects of continuing education programs. However, neither a uniform cause of such job stress nor a universal solution to the problem has been identified.

When Gentry and Parkes (1982) published a perspective on the state of the art of stress recognition and management in critical-care nursing, they reached five general conclusions.

1. There has been a sustained interest in this topic over the last ten years, with a steady increase in the number of articles in medical, nursing, and psychiatric journals.

2. There has been a trend toward studies identifying sources of stress in critical care and analyzing them empirically. This is a step forward from early articles, which tended to be anecdotal.

3. There has been an increasing focus on coping strategies used by nurses.

NURSING RESEARCH NOTE

Knaus W et al.: An evaluation of outcome from intensive care in major medical centers. *Ann Intern Med* 1986; 104:410–418.

Does close collaboration between physicians and nurses really improve ICU patient survival? For years, nurses have believed so; this study now documents the crucial impact of quality nursing care on patient outcome. The study was designed to test the validity of a simplified Acute Physiology and Chronic Health Evaluation (APACHE) in predicting risk of death; its findings about the importance of nurse–physician collaboration were serendipitous.

The researchers prospectively studied treatment and outcome in 5,030 patients in 13 tertiary-care hospitals' intensive care units. Utilizing diagnosis, treatment indication, and APACHE score, they stratified each hospital's patients by individual risk of death; then, using group results as the standard, they compared actual and predicted death rates. (Research methodology in the first step utilized a multiple logistic regression analysis; the second step

utilized a multivariate logistic regression analysis, a *t*-test, and partial chi-square tests. The reader interested in the details of the research methodology should consult the original source.)

One hospital had a significantly lower death rate and one a significantly higher death rate than the others ($p < 0.0001$). Further investigation revealed profound differences in the intensive care in these two hospitals. The hospital with the significantly lower death rate utilized carefully planned clinical protocols, implemented by senior physicians in the unit. Within these protocols, nurses had independent responsibilities; for example, they could cancel surgery if adequate nursing staff were not available. Primary nursing was used, and communications between nurses and physicians were ongoing and respectful. An extensive support system included comprehensive educational programs and clinical specialists with Master's degrees and extensive ICU experience.

In contrast, the hospital with the significantly higher death rate had no dedicated unit physician, centralized

nursing authority, formal educational program, primary nursing, or other provision for continuity of care. Physician and nurse communication was marked by frequent disagreement and an air of distrust. Staff shortages sometimes meant that non–ICU-prepared nurses cared for patients.

The researchers considered a number of possible measurement biases but found none that would have systematically favored one hospital over another. They therefore concluded that the quality of nurse–physician interaction in this sample has a profound influence on patient survival in the ICUs used for the study.

* * *

According to Elizabeth Draper, RN, a senior research scientist in the study, the researchers now are seeking funding for a major national survey to further evaluate the effect of nurse–physician interaction on patient survival. The 5-year study is projected to survey 40 hospitals and 15,000 patients. [*Am J Nurs* (March) 1987; 87:283–284.]

---

4. There continues to be a paucity of research studies assessing nurses' perceptions of the critical-care environment, the nature of the stresses, and the effectiveness of the coping strategies used.

5. The widely held view that critical-care nursing is more stressful than noncritical-care nursing may need reexamination.

Gardner et al. (1980) have described well the stressful nature of working in the critical-care unit:

The critical care unit personnel are constantly confronted by the sight of acutely ill patients who may be unconscious, deformed, and lying in blood and excretions. The unit may have a high mortality rate, presenting the staff with repetitive losses and the necessity to reinvest physical and emotional energy in a new patient before they have adequately mourned the loss of a former patient to whom they have become attached emotionally.

The role that patient death plays in creating stress for critical-care nurses cannot be overestimated. The observations of Gardner et al. were addressed by staff members at the Washington Hospital Center in Washington, D.C., by setting aside a special time to deal with patient death. These sessions, which they call "Time-out," are described by Richmond and Craig (1985). Similar approaches have been employed in units throughout the United States. None of these solutions can be implemented, however, unless and until critical-care nurses acknowledge the stress that is created by patient death in the intensive care unit (ICU).

Bailey et al. (1980) conducted an extensive survey of 1,800 ICU nurses in an attempt to identify the stressors and satisfiers in the critical-care setting. They identified the greatest stressors as management of the unit, interpersonal relationships, and patient care. Using these findings in a smaller study and additionally addressing the question of whether stress is greater for ICU nurses than for non-ICU nurses, Vincent and Coleman (1986) studied the nursing staff at a single institution. Their data indicate that management of the unit and interpersonal relations (conflicts) are the leading problems for both ICU and non-ICU nurses. Such interpersonal conflicts are generic to the nursing profession and emanate from the historical structure and function of nursing in the hospital setting (Ashley 1976; Jervik and Martinson 1979). In the critical-care setting, these conflicts may be intensified by the more closed environment and the smaller number of staff working together. According to Mendenhall (1982), lack of control or effectiveness contributes to the stresses of interpersonal conflicts. Issues of decision-making, autonomy, responsibility, feeling needed and helpful, and recognition and respect from others all relate to the nurse's self-esteem and self-actualization. Christopherson (1986) discusses these stressors within the context of control and power in the critical-care setting. She encourages the nurse to be self-reflective in identifying the extent of control that he or she needs to reduce stresses or resolve conflicts in the critical-care setting. To completely understand and resolve the stress of unit management and interpersonal relations, we may have to change the structure and function of nursing and even that of women in the workplace; burnout is not an exclusive problem of ICU nurses; it is shared by many in the workplace. Freudenberger and North's (1985) work related to burnout in women provides significant information to all nurses at risk for stress/burnout on the job. They identify general risk factors, such as being taken for granted as the "resident" nurturer, feeling alone and lonely, having a sense of powerlessness about one's professional and personal life, and being frustrated by notions of autonomy and dependency. We should, however, continue our research in the ICU setting to identify specific issues of stress and their resolution.

Another identified area of stress for the critical-care nurse relates to expertise and excellence in practice. Such stress and anxiety experienced by the critical-care novice is an important consideration. Mastering skills and developing expert knowledge and practice greatly reduce stress in the critical-care setting. Benner's (1984) work has provided us with much information about the development of expert practice. In particular, the continuing mastery of the ever-changing technology of the critical-care unit does much to reduce the stress experienced by the practicing nurse.

Our discussion of stress and stressors would be incomplete without a discussion of job dissatisfaction and staff turnover in the critical care setting. Though these two factors are a result of stress, they also contribute to stress in the ICU. Dear et al. (1982) found that ICU nurses experienced the same level of job satisfaction as their non-ICU nurse counterparts; dissatisfaction was related more to hospital nursing than to working in the critical-care setting. On the other hand, staff shortages and turnover do contribute to the increased stress levels experienced by ICU nurses. Benner (1984) notes that the need to work with temporary or inexperienced staff alters the quality of care that nurses give to their patients, limits their coping strategies, and decreases the work satisfaction they are able to enjoy. The nurses interviewed by Benner said they felt they had little time for reflection and were performing only "emergency nursing"—that their own learning and growth had stopped. Such a situation of dissatisfaction and turnover can become self-perpetuating; coupled with the ever-increasing nurse shortage in the United States, the stressful nature of working in the critical-care unit is likely to continue.

Stress-Reduction Mechanisms

Critical-care nurses should individually and collectively identify the stressors in their professional practice. Identifying the stressors in one's own practice and identifying ways to resolve them are essential to success as a person and a nurse. Gentry and Parkes (1982) remark that "if adequate staffing is maintained, nurses are able to take all other frustrations in their stride." This, however, may be a simplistic solution to a complicated problem and serves to diminish the rich and complex nature of nursing practice.

As with everyone else, critical-care nurses should identify where the stresses in their lives originate. If they derive from personal life, then individual methods of resolution may be needed. If they stem from work, then professional support and collegiality can serve as a buffer and provide a supportive environment in which to discuss and resolve shared problems. Staying current and competent in one's skills and knowledge can also decrease stress.

Institutional changes may be required to reduce stress for everyone in the critical-care unit. Professionals must work together to implement changes such as altering work schedules (10–12-hour days), not splitting days off (to allow for adequate recovery from work-related stress), utilizing effective methods of nurse staffing (either rotating assignments or primary-care assignments depending on which will better reduce stress), and setting up special staff conferences and programs to deal with both the stress experienced and the causes for the stress.

Some of the problems created by the increasing complexity of critical-care technology, the increasing acuity of our patient population, the decrease in resources because of cost containment, and the predicted increasing shortage of nurses are not easily solved. We may find that redefinition and adaptation of our practice will be necessary as we work towards realistic solutions to delivering quality care in the critical-care unit.

Ethics: Principles and Dilemmas

The delivery of health care has traditionally been directed by ethical principles. From the time of Hippocrates, physician care and practice has been influenced by certain ethical principles; nursing care has similarly been directed by such principles. In the latter half of the twentieth century, however, increasing attention has been paid to ethics in health care. A new term has even been coined to describe this new area of ethics: *bioethics*. The explosion of interest and concern can be attributed to a number of factors, including the extension of life by the development and application of high technology, the rapidly increasing cost of medical care, and growing emphasis on quality of life. In addition, the delivery of medical care and the actions of practitioners are no longer private or mystical. The dissemination of knowledge and information in our modern world is supported by our individual and collective belief in a right to know and understand everything that affects our physical and emotional well-being; modern communication media make information about medical advances and their use accessible to most people in the United States and other Western countries. As the public has gained this information about the state of health care, they have also been introduced to and become a part of the ethical decision-making and dilemmas that health care practitioners and our system are confronting.

This section reviews selected ethical principles that are particularly relevant to the functions of the intensive care unit, the dilemmas that may arise from ethical conflicts, and methods by which such dilemmas may be resolved. Nurses in critical-care units have a vital role in these situations, ranging from their identification to assuring and participating in their resolution.

The principle of *beneficence* is a foundation stone of nursing practice in all settings, including the critical-care unit. *Beneficence* means that our care and actions are directed toward "doing good." Our actions are directed by the belief that the care and interventions we offer patients should be directed toward assuring a positive outcome—saving the patient's life, relieving suffering, preventing complications. When care is guided by the principle of beneficence it is usually active—employing major and minor procedures that lead to a positive benefit to the patient.

The principle of *nonmalefescence* is a corollary to beneficence. *Nonmalefescence* is most simply described as "doing no harm" and is the principle most commonly associated with the Hippocratic Oath. Because of that history and association, it has traditionally been considered the dominant principle of medical/nursing practice. This principle is defined as one of restraint or constraint; when applied to a patient situation, it may prevent the practitioner from carrying out procedures that could cause harm to the patient. How one defines *harm* becomes significant to the interpretation and application of this principle. The harm is generally irreversible and either is associated with an active process (procedure) where it outweighs the benefit, or results from negligence or malpractice on the part of the practitioner. Though we may assume that doing no harm automatically means we will be beneficent, this is not necessarily so. Practicing nonmalefescence prevents harm but does not automatically mean that an active, beneficial process is going on. In the critical-care setting, both principles are simultaneously employed to guide patient care.

Veracity as an ethical principle is "telling the truth." As public awareness and knowledge about health and disease have increased, patients have come to expect to be told the truth about illness, treatments, and the outcome of their disease or condition. The consumer emphasis on health care as a commodity assumes that patients are capable of and will make choices and decisions about their care. For them to do so means that truthful information should be provided by the professional caregiver to the greatest extent possible.

Closely associated with the principle of veracity is the principle of *autonomy*. This modern ethical principle is defined as the individual's right and responsibility to make decisions about all aspects of his or her life to the degree that they do not violate the life and well-being of another. When applied to the medical setting, this principle requires that every patient have the right to make decisions about the care he or she wishes to receive. It further assumes that the patient has the right to accept or refuse care and that the patient's decision is honored (not overruled by another).

The principle of *paternalism* is the one traditionally seen as conflicting with the principle of autonomy. *Paternalism* (perhaps better referred to as *parentalism*) holds that certain individuals are better able and have the right to make decisions for another. In the health care setting, this principle usually is applied to physicians but may easily include nurses as well. Paternalism (parentalism) is practiced in circumstances when we make decisions for patients in non–life-threatening situations or when we attempt to coerce or influence unduly the patient's decision-making to follow the practitioner's objectives.

The principle of *justice* as fairness is a modern ethical principle often applied to our modern health care system. Although not usually applied to individual patient situations, this principle guides and dominates discussions and decisions about the allocation of health care resources, equity in access to care, and delivery of care to certain groups or to all. The usual definition of justice as fairness means providing resources so that all will benefit to the level of equity.

The existence and employment of these ethical principles in the critical-care unit does not necessarily constitute an ethical dilemma. Dilemmas are created when human beings apply differing or conflicting ethical principles in the same situation. These people can be any of the health care professionals, the patient, or any person significant to the patient. Determination of whether an ethical dilemma exists requires first that each person involved be clear about what is creating the conflict, which means that one understands one's own set of values. Ethical principles such as those defined above are often identified as "universals"; many people believe that all persons share a belief in such a principle. In resolving an ethical dilemma, everyone involved must understand the nature and meaning—for each participant—of the relevant ethical principles. Further conflicts may arise if one of the participants does not share a belief in one of the principles (e.g., the patient's autonomy or the veracity of professionals).

When it is clear that a dilemma exists, there are two theoretical methods for resolution. The *deontological ethical method* says that, in any dilemma, there is only one right action that is consistent with ethical principles. If there is conflict between principles, then the higher-level principle should prevail. The second ethical method is the *utilitarian method*. This first defines the problem and alternative solutions. It then assigns—to each solution—a happiness value (best outcome for all) that will be produced by that alternative. The alternative with the highest value is the ethically right choice. (For a more complete discussion of these two methods and their variations, refer to Davis and Krueger 1980). Jonsen et al. (1982) have developed a model of ethical decision-making that is specific to the medical setting; it takes into account the medical situation/indications, patient preferences, quality of life, and external factors.

The actual process of ethical decision-making can be undertaken when everyone is familiar with the meaning of the ethical principles and agrees that a dilemma exists. Finally, the group involved in the decision-making should be familiar with the various theoretical methods by which to arrive at a decision.

Although theoretically this process can be undertaken by any group, ethical dilemmas in the critical-care setting are usually resolved by an experienced group of people from within the unit or hospital. Because of a growing emphasis on ethical dilemmas in hospitals, an increasing number of hospitals has organized bioethics committees and called on experts to assist in resolving ethical dilemmas. There is an increasing amount of literature in nursing, medical, and ethics journals regarding the functions of these bioethics committees.

Critical-care nurses must be familiar with the increasingly important area of bioethics—understanding the principles, recognizing dilemmas, and being actively involved in their resolution. Because ethical dilemmas add to the stress of working in the critical-care unit, it is especially important to critical-care nurses that these dilemmas be appropriately resolved. To assure the quality of patient care in their unit, nurses should insist on being a part of this special process.

Types of Ethical Dilemmas

Critical-care nurses often question the benefit that arises from use of the critical-care environment for certain patients. Such might be asked about the terminally ill patient (very often also elderly) or the patient admitted to the ICU who is not viewed as being critically ill. For the terminally ill patient, the ICU interventions often necessary (beginning with simple procedures such as drawing blood and IV placement) may appear to "harm" the patient more than they benefit. If one works in a unit that carries out research protocols, similar questions may be raised about the perceived conflict between benefit and harm.

The conflicts between paternalism and autonomy still exist in many ICUs. Perhaps expressed more subtly than in the past by practitioners, many still believe *they* know what is "best" for their patients. Recommending procedures and treatments, as well as minimizing discussion about alternatives, is still a typical approach of some physicians. Nurses often witness such practices with patients or families during the stay in critical-care units. Before we identify paternalism as a dilemma, however, we need to be sure that the patient or family identifies it as causing a dilemma. Not all patients and their families feel capable of making decisions about their medical care, choosing instead to rely on the expertise of physicians and nurses during an acute illness.

Requiring them to make difficult decisions may be inappropriate during the critical-care experience. Critical-care nurses must listen closely to patients and their families, however, to determine whether the patient's autonomy is being violated.

We also should be familiar with ways in which patients express their wishes regarding care. *Living wills* have been implemented by many individuals; from state to state, the legality and form of such documents differs, so we should all become familiar with what exists in our particular state. More recently, another form of document has been implemented to ensure a person's autonomy in the medical setting. The *durable power of attorney* allows an individual to assign legal power of attorney to another (not necessarily the legal next-of-kin) to make decisions about medical care when the individual is rendered incapable of doing so. Through education about and implementation of such documents, our current patients and future patients will be able to exercise more autonomy in their medical care.

A typical example of potential conflict between paternalism and autonomy is that related to the order "Do not resuscitate." Patients and families who request such an approach to continuing or terminating care must resolve any potential conflict with the physicians and nurses providing care. Discontinuation of life-extending or life-saving treatment also requires resolving any conflict between the principles of paternalism and autonomy.

The principle of justice as fairness is generally applied to situations involving the entire critical-care unit and general delivery of care (rather than an individual patient situation). This ethical principle is usually cited during discussions of the use and allocation of resources—human, financial, and technologic. The cost of critical care remains a major problem for both patients and third-party payers. In addition, there are continuing discussions regarding the use of critical-care beds for certain patients and the decisions made regarding which patients will receive care in the ICU. Engelhardt and Rie (1986) have described the problems of allocating ICU beds as a distribution issue (under the principle of justice as fairness) by identifying three areas of conflict:

(1) when further admissions to an ICU will jeopardize the standard of health care for all those in the ICU, (2) when those eligible for admission to an ICU (newcomers) appear to show greater promise of benefiting from treatment than those already allocated an ICU bed (early arrivers), or (3) when the investment of resources appears disproportionate given the marginal benefits likely to be obtained.

A study by Strauss et al. (1986) reviewed the issue of decision-making about patient admission and discharge from the ICU. Among other findings, they concluded that, during episodes of bed shortage, patients were generally more severely ill at the time of admission as well as discharge from the unit and had shorter stays in the unit. When there were available beds, severity of illness at the time of admission was less and stays were longer. Of interest is that bed availability had no effect on rates of death in the ICU, after discharge from the ICU, or upon readmission to the ICU.

What impact do these issues have on critical-care nurses? In many facilities, nurses participate actively in the policies and decision-making regarding patient admission to and discharge from the ICU. Nurses should be familiar with the ethical principles that dictate the allocation of ICU resources and should protect the established ICU policies and procedures from frivolous or inappropriate use. Nurses may not be directly involved with families and decision-making regarding admission to the ICU, but they are more frequently involved in explaining the transfer of patients from the ICU. Such interaction means the critical-care nurse should explain fully the reasons for discharge, how it is determined that the patient is able to be discharged, and assurance that care will be adequately and appropriately given by other nursing staff following discharge from the ICU.

Another issue with which critical-care nurses must often deal is that of terminal care being delivered in the critical-care unit when it seems clear that the resources being used will not be able to save the patient's life. This dilemma is further exacerbated by conflicts about resuscitation for these terminal patients. Should such patients be automatically transferred from the ICU? Is transfer seen as abandonment by family members? Or can nurses explain this decision so that families understand its medical intent?

An issue in allocation of ICU resources that has an impact most directly on the critical-care nurse is that of professional staff. The *availability* of critical-care nurses may limit admission of patients to the unit. Establishment and maintenance of appropriate patient–nurse ratios is critical to the continued provision of ICU services to the patient population. Adverse effects of shortages will be felt in a variety of ways by the institution and the patient—lowered quality of care, decreased total patient admissions, changes in types or numbers of patients admitted by physicians if they are not guaranteed quality critical care in that facility at that time, and increased stress on critical-care nurses (see previous discussion). Legal problems may also occur (see next section).

Legal Issues

Critical-care nursing is a high-risk occupation from a legal standpoint. According to Kimberly et al. (1982), nurses are often abysmally ignorant of the situations that place them at legal risk. Nurses face the increasing likelihood of becoming involved in a lawsuit. According to figures from the National Association of Insurance Commissioners (NAIC), nurses in 1978 were codefendents in almost 20% of all malpractice claims. This percentage is very likely to increase. Some of the general legal principles that critical-care nurses should know about are in the area of civil law, specifically tort law. *Tort law* applies to situations in which a person is injured or damaged by another person. In contrast, *criminal law* applies to injury or damage committed against the state or society by violation of statutes (laws). Typical torts cited in cases involving medical care are:

- *Negligence*—when harm comes to someone because the professional has failed to conform to an identified standard of care or practice.
- *Malpractice*—when a negligent act or omission in care or practice causes harm or injury.

The principle of *respondeat superior* is of special interest to nurses; it holds that the employer may be held vicariously liable for the acts of nurses.

Traditionally, nurses employed by an institution have been provided with professional insurance and would be protected and represented by the institution should a legal matter arise. As an employment benefit, insurance coverage is usually provided to full-time nursing personnel. Depending on the nurse's actions (or inactions) in certain situations, the hospital may or may not be obligated to provide legal counsel and support. Nurses should become aware of the limitations to the protection provided by the hospital. It is the nurse's responsibility to know what coverage and services the hospital will provide; any gaps in coverage should be assumed privately by the nurse. The hospital's insurance policy will cover nurses only when they are functioning within the scope of their job description. Moreover, the nurse's memory or viewpoint may differ from that of another employee; if such a conflict occurs, the hospital's attorney may not provide adequate representation. In addition, if the hospital pays a claim because of a nurse's negligence, it has the legal right to sue the nurse for reimbursement (George 1982).

Additional insurance coverage is available and is usually provided through groups such as a specialty organization (AACN), the American Nurses Association (ANA), or the state nurses' association. Nurses who are employed part-time, in a "casual" category, or on per-diem status may not have the insurance coverage afforded the full-time nurse; nurses working in these capacities should determine what insurance coverage they have and what they need. Nurses working via registries also should become cognizant of what coverage, if any, is provided by their agency.

Reasons for Lawsuits

According to Grane (1983), patients usually sue nurses for one of 12 reasons:

1. Failure to observe or monitor a patient adequately.
2. Failure to record or communicate significant changes in the patient's condition.
3. Failure to perform a procedure properly.
4. Failure to follow a physician's order promptly and correctly.
5. Failure to make prompt, accurate entries in a patient's chart.
6. Failure to give medications correctly.
7. Failure to report another professional's deviations from accepted practice.
8. Failure to use equipment properly.
9. Failure to resuscitate a patient properly.
10. Failure to protect the patient from avoidable injuries.
11. Failure to take a complete nursing history.
12. Failure to function within the scope of the nurse's education and job description.

Whether the nurse's behavior and practice in any situation is negligent is determined by comparing it to the acceptable standard of care, defined as that which a reasonably prudent nurse would have applied in the same situation. Standards of practice promulgated by professional organizations (e.g., AACN, ANA) also serve as definitions of standards of care.

Experience indicates reasons why lawsuits are filed against nurses (or physicians and nurses). The most important cause is usually that one has not established rapport or has lost rapport with the family or the patient, who feel they have been treated badly. The actual incident is often secondary and relates to breaks in established techniques or procedures, or a sudden, unexpected negative change in the patient's condition, or an unexpected poor outcome of care.

Protection Against Lawsuits

Nurses often dismiss the possibility of a lawsuit by saying, "It can't happen to me. I am a professional." Assumptions about one's expertise and denial of the possibility are not enough, however. There are specific measures that one can take; some of them follow.

Know your job. Know exactly what job you are supposed to be doing—its scope and its limitations. Know what the job description says that you are to be doing; know that it reflects the current responsibilities and practices of you and your colleagues.

Document promptly, completely, clearly, and accurately. Carefully record the time that events occurred as well as the time of documentation (especially if there has been a time lapse). Any corrections made to your charting should be noted with a single line through the entry and the word "error" and reason for error noted. Never totally obliterate an entry by crossing over or with use of "white-out." Because lawsuits often are filed several years after the event, develop a charting style that you will recognize and perhaps will allow a greater sense of recall about the events. Review physician notes and charting about especially important or problematic incidents and resolve discrepancies with the physician at the time of the event; it is often too late at the time of deposition and trial.

Never be too busy to talk to the patient or family (or significant others). At the end of the crisis or the resuscitation procedure, take a moment to talk to the family; make this the first priority (when you would surely prefer a moment of rest and quiet for yourself). Be as honest as possible about what is happening; do not try to minimize crises or simply dismiss the apparent gravity of the situation. For families and loved ones, events that we consider usual or expected in the critical care setting still remain frightening and unexpected.

Special Legal Problems

There are a number of areas of critical care that may pose potential legal problems for the nursing staff. Legal experts have made recommendations for preventing problems in these areas.

The medically questionable order is one of the most common dilemmas faced by the critical-care nurse and has been the subject of several legal decisions. To pro-

tect yourself, there are several kinds of orders you should question, including ambiguous orders, any order the patient questions, any order that will compromise a preexisting patient condition, and standing or PRN orders if you cannot judge whether they are appropriate for the situation. Finally, always read back verbal orders and ask the physician any questions about them to be sure you have understood and noted them correctly.

Regarding written orders, the courts have clearly indicated that when there is a question about a medical order, the nurse is responsible for contacting the physician who wrote it (Roach 1980). If you disagree with the order and the physician still directs you to carry it out, you have a duty to refuse. When the situation is less clear and you are unclear about the order or its rationale, you can discuss the order with other physicians involved in the case or consult with the medical director of the critical-care unit. Some units require a second nurse to listen to verbal orders. The safest form of documentation would, of course, be to tape record all such telephone orders (Bennett 1981).

"Do not resuscitate" (DNR or no code) orders have already been mentioned as a potential ethical dilemma. Without information provided in writing by the patient, such orders are more difficult to carry out within the ICU. Individual states have made different rulings on such orders, so it is necessary for the nurse to be aware of established case law. The issuance of verbal orders regarding DNR and "slow codes" create even greater dilemmas and should be avoided through procedural mechanisms in the ICU setting.

Withdrawal of life support for the terminal, comatose patient is a more current dilemma which again is being resolved in case law. Often this occurs after transfer from the ICU and thus does not impact as directly on the critical-care nurse. However, it has the potential for creating both ethical and legal dilemmas for the nursing staff.

What to Do if You Are Sued

Being sued is usually an unexpected and emotional traumatic event. By the time you are made aware of a lawsuit, an attorney has been retained by the plaintiff (the patient and/or family) and the patient's medical record has been reviewed by an expert who determined that care was substandard (negligence or malpractice). You will receive a copy of the filed *petition* (complaint) naming you, specifying the allegation, and indicating the amount of money for damages that is being sought. Upon receipt, notify the hospital's attorney through your appropriate supervisory channels and your own insurance company if you have separate coverage. Arrangements will be made for you to give a *deposition* (testimony given under oath and in the presence of both attorneys in response to their questions). This legal testimony is admissible as evidence during a trial. If your lawyer does not volunteer to do so, insist that he or she meet with you to review all the information that has been discovered in the case and to explain fully the process of taking a deposition. Be aware that the plaintiff's attorney may challenge your answers in an attempt to confuse and rattle you—try to keep calm and do not become argumentative. You will have an opportunity to review the deposition for its accuracy. Approximately 80% of all cases are settled out of court (usually immediately before the trial begins); this may occur even if you truly believe you were not at fault. Be prepared for this possibility, so the process will not seem useless or frustrating.

Remaining aware of ways in which legal action can be prevented and ensuring that nursing practice is professional at all times can assist in avoiding lawsuits. In our increasingly litigious society, however, nurses should no longer believe they will not be sued. Nurses individually and collectively are increasingly at great risk. For example, Engelhardt and Rie (1986) reviewed the case of a lawsuit against critical-care nurses and a hospital because of inadequate staffing in the ICU that caused patient complications.

Example: The Case of Organ Donation

The following discussion of the process of organ donation is an example of all the various aspects of critical-care nursing that we have so far discussed—stress and emotional aspects of critical-care nursing, ethical dilemmas and decision-making, and legal considerations of practice—all occurring in a highly technologic environment. While there are a number of issues that could be discussed, organ donation has been chosen because it has a fairly long history of development, many (although not all) of the issues have been resolved, and, most important, it is a universal process—one that can be accomplished in every ICU in the United States.

For purposes of this discussion, organ donation will include the donation of all organs and tissues currently being used for both research and clinical transplants from cadaver donors. The history of organ donation is a long one, with the first solid organs (kidneys) being re-

moved in the 1950s and 1960s (Moore 1964). The development of the ICU, with the use of artificial respirators, made the concept of organ donation a possibility by providing complete respiratory function; without such treatment, brain death would never have become an identified phenomenon (Hopper 1983).

Organ donation is achieved when a number of factors are met through the efforts of a number of people. At the center of the process is an individual (usually young and healthy) who has suffered brain death secondary to an unexpected accident, injury, or disease. The patient's next-of-kin and other loved ones are intimately involved in the donation. Physicians representing a number of specialties are providing medical care to the patient, initially directed toward life-saving treatments and procedures. Critical-care nurses are providing direct care to the patient and share the goal of patient recovery; in addition, they closely interact with the family and other loved ones. Law enforcement officials and medical examiners/coroners are also frequently (although not universally) involved.

Stress of Organ Donation

The stress of caring for the organ donor has been poorly measured and documented. Sophie et al. (1983) measured the responses of critical-care nurses to organ donation. They found that many nurses report this is often a frustrating experience that conflicts with their goals as critical-care nurses. Physicians as well feel these conflicts when their attempts to save a life are negated by brain death. It is not uncommon for physicians to seem to withdraw in such situations, providing necessary supportive care but referring the patient to appropriate transplant agencies/physicians for continued care. Nurses continue to provide direct care to the organ donor and struggle with the issue of caring for someone who is dead. An additional stressor is present in this nursing care: the nurse is the direct protector of the critically important vital organs that will be removed and used for transplantation. The need to provide expert care, to monitor and maintain excellent cardiac, respiratory, liver, and kidney function in a hemodynamically fragile patient is a challenge to the critical-care nurse. A recent article by Goldsmith and Montefusco (1985) outlines in detail these nursing care responsibilities and interventions. The stress is compounded by the frequent need for the nurse to serve as coordinator of all the agencies involved in organ/tissue donation, making the necessary arrangements for the actual recovery of organ and tissues to be accomplished. Lastly, the critical-care nurse is expected to provide emotional and informational support to the family of the organ donor in a way that assures donation will be a positive experience for them.

Ethical Aspects of Organ Donation

The ethical considerations of organ donation and the related transplant seem to parallel the development of bioethics. In conjunction with the problems of those awaiting organ transplants (selection for and treatment with dialysis, death of children and young adults from cardiac or liver disease), organ donation raised issues of beneficence, autonomy, and allocation of resources. These ethical issues and attendant dilemmas continue to emerge in various forms at different times and in different situations, for instance, debates about voluntary or presumed consent for organ donation or which group of patients (citizens vs noncitizens) receive transplants. Even the redefinition of life and death (brain death vs cardiorespiratory death) has required the clarification of values by health professionals and the public.

With the first heart transplant in 1967, everyone had to confront the fact that biological life was dependent on brain function, not cardiac function as tradition had taught. The survival and function of a transplanted heart created conflicts of biology and soul; individuals had to rethink the meaning of life and death. This dilemma of redefinition is continuing through new discussions of the use of anencephalic newborns as organ donors at the time of birth (Harrison 1986).

The ethical principle of beneficence may be achieved through organ donation, albeit indirectly. While the organ donor receives no direct benefit, it is held ethically good that the organs and tissues donated provide life, improve quality of life, and relieve suffering for those who receive the transplants. Benefit is also given to families who are comforted by the knowledge of benefit to the transplant recipients.

The principle of autonomy in organ donation was defined in 1964 with the Uniform Anatomic Gift Act, which provided adults with the right to make decisions regarding organ/tissue donation following their death. The right to sign a donor card as a legal document expressing one's wish about organ donation has stood the test of time. This autonomous decision is rarely overridden by family members; when this occurs, professionals deem it necessary for the psychological well-being of the family not to carry out the wishes of the deceased individual. Changes affecting the autonomy of patients in regard to organ donation have been made; some states allow for the removal of corneas without the donor's express consent (via a donor card) or without consent of the next-of-kin. Caplan (1983) advocates the principle of *presumed consent* for organ donation, which would allow anyone to serve as an organ/tissue donor unless the person had, in writing, expressly indicated opposition to donation.

The principle of justice as fairness usually is applied to organ donation in regard to the maintenance of donors in the critical-care unit; again, the benefit of fairness is assigned to the transplant recipients. When resources are scarce or unavailable, is it appropriate to continue the life support maintenance of the potential organ donor while consent is being obtained, arrangements made, and transplant teams travel to the donor hospital? Does the benefit outweigh the risks to other patients that come from these limited resources? Is the brain-dead patient to be admitted to the busy critical-care unit to receive supportive care until organs can be recovered? These questions are not easily resolved by policy or regulation and create continuing ethical dilemmas for the nurse involved with organ donation.

Legal Aspects of Organ Donation

Consent for organ donation was established by statute, as previously described. That same legislation describes the legal order of consent by next-of-kin. Critical-care nurses should become familiar with the legal order and often are responsible for assuring that the legal next-of-kin is identified for purposes of consent. In some circumstances this is not as simple as it may seem. Careful attention to the legal aspects (as well as donor care) can prevent potential litigation. If questions arise regarding consent for organ donation, the critical-care nurse should consult a member of the transplant team, the organ procurement agency, or the hospital's attorney for expert advice.

The definition of brain death has moved from being a medical diagnosis in the 1960s (Ad Hoc Committee 1968) to becoming a recognized legal definition embodied in state statute. Presently, 38 states and the District of Columbia have statutes recognizing the legality of the diagnosis or pronouncement of brain death. In other states, court decisions have supported the legality of brain death. Medical assessment and testing is performed to determine that total and irreversible cessation of brain function, including the brain stem, has occurred. Though the President's Commission for the Study of Ethical Problems in Medicine and Biomedical and Behavioral Research (1981) recommended uniform legislation for the determination of death (including brain death), such legislation has not been forthcoming. Critical-care nurses should therefore become very familiar with the legal determination of brain death in their state to assure that this process is carried out properly.

Other legal parameters of organ donation may involve traditional state laws about reporting to law enforcement personnel or medical examiners/coroners deaths occurring in the hospital. States have lenient to rigid laws regarding the reporting of unexpected or sudden deaths (even from "natural" causes) as well as those associated with accidents or at the hand of others. Medical examiners/coroners are considered to be the recipients of the patient's body in cases where an autopsy must be performed to determine the legal cause of death. Thus, the procedure of organ donation must be approved by the coroner to assure that the removal of organs will not interfere with or compromise the ability to determine the legal cause of death. Medical examiners/coroners interpret their role in organ donation in very different ways and have established local (county) policies and procedures regarding organ donation. The critical-care nurse should also be familiar with these policies.

Another legal parameter involving organ donation is being adopted by a number of states and will probably be proposed as federal legislation. The concept of *required request* assures that all hospitals and their staffs (including physicians and nurses) inquire about organ/tissue donation at the time of death of every patient. Appropriate documentation of this request is required in the patient's chart. These statutes carry fines and other censure mechanisms for hospitals not in compliance.

In summary, organ donation is a complex procedure carried out in the critical-care unit primarily by nurses. These nurses should have available written materials regarding policies and procedures for organ donation specific to their institution and their county and state. Personnel are also available from the various transplant/organ procurement programs to advise and assist the critical-care nursing staff.

Organ donation is simply one of many of the issues (ethical, legal, and professional) that affect the practice of critical-care nurses. Nurses who work in critical-care settings must be expert practitioners in a variety of specialties and subspecialties. Their expertise is the key to assuring the successful completion of this process and all others that are currently a part of critical care.

REFERENCES

Ad Hoc Committee: A definition of irreversible coma: Report of the ad hoc committee of the Harvard Medical School to examine the definition of brain death. *JAMA* 1968; 205(6):337–341.

Ashley JoAnn: *Hospitals, paternalism, and the role of the nurse.* New York: Teachers College Press, 1976.

Bailey J et al.: The stress audit: Identifying the stressors of the ICU nurse. *J Nurs Ed* 1980; 19:15–25.

Benner P: *From novice to expert: Excellence and power in clinical nursing practice.* Menlo Park, CA: Addison-Wesley Publishing Co., 1984.

Bennett H: The legalities of critical care. *Crit Care Nurse* (March/April) 1981; 54–55.

Caplan L: Organ transplants: The costs of success. *The Hastings Center Report* (December) 1983; 23–32.

Christopherson DJ: Control and power in critical care. *Dimen Crit Care Nurs* 1986; 5(5).

Davis J, Krueger C: *Patients, Nurses, Ethics.* New York: American Journal of Nursing Co., 1980.

Dear M et al.: The effect of the intensive care nursing role on job satisfaction and turnover. *Heart Lung* 1982; 11:560–565.

Engelhardt HT, Rie A: Intensive care units, scarce resources, and conflicting principles of justice. *JAMA* 1986; 255(9):1159–1164.

Freudenberger HJ, North G: *Women's burnout.* Garden City, NY: Doubleday, 1985.

Gardner D et al.: The nurse's dilemma: Mediating stress in critical care units. *Heart Lung* 1980; 9:103–106.

Gentry W, Parkes K: Psychologic stress in intensive care unit and non-intensive care unit nursing. A review of the past decade. *Heart Lung* 1982; 11:43–47.

George J: Malpractice insurance. *J Emerg Nurs* 1982; 6:319–320.

Goldsmith J, Montefusco CM: Nursing care of the potential organ donor. *Crit Care Nurse* 1985; 5(6):22–29.

Grane N: How to reduce your risk of a lawsuit. *Nurs Life* (January-February) 1983; 17–20.

Harrison M: Anencephalic newborns as organ donors. *The Hastings Center Report* (April) 1986; 16(2):21–23.

Hopper S: Science, technology, and organ recovery (Unpublished Paper). 1983.

Jervik DK, Martinson IM: *Women in stress: A nursing perspective.* New York: Appleton-Century-Crofts, 1979.

Jonsen AR et al.: *Clinical ethics.* New York: Macmillan, 1982.

Kimberly R et al.: What do the courts expect from nurses? *Nurs Life* (September/October) 1982; 34–37.

Mendenhall J: Factors affecting job satisfaction/dissatisfaction among critical care nurses. *Focus* (October/November) 1982; 14–18.

Moore FD: *Transplant: The give and take of tissue transplantation.* New York: Saunders, 1964.

President's Commission: *Defining death: Medical, legal and ethical issues in the determination of death.* President's Commission for the Study of Ethical Problems in Medicine and Biomedical and Behavioral Research. Washington, D.C.: U.S. Government Printing Office, 1981.

Richmond T, Craig M: Timeout: Facing death in the ICU. *Dimen Crit Care Nurs* 1985; 4(1):41–45.

Roach W: Responsible intervention: A legal duty to act. *J Nurs Admin* (July) 1980; 18–24.

Sophie LR et al.: Intensive care nurses' perceptions of cadaver organ procurement. *Heart Lung* 1983; 12:261–267.

Strauss MJ et al.: Rationing of intensive care unit services. *JAMA* 1986; 255(9):1143–1146.

Vincent P, Coleman WF: Comparison of major stressors perceived by ICU and non-ICU nurses. *Crit Care Nurse* 1986; 6(1):64–69.

SUPPLEMENTAL READING

Baldwin R: The trial of a medical malpractice case. *Crit Care Nurse* 1986; 6(4):19–21.

Birkholz G: IABP: Legal and ethical issues. *Dimen Crit Care Nurs* 1985; 4(5):285–287.

Cox J: Organ donation: The challenge for emergency nursing. *JEN* 1986; 12(4):199–204.

Cranford RE, Doudera AE (eds): *Institutional ethics committees and health care decision making.* Ann Arbor, MI: Health Administration Press, 1984.

Cranford RE, Van Allen EJ: The implications and applications of institutional ethics committees. *Am Coll Surg Bull* 1985; 70(6):19–24.

Diggs CL: Recognition and nursing care of organ donors. *JEN* 1986; 12(4):205–209.

Galanes S et al.: The intensive care unit population within the prospective payment system. *Heart Lung* 1986; 15(5):515–520.

Goldsmith J, Montefusco CM: Nursing care of the potential organ donor. *Crit Care Nurse* 1985; 5(6):22–29.

Goodman MR, Aung MH: Cerebral death: Theological, judicial, and medical aspects. *Heart Lung* 1978; 7(3):477–483.

Johnson LW: A case for organ donation. (Case Review) *JEN* 1986; 12(4):196–198.

Lipton H: Do-not-resuscitate decisions in a community hospital: Incidence, implications, and outcomes. *JAMA* 1986; 256(9):1164–1169.

Moskowitz LD, Moskowitz S: Autonomy and the critically ill patient: The legal issues. *Heart Lung* 1986; 15(5):520–524.

Questions and answers about organ donation. (Emergency Nursing News) *JEN* 1986; 12(4):24–26.

Vincent P, Coleman WF: Comparison of major stressors perceived by ICU and non-ICU nurses. *Crit Care Nurse* 1986; 6(1):64–69.

Unit 2

COMMUNICATION

3

Communication:
Patient and Family

CLINICAL INSIGHT

Domain: The helping role

Competency: Providing emotional and informational support to patients and families

Critical-care nurses view their constituency as not just patients but families as well. While they are engaged primarily with patients' physiologic crises, they never forget the distraught families desperately in need of nurturing. Accustomed to the hectic, high-technology environment, critical-care nurses nevertheless know how sterile and cold it can seem to families. They are committed to making this forbidding environment understandable and to helping families maintain hope in the face of devastating illness. Because of repeated exposure to the system of care for the critically ill, nurses can help interpret for families the complex organizational network surrounding them, as well as identify when and how the family can best provide emotional support to the patient. Through the simple acts of acknowledging and preserving family bonds, nurses bring humanity and grace to an otherwise nightmarish experience. This is illustrated in the following examplar, from Crabtree and Jorgenson (1986, pp. 118-119).

I feel like every time I go to a patient's room, I say, do you have family? Are there significant others here? I bring them in the room; I go through everything with them. It's just foreign objects to them, and I'm sure it looks like E.T. As you explain all these things, you really alleviate their anxieties. This is a monitor; it's like an electrocardiogram—because they can identify with that. And, this is why we're watching it, not because there's something wrong with your mother's heart, but the rate will tell us lots of things—if the patient's temperature is going up, if they're anxious, if there's any problem with their lungs. I really go through it all, because I give the public credit for knowing a lot. To me, it's amazing; they've all read Readers' Digest.

They know that I'm there for their loved one, period. I convey that some way in communicating. And, I'll keep you informed. And, the things that I have found that I am able to accomplish is that they go home—the families go home. Because, they need permission to go home. And, I tell them, you're in intensive care now. The reason you're here is the nurse is going to be with your mother, your father, whatever, around the clock. We're not going to physically stand at the bedside, but we're monitoring them here and at the desk, and this is the time that you need rest. You've had a hard day, too; and it's okay to go home.

Things can change. Right now everything is stable; the blood pressure is stable; the pulse is stable. I know that you can't communicate because they're on the respirator, and I tell them why they can't communicate. They feel that their mother's never going to talk again, so it's really important to me to tell them when this tube comes out, they're going to be able to talk, and I tell them why they can't talk because air can't get by the vocal cords, etc. They understand it. Tonight we're going to heavily sedate your mother and keep her as comfortable as possible, and this is a good time for you to get rest. Because, when the patient comes out onto the floor situation, there's not going to be as many nurses, and this is when she's going to really need you. I'll give you my phone number. You can call any time.

Communication is the dynamic, multisensory interaction in which a person shares thoughts and feelings with other people in his psychosocial environment. This chapter looks at ways you can alleviate the impact of a critical illness on the psychosocial health of the previously well-adjusted person and family who are now stressed by a situational crisis. It does not address psychiatric or communication disorders requiring specialized assessment and therapy; if you encounter patients with such problems, seek consultation from and/or provide referral to appropriate professionals.

Assessment

Communication consists of both process and content. Your goals in assessing your patient's communications therefore are two-fold: to identify both how and what the patient communicates. A suggested format for assessment is shown in Table 3-1.

Process: History and Physical Examination

In order to communicate, a person must have both motivation and means. Although severe communication difficulties should be evaluated by specialists, you can perform a brief, functional assessment of communicative processes that can be a guide in future interactions with your patient. Most times, attentive observation of the patient will suffice. Occasionally, you may want to supplement observation with questions to the patient or family, or simple tests.

The brain receives three major types of stimuli related to communication: visual, auditory, and tactile. Each input modality requires the person to receive the stimulus, perceive its characteristics, and then associate it with previously integrated stimuli. There also are three ways in which the brain can communicate messages: speech, gestures, and writing. Each output modality requires the person to conceptualize an idea, formulate it into neural stimuli, and express it through motor activity.

Visual Input   You will recall that the retina perceives light rays in a reversed fashion; that is, rays from the right side of the visual field strike the left side of the retina. Nerve fibers from the retina form the optic nerve. The inner halves of the two optic nerves cross in the optic chiasma and rejoin the outer halves to form optic tracts (Figure 3-1). Because of this partial crossing, each optic trace contains fibers from the same half of each eye. For example, the right optic tract has fibers from the right half of each eye (which perceive rays from the left half of each visual field).

The tracts terminate in the thalamus (specifically, in the lateral geniculate bodies). From there, the optic radiations course to the visual portions of the occipital lobes.

Knowledge of this anatomy is important in understanding the various types of blindness. The patient who is blind in one eye but not the other has damage to the retina or optic nerve. *Hemianopia* is visual loss in half of each visual field. Blindness in the temporal field of each eye *(bitemporal hemianopia)* results from a lesion involving the optic chiasma. The patient who is blind in the nasal field of one eye and temporal field of the other eye *(homonymous hemianopia)* is suffering from an injury to the optic tract, optic radiation, or visual cortex. For example, suppose your patient could not see anything in the temporal field of the right eye and the nasal field of the left eye. Light rays from these fields strike the left half of each retina. Because the partial crossing of the optic nerves occurs in the optic chiasma, impulses from the left half of each retina traverse the left optic tract, lateral geniculate body, and optic radiation to the visual cortex, any of which could be the site of the lesion.

When assessing visual input, note whether the patient has any visual deficits. These may be pre-existing (such as blindness, cataracts, or decreased visual acuity) or associated with the current illness (such as hemianopia, which often accompanies hemiplegia). Find out if the person reads Braille, uses glasses, or wears contact lenses. Also estimate the patient's reading level as a guide for future teaching techniques.

TABLE 3-1 COMMUNICATION ASSESSMENT FORMAT

Process

1. History _____

   _____

2. Physical

   Vision _____

   Reading ability _____

   Hearing _____

   Tactile perception _____

   Speech _____

   Writing ability _____

   Gesturing ability _____

3. Diagnostic procedures and laboratory tests _____

   _____

4. Other relevant data _____

Content

1. History _____

   Ethnic background _____

   Religion _____

   Education _____

   Occupation _____

   Usual coping methods

      Pain _____

      _____

      _____

      Anger _____

      Substance abuse _____

   Emotional problems _____

   _____

2. Current information

   Expressed concerns _____

   _____

   _____

   Expectations of hospitalization _____

   _____

   _____

   Significant others _____

   _____

   Role in the family _____

   Apparent stage of adaptation to illness _____

   _____

3. Diagnostic procedures _____

4. Other relevant data _____

   _____

   _____

   _____

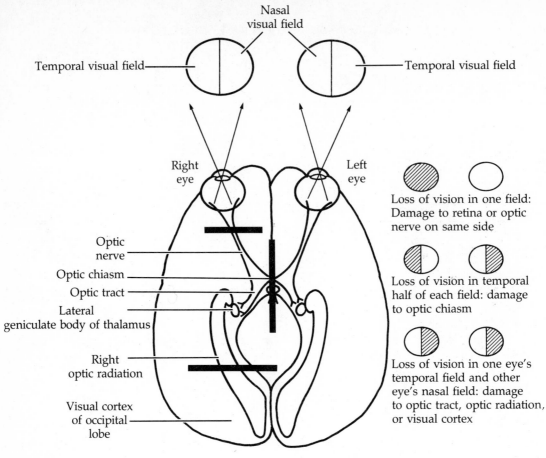

Nasal
visual field

Temporal visual field

Temporal visual field

Right
eye

Left
eye

Loss of vision in one field:
Damage to retina or optic
nerve on same side

Optic
nerve

Optic chiasm

Optic tract

Lateral
geniculate body of thalamus

Loss of vision in temporal
half of each field: damage
to optic chiasm

Right
optic radiation

Visual cortex
of occipital
lobe

Loss of vision in one eye's
temporal field and other
eye's nasal field: damage
to optic tract, optic radiation,
or visual cortex

FIGURE 3-1

Visual pathways.

Auditory Input Auditory impulses are transmitted from the cochlea along the acoustic (eighth cranial) nerve to the brainstem. From there, they ascend to the thalamus and the auditory area in the temporal lobe. If the person fails to respond normally to sound, a conductive or sensorineural hearing loss may be present. A conductive loss results from conditions which block the transport of sound to the middle ear, such as impacted cerumen, middle ear infections, or a perforated eardrum. A sensorineural loss means that the inner ear is unable to transmit sound energy to the brain. An example of sensorineural hearing loss is streptomycin ototoxicity. If the person has a hearing deficit, note whether he or she uses sign language, wears a hearing aid, or can read lips.

Tactile Perception Tactile perception, while a lesser form of stimuli input, nevertheless is important. The person with a tactile deficit may have difficulty sensing objects in contact with him. As a result, he may be unable to distinguish objects by touch, perceive pain, or sense others' emotions expressed through touch. In addition to assessing whether the person perceives tactile stimuli normally, ask whether he or she likes to be touched by others. Some people find it warm and comforting; others experience it as a territorial intrusion.

Expressive Output Output consists of speaking, writing, and/or gesturing. Output difficulties usually are thought of as resulting from a motor disturbance such as paralysis, Parkinsonism, or cerebral palsy. Among the critically ill, however, probably the number-one output problem involves the intubated patient. One ventilator patient, a physician, later described his communication difficulties vividly (Chaney 1975):

I was lying there on my back with the respirator humming away, when I suddenly felt a wave of nausea. I immediately knew I'd developed gastric distention and that I was vomiting and aspirating a lot of gastric fluid. Since I couldn't talk with the endotracheal tube, I frantically signaled the nurse and tried to communicate I was aspirating. She tried to reassure me that I wasn't, but there was no doubt. It felt like it was at least a gallon, and I felt like I was drowning. . . . I still feel that had I been successful in my desperate attempts to pull the bite block and the tube out so I could vomit over the side of the bed, I would've been able to prevent much of the damage. . . . I just lay there waiting for my aspiration pneumonia to develop—which is exactly what happened.

Ventilator patients who are paralyzed with pancuronium bromide or curare are in double emotional jeopardy. In addition to the terror of not being able to speak, which can afflict any ventilator patient, these patients suffer the additional terror of being unable to move. Worse, staff often ignore them or treat them as if they were comatose. Because their eyes are closed, they appear to be sleeping or unconscious. These patients need exceptional emotional support from a caring, sensitive staff and family. They also may benefit from sedation to blunt their perception and combat the panic provoked by paralysis.

Aphasia Aphasia is the loss of verbal comprehension and/or expression. Aphasia often accompanies strokes or head trauma and also may occur with cerebral hemorrhage or embolism.

Comprehension of spoken or written speech is a function of Wernicke's speech area in the temporal lobe. To distinguish a hearing deficit from receptive aphasia, make a loud sound next to the ear—the aphasic will be startled, the deaf person will not. The ability to write or speak is controlled by a premotor area in the frontal lobe, which directs the motor cortex and extrapyramidal system to produce coordinated movements of the muscles of speech or writing. Broca's area, the motor/speech area, is almost always dominant in the left cerebral cortex, regardless of whether a person is right or left handed. Thus, a right-handed person who develops right-sided paralysis usually also loses speech, because both are controlled by the left hemisphere. In contrast, a right-handed person who develops left-sided paralysis usually retains speech, because the paralysis results from a lesion in the nondominant (right) hemisphere.

To summarize: Damage to Broca's area in the frontal lobe results in the loss of motor speech. The patient has unintelligible or garbled speech but understands when spoken to. This type of aphasia is termed *nonfluent aphasia* or *expressive aphasia*. Damage to Wernicke's area in the temporal lobe results in the loss of the ability to understand spoken and/or written language. The patient often can enunciate individual words but does not understand spoken and/or written language. This type of aphasia is termed *fluent aphasia* or *receptive aphasia* (Burns and Halper 1986). Patients with neurologic damage to the frontal and temporal lobes often have a mix of both disorders.

Content

The sections above have described nursing assessment of methods of communication. Equally important is assessment of the thoughts and feelings the patient communicates—in other words, the content of communication. A comprehensive, highly theoretical discussion of communication content is beyond the scope of this book. Instead, this chapter will focus on practical ways you can assess the content of your patient's communications and intervene to assist his adaptation to the crisis of critical illness.

An assessment of content should include both history and current information.

History The patient's ethnic status, religion, education, and occupation provide information about the patient's background. As such, they can provide clues to her or his values and beliefs. They also can help you identify possible problem areas, such as differing health beliefs between the patient's culture and your own. To avoid stereotyping your patient, be sure to validate any suppositions you are tempted to make solely on the basis of background information.

Asking the person how he or she usually copes with stressful situations can help you to interpret more accurately the person's current behavior under stress. It also allows you to identify and support successful coping strategies or suggest alternatives to ineffective ones. Because many people have difficulty expressing pain and anger, be sure to ask how the person usually copes with these feelings. Also ask specifically about the use of alcohol, tranquilizers, sleeping pills, and other mood-altering substances. The replies not only may provide insight into the patient's coping abilities but also may help you anticipate some physiologic problems, such as delirium tremens following the sudden withdrawal of alcohol or convulsions following abrupt cessation or barbiturate abuse.

Inquire, too, about a history of emotional problems, recent or significant lifestyle changes, and the quality of previous health care experiences. Knowledge of past emotional problems, particularly those severe enough to warrant treatment, can be important in prevention and early recognition of psychotic episodes. Descriptions of lifestyle changes can lead to fruitful information about patient and family role dislocations, frustrations, and emotional losses such as the death of a spouse. Descriptions of past health care experiences can help you determine whether there are primarily unpleasant memories, which tend to create a negative set toward hospital care, or mostly positive memories, which create a favorable basis on which to build trusting relationships with health care providers.

Current Information The next section of your assessment should elicit data about the person's current emotional state. There are five areas to assess: expressed concerns, expectations of hospitalization, significant others, role in the family, and stage of adaptation (which are discussed in detail in the following section).

Expressed Concerns A critical illness imposes not only physiologic crises for the patient but also emotional problems for the patient and family. A crisis is defined as the emotional disequilibrium that results from the sudden disruption of one's customary behaviors, beliefs, or values. Each person responds individually in a crisis; elements of a situation that are stressful for one person may not be for another. The patient's emotional crisis may be provoked by an unfamiliar environment, forced dependency, fear of pain, fear of disfigurement or death, or other factors. A family member's crisis may be precipitated by fear of the outcome of the patient's illness, worry about finances, changed roles within the family, an unresolved preadmission argument with the patient, or perhaps conflict between wanting to be with both the patient in the critical-care unit and small children at home.

You can begin to determine what emotional problems are troubling the person through sensitive listening and observation of affect and behavior. If the person can speak, ask what is troubling him or her. If the person is unable to speak, you may have to attempt to deduce his or her feelings from facial expressions or perhaps from "yes/no" answers to questions you frame. In either case, be sure to validate with the person your interpretations of his or her feelings. Evaluate the person's response for its appropriateness to reality by assessing content/affect and verbal/nonverbal congruence.

Expectations of Hospitalization By asking the patient and/or family what they think will happen during and after the hospitalization, you may be able to identify unrealistic expectations or areas of ignorance, denial, or misconception about the plan of therapy. It also is helpful to ask about the experiences of relatives or friends with similar disorders. It is not uncommon, for instance, to discover that your preoperative patient has a positive attitude because a coworker or neighbor was helped by

similar surgery, or alternatively fears the surgery because an acquaintance developed a complication and died.

Significant Others Significant others are those persons who play key roles in the patient's life. Most often they are relatives, though they may include friends, lovers, employers, other patients, and members of the hospital staff. (Throughout this book, the term "significant others" is used interchangeably with "family." "Family" means not just blood relatives but all those who care about and nurture the patient.) Try to identify the nature of their relationships with the patient before illness and their current levels of involvement. There may, of course, be some whose significance lies in negative or unhealthy relationships with your patient, such as an overly critical or demanding spouse. Lastly, try to identify the family's feelings—such as helplessness, fear, anger, grief, guilt—and evaluate their apparent coping levels.

Role in the Family The patient's role in the family is becoming increasingly recognized as an independent factor for successful adaptation to medical crisis (Brandt 1984; Fife 1985; Stryker and Statham 1985). Sudden illness within a family can disrupt established roles and force members to reintegrate positions in order to regain equilibrium. Role theory pertains to the pattern of behavior that occurs within a specific social context. *Role* refers to distinct expectations, responsibilities, and privileges associated with a person's position within a social structure such as the family. Fife (1985) has proposed a model for predicting the adaptation of families to medical crisis. It is based on the premise that families will adjust to a medical crisis using previous coping strategies. Although previous strategies may not always be a viable alternative in a crisis or may be ineffective, family functioning prior to a crisis should provide a measure of how a family might cope with the stress and disruption of having a loved one in an intensive care unit. Some relevant questions to ask when assessing role function within the family are:

How has the family met previous family crises?

Who maintains the roles within the family?

Is there flexibility in the family for role definitions?

How are role expectations within the family expressed and relayed to other family members?

Does one family member assume the primary responsibility for meeting the family's needs?

Since the crisis, have children in the family been expected to inappropriately assume adult roles?

Are financial resources adequate?

How is power distributed among the members?

How are decisions made? (Fife, 1985).

Stage of Adaptation Adaptation to a crisis evolves in four stages: shock, disorganization, reorganization, and resolution. You can identify the patient's stage of adaptation by assessing his or her affect, verbal statements, behavior, sleeping pattern, and gastrointestinal function. The length of time since the onset of the crisis is also an important factor to assess.

1. Shock The shock phase begins with the onset of the crisis and usually lasts 24–36 hours. In this phase the person is stunned by what has happened. The patient may describe feeling numb or extremely calm, or may minimize the severity of what has happened, say he or she is in control of the situation, or ignore it completely. The patient may be inappropriately calm or cheerful, keep interactions on a superficial level, or try to focus conversations on you and your interests, or may attribute the hospital admission to a desire to placate others, such as a spouse or the doctor. All of these behaviors are manifestations of the patient's attempt to protect self by denying reality.

2. Disorganization The stage of disorganization evolves when the person begins to realize what has occurred and its implications for the future. It usually starts within one to two days and lasts a variable period of time, typically two to four weeks. Behavior during this stage may be marked by anxiety, depression, or anger. The anxious person displays signs of emotional agitation, muscle tension, and autonomic nervous system hyperactivity, such as restlessness, fidgeting, shaking, anorexia, nausea, diarrhea, sweaty palms, dry mouth, tachycardia, flushing, clenched hands, or rigid posture. There is often difficulty sleeping, concentrating, or making decisions. The patient may talk almost continuously, failing to respond to cues that normally indicate a transition between topics or the end of a conversation; silence seems intolerable.

The person may also respond with rage at the unfairness of what has happened and the inability to control it. He or she may be demanding or antagonistic, making disparaging remarks about his or her care. Attempts to help the person are greeted with active rejection or passive-aggressive responses such as "Yes, but . . . ." The anger often is displaced onto safer or more available targets. Minor annoyances such as a late visitor may escalate into major confrontations, as the person deliberately provokes arguments in order to release anger.

Withdrawal and depression may characterize the person who is unable to express anger and so turns it inward. The depressed person looks sad and may cry easily and uncontrollably. He or she may move slowly, sleep excessively, eat poorly, and allow grooming to deteriorate. Such persons may curl into a fetal position or slump apathetically in bed. Often, they will not initiate conversation and will ignore others' conversational attempts or respond only with monosyllables.

The period of disorganization is painful but necessary. After the impact of the event has fragmented the person's self-image, there is a need to express anxiety, rage, or depression before one can begin rebuilding a life. Premature (though well-intentioned) interference with these expressions can prolong the period of time the person remains in this stage.

3. Reorganization The next two stages, reorganization and resolution, usually occur after hospital discharge. In the reorganization stage, the person actively begins to identify ways to rebuild life. He or she may question old assumptions and seek suggestions and guidance from others who are more knowledgeable, for instance, physical therapists or members of self-help groups such as ostomy or myocardial infarction clubs. The person may try out new attitudes and behaviors, or may grieve for parts of a lifestyle that cannot be reincorporated, perhaps crying or reminiscing about them. At times, the person may question whether rebuilding life really is worth the effort. These periods of despair may be interspersed with progressively longer bouts of renewed determination.

4. Resolution Resolution is achieved when the person has established a realistic view of self as a person with some limitations. In this stage, his or her activities are appropriate for his or her capabilities. When necessary, the person seeks help in a matter-of-fact rather than self-pitying manner. He or she may even discover new strengths, such as greater compassion for others or a desire to help others facing the same crisis.

5. Overlap The patient may display different stages of adaptation to different problems in life. For example, the MI patient may be undergoing disorganization in relation to job involvement while still denying the infarction's implications for future sexual activity.

The above assessment will help you to identify whether the patient is able to communicate freely, how well he or she is coping psychologically with illness, the degree of assistance needed from you, and the ways you can help most effectively.

The last three diagnoses listed in the following box are quite broad and incorporate information that you may wish to abstract if you choose to use a more specific diagnosis for your patient or his or her family. For instance, incorporated in "ineffective individual coping" are suggestions that are applicable to the patient feeling anxious or powerless; incorporated in "ineffective family coping" are suggestions related to anticipatory grieving.

NURSING DIAGNOSES

As any critical-care nurse can validate, the communication needs of patients and families are numerous and varied. Nursing diagnoses in the broad area of communication are listed in Table 3-2. This chapter examines selected diagnoses that are most commonly encountered in caring for the critically ill and their families:

- Impaired verbal communication
- Sensory-perceptual alteration
- Ineffective individual coping
- Ineffective family coping

Planning and Implementation of Care

Once you have assessed the patient, you are ready to plan and implement nursing measures to foster communication.

TABLE 3-2 NURSING DIAGNOSES RELATED TO COMMUNICATION

Anxiety

Communication, impaired verbal

Coping, ineffective individual

Coping, ineffective family: compromised

Coping, ineffective family: disabling

Coping, family: potential for growth

Family processes, alteration in

Fear

Grieving, anticipatory

Grieving, dysfunctional

Hopelessness

Parenting, alteration in

Posttrauma response

Powerlessness

Social interaction, impaired

Social isolation

Spiritual distress

Violence, potential for

Source: Adapted from McLane A: *Classification of nursing diagnosis: Proceedings of the seventh national conference.* St Louis: Mosby, 1987, pp 418–419.

Impaired Verbal Communication Related to Vision Deficit, Hearing Deficit, or Loss of Speech

It is essential to individualize assistance for the person with process difficulties, taking into account both deficits and remaining abilities. In the following sections are some suggestions for ways to help your patient communicate more effectively.

Input Problems Follow these guidelines to improve patient input.

1. If not already done, have a specialist evaluate severe vision or hearing deficits.

2. Because the hemianopic person has only half a visual field, that person may not see objects on the blind side, such as some food on a plate or obstacles in a pathway. Teach her or him to compensate by turning the head to scan the environment. Always approach from the sighted side.

3. Assist the blind patient by providing auditory and tactile cues for activity. Always identify yourself when you approach. The patient may have preferred ways of orienting to a strange environment; ask the patient or family how you best can help.

4. To communicate with hearing-loss patients, capture their attention, speak directly to them, talk slowly, and augment your speech with gestures. If necessary, write messages or use sign language if you and the patients know it.

Output Difficulties A variety of methods can be used to communicate with the patient able to formulate thoughts but unable to speak. If the loss of speech can be anticipated (for example, laryngectomee or electively intubated patient), discuss with the patient in advance which method is preferred. Follow these guidelines to improve patient output:

1. If the patient can write, use a magic slate or pencil and paper.

2. Develop a set of cards, each of which contains a phrase the patient may want to use frequently. The cards could be personalized for each patient by including the names of family, physician, and so on. The idea also could be adapted for the patient who does not speak English; a bilingual person would write on one side of the card a foreign language phrase and on the other side its English equivalent.

3. Develop a placemat illustrating patients' needs. Van Tassell (1982) has developed a 12-inch by 18-inch placemat with pictures illustrating *activities* of daily living, *primary needs* (such as pain medication and a spiritual counselor), and *rest and recreation*. The 62 illustrated needs are printed on placemats that are laminated for easy cleaning. This clever idea facilitates communication and reduces frustration for the patient, who simply can point to the appropriate illustration.

4. A less desirable alternative is to show the patient an alphabet and have her or him point to the letters of words she or he wants to express. This method is laborious but can be used effectively for unique messages.

5. Sometimes a person is unable to speak, write, or point, for instance if she is paralyzed or intubated with both arms restrained. In this case, use a variation of the yes-and-no method, such as one eye blink for yes and two for no.

It is very important that you remain calm and patient when trying to "talk" to a person with a communication deficit. The patient will pick up readily on your frustration or impatience and may become anxious, confused, or discouraged. Conversely, you can provide a real incentive to communication with an empathic comment such as "This is hard work for us, but I'm glad we can communicate with each other."

Be sure to alert other staff and, if necessary, visitors to the patient's method of communication, as she or he will feel less confused and insecure if others use a consistent approach. This is especially important if the person will be outside the critical-care unit, for instance in the x-ray department or operating room.

Hickey (1986) has offered some useful guidelines for working with the aphasic patient:

Mild Nonfluent (Expressive) Aphasia

- Stimulate conversation by asking open questions.
- Allow the patient time to search and speak words.
- Assure the patient that speech will gradually improve.

Severe Nonfluent (Expressive) Aphasia

- Accept any form of patient communication (e.g., pantomime, pointing).
- Do not pressure the patient, and accept behaviors that indicate frustration.
- Provide a book or board of pictures depicting common objects.
- Assure the patient that speech can improve with time.

Mild Fluent (Receptive) Aphasia

- Speak slowly and distinctly, using simple sentences.

- Repeat or rephrase any instructions, speaking in a normal tone and level of voice.
- Assess the possibility that the patient still understands written language.

Severe Fluent (Receptive) Aphasia

- Use whatever form of communication the patient can still understand (e.g., pantomime, pointing, touch).
- Use only simple sentences or two- or three-word phrases.
- Divide tasks into small units.
- Assess the possibility that the patient still understands written language.

Finally, when you leave your patient, always check that a call bell is within reach. If the patient is conscious but unable to use the call bell and also unable to make any noise to summon help, she or he should not be left alone. Many intubated, paralyzed patients have described the stark terror and loneliness they experienced when they realized their inability to attract others' attention. Fortunately, special sensors are now available that the paralyzed patient can trigger with the head, mouth, or shoulder.

Sensory-Perceptual Alterations Related to Excessive and/or Meaningless Stimuli, Chemical Imbalances, or Drugs

The proportion of patients who suffer sensory disturbances in critical-care units is uncertain. Some reports of postcardiotomy patients reveal the occurrence of sensory disturbances. Their frequent occurrence in other patients is supported by the author's experience in critical-care units and in post-ICU and post-CCU interviews with patients. Many patients probably do not report sensory disturbances because they are not asked specifically about them or are afraid of appearing crazy.

Laboratory studies of sensory deprivation usually are not directly applicable to the critical-care setting because of extreme experimental conditions, such as gloves, opaque eyegoggles, and earplugs. Studies in more hospital-like environments are sparse. One study that does provide some insight is that reported by Downs (1974). Her subjects were 90 male and 90 female adults, 18–35 years old, who were believed healthy, had normal hearing and vision, and were not on drugs. She placed them on bedrest for 2¾ hours in a room that simulated a semiprivate hospital room. Her study was intended to measure the effects of personality and varied auditory input on cardiovascular function, motor activity, and time perception; data on abnormal sensory experiences were not solicited. A fascinating, incidental finding of her study was that at least 20% of her subjects suffered sensory distortions they knew were neither real nor dreams. Among the distortions reported were cooking odors; ceiling lights about to fall down; sensations of floating above the bed; detachment of body parts; and changes in room temperature, light, and sound intensity. Subjects also reported being lonely, bored, unable to concentrate, and irritated by the aimless wandering of their minds. To emphasize, these experiences were suffered by normal, healthy, young adults after less than three hours bedrest!

Patients in critical-care units are subjected to a distressing amalgam of unit noise: beeping sounds from cardiac monitors; whooshing sounds from ventilators; ear-piercing alarms; rattling trays; flushing toilets; snatches of conversation; and hospital pages. They are in unfamiliar beds in unfamiliar rooms that are lit constantly and may have no windows out of which they can look. They are connected by myriad tubes and wires to strange machines that watch them unceasingly. They have regressed to being bathed, fed, and toileted by strangers. They are deprived of undisturbed sleep for more than two or three hour stretches. Their minds may be clouded by their diseases, fluid and electrolyte imbalances, or drugs. All this is at a time when they are trying to cope with life-threatening illnesses that may have been thrust upon them with shocking suddenness. It is a wonder that *all* of them do not report sensory disturbances!

To help your patient maintain accurate sensory processing while on bedrest, use these measures:

1.   Introduce yourself and briefly explain what you will be doing each time you care for a new, confused, or comatose patient. Touch the patient to express warmth and caring and to provide tactile stimulation.

2.   Take a nursing history from the patient (and/ or family). Ask the patient to describe his or her normal pattern of activities and how he or she reacts when it is disrupted significantly. Use this information to duplicate as closely as possible the normal patterns of eating, sleeping, bathing, and toileting.

3.   Orient the patient and family to the unit. Explain the purpose of equipment used and how to summon help. Describe visiting policies, eating facilities for visitors, the location of nearby telephones, and if necessary the locations of possible overnight accommodations.

4.   Encourage family and friends to visit. Suggest that they bring items that would be meaningful to the patient, for instance, snapshots or tape recordings of children too young to visit. Books, magazines, crossword puzzles, etc. can be tangible expressions of affection as well as welcome diversions.

5.   Help the patient remain oriented to time. Place a calendar and clock in the room. Each day, mention the day of the week, any special characteristics of the day (such as holidays), and the weather. Try to perform activities at a consistent time each day.

6.   Reduce unnecessary stimuli. Helpful measures include dimming overhead lights for those patients who do not need continuous observation and placing standby equipment out of the patient's immediate environment. Other ways to reduce disturbing stimuli are to mute the hospital paging system inside critical-care units and to ensure that telephones are answered promptly. A telephone that rings and rings can be a real annoyance for the patient—imagine how aggravating it must be to lie immobile when your urge is to answer the phone!

7.   Enhance the meaningfulness of necessary stimuli. Identify the noises of the cardiac monitor, ventilators, and other equipment the patient and family may hear. Clearly define their relatedness to the patient. It is common for patients after surgery to assume that all nearby noises relate to them, when in fact some of them emanate from equipment used for the patient in the next bed. Always explain to patients the steps of procedures you plan to perform and the sensations they may experience during them.

8.   Provide some visual interest in the unit. An increasing number of critical-care units are being decorated in bright, cheerful colors. Old calendars and magazines are good sources of inexpensive yet interesting pictures.

9.   Provide a pleasant auditory environment. Maintain a sensitive but cheerful attitude; humor can be an excellent antidote to the gloom engendered by confinement in a critical-care unit. Discuss with the patient his or her hobbies, current events, or other topics that may be of interest.

10.   Either involve your patient in conversations or hold them out of earshot. It is dehumanizing to tend to patients' physical needs while you ignore their spirit— particularly if you are chattering or joking with colleagues about personal matters. Avoid conversations just outside a patient's room; patients often decipher such snatches of conversation incorrectly as applying to them. Keep conversations at the nurses' station quiet (especially at change of shift).

11.   An excellent investment of unit funds might be a small tape recorder. Patients could use it to "talk" to faraway loved ones or play messages from them. Family

members could bring in recordings of favorite music or relaxation tapes to soothe patients. Nurses might experiment with it as a supplement to change-of-shift reports or a teaching tool.

12. Alert patients to the possibility that they may experience unusual ideas or feelings because of illness, drugs, or the unfamiliar environment. Tell them these imaginings are common and do not mean they are going crazy. Ask them to tell you or other staff if these experiences occur. Also be alert for nonverbal cues such as a confused or frightened expression, sniffing, unusual body movements, or inappropriate speech. If patients appear to be having sensory disturbances, ask them to describe them, reassure them they are temporary, reorient them to reality, and try to identify and remove the causes.

Ineffective Individual Coping Related to Crisis

Once a communication process is underway, focus on ways to enhance the patient's adaptation to the crisis of critical illness.

Shock Phase To assist the patient through the shock phase, follow these guidelines:

1. To intervene effectively in a crisis, quickly establish rapport by introducing yourself and engaging direct eye contact. Sitting down (if possible) implies you have time to listen to the person. Spontaneous touching also can be very effective in establishing warmth and caring.

2. Orient the person to the milieu. Briefly explain the equipment used in caring for him or her. Ask if the patient has wondered about anything else seen or heard. Patients often are disturbed and frightened by the critical-care environment, especially if they witness a cardiac resuscitation, invasive procedure, or death.

3. Help the patient learn the patient role. The patient unintentionally may fail to report important bits of information or fail to comply with health recommendations because no one has explained their significance. The patient and family will look to you for cues to acceptable behavior.

4. Provide anticipatory guidance. Explain the stages of adaptation, and instill hope that the current stage will not last much longer and that resolution can be achieved. Point out that the adaptive process is not smooth, instead being marked by plateaus, surges, and occasional temporary regression to an earlier stage.

The person may be quite distressed by emotional liability, particularly if the person is one who values self-control and independence.

5. Reduce depersonalization. Observe typical social amenities by introducing the patient to other staff, avoiding demeaning nicknames, and involving the patient in bedside conversations about him or her. Allow the patient to keep favorite personal belongings nearby whenever possible.

6. Respect the person's modesty and need for privacy. Even such a simple courtesy as knocking on the door before entering displays respect for the need to control territorial intrusion.

7. Be sensitive to the role of the patient's hygiene in self-esteem. Help him or her to stay as clean and presentable as possible.

8. Use consistent patient care assignments. It is very difficult to establish a therapeutic relationship when you care for a different patient each day and the patient is exposed to a different nurse each day. (Even with consistent planning, the patient will be cared for by several nurses in one week.) Primary nursing is one promising approach to providing a key person with whom the patient can build a therapeutic relationship. Another approach some critical-care units are trying is the 12-hour shift. Within each 24-hour period, the patient then has two rather than three nurses caring for him or her.

Disorganization Phase To assist the patient through the disorganization phase, follow these guidelines:

1. Provide repeated explanations about aspects of the critical-care environment and the patient's illness. Ask for the patient's perceptions of progress. Solicit feedback so you can clarify any misconceptions that persist.

2. Help the person to identify the causes of his or her feelings. It is much more difficult to cope with free-floating anxiety or anger than that which consciously has been associated with a specific event.

3. Allow the person to experience his or her feelings. Following this recommendation is hard; often we openly or subtly urge the patient to feel differently because of our own discomfort. It is particularly important that you allow him or her to experience denial if present. Because we tend to view denial negatively, we overlook its value as an appropriate, protective response to an inability to alter threatening circumstances. Short-term denial can contribute to the patient's physical and emotional survival, since it conserves energy by obviating the "fight or flight" response and ego disintegration.

4. Be alert to topics the patient does *not* bring up as well as those she or he does. For example, patients often hesitate to raise questions about future sexual functioning because they are afraid they will offend the staff or be viewed as inappropriately or overly concerned with this aspect of life, or because they are afraid of the answers they may hear.

5. Share with the patient updated information on his or her condition. Emphasize even small signs of progress to instill hope. Use future-oriented statements to imply that the person will have a future. To prevent discouragement, point out the temporary aspects of the illness or treatment.

6. Reassure patients who have nightmares that nightmares are common during this stage, do not mean they are going crazy, and usually subside with time. If nightmares are especially disturbing or persistent, consult with a psychiatric nurse clinician or other psychological expert about ways to help the patient.

7. If the patient is receptive, teach him or her focused relaxation techniques. Use guided mental imagery to help the patient visualize getting better, as well as to prepare for coming procedures or surgery. This type of "dress rehearsal" can be very effective in promoting calmness and strength in the patient.

8. If the patient's use of denial leads to life-endangering behavior, some intervention will be necessary. A typical example is the MI patient who repeatedly gets out of bed against orders. In this situation, you often end up threatening the patient, to no avail, and then label him or her as "denying his illness." This label conveniently identifies the problem as the patient's. A more productive response is to examine the staff's role in the problem. For example, perhaps the assumption that patients benefit more from bedrest than from limited out-of-bed activity is unwarranted for this person, and the physician could modify activity restrictions. Alternatively, perhaps the person does not believe the staff when they say activity will be harmful. This can be especially true if the person has been up several times already without apparent physical harm. In this case, you might propose a compromise, such as calling you for assistance when he or she plans to get out of bed.

9. Support the person's self-esteem. Avoid threats, confrontation, and criticism. Praise attempts to adapt. If they are inappropriate, acknowledge the efforts and tactfully suggest more effective means.

10. For suggestions on ways to help the patient concerned about body image or sexuality, see Chapter 20.

Reorganization and Resolution Phases You will usually not encounter these phases during the patient's short stay in the critical-care unit. However, during the time you care for the patient you can facilitate postdischarge adaptation by laying the groundwork for these future phases.

1. Restore some control to the person by developing the care plan together. If joint development is inappropriate for the patient's condition, at least share the care plan with the patient and family. Emphasize ways they can promote the patient's recovery. When you make rounds or give bedside reports to other staff, include the patient and family in your conversation.

2. Begin a teaching and rehabilitation program. In their classic study of psychologic responses following MI, Cassem and Hackett (1973) and Hackett and Cassem (1974) contend that such a program for MI patients should begin no later than the third coronary-care-unit day. This recommendation is based on the timing of psychiatric consultation requests and their observation that the most depressing factor for patients was the feeling of being "all washed up" that was engendered by inactivity. Their suggestions for physical activity include passive range of motion exercises, use of chair rest and bedside commode, and early mobilization. They state that taking a detailed activity history, teaching the patient and family about the metabolic cost of various activities, and clarifying misconceptions about the future are helpful both to dispel depression and to ensure a safe recovery.

3. Encourage patients to participate in performing their care, consistent with physical capabilities and emotional state. If they are in emotional shock or extremely disorganized, they may be very dependent and need specific directions or actual physical assistance with activities of daily living. As emotional immobilization decreases and physical condition allows, gently encourage them to resume self-care. Even such simple activities as washing one's own body can restore some control and power.

4. Help the person to set short-term goals that are both meaningful and manageable. Call attention to achievement of these goals or other manifestations of improvement such as a lowered medication dosage or less need for suctioning.

5. Assist the patient to make necessary and feasible changes in lifestyle. Help him or her identify necessary changes and options for implementing them.

6. Provide clear discharge instructions to the patient and family well in advance of the actual discharge period, which often is too hectic to allow assimilation of information. Solicit feedback on their interpretation of the instructions. Be sure to find out whether the discharge instructions are feasible; if not, modify them (with the physician's knowledge) or refer the person to a social service agency, public health nurse, or other community support group.

7. Expect that transfer from the unit will be a time of renewed anxiety. Beginning soon after admission, prepare the patient by emphasizing the temporary nature of the unit stay. As the time for transfer approaches, reinforce the idea that it is a positive step toward recovery. Explain how other units' routines will be different. If possible, have nurses from the new unit come over to meet the patient prior to the transfer. This enables the patient to begin establishing rapport with the new staff, thus facilitating a reduction in anxiety.

Summary In a crisis, a person may manifest behavior such as confusion, hysteria, or withdrawal, which does not help in coping effectively with the sources of disequilibrium. Such nonproductive activities drain the person's energy and hamper adaptation to the crisis. Your skills at crisis intervention can assist the person to regain emotional equilibrium and energy to cope productively with reality.

Ineffective Family Coping (Compromised or Disabling) Related to Crisis

The bewildered look on the face of a critically ill's loved one is an expression with which any critical-care nurse is familiar. It is at once poignant—appealing to the nurse's desire to nurture—and frightening, because it reminds the nurse that he or she could one day be the dazed person trying to cope with the impact of critical illness on the family.

The needs of family members have received increasing attention in the nursing literature. In their review, Bedsworth and Molen (1982) identified nine types of *threats* faced by spouses of MI patients: (a) loss of the loved one's life; (b) loss of a healthy mate; (c) financial worries; (d) new family roles; (e) change in responsibility for dependents' care; (f) change in own goals or motives; (g) separation from the mate; (h) unfamiliar hospital environment; and (i) fear of recurrence of the MI. Breu and Dracup (1978), in a classic study, delineated the losses and needs of spouses of CCU patients. Feelings of loss, which provoke anticipatory grieving (that

is, grieving before the loss actually happens), included: (a) threat of their mate's death; (b) deprivation of their primary source of social contact, gratification, and self-esteem; (c) interruption of all daily routines, including eating and sleeping; (d) sudden role reversal; (e) involuntary independence; (f) disruption of social contacts; (g) financial instability; (h) disturbed system of interpersonal rewards; and (i) relocation to a strange environment for the majority of the day.

A number of nursing research articles have investigated the needs of other family members (Daley 1984; Leske 1986; Molter 1979; Norris and Grove 1986). Daley (1984) found that families would rather have information about the patient and were least concerned with their own personal needs. Nurses can do several things to eliminate some potential problems often seen during this period of initial hospitalization. The nurse should be with the physician when he or she discusses the case with the family. In this way the nurse would then be able to reinforce pertinent information, validate feelings, and assess the family's comprehension. The nurse, based on this assessment, may ask the physician to speak to the family members, again for the specific purpose of relieving their anxiety, even though the information may not be anything new. In addition, nurses should make it a point to let family members know that they are not too busy to help them, emphasizing that family members are a part of the care plan, as is the patient.

Molter (1979), Daley (1984), and Leske (1986) in validation studies have ranked the needs of family members from most important to least important. The top 30 family needs, in decreasing order of importance, were:

1. To feel there is hope.
2. To have questions answered honestly.
3. To know the prognosis.
4. To know specific facts concerning the patient's progress.
5. To have explanations given in terms that are understandable.
6. To receive information about the patient once a day.
7. To be called at home about changes in the patient's condition.
8. To feel that the hospital personnel care about the patient.
9. To see the patient frequently.
10. To know why things were done for the patient.
11. To have the waitingroom near the patient.

NURSING RESEARCH NOTE

McMahon P: Nurses' perceptions of families' needs compared with families' identification of their needs in critical care units. *Heart Lung* 1987; 16:338.

Faced with the multiple demands of a busy critical-care unit, limited time to spend with family members, and the difficulties inherent when strangers attempt to communicate feelings, critical-care nurses may wonder just how astute they are at assessing families' needs. This study evaluated the congruence between family reports of their needs and nurses' assessments, a topic on which no previous studies were found.

Twenty-nine family members with relatives in the coronary care unit, surgical intensive care unit, and neurosurgical intensive care unit were studied, along with 29 of the relatives' nurses. Each subject completed Molter's 45 Needs Statement questionnaire within 48–72 hours of admission. The ten most important needs and five least important needs identified by the nurse and the family member were determined.

Both groups identified similar top-10 needs. Among the least important needs, family members ranked visitation higher than did nurses. The *t*-tests used to compare family and nurse perceptions revealed no statistically significant differences ($p < 0.01$) in the categories of physical, emotional, spiritual, informational, visitation, or relationship-with-staff needs.

Further studies with groups representing various ethnic groups, economic statuses, and geographic locales are recommended.

12. To be assured that the best care possible is being given to the patient.

13. To know exactly what is being done for the patient.

14. To know how the patient is being treated medically.

15. To visit at any time.

16. To have visiting hours changed for special conditions.

17. To have a place to be alone while in the hospital.

18. To feel accepted by the hospital staff.

19. To have explanations of the environment before going into the critical-care unit for the first time.

20. To talk about negative feelings, such as guilt and anger.

21. To have directions regarding what to do at the bedside.

22. To have visiting hours start on time.

23. To be told about transfer plans while they are being made.

24. To be assured it is all right to leave the hospital for a while.

25. To talk to the doctors every day.

26. To be alone at any time.

27. To have friends nearby for support.

28. To be encouraged to cry.

29. To talk about the possibility of the patient's death.

30. To have a telephone near the waiting room.

Given this somewhat overwhelming list of needs, what can critical-care nurses do to help family members? The nursing research just described leads to the following ideas for practical, realistic ways to alleviate the suffering of family members.

Need to Feel Hope   Family members who speak as if there were no hope seem to cope less successfully and often appear highly anxious, agitated, and angry (King and Gregor 1985). Nurses should be alert to statements that indicate hope, or lack of it, because these are measures of coping ability. A realistic nursing intervention would be to foster realistic hope. Werner-Beland (1980) has suggested that promoting a "perhaps" attitude—"Perhaps things will get better, not all is lost"—allows family members time to absorb the shock of having a loved one in the intensive care unit. In general, nurses provide support and hope by creating an atmosphere of trust and willingness by encouraging questions that otherwise would go unasked and unanswered (Brandt 1984).

Need to Be Informed of the Patient's Condition   Rasie (1980) identified the family's need for medical information and their uncertainty about obtaining it. To help the family, identify the physicians assigned to the patient. Help them sort out which specialist can answer which questions. Clarify the best time to contact the physicians.

The critical-care nurse also is an important source of information for the family. So that you can serve as a link with their loved one, arrange for specific methods of telephone contact with you during the time they are away from the unit. Group meetings between unit nurses and families are very helpful in lessening families' loneliness and staff's need to repeat information. Chandler (1982) recommends that such meetings be held twice a week, just before and just after the weekend. At the meetings, you can provide general information, such as explanations of patient care or locations of the best places to eat or do laundry.

Need for Assurance of Loved One's Comfort
Assure the family that the critically ill person will be kept as comfortable and pain-free as possible. Introduce yourself and reassure the family that you care. Explain that you will be "your father's/mother's/sister's nurse," and that you will be observing your patient closely, implementing necessary treatments, and helping him or her to understand what is going on. Orient the family to the unit layout, the equipment used for their loved one, and the unit routine.

Need to Be with the Patient   Nursing measures to help meet the family's need to be with the patient include finding out where family members can be reached, clarifying unit visiting policies, and arranging flexible visiting hours acceptable to both family and staff. The topic of appropriate visiting hours is controversial among critical-care nurses. In a national survey of 235 hospitals, Kirchoff (1982) discovered that the ritual of hourly visits is most common in hospitals with under 200 beds, with the predominant pattern in larger hospitals being scheduled visits (for instance, 10 A.M., 2 P.M., and 7 P.M.). Another pattern utilized by all sizes of hospitals was the every-2-hour visits. In small, more general units with lesser percentages of coronary beds, visits tend to be short, frequent, for immediate family only, and for one visitor at a time. Larger units, those with larger percentages of beds dedicated to coronary care, and specific coronary-care units tended to allow longer but less frequent visits.

The best pattern of visits remains to be identified. Fuller and Foster (1982) point out that although there are some data suggesting that family visits are stressful and associated with increased dysrhythmias, the reports relate only to CCU patients and compare the effects of interpersonal interactions only to periods of time when the patient is "alone." Their study of 28 surgical intensive care patients used BP and heart rate data, obtained from automatic monitoring devices, and vocal microtremor, a measure of inaudible frequency changes in audiotaped speech. Their findings are preliminary, being based on a small sample, and serve only to indicate areas for further study; nevertheless, they are fascinating. Their data suggest that 15-minute visits were no more stressful than 5-minute visits, that there was no significant change in cardiovascular variables during and after the visits, and that family or friend visits were no more or less stressful than nurse–patient interactions.

Need to Be Helpful   As Rasie (1980) points out, families are caught in a classic dilemma: they want to help but do not know how, so they end up feeling useless and in the way. One valuable nursing intervention in this area is to find out whether family members would like to assist with daily care of the patient. If they would, identify in which areas they would like to be involved, and explain how they can help best.

Need to Ventilate   Rasie (1980) reported that a common recurrent theme in the family members she interviewed was the need to relive in detail the incident that precipitated admission to the critical-care unit. This need probably represents a need to come to grips with the reality of the situation. Help the family ventilate this and other concerns by arranging brief periods of time with them away from the bedside.

Need for Comfort and Support   The first time the family sees their loved one in the ICU is usually a time of extreme stress. Prepare them by describing in advance the appearance of the person and the critical-care environment. Help them to see the patient as a person alive and still needing and loving them. Accompany them into the unit to demonstrate emotional support and to provide physical support and comfort in case they become faint or extremely upset.

The development of complications can be another emotional crisis period during which the patient or family may retreat to an earlier stage of adaptation in an attempt to protect themselves. If the patient's prognosis is poor, you can help him or her and the family begin to adapt to impending death. They may be relieved that the patient's suffering will end soon and may be comforted by their ability to face the end honestly and openly. Alternatively, they may react with rage, despair, or withdrawal.

The care and concern demonstrated by nurses and other health professionals are major sources of comfort and support for the family. Although you may have little time to devote to the family during the initial critical period, some attention to their needs can ease their anguish, enhance their ability to nurture the patient, and establish the foundation for a trusting relationship with the staff. You might offer to call those people to whom the family turns for support—perhaps other family members or spiritual advisors.

Especially during admission and other crisis periods, some family members may become acutely anxious, hysterical, or depressed. Sedatives and tranquilizers may be prescribed but often have the detrimental effect of blunting perception and impairing thought processes, resulting in a sense of unreality and repression of feelings. A more creative and therapeutic response is referral to a crisis-oriented psychologic service, such as an inhospital psychiatric nurse consultant to your critical-care unit, a crisis hotline, or a community counseling service.

Need to Be Aware of and Participate in Discharge Planning Patient survival rates following injury have increased, often with accompanying increase in long-term disability. While patient survival is often the main objective for many families during the acute episode of an ICU hospitalization, families are ill prepared to participate in optimizing the outcome once the patient is being prepared for discharge from the unit (Crittenden 1983; Pfeiffer and Cohen 1982). The Joint Commission on Accreditation of Hospitals views discharge tasks as involving both nursing and social work. Arenth and Momon (1985) found two aspects of the discharge planning process crucial for success: first, how accurately nurses assess patient needs; and second, the extent to which patient/family actively participate in the process.

Discharge planning is therefore a joint effort between patient, family, primary nurse, and social worker. Each participant plays a vital role in the team process. Early communication between these players is increasingly being recognized as important for comprehensive patient care (Mathis 1984; Sherburne 1986). Team responsibilities are delineated along the following guidelines. The primary nurse assesses the patient's activities of daily living, physical limitations, equipment needs, medications, discharge instructions, and referrals to social and community support services. The primary nurse's role involves the four functions of 24-hour accountability, main communication mediator, coordinator of care, and patient/family teacher (Sherburne 1986). The social worker assesses the need for patient/family counseling in the areas of finances, psychologic status of role functioning, clarification of family involvement in the treatment plan, and resolution of previously identified patient/family needs and their relationship to discharge planning and placement (Arenth and Momon 1985).

The patient and family become the primary source for information and validators of the information-gathering process. These tasks might be accomplished by structured interviews with the family and patient or might be accomplished by informal information-gathering sessions summarized in a formal family meeting held before discharge. Many units have devised a take-home family evaluation tool that clearly delineates the patient

and family needs identified and how these needs were met or will be met following discharge from the unit. In this way, continuity of quality patient care is ensured for further or future hospital or community treatment (Pilcher 1986).

Need to Be Informed of Impending Death The impending death of a patient is a difficult time for all involved: patient, family, friends, and staff. The literature on death and dying is extensive, and you may wish to explore it if you are not already familiar with it. Research strongly suggests that anticipatory grieving is a crucial variable in the spouse's future well-being (Forsyth 1982). Johnson (1983) found in her practice and in clinical research on grief reactions that the severity and length of the grief reaction can be estimated by considering the recent stability of the family member's life, the void created by the death, and the amount of time the family member had to prepare for the death. Intense, prolonged reactions are more likely if there have been many changes to which the spouse has had to adapt recently, if the dying person was a major part of the family member's life, or if the death was sudden.

Nurse thanatologist Joy Ufema (1981) has identified several recommendations that can be used to guide what you say and do when a patient is dying. She suggests that you first identify yourself, if the family does not already know you, and then share the news of the impending death in a short, direct statement. If the emergency team is with the patient, tell the family members, and assure them that everything possible is being done to save the patient's life. Alert the team that the family wants news, and serve as a conduit for information from the emergency team to the family while the resuscitation is underway.

If the patient dies, encourage the physician to talk to the family immediately, and, if possible, accompany him or her. If you have established rapport with the family, your presence when they receive news of the death can be very supportive. In addition, your presence can also help support the physician in the difficult task of breaking the news and dealing with the emotional aftermath. Avoid automatic sedation; although the pain of grief is intense, sedating the family often serves only to delay the effects of the death and to contribute to an air of unreality about the death. Offer the family an opportunity to see the patient (after the body is made presentable) and ask them whether they would like you to accompany them to the bedside or whether they would prefer to be alone. You also may want to ask if they wish to assist with portions of postmortem care. Encourage them to call other family members and their spiritual advisor; call these people yourself if the family seem unable to do it. Give family members "permission" to cry if they seem to need it; if you are moved to tears, do not be afraid to share this aspect of your humanness with them. Praise the family and remind them of warm moments they shared with the patient. Finally, remember to say good-bye when the family leaves; doing so helps to bring closure to their experience.

Outcome Evaluation

Evaluate the patient's progress toward satisfactory communication and adaptation to critical illness. By the time of discharge from the critical-care unit, the patient ideally should meet these outcome criteria:

- If conscious but unable to speak, can communicate wants and feelings through an alternate communication process.
- Does not exhibit life-threatening denial of illness.
- If anxious, angry, or depressed, expresses: (1) awareness that such feelings are part of the normal process of adaptation; and (2) ability to cope with such feelings.
- Is receiving preparatory assistance with reorganization and resolution through participation in a beginning teaching and rehabilitation program.
- Is aware of and participating in discharge planning.

Also evaluate the family's progress toward effective coping with their loved one's illness. By the time of the patient's discharge from the critical-care unit, the family ideally should meet these outcome criteria:

- Relief of initial anxiety.
- Adequate time to be with the patient.
- Awareness of specific ways to help the patient.
- Belief that the loved one is being kept as comfortable as possible.
- Knowledge of specific ways in which to keep informed of the patient's condition.
- Opportunity to ventilate feelings.
- Ability to receive comfort and support.
- Awareness of and participation in discharge planning.

REFERENCES

Arenth LM, Momon JA: Determining patient needs after discharge. *Nurs Manag* 1985; 16(9):20–24.

Bedsworth J, Molen M: Psychological stress in spouses of patients with myocardial infarction. *Heart Lung* 1982; 11:450–456.

Brandt M: Consider the patient part of a family. *Nurs Forum* (Jan) 1984; 21:19–23.

Breu C, Dracup K: Helping the spouses of critically ill patients. *Am J Nurs* 1978; 78:51–53.

Burns M, Halper A: Language disorders associated with aging. *Top Geriatr Rehabil* (July) 1986; 1:15–27.

Cassem N, Hackett T: Psychological rehabilitation of myocardial infarction patients in the acute phase. *Heart Lung* 1973; 2:382–388.

Chandler N: How to make a lonely place a little less lonely. *Nurs 82* (October) 1982; 47–50.

Chaney P: Ordeal. *Nurs 75* 1975; 5:27–40.

Crittenden F: *Discharge Planning for Health Care Facilities.* New York: Allied Health Publications, 1983.

Daley L: The perceived immediate needs of families with relatives in the intensive care setting. *Heart Lung* 1984; 13:231–237.

De Ramon P: The final task: Life review for the dying patient. *Nurs 83* (Feb) 1983; 13:44–49.

De Vito A: Critical care patients have families. *Crit Care Nurse* (Sept/Oct) 1981; 8–11.

Downs F: Bed rest and sensory disturbances. *Am J Nurs* 1974; 74:434–436.

Fife B: A model for predicting the adaptation of families to medical crisis: An analysis of role integration. *Image: J Nurs Scholarship* 1985; 27:108–112.

Forsyth D: The hardest job of all. *Nurs 82* (April) 1982; 86–91.

Fuller B, Foster G: The effects of family/friends visits vs. staff interaction on stress/arousal of surgical intensive care patients. *Heart Lung* 1982; 11:457–463.

Hackett T, Cassem, N: Development of a quantitative rating scale to assess denial. *J Psychosom Res* 1974; 18(2):93–111.

Hickey J: Rehabilitation. Pages 196-197 in *The clinical practice of neurological and neurosurgical nursing,* 2d ed., Hickey J (ed). Philadelphia: Lippincott, 1986.

Johnson S: Giving emotional support to families after a patient dies. *Nurs Life* (Jan) 1983; 34–39.

King S, Gregor F: Stress and coping in families of the critically ill. *Crit Care Nurse* 1985; 5:48–51.

Kirchoff K: Visiting policies for patients with myocardial infarction: A national survey. *Heart Lung* 1982; 11:571–576.

Leske J: Needs of relatives of critically ill patients: A follow-up. *Heart Lung* 1986; 15:189–193.

Mathis M: Personal needs of family members of critically ill patients with and without acute brain injury. *J Neurosurg Nurs* 1984; 16(1):36–44.

Molter N: Needs of relatives of critically ill patients: A descriptive study. *Heart Lung* 1979; 8:332–339.

Norris L, Grove S: Investigation of selected psychosocial needs of family members of critically ill adult patients. *Heart Lung* 1986; 15:194–199.

Pfeiffer E, Cohen E: Assessment: The long-term care issue of the 80's. *Coordinator* 1982; 2(6):16–17.

Pilcher M: Postdischarge care: How to follow up. *Nurs 86* (August) 1986; 50–51.

Porch B: Communication. In *Rehabilitation: A Manual for*

Care of the Disabled and Elderly, 2d ed., Hirshberg G, Lewis L, Vaugh P (eds). Philadelphia: Lippincott, 1976.

Rasie S: Meeting families' needs helps you meet ICU patients' needs. *Nurs 80* (July) 1980; 32–35.

Sherburne E: A rehabilitation protocol for the neuroscience intensive care unit. *J Neurosurg Nurs* 1986; 18(3):140–145.

Stryker S, Stratham A: Symbolic interaction and role theory. In *Handbook of Social Psychology,* 3d ed., Lindzey G, Aronson E (eds). Reading, MA: Addison-Wesley, 1985.

Ufema J: Grieving families. *Nurs 81* (Nov) 1981; 81–83.

Van Tassell G: Placemats show patients' needs. *Nurs 82* (Sept) 1982; 81.

Werner-Beland J: Nursing and the concept of hope. In *Grief responses to long-term illness and disability: Manifestations and nursing interventions,* Werner-Beland J (ed). Reston, VA: Reston, 1980.

SUPPLEMENTAL READING

Abrams R: When death do us part. *Am J Nurs* (Jan) 1983; 83:90–93.

Bozett F, Gibbons R: The nursing management of families in the critical care setting. *Crit Care Update* 1983; 10:22–27.

Bullock-Loughran P: Territoriality in critical care. *Focus on AACN* (Oct/Nov) 1982; 19–21.

Elliott S: Denial as an effective mechanism to allay anxiety following a stressful event. *J Psychiatr Nurs* (Oct) 1980; 18:11–15.

Heidt P: Effect of therapeutic touch on anxiety levels of hospitalized patients. *Nurs Res* 1981; 30:32–37.

Hodovanic B et al.: Family crisis intervention program in the medical intensive care unit. *Heart Lung* 1984; 13:243–249.

Kitto J, Dale B: Designing a brief discharge planning screen. *Nurs Manag* (Sept) 1985; 16(9):28–30.

Lust B: The patient in the ICU: A family experience. *CCQ* (March) 1984; 6:49–57.

McGee RF: Hope: A factor influencing crisis resolution. *ANS* (July) 1984; 6:34–44.

Moulton PJ: Chronic illness, grief, and the family. *J Comm Health Nurs* 1984; 1(2):75–88.

Noble M: *The ICU Environment.* Reston, VA: Reston, 1982.

Obleu L, Knoefel J: The effects of normal aging on speech, language, and communication. *Top Geriatr Rehabil* (July) 1986; 1:5–13.

Scalzi CC: Nursing management of behavioral responses following an acute myocardial infarction. *Heart Lung* 1973; 2(1):62–69.

Smitherman C: Dealing with the patient's denial: What should you do? *Nurs 81* (Dec) 1981; 70–71.

Stanitis M, Ryan J: Noncompliance: An unacceptable diagnosis? *Am J Nurs* 1982; 82:941–942.

Thomas S et al.: Denial in coronary patients: An objective reassessment. *Heart Lung* 1983; 12:74–80.

Vanson R et al.: Stress effects on patients in critical care units from procedures performed on others. *Heart Lung* 1980; 9:494–496.

Warmbrod L: Supporting families of critically ill patients. *Crit Care Nurse* (Sept/Oct) 1983; 49–52.

Wright L, Leahey M: *Nurses and families: A guide to family assessment and intervention.* Philadelphia: Davis, 1984.

Unit 3

STIMULATION

4

Stimulation Assessment

CLINICAL INSIGHT

Domain: The diagnostic and monitoring function

Competency: Anticipating problems: future think

Diagnostic and monitoring skills are vital components of critical-care nursing that permeate all phases of the nursing process. Nurses become connoisseurs of even minor physical and emotional changes and search among multiple possibilities for their cause. As such, they become masters at interpreting subtle shifts. They must react promptly to insignificant changes—yet not overreact to minor ones. Learning to differentiate the two requires continual awareness of what could be happening with a particular patient—not just what happens with nine of ten other patients, but, given this patient's history, what's reasonable for this one. Caring for unstable patients also requires an ability to titrate interventions so that precursors of catastrophe remain detectable. In the following exemplar, from Benner and Tanner (1986, pp. 26–27), an expert nurse elegantly describes the tightrope walk involved in anticipating critical-care problems.

Vasospasm can be devastating. It is like a stroke. Everybody is so individual. If they have severe subarach-

noid hemorrhages and are agitated, restless, and combative, their blood pressures go up, and then they get very quiet and their blood pressures drop down. You are worried about bleeding, and then you are worried about their stroking. You just play a game. And you play with these drugs and you try to keep it within the limits as well as you can.

Most of the time, if the bleed is bad enough, the people are pretty confused and agitated. So they are combative, and there is not anything you can really do for that. You don't want to snow them because you don't want to put them out, even enough to keep them quiet, because you won't know if the quietness is neurological, an indication of a rebleed, or whatever. It's very difficult.

The ability to anticipate problems rests on a solid foundation of assessment skills and rich background experience. This chapter presents the information a nurse should have at his or her command to assess a person's ability to receive, interpret, and integrate impulses into a unified response—the process called *stimulation* in the FANCAS system (Swendsen 1975).

Stimulation is mediated by the nervous system, a wondrously complex constellation of structures. These structures can be divided anatomically into those inside the skull and vertebral column—that is, the central nervous system (CNS), consisting of the brain and spinal cord—and those outside the bony structures—that is, the peripheral nervous system, consisting of the cranial, spinal, and autonomic nerves. The nervous system can be subdivided functionally into voluntary versus involuntary functions and sensory versus motor functions. Although these distinctions are helpful in developing a cognitive framework for understanding the nervous system, they blur in practical application to patient assessment. The assessment plan that follows is one of several ways to organize a practical, convenient assessment of a system that defies neat compartmentalization.

Before proceeding, however, we need to fix in mind the reason for nursing assessment. Mitchell et al. (1984) compared medical and nursing evaluation. They report that the purpose of medical evaluation is to diagnose and treat disease, whereas the purpose of nursing evaluation is to assess the actual or potential changes in activities of daily living related to the health problem and assist the person to cope effectively. In the critical-care environment, medical and nursing assessment have the common goal of detecting and preventing life-threatening disorders. Therefore, when evaluating a patient, one should consider whether a patient is stable, improving, or deteriorating. The patient's condition then dictates the extent of the initial examination.

History

History-taking in the patient with neurologic dysfunction may be difficult due to an altered level of consciousness, communication problems, or memory impairment. Patient interviewing should be done to the extent possible. Questioning should elicit presenting symptoms and their interference with activities of daily living. Particularly note any history of loss of consciousness (onset, duration, behavior after regaining consciousness), seizure activity, behavioral changes, headache, pain, visual abnormalities, dizziness, weakness, decreased level of consciousness, memory loss and impaired speech. If information is unobtainable from the patient or there is any question of memory loss, interview family members or others who have observed the patient.

Physical Examination

Assessment of stimulation is divided into general areas that test integrated neuromuscular functions: (a) level of consciousness; (b) mentation; (c) head and neck; (d) cranial nerves; (e) sensorimotor function; (f) reflexes; (g) coordination; and (h) vital signs. The following sections present the neurologic physical examination in detail, to facilitate comprehension of its components and related neuroanatomy.

Often, the critically ill patient will require rapid, frequent neurologic nursing assessment. An abbreviated neurologic examination ("neurochecks") usually consists of:

- Level of consciousness.
- Pupil responses.
- Motor function.
- Vital signs.

Noting subtle changes and reporting them promptly is particularly important in the critically ill neurologic or neurosurgical patient. To simplify documentation and evaluation, a flow sheet may be used. A sample is shown in Table 4-1.

Assessment of the Level of Consciousness

Key Brain Structures The key structures of the brain are shown in Figure 4-1.

The major divisions of the brain are the cerebral hemispheres, the diencephalon, the brainstem, and the cerebellum. The *cerebrum* consists of two hemispheres (connected by the corpus callosum). The outer layer of each hemisphere, the *cerebral cortex,* is subdivided into four lobes: the frontal, parietal, temporal, and occipital. The interior of the cerebrum consists of bundles of nerve fibers called *cerebral tracts.* Near the thalamus and basal ganglia, a group of sensory and motor tracts form a large mass known as the *internal capsule.* Deep inside the cerebral hemispheres are islands of gray matter called *basal ganglia.*

The *diencephalon* is the part of the brain located between the cerebrum and midbrain. It contains several structures around the third ventricle, the most important ones being the *thalamus* and the *hypothalamus.*

The next major part of the brain is the *brainstem,* which consists of the *midbrain, pons,* and *medulla oblongata.*

The *cerebellum* sits below the occipital lobes and partially covers the brainstem. It, too, has two hemispheres, which are connected to each other and the brainstem by tracts called *cerebellar peduncles.* The functions of the various parts of the brain will be explained as the assessment plan progresses. For easy reference, the functions of brain structures are summarized in Table 4-2.

TABLE 4-1 NEUROLOGIC FLOW SHEET

ST. FRANCIS MEDICAL CENTER
La Crosse, Wisconsin
Neurologic Flow Sheet

92-626   Nurse's Signature and Initials

Pt. Name Plate

C O M A S C A L E		Date and Time														**C =** Eyes Closed by Swelling
	Eyes Open	Spontaneously	4													
		To Command	3													
		To Pain	2													
		No Response	1													
	Best Motor Response	Obeys Commands	6													Record Best Arm Response
		Localizes Pain	5													
		Flexion-Withdrawal	4													
		Flexion (abnormal)	3													
		Extension (abnormal)	2													
		No Response	1													
	Best Verbal Response	Oriented	5													**T =** Endo-tracheal Tube or Tracheos-tomy **A =** Aphasia
		Confused	4													
		Inappropriate Words	3													
		Incomprehensible Sounds	2													
		No Response	1													
TOTAL SCORE																
P U P I L S	Size	R														**B =** Brisk **S =** Sluggish **N =** No Reaction **C =** Closed
	Reaction															
	Size	L														
	Reaction															
L I M B M O V E M E N T	Grade Limb Movement Spontaneous or to Command, Do Not Rate Reflex Movement	RA														Use Limb Movement Scale To Grade
		RL														
		LA														
		LL														
V I T A L S	Blood Pressure															Respiration Type **N =** Normal **CS =** Chayne Stokes **SH =** Sustained Hyperventilation **U =** Uncoordinated
	Pulse															
	Temperature															
	Respiratory Rate															
	Respiratory Type															
	Nurse's Initial															

Limb Movement Scale
0-No response
1-Flicker of Trace of Contraction
2-Active Movement with Gravity Eliminated
3-Active Movement Against Gravity
4-Active Movement Against Gravity and Resistance
5-Normal Power

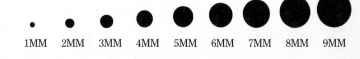

1MM   2MM   3MM   4MM   5MM   6MM   7MM   8MM   9MM

Source: Davenport-Fortune P, Dunnum L: Professional nursing care of the patient with increased intracranial pressure: planned or 'hit and miss'? *J Neurosurg Nurs* 1985; 17:367–370.

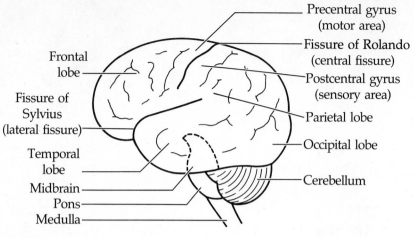

FIGURE 4-1

Lateral view of the brain.

Consciousness Consciousness is mediated by the reticular activating system (RAS), which originates in the brainstem and terminates in almost all areas of the diencephalon and the cerebrum. Changes in the level of consciousness are the most important indicator of overall CNS function (Figure 4-2). The following description of this system is based on Guyton (1986).

The brainstem reticular activating system receives input from sensory stimuli via ascending tracts from the spinal cord and brainstem. Retrograde stimulation of the RAS by the cerebrum is mediated through direct fiber pathways into the reticular formation from (1) the somatic sensory cortex, (2) the motor cortex, (3) the frontal cortex, (4) the basal ganglia, (5) the hypothalamus, and (6) the hippocampus and other limbic structures. The brainstem reticular formation integrates these stimuli and transmits them over discrete pathways to the diencephalon and the cerebrum. The RAS is believed to be responsible for arousal and wakefulness; when it is stimulated, it causes diffuse activation of the entire brain. For full consciousness, the person must have both a functioning reticular activating system

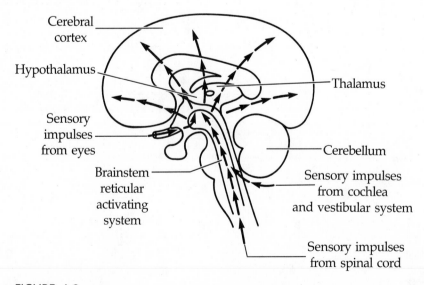

FIGURE 4-2

Reticular activating system.

TABLE 4-2 FUNCTIONS OF BRAIN STRUCTURES

STRUCTURE	FUNCTIONS
Cerebrum	Gray and white matter with sensory, motor, and integrative functions
A. Cerebral cortex	Outer layer consisting of gray matter
1. Frontal lobe	Complex intellectual functions such as memory, judgment, and problem solving; personality
Precentral gyrus	Primary motor area
2. Temporal lobe	Primary auditory area; taste, smell; comprehension of speech
3. Parietal lobe (specifically, postcentral gyrus)	Primary somatic sensory area
4. Occipital lobe	Primary visual area
B. Internal capsule	White matter; sensory and motor tracts, located between thalamus and basal ganglia
C. Basal ganglia	Gray matter deep in each hemisphere; coordination of muscular activity; automatic movements of expression
Diencephalon	Gray matter between cerebrum and midbrain; structures around third ventricle, particularly thalamus and hypothalamus
A. Thalamus	Gray matter located against lateral walls of third ventricle; reception of sensory impulses; participation in arousal mechanism; conscious awareness of crude sensations; relay of sensations to cortex for fine discrimination
B. Hypothalamus	Regulation of activity of autonomic nervous system; secretion of hormonal releasing factors, antidiuretic hormone and oxytocin; participation in arousal mechanism; control of appetite and body temperature
Brainstem	
A. Midbrain (mesencephalon)	White and gray matter connecting cerebrum and pons; contains nuclei of third cranial nerve (including the pupillary reflex center) and nuclei of fourth and part of fifth cranial nerves
B. Pons	White matter and nuclei of fifth to eighth cranial nerves; participation in regulation of respiration; projection tracts between brain and spinal cord
C. Medulla oblongata	Mostly white matter and nuclei of ninth to twelfth cranial nerves; cardiac, vasomotor, and respiratory reflex centers; also reflex centers for sneezing, coughing, vomiting, swallowing; projection tracts between brain and cord
D. Reticular activating system	Diffuse gray and white matter in brainstem core; relays impulses from cord and specialized sensory tracts to thalamus and then to cortex; portion rostral to midpons functions to arouse cerebral cortex and to maintain consciousness
Cerebellum	Coordination of muscular activity; maintenance of muscle tone, equilibrium, and posture

and relatively intact cerebral hemispheres (Plum and Posner 1980).

General Descriptions Describe the level of consciousness in general terms only if those terms are known and agreed upon by all staff with whom you communicate. Mitchell (1984) recommends the following descriptions for acute alterations in consciousness (arousal):

- *Clouding of Consciousness:* Reduced wakefulness and decreased attention.
- *Confusional State:* Disorientation, poor memory.
- *Delirium:* Disorientation, fearfulness, irritability, misperception of sensory stimuli, visual hallucination.
- *Obtundation:* Mental blunting, decreased alertness, decreased interest in environment.
- *Stupor:* Deep sleep, arousable only by vigorous and repeated stimulation.
- *Coma:* Unarousable by any stimulus, psychologic unresponsiveness.

Glasgow Coma Scale The Glasgow coma scale was designed to measure effectively the functional state of the brain as a whole, since the unconscious state may be brought on by focal or diffuse pathology. It is general enough to assess all gradations of the continuum, from full consciousness to coma, yet is objective enough that interrater reliability is high. The scale relates consciousness to three parameters: *eye opening, verbal response,* and *motor response.* Points are assigned to each level of response and the total score computed. The fully alert, responsive patient will score 15; the comatose patient will score 7 or less. When assessing a patient, always observe for spontaneous activity before stimulating the patient. If spontaneous activity is not present, then proceed to verbal stimulation and ultimately to tactile (painful) stimulation, if necessary. The Glasgow coma scale may be incorporated in ICU and ED flow sheets to detect early changes in neurologic function (see Table 4-1). The score is also used as a predictor of the degree of recovery to be expected.

Drawbacks of the Glasgow coma scale include the difficulty for use with very young or very old patients, and the possibility of a falsely low score with deaf, intoxicated, or uncooperative patients or those who cannot speak English. The scale, therefore, should be viewed as a rapid method for assessing consciousness, to be followed by history-taking, a more thorough neurologic examination, and diagnostic testing.

Assessment of Mentation

Mentation can be defined as the content of consciousness. It reflects general cerebral function and is evaluated with a mental status examination. The components of this examination are: (a) general appearance and behavior; (b) mood and affect; and (c) cognitive functions. To assess general appearance, note the person's dress and grooming. In evaluating behavior, note speech patterns, body language, and the appropriateness of behavior. Next, note mood and affect, that is, the appropriateness, diversity, and speed of change of the person's emotions. Finally, evaluate cognitive functions. These include orientation, attention and concentration, memory, ability to reason, insight, judgment, and thought content.

To evaluate *orientation,* ask the person questions to test awareness of person, place, and time. Test *attention* and *concentration* by asking the person to repeat a series of numbers forward and backward. Most people can remember five to eight numbers in a forward series, and four to six in a backward series (Mitchell et al. 1984).

Memory consists of short-term, recent, and remote memory. Evaluate *short-term memory* by asking the patient to repeat a phrase given a few minutes earlier. Evaluate *recent memory* by asking what brought the patient to the hospital. Ask about events that occurred several years ago to test *remote memory.*

Test *abstract thinking* by asking the person to identify similarities in two objects and to interpret a proverb or solve a problem appropriate to her or his education level. Evaluate *insight* and *judgment* by asking about the cause of the patient's illness and what she or he would do in a given situation, such as discovering a fire. To assess *thought,* note the clarity, content, and flow of thought. Especially note hallucinations, delusions, and suicidal ideation. For example, you might ask the person whether she or he has had any problem with thinking or had any experiences recently that he or she cannot explain (Hickey 1986).

Examination of the Head and Neck

Bones The skull is formed of many bones, the major ones of which are the frontal, parietal, temporal, occipital, and sphenoid bones and the cribriform plate. Disruption of these bones implies potential damage to the underlying structures.

The interior floor of the skull is divided into three areas. The anterior fossa contains the frontal lobes of the brain. The middle fossa contains the temporal lobes, the upper brainstem, and the pituitary gland. The posterior fossa contains the brainstem and cerebellum. At the base of the skull is an opening, called the *foramen magnum,* through which the spinal cord emerges. Other openings in the skull provide passageways for the cranial nerves.

Meninges Between the skull and the brain, and between the vertebral column and spinal cord, are membranes called *meninges.* The outermost layer, the *dura mater,* is a tough membrane that adheres to the skull though not to the vertebral column. The middle layer is the *arachnoid.* The innermost membrane, the *pia mater,* adheres to the brain and cord.

Folds of the dura support the brain. The midsagittal fold that divides the cerebral hemispheres is known as the *falx cerebri.* Its posterior portion swoops out laterally and anteriorly to form the *tentorium cerebelli,* which separates the middle from the posterior fossae, that is, the temporal and occipital lobes from the cerebellum and most of the brainstem. Structures contained in the anterior and middle cranial fossae thus are described as *supratentorial,* while those in the posterior fossa are *infratentorial.*

The spaces outside and between the meninges are named for their locations: between the skull and dura is the *epidural* space; between the dura and arachnoid is the *subdural* space; and between the arachnoid and the pia is the *subarachnoid* space. The larger subarachnoid spaces are called *cisterns,* with the largest, the *cisterna magna,* being located between the foramen magnum and the first cervical vertebra.

The meninges provide spaces for the potential accumulation of blood and cerebrospinal fluid. Cerebrospinal fluid (CSF), which circulates in the subarachnoid space, will be discussed in detail later in the chapter. While inspecting and palpating the cranial bones, look for cerebrospinal fluid leaks, which usually appear as clear, colorless fluid oozing or dripping from the ear *(otorrhea)* or nose *(rhinorrhea)* or down the posterior pharynx. To differentiate this fluid from mucus, test it for glucose—CSF contains glucose, but mucus does not. The presence of blood in the fluid will invalidate this assessment tool, because blood, too, contains glucose.

While examining the skull, note also whether the person can touch chin to chest or whether *nuchal rigidity* (a sign of meningeal irritation) is present. (Do not flex the neck if trauma to the cervical spine is suspected.)

Blood Supply The arterial blood supply to the brain arises from the two internal carotid arteries anteriorly and the two vertebral arteries posteriorly (Figure 4-3). You may recall that the first three branches of the aorta are the brachiocephalic (which subdivides into the right common carotid and right subclavian arteries), the left common carotid, and the leftsubclavian arteries. The common carotid arteries give rise to the internal carotid arteries, which enter the skull through the cranial floor. The subclavian arteries give rise to the vertebral arteries, which travel up through the transverse processes of cervical vertebrae and through the foramen magnum to unite into the basilar artery. The internal carotid arteries and basilar artery join at the base of the brain in the circle of Willis. The internal carotid arteries give rise to the anterior and middle cerebral arteries. The basilar artery gives rise to the posterior cerebral arteries. The circle of Willis provides for collateral circulation among all of these intracranial arteries so that, even if one of the internal carotid or vertebral arteries becomes occluded, blood supply to the brain is maintained.

The anterior cerebral artery serves the anterior and middle portions of the brain tissue along the falx cerebri, that is, part of the frontal and parietal lobes and the corpus callosum. The middle cerebral artery nourishes the lateral part of the hemisphere, that is, portions of the frontal, parietal, and temporal lobes, and supplies branches to nourish the deep structures such as the basal ganglia. The posterior cerebral artery serves the posterior surface of the hemisphere, that is, part of the temporal lobes and all of the occipital lobes. Branches of the vertebral and basilar arteries nourish the cerebellum and brainstem.

Branches of the external carotid arteries give rise to the meningeal arteries, which course between the skull and dura and nourish the dura. The pia and arachnoid are nourished from branches of the internal carotid and vertebral arteries.

The veins draining the cortex travel mostly in the subarachnoid space. They empty into the superior and inferior sagittal sinuses and other sinuses, all of which eventually empty into the internal jugular vein and thus to the right atrium. Trauma to the cranium may lead to arterial or venous bleeding, depending upon the location of the injury.

Assessment of the Cranial Nerves

Twelve pairs of cranial nerves emanate from the brain (Figure 4-4). The critical-care nurse may perform a screening evaluation of cranial nerves, particularly focusing on those whose dysfunction may indicate life threats or seriously interfere with activities of daily living (Table 4-3). The cranial nerves of primary importance to the critical-care nurse thus are the optic (II), oculomotor (III), trigeminal (V), facial (VII), glossopharyngeal (IX), and vagus (X).

Eye examinations are particularly important in critical care. When examining the eyes, assess their resting position, movement, size, shape, equality, response to light, and accommodation.

Eye Position and Movement In the resting state, the eyes normally are in midposition. Deviation may in-

TABLE 4-3 A PRACTICAL ICU SCREENING TEST FOR CRANIAL NERVE FUNCTION

NERVE		TEST PROCEDURE
II	Optic	Shine a light into each eye and note whether the pupil on that side constricts *(direct light reflex).* Then shine a light into each eye and note whether the opposite pupil constricts *(consensual light reflex).*
III	Oculomotor	
V	Trigeminal	Touch the cornea with a cotton wisp. (Approach the eye from the side, and avoid the eyelashes.) Note whether a blink reflex is present.
VII	Facial	
IX	Glossopharyngeal	Touch the back of the throat with a tongue blade and note whether a gag reflex is present.
X	Vagus	

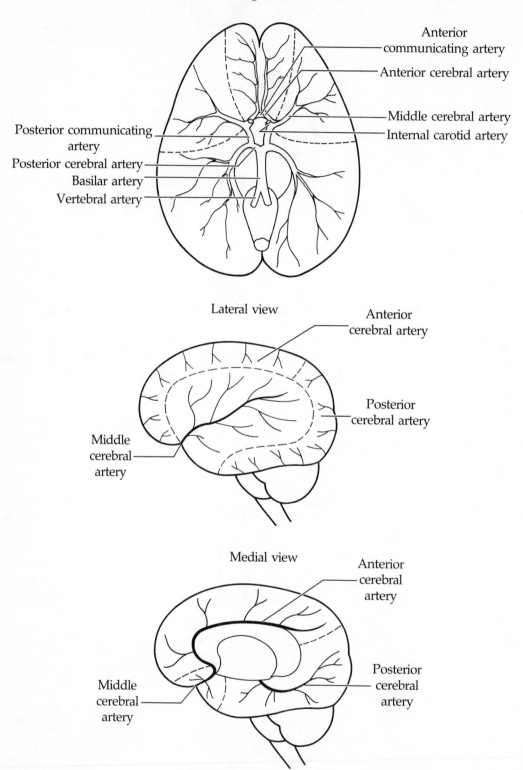

FIGURE 4-3

Major cerebral arteries and their areas of distribution.

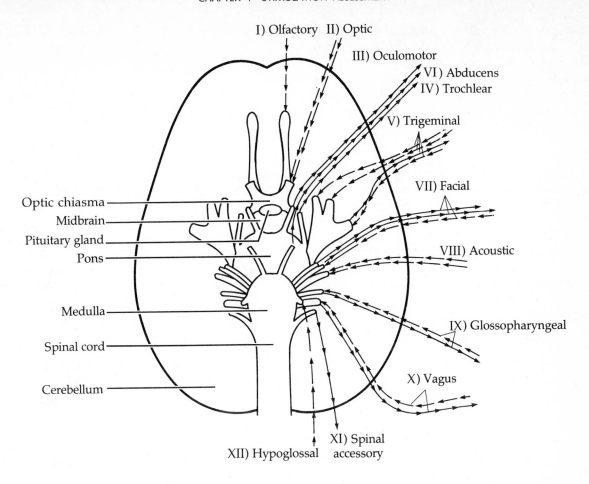

Nerve	Type	Major functions
I) Olfactory	Sensory	Smell
II) Optic	Sensory	Vision
III) Oculomotor	Motor	Eye movements (except those mediated by fourth and sixth cranial nerves), pupil size, and accommodation
IV) Trochlear	Motor	Eye movements (superior oblique muscle)
V) Trigeminal	Sensorimotor	Sensations from face, cornea, teeth, tongue, nasal and oral mucosa; mastication
VI) Abducens	Motor	Eye movements (lateral rectus muscle)
VII) Facial	Sensorimotor	Taste from anterior two-thirds of tongue, facial expressions, and salivation
VIII) Acoustic	Sensory	Hearing and equilibrium
IX) Glosso-pharyngeal	Sensorimotor	Taste from posterior third of tongue, pharyngeal sensations, swallowing, salivation, reflex control of blood pressure and respirations
X) Vagus	Sensorimotor	Sensation and movement of pharynx, larynx, thoracic and abdominal viscera
XI) Spinal accessory	Motor	Movements of head, neck, and shoulders
XII) Hypoglossal	Motor	Movements of tongue

FIGURE 4-4

Cranial nerves.

dicate lesions in the frontal lobe, pons, or third or sixth cranial nerve (Hickey 1986). There normally are either no spontaneous movements or slow, roving movements. Abnormalities include nystagmus and jerking of one eye.

Extraocular movement can be tested in the conscious patient by having him follow the movement of your finger. If the eyes move as a pair, *conjugate* eye movement is present. If they move in different directions, *dysconjugate* eye movement is present, indicating abnormal function of the third, fourth, or sixth cranial nerve.

Pupil Size and Shape   Next assess pupil size and shape. Pupils should be equal in size, unless a congenital disparity exists or constricting or dilating eyedrops have been used in one eye. Anisocoria (unequal pupils) is probably unimportant unless other evidence of a third cranial nerve lesion exists, such as sluggish pupil constriction or diminished medial rectus function (inability to move the eye toward the nose). To enhance accuracy in communication, it is best to specify pupil size in millimeters and also specify the degree of light in which you observed the eyes; for example, "dilated pupils" is less informative than "pupils 8 mm in brightly lit room." Normal pupils are 2–6 mm in diameter, round, and with smooth edges.

Pupillary Responses   Testing pupillary response to light involves testing both the optic and oculomotor nerves. The following testing procedure is recommended. Darken the room if possible. If the patient is conscious, ask him or her to focus on a distant point. This will minimize the reflex constriction that occurs with focusing on a nearby point.

Place the edge of your hand along the patient's nose (to avoid the consensual response, explained below). Shine a bright light into one eye and observe the speed with which it constricts (direct light reflex). Repeat the procedure with the other eye. Each eye should constrict briskly. Next, shine the light in one eye and observe whether the other eye constricts; then test the other eye. When one eye is stimulated, the other should constrict (*consensual light reflex*). The reason this occurs is that one eye perceives the light and transmits impulses to the brain via the optic system; the brain, however, stimulates both oculomotor nerves.

To test accommodation, hold your finger 8–12 inches from the bridge of the patient's nose. Have the patient focus on your finger as you move it toward the patient's nose. As you approach the nose, the pupils should constrict and the eyes converge bilaterally and equally to maintain a clear visual image.

The normal pupil response is recorded as **PNERLA**—Pupils Normal (size and shape), Equal, and Reactive to Light and Accommodation.

Abnormal Pupils   Some important pupillary abnormalities are shown in Figure 4-5 (Plum and Posner 1980). *Small reactive pupils* often are seen in (1) bilateral diencephalic damage during rostral-caudal deterioration in supratentorial lesions, and (2) metabolic encephalopathies.

Large (5–6 mm), *fixed pupils* that spontaneously fluctuate in size and may show spasmodic contractions (hippus) result from lesions in the tectal area (roof) of the midbrain.

Midposition (4–5 mm), *fixed pupils* that are often slightly irregular and unequal are caused by midbrain lesions that interrupt both sympathetic and parasympathetic innervation of the eye. They usually are caused by midbrain damage from transtentorial herniation, but also are seen with midbrain tumors, hemorrhages, or infarcts.

Pinpoint pupils are seen with pontine hemorrhage, which interrupts sympathetic pathways to the eye and produces bilaterally small pupils, and with opiate overdose.

A *dilated, fixed ("blown") pupil* is seen with third cranial nerve damage when uncal herniation compresses the oculomotor nerve against the tentorial edge. Recall that a fold of dura, the tentorium, separates the cerebral hemispheres from the cerebellum. An opening in it, called the *incisura* or *tentorial notch,* allows the upper brainstem and its nerves and blood vessels to pass through. When supratentorial pressure increases, the structures near the notch become compressed. One of these structures is the third cranial (oculomotor) nerve. This nerve contains motor fibers (for eye movement) in the center and parasympathetic fibers (for pupillary constriction and eyelid elevation) on the outside. Compression of one oculomotor nerve causes loss of parasympathetic stimulation to the eye on the same side. Sympathetic stimulation continues unopposed, because the sympathetic fibers are not compressed. (The sympathetic pathway originates in the hypothalamus and courses through the brainstem to the upper three segments of the thoracic spinal cord, where the sympathetic nerves to the eye originate.) The result is pupillary dilation and loss of the reflex response to light on the same side as the compression. Associated symptoms may include lateral, downward deviation of the eye and ptosis.

Bilaterally *wide, fixed pupils* are seen in profound hypoxia, such as cardiac arrest, and in anticholinergic poisoning.

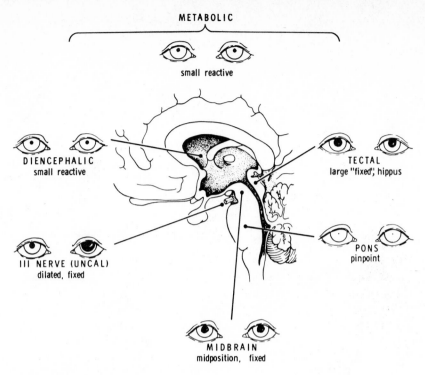

FIGURE 4-5

Pupils in comatose patients. (From Plum F, Posner J: *The diagnosis of stupor and coma,*
3d ed. Philadelphia: Davis, 1980.)

Corneal Reflex When first examining a patient's eyes, note whether a corneal reflex is present. If the person does not blink spontaneously, test the reflex. With a fine wisp of cotton, approach the eye from the side. Avoid the eyelashes and touch the cornea lightly. Normally, this sensation is perceived by the trigeminal nerve and provokes intense blinking. If this reflex is absent, the cornea may become inflamed or ulcerated due to dryness, scratches, or particles that get in the eye. These conditions can deteriorate into inflammation of the iris and blindness. To prevent damage, lubricate the eye with artificial tears and cover with an eye shield. Periodically remove the shield, clean the eye area, and check for inflammation.

Oculocephalic Reflex In addition to testing the pupillary and corneal reflexes, you also should understand the significance of two additional tests the physician may perform to evaluate the intactness of the brainstem: the *oculocephalic reflex (doll's eyes phenomenon)* and the *oculovestibular reflex (ice water calorics).*

To test for the doll's eyes phenomenon, the physician holds the patient's eyelids open and rotates the head from side to side. In the normal (awake) patient,

reflex eye movement cannot be elicited consistently because the patient can exert cortical control of eye movement. In the comatose patient, this maneuver sometimes will cause both eyes to move laterally in the direction opposite to the head rotation (Figure 4-6). This conjugate (parallel) lateral gaze is labeled a positive, normal, or intact doll's eyes response. To understand the significance of this response, recall that the vestibular apparatus transmits information about head position along the acoustic nerve to the pons. The nerves controlling lateral gaze are the sixth cranial nerve from the pons and the third cranial nerve from the midbrain. A positive doll's eyes response indicates that information enters the lower pons, ascends to the upper pons and midbrain, and exits the appropriate cranial nerves, in other words, the brainstem is intact. A positive doll's eyes response thus means the coma-producing lesion is either supratentorial or metabolic. An absent (negative) doll's eyes reflex in a comatose patient usually indicates that the lesion is in the brainstem itself. An exception is the negative doll's eyes response seen in sedative drug intoxication (the only metabolic encephalopathy in which negative doll's eyes is seen). This exception is important to remember, since drug-

Head in neutral position   Head rotated to patient's left

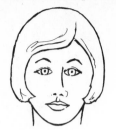 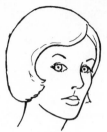 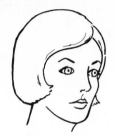

Eyes midline

Positive response:
eyes move in
relation to head

Negative response:
eyes do not move
in relation to head

FIGURE 4-6

Doll's eyes phenomenon.

induced coma is very common. (The author is indebted to Dr. Roger Simon, Assistant Professor of Neurology at the University of California, San Francisco, for a delightful way to remember the information about doll's eyes responses. He points out that expensive china dolls, such as his mother's, have eyes suspended on weights so that they move back and forth as the head is turned. Cheaper, "junky" dolls have painted-on eyes that remain fixed in the position of the head. Thus, eyes that remain fixed in midposition during head turning = junky doll = bad; eyes that move from the midline during head rotation = expensive china doll = mother = good!)

Oculovestibular Reflex Ice water stimulation (ice water calorics) is a maneuver that is physiologically identical to the doll's eyes maneuver but more powerful in inducing eye movements. The following descriptions are based on Plum and Posner (1980). After examining the ear for intactness of the tympanic membrane, the physician places the patient with the head elevated 30 degrees above the horizontal to provide maximal stimulation of the semicircular canal. He or she then uses a large syringe, filled with ice water, and a small catheter to slowly irrigate the canal until nystagmus or ocular deviation occurs (or 120 ml of water have been used). The response in the normal awake patient is nystagmus after 20–30 seconds, with slow movement toward the irrigated ear and rapid movement away. In the comatose patient, you may see the eyes move slowly toward the irrigated ear and remain there for 2–3 minutes; the fast return to midline (quick phase) has disappeared. This response indicates that the lesion is supratentorial or metabolic. If you see an extremely abnormal re-

sponse, such as downward deviation and rotary jerking of one eye, the lesion is in the brainstem. An absent caloric response indicates severe brainstem damage or depression.

Assessment of the Sensorimotor Function

Sensation As a critical-care nurse you usually will not perform a separate, systematic test of various sensations in all parts of the body. It is helpful, however, to have a basic knowledge of sensory function to understand the various pathologies with which patients may present. Such knowledge requires not only comprehension of cranial function but also awareness of spinal cord function.

The vertebral column is made up of seven cervical, twelve thoracic, and five lumbar vertebrae plus the sacrum and coccyx. Central openings in the vertebrae form the spinal canal, which contains the spinal cord. The cord proper extends from the base of the brainstem through the foramen magnum to the second lumbar vertebra, from which a fibrous band attaches to the coccyx. Between the vertebrae and the spinal cord are the spinal meninges (dura, arachnoid and pia). The cord is supplied by the anterior and posterior spinal arteries, which arise from the vertebral arteries at the foramen magnum, and by the lateral spinal arteries. Cerebrospinal fluid circulates between the arachnoid and the cord.

Sensory information reaches the spinal cord and brain from a variety of sources. Impulses pass from a sensory receptor to a peripheral nerve, which carries

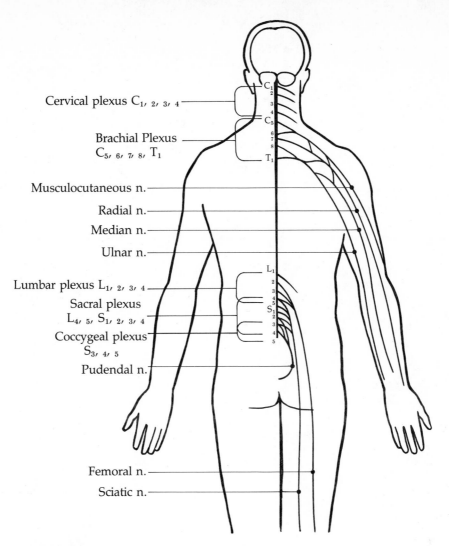

Cervical plexus $C_{1, 2, 3, 4}$

Brachial Plexus
$C_{5, 6, 7, 8}$, T_1

Musculocutaneous n.

Radial n.

Median n.

Ulnar n.

Lumbar plexus $L_{1, 2, 3, 4}$

Sacral plexus
$L_{4, 5}$, $S_{1, 2, 3, 4}$

Coccygeal plexus
$S_{3, 4, 5}$

Pudendal n.

Femoral n.

Sciatic n.

FIGURE 4-7

Spinal nerve plexes and major peripheral nerves arising from them.

sensory, motor, and autonomic fibers from a fairly wide area of the body. The peripheral nerves are regrouped closer to the spinal cord into nerve plexes (Figure 4-7) and then into 31 pairs of spinal nerves. The pairs of spinal nerves correspond to the 31 spinal segments (eight cervical, twelve thoracic, five lumbar, five sacral, and one coccygeal). Near the cord, the spinal nerves split into posterior and anterior roots (Figure 4-8). The roots connect with gray matter shaped like two pairs of horns within the spinal cord. The posterior (dorsal) root carries sensory fibers into the cord. The anterior (ventral) root carries motor fibers out from the cord. Specific skin segments innervated by the sensory roots are called dermatomes. Dermatomes overlap each other considerably; a simplified diagram appears in Figure 4-

9. Knowledge of dermatome innervation aids the physician or nurse in localizing a lesion causing a sensory abnormality.

Synapses within the cord enable sensory impulses to: (1) enter a spinal reflex arc back to the motor root; and/or (2) ascend the spinal cord to the cerebellum via the spinocerebellar tract; and/or (3) ascend the spinal cord to the cortex. To reach the cortex, impulses travel up spinal tracts to the thalamus and pass through the internal capsule to the sensory cortex, which is located behind the fissure of Sylvius in the parietal lobe. Different types of sensory information ascend different spinothalamic tracts (Figure 4-10). Only the most important tracts are discussed here.

Almost all of the sensory information from the body's

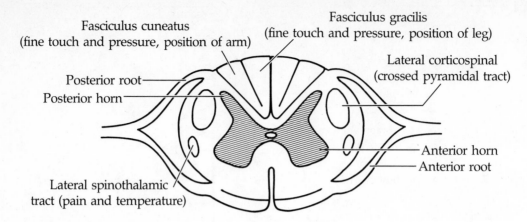

FIGURE 4-8

Spinal cord in cross-section.

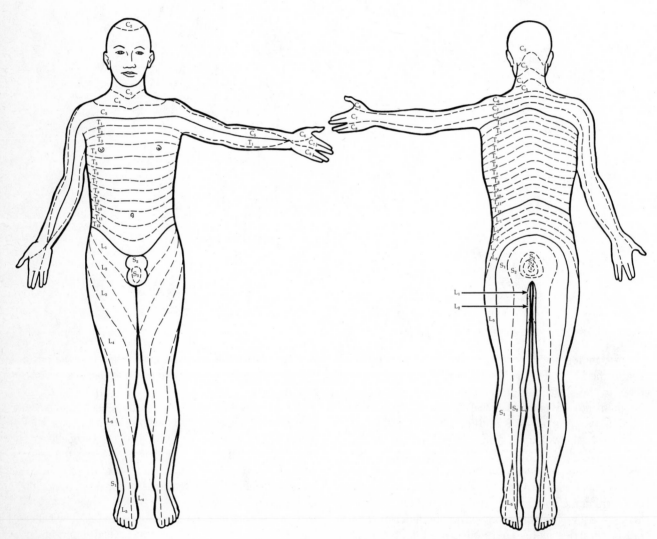

FIGURE 4-9

Dermatomes.

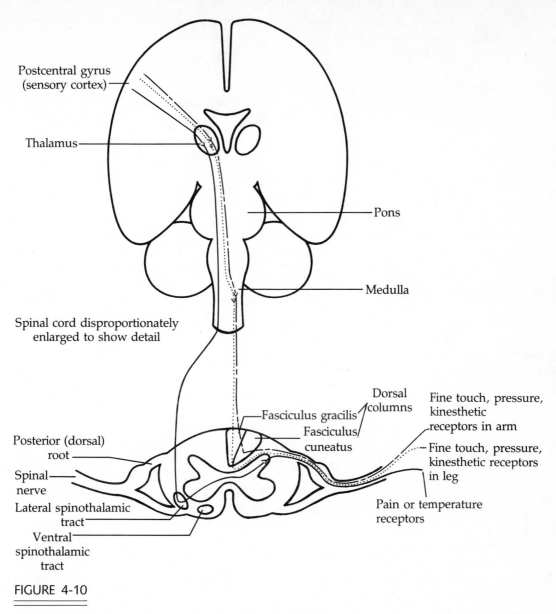

FIGURE 4-10

Sensory (ascending) tracts for sensations from the left side of the body.

somatic segments enter the cord through the posterior roots. After entering the cord, the sensory signals are carried through one of two pathways: the dorsal-column–lemniscal-system (made up of the dorsal column and the spinocervical pathways in the dorsolateral columns) and the anterolateral spinothalamic tracts (Guyton 1986).

The anterolateral spinothalamic tracts carry information about pain, temperature, crude touch, and pressure. Pain and temperature impulses ascend the lateral spinothalamic tract; crude touch and pressure impulses ascend the ventral (anterior) spinothalamic tract. In each case, the fibers carrying the impulses enter the

dorsal root and synapse with another neuron. This neuron crosses to the opposite side of the cord and ascends the appropriate tract to the thalamus. In the thalamus, the crude sensation is perceived and the neuron synapses with a third neuron. This third neuron travels through the internal capsule to the sensory cortex, where the stimulus is discriminated and localized.

In contrast to the broad range of crude sensations transmitted by the anterolateral tract, the dorsal columns transmit only mechanoreceptive stimuli (Guyton 1986). Fibers carrying fine touch and pressure impulses from the skin, and position and vibration impulses from muscles, tendons, and joints enter the cord and ascend uncrossed in the dorsal columns (posterior tract) to the medulla. (Impulses from the arm and upper body ascend in the column called the fasciculus cuneatus, those from the leg and lower body in the fasciculus gracilis.) In the medulla, they synapse with another neuron. This neuron crosses within the medulla and ascends to the thalamus, which again perceives the general sensation. From the thalamus, a third neuron passes through the internal capsule to the sensory area in the parietal lobe.

Voluntary Motor Activity   Proceed with your examination by assessing the patient's motor function. Motor function can be classed conveniently into voluntary and involuntary activity.

Assess *voluntary* motor activity in the upper extremities with handgrips, by asking the patient to grip the second and third fingers of your hands. Note whether she or he is able to do so, and compare the strength of the grip bilaterally. In the patient with an altered level of consciousness, it is important to differentiate a grasp to command from a grasp reflex. To do so, command the patient to release your fingers. If the patient does not release on command, the grasp is a reflex grasp. In addition, ask the patient to close the eyes and extend the arms upright, with the hands supine, for a few seconds. A drifting arm is an early sign of weakness. Assess voluntary motor activity in the legs by asking the patient to push her or his feet against your hands. Note spontaneous movement in those patients unable to obey commands.

Most voluntary activity originates in the primary motor cortex (precentral gyrus), which is a narrow strip in each frontal lobe, anterior to the fissure of Sylvius. Specific body parts are represented in a definite pattern, with the toes on the medial aspect closest to the top part of the hemisphere and the fingers closest to the fissure of Sylvius (lateral fissure). Body parts are represented according to the discreteness of their movement; for example, the hand is more highly represented than the elbow.

From each motor cortex, fibers pass through the internal capsule on the same side. The fibers continue to the medulla, where they are grouped to form the corticospinal (pyramidal) tracts (Figure 4-11). In the medulla, most pyramidal fibers cross to the opposite side and continue down the cord as the crossed pyramidal (lateral corticospinal) tract. Motor impulses leave the cord via the anterior (ventral) horn and traverse spinal nerves, peripheral nerves, and neuromuscular junctions before they reach the muscle itself.

Because the fibers cross in the medulla, voluntary movement initiated by the motor cortex is manifested on the opposite side of the body. Thus, if your patient has lost voluntary movement on one side of his body, it could have resulted from damage to the motor cortex, internal capsule, or medulla on the opposite side of the body.

Involuntary (Reflex) Motor Activity

Posturing   If the person does not display voluntary motor activity, pressure or pain should be used to elicit reflex activity. Avoid pinching the patient, as repeated pinching will bruise the patient. Instead, try light pressure by stroking the extremity; if no response, try deep pressure by pressing intensely on the sides of the fingertips or toes, the Achilles tendon, the supraorbital ridge, the trapezius muscle, or the sternum. Note any specific response and evaluate it as appropriate, inappropriate, or absent. Appropriate responses include pushing your hand away or withdrawing from the stimulus. They indicate that sensory function is intact and motor function from the cortex to the muscle is present to some degree. Inappropriate responses include unilateral or bilateral decorticate or decerebrate postures (Figure 4-12). The following information on these postures is from Plum and Posner (1980). If the patient's response is to bring the arm next to the body; flex his or her fingers, wrist, and arm; and extend his or her leg, rotate it internally, and plantar flex his or her foot, then the patient is showing *decorticate posturing* (abnormal flexion) (Figure 4-12 *a, b*). This response is typical of the interruption of corticospinal pathways produced by a lesion in the motor cortex or internal capsule. If the patient's response is to rigidly extend the arms and legs, bring his or her arms close to the body and hyperpronate them, plantar flex the feet, and sometimes to arch the back (opisthotonus), then the patient is displaying *decerebrate posturing* (abnormal extension) (Figure 4-12c). This sign indicates a more life-threatening situation than decorticate posturing. It indicates a cerebral lesion that is compressing or destroying the lower thalamus and midbrain, or all the brainstem above the middle of the pons. Decerebrate changes in the arms with flaccidity or weak flexor responses in the legs are primitive reactions seen in patients with extensive brainstem damage (Figure 4-12d).

There are some important points to remember about decorticate and decerebrate postures. The above descriptions are of full-blown responses; often, you will see only fragments of a posture, such as flexion of one arm. These fragments are important to note and report to the physician, as they are early indicators of abnormal responses. The postures may occur with or without your stimulation, and may be intermittent or continuous.

Spinal Reflexes   Spinal reflexes include superficial and deep tendon reflexes. Superficial reflexes are tested by

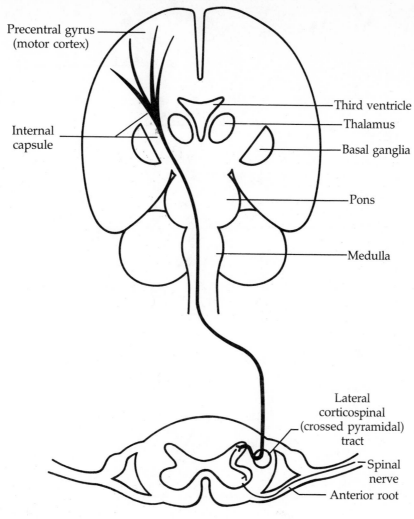

Precentral gyrus
(motor cortex)

Internal
capsule

Third ventricle

Thalamus

Basal ganglia

Pons

Medulla

Lateral
corticospinal
(crossed pyramidal)
tract

Spinal
nerve

Anterior root

FIGURE 4-11

Motor (descending) tracts for movement of the left side of the body.

stroking the skin. One superficial reflex you may have observed in males is the cremasteric reflex: your stroking the inner thigh skin (such as when you manipulate a urinary catheter) causes testicular elevation on the same side. Critical-care nurses evaluate superficial reflexes when they use light pressure to evoke a withdrawal response in a patient who does not respond to simple commands or when they check the plantar reflex for the Babinski sign.

To evaluate the plantar reflex, use a semisharp object such as a pen. Start at the outer edge of the heel. Stroke up the outer side of the sole and across the ball of the foot. Normally, the person will plantar flex the big toe. The abnormal response of dorsiflexing the big toe (and sometimes flaring the other toes) is called a *positive Babinski sign* and indicates damage to the pyramidal tract (Figure 4-13).

Deep reflexes usually are not tested by the critical-care nurse; the physician tests them by briskly striking a partially stretched tendon or bony prominence with a reflex hammer and evaluating the resulting muscular contraction. Examples are the biceps and patellar reflexes.

The scale on which deep tendon reflexes are graded is:

0^+ denotes no response.

1^+ denotes a reflex weaker than average.

2^+ denotes an average reflex.

3^+ denotes a reflex stronger than average.

4^+ denotes a hyperactive reflex.

A value of 1^+, 2^+, or 3^+ may be a normal reflex for the patient. An intact deep tendon reflex requires a

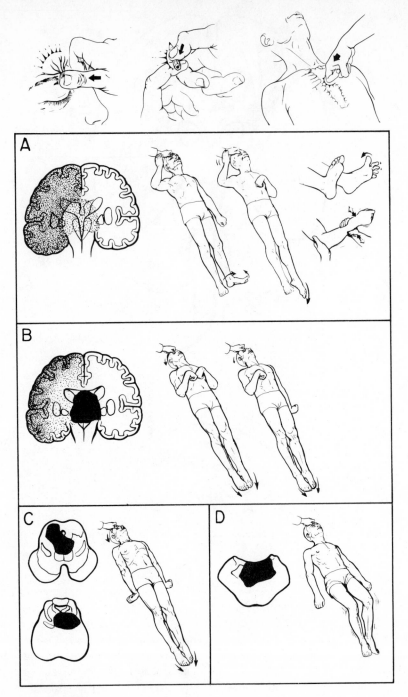

FIGURE 4-12

Motor responses to noxious stimulation in patients with acute cerebral dysfunction. Noxious stimuli can be delivered with minimal trauma to the supraorbital ridge, the nail bed, or the sternum, as illustrated at top. Levels of associated brain dysfunction are roughly indicated at left. The text provides details. (From: Plum F, Posner J: *The diagnosis of stupor and coma,* 3d ed. Philadelphia: Davis, 1980.)

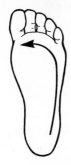
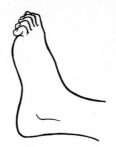
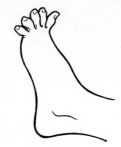

Stroke up sole of foot
and across ball

Normal response—plantar
flexion of all toes

Abnormal response—dorsiflexion
of big toe with or without
fanning of other toes

FIGURE 4-13

Babinski sign.

healthy peripheral sensory nerve, spinal nerve, dorsal root, cord synapse, motor root, motor nerve, neuromuscular junction, and muscle. Reflex activity does not depend upon pyramidal or extrapyramidal tracts or the cerebellum, but the intensity and smoothness of a reflex may be influenced by them.

Motor Neuron Lesions Disorders causing loss of voluntary or reflex movement commonly are described as upper motor neuron or lower motor neuron lesions. As mentioned earlier, peripheral nerves can carry motor and sensory fibers. The motor fibers eventually subdivide so that one motor fiber serves one muscle fiber. This last motor neuron innervating a muscle fiber is called the final common pathway because all motor impulses must pass through it to the muscle fiber.

Motor neurons serving the final common pathway are of two types. Those between the cerebral cortex and the motor nuclei of the brainstem or spinal cord are called upper motor neurons. Those between the motor nuclei of the brainstem (for cranial nerves) or the anterior horn cell in the spinal cord (for spinal nerves) and the muscle are called lower motor neurons.

Upper motor neuron lesions produce hyperactive reflex activity: while the reflex arc remains intact, cortical inhibition is lost. Although reflex activity is retained, voluntary motor function is lost (spastic paralysis). An example of an upper motor neuron lesion is hemiparesis following a cerebrovascular accident. Lower motor neuron lesions produce hypoactive reflexes, loss of voluntary movement, and muscle atrophy (flaccid paralysis). An example is anterior poliomyelitis.

Extrapyramidal System Background muscle tone, automatic movements (such as those that maintain pos-

ture), equilibrium, smoothness, and coordination of muscular activity are controlled by the extrapyramidal system. This system consists of the cerebellum, basal ganglia (gray matter deep in the cerebrum), and extrapyramidal pathways in the spinal cord.

The cerebellum, located below the occipital lobes of the cerebrum, consists of two hemispheres. Tracts (peduncles) connect the hemispheres to each other and to the brainstem. The cerebellum receives input from the motor cortex, brainstem, and peripheral areas. It modifies motor activity in numerous ways, which can be grouped into regulation of muscle tone, coordination of muscle movements, and maintenance of equilibrium.

The basal ganglia are bodies of gray matter found deep in the cerebral hemisphere. They are a major center of the extrapyramidal motor system and influence muscle tone, motor integration, and postural reflexes (Rudy 1984).

Impulses from the cerebellum and basal ganglia are transmitted to the muscles via extrapyramidal pathways in the spinal cord. During your assessment of motor activity, note whether movements are smooth and coordinated. Specific tests of cerebellar function (such as finger-to-nose, heel-to-shin, and rapid alternating movements, to test coordination; heel-to-toe walking to evaluate gait; and the Romberg test to assess balance) are part of the comprehensive neurologic examination of the ambulatory patient but not the patient with an acute neurologic problem. Loss of smoothness and coordination can result from damage to the cerebellum, basal ganglia, and/or extrapyramidal pathways in the cord.

Patterns of Pathology So far, correlation of signs and symptoms and sites of dysfunction has been presented beginning with the symptom and then identifying

TABLE 4-4 PATTERNS OF PATHOLOGY

TYPE OF LOSS	LOCATION OF LESION
Sensory	
1. Decrease or loss of all sensation in area served by peripheral nerve	Peripheral nerve
2. Decrease or loss of all sensation in dermatome	Sensory (dorsal) root
3. Decrease or loss of pain and temperature sensation on one side of body	Lateral spinothalamic tract on opposite side of body
4. Decrease or loss of fine touch discrimination, vibration awareness, awareness of limb position	Dorsal column (fasciculus gracilis or cuneatus) on same side of body
5. Decrease or absence of all sensation on one whole side of body	Thalamus on opposite side of body
6. Retention of crude sensation with loss of fine discrimination on one whole side of body	Sensory cortex on opposite side of body
Motor	
1. Loss of voluntary activity below level of lesion with retention of reflex activity (spastic paralysis)	Corticospinal (pyramidal) tract (upper motor neuron); side of body depends on level of lesion
2. Loss of voluntary and reflex activity below level of lesion (flaccid paralysis)	Lower motor neuron on same side of body
3. Decrease or loss of fine sensation and voluntary movement on entire side of body, with retention of crude sensation and reflex activity	Internal capsule
4. Decrease of muscle tone; inability to synchronize movements, gauge distance and speed, alternate movements quickly; intention tremor; poor equilibrium; voluntary and reflex motor activity present	Cerebellum
5. Rigidity, resting tremor, involuntary movements such as in Huntington's chorea; voluntary and reflex motor activity present	Extrapyramidal system

possible sites. As you have seen, most symptoms can be due to lesions in a variety of sites. The differential diagnosis of pathology requires extensive education and experience in neurology and is based upon the level and extent of symptomatology and a knowledge of the patterns of findings produced by lesions in different sites. Some patterns of pathology you may observe are presented in Table 4-4. It is useful to acquaint yourself with them, both to understand how a neurologist identifies the site of a lesion and to predict a patient's deficits from a medical diagnosis so you can better plan nursing care.

Examination of the Vital Signs

Vital signs can provide valuable clues to nervous system function but must be interpreted with caution due to the multiplicity of factors that influence them. It is also important to remember that changes in level of consciousness are earlier, more sensitive indicators of central nervous system dysfunction than are vital sign changes.

Autonomic Nervous System Although vital signs can be affected by the voluntary nervous system, they are controlled primarily by the involuntary or autonomic nervous system (ANS). This complex system is responsible for unconscious control of involuntary muscles and most glands. It therefore regulates vital signs, fluid intake and output, appetite, gastrointestinal activity, carbohydrate and fat metabolism, sleep, and sexual functioning. Its effects are widespread because they are exerted both by nerves and by chemical mediators.

Overall control of the ANS resides in the hypothalamus. From the hypothalamus, neurons descend through the brainstem and spinal cord and end in three groups. One group of neurons is clustered in the brainstem (around the nuclei of the third cranial nerve in the midbrain and the seventh, ninth, and tenth cranial nerves in the medulla). Another group of neurons is located in the cord around the thoracic and upper lumbar vertebrae, and the last group is centered around the sacral portion of the cord (Figure 4-14). The thoracolumbar group gives rise to the *sympathetic* division of the ANS, and the cranial and sacral groups form the *parasympathetic* division.

Neurons from the thoracic and lumbar area leave the cord through its anterior roots and form an interconnected chain of ganglia on either side of the vertebral column and along its complete length. Since these sympathetic ganglia are close to the cord, fibers between

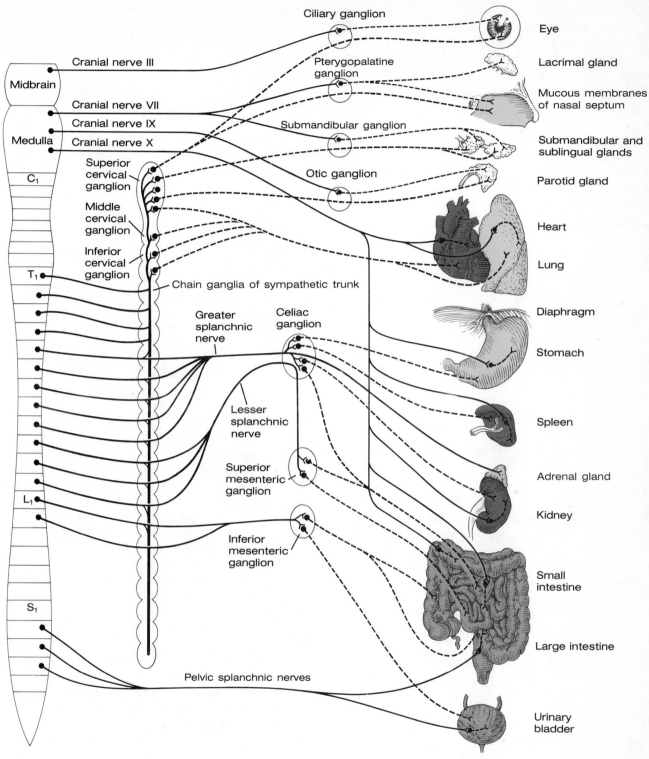

FIGURE 4-14

Autonomic nervous system. (From Spence AP, Mason EB: *Human anatomy and physiology*, 3d ed. Menlo Park, CA: The Benjamin/Cummings Publishing Company, 1987, p. 418.)

the cord and the ganglia (preganglionic fibers) are short, whereas those between the ganglia and effector organs (postganglionic fibers) are long. The primary chemical mediator secreted by sympathetic postganglionic endings is norepinephrine (noradrenalin); drugs that mimic its effects are called *adrenergic* or *sympathomimetic* agents.

In contrast to the sympathetic system, neurons from the cranial and sacral parts of the ANS form parasympathetic ganglia near the effector organs. Their preganglionic fibers thus are long and their postganglionic fibers short. The parasympathetic postganglionic endings primarily secrete acetylcholine, and drugs mimicking its effects are known as *cholinergic* agents.

The distribution of fibers to effector organs does not necessarily follow the distribution of spinal nerves and is determined partially by the embryonic origin of the organ. Most muscles and glands are innervated by both sympathetic and parasympathetic fibers; their effects are antagonistic but balanced.

Temperature Changes Although temperature is regulated by the hypothalamus, changes in temperature more often reflect infection in other body sites than hypothalamic dysfunction. Metabolic coma, exposure to extreme cold, and hypothalamic disorders may produce a temperature drop (Plum and Posner 1980), whereas a rise may occur with cerebrospinal fluid infection, blood in the CSF, dehydration, or exposure to extreme heat.

Blood Pressure Changes Blood pressure is influenced by the vasomotor center in the lower pons and upper medulla. This center exerts its effects on blood vessels through the sympathetic vasoconstrictor system, which contains fibers to all blood vessels except capillaries. The lateral portions of the vasomotor center excite the sympathetic vasoconstrictor fibers, whereas the medial portion inhibits them. The vasomotor center responds to a variety of stimuli, including input from the cerebral cortex, hypothalamus, and reticular substance of the pons, midbrain, and diencephalon; central and peripheral chemoreceptors which sense changes in CO_2 concentration of the CSF and arterial blood; and peripheral baroreceptors that sense changes in blood pressure. Because of the influence of peripheral reflexes and other factors, the cardiovascular system adjusts pumping independent of central nervous system regulation. Blood pressure changes do occur with posterior fossa lesions, hypertensive encephalopathy, and following subarachnoid hemorrhage, but otherwise appear inconsistently or not at all. As a result, blood pressure changes are not very useful as indicators of neurologic status.

Pulse Rate and Volume Changes As with blood pressure, pulse rate and volume are under both peripheral and central control. The pulse is influenced by the vasomotor center in the lower pons and upper medulla. The lateral portions send excitatory impulses via the sympathetic nerves to the heart, thus increasing pulse rate and myocardial contractility. The medial portion sends inhibitory impulses to the heart via the vagus nerves (part of the parasympathetic system), thus slowing the heart rate. Dysrhythmias may occur due to pressure on the vasomotor center or more commonly, blood gas alterations that accompany brain disorders.

Respiratory Changes Respiration is influenced by many levels of the brain and cannot occur without central nervous system regulation of skeletal muscles. Since respiration also is influenced by metabolic factors, they must be ruled out before one assumes a neurologic basis for abnormal respiration.

The main respiratory center consists of the dorsal and ventral neurons in the medulla and the pneumotaxic center in the pons (Guyton 1986). The basic rhythm of respiration is generated in the dorsal neurons of the medulla. The pneumotaxic center functions to limit the duration of inspiration and to increase the respiratory rate. An apneustic center in the lower pons also may provide extra inspiratory drive. It does not influence normal respiration because it is overridden by the pneumotaxic center. Influences from stretch receptors in the lung, peripheral and central chemoreceptors, the spinal cord, midbrain, and cerebral cortex also modify respiratory rate, depth, and pattern.

As explained in Chapter 16, the most potent stimulus to respiration is the CO_2 concentration or pH of cerebrospinal fluid bathing the respiratory center. The CSF in turn is influenced by changes in CO_2 concentration or pH in arterial blood. Increased CO_2 concentration (decreased pH) causes the rate and depth of respirations to increase (hyperventilation); decreased CO_2 concentration (increased pH) causes the respiratory rate and depth to decrease. Plum and Posner (1980) state that when hyperventilation reduces arterial CO_2 tension below its normal resting level, the stimulus that causes rhythmic breathing appears to arise from the forebrain. In other words, rhythmic breathing due to normal variation in CO_2 appears to originate in the respiratory center in the medulla, whereas that following hyperventilation appears to originate in the forebrain.

Respiratory patterns thus can be used as a reliable guide to the level of neurologic involvement once metabolic causes (such as diabetic ketoacidosis) have been ruled out. Following are the most common respiratory changes in neurological patients, based on Plum and Posner's descriptions (Figure 4-15).

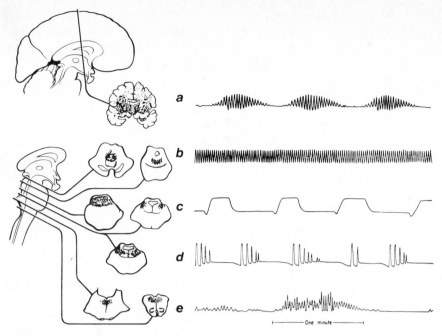

FIGURE 4-15

Abnormal respiratory patterns associated with pathologic lesions (shaded areas) at various levels of the brain. Tracings by chest-abdomen pneumograph, inspiration reads up. **a,** Cheyne-Stokes respiration; **b,** central neurogenic hyperventilation; **c,** apneusis; **d,** cluster breathing; **e,** ataxic breathing. (From Plum F, Posner J: *The diagnosis of stupor and coma,* 3d ed. Philadelphia: Davis, 1980.)

After taking five or six deep breaths, the normal person experiences either no apnea or apnea of less than 10 seconds; presumably, the lowered arterial CO_2 tension produced by this hyperventilation has been followed by a forebrain respiratory stimulus. If breathing ceases for more than 12 seconds after this maneuver (posthyperventilation apnea), forebrain response is lacking and the person will resume breathing only when the CO_2 accumulating in the blood again stimulates the respiratory center. Posthyperventilation apnea indicates a diffuse process affecting both cerebral hemispheres, such as metabolic disease.

Smoothly alternating crescendo/decrescendo breathing followed by apneic periods is known as *Cheyne-Stokes respiration.* It results from the combination of an increased respiratory center response to CO_2 stimulation (which produces the hyperpnea) and a decreased cortical response to lowered CO_2 (which produces the apnea). The neurologic cause usually is bilateral lesions deep in the cerebral hemispheres or diencephalon. (Cheyne-Stokes respiration may occur in other disorders, most often in profound cardiac failure, where it probably results from prolonged circulation time between the lungs and brain. This delay allows

large changes in blood gas concentration to occur before the respiratory center detects and reacts to them.)

A pattern of prolonged, rapid hyperpnea occurs in some patients with lesions in the low midbrain and upper pons, and many patients in whom cerebral hemorrhage has caused herniation through the tentorial notch and resulting midbrain compression. Evidence indicates that true central neurogenic hyperventilation is rare. Instead, the hyperventilation so often seen in unconscious patients probably results from pulmonary congestion due to aspiration, dependent congestion, and infection.

Brief (2–3-second) pauses at the end of inspiration characterize *apneustic breathing.* Expiratory pauses and other irregularities may be present as well. This pattern indicates extensive pontine lesions.

Varying groups of breaths with irregular in-between pauses *(cluster breathing)* typify lesions in the lower pons or upper medulla.

Totally irregular respiration indicates damage to the respiratory center in the medulla, such as that produced by downward herniation, upward herniation from rapidly expanding posterior fossa lesions, or pontine or medullary hemorrhage. Called *ataxic breathing* (Biot's respirations), this type consists of random shallow and deep breaths with irregular apneic pauses. It indicates disrupted coordination between inspiratory and expiratory neurons in the medulla. With respiratory center damage, the patient is more susceptible to depressant drugs and less susceptible to usual chemical stimulation than normal, so that respiratory depressants or sleep may produce apnea. This type of breathing necessitates mechanical ventilation if the patient is to survive.

Diagnostic Procedures

Numerous diagnostic procedures are available to aid the physician and you in assessing the location and extent of neurologic damage and the prognosis for recovery. The ones to be reviewed are: cerebrospinal fluid sampling, electroencephalography, computerized tomography, cerebral arteriography, and magnetic resonance imaging. Intracranial pressure monitoring is discussed in the next chapter.

Cerebrospinal Fluid Sampling

Cerebrospinal fluid (CSF) is secreted from blood primarily by the choroid plexus. The plexus consists of tufts of capillaries and epithelium lining the brain's ventricular system. The ventricular system is composed of two lateral ventricles, a central third ventricle, a fourth ventricle located between the brainstem and cerebellum, and interconnecting canals (Figure 4-16).

One lateral ventricle sits in each cerebral hemisphere

and consists of an anterior horn in the frontal lobe, a body in the parietal lobe, a posterior horn in the occipital lobe, and an inferior horn in the temporal lobe. From each lateral ventricle, CSF passes through a foramen of Monroe into the third ventricle and then through the aqueduct of Sylvius into the fourth ventricle. It then passes through openings in the fourth ventricle (foramens of Luschka and Magendie) into the subarachnoid space. After flowing over the brain and down around the spinal cord, it is drained from the subarachnoid space through the arachnoid villi, which project into the superior sagittal sinus, the large superficial midline sinus of the dura mater.

CSF functions to cushion and nourish the brain. It is formed and absorbed constantly, at the rate of 400–500 ml in 24 hours; at a given moment, about 140 ml is circulating. It is clear, colorless, and odorless and normally contains no red cells and a few white cells. Glucose content varies with the serum glucose level, averaging about 60% of the serum glucose. The normal value is approximately 50–75 mg/100 ml. Protein concentration varies with the sampling site, normally measuring 5–15 mg/100 ml in the ventricles, 15–25 mg/100 ml in the cisterna magna, and 15–45 mg/100 ml in the spinal canal. Normal specific gravity is 1.007. Opening pressure is up to 180 mm H_2O recumbent.

Samples of CSF can be obtained from the lumbar subarachnoid space of the spinal canal, the cisterna magna (the large subarachnoid space below the occipital bone), and the lateral ventricles. For sampling at any site, the patient and/or family should be prepared psychologically with a description of the benefits and risks, steps in the procedure, and normal sensations. An informed consent should be signed and the patient sedated if necessary. Lumbar and cisternal punctures may be done in the critical-care unit; ventricular punctures

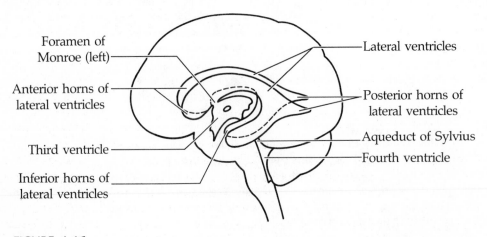

Foramen of
Monroe (left)

Anterior horns of
lateral ventricles

Third ventricle

Inferior horns of
lateral ventricles

Lateral ventricles

Posterior horns of
lateral ventricles

Aqueduct of Sylvius

Fourth ventricle

FIGURE 4-16

Ventricular system (left lateral view).

usually are performed in surgery or in some cases on the unit. The following descriptions of the various procedures are based on Hickey (1986) and Rudy (1984).

A lumbar puncture, the most common, may be done to measure CSF pressure, sample CSF, remove CSF to lower intracranial pressure, or inject contrast media or medications. Contraindications to a lumbar puncture are inflammation at the proposed injection site, a subarachnoid block, or greatly increased intracranial pressure; in the latter case, removal of CSF from the spinal canal could precipitate brain herniation. To assist with a lumbar puncture, explain to the patient that the procedure will last only a few minutes and usually is not painful; that the doctor will give a local anesthetic to reduce the feeling of pressure from the needle insertion; that he or she will lie on the side and should stay very still; and that short pains in the legs or pelvis may be experienced if the needle brushes nerves to those areas. Bring to the bedside a lumbar puncture tray, local anesthetic, sterile gloves, and a bandaid. Place the patient on his or her side with the back at the edge of the bed and the spine curved; or have the patient sit up and bend over a bedside table. You may need to hold a restless patient. The physician will clean the skin and infiltrate it with a local anesthetic. She or he then will insert the needle and stylet at the level of the iliac crests. Insertion of the needle at this level places its tip in the spinal canal below the termination of the cord. After removing the stylet, the physician will connect the manometer, measure opening pressure, drain off fluid into laboratory tubes, measure closing pressure, remove the needle, and cover the puncture site with a small bandage. During the procedure, reassure the patient, remind him or her not to move, and observe for a change in the level of consciousness, which may signify herniation. After the procedure, observe for changes in the level of consciousness or vital signs, meningeal irritation, edema or hematoma at the puncture site, and motor power in the lower limbs. Headache is common and may be eased by (1) having the patient remain lying flat for 1–6 hours, (2) increased fluid intake, and (3) analgesics. Transient back and leg pain may result from nerve root irritation.

A puncture of the cisterna magna may be done if a lumbar puncture is contraindicated or a subarachnoid block is present. The procedure is more dangerous than lumbar puncture because the needle is inserted close to the brainstem. Contraindications to a cisternal puncture are posterior fossa pathology or greatly increased intracranial pressure. To assist with a cisternal puncture, explain the procedure to the patient. Shave the nape of the neck and place the patient on the side with the back at the edge of the bed and a sandbag under the head. Bend the patient's head slightly forward and hold it firmly. The physician will clean and anesthetize the skin

and insert the needle below the occipital bone in the midline. The test proceeds as does a lumbar puncture, and observations are the same (with the exception of back and leg pain, which do not occur with a cisternal puncture). Headache usually does not follow a cisternal puncture. Postprocedure care is the same as for lumbar puncture.

A ventricular puncture is done if lumbar and cisternal ones are contraindicated or if ventricular drainage is necessary for increased intracranial pressure. In the critical-care unit, ventricular puncture most likely will be done to monitor intracranial pressure. For details, see the section in Chapter 5 on measuring intracranial pressure. Nursing care following a ventricular puncture consists of 10–15 degree elevation of the head; bedrest for 24 hours; neurologic checks every 30–60 minutes until stable; and maintenance of a dry, sterile dressing over the sutured skin incisions. The patient should be watched closely, as she or he may develop a headache, respiratory distress, convulsions, or increasing intracranial pressure.

Electroencephalography

In this procedure, the electrical activity of the brain is recorded from scalp electrodes. The electroencephalogram (EEG) is used to diagnose disorders that cause changes in electrical patterns, such as epilepsy, tumors, and brain death.

Other than an explanation to the patient, no particular preparation is necessary. Either the patient will be taken to a soundproofed, electrically shielded room or, if he or she is too sick to be moved, the EEG will be recorded at the bedside. Electrodes are applied with paste or needles to the scalp over the various lobes, and the tracing is recorded while the patient remains relaxed and still to avoid creating electrical artifacts. The EEG may take up to 2 hours and will be interrupted periodically so the patient can change position. Alert the patient in advance that he or she will be asked to hyperventilate for a short time to provoke any abnormal discharge and can anticipate transient lightheadedness or dizziness during this hyperventilation.

An EEG is not painful and does not produce any postprocedure complications.

Computerized Tomography (CT)

Computerized tomography (CT) scanning is a neurodiagnostic procedure that utilizes a computer to analyze x-ray data. Although a beam of x-ray photons is used, the data are recorded numerically rather than in a conventional x-ray. CT scanning shows horizontal cross-sections of the brain. CT scans are much more sensitive than conventional x-ray studies, and they are highly accurate.

Patient preparation for a CT scan should include a brief description of the equipment and procedure. The patient must hold very still, as even small movements induce artifact. If the patient is unable to hold still, sedation may be necessary. The scan is safe and painless; the only unpleasant sensation the person might experience is a brief burning sensation if contrast media are used. Clicking sounds normally are heard from the scanner.

The reference line for the planes of scanning is the orbitomeatal line, the line between the outer angle of the eye and the external auditory meatus. The patient lies on a table with his or her head positioned within the section of the scanner containing the x-ray tube. The x-ray tube rotates 360° around the head, transmitting an x-ray beam (a scan) through the head.

A *slice*—the thickness of a scanner layer—varies from 1.5 mm to 15.0 mm, depending on the resolution desired. Both the level and angle of the scans can be varied and recorded so that lesions can be localized exactly. The duration of the scan is about 10 minutes without contrast medium, and 25 minutes with contrast medium.

After each scan, the table moves so the patient's head is progressively withdrawn from the apparatus. On the opposite side of the head from the beam is a crystal detector that reads the transmission. The readings form the basis of complex equations that the computer solves and transforms into absorption coefficients indicating the density of predetermined volumes of brain tissue.

The data from the scan are available in three forms: a computer printout, cathode ray (television) tube display, and hard-copy print on standard x-ray film or polaroid film.

The computer constructs a picture based on the density values and displays it on a screen. The picture varies in light intensity from white (high-density structures) to black (low-density structures). The structures are shown as if you were looking from above at a transverse slice of the brain. Major anatomical structures are identified by size, shape, and location. Easily identified structures are white matter, gray matter, Sylvian fissures, fissure of Rolando, lateral ventricles, third ventricle, choroid plexuses, and calcified pineal body. For detailed study, areas of display can be enlarged.

Abnormalities are detected by deviations from normal density and sometimes also by displacement of normal structures. Lesions that can be located by CT are tumors, cysts, abscesses, hematomas, infarctions, aneurysms, and arteriovenous malformations.

Since the amount of radiation exposure is relatively low, serial CT scans can be taken to follow the resolution of cerebral disorders. Although CT scans have reduced the use of cerebral arteriography for tumor screening, the cerebral arteriogram is more precise than the scan for visualizing vascular anatomy and abnormalities such as aneurysms and occlusions.

No special physiologic care is necessary after a scan without contrast medium. If contrast medium is used, observe for a possible allergic reaction.

Cerebral Arteriography

In this diagnostic maneuver, contrast medium is injected into the cerebral circulation to visualize the arteries and veins. It is used to detect aneurysms, occlusions, hematomas, tumors, and other lesions sizable enough to destroy cerebral vessels.

Before the procedure, assist the physician in explaining its benefits and risks and secure informed consent. Particularly prepare the patient for the sequence of steps and the intense burning sensation that may be experienced when dye is injected. This sensation is normal and lasts 20–30 seconds.

Preprocedure preparation usually includes a sedative the night before, nothing by mouth for 8 hours before the procedure, and shaving of the proposed injection site. Just before the patient leaves the unit, you should record a current neurologic assessment and *then* premedicate.

The patient will be taken to the neuroradiology department and placed on a movable x-ray table. Depending upon the anticipated site of pathology, the physician will plan to inject either the carotid artery (to visualize the anterior, middle, and posterior cerebral arteries) or the vertebral artery (to visualize it and the basilar artery). The carotid and vertebral arteries can be punctured directly or reached by a catheter advanced from other arteries, such as the femoral or brachial. The physician will prepare the skin, inject local anesthesia, make a percutaneous entry into the vessel, introduce and advance a catheter under fluoroscopic examination, and inject radiopaque dye while repeated x-rays are taken. During this time, the patient will be monitored closely for an anaphylactic reaction and signs of increased intracranial pressure.

After the procedure is completed, the patient will be returned to his or her room. Perform neurologic checks every 30 minutes to 4 hours, depending upon the patient's stability. Also follow the measures outlined in the section on cardiac catheterization (Chapter 11) for potential complications after catheterization. Patients usually recover from this procedure in a few hours and without severe reactions.

To experience cerebral arteriography vicariously, talk with patients who have undergone the procedure. Seeking this information will sensitize you to the concerns of patients and help increase your ability to alleviate their worries.

Magnetic Resonance Imaging (MRI)

Magnetic Resonance Imaging is a noninvasive, painless procedure that has proven especially effective for imaging the nervous system. MRI utilizes a magnetic field and radiofrequency to generate body organ images of such quality and precision that you feel you are looking at the anatomical specimen. Due to high reliability and minimal patient risk, the use of CT and/or MRI has almost eliminated the need to perform pneumoencephalograms or ventriculograms.

Certain features, described below, prevent the use of MRI with acutely unstable patients. Despite this, the critical-care nurse still needs to understand the technique, indications, and special considerations, since many patients will be nursed in a critical-care unit following procedures based on MRI.

The principles of MRI, according to Rudy (1985), Lee (1986), and James (1985), are based on the interaction between a magnetic field and the nuclei of a selected atom. The atom to be studied must possess an odd number of protons and neutrons, thereby giving it magnetic properties. Atoms having nuclei with magnetic properties include hydrogen, carbon 13, fluorine 19, sodium 23, and phosphorus 31. Present imaging techniques measure the absorption and remission of units of energy from the hydrogen atom, since it is most abundant in human tissue and has a relatively strong signal.

The magnet used is in a housing similar to that for CT scanning (Figure 4-17). When the patient is placed inside the unit and the magnet is turned on, the magnet aligns, or polarizes, the hydrogen protons. Radiofrequency (RF) waves are then transmitted into the magnetic field, causing the protons to change alignment, or depolarize. Termination of the RF waves allows the protons to return to their original state. The energy emitted and the speed with which the protons return to their polarized state differentiate healthy tissue from diseased tissue.

Based on this information, the computer constructs

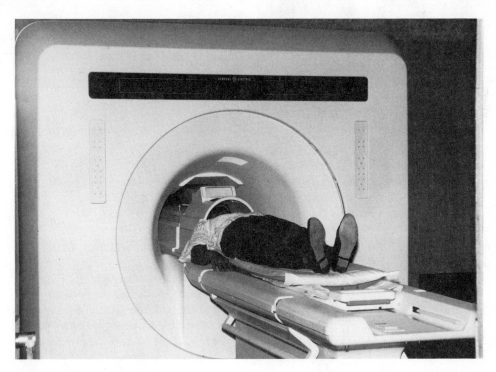

FIGURE 4-17

MRI housing unit, showing a patient lying on a pallet with head inside the bore. (Photo courtesy of Santa Barbara Cottage Hospital, Glenn Dubock photographer.)

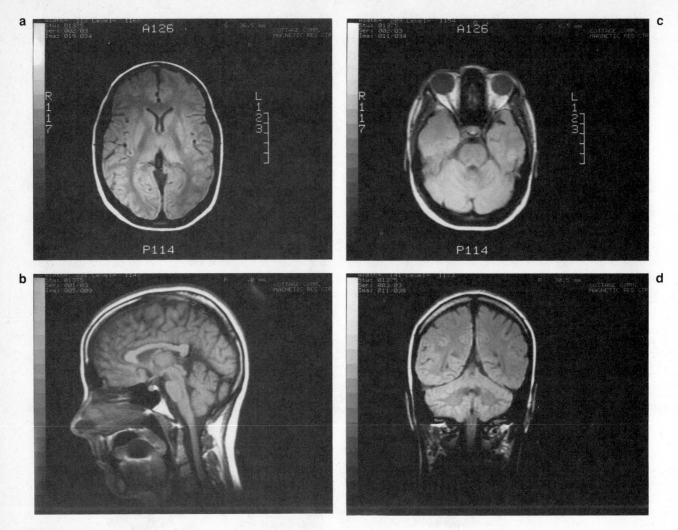

FIGURE 4-18

Magnetic resonance images. **a,** Axial view at midthalamic level; **b,** midline sagittal image; **c,** axial image at level of upper pons; **d,** coronal image through occipital lobe and cerebellum. (Photos courtesy of Cottage Community Magnetic Resonance Center.)

an image of the tissue in one of three projections—axial, coronal, or sagittal—depending on the program. (See Figure 4-18.) All planes can be obtained in approximately 35 minutes, with each plane consisting of 20 slices. Still images are permanently recorded on x-ray–type film.

Use of magnetic resonance imaging is indicated when lesions are poorly demonstrated on CT scan or patients are allergic to iodinated contrast media. Sequential exams may be carried out with minimal patient risk, since MRI does not employ ionizing radiation. MRI appears to be more sensitive than CT in detecting: (1) demyelinization associated with multiple sclerosis, and (2) lesions

located in the brainstem, craniocervical junction, or spinal cord.

The major disadvantage of MRI results from the use of a strong, static magnetic field. Since the magnetic field attracts ferromagnetic devices, sheet metal workers (who may have metal slivers imbedded in their tissues) and patients with prosthetic devices such as cardiac valves, aneurysm clips, and orthopedic pins are excluded from MRI screening due to the potential danger to the patient. The physical environment of the room housing the MRI scanner must also be free of ferromagnetic objects. Pens, scissors, gurneys, and emergency equipment are all attracted to the magnet, thus presenting a hazard to the patient and health care worker. The hazard is particularly significant for cardiac pacemakers. Magnets are used to close the reed switch on permanent pacemakers. This closure changes the mode of operation from synchronous (demand) to asynchronous (fixed rate). Fixed-rate pacing in the presence of an intrinsic rhythm sets up the potential for competition and dysrhythmias. Before ordering MRI for the patient with a pacemaker, the physician should weigh carefully its diagnostic benefits against the risk.

Patient education focuses on the potential problems related to the MRI housing unit and the magnetic environment. The table the patient lies on and the opening (bore) in the housing unit are narrow (see Figure 4-17). When the pallet moves inside the unit, the patient may experience claustrophobia. To minimize this feeling, most units have mirrors so the patient can see out into the room and not feel so enclosed. Also, the technicians move the pallet slowly into the unit so the patient can adjust to the space. Although the technicians must be out of the room while the test is in progress, the patient can still communicate with them. Assure the patient that it is normal to hear a continuous knocking sound during the test.

Make sure that the patient, prior to entering the magnetic area, removes any items that might be ferromagnetic, including nondigital watches, rings, bobby pins, hair clips, eyeglasses, and any articles of clothing with metal snaps, zippers, or buckles.

REFERENCES

Guyton A: *Textbook of medical physiology,* 7th ed. Philadelphia: Saunders, 1986.

Hickey JV: *The clinical practice of neurological and neurosurgical nursing.* Philadelphia: Lippincott, 1986.

Jacob S et al.: *Structure and function in man,* 5th ed. Philadelphia: Saunders, 1982.

James AE et al.: Current status of magnetic resonance imaging. *Southern Medical Journal* (May) 1985; 78:580–596.

Lee B: Magnetic resonance imaging of the central nervous system. *Hosp Med* (Mar) 1986; 199–216.

Mitchell PH et al.: *Neurological assessment for nursing practice.* Garden City, NY: Prentice-Hall, 1984.

Oldendorf WH, Oldendorf W Jr: Modern diagnostic imaging techniques in medicine, Part I: CT scan methods. *Am J Cont Ed Nurs* 1986; 1(2–3):26–30.

Plum F, Posner J: *The diagnosis of stupor and coma,* 3d ed. Philadelphia: Davis, 1980.

Ricci MM (ed): *Core curriculum for neuroscience nursing,* 2d ed. Chicago: American Association of Neuroscience Nurses, 1984.

Rudy EB: *Advanced neurological and neurosurgical nursing.* St Louis: Mosby, 1984.

Rudy EB: Magnetic resonance imaging: New horizon in diagnostic techniques. *J Neurosurg Nurs* (Dec) 1985; 17:331–337.

Swendsen L: FANCAS: A framework for nursing assessment. University of California School of Nursing. (Course syllabus, 1975)

SUPPLEMENTAL READING

Blackburn D, Peterson L: Oculoplethysmography. *Nurs* (Oct) 1982; 76–78.

Boss B, Stowe A: Neuroanatomy. *J Neurosci Nurs* (Aug) 1986; 18:214–230.

Engler MB, Engler, MM: The hazards of magnetic resonance imaging. *Am J Nurs* 1986; 86:650.

Knight RL: The Glasgow coma scale: Ten years after. *Crit Care Nurse* 1986; 6(3):65–71.

Konikow NS: Alterations in movement: Nursing assessment and implications. *J Neurosurg Nurs* 1985; 17(1):61–65.

Marchette L, Holloman F: A first-hand report on the new body scanners. *RN* (Nov) 1985; 28–31.

Norman S: The pupil check. *Am J Nurs* 1982; 588–591.

Ozuna J: Alterations in mentation: Nursing assessment and intervention. *J Neurosurg Nurs* 1985; 17(1):66–70.

Price M, DeVroom H: A quick and easy guide to neurological assessment. *J Neurosurg Nurs* (Oct) 1985; 17:313–320.

Ricci M: Neurological examination and assessment of altered states of consciousness. In *The critically ill neurosurgical patient,* Nikas D (ed), pp 1–27. New York: Churchill Livingstone, 1982.

Ropper A et al.: Computer-guided neurological assessment in the neurologic intensive care unit. *Heart Lung* 1981; 10:54–60.

Rudy E: Brain death. *Dimen Crit Care Nurs* 1982; 1:178–184.

Rudy E: Glasgow coma scale. *Health Care Quart Rev* 1982; 1:10–13.

Seago K: MRI's place in imaging. *Applied Radiology* (Mar/Apr) 1986; 25–33.

Walleck C: A neurologic assessment procedure that won't make you nervous. *Nurs 82* (Dec) 1982; 50–57.

5

Stimulation Disorders

CLINICAL INSIGHT

Domain: Administering and monitoring therapeutic interventions and regimens

Competency: Combating the hazards of immobility: preventing and intervening with skin breakdown, ambulating and exercising patients to assure maxium mobility and rehabilitation, preventing respiratory complications

Combating hazards of immobility requires not just deciding what activity a patient needs but also inspiring the patient to exercise despite pain and fatigue, controlling any pain provoked by the activity, and, when necessary, setting and enforcing limits. In the following exemplar, from Crabtree and Jorgenson (1986, pp. 112–114), a nurse reflects on the challenge presented to her and a second nurse by Liz, a 16-year-old Guillain-Barré patient whose natural adolescent limit-testing was exacerbated by her months-long hospitalization in the critical-care unit. After being completely dependent—mechanically ventilated and unable even to open her eyes—Liz gradually regains muscle function. Unfortunately, Liz has become both manipulative in response to her forced dependency and addicted to narcotics. Recognizing that Liz desperately needs some control restored to her life, the two nurses become instrumental in using behavior

modification to manage her acting out—and try to enlist her parents' support.

We had care conferences on Liz. Her mother came to the first one we had, although we talked to both of her parents, but she was there during the day more. They always stated they were aware of it (referring to giving in to Liz), but they just couldn't stop themselves. You know, they always said that they would try, and then her father would take that role and be stern and say, this is what you do; the nurses are telling you to do this, but then Liz would cry. And, her dad would fall apart. And, so, it was like being that intimate with her father; he couldn't do it. He could do it until Liz cried, he fell apart, and then he turned around and took back everything he'd said and said, okay, I'll go get the nurses to put you back to bed. And, Liz knew it! She knew that, if she didn't like her parents' behavior, all she had to do was cry and that would change everything.

Recognizing that soliciting the parents' support in setting limits was unsuccessful, the two nurses assume a more parental role. Liz's crying has been effective in interrupting badly needed physical activity, until . . .

. . . she hit up with Chris and I, and then it didn't work any more—and we did not back down; that was

the biggest thing. We did not back down. If you want to cry, you cry then. But, you're still going to sit in the chair, and I'll draw the curtain so that you can sit in here and cry, and you don't have to feel like everybody walking by is watching you cry, but you're going to stay in the chair. You know? And, yes, I do feel sorry for you, but crying doesn't put you back in bed.

As the months pass, the nurses use the reward of walking outside, which Liz loves, for sitting in the chair, which she dislikes.

Basically, we only went out the door. But, that worked then. She loved to be outside. It worked remarkably. We had a changed young lady by April, by the time we transferred her out to the floor. She was very motivated when she went to rehabilitation in April. She was motivated to work; she was up walking in days after she started her rigorous physical therapy. She was up in the wheelchair independently by herself very quickly once she transferred down there. And Chris and I, the other nurse who co-primaried her, we transferred that information to rehabilitation, and they continued it.

Though Liz struggled against the limits, it was the nurses' very act of setting them that allowed her to grow beyond adolescent limit-testing in dealing with her devastating illness.

She's come back to visit several times, and she said, you know, I hated you with a passion. But, she said, if I ever really wanted anything or needed anything, I knew you two would do it. You know, you wouldn't put up with the bullcrap, but if I really needed something, you'd be there. And, it got to a point when she's come back to visit and said, it was the two of you who sorted through that constantly for me, what was real and what was not real.

Stimulation (neurologic) disorders present challenging problems to nurses, particularly disorders that are chronic or marked by prolonged recovery. This chapter reviews not only acute disorders of stimulation—increased intracranial pressure, herniation syndromes, and status epilepticus—but more chronic ones as well—stroke, Guillain-Barré syndrome, and myasthenia gravis. As the Clinical Insight demonstrates, nurses can be instrumental in helping a patient adjust to the pervasive life changes necessitated by these disorders.

Increased Intracranial Pressure

The intracranial contents consist of brain tissue and extracellular fluid (subdivided into blood, cerebrospinal fluid, and interstitial fluid). Because the amount of interstitial fluid is negligible, for practical purposes the *intracranial volume (ICV)* equals the sum of *brain volume (BV)*, *cerebrospinal fluid volume (CSFV)*, and *cerebral blood volume (CBV)*; that is,

$$ICV = BV + CSFV + CBV$$

The volume within each intracranial compartment exerts pressure. Since the easiest pressure to measure is that of CSF, this is the pressure commonly referred to as *intracranial pressure (ICP)*.

Assessment

Risk Conditions Be alert for patients with actual or potential increases in intracranial pressure. Because cranial contents consist of tissue mass, cerebral blood volume, and cerebrospinal fluid, it is convenient to group risk conditions for increased ICP according to these three categories. Conditions increasing the patient's risk include: mass lesions such as cranial tumors, hematomas, and brain swelling; cerebral vascular congestion due to vasodilation, loss of autoregulation, or increased systemic venous pressure; and diminished CSF absorption, such as when the meninges are covered with blood breakdown products *(subarachnoid hemorrhage)* or exudates *(meningitis)* or when there is a blockage of CSF pathways *(obstructive hydrocephalus)*.

A common misconception is that increased intracranial pressure always is harmful to the patient. As Mitchell (1982) points out, many everyday activities such as sneezing, coughing, and straining at bowel movements cause spikes of pressure far above normal levels. Moreover, patients with benign intracranial hypertension (caused by jugular venous or vena caval obstruction) can have extremely high intracranial pressures that nevertheless are well tolerated.

Although these exceptions are important, it is imperative to realize that acute increases of intracranial pressure (especially focal increases) can be lethal for patients in critical-care units. This section focuses on methods you can use to anticipate, prevent, and ameliorate detrimental increases in intracranial pressure (ICP).

Intracranial Dynamics According to the Monroe-Kellie hypothesis, when the volume of one compartment increases, the total pressure will increase also unless there is a reciprocal change in another compartment. Fortunately, although the skull is a nondistensible structure, it has openings for the spinal cord, cranial nerves, and blood vessels. Cranial contents can escape through these openings, thus lowering intracranial pressure. The major pressure buffer is CSF, for two reasons: (1) the dura covering the spinal cord is loosely attached and can expand readily to accommodate CSF leaving the cranial subarachnoid space; (2) CSF absorption by the arachnoid villi is partially dependent on CSF pressure. The ability of CSF to buffer pressure changes is compromised when an expanding mass blocks subarachnoid pathways or when CSF absorption is diminished.

Both systemic arterial pressure and intracranial pressure strongly influence cerebral perfusion. Cerebral perfusion pressure (CPP) is the difference between cerebral arterial and venous blood pressures. Cerebral arterial pressure approximates mean systemic arterial pressure (SAP), and cerebral venous pressure approximates intracranial pressure when ICP is elevated, so CPP = SAP − ICP. To estimate CPP, first note the systolic systemic BP and the diastolic systemic BP, preferably from an arterial monitoring line. Subtract the diastolic BP from the systolic BP; take one-third the difference, and add it to the diastolic BP to get the mean systemic arterial pressure. From the mean systemic arterial pressure, subtract the intracranial pressure to get the approximate cerebral perfusion pressure:

$$\text{Mean SAP} = \frac{\text{Systolic BP} - \text{Diastolic BP}}{3}$$
$$+ \text{ Diastolic BP}$$
$$\text{CPP} \approx \text{Mean SAP} - \text{ICP}$$

Normal CPP is 80–90 mm Hg (Robinet 1985). CPP can be reduced by either a drop in SAP or a rise in ICP. As ICP increases and cerebral blood flow slows, compensatory cerebral vasodilation occurs *(autoregulation)*. Although this compensation increases cerebral blood flow (CBF), it also increases ICP; the net result is a decrease in CPP. Most authorities recommend maintaining a minimum CPP of at least 60 mm Hg in critically ill patients with injured brains (Hickey 1986).

At a mean SAP of 50–150 mm Hg, the diameter of cerebral blood vessels (and therefore their resistance) alters automatically to maintain a constant CPP. This type of automatic regulation is known as *pressure autoregulation* and is essential in avoiding drastic changes in CBF. Pressure autoregulation combined with an ICP less than 30 mm Hg will maintain CPP within the range of 50 mm and 150 mm Hg (Hickey 1986).

Intracranial hypertension exists when mean ICP is 15 mm Hg or higher. Autoregulation is believed to fail when ICP exceeds approximately 30 mm Hg (Mitchell et al. 1981), mean SAP falls below 50 mm Hg, or CPP drops below 50 mm Hg (McGillicuddy 1985). When autoregulation fails, CBF no longer alters appropriately with pressure or metabolic needs; instead, CBF fluctuates directly with systemic BP. Increases in mean SAP pound more blood into cerebral vessels, further elevating ICP and increasing cerebral edema. Conversely, decreases in mean SAP increase cerebral ischemia. In this situation, even the brain's desperate needs for O_2 and removal of CO_2 and lactic acid cannot provoke improved CBF.

Signs and Symptoms Maintain a high index of suspicion for signs and symptoms of increased ICP. Early findings as described by Hickey (1986) include: change in level of consciousness, pupillary dysfunction, paresis/paralysis, and headache. Later findings include: continued decrease in level of consciousness, changes in respiratory pattern, abnormal posturing, vomiting, alterations in vital signs, and impaired brainstem reflexes. See Chapter 4 for a discussion of various respiratory patterns and pupillary changes that may be seen.

It has been established that clinical signs do not always correlate with the ICP, since it is dynamic and affected by many variables. Therefore, patients likely to suffer acutely increased ICP ideally should have the benefit of direct monitoring of CSF pressure. Such monitoring does not, however, eliminate the need for astute bedside physical assessment.

Measuring Intracranial Pressure The following sections describe techniques of intracranial pressure monitoring.

Types of Pressure Monitoring Although CSF pressure can be evaluated by lumbar punctures, such readings are isolated and inaccurate in the presence of subarachnoid block. More importantly, lumbar punctures present a danger of herniation in those patients who most need pressure evaluation. In contrast, an intracranial transducer, ventricular catheter, or subarachnoid screw can monitor intracranial pressure accurately and continuously, without danger of herniation through the foramen magnum. The three cranial areas monitored most frequently are the epidural space, the subarachnoid space, and the lateral ventricle (Figure 5-1).

Epidural monitoring is done with an intracranial transducer or with an intracranial balloon connected to an external transducer. The dura is not opened, so

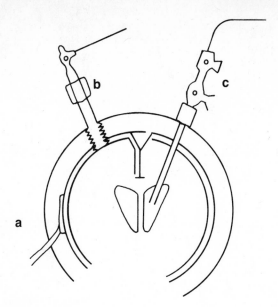

FIGURE 5-1

Three methods of monitoring intracranial pressure. **a** is an epidural transducer, placed against the dura. **b** is a subarachnoid bolt, threaded into the skull and contacting the subarachnoid space. **c** is the intraventricular cannula, traversing both skull and brain tissue to reach a lateral cerebral ventricle. (From: Nikas D (ed): *The critically ill neurosurgical patient.* New York: Churchill Livingstone Inc., 1983, p. 38.)

there is less danger of cranial infection than with other methods. The internal transducer reduces the danger further, but it is affected by heat and cannot be recalibrated. Epidural monitoring does not allow for CSF drainage or testing of intracranial compliance, so most head trauma centers do not use it.

The ventricular catheter is inserted under local anesthesia, through a drill hole in the skull and a puncture of the dura, into the frontal horn of the lateral ventricle in the nondominant hemisphere. Advantages include the abilities to drain CSF, recalibrate the transducer, test compliance, and instill contrast media for visualization of the size and patency of the ventricular system. Disadvantages include the technical difficulty of insertion in the presence of marked cerebral edema and the potentials for infection, CSF loss, and blockage of the catheter by blood clots.

The subarachnoid screw is a small, hollow screw whose tip sits in the cranial subarachnoid space. Advantages include ease of insertion, ability to recalibrate the transducer as necessary, and potential for draining CSF. Disadvantages are possible infection, CSF loss, inability to instill contrast media, and possible blockage of the screw by brain tissue.

Because the ventricular catheter and the subarachnoid screw are used more frequently, the remainder of this section on ICP monitoring is devoted to the care of patients being monitored by these methods.

Insertion of the Ventricular Catheter or Subarachnoid Screw To prepare the patient and family before insertion, explain that monitoring is a temporary measure to enable the nurses and doctors to detect the onset of increased intracranial pressure and intervene early to prevent or ameliorate its detrimental effects. Explain that the scalp will be numbed with local anesthesia and that the insertion itself will be painless. Briefly explain the setup and monitor so that the family will not be horrified by the tubes and wires connected to their loved one's brain. Ideally, the ICP monitoring device is inserted under sterile conditions in the operating room. If transport to the OR is not feasible, then the following protocol may be followed.

Gather the equipment necessary for the monitoring: the catheter or screw; an insertion tray containing a syringe and needle for anesthesia, scalpel, drill, sutures, and dressing supplies; skin preparation solution; local anesthetic; sterile gloves; monitor; and monitoring system. Assemble the equipment sterilely before the catheter or screw is inserted. Details of setting up the monitoring system vary according to unit. One typical setup is shown in Figure 5-2. Preassembled, presterilized monitoring sets also are available.

Assist the physician in inserting the catheter or screw. The physician will shave, clean, and infiltrate the insertion site with a local anesthetic. He or she then will incise the scalp, drill a hole, puncture the dura, and insert the catheter or screw. Remove the cap covering the stopcock side port and connect to the catheter or screw. At this point, you should see a waveform on the oscilloscope. The physician will suture the incision and apply a sterile dressing.

Nursing Care Responsibilities The following sections describe nursing responsibilities related to intracranial pressure monitoring.

Obtain Accurate Pressure Measurements Follow these steps each time you measure the pressure.

1. Place the patient in the baseline position, which is usually 20 to 30 degrees of head elevation. False pressure changes will occur if the level of the head has changed in relation to the transducer. The internal reference for ICP monitoring is the foramen of Monroe. The external reference points that have been used are the outer canthus of the eye (Smith 1983), top of the ear (Horner 1985), and the external auditory meatus. The most important aspect is to always verify that the

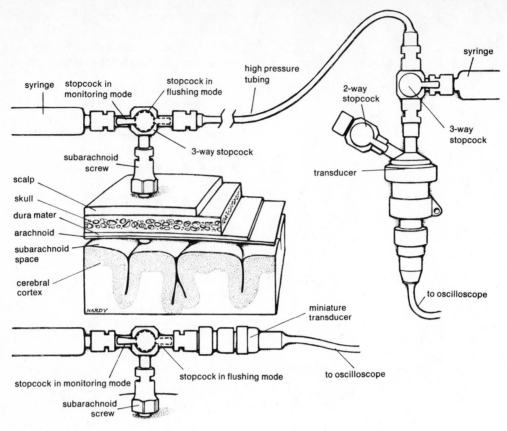

FIGURE 5-2

Intracranial pressure monitoring with a subarachnoid screw. (From Johnson M, Quinn J: The subarachnoid screw. © March 1977, The American Journal of Nursing Company. Reproduced with permission of artist Neil O. Hardy and publisher, from the *American Journal of Nursing* 77:3.)

transducer is level with the external reference point used. Pole-mounted transducers require a carpenter's level to assure proper alignment. Large transducers may also be secured on a towel roll and kept at the reference level. Miniature transducers can be taped directly to the head to preclude measurement error.

2. Observe the waveform of the oscilloscope to verify patency of the line. A flattened (dampened) waveform can result from kinked tubing, an air bubble or other blockage in the system, collapse of the ventricle or dura against the tip of the monitoring device, or herniation of brain tissue into the catheter or screw. First check for kinks, and remove any that are present. Inspect the system for air bubbles. If bubbles are present, turn off the stopcock closest to the patient, open the 2-way transducer stopcock, and gently flush the system with a saline-filled syringe. Then close the 2-way stopcock, open the stopcock closest to the patient to reconnect the monitoring device and the transducer, and ob-

serve the waveform. If it still appears dampened, consult the physician. Many physicians do not want the monitoring device flushed. If the physician does want you to flush the system, proceed as he or she recommends. One flushing method follows. Fill a syringe only with the amount of flush solution specified by the physician (usually 0.1 ml of preservative-free saline). Connect it to the 3-way stopcock attached to the catheter or screw. Turn the stopcock so it is off to the transducer, that is, so the syringe and catheter or screw are connected. *Slowly* flush the catheter or screw. (Do not aspirate first, as you would with a line for monitoring vascular pressure. Aspiration may suck brain tissue into the screw.) Turn the stopcock so the catheter or screw and transducer are reconnected. Again observe the waveform. If it remains dampened, notify the physician.

3. Do not measure the pressure when the patient is moving, coughing, sneezing, using abdominal muscles to inspire, or has his or her head turned, since these actions will cause temporary increases in intracranial pressure.

4. Horner (1985) recommends balancing and calibrating the transducer every 4 hours. To assure accurate readings, the transducer must be leveled and re-zeroed to the external reference point whenever the head position is changed.

Analyze the Pressures Critically Following are guidelines for pressure analysis.

1. Evaluate the recorded ICP value. Remember that the trend is more significant than any isolated reading. Compare the readings to the patient's norm rather than to an arbitrary standard; the patient with chronically increased intracranial pressure will have a higher "normal" value than the patient being monitored to detect the onset of increased pressure. Reported normal ranges are 0–10 mm Hg or 0–136 mm H_2O (Mitchell et al. 1981). Pressures normally fluctuate with cardiac pulsations (transmitted to the CSF through the choroid plexus) and changes in the thoracic and abdominal pressures (transmitted to the CSF through the vena cava and the jugular veins).

2. Monitor CPP by subtracting ICP from MAP. Again, the trend is more significant than individual values.

3. In addition to evaluating absolute pressure values, note the morphology and amplitude of the waveform. As mentioned above, changes in cardiac pulsations are transmitted to the CSF through the choroid plexus. Normally, as cranial blood pressure rises and falls, blood and CSF escape and return through patent outflow channels in the foramina at the base of the skull. These compensatory mechanisms, along with intact autoregulation, keep the amplitude of each pulsation trans-

mitted from the arterioles throughout the brain and CSF small. Price (1981) describes the pulse wave as resembling an arterial blood pressure wave with a sharp initial inflection that then slopes back to baseline. Loss of compensatory mechanisms or autoregulation results in an increased pulse pressure leading to an increased CSF pulse. Progressively larger, more-rounded waves may be an early indicator of changing intracranial dynamics.

4. Look also for spontaneous abnormal variations in pressure called *pressure waves* (Figure 5-3). In a classic article, Lundberg (1960) described three types of pressure waves. B waves are sharp, rhythmic waves with a sawtooth appearance. They occur every 30 seconds to 2 minutes and raise intracranial pressure up to 50 mm Hg. C waves are smaller rhythmic waves that occur every 4–8 minutes and raise intracranial pressure as much as 20 mm Hg. B and C waves coincide with rhythmic variations in respiration and BP, but they are not clinically significant. More important are A waves, commonly called *plateau waves*. These waves raise intracranial pressure 50–100 mm Hg and last for 5–20 minutes (Smith 1983). These sustained pressure elevations occur on an already elevated mean intracranial pressure baseline exceeding 20 mm Hg. Plateau waves are believed to be significant because they may reduce cerebral perfusion pressure and contribute to brain cell hypoxia. Supporting this assumption is Lundberg's observation that transient displays of the classic signs of increased pressure most often occurred at the peak of plateau waves. Of particular importance to nursing is his observation that above a baseline pressure of 20 mm Hg, transient pressure rises may summate into plateau waves.

5. Assist the physician with testing intracranial

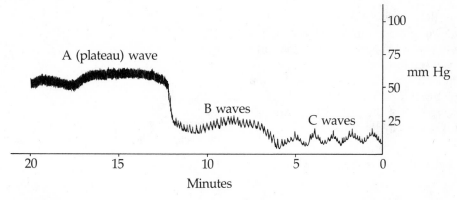

FIGURE 5-3

Intracranial pressure waves. Composite diagram of A (plateau) waves, B waves, and C waves. See text for discussion.

compliance (ability to compensate for a volume change without a large pressure increase). The compensatory mechanism can be evaluated with ventricular monitoring systems by introducing a known amount of fluid (1 cc preservative-free normal saline) into the ventricle and noting the ICP. If the patient's ICP is relatively normal and compensatory mechanisms are working, instilling a small amount of fluid causes only slight increases in ICP and amplitude. If the ICP is increased significantly and compensatory mechanisms are ineffective, the pressure will rise dramatically and the amplitude will increase considerably. Price (1981) states that the volume/pressure test is positive if a pressure increase of greater than 5 mm Hg occurs. Awareness of the brain's compensatory status may influence nursing interventions. Because this procedure can cause decompensation, you must be prepared to drain CSF and support ventilation immediately if necessary.

Anticipate and Prevent Complications of Monitoring Implement the following measures for patients on ICP monitoring.

  1. *Avoid infection* by scrupulous aseptic technique. Breaks in technique are particularly likely when you are setting up the system and when you are preparing to flush the system. Good handwashing and cleaning around parts with betadine prior to changing syringes will decrease the chance of infection. When zeroing the system, a hydrophobic millipore filter should be used. It allows air to communicate with the transducer dome but not bacteria. Horner (1985) and Hickey (1986) recommend that the dressing be changed every 24–48 hours; on the other hand, Robinet (1985) advocates leaving the head dressing in place, without being changed, for as long as the intraventricular catheter is in place. If the dressing becomes soiled or wet, the physician should be notified to change it.

  2. *Observe* the system *for CSF leaks,* which are dangerous because they allow a pathway for infection and because they lower the pressure in the system and allow brain tissue to be sucked against or into the catheter or screw. If you see fluid on the stopcocks or tubing, tighten or replace them. If you are unable to stop the leak, turn the stopcock attached to the catheter or screw off to the direction of the leak, cover the leak with a sterile towel, and notify the physician.

Planning and Implementation of Care

Many maneuvers that nurses commonly use in caring for critically ill patients may have deleterious effects on patients already suffering from increased ICP. To un-

---

> ### NURSING DIAGNOSES
>
> **ALTERED TISSUE PERFUSION (CEREBRAL)**
> This is a nursing diagnosis that is formally accepted by the North American Nursing Diagnosis Association (NANDA). You might want to use it to phrase the diagnosis if your patient has increased ICP.

derstand why, it is helpful to review intracranial dynamics briefly.

Oxygenation and Ventilation Cerebral blood flow varies in response to metabolic changes, specifically the arterial partial pressures of CO_2 (P_aCO_2) and O_2 (P_aO_2) and the level of lactic acid. Within the normal range of P_aCO_2 (35-45 mm Hg), changes in CO_2 level exert more effect on CSF than do changes in O_2 level. *As P_aCO_2 increases,* cerebral vessels dilate; because their resistance decreases, cerebral perfusion pressure and blood flow increase. P_aO_2 affects cerebral blood vessels when it drops below 50 mm Hg (Mitchell 1982). *As P_aO_2 decreases,* cerebral vessels dilate and CBF increases. Lactic acid accumulation also causes vasodilatation. To summarize, *hypercapnia, hypoxemia,* and *lactic acidemia* all cause cerebral blood vessels to *dilate.*

When intracranial pressure rises, venous outflow and therefore cerebral blood flow decrease. As a result, more CO_2 accumulates in cerebral vessels, and less oxygen than normal is available to the cells. The CO_2 excess and oxygen deficit both cause vasodilatation, which reduces resistance and increases cerebral blood flow toward normal (metabolic autoregulation). Unfortunately, the increased blood flow tends to increase intracranial pressure even more. The following sections describe ways of maintaining oxygenation and ventilation to lessen this vicious cycle.

Airway Patency Establish and maintain a patent airway. This may be accomplished simply with oral or nasal airways, or it may necessitate endotracheal intubation.

Hypoxemia and/or Hypercapnia Avoid hypoxemia and/or hypercapnia, either of which can cause vasodilatation with a resultant further increase in ICP. Particularly important measures are close monitoring of arterial blood gases, preoxygenating and hyperventilating before suctioning, and limiting suction to 10–15 seconds in the apneic patient to minimize CO_2 accumulation. The administration of xylocaine 50 mg IVP, 5 minutes prior to

NURSING RESEARCH NOTE

Metcalf C, Mitchell P: The effects of pre-suctioning and postsuctioning treatment on intracranial pressure: Hyperoxygenation versus combined hyperinflation and hyperoxygenation. *Heart Lung* 1987; 16:327–328.

Currently accepted practice for suctioning a mechanically ventilated patient includes combined hyperoxygenation and hyperinflation before and after suctioning, yet few studies indicate whether this procedure is safe for patients with intracranial pathology. Specifically, how does this recommended practice affect mean intracranial pressure (MICP) and cerebral perfusion pressure (CPP)?

A convenience sample of six artificially ventilated patients with intracranial disease was studied. Each patient had a Richmond subdural bolt for monitoring ICP and an arterial line for monitoring mean arterial blood pressure. Following a repeated-measures quasiexperimental design, one to two randomized presuction and postsuction trials of two methods were administered to each patient (hyperoxygenation alone or combined with hyperinflation). The trials were delivered by ventilator, and hyperoxygenation before and after suctioning was held constant. MICP and CPP were determined every 15 seconds during each suctioning procedure.

Data were analyzed using analysis of variance with repeated measures (α at 0.05). Analysis revealed no signficant difference between the two methods. MICP changed transiently, but suctioning-associated increases in mean arterial pressure ($p < 0.001$) counterbalanced the effect of increased MICP on CPP. Although the small sample size limits generalization, the research outcomes suggest that nurses can utilize the intracranial disease patient's pulmonary needs to guide the selection of an appropriate endotracheal suctioning method.

suctioning, is effective in limiting elevations of ICP by preventing coughing. For other measures to maintain oxygenation and ventilation, see Chapter 9.

Prevention of Obstructions to Venous Outflow

Try to prevent obstructions to venous outflow from the brain. Such obstructions not only increase pressure in the capillary bed (predisposing toward cerebral swelling) but also diminish absorption of CSF. Because CSF is absorbed by the arachnoid villi into the sagittal sinus and then into the jugular veins, pressure resulting from compression of the jugular veins will be transmitted back into the brain. A continuing rise in pressure may precipitate reduction in one of the other volumes. Blood volume may decrease, causing ischemia, or brain tissue may herniate.

Unless specifically ordered by the physician, do not place the patient with increased ICP flat or in Trendelenburg's position. Instead, keep the head of the bed elevated to increase the pressure gradient between the brain and heart. Although 30° is a common elevation, the degree of elevation often must be individualized. Researchers have found that ICP can be reduced significantly by placing the patient in a semisitting or sitting (>35°) position (Parsons and Wilson 1984).

Position the head and neck midline to avoid jugular venous compression. Also, maintain a neutral position, avoiding both extreme neck flexion and extension. Recent research indicates that extreme hip flexion also elevates ICP and should be avoided. For example, if you must catheterize a female with increased ICP, flex the legs as little as possible.

Prevention of Increases in Intrathoracic Pressure   Prevent avoidable increases in intrathoracic pressure. If the physician plans to insert a jugular venous catheter, you should modify your usual preparation of the patient. Avoid placing the patient in Trendelenburg's position and having him or her execute a Valsalva maneuver, as you do with other patients to minimize the danger of air embolism due to negative intrathoracic pressure. Instead, the physician should prevent air being sucked into the catheter during insertion by maintaining suction on the catheter with a syringe.

Take actions to avoid other Valsalva maneuvers. For example, teach the patient to exhale when moving his or her bowels; assist him or her to turn; and keep fecal contents soft through diet, fluid intake, and/or stool softeners. Though a Valsalva maneuver alone may not be sufficient to cause a plateau wave, in combination with other pressure-increasing actions it can cause a sustained increase in intracranial pressure.

PEEP can cause increased intrathoracic and intracranial pressure. Monitor patients on PEEP particularly closely and try to avoid doing more than one activity that increases ICP at a time. For example, you should avoid turning a patient if you have just finished suctioning her.

A study reported by Mitchell et al. (1981) compared the effects of eight nursing care activities on increased intracranial pressure in 18 neurologic and neurosurgical patients with ventricular drainage. Their findings supported empirical observations that nursing activities do in fact influence ICP and that these effects are potentially dangerous in some patients. The measures evaluated were: (a) turning the body to four positions (supine to right, right to supine, supine to left, left to supine); (b) two passive range of motion exercises (arm extension and hip flexion); and (c) two head rotations (right and left). The passive exercises did not provoke clinically significant changes in ventricular pressure in most patients. Large increases in ICP occurred in the five patients who had head rotations. Turning in any direction caused more variability in ventricular pressure than the head rotations or passive exercises. Activities spaced 15 minutes apart, regardless of their nature, caused a cumulative increase in ICP; those spaced an hour apart did not. Although nurses usually are encouraged to group care activities together, doing so may worsen increased ICP. In particular, performing closely spaced activities with the patient supine may be most apt to increase ICP. The authors recommend spacing procedures known to increase ICP, such as suctioning, after the patient has been resting for some time and perhaps with the person in the lateral position.

Minimizing Arterial Hypo- or Hypertension

Many nursing care activities cause an arousal response accompanied by increased systemic blood pressure. Among the stimuli that can provoke this arousal response are an endotracheal tube, suctioning, chest physiotherapy, and pain. Use BP and intracranial pressure monitors to evaluate your patient's response to these circumstances and adapt your care accordingly. For instance, try timing suctioning or chest PT for intervals of peak sedation; check with the physician about using topical anesthesia if suctioning provokes hypertensive episodes; use muscle relaxants as ordered by the physician if repeated explanations are ineffective in calming the patient fighting an endotracheal tube and if your evaluation reveals he or she is not hypoxic. Decrease the occurrence of painful stimuli or any other nonspecific stimuli that provoke the hypertensive response in your particular patient.

Also try to reduce the risk of small pressure increases summating into plateau waves. If you must do two activities each of which causes a pressure increase, time your care judiciously so that pressure can diminish after the first activity before you institute the second.

Prevention of Infection Infection can be catastrophic in patients on ICP monitoring. Meticulous sterile technique and prompt antibiotic therapy if signs of infection appear may protect the patient against meningitis or full-blown sepsis. Because sepsis can lead to increased cardiac output and vasodilatation, it can contribute to a dangerous rise in intracranial pressure.

Implementing Medical Therapy An important aspect of nursing the patient with increased ICP is implementing the plan of medical therapy. Definitive therapy, of course, varies with the cause. General therapeutic measures include hypertonic agents, assisted ventilation with hyperventilation, corticosteroids, CSF drainage, sedation, surgical decompression, and barbiturate coma.

Hypertonic Agents Hypertonic agents are used to reduce cerebral edema by drawing fluid out of brain cells into the hypertonic blood. Hypertonic agents are only temporary measures that bide time for more definitive treatment. Commonly used agents include mannitol (the drug of choice), urea, and glucose. When hypertonic agents are used, be alert for the development of congestive heart failure. Also watch for increasing cerebral edema, which may occur when these drugs pass through the disrupted blood–brain barrier and raise brain osmolality. To reduce the risk of ICP rebound, only a portion of the volume lost during diuresis should be replaced. Mannitol is always administered intravenously through a filter because it crystallizes; failure to use a filter can cause microemboli to be introduced into the patient's bloodstream. Potential complications of mannitol administration are hyperosmolality and hyperkalemia.

Continuous Hyperventilation Continuous hyperventilation may be tried if drug therapy is ineffective. Lowering the P_aCO_2 to 25–30 mm Hg constricts the cerebral vasculature and therefore lowers ICP and improves compliance. Unfortunately, this effect depends upon retained CO_2 responsiveness, which often is lost if extensive tissue is diseased or the brain has suffered an anoxic insult.

Corticosteroids The corticosteroids most often used are *dexamethosone* (Decadron) and *methylprednisolone* (Solumedrol). Although they remain in widespread use, their value in treating cerebral edema resulting from trauma is controversial.

CSF Drainage CSF drainage is particularly helpful when the cause of increased intracranial pressure is decreased CSF absorption. It is safest when done against positive pressure to decrease the risk of ventricular collapse. To provide positive pressure, the drainage reservoir is set at a specified level above the ICP reference point. CSF then drains only when the pressure exceeds the specified level. It is imperative that the level of the head of the bed *not* be altered while a CSF drain is open.

Surgical Decompression   Surgical decompression may be used in severe cerebral edema to "buy time" and prevent herniation while other therapies reduce swelling. To allow the swollen brain to expand, a flap of bone is removed.

Barbiturate Coma   Barbiturate coma is the induction and maintenance of coma by continuous administration of pentobarbital or thiopental. It is used with severe, persistent intracranial hypertension that is refractory to other therapies. The exact mechanism of action is unclear; possible explanations include cerebral vasoconstriction, reduced responsiveness to stimuli, and reduced cerebral metabolic demand. Barbiturate coma necessitates extremely close nursing supervision. The patient must be intubated and on a ventilator. Monitoring devices must include an ICP monitor, cardiac monitor, arterial line, PA line, nasogastric tube, and urinary catheter. The blood barbiturate level must be monitored daily.

Because barbiturates may lower SAP, vasopressor and/or colloid administration may be necessary.

Outcome Evaluation

Evaluate the patient's progress according to these outcome criteria:

- Return to premorbid level of consciousness
- Pupils of normal and equal size that accommodate briskly to light
- BP, pulse, respirations, and temperature WNL for the patient
- Appropriate responses to stimuli
- Arterial blood gases WNL for the patient
- If monitored, ICP and CPP WNL for the patient

Herniation Syndromes

Herniation may be defined as the protrusion of a portion of the brain through the openings of the cavity sur-

rounding it. There are three main patterns of *supratentorial* herniation. Herniation of the cingulate gyrus of the cerebrum can occur under the midline dural fold known as the *falx cerebri*. This type of herniation is referred to as *cingulate* or *transfalcian* herniation. *Central* or *transtentorial* herniation is the compression and movement of the diencephalon through the tentorial notch due to downward displacement of the cerebral hemispheres. In the third pattern, called *uncal herniation,* a laterally located expanding lesion results in a shift of the uncus of the temporal lobe towards the midline and pushes it under the tentorial notch. The type of herniation does not correlate consistently with the site of the lesion. Uncal herniation is more common than central herniation in neurologic emergencies. Central herniation is more common in subacute and chronic disorders.

Assessment

Risk Conditions   Risk conditions for herniation include tumors, intracerebral and extracerebral hemorrhage, infections, and cerebral edema. Increased ICP in itself does not lead to herniation unless it increases so rapidly that it causes a mass effect.

Signs and Symptoms   Assessment of the patient at risk for herniation includes evaluating level of consciousness, sensorimotor function, respiratory patterns, eye function, and vital signs. Because supratentorial herniation generally progresses in a head-to-toe *(rostral-caudal)* fashion, upper-brain functions are affected first and brainstem functions last. Thus, level of consciousness is the earliest category of brain function to deteriorate, whereas vital signs are the last.

Cingulate herniation will be considered with central herniation because a disorder causing the former also is likely to produce the latter.

Central and uncal herniation produce distinctly different clinical pictures early in their courses. Nurses should learn to recognize these changes so medical intervention can be instituted rapidly. Once the midbrain and lower levels are involved, the clinical picture is the same for both, and the patient's chance for complete recovery diminishes. The following descriptions are taken from Plum and Posner (1980).

Central Herniation   In central (transtentorial) herniation, an expanding lesion forces the hemispheres and basal nuclei downward. The progressive compression displaces the diencephalon and midbrain downward through the tentorial notch. Displacement of branches

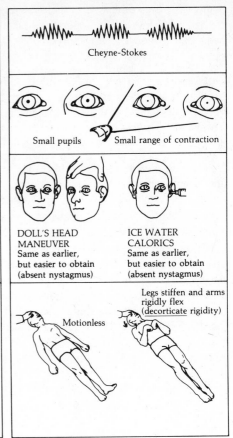

FIGURE 5-4

Signs of central transtentorial herniation. Adapted from McNealy, D., Plum, F.:
"Brainstem Dysfunction with Supratensorial Mass Lesions" from *Archives of Neurology*,
July, Volume 7:10–32. Copyright 1962, American Medical Association.

of the basilar artery causes ischemia and severe brainstem deterioration. Central herniation also can block the aqueduct of Sylvius, between the third and fourth ventricles. This blockage, which cannot be diagnosed clinically, robs the brain of its ability to displace fluid from the ventricular system to compensate for increased brain volume and causes a severe rise in supratentorial pressure. However, impaired CSF circulation probably is less instrumental in causing herniation than the factor initially causing the increase in intracranial pressure.

Central herniation generally causes ischemia to advance in a rostral-caudal direction. Plum and Posner (1980) describe manifestations typical of four stages of progression: early diencephalic, late diencephalic, midbrain–upper pontine, and lower pontine–upper medullary. These changes are shown in Figure 5-4.

The earliest sign in the *diencephalic stage* is diminished alertness characterized by difficulty in concentration, memory lapses, lethargy, and stupor. Pupils are small (1–3 mm). Although on superficial examination they may appear not to react to light, a closer look reveals that they react rapidly but only within a small range of contraction. The doll's eyes reflex is present. The ice water caloric test provokes normal slow movement but diminished or absent fast movement. Respirations may be a relatively normal pattern interspersed with yawns, sighs, and pauses, or Cheyne-Stokes breathing. There often is a preexisting hemiparesis or hemiplegia on the opposite (*contralateral*) side of the body from the lesion, which may become more severe as this stage develops. In addition, the extremities on the same side of the body (*ipsilateral*) to the lesion develop paratonic resistance, although they continue responding appropriately to noxious stimuli. Bilateral positive Babinski signs are present, although they are weaker on the ipsilateral side. Later, resistance to passive stretch increases and grasp reflexes emerge.

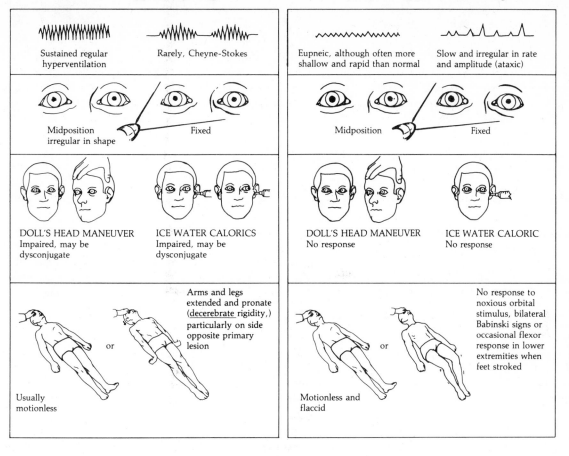

Mid-brain-upper pons stage

Sustained regular hyperventilation

Rarely, Cheyne-Stokes

Midposition irregular in shape

Fixed

DOLL'S HEAD MANEUVER Impaired, may be dysconjugate

ICE WATER CALORICS Impaired, may be dysconjugate

Usually motionless

or

Arms and legs extended and pronate (<u>decerebrate</u> rigidity,) particularly on side opposite primary lesion

Lower pons-upper medulla stage

Eupneic, although often more shallow and rapid than normal

Slow and irregular in rate and amplitude (ataxic)

Midposition

Fixed

DOLL'S HEAD MANEUVER No response

ICE WATER CALORIC No response

Motionless and flaccid

or

No response to noxious orbital stimulus, bilateral Babinski signs or occasional flexor response in lower extremities when feet stroked

---

Finally, decorticate posturing appears, first on the contralateral side and then bilaterally.

In the *midbrain–upper-pontine stage,* pupils become somewhat dilated (3–5 mm), fixed in midposition, and unresponsive to light. Their shape often is irregular. The doll's eyes response becomes impaired, and the ice water caloric response becomes harder to provoke. Respirations may change from Cheyne-Stokes to sustained hyperventilation. Decerebrate posturing occurs in response to painful stimuli or spontaneously. Wide swings of body temperature are common.

In the *lower-pontine–upper-medullary stage,* the pupils remain fixed in midposition and unresponsive to light. Both the doll's eyes and ice water caloric responses are absent. Respirations become more or less regular but rapid and shallow. The patient remains flaccid with bilateral Babinski reflexes and occasionally nonpurposeful flickers of movement in response to painful stimuli.

In the terminal medullary stage, medullary ischemia causes ataxic respirations, varying pulse rates, hypotension, dilated pupils, and respiratory arrest.

The authors point out two exceptions to the generalization of rostral-caudal progression in untreated supratentorial lesions: (1) acute cerebral hemorrhage, and (2) lumbar punctures in patients with impending herniation. In both cases, sudden medullary failure may occur. In acute cerebral hemorrhage, structures around the fourth ventricle are compressed by hemorrhage into the ventricular system. In the second case, the extraction of spinal fluid apparently removes support from the brain, allowing it to herniate into the foramen magnum.

Uncal Herniation The uncus, a medial portion of the temporal lobe, overhangs the edge of the tentorial notch. Expanding lesions in the temporal lobe or lateral middle fossa can force the uncus over the edge of the incisura. This uncal herniation compresses the midbrain (which passes through the notch) and opposite cerebral peduncle up against the opposite edge of the tentorial opening. It compresses the oculomotor nerve and pushes the posterior cerebral artery down, trapping it against the incisural edge. Compression of the oculomotor nerve is discussed below. Posterior cerebral artery compromise can provoke occipital ischemia, edema and infarction. Uncal herniation also can compromise CSF circulation by compressing the aqueduct of Sylvius, with the results indicated above under central herniation.

Because of the anatomical location of the uncus, uncal herniation produces early stages that are different from central herniation: the *third nerve stage* and the *midbrain–upper-pontine stage* (Figure 5-5). The earliest consistent sign is not the level of consciousness (which may vary from diminished alertness to coma) but rather a unilaterally dilating pupil.

In the early third nerve stage, compression of the third cranial nerve first affects the pupillary parasympathetic fibers that make up the outer portion of the nerve, causing a unilaterally dilated pupil on the affected side. When you flash a light in that eye, the pupil will react sluggishly or not at all, although the other eye will respond consensually. Similarly, a light flashed in the nonaffected eye will provoke a normal direct reflex in it but a sluggish or absent consensual response in the affected eye. This pupillary abnormality may be the *only* sign of early uncal herniation. Early motor signs may consist of contralateral paratonic resistance and extensor plantar reflex due to compression of the ipsilateral cerebral peduncle.

In the late third nerve stage, increasing pressure next affects the fibers in the center of the third cranial nerve that control oculomotor-mediated eye movement. As a result, diplopia and ptosis appear, and the eye (when resting) looks downward and outward due to the unopposed action of the sixth cranial nerve. The patient becomes deeply stuporous and then comatose. Oculocephalic reflexes show absent or dysconjugate doll's eyes. Oculovestibular responses rapidly become sluggish and disappear. Because the opposite cerebral pe-

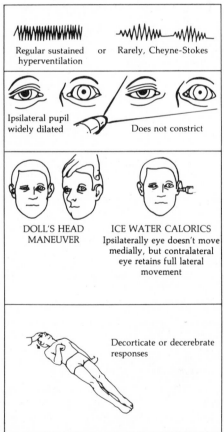

FIGURE 5-5

Signs of uncal herniation. Adapted from McNealy, D., Plum, F.: "Brainstem Dysfunction with Supratensorial Mass Lesions" from *Archives of Neurology,* July, Volume 7:10–32. Copyright 1962, American Medical Association.

duncle becomes compressed against the opposite tentorial edge, hemiplegia develops on the ipsilateral side as the lesion. Bilateral motor signs develop, and noxious stimuli elicit abnormal extension of the extremities.

Uncal herniation is particularly dangerous because it tends to progress rapidly to produce irreversible midbrain–upper-pontine damage. In this stage, pressure on midbrain corticospinal and other tracts results in bilateral decerebrate rigidity. The opposite pupil may dilate widely and be fixed to light; eventually both pupils fix in midposition (5–6 mm). Doll's eyes and ice water responses are abnormal, and the respiratory pattern shows sustained hyperventilation. After this stage, the uncal syndrome progresses in the same fashion as the lower-pontine–upper-medullary stage of central herniation.

NURSING DIAGNOSIS

The most appropriate nursing diagnosis for this disorder may be phrased as: "Altered tissue perfusion (cerebral) related to impending (or actual) herniation."

Planning and Implementation of Care

The above descriptions of downward brain herniation accentuate the importance of conscientious physical examinations by nurses and prompt reactions at the *first* signs of possible impending herniation. Alert the physician if you observe *any* signs of possible incipient herniation, even if they are transient or equivocal.

For the patient on continuous intracranial pressure monitoring, notify the physician promptly if there is a consistent rise in ICP, plateau waves, or widening of the pulse pressure, so that CSF drainage, mannitol administration, or other therapy can be instituted.

Should you suspect imminent herniation, immediately summon medical assistance. Meanwhile, hyperventilate the patient to reduce the P_{CO_2}. This action will constrict the cerebral vessels and temporarily decrease intracranial pressure and may avert herniation long enough for more definitive medical therapy to be instituted.

Outcome Evaluation

The following outcome criteria are ideal:

- Return to premorbid level of consciousness

- Pupils of normal size, bilaterally equal and briskly responsive to light
- Vital signs WNL
- Normal motor response (no posturing, normal Babinski reflex)

Status Epilepticus

Status epilepticus is one of the most common neurologic emergencies encountered by the critical-care nurse. *Status* is defined as seizure activity of 30 minutes' or more duration caused by a single seizure or a series of seizures in which there is no return of consciousness between seizures (Wittman 1985). Status epilepticus can occur with any type of seizure activity (see Table 5-1). The most common and most dangerous form of status epilepticus is generalized grand mal (tonic-clonic)

TABLE 5-1 INTERNATIONAL CLASSIFICATION OF EPILEPTIC SEIZURES

1. **Focal or partial seizures**

    Simple (general without an impairment of level of consciousness)

    - Motor (eg, Jacksonian seizures)
    - Sensory or somatosensory
    - Autonomic

    Complex (the spread of simple or partial to a generalized convulsive form such as temporal lobe or psychomotor)

II. **Generalized seizures (without a local onset, bilaterally symmetric)**

    Absences (petit mal)

    Tonic-clonic (grand mal)

    Infantile spasms

    Bilateral massive myoclonus

    Clonic seizures

    Tonic seizures

    Atonic seizures

    Akinetic seizures

III. **Unilateral seizures**

IV. **Unclassified seizures (when complete data is not available)**

V. **Classification of paroxysmal forms**

    Benign febrile seizures

    Convulsive equivalent syndrome

    Breath-holding spells

Source: Kneisl C, Ames SA: Adult health nursing: A biopsychosocial approach. Menlo Park, CA: Addison-Wesley Pub. Co., 1986, p. 116.

caused by paroxysmal, uncontrolled electrical activity that spreads across the brain (O'Neill 1984). If not treated promptly, permanent neurologic sequelae may develop or death from cardiovascular failure, respiratory depression, or cerebral edema may intervene. Prognosis depends on the cause of the seizures and the period of time between onset and cessation.

Assessment

Risk Conditions Grand mal status epilepticus occurs in up to 10% of all epileptics (Hickey 1986) but can occur in people without a history of epilepsy. There are numerous causes for status epilepticus. The most common cause is insufficient serum levels of anticonvulsant drugs caused by the individual's deliberate or inadvertent stopping the drug or by inadequate therapy. Other causes include changing anticonvulsant agents, metabolic imbalances, drug withdrawals, trauma, neoplasm, and acute cerebral edema (Table 5-2). The most serious

TABLE 5-2 COMMON CAUSES OF SEIZURES AND STATUS EPILEPTICUS

Insufficient serum levels of anticonvulsant agents
- Noncompliance: deliberate or inadvertent
- Inadequate prescribed therapy

Metabolic disturbances
- Hyperglycemia vs hypoglycemia
- Hypoxia
- Drug or alcohol withdrawal
- Electrolyte imbalances
- Low magnesium, calcium, or phosphorus serum levels
- High Pco_2 serum levels
- Hyperpyrexia

Infections

Structural CNS Lesions
- Concussion
- Infarctions
- Cerebral or Subdural Hematoma
- Subarachnoid Hemorrhage
- Undetectable structural lesion

Familial predisposition

Idiopathic

Life-threatening dysrhythmias

Focal brain trauma

Environmental stimuli (lights, sounds)

Cerebral neoplasm

Stress

High aspartame intake (Nurses' Drug Alert 1986)

Acute cerebral edema

complications of status epilepticus are neurologic sequelae and death. The patient is twice as likely to develop neurologic deficits as to die (Wittman 1985). Neurologic sequelae can range from focal neurologic deficits, behavior disorders, and chronic epilepsy to mental retardation and brain atrophy.

Signs and Symptoms There are four distinct phases during tonic-clonic seizures. The *preictal phase*, or *aura*, may or may not be apparent to the patient. The aura may consist of subtle, unusual sensory illusions (smells or patterns of light), mood changes, or focal motor activity. Origin of the seizure may be pinpointed by the characteristics of the aura.

Nursing staff may not be aware of the aura but will note the sudden shrill cry or moan at the beginning of the *tonic phase*. This cry or moan is caused by air being forced past the closed glottis and larynx by the contraction of thoracic and abdominal muscles. Some muscle groups contract; others become flaccid. The person will lose consciousness and instantly collapse, increasing the potential for injury (O'Neill 1984). Rigid, intense muscle contractions are exhibited by extended extremities, arched spine, and clamped jaw (Rudy 1984). Apnea ensues for 10–15 seconds (O'Neill 1984) but can last up to 1 minute (Rudy 1984). A concurrent increase in saliva production with sequestering in the mouth and throat increases the potential for aspiration (O'Neill 1984). The saliva may turn bloody if the tongue was bitten as the jaw snapped shut. Pupils become dilated and nonreactive to light and deviate conjugately or rove due to severe hypoxia (Rudy 1984). This deviation is not considered as pointing to the seizure focus (Rudy 1984). Heart rate slows secondary to parasympathetic, vagal stimulation (Rudy 1984). There is an abrupt end to the tonic phase as the clonic phase begins (O'Neill 1984).

The muscles begin violent jerking at the onset of the *clonic phase* (O'Neill 1984). This bilateral, global jerking gradually decelerates until it fades when the nutrition and potassium of the brain cells are depleted (Rudy 1984). There is violent facial grimacing, profuse diaphoresis, and usually incontinence (O'Neill 1984). Respirations become irregular and noisy, with frothing at the mouth from accumulated saliva (O'Neill 1984). Pupil size and reactivity may or may not change. Bradycardia or tachycardia may be present (Rudy 1984). Clonus usually lasts 2–5 minutes (Rudy 1984) and ends with a deep breath followed by irregular, shallow respirations (O'Neill 1984).

Clonus is then replaced by the *postictal phase* of muscle flaccidity and deep sleep than can last from 5 minutes up to several hours (O'Neill 1984). This deep sleep is due to brain and muscle exhaustion from severely depleted cellular glucose and oxygen supplies (Rudy 1984). Respirations gradually become deep and regular (O'Neill 1984). Pupils react to light (Rudy 1984). The patient awakens confused and amnesic and may complain of headache, muscle aches, and fatigue (Rudy 1984).

These stages of activity are common in all grand mal seizures. In the status epilepticus patient, the postictal phase may be brief or not apparent with the onset of another seizure. The resulting prolonged apnea can cause severe neurologic deficits or death.

Significant reductions in cerebral cortical oxygenation and insufficient regional oxygenation occur within 20 minutes of seizure onset (Wittman 1985). The intense electrical activity causes a marked increase in cerebral metabolic rate, oxygen and glucose utilization, glycolysis, rapid depletion of adenosine triphosphate bonds (the energy source for cells), and consumption of neurotransmitter substances (Lovely and Ozuna 1982). Cerebral blood flow may increase to as much as five times normal (Meldrum 1976) due to increased arterial pressure and vasodilation resulting from CO_2 and lactic acid accumulation. As status epilepticus continues, autoregulation is lost, cerebral vessels dilate, arterial pressure falls, and cerebral perfusion pressure is jeopardized (Meldrum 1976).

During the first 30 minutes of status epilepticus, arterial BP rises, probably due to vasoconstriction resulting from vasomotor center stimulation, mediated by hypoxic or hypercarbic stimulation of aortic arch and carotid body chemoreceptors (Lovely and Ozuna 1982). After the first 30 minutes, mean arterial BP usually falls below normal and may stay depressed in the postictal period (Meldrum and Brierly 1973).

Permanent cellular damage can occur in the medullary, cerebral, thalamic, and middle cortical layers by 60–90 minutes (Wittman 1985). Severe metabolic imbalances (including hypoxia, hypotension, hypoglycemia, hyperkalemia, and hyperpyrexia) and increased intracranial pressure create an imbalance between supply and demand for glucose and oxygen for which the body may be unable to compensate (Wittman 1985).

Planning and Implementation of Care

Ineffective Airway Clearance Related to Airway Occlusion by Tongue, Bronchoconstriction, or Increased Secretions Maintenance of a patent airway and adequate ventilation are the first priority in status epilepticus. Turn the patient on the side to facilitate drainage of secretions. Use low, gentle oropharyngeal suction as needed to aspirate secretions. Do not try to place an oral airway when the jaw relaxes unless there is airway obstruction. The patient may start to seize again and injure self or the nurse. Also, airway placement could stimulate vomiting (Rich 1986) and increase the chance of aspiration. Possible insertion of a soft airway such as gauze sponges or a washcloth before the onset of tonus is recommended by Cline and Fisher (1984). Side positioning or chin-lift–jaw-thrust maneuver will usually maintain a patent airway.

Ineffective Breathing Pattern Related to Apnea, Brainstem Depression, or Overmedication Carefully monitor and evaluate the respiratory pattern, rate, and depth for signs of insufficiency. Loosen tight clothing on the chest if necessary. Anticipate intubation when respiratory distress is present and place an intubation tray at bedside. There are no clear-cut guidelines regarding mechanical ventilation; an individual decision must be made by the physician on the basis of ventilatory pattern and arterial blood gas values.

Impaired Gas Exchange Related to Excessive Oxygen Demand or Aspiration Administer supplemental oxygen by nasal prongs as a mask may impede clearance of emesis. Monitor oxygenation and acid–base status via arterial blood gas sampling. If the status epilepticus does not respond readily to therapy, insert a nasogastric tube, per physician's order, to prevent chemical pneumonitis caused by aspiration of gastric contents or vomitus.

Potential Altered Tissue Perfusion Related to Decreased Blood Pressure or Cardiac Output Monitor vital signs closely. Place the patient on continuous ECG monitoring. Establish an intravenous line at

---

NURSING DIAGNOSES

The life-threatening nature of status epilepticus makes prompt nursing diagnosis and intervention crucial. The nursing diagnoses for a patient in status epilepticus include:

- Ineffective airway clearance
- Ineffective breathing pattern
- Impaired gas exchange
- Potential altered tissue perfusion
- Potential for injury
- Potential ineffective individual coping
- Sensory-perceptual alteration

a TKO ("to keep open") rate. To avoid cerebral edema, isotonic solutions such as lactated Ringer's or N.S. are preferred; glucose-containing solutions, such as 5% dextrose in lactated Ringer's, frequently are used to provide glucose to the brain (Rich 1986).

Potential for Injury Related to Tonic-Clonic Movements and Repeated Seizures Never leave the patient unattended during a seizure. Protect the patient from injury by removing any nearby objects. Moving the patient is not advised unless a potentially damaging nearby object cannot be removed. Never try to force anything into the mouth or try to restrain the extremities, because this could tear or stretch the muscles. Gentle guiding of the extremities is acceptable.

If the patient is in a chair, gently lower him or her to the floor. Once the patient is on the floor, place a pad, rolled cloth, or pillow under the head to prevent trauma. When the patient is in bed, lower the head and raise the side rails. Pad the side rails and head and foot boards with special pads or pillows. Remember, though, that raised bedrails and padding may be embarrassing to the patient. Active listening and explanation of the need to be protected from injury may help the patient accept these measures.

Potential Ineffective Individual Coping Related to Loss of Privacy The patient's privacy should be maintained at all times. With screens or polite requests to leave, shield the patient from any nearby onlookers. If you are alone, discreetly notify coworkers of your need for assistance and have them call the physician. Since the patient's hearing may be unaffected by the seizure, use a soft, calm, normal voice to explain what is happening to the patient. When the seizure is over, cover the patient with a blanket. Gently remove the patient to a private place when necessary. Efficient cleansing of the patient for incontinence is important and must be done in complete privacy. The nurse's unbiased attitude toward seizure care and protection of privacy will help the patient accept the illness and learn to deal positively with it.

Sensory-Perceptual Alteration Related to Postictal Phase The patient may awaken confused, disoriented, or amnesic. Attempts at reorientation will probably not be effective until the patient is fully alert. Be careful not to speak loudly or make sudden, jerking movements with the patient as this may stimulate another seizure. When clearing the airway, gentle suctioning of the mouth and oropharynx should reduce the risk of this hazard. The patient may be safely left with the

family in attendance once reoccurrence of seizure activity is abated.

Monitor general neurologic status between seizures. Neurochecks should include level of consciousness, pupil size and reaction, and sensorimotor function. Carefully observe seizure characteristics, particularly noting its onset, progression and length, any pupil changes, and any lateralizing signs.

Draw blood samples for laboratory studies, including complete blood count, serum electrolytes, blood glucose, and toxicology screen. If the patient has been on anticonvulsant therapy, a serum sample should be drawn for determination of baseline blood level of the particular drug(s).

Implement drug therapy as ordered by the physician. Selection of pharmacologic agents may vary with the individual physician as well as the patient's condition. The drugs used most often are diazepam, phenytoin, and phenobarbital.

Diazepam (Valium) is regarded as the initial drug of choice by most physicians. Intravenous diazepam is a rapid-acting, short-lived anticonvulsant; thus, the dose can easily be titrated according to the patient's response. Seizure activity usually stops during or immediately after the injection. The patient should be monitored closely, as respiratory depression, hypotension, and further decreases in level of consciousness may occur. Also observe the patient without an artificial airway for possible airway obstruction by the tongue due to diazepam's marked muscle relaxation. Because diazepam provides only short-term cessation of seizure activity, a longer-acting anticonvulsant also should be administered.

Phenytoin (Dilantin) is used for longer-term control of seizure activity. Disadvantages include a slow (15-minute) onset of activity, potential cardiotoxicity, and tendency to crystallize in glucose. Phenytoin often is given in conjunction with diazepam to provide both immediate and long-range control of seizures. Phenytoin should be avoided or used only with extreme caution in patients with sinus bradycardia, SA or AV block, hypotension, or severe myocardial failure. A patient receiving intravenous phenytoin should be under constant ECG surveillance. The drug should be given no faster than 50 mg/min in a normal saline solution. Side effects, usually due to excessively rapid administration, include hypotension, conduction disturbances, and cardiorespiratory arrest.

Phenobarbital is a barbiturate long used to control status epilepticus. Intravenous administration provides long-range (24-hour) control, similar to phenytoin. It is the preferred drug in status epilepticus due to barbiturate withdrawal. Side effects include marked sedation, respiratory depression, and hypotension. Be particularly alert when a patient is given both diazepam and phenobarbital; their interaction may cause severe cardiorespiratory depression.

Phenobarbital and diazepam are not the only anticonvulsant drugs that interact, however. Most of the anticonvulsant drugs interact with each other in some manner as well as with many other drugs given to critically ill patients.

Refractory status epilepticus is present when the patient does not respond to the usual therapy. It may be treated with paraldehyde, neuromuscular blocking drugs, or general anesthesia. Neuromuscular blockade stops motor manifestations of the seizure but not the cerebral seizure activity itself. It requires intubation and mechanical ventilation because of respiratory muscle paralysis. General anesthetics suppress cerebral seizure activity but also require extensive ventilatory support. Other problems with neuromuscular blockage and general anesthesia therapies are the difficulty of determining how long to continue therapy, no guarantee for complete suppression of the seizure activity, and the fact that anesthesia requires full operating room support (Wittman 1985). Recent research findings in the concomitant use of hypothermia and barbiturate coma in the treatment of children may be instituted for adults in the future (Wittman 1985).

Outcome Evaluation

Desirable outcome criteria for a patient with status epilepticus are:

- Control of abnormal seizure activity
- Minimal or no loss of privacy during seizure
- Vital signs WNL
- Arterial blood gas values WNL
- Return to a normal level of consciousness

Vascular Disorders

Stroke as a sydrome is characterized as a sudden, rapid onset of neurologic deficits related directly or indirectly to a deficiency of the cerebral blood supply (Hickey 1986).

It is the third leading cause of death in America, exceeded only by heart disease and cancer. Approximately 500,000 people in the United States suffer from stroke each year (Rudy 1984). The morbidity associated with stroke leads to chronic disability. Kneisl and Ames (1986) report that stroke occurs more frequently in men than in women and in blacks than in whites. The elderly, ages 75 to 85 years, have the highest incidence of stroke; for people under the age of 65, stroke occurs in one out of seven individuals.

Arterial Syndromes

Two arterial systems form the cerebral circulation, the carotid and the vertebrobasilar. The reader is referred to Chapter 4 to review the cerebral circulation. Interruption of blood supply for whatever reason will produce symptoms related to the location of the lesion in the arterial tree and the portion of brain supplied (Table 5-3).

Stroke Classification

Occlusive stroke and hemorrhagic stroke are the two major kinds of stroke. Based on mechanism, occlusive stroke is subdivided into thrombotic and embolic. Cerebral thrombosis accounts for over 50% of all stroke cases, intracranial hemorrhage 10–25%, and cerebral embolism around 5% (Rudy 1984).

Occlusive Stroke

Thrombotic Stroke Thrombotic stroke causes a lack of blood supply due to thrombosis of the vessel, which leads to ischemia and infarction. Atherosclerosis is the most common cause of ischemic stroke. It affects the carotid vessels five times more often than the vertebrobasilar arteries (Samuels 1986). Atherosclerotic plaques form at the branching of the blood vessels and cause narrowing of the vessel lumen. Thrombotic stroke is progressive in nature, from partial to total obstruction of the vessel. The resulting clinical picture is evolutionary—from initial warning signs to completed stroke.

A transient ischemic attack (TIA) is an abrupt onset of neurologic dysfunction lasting less than 24 hours and with complete resolution of symptoms. TIAs more commonly present with anterior circulation symptoms that may be traced to internal carotid artery obstruction. TIAs are a warning event in 80% of thrombotic ischemic strokes (Samuels 1986).

The thrombotic stroke-in-evolution causes symptoms that progress over hours to days. The completed stroke is the residual neurologic deficit. Taylor (1985) reports

TABLE 5-3 BODY LOCUS OF STROKES AND ASSOCIATED SYMPTOMS

Anterior Circulation

Internal Carotid Artery Syndrome

- Ipsilateral amaurosis fugax (fleeting blindness)
- Contralateral hemiparesis
- Contralateral hemisensory changes
- Dysphasia (dominant hemisphere)

Middle Cerebral Artery Syndrome

- Contralateral hemiplegia (face, arm, and leg)
- Contralateral sensory impairment
- Homonymous hemianopsia
- Aphasia
- Decreased level of consciousness

Anterior Cerebral Artery Syndrome

- Contralateral paralysis of foot and leg
- Contralateral paresis of upper extremity
- Sensory impairment of foot and leg greater than that of arm
- Mental status impairment (apathy, flat affect, slowness, amnesia, confusion, decreased intellectual function)
- Urinary incontinence

Posterior Circulation

Vertebrobasilar Syndrome

- Dysarthria, dysphagia
- Vertigo, nausea, syncope
- Ataxia
- Drop attacks
- Double vision, homonymous hemianopia
- Alternating hemiparesis

Posterior Cerebral Artery Syndrome

- Visual field deficit
- Hemihypalgesia
- Impaired recent memory
- Dysphasia
- Hemiplegia (sometimes)

Posterior Inferior Cerebellar Artery Syndrome

- Dysphagia and dysarthria
- Ataxia and vertigo
- Loss of pain and temperature sensation on ipsilateral side of face and contralateral side of body
- Ipsilateral Horner's syndrome

that high blood pressure and diabetes are the most common risk factors for thrombotic stroke. Those in the critical-care unit should be especially cognizant of conditions leading to inadequate cerebral perfusion, such as hypotension and dehydration, since these factors may increase the risk of thrombosis.

Embolic Stroke Embolic stroke leads to ischemia and infarction due to an embolus that travels via the bloodstream and lodges in a cerebral vessel. Symptoms develop rapidly without any warning signs. The neurologic deficit relates to the area of brain lacking blood supply. Embolic stroke tends to occur during activity, whereas thrombotic stroke often develops at rest.

Sources of cerebral emboli include the heart, aorta, neck vessels, foreign substances, and increased blood coagulation. Calcified plaques in the aorta, carotids, or vertebrals may break loose and embolize. Cardiac conditions such as myocardial infarction, endocarditis, rheumatic heart disease, and postcardiac surgical procedures all bear the potential to produce an embolus. Kneisl and Ames (1986) report that the risk of embolic stroke for patients with atrial dysrhythmias is five times greater than for those without. Air embolus may be associated with a disconnected central line or a complication of posterior fossa surgery in the sitting position. Fat emboli may occur after traumatic injury with multiple fractures. Conditions such as polycythemia, sickle cell disease, use of oral contraceptives, or hypercoagulable states all carry a risk for embolization.

Hemorrhagic Stroke Hemorrhagic stroke results from the rupture of blood vessels, with blood extravasation into brain tissue. Common causes of hemorrhagic stroke are ruptured cerebral aneurysm, hypertensive intracerebral hemorrhage, and ruptured arteriovenous malformation. Hypertension and abnormalities of the cerebral vessels are major risk factors. Subarachnoid hemorrhage (SAH) is bleeding into the subarachnoid space subsequent to a hemorrhagic stroke.

Cerebral Aneurysm A cerebral aneurysm is a localized dilatation of a blood vessel. Congenital weakness in the media of the cerebral vessel allows for a saccular or fusiform aneurysm to develop. Because saccular aneurysms resemble a berry with a stem, they are referred to as *berry aneurysms*. The majority of aneurysms are located around the anterior portion of the circle of Willis.

The incidence of SAH from rupture of an aneurysm is approximately 12 per 100,000 population (Heros and Kistler 1983). Roughly 50% of these patients die or become permanently disabled due to the initial bleed. Warning symptoms precede major aneurysmal rupture 40% of the time. Warning symptoms are attributed to expansion of the aneurysm or minor bleed. Enlargment of the aneurysm may produce symptoms of localized headache, cranial nerve palsies (especially third nerve), and visual deficits. A minor bleed can cause a generalized headache, malaise, neck pain, and photophobia. Careful history-taking will assist in identifying the patient at risk for a major bleed.

A major subarachnoid bleed is preceded by a sudden, severe headache, often described by the patient as "explosive" and like no other headache ever experienced.

Visual disturbances, nausea and vomiting, motor deficits, or loss of consciousness may follow the headache. Meningeal irritation from blood in the subarachnoid space causes nuchal rigidity, photophobia, irritability, and low-grade fever. A grading system based on clinical findings is used as a prognostic indicator and as a guide for surgical intervention. See Table 5-4 for the Botterel scale.

Three major complications of ruptured cerebral aneurysms are rebleeding, cerebral vasospasm, and communicating hydrocephalus. According to Jane (1985), the risk of *rebleed* is highest immediately after rupture, diminishes to 30% at 15 days, and stabilizes at 3% per year after 6 months. Rebleed carries significant mortality and morbidity. To prevent rebleed, patients are placed on bedrest in a quiet environment. Blood pressure is controlled with hydralazine hydrochloride (Apresoline), methyldopa (Aldomet), reserpine, or a beta blocker. Aminocaproic acid (Amicar) is an antifibrinolytic agent used to prevent clot lysis. Usual dosage is 24–36 g daily. Potential complications of Amicar, such as dysrhythmias and pulmonary emboli, limit its use.

Jackson (1986) defines *cerebral vasospasm* as the an-

giographically demonstrable narrowing of portions of the arteries comprising the circle of Willis and its major branches. Vasospasm can result in cerebral ischemia and infarction. The exact cause of vasospasm remains unknown, but there is a high correlation between the existence of blood clots around the vessels at the base of the brain and the development of spasm. Clinical deterioration from vasospasm occurs between the fourth and twelfth day after initial bleed (Kim and Tew 1985). Its onset is gradual, with increasing symptomatology depending on the arterial territory. Confusion, disorientation, hemiparesis, or aphasia may be exhibited.

A primary objective in the management of cerebral vasospasm is the prevention of cerebral ischemia, by elevating the cerebral perfusion pressure. This is achieved by expanding intravascular volume and/or using vasopressors to keep the patient hypertensive. These therapies are risky: in the patient whose aneurysm has not been surgically repaired, maintaining the hypervolemic/hypertensive state increases the risk of rebleed. Another treatment modality being studied is the use of calcium channel blockers. Nimodipine, a compound similar in structure to nifedipine, has been found more selective, more potent, and more lipid-soluble than nifedipine. Studies suggest it may benefit patients who manifest cerebral ischemia due to subarachnoid hemorrhage (Kim and Tew 1985).

Communicating hydrocephalus as a complication of subarachnoid hemorrhage can occur with the initial bleed or weeks later. The products of blood breakdown plug the arachnoid villi, preventing the absorption of CSF into the venous sinuses. Hydrocephalus produces a generalized increase in intracranial pressure. Presenting symptoms in the acute stage include changes in level of consciousness and mental status and may progress to respiratory, pupillary, and motor involvement if not recognized. CT scan confirms hydrocephalus. Temporary relief may be obtained by insertion of an ICP monitoring catheter into a ventricle and draining off some CSF. If the situation does not resolve on its own, long-term management requires ventriculoperitoneal shunt.

Diagnosis of Stroke

Patient history is extremely valuable in identifying the onset of symptoms and risk factors. Physical examination may reveal localizing signs, indicating the involved area of the brain.

Occlusive stroke will demonstrate necrotic areas on the CT scan. CT scan will show intracerebral bleeding or blood in the subarachnoid space at the base of the brain indicative of hemorrhagic stroke. Magnetic resonance imaging may be used in the stable patient.

TABLE 5-4 THE BOTTEREL SCALE FOR GRADING RUPTURED CEREBRAL ANEURYSMS

CATEGORY	CRITERIA	SURVIVAL RATE
Grade I (minimal hemorrhage)	Client alert, neurologically intact, with a minimal headache and slight nuchal rigidity	65%
Grade II (mild hemorrhage)	Client alert, with minimal neurologic deficits, such as CN III palsy (eg, ptosis, diplopia), with a mild to severe headache and nuchal rigidity	55%
Grade III (moderate hemorrhage)	Client has definite change in level of consciousness, is drowsy or confused; nuchal rigidity is present, with mild focal deficits	45%
Grade IV (moderate to severe hemorrhage)	Client stuporous or semi-comatose, with mild to severe hemiparesis, nuchal rigidity, and possible early decerebration	30%
Grade V (severe hemorrhage)	Client decerebrate, comatose, with a moribund appearance	5%

Source: Kneisl CR, Ames SW: *Adult health nursing: A biopsychosocial approach.* Menlo Park, CA: Addison-Wesley, 1986, p. 1156.

Cerebral angiography is the definitive diagnostic tool. Visualization of the cerebral vessels, including carotid and vertebrobasilar, will locate an aneurysm, arteriovenous malformation, thrombosis, vascular narrowing, or vasospasm. Angiography is not without risk to the patient. When or when not to do it is a critical decision made by the physician.

Lumbar puncture may be performed as part of the diagnostic workup. If increased intracranial pressure is suspected, it should be done only by an experienced person. Grossly bloody cerebrospinal fluid is suggestive of a hemorrhagic stroke.

Noninvasive blood flow studies such as Doppler imaging, carotid phonoangiography, and oculoplethysmography are also used to diagnose disease in the extracranial vessels. Early recognition of lesions in the carotids can guide therapy and may prevent a stroke from occurring.

Management of Stroke

Medical Management The main goal in the acute phase of stroke is to preserve viable brain tissue. Attention to the basic ABCs is imperative. Measures to prevent hypoxemia and hypercarbia should be instituted. Antihypertensive medications to control the blood pressure may be indicated. Since hypotension may lead to inadequate cerebral perfusion and cause ischemia, the blood pressure should be optimized for the individual. Hyperosmolar drugs and steroids are administered to combat edema and the resultant increased intracranial pressure.

Anticoagulant and antiplatelet aggregation therapy is controversial. It is beneficial in treating patients with TIAs to reduce the risk of further TIAs and subsequent stroke. Obviously, anticoagulant therapy is contraindicated in hemorrhagic stoke. Therefore the challenge faced by the physician is to accurately diagnose the type of stroke. The treatment of stroke caused by emboli should also be directed at the causative factor. Patients who have mitral stenosis and atrial fibrillation or a prosthetic mechanical heart valve should be placed on anticoagulant therapy.

Seizures frequently occur with thrombotic occlusive stroke. Anticonvulsive drugs may be employed prophylactically or when a seizure occurs.

Surgical Management

Carotid Endarterectomy Carotid endarterectomy is the surgical removal of a plaque obstructing the carotid artery. Immediate postoperative concerns are to maintain a patent airway and control the blood pressure.

Bleeding from the operative site may lead to hematoma formation, which compresses the upper airway. The patient should be watched closely for signs indicating airway obstruction. Also, the operative site should be examined for evidence of swelling. The physician should be notified if either occurs.

Manipulation of the carotid body during the surgical procedure causes blood pressure and pulse changes postoperatively. Hypertension should be aggressively controlled to prevent stroke or bleeding at the operative site. On the other hand, hypotension should be avoided, as the hypoperfusion state may also cause stroke. Frequently, these patients are bradycardic. Junctional or ventricular escape beats or ventricular ectopics occur due to the slow rate. Atropine may be necessary to maintain an adequate rate to suppress ectopy.

Neurologic checks should be done and compared to the preoperative assessment. During the operative procedure, stretching of cranial nerves may lead to temporary or permanent deficits. Especially assess the patient for facial drooping, tongue deviation, hoarseness, and the abilities to swallow and turn the head from side to side. Because deteriorating neurologic signs may result from operative complications or an intracranial event, any changes should be documented and the physician notified.

Craniotomy Surgical clipping of the aneurysm, if approachable, is the definitive treatment modality. The operating microscope and improved anesthetic techniques have greatly assisted the surgeon in reducing operative mortality. The operative procedure involves exposing the aneurysm. Then, while using controlled hypotension, the surgeon applies a self-closing spring clip to the neck of the aneurysm. Aneurysms that cannot be clipped may be wrapped with a gauze material and coated with an acrylic substance.

Postoperative nursing care is similar to that for any patient after craniotomy. For specifics, the reader is referred to the section on craniotomy in Chapter 6. Of major concern is neurologic deterioration due to vasospasm. Early recognition and reporting of decreasing LOC or focal deficits optimizes time for discovering the cause and instituting treatment.

The timing of surgery is controversial. Proponents of early surgery, that is, within 48–72 hours of rupture, argue that it: (1) prevents rebleed, (2) allows for removal of extravasated blood from the subarachnoid space, thereby minimizing vasospasm, (3) allows for hypervolemic/hypertensive treatment of vasospasm if it occurs, and (4) reduces the risk of medical complications that occur while waiting for surgery (Kim and Tew 1985).

NURSING DIAGNOSES

The following nursing diagnoses may be utilized to guide patient care for strokes.

- Ineffective airway clearance
- Fluid volume deficit
- Ineffective breathing pattern
- Impaired gas exchange
- Altered cerebral perfusion
- Alteration in comfort: headache, stiff neck, neck pain, photophobia
- Impaired verbal communication
- Sensory-perceptual alteration
- Impaired physical mobility

Planning and Implementation of Care

Stroke patients may present with minimal to severe neurologic dysfunction. The most common clinical presentation is the middle cerebral artery syndrome. Their actual or potential problems range from airway and blood pressure control to sensory-perceptual alterations. Many of the nursing diagnoses related to aeration and fluid balance apply to the stroke patient. These are discussed in the sections on increased intracranial pressure and head trauma, so they will not be repeated here. Instead we will focus on some of the deficits that interfere with the patient's ability to perceive sensory information, communicate, or be physically active.

A sample nursing care plan addressing specific needs of the patient with ruptured cerebral aneurysm is found on p. 102.

Impaired Verbal Communication Related to Cerebral Injury Language is a highly integrated function that involves multiple areas of the brain. The primary centers that control speech are located in the left cerebral hemisphere. *Fluent dysphasia,* a disturbance in Wernicke's area, is a condition in which the patient lacks comprehension of the spoken word and may paraphrase, invent new words, or repeat words over and over. The patient's speech is "fluent" but not related to the conversation. *Nonfluent dysphasia* results from an insult to Broca's area. Comprehension of the spoken word is usually intact, but there is an inability to verbalize. *Dysarthria* is the inability to articulate and phonate due to the primary loss of neuromuscular control of speech. Speech may be slurred and thick or jerky and irregular.

To evaluate the extent of language dysfunction, assess the patient's ability to understand yes/no questions, follow simple verbal directions, follow visual cues, name objects, repeat words, and understand the written word. The speech pathologist is a key person to assist you in communicating effectively with the patient.

When caring for patients with *left hemisphere damage* remember to speak slowly, avoid shouting, keep verbal instructions simple and concise, and use gestures, nonverbal cues and pantomime. Promote language stimulation by naming objects in the environment and encouraging the patient to repeat the names.

Verbal rambling and use of excessive detail characterize the speech of a patient with *right hemisphere damage.*

Sensory-Perceptual Alteration Related to Cerebral Insult Although sensory-perceptual deficits may occur when either hemisphere is involved, they are more pronounced in the patient with a right hemisphere stroke. The right cerebral hemisphere is developed for visual/spatial perception, appreciation of nonverbal information, and music appreciation. Assess the patient's ability to: recognize objects in both visual fields; orient self in space; identify objects by sight, sound, or touch; identify sensations of pain, touch, and temperature; recognize own body parts; and distinguish right from left.

Visual field deficits may occur with right or left hemispheric stoke. Stroke involving the right or left middle cerebral artery may result in homonymous hemianopia (refer to back to Chapter 3 and Figure 3–1). Patients with visual field deficits should be reminded to scan their environment. Place commonly used items on the unaffected side. Position the patient's bed so he or she can see the "action." Be sure the patient does not miss the best part of the meal tray. Impaired sensory interpretation may be handled by presenting the patient with various items to touch while you name them. Sensory-perceptual deficits specific to left hemisphere damage include poor abstract thinking and short attention span. When working with these patients, be precise and concise. Difficulty with visual-spatial relationships, bodily perception and orientation in space, and impaired judgement characterize the patient with a right hemisphere stroke. Reinforce bodily parts to the patient, and distinguish left from right for them. Provide a safe environment and assist them to recognize body position.

Impaired Physical Mobility Related to Neurologic Dysfunction Strokes involving the motor cortex or internal capsule will produce contralateral hemiparesis or hemiplegia. Arm involvement is usually greater than leg involvement. Flaccid paralysis may be evident at first. Since the stroke causes an upper motor neuron

SAMPLE NURSING CARE PLAN

Ruptured Cerebral Aneurysm, Acute Phase

NURSING DIAGNOSIS	SIGNS AND SYMPTOMS	NURSING ACTIONS	DESIRED OUTCOMES

Altered cerebral perfusion related to:
• Ruptured aneurysm
• Increased intracranial pressure
• Cerebral edema
• Vasospasm
• Hydrocephalus
	• Abnormal respiratory pattern:
	  - Cheyne-Stokes
	  - Central hyperventilation
	  - Apneustic
	  - Cluster
	  - Ataxic
	• Elevated P_{CO_2}
	• Decreased P_{O_2}
	• Increased blood pressure
	• Neurologic deficits:
	  - Decreased LOC
	  - Confusion
	  - Agitation
	  - Cranial nerve palsies
	  - Pupil changes
	  - Paresis or paralysis
	  - Abnormal flexion or extension of extremities
	  - Seizure
	• Rhythm and EKG changes
	• Hyperthermia
		1. Establish airway and assess respiratory pattern.
		2. Administer oxygen.
		3. Obtain ABGs.
		4. Monitor vital signs and perform neurologic checks.
		5. Provide for complete bedrest in quiet, nonstimulating environment.
		6. Administer drugs as ordered:
		  • Antihypertensives
		  • Hyperosmolar agents
		  • Steroids
		  • Diuretics (usually Lasix)
		  • Aminocaproic acid
		  • Analgesics
		  • Sedatives
		  • Stool softeners
		  • Laxatives
		7. Notify physician immediately of new or worsening neurologic deficits.
		8. Implement continuous EKG monitoring.
		9. Administer antidysrhythmics as ordered.
		10. Monitor temperature.
		11. Control temperature with antipyretics and/or hypothermia blanket.
		12. Institute seizure precautions.
		13. Administer anticonvulsants as ordered.
			• Normal respiratory pattern
			• ABGs WNL for patient
			• Systolic blood pressure WNL for patient
			• Absence of neurological deterioration
			• Compliance with restricted activities
			• Normal cardiac rhythm
			• Afebrile
			• Absence of seizure activity

Alteration in comfort: headache related to cerebral hemorrhage; stiff neck and pain in neck related to meningeal irritation	• C/o headache and neck pain • Limited movement, and pain on neck flexion	1. Assess headache for severity and location. 2. Administer analgesics as ordered. 3. Evaluate response to analgesics. 4. Avoid undue neck and head movement. 5. Support head when turning.	Verbalizes relief of headache and minimal neck discomfort.
Alteration in comfort: photophobia related to meningeal irritation	• C/o discomfort with bright light • Keeps eyes closed	1. Minimize direct lighting; pull curtains or shades. 2. Limit time taken assessing pupils so as not to prolong direct light in the eye. 3. Provide nightshades if patient desires.	Verbalizes less discomfort.

lesion, reflexes will reappear. Spasticity then becomes a problem. Prevention of contractures and loss of muscle tone is key in rehabilitating the patient to an independent lifestyle. The affected extremities should be passively exercised and put through full range of motion. This activity is the responsibility of not only the physical therapist but the nurse as well. The patient and family should be taught early, since exercising will need to be continued in the home setting. Patients should be taught how to use the stronger extremity to move the weaker. Remind patients to look at their weak extremities and get them in position before moving. Also, instruct patients to maintain their weight on the stronger side while pivoting.

Outcome Evaluation

The patient's progress should be evaluated according to these outcome criteria:

- Expresses needs/feelings
- Understands and follows direction
- Recognizes body parts
- Knows left from right
- Assists with ADLs
- Has motor function that is the same or improved
- Assists with exercising of extremities
- Utilizes adaptive equipment for ADLs and mobility

AUTOIMMUNE DISORDERS

Autoimmune diseases currently are in the forefront of medical research. Several neurologic diseases have autoimmune components, but Guillain-Barré syndrome and myasthenia gravis are the ones most often encountered in the critical-care unit.

Guillain-Barré Syndrome

Guillain-Barré syndrome is a disease of the peripheral nervous system typically characterized by an acute, rapidly progressing, ascending, symmetric motor weakness with associated sensory disturbances. Recovery is spontaneous and may occur within one to several months or can take up to a year or more depending on the extent of nerve involvement. Severity varies widely. If the diaphragm becomes involved, the disease can be life-threatening. The disease has been known variously as Landry-Guillain-Barré-Strohel syndrome, acute polyradiculoneurophathy, infectious polyneuritis, Landry's acute ascending paralysis, ascending transverse myelitis, and schwannosis (Barnes 1984; Griswold and Ropper 1984).

Assessment

Risk Conditions Guillain-Barré syndrome can occur at any age and is nonspecific to gender, race, season, or environment. It is the most common cause of acute weakness in people under age 40 and occurs at the rate of 1.7 per 100,000 population (Miller 1985). The syndrome is more severe in pregnancy and in the young and the elderly (Kneisl and Ames 1986). In 50–65% of cases, viral illness commonly associated with the respiratory or gastrointestinal tract precedes the syndrome by several weeks (Barnes 1984; Jones 1985; Rudy 1984). Less common preceding problems are immunization (swine flu vaccine in 1977), animal bites, and surgery. Guillain-Barré also may occur during the course of lymphoma or systemic lupus erythematosus (Jones 1985). Prompt recognition and intervention has kept the mortality rate at 1.5% (Miller RG 1985). Mortality is usually due to complications from pulmonary or urinary infections and sepsis. Occasionally, deaths may be due to pulmonary embolus, delayed treatment of respiratory failure, or severe hypotension (Griswold and Ropper 1984).

In order to comprehend the progression of Guillain-Barré, one needs to understand normal nerve conduction. The peripheral nerve is an axon enveloped by a myelin, lipid sheath produced by the Schwann cell. Motor and proprioceptive sensory nerves are the most heavily myelinated, with the myelin sheath proportional to the nerve diameter (Griswold and Ropper 1984). The sheath insulates the nerve fiber and limits ion exchanges or impulse conduction along the axon (Guyton 1986). A break in the sheath occurs approximately every millimeter. These nonmyelinated areas, called *nodes of Ranvier,* allow impulses to "jump" along the sheath, resulting in faster impulse conduction than nerve fiber or myelin sheath conduction. This saltatory conduction, jumping along the gaps, also conserves energy by making impulse conduction possible with less ion shifts at the cell membrane (Guyton 1986).

Diffuse, intense inflammation and demyelination of

the peripheral nerves at any level between the nerve's root and distal end is the reason for the progressive muscle weakness. Segmental destruction of myelin between the nodes of Ranvier without axonal destruction is the typical pattern (Griswold and Ropper 1984), but secondary axonal damage does occur in severe cases (Miller RG 1985). The exact mechanism causing the demyelination is unknown. It may be an autoimmune attack on a component of the peripheral myelin sheath mediated by macrophages and possibly by T-cell lymphocytes (Miller RG 1985). Another explanation is that an immune response to several antigens produces a demyelinating antibody that has a direct toxic effect on the nerves or can stimulate an intracellular mechanism that destroys the myelin sheath (Griswold and Ropper 1984).

Signs and Symptoms Typically, symmetric weakness, numbness, and tingling begin in the legs and quickly ascend to the trunk and arms, resulting in a generalized limb weakness usually accompanied by areflexia. Atypical patterns of Guillain-Barré syndrome occur and are summarized in Table 5-5. Pain, skin hypersensitivity (Barnes 1984), or stiffness in the limbs (Griswold and Ropper 1984) is present in about 50% of patients (Miller RG 1985). Two-thirds of the patients experience distal paresthesia in a "glove and stocking" pattern (Jones 1985). Since the cranial nerves are part of the peripheral nervous system, facial weakness, dysphagia, dysarthria, diplopia, ocular paralysis, and papilledema are not uncommon (Miller RG 1985). There usually is a sharp demarcation of sensory level and frequently bowel and bladder problems (Miller RG 1985).

Although all of these symptoms are distressing to the patient, except for dysphagia Guillain-Barré is not life-threatening until the respiratory musculature becomes involved. Serial pulmonary function tests (PFTs) show a gradual or sometimes sudden drop in values for spontaneous and forced vital capacity, inspiratory force, and spontaneous tidal volume. Griswold and Ropper (1984) specify this as the reason Guillain-Barré patients must be monitored in a critical-care unit. Labile autonomic function is another reason for close monitoring. Demyelination of the vagus nerve gives rise to autonomic dysfunction manifested by bradycardia, tachycardia, hypertension, postural hypotension, and/or diaphoresis (Barnes 1984).

Recovery from Guillain-Barré syndrome is spontaneous, and the typical pattern is descending or opposite the pattern of function loss. The extent of underlying axonal damage determines the extent and length of the recovery phase. Recovery can start once deterioration has stopped, usually 1–3 weeks after the onset of

TABLE 5-5 VARIANTS OF GUILLAIN-BARRÉ SYNDROME

VARIANT	CHARACTERISTICS
Ascending (typical)	• Starts in lower extremities • Ascending motor loss • Ascending mild distal sensory loss (stocking and glove paresthesia) • Late respiratory failure in 50% of patients • Facial weakness • DTRs diminished or absent
Descending	• Starts in face or bulbar muscles • Descending motor loss • Distal sensory loss (usually starts in hands) • Early respiratory failure • Ophthalmoplegia occasionally • DTRs diminished or absent
Pure motor	• Same as for Ascending, but without sensory loss • Rare pain problems
Inflammatory cranial neuropathies	• Restricted to cranial nerves (usually CN III) • Diminished or absent reflexes • Diplopia common • Paresthesia of face and tongue • Elevated CSF protein
Miller-Fisher	• Ophthalmoplegia • Areflexia • Profound ataxia • Nonreactive pupils • Rare respiratory involvement • Rare sensory loss • Rare motor deficits
Relapsing or chronic progressive	• Slow, progressive course rather than acute course • Less than 8% of patients have relapse

Source: Griswold K, Ropper AH: An approach to the care of patients with Guillain-Barré syndrome. *Heart Lung* 1984; 13:66–72. Reprinted by permission of the C.V. Mosby Company.

symptoms. A plateau phase of no discernible change can last several days to weeks before improvements are noted. Full recovery correlates with remyelination and axonal regeneration and usually takes 4–6 months but sometimes up to 2 years (Griswold and Ropper 1984).

Diagnostic Procedures Since there is no one cause for Guillain-Barré syndrome, there is no specific test to identify it. Clinical signs and health history are the most important factors (Barnes 1984). However, Guillain-Barré syndrome must be differentiated from other neuromuscular disorders, botulism, hysteria, tick paralysis, and acute toxic neuropathy (Miller RG 1985). Elevated protein with normal cell counts and pressure in cerebrospinal fluid is common but does not occur until 1–2 weeks after the onset of symptoms (Griswold and Ropper 1984). The presence of mononuclear leukocytes in CSF points to Guillain-Barré syndrome, whereas polymorphonuclear leukocytes in CSF are not associated with Guillain-Barré (Miller RG 1985).

Electrophysiology studies reveal nerve conduction velocity decreased by 40% in most Guillain-Barré patients (Jones 1985). The majority of patients exhibit the characteristic changes of segmental slowing in patchy areas of several nerves and multifocal conduction blocks (Miller RG 1985). However, this testing does not correlate well with the severity of clinical symptoms (Griswold and Ropper 1984). Electromyography (EMG) studies do reflect the degree of underlying neuronal damage (Jones 1985). EMG studies demonstrate the muscle's electrical activity and reflect nerve function (Griswold and Ropper 1984). It typically takes 4 weeks or more before any changes are seen (Miller RG 1985). If EMG findings are close to normal, the recovery tends to be quick. When testing shows fibrillation of the muscle, the recovery period is usually prolonged (Jones 1985).

NURSING DIAGNOSES

Guillain-Barré syndrome can be life-threatening when respiratory muscles are involved. Therefore sophisticated nursing management with prompt effective nursing interventions can be life-saving. Pertinent nursing diagnoses for Guillain-Barré syndrome patients include:

- Ineffective airway clearance
- Ineffective breathing pattern
- Inadequate nutrition
- Impaired verbal communication
- Impaired physical mobility
- Impairment of skin integrity
- Potential for infection
- Potential for injury to peripheral muscles and nerves
- Alteration in comfort: pain
- Bowel and bladder dysfunction (altered bowel elimination: incontinence; altered bowel elimination: constipation; total (urinary) incontinence; urinary retention)
- Anxiety, fear, powerlessness
- Ineffective family coping

Planning and Implementation of Care

Ineffective Airway Clearance Related to Respiratory Muscle Weakness As the syndrome progresses and ascending muscle weakness begins affecting the respiratory muscles, the patient will be unable to effectively clear the respiratory tract. Close monitoring for signs of mucus accumulation is necessary to prevent hypoxia, atelectasis, and pneumonia. Listen frequently to breath sounds (anteriorly, laterally, and posteriorly) for signs for compromised air exchange. Suction with aseptic technique to remove secretions when necessary. Encourage deep breathing, holding inspiration, and coughing to prevent atelectasis (Griswold and Ropper 1984). Anticipate intubation if the patient is unable to clear secretions. Keep the physician informed of airway patency.

Ineffective Breathing Pattern Related to Respiratory Muscle Weakness Monitor lung sounds, chest excursion, respiratory muscle activity, and ease of breathing at least every 2 hours (more frequently if changes occur). Perform PFTs every 2 hours and as needed for any change. Be alert to the signs of respiratory failure, e.g., confusion, disorientation, tachycardia, dyspnea; see Chapter 8 for further details. Position the patient for maximal lung expansion: upright, semi-Fowler's, or side positioned with the upper arm off the chest.

Remember, respiratory dysfunction can be either gradual or sudden in these patients. The pregnant Guillain-Barré patient presents a more difficult assessment, especially in the last trimester, when respiratory function is normally diminished. Anticipate intubation when pulmonary function values begin dropping, especially in pregnancy. Also remember that early controlled intubation is less traumatic to the patient than late emergent intubation. Alert the physician to any change in respiratory status.

Inadequate Nutrition Due to Impaired Swallowing Related to Poor Neuromuscular Transmission Adequate intake of essential amino acids, fats, and carbohydrates is mandatory for health maintenance and injury healing. Be aware of the patient's fluid and nutritional status, and notify the physician early of potential needs. This is especially important with severe Guillain-Barré syndrome, which produces neuromuscular dysfunction for several months.

Monitor the swallowing function. Position the patient on his or her side when resting and upright during eating to prevent aspiration. Encourage soft foods instead of liquids, to minimize choking. Monitor the fluid status of patients with low oral intake. Assess gastrointestinal function daily. Anticipate enteral feeding to maintain adequate nutrition and gastrointestinal function. Remember, large feeding tubes are associated with a higher incidence of aspiration. Anticipate total parenteral nutrition therapy when gastrointestinal dysfunction is present.

Impaired Verbal Communication Related to Poor Neuromuscular Transmission When the cranial nerves are involed, the patient may lose the ability to speak, blink the eyes, or move the head to communicate with staff. Effective communication concerning likes, dislikes, comfort positions, effective interventions for pain, and so on *before* the patient becomes uncommunicative will promote consistent, individualized care. If the patient is unable to communicate when admitted to critical care, talk to the family and/or friends to obtain this information. Patients will still be frustrated but may be comforted by the nurses' attempts to make them comfortable. As the patient recovers partial motor ability, different levels of communication can be established, such as blinking the eyes, squeezing the hands, moving the toes, or use of an alphabet board or word list. The patient may develop a unique communication style using whatever gross motor movements he or she possesses. Place a soft-pressure-activated nurse call bell within the patient's limited reach for easy notification. Explain all procedures to the patient before starting. Continually orient the patient to the time of day, the week, the month, and so on. Use television or radio to keep the patient updated to current events. Encourage the family to talk with the patient about everyday family happenings to promote a sense of belonging.

Impaired Physical Mobility Related to Generalized Muscle Weakness Assess motor functions on admission and every shift change thereafter to evaluate the progression of the syndrome. When motor abilities are deteriorating, check motor strength more frequently as needed. Do passive range of motion exercises to maintain joint function and prevent contractures. Reposition every 2 hours or more frequently to prevent pneumonia, skin breakdown, and pressure to peripheral nerves. Monitor extraocular muscle function and suggest eye care to the physician when needed. Rotate eye patch if such is used to treat diplopia. Explore the use of prism glasses to see if vision can be improved.

Impairment of Skin Integrity Loss of mobility, poor nutrition, and inability to communicate physical needs all can lead to skin problems. Timely, proficient cleansing during daily bathing and after incontinence is necessary to prevent skin breakdown. Oral hygiene, skin massage, use of specialized mattresses to decrease pressure areas, and joint protectors are only a few of the interventions available. Hair washing will not only maintain skin integrity but also promote psychologic well-being in the patient. If antiemboli stockings are ordered, remove them every 8 hours for at least 30 minutes.

Potential for Infection Immobility, inadequate nutrition, sequestering of pulmonary secretions, dysphagia with aspiration, steroid therapy, skin breakdown, bowel and bladder dysfunction, and numerous invasive lines are some of the potential causes of infection in Guillain-Barré patients. Monitor closely for signs of local infection from any invasive line. Maintain circulation to the skin and extremities to prevent local hypoxia, tissue destruction, and subsequent opportunistic infection. Observe all drainage from the skin, orifices, and tubes for color or odor changes that suggest infection. Obtain specimens for culture per unit protocol or physician's orders. Evaluate vital signs and general progress for subtle signs of systemic infection. Investigate any areas of tenderness. Maintain current records for dates of invasive-line changes. Notify the physician of any suspicion of infection.

Potential for Injury to Peripheral Muscles and Nerves Related to Immobility and Communication Deficits Range of motion exercises are performed to maintain joint mobility, and frequent repositioning is done to prevent numerous problems. If either of these procedures is done incorrectly, the peripheral muscles and nerves may be damaged. During the acute phase of Guillain-Barré syndrome, active range of motion exercises should be avoided. Active participation and overzealously done passive exercises can stretch the muscles and tendons, causing damage and prolonging recovery. This could also happen while turning the patient with inadequate support to the extremities. Also, active range of motion exercises overzealously done by the recovering patient may tire his or her muscles, prolong recovery, and lead to frustration and depression from perceived "poor progress."

Peripheral nerve damage can prolong recovery periods or cause the permanent loss of function in the affected extremity. Throughout hospitalization, care must be taken to avoid pressure to extremities and joints. This is especially important when the patient is unable to communicate. Using pillows or foam pads to decrease pressure and splints to maintain proper alignment is common.

As activity increases, care should be exercised when

first sitting the patient upright. Postural hypotension may be a problem, especially in patients with autonomic dysfunction. Avoid back-muscle injury from premature chair-sitting with weakened muscles.

Alteration in Comfort: Pain Related to Sensory Nerve Dysfunction Hypersensitivity of the skin is common in the arms, legs, back, and buttocks. Bathing and repositioning become a real challenge because even gentle touch can cause pain. Remember, the paralyzed patient may be unable to communicate the extent of that pain. Mild analgesic agents are usually adequate for pain control. If the patient complains of inadequate pain relief with nonnarcotic analgesics, investigate for a hidden cause of the pain. If no covert cause is found for the unrelieved pain, explore the possibility of a negative psychologic response to the patient's present dependence on others and to prolonged recovery. It may be that the patient prefers the "high" of a narcotic analgesic to the reality of present circumstances.

Bowel and Bladder Dysfunction Related to Autonomic Nervous System Dysfunction Autonomic nervous system dysfunction increases the potential for bowel or bladder incontinence in the acute stage, and for bladder distention or bowel impaction during the recovery phase. Monitor bowel and bladder function closely. Assess frequently for incontinence, and cleanse the skin thoroughly after incontinence. Insert an indwelling catheter per physician's orders in the acute phase. Anticipate bowel and bladder training once the acute phase is over. Be alert to signs of autonomic dysreflexia as this can be life-threatening. (See the section on "Spinal Cord Injuries" in Chapter 21 for information on autonomic dysreflexia.)

Anxiety, Fear, Powerlessness Related to Sudden Debilitating Disease The very nature of a sudden, progressive loss of motor function, inadequate breathing, and communication disability leads to feelings of fear, anxiety, and powerlessness. The fact that no health care provider can quantify the extent of disease or length of recovery only magnifies these feelings. Closely monitor the patient during the acute stage not only for signs of disease progress but also to decrease the patient's anxiety and fear of abandonment. Communicating about normal living activities and keeping the patient advised of current events will promote interest outside the self, thereby helping to distract the patient from any anxiety and fear. Another way to diminish anxiety in the patient undergoing prolonged recovery is to perform daily neurologic checks with the physician, thereby decreasing the number of times per day that the patient is reminded of motor deficits.

As paralysis spreads, the patient's feelings of powerlessness increase. Allowing the patient as much control over daily activities as possible will conteract this. Listen to the patient, encourage verbalization of feelings, and offer moral support. Acknowledge improvements, and emphasize that function will return with time and physical therapy.

Ineffective Family Coping Related to Sudden Debilitating Disease The patient's family is usually shocked by the sudden, progressive loss of function in their loved one. Active listening, close monitoring, and emphasizing the expected regain of function should help. If the patient is the main source of income for the family, additional worries of financial concern may produce feelings of frustration, possibly manifested as anger toward the health care providers for not making the patient better faster. For patients undergoing prolonged recovery, there is significant disruption of family life. Active listening to the family will alert the nurse to problems that may need intervention. Collaboration with the physician and social worker about immediate and long-term needs early in the patient's hospitalization will promote open communication and trust.

The majority of the treatment for Guillain-Barré syndrome is supportive and symptomatic. Thus, the nurse and physician plan the patient's care with the goals of early recognition, prevention of potential problems, and minimizing the impact of the symptoms.

Some therapies are controversial. Steroids have been used, but there are no data to support their efficacy (Jones 1985). Furthermore, some experts believe that corticosteroids prolong recovery and increase the chance of relapse (Miller RG 1985). Recently, plasma exchange has been used during the acute phase, with some dramatic improvements noted. However, no consistent guidelines for use have been established (Miller RG 1985).

Outcome Evaluation

Desirable outcome criteria for Guillain-Barré syndrome patients are:

- Return to previous level of sensorimotor function
- Vital signs within normal limits for the patient
- Verbalization of fears and anxiety
- Prevention of complications during disease process

Myasthenia Gravis

Myasthenia gravis is a progressive, deteriorating autoimmune disease involving the postsynaptic membrane of the myoneural junction. The occurrence of myasthenic or cholinergic crisis is the usual reason for admission to critical care. During crisis, the patient is unable to breathe due to either inadequate neuromuscular transmissions (myasthenic crisis) or to overstimulation by neuromuscular transmittors and resultant muscle fatigue (cholinergic crisis). Without immediate intervention, the patient will die of respiratory failure.

Assessment

Risk Conditions Myasthenia gravis can strike a person of any age or gender, although two-thirds of stricken women are under 40 and two-thirds of stricken men are over 40 (Herrmann 1985). No specific genetic link has been found, but familial frequency has been noted (Herrmann 1985). A transient form has been noted in neonates of myasthenic mothers. No racial or geographic determinants have been discovered (Seybold 1986). Factors precipitating the onset or exacerbation of the disease include bright sunlight, heat, emotional stress, initiation of corticosteroid therapy, infection, surgery, menses, pregnancy, thyrotoxicosis, and inadequate medication or overmedication.

Sign and Symptoms Myasthenia gravis is characterized by intermittent, abnormal skeletal muscle fatigue that increases with activity and partially reverses with rest. The cause of the muscle weakness is believed to be an autoimmune process.

Normally the myelinated nerve branches stimulate muscle fibers by releasing neurotransmittors across the neuromusculor junction. The terminal end of the nerve on a skeletal muscle is called the *end-plate*. This end-plate burrows into the muscle fiber, creating a synaptic trough and cleft, the space between the nerve and muscle. The neurotransmittor acetylcholine is released from the nerve's terminal vesicles into the synaptic cleft and stimulates the muscle fiber membrane at specific receptor sites (Guyton 1986). Each receptor site is formed by glycoprotein subunits: two alpha and three other types (see Figure 5-6). The alpha-subunits contain the acetylcholine binding sites (Seybold 1986). These receptor sites surround ion-specific channels that open and allow the influx of sodium and calcium ions to enter the muscle and cause depolarization. Acetylcholine is then rapidly destroyed by acetylcholinesterase to prevent further muscle depolarization (Guyton 1986). The acetylcholine receptor sites are regularly removed by endocytosis every 6–13 days and replaced with new receptor sites (Seybold 1986).

The problems in myasthenia are that the receptor sites are destroyed more rapidly than they are replaced and the synaptic cleft is deformed and widened. Several theories currently explain the autoimmune process believed to cause this destruction. Antibodies attach to the acetylcholine binding site or other areas of the receptor site and prevent normal binding or opening of the ion channel (Seybold 1986). The antibody may cross-link with the receptor site and increase the rate of receptor degradation, resulting in too few receptor sites to propagate depolarization (Seybold 1986). Complement-mediated focal lysis of the acetylcholine binding sites may be the cause (Herrmann 1985). Thus, neurotransmission is unsuccessful, especially after repeated nerve impulses (Herrmann 1985). Weakness appears to be proportional to the amount of receptor site loss (Seybold 1986).

Onset of symptoms may be sudden or gradual, and their severity varies during the day and from day to day. There are numerous classifications (see Table 5-6), since the course of the disease is unpredictable and spontaneous remissions do occur. It may begin with ocular symptoms and may or may not progress to generalized weakness; or the disease may manifest itself with generalized weakness of mild to moderate severity. Neurologic deficits such as sensory loss, coordination problems, and abnormal reflexes are not associated with myasthenia gravis (Seybold 1986).

The initial symptoms are usually ocular, diplopia and ptosis. Pupillary reaction remains normal. Progression is manifested by facial weakness, loss of expression, and a nasal twang to speech. One characteristic is a snarl when attempting to smile (Jones 1985). There is weak chewing and swallowing with nasal regurgitation, which can lead to weight loss (Kess 1984) or aspiration (Seybold 1986). The mouth hangs open, and it is difficult to hold the head erect due to weak neck flexor muscles (Jones 1985). Intermittent dyspnea or increases in dyspnea herald respiratory muscle involvement. Extremity-muscle involvement is mostly proximal, but distal involvement is present (Jones 1985). Shoulder girdle weakness is manifested by difficulty in combing hair or shaving (Seybold 1986). Lower-limb muscle weakness is seen in difficulty in climbing stairs or in rising from a seated position (Kess 1984) or as sudden falls (Seybold 1986). There is no associated muscle atrophy or muscular pain (Kess 1984). Since stress is the precipitating factor in approximately 30% of cases, a psychiatric diagnosis such as depression, hypochondriasis, or hysteria is not uncommon and can be life-threatening (Kess 1984). These diagnoses seem to

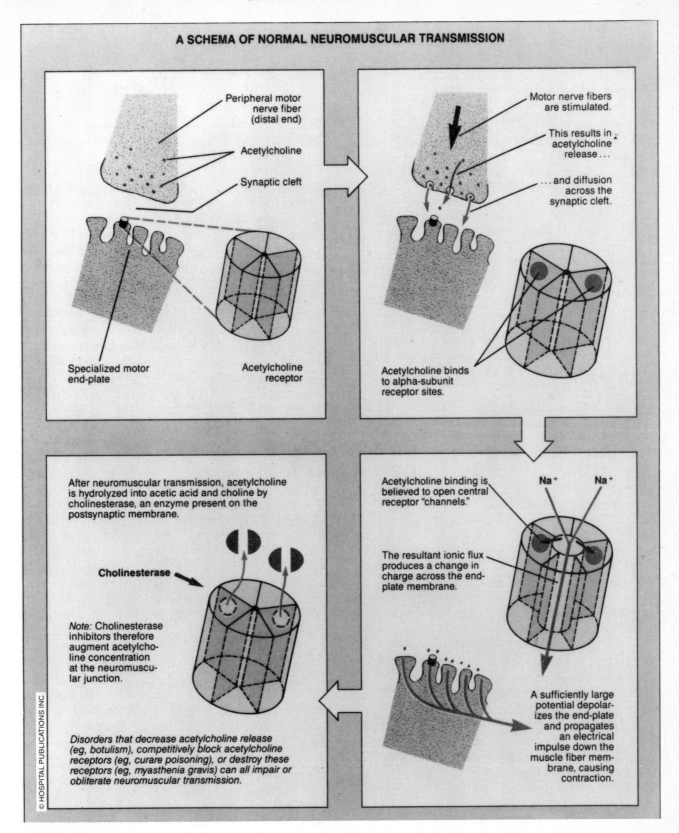

A SCHEMA OF NORMAL NEUROMUSCULAR TRANSMISSION

Peripheral motor nerve fiber (distal end)

Acetylcholine

Synaptic cleft

Specialized motor end-plate

Acetylcholine receptor

Motor nerve fibers are stimulated.

This results in acetylcholine release . . .

. . . and diffusion across the synaptic cleft.

Acetylcholine binds to alpha-subunit receptor sites.

After neuromuscular transmission, acetylcholine is hydrolyzed into acetic acid and choline by cholinesterase, an enzyme present on the postsynaptic membrane.

Cholinesterase

Note: Cholinesterase inhibitors therefore augment acetylcho-line concentration at the neuromuscu-lar junction.

Disorders that decrease acetylcholine release (eg, botulism), competitively block acetylcholine receptors (eg, curare poisoning), or destroy these receptors (eg, myasthenia gravis) can all impair or obliterate neuromuscular transmission.

Acetylcholine binding is believed to open central receptor "channels."

Na$^+$ Na$^+$

The resultant ionic flux produces a change in charge across the end-plate membrane.

A sufficiently large potential depolar-izes the end-plate and propagates an electrical impulse down the muscle fiber mem-brane, causing contraction.

© HOSPITAL PUBLICATIONS INC.

FIGURE 5-6

A Schema of Normal Neuromuscular Transmission From Seybold ME: Myasthenia Gravis. *Hosp Med* (May) 1986; 143. © 1986 Reproduced from *Hospital Medicine* May 1986, with permission of Hospital Publications, Inc.

TABLE 5-6 CLASSIFICATIONS OF MYASTHENIA GRAVIS

TYPE	CHARACTERISTICS
Ocular	• Cranial nerves III, IV, VI involvement • Only extraocular movements affected • Visual disturbances
Generalized Mild	• General muscle involvement • No respiratory involvement • Slow onset
Moderate	• General muscle involvement • Bulbar* and respiratory involvement • Gradual onset
Acute fulmi- nating	• Severe bulbar involvement • Early respiratory involvement • General muscle involvement • Rapid onset
Neonatal	• Bulbar involvement • Generalized weakness • Transient in 20% maternal myasthenia • Spontaneous improvement after one month
Congenital	• Structural abnormality at neuromuscular junction • No evidence of autoimmune disease or maternal myasthenia • Rare
Drug-induced	• Penicillamide • Trimethadione • Phenytoin

*Bulbar = swallowing and respiratory muscle involvement.

occur more frequently with young women (Kess 1984).

Crisis is characterized by severe muscle weakness that interferes with the patient's ability to maintain a patent airway. This may be due to difficulty in clearing secretions, inadequate air exchange, or both (Herrmann 1985). Whether the cause is myasthenic or cholinergic crisis, the initial treatment is the same: maintain a patent airway and support ventilation (Adams et al. 1984).

Older patients in a more fragile state of health are more likely to experience crisis than the younger myasthenic patient (Getting Myasthenic Patients 1986). Crisis is also common in summer heat (Jones 1985). Other precipitating factors include infections, emotional stress, cardiovascular or pulmonary problems, recent initiation or withdrawal of corticosteroids, drug interactions, alcohol intake, and pregnancy (Jones 1985; Getting Myasthenic Patients 1986).

Myasthenic crisis occurs in the severe myasthenia patient who is either not under treatment, receiving inadequate medications, or drug resistant (Adams et al. 1984). Signs and symptoms may be subtle at first, with no obvious respiratory distress and normal arterial blood gases. Usual signs of respiratory distress such as nasal flaring and accessory muscle use may not be present. Apprehension and insomnia may be the first signs of problems. Eventually chest excursion and air movement will diminish. Dysphagia, dysarthria, dysphonia, and pooled secretions increase the risk of aspiration. Respiratory insufficiency becomes obvious very late, and apnea may be sudden (Kess 1984).

Cholinergic crisis is caused by an overdose of anticholinergic medication due to either overmedication or secondary to occasional remissions (Adams et al. 1984). Signs of cholinergic overmedication can be muscarinic or nicotinic (Hickey 1986). Muscarinic signs include excessive secretions (salivation, tearing, diaphoresis) and pulmonary abdominal cramping, blurred vision, diarrhea, dyspnea, pulmonary edema, and bowel or bladder incontinence (Kess 1984). Nicotinic signs are demonstrated by muscle fasciculations, twitching, and cramps resulting in fatigue, weakness, and paralysis (Hickey 1986). Thus, except for excessive secretions, the weak, dyspneic patient in cholinergic crisis does not look different from the weak, dyspneic patient in myasthenic crisis. It is the physiologic cause that is different and demands different treatment for successful resolution.

Diagnostic Procedures Injection of 2–10 mg edrophonium chloride (Tensilon) is the classic test for myasthenia gravis (Jones 1985). It is a short-acting anticholinesterase that blocks the breakdown of acetylcholine (Rudy 1984). With more acetylcholine to stimulate receptor sites, a transient increase in muscle strength is noted within 5 minutes (Jones 1985). The test also may be used to differentiate myasthenic from cholinergic crisis. If the patient improves after a cautious injection of Tensilon, it is considered a myasthenic crisis; if the patient shows no improvement or symptoms worsen, it is considered a cholinergic crisis (Adams et al. 1984).

Repetitive electrical stimulation of a nerve shows an initial decrease in muscle response by the second stimulation. By the fifth electrical stimulation, this has fully developed to a drop of 8–10% from the initial muscle response (Jones 1985). Single-fiber electromyography (EMG) measures the time-interval difference between the action potentials of two single, adjacent muscle fibers when their common nerve is stimulated. This difference normally is constant. Variability in the time intervals produces "jitters" on the EMG. The jitters are significantly increased in myoneural junction disorders (Herrmann 1985).

Serum studies show an elevated number of acetylcholine receptor antibodies in myasthenia gravis. They do not correlate with the clinical course and may be normal in some patients (Herrmann 1985). Other abnormal serum tests may include sedimentation rates, antinuclear antibodies, thyroid function studies, and creatine phosphokinase (Rudy 1984).

Thymomas are present in 15% of myasthenia patients and are diagnosed by chest x-rays, mediastinal tomography, and, recently, magnetic resonance imaging (Mulder et al. 1986). Serum striated-muscle antibodies are present in 95–100% of patients with thymomas (Herrmann 1985).

NURSING DIAGNOSES

Some of the nursing diagnoses appropriate to myasthenia gravis and the life-threatening nature of crisis include:

- Ineffective airway clearance
- Ineffective breathing pattern
- Impaired verbal communication
- Impaired swallowing
- Potential for infection
- Activity intolerance
- Impaired physical mobility
- Sensory-perceptual alteration: vision
- Potential for injury
- Bladder and bowel dysfunction
- Ineffective coping
- Knowledge deficit

Planning and Implementation of Care

Ineffective Airway Clearance and Breathing Pattern Related to Respiratory Muscle Dysfunction These problems are the reason most myasthenia patients are admitted to critical-care units. Closely monitor for respiratory insufficiency. Assess lung expansion, pulmonary function, and breath sounds every 2 hours–or more frequently with changing values. Pulmonary secretions are a problem for two reasons. Anticholinesterase drugs increase secretions. Cholinergic crisis will further increase secretions, which the patient is unable to clear, since the patient cannot cough and deep breathe. Perform chest physiotherapy and suction audible secretions as needed. Monitor pulmonary function tests: respiratory rate and depth, vital capacity, tidal volume, and inspiratory force. Check vital

capacity by having the patient take a deep breath and count for as long as possible before taking another breath. Normally, counting reaches 40 to 50 (Kess 1984). Assess for subtle signs of muscle weakness, since early signs of respiratory insufficiency may not be present (Kess 1984). Anticipate a decrease in pulmonary function with the initiation of or withdrawal from steroid therapy. Give anticholinesterase medications on time. Being even 5 minutes late may decrease the blood level, increase muscle weakness, and exacerbate existing pulmonary problems because of rapid drug metabolism (Noroian 1986). Be aware of drugs that exacerbate myasthenia (see Table 5-7). Listen to the patient, who is the expert and can warn you of impending crisis. Anticipate respiratory arrest, intubation, and mechanical ventilatory support as pulmonary status deteriorates.

TABLE 5-7   DRUGS THAT MAY EXACERBATE MYASTHENIA GRAVIS*

Steroids

Antibiotics

Cardiovascular Drugs
   Quinidine
   Class I antiarrhythmics
   Beta-blockers
   Trimethaphan

Anticonvulsants
   Phenytoin
   Diphenylhydantoin (theoretically)
   Ethosuximide
   Trimethadione toxicity
   Magnesium sulfate (toxemia)

Psychotropic agents
   Chlorpromazine
   Lithium carbonate
   Amitriptyline

Narcotic Analgesics

Ophthalmic Solutions
   Timolol
   Ecothiopate

General anesthetics

Neuromuscular blocking agents

Antirheumatic Agents

Miscellaneous
   Thyroid replacement
   Sodium lactate solutions
   Diuretics
   Muscle relaxants (possible)
   CNS depressants
   Antimalaria drugs
   Quinine

*Partial list.

Adapted from Adams SL et al.: Drugs that may exacerabate myasthenia gravis. *Ann Emerg Med* 1984; 13:532–538.

Impaired Verbal Communication Related to Poor Neuromuscular Transmission Dysphonia may be an early, subtle sign of impending crisis. Be alert to changes in the patient's speech pattern, which can vary from nasal quality to an imperceptible whisper. Request other staff familiar with the patient to corroborate any suspected changes. Encourage the patient to develop and use an individual means of communication with staff. Detail the communication system in the Kardex for other staff members to use. Talk to the patient, and keep him or her informed of all procedures, plans of action, and current events. Allow the patient plenty of time to speak. Have the patient use a radio for orientation to current events, since diplopia interferes with reading and with watching television.

Impaired Swallowing Related to Poor Neuromuscular Transmission Dysphagia should alert the nurse to the potential for aspiration and impending respiratory arrest. Encourage the largest food intake in the morning, to coincide with the normal time of maximal muscle strength. Administer medications 1 hour before meals for best muscle strength. Assist eating by providing mechanically soft foods that require less work to consume. Suggest small amounts of food with frequent rest periods. Be ready to reheat food so it remains appetizing. Encourage liquids to maintain fluid balance. To improve swallowing ability, trigger the swallow reflex with liquids or hot food (Noroian 1986). Keep the patient in high Fowler's position during meals to reduce the chance of aspiration. If the patient is unable to swallow, suction as needed and/or catch pooled secretions with a towel (change frequently). Anticipate use of enteral feeding tubes to maintain nutritional status when oral intake is inadequate.

If the patient enters critical care debilitated from previous nutritional deficits, anticipate total parenteral nutrition to prevent muscle wasting and increased potential for infection. Follow standard precautions and unit protocols when using enteral or parenteral feedings.

Potential for Infection Related to Poor Nutrition, Communication Impairment, Muscle Weakness, Medications, and Invasive Maneuvers Myasthenia gravis patients are bombarded by a multitude of factors that increase their potential for infection. Immunosuppressive agents and steroids are frequently used in the treatment of myasthenia and more recently in the treatment of crisis (Seybold 1986). Recent thymectomy or current plasma exchange also heighten the chance of infection (Noroian 1986). Poor respiratory function and pooled secretions increase the potential for pneumonia. Poor nutrition diminishes the body's normal mechanisms of defense.

Assess the patient, including sites of all invasive lines and any drainage, for signs of infection every 4 hours or more frequently as needed. Alert the physician to any suspicion of infection. Replace all suspicious lines per physician's orders or unit protocol. Use common infection control techniques. Wash your hands between patients. Use meticulous sterile technique when needed. Reposition the patient every 1–2 hours to prevent skin breakdown and pneumonia.

Activity Intolerance Related to Neuromuscular Dysfunction Schedule the patient's activities to coincide with maximal muscle strength. Plan the heaviest activity in the morning, and allow periodic rest periods. Suggest rest periods for after medication administration. The patient then benefits from the effects of both rest and peak drug effect before engaging in activity. Encourage self-care as much as possible. Assist the fatigued patient. Convey signs of improvement.

Impaired Physical Mobility Related to Neuromuscular Dysfunction During crisis, patients are either partially or fully paralyzed until their medications are adjusted to their individual needs. Assess motor functions on admission and every shift change thereafter to evaluate progress. When motor abilities are deteriorating, check motor strength more frequently. Do passive range of motion exercises to maintain joint function and prevent contractures. Reposition every 2 hours or more frequently to prevent pneumonia and skin breakdown.

Sensory-Perceptual Alteration in Vision Related to Neuromuscular and Cranial Nerve Dysfunctions Ocular symptoms are frequently the initial signs of myasthenia gravis. During crisis, patients have ptosis, diminished eye movements, eye deviation, or inability to open the eyes. Assess visual acuity and EOMs. Keep the patient informed of what you are doing. Try experimenting with various methods aimed at restoring the patient's sight. If a patient is unable to open the eyes, tape one eye open while you are present. (Taping both eyes open would result in diplopia.) For the patient who can open the eyes, manage the problem of diplopia with eye patches. Alternate the patch to prevent eye strain. Anticipate use of artificial tears with incomplete lid closure to prevent corneal damage. Use glasses with an eyelid crutch, when available, for patients unable to open their eyes (Noroian 1986).

Potential for Injury Related to Trauma Assess the patient for skin breakdown or hidden fractures secondary to sudden falls. Anticipate the possible need for support during walking, when increasing activity, or when medications or dosages are changed. Encourage the patient to continue activity. Remind the patient of progress when exhibited.

Bladder and Bowel Dysfunction Related to Medications or Neuromuscular Dysfunction Remember, bowel and bladder incontinence can be signs of cholinergic crisis. Anticipate reduction or discontinuance of anticholinesterase medications. Investigate other causes. Maintain hygiene with immediate, thorough skin cleansing.

Ineffective Individual Coping Related to Acute and/or Chronic Disease Deteriorating pulmonary function is the primary reason for anxiety in crisis patients. Diplopia, dysphonia and dysarthria, misdiagnosis prior to hospitalization, and fear of the unknown could also be causes. Due to facial muscle weakness, the patient does not look anxious. This calm appearance can lead the health care professional to disbelieve the anxious patient. Sensing this disbelief, the patient becomes more anxious. Explain everything you do and plan to do for the patient in a calm, confident manner. Repeated hospitalizations and lifestyle changes also can cause anxiety and feelings of vulnerability. Active listening may clue the nurse into possible interventions.

Myasthenia gravis disrupts a person's normal lifestyle. In crisis, it places the formerly independent person in a position of complete dependence on health care professionals. Assess the patient's psychologic adjustment to the disease. Evaluate whether the patient is in the shock, denial, anger, depression, or acceptance stage (see Chapter 3). Look for clues such as forgetting to take medication, delaying physician referral until symptoms are severe, refusing to curtail activity, or complaining of poor medical care. Having the newly diagnosed myasthenia patient talk with a longer-diagnosed, independent patient could decrease uncertainty and facilitate coping. Adjusting to a new self-image (e.g., expressionless face, scars from surgery, and steroid changes) may take months or years. The nurse can help by directing the patient to supportive outpatient services.

Knowledge Deficit: Disease Process How long the patient has had myasthenia and how well he or she has accepted the diagnosis will determine how much teaching the nurse needs to do. Remember, the patient must at least partially accept the reality of lifestyle changes before teaching can be effective. Including the family or close friends in such teaching is important, because it promotes the family unit, keeps the patient from feeling alone, and is a more efficient use of teaching time. Discuss the signs and symptoms of myasthenic and cholinergic crisis, medication side effects and potential interactions, precipitating factors, and emergency procedures. Practical information on coughing and deep breathing exercises, sighing, chest physiotherapy, suctioning, circumventing swallowing problems, and the care of feeding tubes or tracheostomy will help the patient and family cope with the problems of chronic illness.

Supply written material for future reference. In fact, reading about the disease may be the patient's first step toward acceptance. Stress the need to wear a medic-alert tag to speed emergency care. Encourage the patient and family to contact the Myasthenia Gravis Foundation.

The treatment of myasthenia is control of symptoms. The patient must understand that no drug will completely restore muscle strength (Kess 1984). Traditionally, control has been accomplished with anticholinesterase medications. Pyridostigmine bromide, neostigmine bromide, and ambenonium chloride are those most frequently used (Seybold 1986). Medications must be tailored to the individual patient to control symptoms and prevent cholinergic side effects. When patients are unable to tolerate the cholinergic side effects, atropine is sometimes included. The nurse should be alert to the fact that atropine will mask the symptoms of cholinergic toxicity.

Thymectomy is performed on any patient with thymoma. Although recently promoted as a therapeutic measure, thymectomy in patients without thymomas is highly controversial. The rationale is that there is an assumed thymus gland role in antibody formation and removal of the thymus gland leads to improvement in some patients. In one center a 51% remission rate and a 36% improvement in status was achieved (Mulder et al. 1986).

Another controversial recent therapy is plasma exchange. It has been used for ventilator-dependent patients, for patients on the brink of crisis (Herrmann 1985), and preoperatively to improve the patient's status (Seybold 1986). Some correlation has been noted between the decline in antibody titer and the dramatic improvement of symptoms (Gracey et al. 1984a). Three to five exchanges, each removing 2–4 liters, are usually done over 8–10 days (Gracey et al. 1984a). Frequently, immunosuppressive agents are used adjunctively to prolong the short-term improvement produced by the exchange (Gracey et al. 1984a).

Corticosteroids are used as an adjunct to anticholinesterase medications when the latter have been unsuccessful (Seybold 1986). In myasthenia patients, steroids have the unique effect of transiently increasing weakness whenever started, increased, or withdrawn

(Herrmann 1985). Intensive high-dose therapy versus gradually increased low-dose therapy are currently being debated as the best initial approach. Intensive-therapy patients must be monitored in the hospital during the first 2–3 weeks (Herrman 1985). Most authorities agree that maintenance with a moderate dosage every other day for several months followed by a tapered decrease in dosage to a lower level is applicable for all but the most severe patients. Most patients remain on alternate-day prednisone therapy indefinitely.

Azathioprine, another immunosuppressive agent, has been used in patients unable to take steroids or as an adjunct to medications (Seybold 1986) and more recently to plasma exchange (Gracey et al. 1984a). As with all immunosuppressive therapy, the risk of infection is increased. Other side effects include alopecia and liver toxicity (Seybold 1986). Other therapies less frequently utilized include cyclophosphamide, gamma globulin, antilymphocyte antiserum, and splenic or whole-body radiation (Seybold 1986).

Outcome Evaluation

Outcome criteria appropriate for the patient with myasthenia gravis include:

- Ability to clear airway and maintain normal breathing
- Normal communication abilities
- Adequate nutritional status
- Lack of infection
- Established schedule to maintain self-care with minimal muscle fatigue
- Near-normal mobility
- Regain of visual acuity with or without supportive devices
- Return of normal bowel and bladder function
- Diminished anxiety and improved coping mechanisms
- Knowledge of disease, medications, and available support

REFERENCES

Acute weakness. *Emerg Med* (Oct) 1984; 16:80–84, 88–92, 94–96.

Adams SL et al.: Drugs that may exacerbate myasthenia gravis. *Ann Emerg Med* 1984; 13:532–538.

A last resort for seizures. *Emerg Med* (Oct) 1985; 17:47–48.

Alspach JG, Williams SM: *Core curriculum for critical care nursing.* Philadelphia: Saunders, 1985.

Anderson D et al.: 119 days in the ICU: Nursing Buster back from the brink. *RN* (Jan) 1985; 48:30–36.

Barnes PH: Guillain-Barré syndrome. *Crit Care Nurse* (Jan/Feb) 1984; 4:68–71.

Beyerman K: Bring back the dream lady . . . *Am J Nurs* 1986; 86:1034.

Bohannon RW, Dubuc WE: Documentation of the resolution of weakness in a patient with Guillain-Barré syndrome: A clinical report. *Phys Ther* 1984; 64:1388–1389.

Boortz-Marx R: Factors affecting intracranial pressure: A descriptive study. *J Neurosurg Nurs* 1985; 17:89–94.

Bruya MA: Planned periods of rest in the intensive care unit: Nursing care activities and intracranial pressure. *J Neurosurg Nurs* 1981; 13:184–194.

Cline B, and Fisher M: The patient with a seizure disorder. In Rudy E (ed): *Advanced neurological and neurosurgical nursing,* pp. 320–344. St Louis: Mosby, 1984.

Conomy JP: Management of patients with intractable seizures. *Postgrad Med* 1985; 77:138, 140, 142.

Dau PC: Respiratory failure in myasthenia gravis: Use of plasmapheresis. *Chest* 1984; 85:721–722.

de la Monte SM et al.: Risk factors for the development and rupture of intracranial berry aneurysms. *Am J Med* 1985; 78:957–964.

Edwards R: Maternal Guillain-Barré syndrome. *J Neurosurg Nurs* 1984; 16:306–312.

Eisner FR et al.: Efficacy of a "standard" seizure workup in the emergency department. *Ann Emerg Med* (Jan) 1986; 15:33–39.

Gary R et al.: Stroke: How to contain the damage. *RN* (May) 1986a; 49:36–42.

Gary R et al.: Stroke: How to start the long road back. *RN* (June) 1986b; 49:49–55.

Getting myasthenic patients through a crisis. *Emerg Med* 1986; 18:110, 112–113.

Goetter W: Nursing diagnoses and interventions with the acute stroke patient. *Nurs Clin North Am* 1986; 21:309–319.

Gorelick PB: Cerebrovascular disease: Pathophysiology and diagnosis. *Nurs Clin North Am* 1986; 21:275–288.

Gracey DR et al.: Plasmaphoresis in the treatment of ventilator-dependent myasthenia gravis patients: Report of four cases. *Chest* 1984a; 85:739–743.

Gracey DR et al.: Postoperative respiratory care after thymectomy in myasthenia gravis: a 3-year experience in 53 patients. *Chest* 1984b; 86:67–71.

Grant L: Hydrocephalus: An overview and update. *J Neurosurg Nurs* 1984; 16:313–318.

Griswold K, Ropper AH: An approach to the care of patients with Guillain-Barré syndrome. *Heart Lung* 1984; 13:66–72.

Guyton AC: *Textbook of medical physiology,* 7th ed. Philadelphia: Saunders, 1986.

Habermann-Little B: Research shorts: Therapeutic touch and tension headaches. *J Neurosci Nurs* 1986; 18:302.

Hartshorn JC: Aneurysm! Keeping your patient alive until surgery. *RN* (Jan) 1984; 47:30–33.

Hartshorn JC, Hartshorn EA: Nursing interventions for anticonvulsant drug interactions. *J Neurosci Nurs* 1986; 18:250–255.

Heros RC, Kistler JP: Intracranial arterial aneurysm: An update. *Stroke* 1983; 18:1–5.

Herrmann C Jr.: Myasthenia gravis—Current concepts. Clinical conference, *West J Med* 1985; 142:797–809.

Hickey JV: *The clinical practice of neurological and neurosurgical nursing.* Philadelphia: Lippincott, 1986.

Horner AJ, Mechsner WK: Bedside insertion of ICP monitoring devices. *Crit Care Nurse* (July–Aug) 1985; 5:21–27.

Jackson LO: Cerebral vasospasm after an intracranial aneurysmal subarachnoid hemorrhage: A nursing perspective. *Heart Lung* 1986; 15:14–21.

Jane JA et al.: The natural history of aneurysms and arteriovenous malformations. *J Neurosurg* 1985; 62:321–323.

Johnson M, Quinn J: The subarachnoid screw. *Am J Nurs* 1977; 77:448–450.

Jones HR Jr.: Diseases of the peripheral motor-sensory unit. *Clin Symposia* 1985; 37(2):2–32.

Kasuya A, Holm K: Pharmacologic approach to ischemic stroke management. *Nurs Clin North Am* 1986; 21:289–296.

Kenning I et al.: Upright patient positioning in the management of intracranial hypertension. *Surg Neurol* 1981; 15:148–152.

Kess R: Suddenly in crisis: Unpredictable myasthenia. *Am J Nurs* 1984; 84:994–998.

Kim LYS, Tew JM: Saccular aneurysms, subarachnoid hemorrhage, and the timing of surgery. *Heart Lung* 1985; 14:68–74.

Kneisl CR, Ames S: The client with nervous system dysfunction. Unit 6 in *Adult health nursing: A biopsychosocial approach.* Menlo Park, CA: Addison-Wesley, 1986.

Lipe HP, Mitchell PH: Positioning the patient with intracranial hypertension: How turning and head rotation affect the internal jugular vein. *Heart Lung* 1980; 9:1031–1037.

Lovely M, Ozuna J: Status epilepticus. In *The critically ill neurosurgical patient*, Nikas D (ed). New York: Churchill Livingstone, 1982.

Lundberg N: Continuous recording and control of ventricular fluid pressure in neurosurgical practice. *Acta Psychiatr Neural Scand* 1960; 36 (Supplement 149):7–12.

Mauldin R, Coleman L: Intracerebral herniation. *J Neurosurg Nurs* 1983; 15: 287–290.

McGillicuddy JE: Cerebral protection: Pathophysiology and treatment of increased intracranial pressure. *Chest* (Jan) 1985; 87:85–93.

Meldrum B: Neuropathology and pathophysiology. In *A textbook of epilepsy*, Laidlaw J, Richens A (eds). New York: Churchill Livingstone, 1976.

Meldrum B, Brierly J: Prolonged epileptic seizures in primates. *Arch Neurol* 1973; 28:10–17.

Miller JD: Intracranial pressure monitoring. *Arch Neurol* 1985; 42:1191–1193.

Miller RG: Guillain-Barré syndrome: Current methods of diagnosis and treatment. *Postgrad Med* (May) 1985; 77:57–59, 62–64.

Mitchell PH: Intracranial pressure: Dynamics, assessment and control. Chapter 2 in *The critically ill neurosurgical patient*, Nikas D (ed). New York: Churchill Livingstone, 1982.

Mitchell PH et al.: Moving the patient in bed: Effects on intracranial pressure. *Nurs Res* 1981; 30:212–218.

Mulder DG et al.: Thymectomy: Surgical procedure for myastenia gravis. *AORN* 1986; 43:640–646.

Muwaswes M: Increased intracranial pressure and its systemic effects. *J Neurosurg Nurs* 1985; 17:238–243.

Noroian EL: Myasthenia gravis: A nursing perspective. *J Neurosurg Nurs* 1986; 18:74–80.

Nurses' Drug Alert: Seizure and mania due to high aspartame intake? *Am J Nurs* 1986; 86:1145.

Oertel LB: The dilemma of cerebral vasospasm treatment. *J Neurosurg Nurs* 1985; 17:7–13.

O'Neill S: Dealing with seizures. *RN* (Sept) 1984; 47:39–41.

Parsons L, Wilson M: Cerebrovascular status of severe closed head injured patients following passive position changes. *Nurs Res* (March/April) 1984; 33:68–75.

Peck S: Calcium blocking agents for treatment of cerebral vasospasm. *J Neurosurg Nurs* 1983; 15:123–126.

Plum F, Posner JB: *The diagnosis of stupor and coma.* Philadelphia: Davis, 1980.

Price MP: Significance of intracranial pressure waveform. *J Neurosurg Nurs* 1981; 13:202–206.

Rich J: Action STAT! Generalized motor seizure. *Nurs 86* (Apr) 1986; 16:33.

Robinet K: Increased intracranial pressure: Management with an intraventricular catheter. *J Neurosurg Nurs* 1985; 17:95–104.

Rochan EH: Research shorts: Discontinuing antiepileptic medications. *J Neurosci Nurs* 1986a; 18:159.

Rochan EH: Research shorts: Exacerbation of seizures. *J Neurosci Nurs* 1986b; 18:159.

Rudy EB: *Advanced neurological and neurosurgical nursing.* St Louis: Mosby, 1984.

Samuels MA: All about stroke. *Emerg Med* (March) 1986; 95–117.

Seybold ME: Myasthenia gravis. *Hosp Med* 1986; 22:139–140, 143, 147–148.

Sjogren ER: Amicar. *Crit Care Nurse* (Mar/Apr) 1984; 4:56–57.

Smith SL: Continuous intracranial pressure monitoring: Implications and applications for critical care. *Crit Care Nurse* (July/Aug) 1983; 3:42–51.

Stanley M: Cerebral vasospasm: Pathophysiology and nursing care. *Crit Care Nurse* (Nov/Dec) 1984; 4:39–42.

Taylor JW: Nursing management of stroke: Acute care—Part I. *Cardiovas Nurs* 1985a; 21:1–5.

Taylor JW: Nursing management of stroke: Acute care—Part II. *Cardiovasc Nurs* 1985b; 21:7–12.

Toole J: *Cerebrovascular disorders*, 3d ed. New York: Raven Press, 1984.

Webster M: Trends and controversies in head-trauma care. *Nurs Life* 1984;4(6):46–51.

Wittman B: Research shorts: Refractory status epilepticus. *J Neurosurg Nurs* 1985; 17:138–140.

Yukioka H et al.: Intravenous lidocaine as a suppressant of coughing during tracheal intubation. *Anesth Analg* 1985; 64:1189–1192.

Zegeer LJ: Systemic cardiovascular effects of intracranial disorders: Implications for nursing care. *J Neurosurg Nurs* 1984; 16:161–167.

SUPPLEMENTAL READING

Bader T: Telling pseudoseizures from true. *Emerg Med* (July) 1985; 17:41, 45, 49.

Blanco K et al.: From the other side of the bedrail: A personal experience with Guillain-Barré syndrome. *J Neurosurg Nurs* 1983; 15:355–359.

Burokas L: Factors affecting nurses' decisions to medicate pediatric patients after surgery. *Heart Lung* 1985; 14:373–379.

Davenport-Fortune P, Dunnum LR: Professional nursing care of the patient with increased intracranial pressure: Planned or "hit and miss"? *J Neurosurg Nurs* 1985; 17:367–370.

Habermann B: Research shorts: The treatment of intractable epilepsy. *J Neurosurg Nurs* 1984a; 16:171.

Habermann B: Research shorts: Prophylactic anticonvulsants following neurosurgery. *J Neuro Nurs* 1984b; 16:283–284.

Johnson LK: If your patient has increased intracranial pressure, your goal should be: No surprises. *Nurs 83* 1983; 83:58–64.

Mitchell PH: Decreased adaptive capacity, intracranial: A proposal for a nursing diagnosis. *J Neurosurg Nurs* 1986; 18:170–175.

Owens ME: A crying need. *Am J Nurs* 1986; 86:73–74.

Price AS, Wilson LM: *Pathophysiology: Clinical concepts of disease processes*. New York: McGraw-Hill, 1986.

Saul TG, Ducker TB: Intracranial pressure monitoring in patients with severe head injury. *Am Surgeon* (Sept) 1982; 49:477–480.

6

Stimulation Treatment Techniques and Pain Management

CLINICAL INSIGHT

Domain: The teaching-coaching function

Competency: Providing an interpretation of the patient's condition and giving a rationale for procedures

The complex, high-technology world of the intensive care unit can seem foreign and forbidding to patients and their families. The need to make crucial decisions in such an environment can be paralyzing, yet patients and families often must choose among treatment options that all seem fraught with peril. Expert nurses are committed to demystifying these choices by translating the esoteric language in which they may have been presented into understandable options. In this paradigm, the nurse demonstrates that expert teaching in the ICU is more than simply giving information. By making herself or himself available to the patient, the nurse thoughtfully helps that patient face a potentially devastating choice of treatment, as the following exemplar shows (Benner 1984, pp. 87–88):

It was a typical morning with doctors coming and going, patient going off to tests, etc. when I walked into one of my patients' rooms. A vascular surgeon and a neurosurgeon had just come out. . . . The pa-

tient was slowly going blind due to an aneurysm at the optic chiasma . . . . The patient was quite jittery—the surgery planned was a bypass of cranial arteries followed by a craniotomy to remove the aneurysm—after the pressure had been released around it.

Her first words were, "Should I have the surgery? Do you think it is safe?" She took a deep breath and began to express her many fears and concerns about the surgery. She expressed the thought that if she didn't have the surgery she would only get progressively more blind but still live. If she had the surgery she could die, she could go completely blind, she could be permanently disabled, or she could live with the remaining part of her vision. . . . I asked her if she would like me to explain what would be going on, to which she agreed. I took in Ichabod Crani—a plastic puzzle of the head with removable parts and identification of all the parts—brain, bone, veins, arteries, etc. In the next hour we played with the parts, and I answered her questions. By the end of the hour the patient had decided that since she had come all this way, she would go ahead with the surgery.

When I finally left the room, I felt that the patient had made the right decision but that she had made it on her own. I felt good because I had given her a very descriptive account, in terms she could understand, of what was to happen to her. I had tried to remain unbiased and open and answer her questions accord-

ingly. It was a very positive experience and it seemed to be for her. . . . She eventually got better, with lots of care, and is now at a rehab hospital and recuperating remarkably well.

In order to provide the degree of teaching evidenced in this paradigm, the nurse must have a thorough understanding of various therapies. The following chapter discusses nursing care related to craniotomy, ventricular shunts, and pain management.

Technology has revolutionized surgical intervention for intracranial lesions. Improved neurosurgical techniques are a result of the introduction of the operating microscope, microinstrumentation, and the surgical laser.

Craniotomy

Assessment

Intracranial lesions requiring surgical treatment include tumors, aneurysms, hematomas, abscesses, arteriovenous malformations, hydrocephalus, and seizure focus.

Common Operative Procedures   The particular neurosurgical procedure performed depends on the type and location of the lesion.

Burr Hole   A burr hole is a small circular opening drilled in the skull. Evacuation of extracerebral hematomas or brain biopsies may be done through a burr hole.

Craniotomy   A craniotomy is a surgical opening in the skull large enough to allow for visualization of the intracranial lesion. The bone flap created to allow access for removal of injured brain, tumor, or a vascular lesion is replaced at the end of the procedure.

Craniectomy   Removal of a portion of the skull without replacing it is a craniectomy. This procedure may be done to decompress a bruised, swollen brain.

Craniotomies often are described as supratentorial or infratentorial. The *tentorium* is the dural sheath that separates the posterior fossa from the rest of the brain. *Supratentorial* craniotomies provide access to the cerebral hemispheres. The brainstem and cerebellum are approached via an *infratentorial craniotomy*.

Operating Room Protocol   Awareness of events in the operating suite provides the nurse with a more comprehensive understanding of the neurosurgical patient.

Preparation   Upon arrival in the operating suite, the patient is prepared as for any major surgery. Vascular access for fluid and drug administration is accomplished with insertion of peripheral and central lines. EKG and temperature are monitored continuously. Placement of an arterial line and central venous pressure line or pulmonary artery catheter is done to track hemodynamics.

Once the patient is intubated and anesthesia is initiated, the head is shaved. Great care is taken to avoid cuts, which could be a source of infection. The head is then prepped and supported in a pinned headrest (see Figure 6-1). At the same time, the patient is positioned according to the surgical procedure to be performed.

Adjuncts to Surgery   Measures employed to enhance the surgical repair are controlled hyperventilation, hypotension, and hypothermia. *Hyperventilation* is a quick and effective means of decreasing intracranial pressure by reducing brain bulk. Driving the PCO_2 down to 25–30 mm Hg causes cerebral vasoconstriction and reduced cerebral blood flow. Brain bulk is further reduced with the administration of intravenous mannitol. The combined effect is to provide precious space for the neurosurgeon's work. Controlled *hypotension* is utilized when vascular lesions are being repaired. It also may be employed when unexpected bleeding occurs. Deepening anesthesia by using more Enflurane may lower the

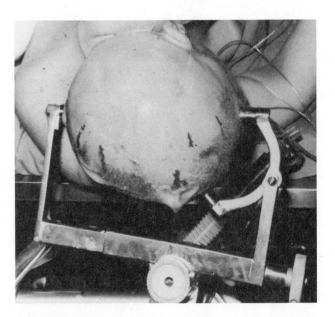

FIGURE 6–1

Head supported in pinned headrest device prior to draping. The clamp is applied to the head and tightened until the pins penetrate the outer table of the skull. Kaminski, D.: *Surgical approaches to nervous system dysfunction in adult health nursing: A biopsychosocial approach.* Kneisl, C. and Ames, S.: 1986: Menlo Park, Ca: Addison-Wesley.

blood pressure. Nitroprusside may also be used to rapidly lower blood pressure. *Hypothermia* may occur secondary to the cold operating room environment and anesthesia. Intentional induction can be done using a cooling blanket. In theory, there is a 6% reduction in oxygen consumption by the brain for every degree lowered from 37°C to 25°C (Hickey 1986). Practically, the problems encountered—such as shivering and drift—contribute to intentional hypothermia's not being used commonly.

NURSING DIAGNOSES

PREOPERATIVE

Two major preoperative concerns for the nurse are (1) the patient's emotional needs and (2) establishing a baseline neurologic assessment to monitor for impaired cerebral perfusion. Appropriate nursing diagnoses are:

- Anxiety and fear
- Potential altered cerebral perfusion

POSTOPERATIVE

Critical parameters to be monitored in the immediate postoperative period are airway, neurologic checks, vital signs, and fluid and electrolyte balance. Potential nursing diagnoses that may be identified include:

- Ineffective airway clearance
- Impaired gas exchange
- Ineffective breathing pattern
- Altered cerebral perfusion
- Altered cardiac performance*
- Imbalance of fluid and electrolytes*
- Potential for injury

*Diagnosis developed by contributor.

Preoperative Planning and Implementation

Anxiety and Fear Related to Impending Surgery Patients should be prepared for craniotomy according to established hospital protocol. This includes ensuring that the informed consent form has been signed and routine laboratory tests have been done. Markin (1986) identifies the following patient concerns prior to craniotomy: (1) loss of function, (2) return of function, (3) current disability, (4) physician's ability, (5)

the operation, and (6) prognosis. Every patient should be treated as a unique person with specific needs. Provide time for the patient to express his or her concerns. Reinforce explanation about pre- and postoperative care that will be administered. Help clarify any misconceptions the patient or family might have related to the procedure. Utilize other health team members as needed to provide emotional support.

Potential Altered Cerebral Perfusion Related to Intracranial Lesion Neurologic examination is an ongoing process, from admission to discharge. An in-depth neurologic assessment should be completed and documented *before* the patient goes to surgery. At any time, should the neurologic assessment indicate deterioration, the physician needs to be called immediately. The preoperative and postoperative neurologic assessments should be compared to quickly establish if the patient's neurologic status is the same, improved, or worse.

Postoperative Planning and Implementation

Potential Ineffective Airway Clearance Related to Neurologic Deficits and/or Altered Level of Consciousness
Impaired Gas Exchange Related to Altered Level of Consciousness
Potential Ineffective Breathing Pattern Related to Interruption of Centers Controlling Respiration The cerebral vasodilating effects of an elevated P_{CO_2} and decreased P_{O_2} are discussed in Chapter 5's section on increased ICP. The nurse should be especially careful to prevent hypercapnia and hypoxemia, since the occurrence of either is detrimental to the patient. The best way to optimize gas exchange is to provide a patent airway and ensure an effective respiratory pattern. If the patient has good respiratory effort, only supplemental oxygen is needed. Altered levels of consciousness may be accompanied by the patient's inability to maintain a patent airway or may be associated with a change in respiratory pattern. Recognition of either should prompt immediate assessment of the respiratory system, including ABGs. An artificial airway and controlled ventilation may be necessary.

Potential Alteration in Cerebral Perfusion Related to Intracranial Lesion, Cerebral Edema, Increased Intracranial Pressure, or Brain Herniation The reader is referred to the Chapter 5 sections on increased ICP and herniation syndromes. Cerebral edema reaches its peak 24–72 hours after craniotomy. It is a major cause of increased intracranial pressure. Control of cerebral edema can best be accomplished by:

- Maintaining the head of the bed at 30 degrees elevation
- Close monitoring of intake and output
- Adhering to fluid restriction as ordered
- Administering Decadron, Mannitol, or Lasix as ordered

Potential Altered Cardiac Performance Related to Hypothalamic Dysfunction or a Complication of Surgery Hypothalamic dysfunction may be related to the primary lesion, surgical manipulation, or increased intracranial pressure. Sympathetic stimulation produces marked hypertension and is associated with lowering of the ventricular fibrillation threshold. Parasympathetic stimulation causes bradycardia and hypotension. Blood pressure should be monitored and measures implemented per medical orders to treat hyper- or hypotension. Cardiac monitoring may reveal dysrhythmias. Whenever a change in rhythm occurs, the patient should be assessed for its effect on cardiac performance. Bradycardia associated with hypotension or frequent ventricular premature beats should be treated with atropine. Frequent ventricular premature beats or ventricular tachycardia need to be treated with lidocaine.

The 12-lead EKG may show ST-segment elevation or depression, T-wave inversion, prominent U waves, or a prolonged Q-T interval. If a long Q-T interval is documented, the nurse should review the present drug regimen. Drugs that prolong the Q-T interval include quinidine, disopyramide, and amiodarone. If the patient is not on any of the antidysrhythmics that prolong the Q-T interval, then the prolongation is presumed to be due to the intracranial event. The patient should be closely monitored for the development of polymorphic ventricular tachycardia.

Potential Imbalance of Fluid and Electrolytes Related to Surgery or Hypothalamic Dysfunction Monitoring of intake and output, serum electrolytes, and osmolality is necessary to detect fluid and electrolyte imbalance. Hypothalamic dysfunction may manifest as over- or underproduction of antidiuretic hormone (ADH). *Diabetes insipidus* occurs when ADH is not secreted in sufficient quantity. This is recognized when urine output exceeds 200 cc per hour for 2 hours and no diuretic has been administered. Dehydration and hypernatremia can occur if the condition is not recognized by the nurse and reported to the physician. Treatment consists of fluid replacement and administration of vasopressin (Pitressin).

The *syndrome of inappropriate antidiuretic hormone (SIADH)* is due to oversecretion of ADH. Urine output less than 30 cc per hour and hyponatremia are suggestive of "water intoxication." SIADH is treated by restricting water intake. If the hyponatremia is severe, administration of sodium chloride may be necessary. For further discussion of DI and SIADH, see Chapter 16.

Potential for Injury Related to Improper Positioning or Cranial Nerve Deficits

Supratentorial versus Infratentorial Craniotomy Nursing management is influenced by whether the patient has had a supratentorial or infratentorial craniotomy. Specific areas of concern deal with positioning, ambulation, and the potential for cranial nerve deficits.

Positioning The patient with a supratentorial craniotomy should be positioned with the head of the bed raised to 30 degrees. This promotes venous drainage, thereby decreasing cerebral edema and decreasing intracranial pressure. Positioning after infratentorial surgery may be with the head of the bed up to 15–30 degrees or flat. This seems contradictory, but differences of opinion exist. The rationale for elevating the head of the bed is to prevent distention of venous sinuses and resultant increased pressure in the posterior fossa. Advocates for the head-flat position feel this prevents downward pressure on the brainstem and dizziness. Follow the physician's orders about position. Clearly label the head of the bed with the head position so all can see it. The patient with an infratentorial craniotomy should not flex the neck, as this puts stress on the suture line and is very painful. Be very gentle when turning the head, to prevent patient discomfort. If a craniectomy has been performed, the patient should not lie on the operative site.

Ambulation Ambulation after supratentorial craniotomy generally progresses fairly rapidly, limited only by the patient's general condition and response to surgery. After infratentorial surgery, patients have problems with dizziness and ataxia. Ambulation progresses more slowly. The patient should not be moved quickly. When getting the patient up, place the patient's feet on a stool, or be sure they firmly touch the floor. This stimulates the posterior columns and helps to orient the patient in space.

Cranial Nerve Deficits Cranial nerve deficits are more likely to occur with infratentorial craniotomies, because the cranial nerves exit through the brainstem. Lesions in the posterior fossa, surgical trauma, or edema have the potential to compromise cranial nerve function. Assess the patient's gag reflex and ability to swallow and cough. Dysarthria and dysphagia may be present. Suction equipment should be at the bedside at all times. The patient should be positioned upright for meals. Speech and dietary consultations are needed for patients with significant feeding problems. Diplopia and loss of the corneal blink reflex may occur. Absence of the corneal blink reflex makes the eye vulnerable to injury. Opthalmic drops/ointment are used along with an eye shield. An eye-patching routine is established if diplopia is present.

Outcome Evaluation

The patient's progress should be evaluated according to these outcome criteria:

- Expresses concerns regarding surgery.
- Can describe what to expect in the postoperative phase.
- Neurologic status is the same or improved.
- Normal respiratory effort.
- ABGs WNL for patient.
- Vital signs WNL for patient.
- Absence of signs and symptoms of increased ICP.
- Fluid and electrolytes WNL.

Ventricular Shunts

Assessment

Risk Conditions Ventricular shunts are used in the treatment of hydrocephalus. *Hydrocephalus* is a progressive accumulation of excess cerebrospinal fluid (CSF) in the cerebral ventricular system due to congenital or acquired conditions (Grant 1984). This is a clinical syndrome, not a disease entity (Hickey 1986). Hydrocephalus is classified as communicating vs noncommunicating, or as high-pressure vs normal-pressure. Hydrocephalus is caused by faulty reabsorption of CSF (the most frequent cause in adults), obstruction in the ventricular system, overproduction of CSF (very rare), or impaired venous reabsorption (Grant 1984).

Types of Hydrocephalus *Communicating hydrocephalus* is characterized by free flow of CSF within the ventricular system and the subarachnoid space coupled with either overproduction of CSF (Grant 1984) or not enough functional arachnoid villi to reabsorb the CSF (Hickey 1986). Communicating hydrocephalus is commonly caused by subarachnoid hemorrhage or exudate from meningitis (Hickey 1986).

Noncommunicating hydrocephalus, or obstructive hydrocephalus, is characterized by an obstruction within the ventricular system or proximal to the subarachnoid space outflow tracts (the foramens of Luschka and Magendie) from the fourth ventricle (see Figure 4–16) (Grant 1984). It commonly is caused by tumors in or adjacent to the ventricular system, congenital stenosis of the aqueduct of Sylvius, or inflammatory processes (Hickey 1986).

High-pressure hydrocephalus is exactly what its name says. There is ventricular enlargement with elevated intracranial pressure (ICP). It usually is caused by obstruction of CSF flow due to tumors within the ventricular system or in the adjacent brain tissue (Youmans 1982). Other causes may be nonneoplastic masses (cysts, abscesses, hematomas), subarachnoid pathway obstruction, or congenital stricture of the aqueduct, which is symptomatic only in adults (Youmans 1982). Clinical symptoms usually start with morning, bifrontal headaches that progressively worsen until they are generalized and continuous, sometimes awakening the individual in the night (Youmans 1982). Neck pain may be present and is possibly due to protrusion of the cerebellar tonsils into the foramen magnum (Youmans 1982). Vomiting, visual disturbances, incontinence, and generally diminished mental and motor functions also may be present (Youmans 1982). As pressure increases, the person exhibits more confusion and papilledema is noted (Youmans 1982). Gait disturbances resembling ataxia or spastic paraparesis are later symptoms (Youmans 1982). Deep tendon reflexes (DTRs) generally are increased, and plantar extensor reflex is present (Youmans 1982). Cranial nerve dysfunctions or focal neurologic signs can suggest the site of obstruction (Youmans 1982). These symptoms may be gradual or acute, depending on how rapidly ICP increases (Youmans 1982).

Normal-pressure hydrocephalus (NPH) also is what its name implies. NPH can be caused by inflammatory processes involving the dura, arachnoid or brain tissue, subarachnoid hemorrhage, head trauma, thrombosis of the superior sagittal sinus (Hickey 1986), aqueductal stenosis, hypertensive ectasia of the basilar artery with aqueductal kinking, or tumors or cysts obstructing ventricular flow, or can be idiopathic (Meyer et al. 1985). Idiopathic NPH frequently is seen in 60–70-year-olds (Hickey 1986). Clinical symptoms are the triad of dementia, apraxia or other gait disturbance, and urinary incontinence (Meyer et al. 1985), which are insidious or slow to develop (Hickey 1986). The initial forgetfulness can progress to an unmanageable state (Hickey 1986). Gait disturbances start with a slowed pace, a wide base, and a zigzag step that makes the person prone to falls and trauma (Hickey 1986). Urinary incontinence, usually a late symptom (Hickey 1986; Meyer et al. 1985), may be due to forgetfulness and lack of social inhibition (Hickey 1986). Unexplained nystagmus frequently is seen (Hickey 1986), but headache and papilledema are not (Youmans 1982). Late symptoms may include positive Babinski, grasp, and sucking reflexes (Hickey 1986). Unfortunately these symptoms frequently are misinterpreted as artifacts of the normal process of aging. NPH, however, is a reversible dementia, although when untreated it can lead to total disability and death (Meyer et al. 1985).

Pathophysiology Regardless of the type of hydrocephalus, the basic problem is an imbalance between the production and reabsorption of CSF that results in an increase in ICP (Grant 1984). Compensatory mechanisms will allow normal brain function, up to a point, but beyond that point the clinical signs and symptoms of increased ICP are seen (Grant 1984). Initially the brain acts like a sponge and responds to the increasing pressure by decreasing venous capacity and extracellular space (Youmans 1982). The effective CSF pressure, or gradient between intraventricular CSF pressure and venous blood pressure, remains less than the elasticity of the brain parenchyma (Youmans 1982). As CSF accumulates and stretches the ventricles, the effective pressure rises until the brain parenchyma gives way and fluid is lost intracellularly (Youmans 1982). The periventricular region receives the greatest stress and yields as the ventricles enlarge (Youmans 1982). This is readily demonstrated on CT scan as enlarged ventricles (Hickey 1986) and as decreased cerebral blood flow in the periventricular area on CT scan with xenon gas contrast (Meyer et al. 1985). Cisternogram can indicate NPH (Hickey 1986). After injection of radioactive isotope by lumbar puncture or cisternal puncture the patient should lie flat for 2–3 hours. With NPH, periodic scans taken over the next 72 hours will demonstrate isotopes in the ventricles but little or no isotopes around the cerebral hemispheres and the presence of isotopes after 48 hours (Hickey 1986).

Rationale for Shunt Insertion Treatment of hydrocephalus is to decrease CSF pressure by unblocking the normal drainage pathways (which can happen spontaneously), opening new pathways, or improving the absorption of CSF (Youmans 1982). Currently the most reliable method of reducing CSF pressure is with a ventricular shunt. The shunt diverts excess CSF to another part of the body, where it is absorbed (Kneisl and Ames

1986). The type of shunt inserted will depend on the patient's age and any previous or existing disease (Hickey 1986).

Ventricular shunting is indicated when increased intracranial pressure or volume depresses normal neurologic function. Occasionally it is used as an intermittent device to lower ICP and stabilize the patient's medical or nutritional status before surgical removal of a lesion (Kneisl and Ames 1986). Less commonly, shunts are used to provide access to the ventricular system for direct administration of chemotherapeutic or antibiotic agents or periodic sampling of CSF via the reservoir (Kneisl and Ames 1986).

Operative Approaches The ventricular shunt is composed of a ventricular catheter, a one-way valve unit, and a distal catheter. A reservoir is added to this basic structure for some patients. The systems may be one-piece or constructed from components. Using components, the surgeon can construct a system specific to the patient's needs (Kneisl and Ames 1986). The ventricular catheter usually is placed in the right lateral ventricle (frontal or occipital horn), since this is the nondominant hemisphere for most people (Kneisl and Ames 1986). If a frontal approach is used, the incision is placed behind the hairline and a frontal burr hole is made (Youmans 1982; Kneisl and Ames 1986). The catheter then is threaded 5–6 cm into the ventricle (Youmans 1982). With the occipital approach, the incision is made above and behind the ear, where the occipital burr hole is made (Grant 1984). The catheter then is threaded 11–12 cm into the ventricle (Youmans 1982).

The distal catheter is placed in either the venous system or the peritoneal cavity. Ventricular–atrial or ventricular–venous catheters (see Figure 6–2) are inserted into the right facial or jugular veins via a small incision along the upper anterior border of the sternocleidomastoid muscle (Youmans 1982; Grant 1984; Kneisl and Ames 1986). The catheter then is threaded into position in the superior vena cava or right atrium (Youmans 1982; Grant 1984; Kneisl and Ames 1986). Ventricular–atrial catheters are contraindicated when there is evidence of cerebrovascular or cardiopulmonary disease, bacteremia, septicemia, meningitis, ventriculitis, or skin infection (Kneisl and Ames 1986).

Ventricular–peritoneal catheters are inserted into the peritoneal cavity via a small midline incision above the umbilicus and small opening in the peritoneum (Youmans 1982). The catheter then is advanced 18–20 cm and the flow checked (Youmans 1982). Ventricular–peritoneal catheters have recently gained favor due to the complications of ventricular–venous catheters (venous thrombosis, fibrin accumulation at catheter tip, embolus phenomenon) (Kneisl and Ames 1986). Ven-

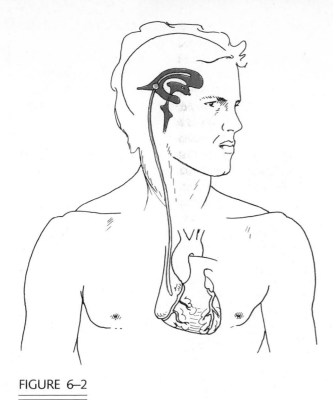

FIGURE 6–2

Ventricular–atrial shunt. (From Kneisl CR, Ames SW: *Adult health nursing: A biopsychosocial approach.* Menlo Park, CA: Addison-Wesley, © 1986, p. 1253.)

tricular–peritoneal catheters are contraindicated in patients with peritonitis (Kneisl and Ames 1986).

Positions of both ventricular and systemic catheters are verified with fluoroscopy or x-ray by visualization of radiopaque bands or injected dye (Youmans 1982; Kneisl and Ames 1986). Once correct position is obtained, the peritoneal catheter is secured to the peritoneum and/or the abdominal muscles (Youmans 1982). Then both catheters are tunneled subcutaneously toward each other and connected with the valve system (Youmans 1982; Grant 1984; Kneisl and Ames 1986).

Shunt Function   Current valve systems are pressure regulated and preset to low, medium, or high pressure (Grant 1984). The valve itself is one-way, to prevent backflow into the ventricles (Hickey 1986). When CSF pressure falls below valve pressure, the valve closes and there is no forward or backward flow through the valve (Kneisl and Ames 1986). The valve may have a reservoir attached to it. Reservoirs are used for easy sampling of CSF, injection of radiopaque or medicinal agents into the ventricles, or "pumping" (Hickey 1986) the system (Youmans 1982; Grant 1984; Kneisl and Ames 1986). The reservoir is placed under the scalp, either close to the burr hole site or along the mastoid

bone (Youmans 1982; Grant 1984; Kneisl and Ames 1986; Hickey 1986). Mastoid bone reservoir placement is used for "pumping" the system, to check patency and to flush the system of exudates (Hickey 1986). Pumping is never done without a physician's order directing the frequency of pumping and the number of times to press the reservoir (Hickey 1986). The nurse should lightly palpate the bone until the reservoir is felt, a "bouncy feel" (Hickey 1986). Then, using the index and middle fingers or the thumb, the nurse presses and gently releases the reservoir the specified number of times (Hickey 1986).

Insertion Procedure   The relatively short procedure for shunt insertion is done under aseptic technique and with general anesthesia (Kneisl and Ames 1986). Minimal monitoring and preparation are needed. An intravenous line, cardiac monitor, possibly prophylactic antibiotics, and skin preparation to the head, neck and/or abdomen are all that is usually necessary preoperatively (Kneisl and Ames 1986). Intraoperatively, some surgeons double-glove at the time of ventricular catheter insertion to decrease the chance of skin flora contamination (Grant 1984).

The complication rate for shunts is 10–40% (Meyer et al. 1985), with infection being the major risk (Grant 1984). Other complications include shunt malfunction or failure, subdural effusions, subdural or intracerebral hematoma, seizures, excess drainage of CSF, and foreign-body reaction (Youmans 1982; Grant 1984; Meyer et al. 1985, Kneisl and Ames 1986; Hickey 1986).

Effects of Insertion   Patient response to shunt insertion will depend on age, type of hydrocephalus, and any underlying disease process. The degree of improvement has no relationship to preshunt ventricular size (Meyer et al. 1985). However, chronic hydrocephalus and extreme ventricular dilation show poor improvement (Meyer et al. 1985). Improvement is manifested by: less dementia, incontinence, and gait disturbances; an increase in the patient's participation in activities of daily living; increased rates of cerebral blood flow, or decreased ventricular size (Meyer et al. 1985). Shunting may decrease CSF pressure without the ventricles returning to normal size, because the increase in surface area is capable of maintaining itself even with some decrease in pressure (Youmans 1982). Continence usually returns after 2 months; mental functions may return quickly or in 3–7 months (Meyer et al. 1985). Gait disturbances usually take several months to improve, depending on the preshunt severity, and may not completely disappear (Youmans 1982).

Idiopathic hydrocephalus response to shunt is difficult to determine, since improvement may be spontaneous (Youmans 1982). Best results are seen when gait disturbances with or without mental changes are the symptoms (Youmans 1982). Hydrocephalus occurs in 40–50% of patients several weeks after subarachnoid hemorrhage. Trauma tends to cause only a slight increase in ICP. Symptoms of hydrocephalus usually occur several weeks or months later and may be due to scarring of the basal cistern or, rarely, to blockage of the major venous sinus, third ventricle, or aqueduct (Youmans 1982). Striking improvement can occur with shunt insertion in posttrauma patients (Youmans 1982). The signs and symptoms of NPH are frequently seen with tumors, aqueductal stenosis, and, rarely, meningitis (Youmans 1982). In well-controlled studies, the improvement rate for NPH with shunt insertion is 60–85% (Meyer et al. 1985). Less improvement is noted when NPH is associated with degenerative disease, Alzheimer's disease, multiinfarct dementia, alcoholic dementia, chronic hydrocephalus, or technical complications with the shunt insertion (Meyer et al. 1985).

Signs and Symptoms Postoperatively, the care of the shunt patient is the same as for any craniotomy patient, but with a few changes (see "Craniotomy" for the care of these patients). The nurse should systematically assess the patient for signs of infection and malfunction (Grant 1984). Frequent neurologic checks are necessary. It is extremely important to promptly report to the physician any negative change in neurologic status or signs of increased ICP. Unlike the situation for most other neurologic or neurosurgical patients, the head of the bed is kept flat to slowly decompress the ventricles and prevent siphonage of CSF (Kneisl and Ames 1986). The head of the bed is elevated according to the physician's order and the patient's response (Kneisl and Ames 1986). A different problem that can be caused by siphonage is subdural hemorrhage. This is especially true when there has been long-standing hydrocephalus, increased ICP, or extensive cortical atrophy (Kneisl and Ames 1986). Subdural hemorrhage results from tearing of the fragile bridging vessels and usually does not manifest itself for several days (Grant 1984). The nurse should be alert to subtle changes in behavior and in level of consciousness (LOC) (Kneisl and Ames 1986).

Infection is the major complication for shunts and is reported in 2–39% of cases within 2 months postoperatively (Meyer et al. 1985). Systematic assessment for the signs of infection includes evidence of neck stiffness, symptomatic fever with other causes ruled out (Grant 1984), irritability, or redness, swelling, or tenderness anywhere along the shunt pathway (Kneisl and Ames 1986). Some authors consider infection an inherent though infrequent problem in adults and recommend prophylactic systemic antibiotics preoperatively and/or postoperatively. Others recommend additional antibiotic

soaking of the shunt before insertion (Youmans 1982; Grant 1984; Meyer et al. 1985; Kneisl and Ames 1986; Hickey 1986). Presence of a reservoir allows for culturing of CSF samples. Documented infection mandates removal of the shunt, antibiotic therapy, and insertion of a new shunt once the infection has been eliminated (Grant 1984). A temporary external catheter drainage system may be necessary during antibiotic therapy for both CSF drainage and antibiotic instillation (Grant 1984).

Shunt malfunction or failure is the next most common complication and should be suspected any time symptoms recur (Meyer et al. 1985). Malfunction can occur for a variety of reasons. Disconnection or kinking anywhere along the system will be hallmarked by swelling along the subcutaneous tunnel (Kneisl and Ames 1986). Subtle behavioral changes may be the clue to malfunction. Although it is a very rare occurrence, a disconnected distal catheter can float through the venous system or peritoneal cavity, with the potential to cause perforation of organs, dysrhythmias, or infection (Kneisl and Ames 1986). Obstruction can result when the tip of the catheter rests on the choroid plexus or in brain tissue or can be caused by blood clot or elevated protein levels in the CSF (Kneisl and Ames 1986). In addition, obstruction can result from faulty initial placement or decreased ventricular size after decompression (Kneisl and Ames 1986).

Subdural effusions, intracerebral hematoma, and seizures are rare complications of shunts (Youmans 1982; Kneisl and Ames 1986; Hickey 1986). Excess drainage of CSF usually results when the preset valve pressure is too low for the individual (Kneisl and Ames 1986). Symptoms of excess drainage include low-pressure headaches, nausea, tachycardia, and diaphoresis (Kneisl and Ames 1986). Persistence of symptoms or neurologic deterioration may necessitate changing the valve (Kneisl and Ames 1986). Immunologic reaction to a foreign body can cause valve malfunction, fibrin accumulation on the catheter tip, or venous thrombosis with subsequent embolic phenomenon (Kneisl and Ames 1986).

Diagnostic Procedures Diagnostic procedures to access the patency and normal function of the shunt system are the same as those used in determining hydrocephalus. CT scan is used to visualize the ventricular size and any shifts in the normal structure of the brain tissue. Isotope studies can be conducted through the reservoir to check shunt patency or as previously described to measure cerebral blood flow. When infection is suspected, CSF samples for culture can be obtained via the shunt. Pneumoencephalogram and angiography may be utilized if CT scan suggests their use, but currently CT scan usually makes both tests unnecessarily invasive (Youmans 1982; Grant 1984; Meyer et al. 1985; Kneisl and Ames 1986).

NURSING DIAGNOSES

The following nursing diagnoses are pertinent to the care of a patient with a ventricular shunt device.

- Potential for infection
- Potential for neurologic status deterioration*
- Patient and family knowledge deficit about signs and symptoms of shunt malfunction

*Diagnosis developed by contributor.

Planning and Implementation of Care

The care of the postcraniotomy patient is pertinent to the ventricular shunt patient. Please review the nursing diagnoses and planning and implementation under "Craniotomy" for specific information in addition to that discussed in the following sections.

Potential for Infection Related to Shunt Infection It is imperative that the nurse systematically assess the patient for signs of shunt infection. Tools to evaluate the potential for infection include: inspection of all incisions along the pathway; palpation and inspection of the subcutaneous tunnel for the catheters, valve and reservoirs; and evaluation of vital signs and laboratory data. Aseptic dressing changes immediately after surgery will reduce the chance of infection. Documenting and promptly notifying the physician of any wound drainage or other signs of infection will ensure timely therapy for the patient. Sampling of CSF fluid from the reservoir using aseptic technique will ensure uncontaminated samples and reduce the risk of introducing infection into the shunt.

Potential for Neurologic Status Deterioration Deterioration in neurologic status can result from shunt malfunction or failure, siphonage of CSF, or subdural hematoma. Frequent neurologic checks with vital signs are important for correct assessment of the postoperative shunt patient. Immediate notification of the physician about any deterioration is mandatory. Monitor the patient for signs of increased intracranial pressure (see Chapter 5's section on increased intracranial pressure

for a complete description), such as diminished level of consciousness, focal neurologic deficits, and pupillary reaction changes. Analyze the patient for subtle behavioral changes that could be clues to shunt malfunction or subdural hematoma, such as restlessness, drowsiness, lethargy, any change in orientation, or irritability (Kneisl and Ames 1986). Inspect the entire length of the system pathway for swelling that would result from the system's becoming disconnected. Immediately notify the physician of any x-ray findings of disconnected or free-floating catheters in the vascular system or peritoneum. Anticipate a return to surgery for malfunction or infection, and prepare the patient and family for this once such a decision is made by the surgeon.

To maintain patency, follow specific physician orders for pumping the shunt. Notify the physician of any change in the feel of the reservoir (which should be bouncy) or of difficulty in pumping the reservoir. Be alert to the signs of CSF overdrainage: headache, nausea, tachycardia, and diaphoresis. Maintain the head of the bed flat until the physician orders its elevation. Keeping the patient flat in bed may necessitate soft restraints for the confused, disoriented, restless, or combative patient. Monitor the patient closely for signs of siphonage while gradually elevating the head of the bed. If these signs appear, halt the procedure and notify the physician of patient progress.

Patient and Family Knowledge Deficit About Signs and Symptoms of Shunt Malfunction Patient and family teaching concerning the signs and symptoms of increased intracranial pressure is one of the most important nursing interventions for the ventricular shunt patient. Explain to the family in the immediate postoperative period about the expected gradual return of function seen with decompression of the ventricles. This will help to reduce anxiety if the patient has a slow recovery. Once the patient is able to understand, start teaching him or her and the family about the signs of increased intracranial pressure. Supply written material for reinforcement and learning at the patient's own pace. Include a review of the signs of shunt infection and disconnection. Review the need to have ready access to sophisticated medical care at all times in case of shunt malfunction, infection, or failure, since prompt medical care could save the patient's life. Impress on the patient the need for regular medical checkups once he or she has been discharged from the hospital. Suggest the use of a wallet card to inform medical personnel of shunt insertion. This could be helpful should the patient be alone when shunt malfunction occurs or involved in an accident and unable to communicate this information.

Assess the family's understanding of hydrocephalus,

or "water on the brain," and address any preconceived notions they may have (Grant 1984). Include the family when teaching the signs of shunt infection or malfunction and increased ICP. Stress the need to understand that the shunt is not a cure but simply a treatment for hydrocephalus. Help the family understand that the degree of recovery may depend on the underlying disease process and general health of the patient.

Perhaps some of the problems with ventricular shunts will be solved when better techniques are developed to treat hydrocephalus. The development of a flow-regulated valve to replace the pressure-regulated valve may decrease the potential for debris and protein to accumulate around the valve (Grant 1984). Perhaps development of drugs that decrease CSF production will be successful. Currently, a carbonic anhydrase inhibitor (Diamox) is producing a 50% decrease in CSF production in animal studies (Grant 1984). Cardiac glycosides have the potential for reducing CSF production, but their systemic and cardiac effects—especially in the older population—have significant drawbacks (Grant 1984).

Outcome Evaluation

Evaluate the patient with a ventricular shunt according to the following criteria:

- Return to normal neurologic status.
- Prevention of complications.
- Patient and family able to list the signs of increased ICP and shunt disconnection and appropriate response.

Pain

The critical-care nurse encounters patients in pain every day. To a large extent, responsiveness to these patients depends on the nurse's understanding of pain, cultural values related to pain, and ability to either relieve pain or tolerate its expression. The subject of pain is virtually neglected in critical-care texts; an average of less than one page per book is devoted to current knowledge about pain—this for a phenomenon with which the critical-care nurse must cope every day! The purpose of this section is to help the critical-care nurse

become more empathetic and effective in pain management by reviewing current pain causation theories and effective pain relief measures.

Assessment

Risk Conditions With the possible exception of the comatose, completely unresponsive patient, *every* critically ill patient is at risk for experiencing pain.

Recent research has improved the understanding of pain as a complex phenomenon. The pain stimulus is initiated in the peripheral nervous system in *nociceptors* (pain receptors) (Rudy 1984). Both small-diameter and large-diameter peripheral nerve fibers are activated by the pain stimulus (Guyton 1986). Small-diameter type-A fibers conduct impulses rapidly, and these signals are perceived as sharp or acute pain (Guyton 1986). Large-diameter type-C fibers conduct impulses more slowly, and these signals are perceived as dull or chronic pain (Guyton 1986) (Figure 6–3). Both types of fibers are activated by heat, pressure, electrical stimulation, or the chemical mediators of inflammation (Bray 1986). These mediators include histamine, bradykinin, prostaglandins, acids, potassium ions, acetylcholine, proteolytic enzymes, and hydrogen ions (Guyton 1986). The chemical mediators have a synergistic effect, causing longer-lasting pain than other stimuli, due to lowered pain thresholds from repetitive stimulations (Guyton 1986). The actions of nonsteroidal antiinflammatory

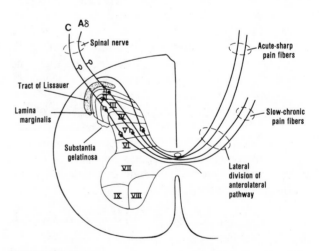

FIGURE 6–3

Transmission of both "acute-sharp" and "slow-chronic" pain signals into and through the spinal cord on the way to the brainstem. (From Guyton A: *Textbook of medical physiology*, 7th ed. Philadelphia: Saunders, 1986, p. 595.)

agents and acetylsalicylic acid inhibit the metabolism of arachidonic acid into prostaglandin at the nociceptors, thus reducing inflammation and pain (Fields and Levine 1984). Catecholamines exacerbate pain stimuli, and interruption of catecholamine influence is believed to be the reason sympathectomies have been successful in the past (Levine 1984). Substance P is a neurotransmitter in the small-diameter fiber pathway of the pain transmitter system. It is synthesized in the dorsal root, released into the spinal cerebrospinal fluid, and transmitted to the peripheral nociceptor (Levine 1984). Experimental blockage of substance P decreases pain (Levine 1984), and antagonists are currently being investigated.

Pain fibers enter the dorsal root and travel along the tract of Lissauer to the dorsal horn in the spinal cord gray matter (Guyton 1986). Sensory fibers for touch and proprioception enter the ventral roots but end up mainly in the superficial layers of the dorsal horn in the spinal cord, near the pain fibers (Levine 1984). Stimulation of the sensory fibers inhibits the ascending pain-transmission pathways (Guyton 1986). This is believed to be the reason that transcutaneous electrical nerve stimulation (TENS), acupuncture, liniments, and massage are effective in pain management (Guyton 1986).

Type-A pain fibers enter the spinal cord gray matter and synapse with second-order neurons before they cross to the opposite, contralateral, side of the cord. These fibers then ascend along the spinothalamic tracts to the brain (Guyton 1986). Type-C pain fibers enter the cord and synapse in the substantia gelatinosa before most of them cross to the contralateral side of the cord and ascend. Some of the type-C fibers do not cross, and they ascend ipsilaterally to the brain (Guyton 1986).

The lateral spinothalamic tract fibers terminate in the somatosensory cortex via the thalamus and are responsible for the sensation of pain and touch (Bray 1986) and for localizing pain (Guyton 1986). The ventral spinothalamic tract fibers terminate in the reticular formation of the brainstem and proceed to the thalamus and limbic system. These fibers than activate the entire brain and arouse the organism with a sense of urgency (Guyton 1986). It also is believed that the reticular formation fibers are where the emotional components of pain originate (Bray 1986) (Figure 6–4).

The variety of responses to pain seen by nurses may be partially due to the descending pain-modulating system or analgesia system (Guyton 1986). This system has three main components (Guyton 1986). CNS neurons in the periaqueductal gray area along the aqueduct of Sylvius are stimulated and then send signals to the raphe magnus nucleus in the lower pons and upper medulla (Figure 6–5). The signals then are sent via de-

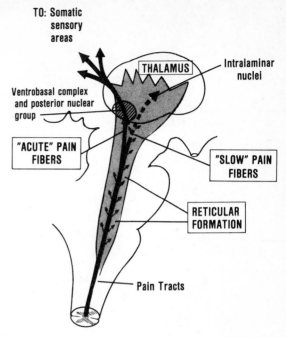

FIGURE 6–4

Transmission of pain signals into the hindbrain, thalamus, and cortex via the "pricking pain" pathway and the "burning pain" pathway. (From Guyton A: *Textbook of medical physiology,* 7th ed. Philadelphia: Saunders, 1986, p. 595.)

scending fibers to the pain inhibitory complex in the dorsal horn of the spinal cord, near the ascending pain fibers.

Specific neurotransmitters have been associated with the pain modulator system (Bray 1986). *Enkephalins* are secreted at many descending nerve fiber endings (Guyton 1986). Enkephalins are believed to exert an inhibitory effect on incoming pain fiber impulses in the dorsal horn (Guyton 1986). Serotonin is secreted at the nerve fiber endings in the dorsal horn, stimulates the secretion of enkephalins there, and may have an analgesic effect. Tricyclic antidepressants used in the treatment of chronic pain block the removal of serotonin at the synaptic cleft, thereby prolonging and enhancing analgesia (Fields 1984).

The periaqueductal gray area of the brainstem is important because of the accumulation there of opiatelike substances that can virtually suppress pain. Thus far, nine of these substances have been found (Guyton 1986) and have been given the generic name of *endorphins* (Fields 1984). Endorphins are believed to act at specific receptor sites along the descending pain-modulating pathway, by either producing potent analgesia or enhancing narcotic analgesia. In animals, local applica-

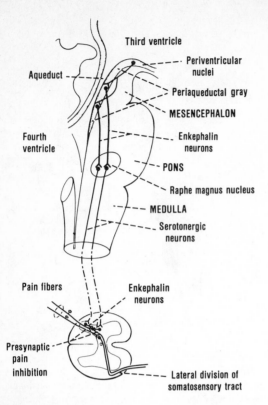

Third ventricle
Periventricular nuclei
Aqueduct
Periaqueductal gray
MESENCEPHALON
Fourth ventricle
Enkephalin neurons
PONS
Raphe magnus nucleus
MEDULLA
Serotonergic neurons
Pain fibers
Enkephalin neurons
Presynaptic pain inhibition
Lateral division of somatosensory tract

FIGURE 6–5

The analgesia system of the brainstem and spinal cord, showing inhibition of incoming pain signals at the cord level. (From Guyton A: *Textbook of medical physiology,* 7th ed. Philadelphia: Saunders, 1986, p. 596.)

tion of small doses of morphine at the opiate receptor sites in the dorsal horn can produce analgesia for up to 24 hours (Fields and Levine 1984). It is this mechanism that initiated the recent use of intrathecal and epidural narcotic administration in postoperative, labor, and cancer patients (Fields 1984). Implantable epidural infusion pumps now are being used for long-term pain control in cancer patients (Fields and Levine 1984).

The last—but certainly not the least important—component to pain perception is the psychogenic aspect. Individual perception of pain is a complex, unique combination of past experiences, expectations, and judgments (Bray 1986). Preoperative patient teaching may help decrease anxiety that normally accompanies surgery and aggravates acute pain (Bray 1986). In the treatment of chronic pain, a multidisciplinary, behaviorally oriented therapy is being used successfully at pain clinics across the United States (Fields and Levine 1984). Patients are taught how to decrease pain through behavioral modification techniques, hypnosis, psycho-

therapy, and biofeedback, ultimately returning to a productive life (Fields and Levine 1984).

Signs and Symptoms Signs and symptoms of pain are highly individual. Pain can be crudely classified as superficial or deep. *Superficial,* or *cutaneous, pain* arises from structures in the skin and subcutaneous tissues. It is often described as sharp or burning in nature and is relatively short in duration. It also is relatively easy to localize. Superficial pain frequently is associated with quick, brisk movements and a sense of increased alertness. In contrast, *deep pain* arises from ischemia, stretching, or unusual contractions of deep body structures. It usually is described as dull or aching. Deep pain is longer-lasting and harder to localize than superficial pain. Deep pain often is accompanied by autonomic symptoms such as nausea, vomiting, diaphoresis, pallor, syncope, and, sometimes, bradycardia and hypotension. In contrast to the patient with superficial pain, whose activity increases, patients in deep pain tend to be very still (think for a moment about the number of times you have been alerted to a patient with ischemic cardiac pain by his or her unnatural stillness).

NURSING DIAGNOSES

There are two NANDA diagnoses pertaining to pain:

• Alteration in comfort: pain
• Altered comfort: chronic pain

Planning and Implementation of Care

Although nurses are most familiar with pain relief through the use of analgesic medications, there are many other nursing activities that can afford the patient relief from pain. Following are some of the techniques found useful for alleviation of pain.

1. Recognize that a person's perception of pain is affected not only by physiologic injury but also by energy level, sociocultural factors, and personal experiences.

2. Recognize that degree of pain correlates poorly with expression of pain.

3. Accept the patient's statement that he or she is in pain. Be alert not to let your own perceptions

TABLE 6-1 SEVEN MYTHS ABOUT PAIN RELIEF

MYTH	COMMENT
1. "Pain caused by anxiety doesn't require treatment."	All pain has physiologic and psychologic components.
2. "I've worked with enough patients to know which ones are *really* in pain."	Nurses and doctors judge the authenticity and severity of "real" pain. The patient is expected to prove they have pain. This generates distrust of the health care provider.
3. "One way to determine if the patient is faking is to give a placebo."	This causes complete distrust of the health care provider when the patient finds out what has happened. The placebo may stimulate the endogenous endorphins and cause analgesia.
4. "When a patient asks for pain medication every 4 hours on the dot, I know I've got a potential addict on my hands."	Patient clock-watching usually means inadequate medication for pain relief.
5. "The patient who needs increasing doses of narcotics to control pain is becoming addicted."	Rarely does a patient develop addiction in the hospital setting. Rather, it is drug tolerance or physiologic dependence that causes the need for higher drug doses.
6. "Giving analgesics only on demand is the best way to prevent abuse."	Studies show that the patient on routine pain medication needs less medication than patients on PRN schedules.
7. "The best injectable narcotic for pain relief is meperidine."	Although meperidine may be the analgesic most popular among health care providers, it is the shortest-acting analgesic in young people since it is metabolized within 2 hours.

Published in *RN* December 1983; 46:30–31. Copyright (c) 1983 Medical Economics Company, Inc., Oradell, JH. Reprinted by permission.

about pain interfere with accepting your patient's complaints about pain. See Table 6–1 (Seven Myths about Pain Relief).

4. Assess the patient's pain systematically. The PQRST mnemonic (described in Chapter 10) is helpful in assessing the history of any type of pain. Also observe for objective signs of pain, such as pallor, diaphoresis, and tachycardia. Finally, note the person's behavioral responses, such as withdrawal, writhing, and grimacing.

5. Attend to basic comfort needs. Patients in severe pain may be too absorbed in coping with it to keep themselves warm and dry. Particularly if the patient is having profuse diaphoresis, changing the patient's gown and sheets and providing blankets for warmth can be simple yet powerful comfort measures.

6. Reduce the impact on pain of fear of the unknown. Before a painful procedure, familiarize the patient with sensations that may be experienced and suggest effective ways to cope with them. For instance, if the patient is having an angiogram, explain that a local anesthetic will be used at the insertion site and that some pressure may be felt as the catheter is inserted, but that he or she should alert the health care team if pain is felt so that additional anesthetic can be used.

7. Help the person obtain adequate rest. Exhaustion significantly depletes a patient's ability to cope with pain.

8. If you must perform or assist with a painful procedure, time the procedure to coincide with the peak effectiveness of analgesic premedication.

9. Use ice packs or hot water bottles for pain relief. Or try local applications of analgesic ointments, such as mentholated ointments, for superficial pain.

10. Use distraction. Obtain a battery-operated tape recorder, headset, and cassettes of music the patient likes. Loud, fast music can distract the person during episodes of pain, whereas slower, melodic music can aid relaxation in between episodes. One useful technique is to tell the patient to increase the loudness if the pain increases. In addition to accentuating the distraction, this technique also gives the patient a sense of control—if not over the pain itself, at least over the response to it.

11. Have the patient sing, either out loud or to self. This technique is especially useful with children.

12. Have the person massage the painful part. Providing cutaneous stimulation actually decreases the patient's perception of pain by inhibiting the transmission of pain impulses at the spinal cord level.

13. If the painful area cannot be massaged, try contralateral stimulation (DeCrosta 1984). Stimulate the side of the body opposite the painful part, using ice packs, a hot water bottle, or massage.

14.   Coach the person on how to breathe slowly and rhythmically. For the patient in severe pain, merely telling him or her to breathe slowly and deeply often is insufficient. To maximize the effectiveness of this technique, establish eye contact and have the patient follow your pattern of breathing. Tell the patient to concentrate on feeling the air move in and out of the lungs as he or she breathes slowly and deeply.

15.   Capitalize on the power of suggestion. For example, any time you suggest a pain-relief technique, speak in positive terms and imply that the technique will be successful. You can also give the patient direct suggestions to relieve pain. For example, tell the newly admitted patient in pain that although an IV insertion is uncomfortable, he or she will relax and feel the pain recede as he or she allows himself or herself to be placed "in safe hands" and to trust the people caring for him or her.

16.   Familiarize yourself with the wide variety of analgesics available on the market. These include narcotic, nonnarcotic, and adjunctive agents such as tranquilizers. If you are not familiar with the merits and disadvantages of the various agents, consult a pharmacology text.

17.   Encourage the patient who has chronic pain to learn behaviorally oriented pain reduction techniques, such as biofeedback and hypnosis.

18.   Patients with severe and/or chronic pain should be referred to a pain clinician if possible. Among techniques that can be tried are dorsal column stimulation and transcutaneous electrical nerve stimulation (TENS), both of which can reduce pain by providing competing sensations for transmission by the large fibers to block incoming pain impulses from the small fibers.

19.   Teach the patient how to use patient-controlled analgesic devices to decrease postoperative pain. These mechanical devices enhance the patient's feeling of control over pain by allowing administration of pain medication without the anxiety of waiting for a nurse to give the drug. Overmedication is prevented by specific dosage and timing controls fed into the device by the nurse following the physician's orders (Rudy 1984).

20.   Recognize the benefits and potential problems of epidural and intrathecal medication administration. Small doses of epidural or intrathecal analgesic agents given close to the endogenous endorphin receptor sites deliver potent pain control without the side effects of systemic analgesic agents. Use of commercial morphine or meperidine via these routes is contraindicated due to meningeal irritation from the preservative used to stabilize the drugs. Recognition of correct dosage orders for central narcotic administration is mandatory, since parenteral dosages could be life-threatening if delivered via epidural or intrathecal spaces. Concomitant parenteral analgesic medication dosage must be substantially reduced or deleted due to the potency of central narcotic administration. Specific care and maintenance of the various indwelling epidural catheters and knowledge of the signs and symptoms of catheter displacement to the intrathecal space are necessary for effective nursing intervention (Baggerly 1986).

21.   Patient and family teaching about the care and maintenance of epidural catheters, the signs and symptoms of overmedication, and troubleshooting techniques will be needed if the patient goes home with these devices.

Outcome Evaluation

Evaluate the patient according to these desirable outcome criteria:

- Verbal expression of absence of pain.
- Relaxed body position.
- Relaxed facial expression.
- Vital signs WNL.

REFERENCES

Arsenault L: Selected postoperative complications of cranial surgery. *J Neuro Nurs* 1985; 17:155–163.

Baggerly J: Epidural catheters for pain management: The nurse's role. *J Neuro Nurs* 1986; 18:290–295.

Bagley CS: Pain assessment: Helping patients where it hurts. *Nurs 85* (July) 1985; 15:16F, 16H, 16L.

Benner P: *From novice to expert.* Menlo Park, CA: Addison-Wesley, 1984.

Bray CA: Postoperative pain: Altering the patient's experience through education. *AORN* 1986; 43:672, 674–675, 677.

Cammermeyer M: Research shorts: Intrathecal morphine following lumbar spine surgery. *J Neuro Nurs* 1986; 18:101.

Cramer FE: First make the patient a believer. *Nurs 84* (July) 1984; 84:36–38.

Crowel RM: Surgical management of cerebrovascular disease. *Nurs Clin North Am* 1986; 21:297–308.

DeCrosta T: Relieving pain: Four noninvasive ways you should know more about. *Nurs Life* (Mar/Apr) 1984; 4:28–33.

Elul R: Principles of clinical management of pain. *Am J Cont Ed Nurs* 1986; 1:31–40.

Fields HL: Neurophysiology of pain and pain modulation. *Am J Med* (September) 1984; 77:2–8.

Fields HL, Levine JD: Pain—Mechanisms and management. *West J Med* 1984; 141:347–357.

Grant L: Hydrocephalus: An overview and update. *J Neurosurg Nurs* 1984; 16:313–318.

Guyton A: *Textbook of medical physiology,* 7th ed. Philadelphia: Saunders, 1986.

Hickey J: *The clinical practice of neurological and neurosurgical nursing,* 2d ed. Philadelphia: Lippincott, 1986.

Jacob S: Smoothing the ragged edges of pain—Bring on the music . . . *Am J Nurs* 1986; 86:1034.

Kneisl CR, Ames SW: *Adult health nursing: A biopsychosocial approach.* Menlo Park, CA: Addison-Wesley, 1986.

Levine J: Pain and analgesia: The outlook for more rational treatment. *Ann Intern Med* 1984; 100:269–276.

Markin DA: Preoperative concerns of the patient undergoing craniotomy. *J Neuro Nurs* 1986; 18:275–278.

McCash AM: Meeting the challenge of craniotomy care. *RN* (June) 1985a; 48:26–33.

McCash AM: Controlling ICP after a craniotomy. *RN* (July) 1985b; 48:23–25.

McGuire L: Seven myths about pain relief. *RN* (Dec) 1983; 46:30–31.

Mense S: Basic neurobiologic mechanisms of pain and analgesia. *Am J Med* (Nov) 1983; 75:4–14.

Meyer JS et al.: Evaluation of treatment of normal-pressure hydrocephalus. *J Neurosurg* 1985; 62:513–521.

Moseley JR: Alterations in comfort. *Nurs Clin North Am* 1985; 20:427–438.

Rudy EB: *Advanced neurological and neurosurgical nursing.* St Louis: Mosby, 1984.

Savoy SM: The craniotomy patient. *AORN* 1984; 40:716–724.

Youmans JR: Hydrocephalus in adults. Pages 1423–1435 in *Neurological surgery,* Vol. 3. Philadelphia: Saunders, 1982.

Unit 4

AERATION

7

Aeration Assessment

CLINICAL INSIGHT

Domain: The diagnostic and monitoring function

Competency: Assessing the patient's potential for wellness and for responding to various treatment strategies

The patient's emotional energy to help himself or herself is of paramount importance to recovery. Stunned and overwhelmed by critical illness, the patient still somehow must muster the energy to respond to treatment in order to become well again. But how do nurses assess the presence of such an ineffable state? Listen to this expert nurse (Benner and Tanner 1987, p. 25):

I am able to tune into patients. For example, a woman came in yesterday with respiratory distress, emphysema history, heart-failure problems. Her P_{CO_2} was 80 when she arrived. . . . This problem had perhaps been exacerbated by the news that her daughter, who had been hospitalized for a heart attack, had just died. So we talked a little bit about it. . . . I was just listening, commenting, "She sounds very special."

I let her know that she didn't have to worry and

that I was going to take care of her, so she could let go a little bit; she trusted me.

She did well until her family came in early in the evening. Then, she got upset because suddenly maybe she could see their grief, I guess. She was intubated about midnight. This morning she was in discomfort and scared but she looked as if she could go through it. She had some strength and energy and was willing to participate in her illness. It seemed that she was going to cooperate with what was going on. I was looking for clues: Had this lady really lost it in her grief? Was she so emotional she was not going to be able to be coached along through this illness? Was she going to be so uptight that we were never going to be able to get her comfortable or maybe achieve some things we could in terms of rest and relaxation, and giving her breathing treatments and suctioning today? Was she going to be available?

You could see it in her eyes. She focused. She looked at me when I said, "Good morning. It looks as if you've had a rough night." Here is an instance of recognizing that a patient is resourceful and going to be all right, at least in the near future. If it's something we can get through then she can get through it. She's got some energy there. She has some energy to help herself and that is one of the basic things we need, one of the predominant things we need.

In the clinical insight, the nurse eloquently describes the process of "tuning in" to patients. Although the patient has problems with aeration, tuning in applies to all types of patients and in all stages of the nursing process.

In addition to the assessment of coping energy, the nurse will need to assess many other factors to judge a patient's aeration capability.

Aeration is a process that includes four major phases. The first phase, *ventilation,* is the movement of air into and out of the alveoli. The second phase is the exchange of gases between the alveoli and pulmonary capillaries, called *alveolar–capillary diffusion.* The third phase is the *transport of gases* in the blood, to and from the cells, and the fourth is *capillary–tissue diffusion.*

Your ability to assess the adequacy of your patient's aeration is vital in assisting that patient to maintain adequate oxygenation and ventilation. Table 7–1 suggests a format for nursing assessment of aeration.

History and Physical Examination

The scope and depth of your history-taking in the critical-care setting depend on the urgency of the situation and whether the physician has already examined the patient. Pertinent factors to note include smoking history, exposure to inhaled toxins, chest trauma, past respiratory illnesses, thoracic surgery, and development of

TABLE 7–1 AERATION ASSESSMENT FORMAT

1. History _____
   _____

2. Physical
   A. Inspection
      Patient position _____ Sputum _____
      Thoracic shape _____ Cyanosis _____
      Respirations: rate/rhythm _____ Clubbing _____
      Chest expansion _____ Use of accessory muscles _____
   B. Palpation
      Trachea _____ Tactile fremitus _____
      Subcutaneous emphysema (crepitus) _____
   C. Percussion _____
   D. Auscultation
      Breath sounds _____
      _____
      Adventitious sounds _____
      _____
      Voice and whispered sounds _____
   E. Dyspnea, chest pain, cough _____

3. Diagnostic procedures and laboratory tests
   Arterial blood gases: F_IO_2 _____ P_aO_2 _____ A–a gradient _____
   pH _____ PCO_2 _____ HCO_3 _____
   Chest x-ray _____ Sputum _____
   Pulmonary function tests _____
   Inspiratory force _____ Compliance _____
   FEV_1/FVC (%) _____ TV _____ RV _____
   FRC _____ TLC _____ VC _____
   V_D/V_T ratio _____
   Other _____
   Other _____

symptoms such as easy fatigability, dyspnea, and hemoptysis.

The physical examination provides information about the patient's current aeration status. The following sections describe in detail aeration physical assessment skills useful for the critical-care nurse.

The Lungs and Thorax

The physical examination must be based on a clear understanding of the relationships between external chest landmarks and the underlying respiratory structures. Figure 7–1 illustrates the relationship of the lungs to the bony thorax. The apices of the lungs extend above the clavicles, anteriorly. The bases extend to the diaphragm, anteriorly between the fifth and sixth rib on expiration and posteriorly to the level of the tenth thoracic spinous process on expiration.

The right lung has three lobes: the upper and middle lobes separated by the minor fissure and the lower lobe separated by the major fissure. The left lung has only an upper lobe and a lower lobe, also separated by a major fissure. It is important to note in Figure 7–1 that the upper lobes (and right middle lobe) are primarily anterior structures, whereas the lower lobes are primarily posterior structures. The lobes are further subdivided into ten segments in the right lung and eight in the left.

Figure 7–2 illustrates the way in which human airways branch from the trachea into the right and left mainstem bronchi and then into bronchioles, terminal (nonrespiratory) bronchioles, respiratory bronchioles, alveolar ducts, and alveolar sacs. The airways from the nasal passages down to the terminal bronchioles serve to conduct air but do not participate in gas exchange.

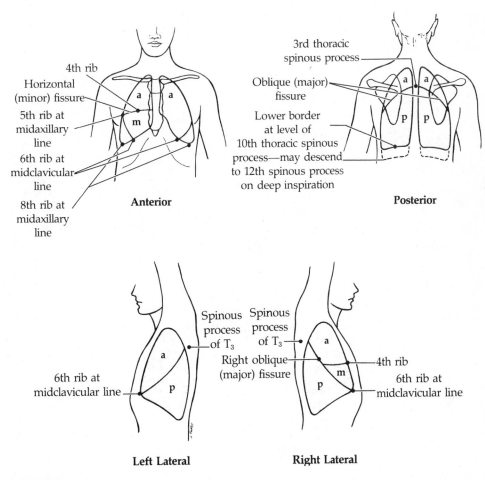

FIGURE 7–1

Lung boundaries. (Adapted from Bates B: *A guide to physical examination.* Philadelphia: Lippincott, 1983.) A = anterior lobe; M = middle lobe; P = posterior lobe.

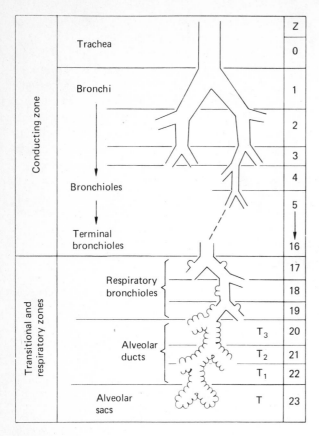

		Z
Trachea		0
Bronchi		1
		2
		3
Bronchioles		4
		5
Terminal bronchioles		16
Respiratory bronchioles		17
		18
		19
Alveolar ducts	T_3	20
	T_2	21
	T_1	22
Alveolar sacs	T	23

Conducting zone

Transitional and respiratory zones

FIGURE 7–2

Idealization of the human airways according to Weibel. Note that the first 16 generations (*Z*) make up the conducting airways and the last 7 the respiratory zone (or the transitional and respiratory zone). (From Weibel ER: *Morphometry of the human lung.* Berlin: Springer-Verlag, 1963, p. 111.)

This area is collectively referred to as *dead space,* or *wasted ventilation.* Gas exchange occurs *only* from the respiratory bronchioles to the alveoli. These areas participating in gas exchange are collectively referred to as an *acinus* and include respiratory bronchioles, alveolar ducts, alveolar sacs, and alveoli. Each acinus contains about five primary lobules. A primary lobule consists of a single respiratory bronchiole; its alveolar ducts, sacs, and alveoli; and its vascular supply structures.

Accompanying the respiratory bronchiole into the lobule are a branch of the bronchial artery carrying oxygenated blood to the tissues and a branch of the pulmonary artery carrying unoxygenated blood that participates in gas exchange. After it is oxygenated, the blood enters a branch of the pulmonary veins, which all ultimately empty into the left atrium.

Description of Examination Findings   Describe the location of your findings in reference to the closest intercostal space or rib and the imaginary chest reference lines. Anteriorly, it is fairly easy to number ribs and spaces by using the angle of Louis as the reference point. (See Chapter 10 if you wish to review the technique.) Remember that only the costal cartilages of ribs 1–7 attach to the sternum. Those of ribs 8–10 attach to the cartilage immediately above each of them, and ribs 11 and 12 have free anterior tips. The reference lines on the anterior chest are the midsternal and midclavicular; on the lateral chest, the anterior, mid, and posterior axillary lines.

Posteriorly, numbering ribs is difficult, since the spinous processes of T_4–T_{11} overlie the vertebral body of the next lower rib (for example, the T_7 spinous process is near the attachment of the eighth rib). It is possible to number the ribs by having the patient flex the neck; the prominent bump at the base of the neck usually is the seventh cervical spinous process. From there down you can palpate and count the thoracic processes. The imaginary reference lines on the posterior chest are the vertebral and midscapular.

Inspection

Thoracic Shape   The normal thoracic shape is symmetric, with the anteroposterior (AP) diameter less than the lateral diameter. When the AP diameter is equal to or greater than the lateral diameter, the patient is said to have a barrel chest, which frequently is seen in chronic pulmonary disease. Other important observations include curvature of the spine and asymmetry of the chest wall.

Respiratory Rate and Rhythm   The rate and rhythm of respiration are controlled by the respiratory center. According to Guyton (1986), the respiratory center consists of three neuronal groups dispersed in the medulla and pons. The first group, located along the length of the dorsal medulla, is responsible for inspiration and are collectively referred to as the *inspiratory area.* Their property of intrinsic excitability allows them to stimulate inspiration with repetitive discharges. A second group of neurons located in the upper pons is referred to as the *pneumotaxic area.* These neurons continually transmit impulses to the inspiratory area to control the duration of inspiration, thereby increasing or decreasing the respiratory rate. The third group of neurons is located in the ventral medulla and is inactive during normal, quiet breathing. When respiratory drive is increased, however, these neurons respond by stimulating ventilation.

The apneustic center, located in the lower pons, is not involved in normal ventilation. Normally overridden by the above centers, its pattern is one of excessive inspiration with short expiratory pauses. This pattern occasionally is observed in neurologic patients.

Various receptors are involved in the regulation of respiration: central and peripheral chemoreceptors and intrapulmonary receptors. The most potent stimulus to respiration is the partial pressure of carbon dioxide (P_aCO_2). This stimulus is mediated primarily by *central chemoreceptors* in the medulla and secondarily by *peripheral chemoreceptors* in the aorta and carotid bodies.

CO_2 affects the central chemoreceptors through its influence on the acidity of cerebrospinal fluid, which bathes the medulla. CO_2 diffuses freely across the blood-brain barrier. It then combines with water to form carbonic acid, which dissociates into a hydrogen ion (H^+) and a bicarbonate ion. The increased H^+ concentration lowers the pH of cerebrospinal fluid. The resulting stimulation of the respiratory center causes an increase in the rate and depth of ventilation *(hyperventilation)*. Similarly, a decrease in P_{CO_2} causes a decrease in ventilation *(hypoventilation)*. Peripheral chemoreceptors are sensitive to P_{CO_2} and pH of arterial blood, although their primary role is ventilatory regulation mediated by changes in arterial P_{O_2}.

The partial pressure of oxygen in arterial blood (P_aO_2) probably is not a strong stimulus to respiration within the normal P_aO_2 range (70 mm Hg or above). As P_aO_2 drops, the chemoreceptors in the aortic and carotid bodies become excited and stimulate the respiratory center by reflex action. Below a P_aO_2 of about 50 mm Hg, the respiratory centers become hypoxic and depressed.

There are three groups of *intrapulmonary receptors*: stretch (Hering-Breuer), irritant, and "j" receptors. *Stretch receptors,* located in the walls of bronchi and bronchioles, are only stimulated with excessive inspiration (tidal volumes over 1.5 liters) and therefore do not play a significant role in normal adult respiration (Guyton 1986). *Irritant receptors* are located in the airways, and *"j" receptors* are located in the alveolar interstitium. They respond to changes such as pulmonary congestion with an increase in respiratory rate (Carrieri et al. 1984).

The respiratory rate normally is 8–16 breaths a minute. The rhythm should be regular, with inspiration slightly shorter than expiration, that is, an I:E ratio of 1:1.5 or 1:2. Abnormal rhythms and their physiologic causes are discussed in detail in Chapter 4 on assessment of stimulation.

Chest Expansion Next, inspect chest expansion to evaluate the muscular work of breathing. Muscular movement depends both on the adequacy of neural impulses from the respiratory center to the muscles and on the integrity of the muscles and bones of the thorax. The chief nerves involved in inspiration are those innervating the external intercostal muscles, and the phrenic nerve, which innervates the diaphragm. Motor stimuli from the respiratory center cause these muscles to contract. Contraction of the dome-shaped diaphragm causes it to flatten, thus expanding the thorax downward. The diaphragm performs 80% of the work of breathing. Contraction of the external intercostals elevates the ribs, expanding the chest laterally.

The lungs expand because their coverings (the *visceral pleura*) closely approximate the lining of the chest (the *parietal pleura*). The space between the visceral and parietal pleurae is a potential space, with a thin layer of pleural fluid to allow gliding movement between the pleural layers. It is important to remember that each lung has a separate pouch of pleura (and pleural space) that surrounds it except at its attachment to the mainstem bronchi and pulmonary vessels (its hilum). Expiration normally occurs passively due to the elastic recoil of the lungs, chest wall, and abdominal musculature.

While inspecting the chest, note whether breathing is thoracic, abdominal, or both. Normally, inspiration causes both expansion of the thorax and outward movement of the abdomen. Predominantly thoracic breathing may be either normal (as in late pregnancy) or abnormal (as in abdominal pain or distention). Predominantly abdominal breathing also may be either normal (as in healthy males) or abnormal. Chronic obstructive lung disease patients often use a mixture of thoracic and abdominal breathing, with upper thoracic effort prominent on inspiration. They may use forceful abdominal contraction on exhalation, because the diaphragm is depressed and relatively immobile, and in some cases (emphysema), the lung has lost its elastic recoil.

Observe, too, for signs of increased work of breathing, such as the use of accessory muscles in the neck or upper chest, retraction or bulging of the intercostal muscles, and active contraction of the abdominal muscles.

Nasal flaring, pursed-lip breathing, and coughing are also signs of respiratory distress. If sputum is present, it should be assessed as to quantity, color, and odor.

Also note whether the ribs and sternum move symmetrically. One abnormal sign is *paradoxical movement;* that is, one part of the chest wall moves in on inspiration and out on expiration. Such movement can be a sign of underlying pleural disease. *Flail chest,* the term for an unstable chest wall, results from double fractures of three or more adjacent ribs and causes severe respiratory distress.

The depth of chest expansion can be classified only crudely by inspection as normal, increased, or decreased. Accurate evaluation of the degree of expansion must be made with a spirometer.

Cyanosis One of the extrathoracic signs of respiratory distress is cyanosis. Cyanosis results from the presence of at least 5 g of desaturated hemoglobin (Hgb) per 100 ml of blood. In the normal person, this amount is equivalent to about one-third of the hemoglobin; however, cyanosis is due not to the proportion of unsaturated Hgb but to the absolute amount. For this reason, the anemic patient may not show cyanosis because he or she does not have enough hemoglobin to accumulate five desaturated grams; the polycythemic patient may display cyanosis even when he or she has an adequate oxygen content. Thus, cyanosis is an unreliable indicator of the degree of oxygen deficit.

There are two basic types of cyanosis: peripheral and central. In the first type, Hgb is saturated normally but flow to the periphery is slowed due to cold, nervousness, or low cardiac output resulting in peripheral cyanosis of extremities and nailbeds. In the second type of cyanosis, the lips, oral membranes, and tongue appear blue-tinged, indicating hypoxemia due to inadequate Hgb saturation with oxygen. Central cyanosis is more serious, since it indicates an oxygen saturation of about 75–80%.

Clubbing Clubbing may be seen in the terminal phalanges of the fingers and toes. To recognize it, examine the angle between the base of the nail and the skin. The normal angle is about 160°; the increase of this angle to 180° or more is called clubbing. The cause of this increase in soft tissue is a combination of proliferation of fibroelastic tissue, interstitial edema, and dilatation and engorgement of the arterioles and venules (Cherniack and Cherniak 1983).

Palpation, Percussion, Auscultation

The remaining steps of palpation, percussion, and auscultation enable you to assess the vibrations transmitted by the thoracic contents. You will recall that air enters the lungs through the nose and mouth, which filter, humidify, and warm it. It then passes through the glottis to the trachea, which is highly vascular and supported by C-shaped cartilaginous rings. The trachea bifurcates into the mainstem bronchi at the carina, located anteri-

orly at the level of the angle of Louis and posteriorly at the level of T_4. The right mainstem bronchus is shorter, wider, and at a greater angle to the trachea than the left mainstem bronchus. The bronchi then subdivide repeatedly into the smaller airways.

In palpation, you will use your hands to feel the vibrations created by the movement of air through the airways when the patient speaks. In percussion, you will feel the vibrations created when you tap on the chest. In auscultation, you will use a stethoscope to exclude extraneous noise while you listen to the vibrations created by patient's breathing or speaking.

Sound Transmission While performing these steps, it is useful to remember some principles of sound transmission. Solid structures conduct sound better than air, unless they are too big or too compressed to respond to sound. Air in the pleural space will conduct sound very poorly.

Sounds are described according to their intensity, pitch, quality, and duration. *Intensity* refers to loudness, and *pitch* to the frequency of vibrations. *Quality* refers to the unique characteristics of a sound that enable you to identify it again once you have heard it, such as the quality of a fingernail scraping a blackboard.

To date, different authorities have used a bewildering array of terms to describe findings on palpation, percussion, and auscultation. This chapter presents the terms currently used by most practitioners as well as the simplified pulmonary labels recommended by the American Thoracic Society (Murphey and Holford 1980).

Palpation To continue the examination, palpate the chest to assess the position of the trachea, chest expansion, tactile fremitus, tenderness, and the presence of crepitus. The trachea should be midline; tracheal deviation can result from such conditions as pneumothorax and atelectasis. To evaluate chest expansion further, stand in back of the patient and place your hands on the lower rib cage so that you grasp the lateral ribs. Instruct the patient to exhale completely and then inhale deeply (using his abdominal muscles) to try to move your hands. As the patient breathes in, note whether your thumbs move apart equally.

Tactile fremitus is the name given to palpable vibrations caused by speaking. To palpate for fremitus, use the most sensitive part of your hands—either the pads of your fingertips or the part of your palm that overlies the heads of the metacarpal bones. Ask the patient to say "ninety-nine" several times while you palpate the chest wall bilaterally. Normally, you will be able to feel vibrations like the purring of a cat over the trachea and bronchi. These vibrations should be equal bilaterally, except over the heart. Since solids conduct vibrations better than air, any condition that consolidates the lung close to the chest wall will increase fremitus. Decreased or absent fremitus occurs when a condition blocks the passage of air (such as an obstructed bronchus) or moves the lung tissue away from the chest wall (such as a pneumothorax). *Crepitus,* or air leaking from the lung into the subcutaneous tissue, is particularly important to assess in the trauma patient or any patient with chest tubes in place. As the chest wall is palpated a crackling sensation is felt under your fingertips.

Percussion   Next, percuss the chest, to evaluate the density of structures just below the chest wall. To do this, press the terminal phalanx of your middle finger on the chest wall and strike it on the knuckle with the tip of your other middle finger. (Be sure to press only the terminal phalanx on the chest wall; if you allow contact between the rest of your hand and the chest, it will damp the vibrations.) Strike the phalanx quickly at almost a 90° angle by cocking your wrist.

There are five sounds you may hear; you can learn four of them by percussing your own body. The sound normally heard over the lungs is medium loud, low-pitched, and relatively long; it is called *resonant.* Increased density of the lungs (as in pulmonary edema or pleural effusion) produces dull or flat sounds. A *dull* sound results from a moderate increase in density. It is soft, short, and high-pitched and is the sound heard when you percuss the liver. A *flat* sound is due to a severe increase in density. It is soft, high-pitched, and very short; you can reproduce it by percussing your thigh. Decreased density (such as in pneumothorax or emphysema) causes either *hyperresonant* or *tympanitic* sounds. A moderate decrease in density produces a loud sound that is lower-pitched and longer than resonance, called hyperresonant; you cannot reproduce this sound in yourself, although you can mimic it somewhat by percussing your chest while you hold a deep breath. A large decrease in density produces a loud, long, high-pitched, drumlike sound described as tympanitic; you can reproduce it by percussing over your stomach. This term usually is not used in describing findings on lung percussion since it is heard commonly over air in an enclosed space.

Begin at the apices and percuss side to side down the chest until you reach the diaphragm. Listen for the sounds and feel for the vibrations produced.

Normally on percussing the chest you will hear resonance, except in a few locations. On the posterior chest, you will hear dullness over the vertebrae, scapulae, and below the diaphragm. On the anterior chest, you will hear dullness over the sternum and heart; dullness starting at about the fifth or sixth intercostal space on the right (the upper border of the liver); and tympany at about the sixth rib on the left, where the stomach begins.

If you hear an abnormal percussion note, localize the finding by percussing from an area of resonance to the abnormal area.

Auscultation   Finally, use the diaphragm of a stethoscope to auscultate the chest from side to side. Ask the person to breathe through the mouth a little more deeply than normal.

Listen first for breath sounds. There are basically three types: bronchial, vesicular, and bronchovesicular. *Bronchial* breath sounds normally are heard over the trachea and are hollow, tubular, and close to the ear and have a short inspiration, pause, and a longer, louder expiration. It is abnormal to hear this tubular breath sound elsewhere (such as the bases). Any condition that consolidates (solidifies) the lung, such as pneumonia or atelectasis, will increase sound transmission to the chest wall, creating bronchial or increased breath sounds. *Vesicular* breath sounds are those heard in the periphery of the lung over smaller airways and are soft, with a long inspiration, no pause, and a shorter, softer expiration. Sounds heard over medium-sized airways are referred to as *bronchovesicular* and have inspiratory and expiratory phases equal in loudness and length. Decreased or absent breath sounds are caused by any condition that reduces air flow (such as an obstructed bronchus) or moves the lungs away from the chest wall (such as pneumothorax or pleural effusion). Because interpretation varies with the listener, it is recommended that breath sounds be described only as normal, decreased, absent, or bronchial.

Next, listen for abnormal (adventitious) sounds, which are superimposed on breath sounds. Listen carefully to determine if the sound is continuous or discontinuous and high- or low-pitched and whether it occurs during inspiration or expiration. The American Thoracic Society recommends the use of four terms: two different discontinuous sounds referred to as coarse crackles and fine crackles (previously referred to as *rales*), and two continuous sounds—high-pitched wheeze and low-pitched rhonchus. *Crackles* (rales) result from either the sudden opening of closed alveoli, as in pulmonary fibrosis, or from air bubbling through fluid in the airway, as in pulmonary edema. Crackles may be heard during inspiration only or during both inspiration and expiration. A high-pitched continuous sound, or *wheeze,* results from air passing through a narrowed airway, as in bronchospasm, airway edema, foreign body, or tumor. If this high-pitched continuous sound is heard only during inspiration, it is called *stridor* (Murphey and Holford 1980). A low-pitched continuous sound, or *rhonchus,* is often associated with secretions and may clear following coughing or suctioning. A pleural friction rub may also be detected as a grating, continuous sound that results from pleural inflammation and varies with breathing. At present, to avoid misinterpretation by others, report your findings by describing their characteristics rather than just by labeling them.

Abnormal voice and whispered sounds rarely are checked in a screening examination by the critical-care nurse. They are included here primarily so you will understand their significance when noted in a thorough workup. Voice sounds are the auscultatory equivalent of the vibrations palpated during tactile fremitus. The patient is asked to say "ninety-nine" repeatedly. Normally, the sounds are heard indistinctly over the large airways and are equal bilaterally. Absent voice sounds occur when air flow is blocked (as in an obstructed bronchus) or the lung and chest wall are separated (as in a pneumothorax). Increased voice sounds are due to consolidation (solidification) of the lung. Increased sounds are detected when the syllables are heard more clearly than normal although still muffled; this finding is called *bronchophony*. A related finding, also due to consolidation, occurs when the patient's spoken E is heard as A; this phenomenon is called *egophony*. Whispered sounds normally are heard only faintly over the mainstem bronchi. In consolidation they are heard clearly; this occurrence is called *whispered pectoriloquy*. The American Thoracic Society recommends a much simpler classification. It suggests that findings be reported as *voice or whispered sounds that are normal; decreased or absent; or increased in intensity or clarity.*

Significance of Findings   To interpret the significance of your findings from inspection, palpation, percussion, and auscultation, consider them in association with each other; some of the common groupings are included in Table 7–2.

When you assume responsibility for a patient, it is useful to at least inspect and auscultate the chest so you have a basis for comparison as you later evaluate the effects of your nursing care. For instance, when you come on duty you might note that your patient is restless and slightly tachycardic. Auscultation might reveal diffuse crackles and rhonchi. After chest physiotherapy and suctioning, you would again auscultate the chest; the absence of the adventitious sounds would indicate the effectiveness of your intervention to improve oxygenation. Your skill at chest diagnosis can be a valuable tool in assessing, diagnosing, planning, implementing, and evaluating the care you give patients.

Other Signs of Respiratory Failure   Cough, dyspnea, and chest pain are three common features of respiratory disease that should be assessed. Frequency, productivity, and changes in cough and sputum production give information as to the onset of retained secretions, congestive failure, etc. Dyspnea, or the patient's subjective feelings of breathlessness, is seen in both cardiac and pulmonary dysfunction. You should elicit from your patient what makes his or her dyspnea worse and what he or she does at home to decrease it. It is important to localize chest pain, for it may indicate viral infection, pulmonary embolism, pulmonary hypertension, pleurisy, pneumothorax, subdiaphragmatic processes, rib fractures, or myocardial ischemia (Luce et al. 1984).

Confusion and disorientation may be seen in hypoxia or CO_2 retention; drowsiness and headache may indicate CO_2 retention. Peripheral edema, jugular venous distention, and liver tenderness may be seen in cor pulmonale.

Atrial and supraventricular dysrhythmias are common in the patient with COPD due to cor pulmonale. In COPD and other respiratory disorders, hypoxia and blood-gas–related electrolyte disturbances can result in tachycardia, ectopy, and blood pressure changes.

Pulmonary Function Tests

A basic understanding of frequently performed pulmonary function tests is essential for the critical-care nurse. With an increasingly older patient population, many of whom still smoke, it is not unusual to have pulmonary function tests available for the patient in chronic respiratory failure as well as the patient with COPD undergoing open heart surgery. Identifying the patient at risk for developing postoperative respiratory failure can help you plan, implement, and evaluate your nursing care.

Lung Volumes and Capacities

The air in the lungs can be subdivided into several volumes and capacities. A lung *volume* cannot be subdivided further. Two or more volumes combine to make a *capacity*. Figure 7–3 presents the volumes and capacities graphically and gives examples of normal values. It must be stressed that these normal values are variable and are predicted on the basis of sex, age, height, weight, activity, and barometric pressure. The "normal" values given here apply only to a healthy young male lying at rest and breathing air at sea level. They are taken from Guyton (1986).

TABLE 7–2 TYPICAL ASSESSMENT FINDINGS

CONDITION	INSPECTION	PERCUSSION	PALPATION	AUSCULTATION
COPD	Patient sitting up-right, leaning forward Pursed-lip breathing Barrel chest Using neck muscles Copious sputum (often green-tinged)	Hyperresonance ↓ diaphragm movement	↓ chest excursion	Decreased breath sounds Faint expiratory wheezes Decreased voice sounds
Pulmonary edema	Patient sitting up-right Shallow, rapid respirations Distended neck veins Copious frothy sputum	Resonance	↓ chest excursion	Coarse crackles (inspiration and expiration) S_3 or S_4 gallop Often, irregular heart rhythm
Pneumothorax	Asymmetrical chest excursion	Hyperresonance	Trachea midline or shifted away from pneumothorax ↓ chest movement	Absent breath sounds Decreased fremitus Decreased voice sounds
Consolidation (pneumonia)	Tachypnea Purulent rust-colored sputum	Dullness		Bronchial breath sounds Increased fremitus Increased voice sounds
Atelectasis	Tachypnea (+/−)	Dullness	↓ chest movement on affected side (if severe) Trachea midline or deviated towards affected side	Decreased breath sounds* Decreased fremitus Decreased voice sounds
Pleural effusion	Tachypnea	Dullness	↓ chest movement on affected side (if large) Trachea deviated away from affected side	Decreased breath sounds Decreased fremitus Decreased voice sounds

*May hear bronchial breath sounds if lobe collapsed and bronchus open.

Tidal Volume, Inspiratory Reserve Volume, and Expiratory Reserve Volume *Tidal volume* (V_T) is the amount of gas inspired or expired with a normal breath. It is measured with a spirometer. Its normal value is 500 ml. *Inspiratory reserve volume* is the volume that can be inspired above tidal volume; the normal value is about 3,000 ml. *Expiratory reserve volume* is the amount that can be expired below tidal volume; the normal value is about 1,100 ml. These two reserve volumes provide little information about pulmonary function.

Residual Volume, Functional Residual Capacity, and Total Lung Capacity *Residual volume* is the amount of gas that always remains in the lungs, that is, that cannot be expelled even with a maximal expiration. It cannot be measured directly. Instead, the patient breathes in a known percentage of an insoluble gas. Expired gas is collected for several minutes and analyzed for the amount of expired air and concentration of the gas. The residual volume can then be calculated; a normal value is 1,200 ml. This test measures only the air in parts of the lung that communicate well with the airways. It is not accurate for completely trapped gas, as

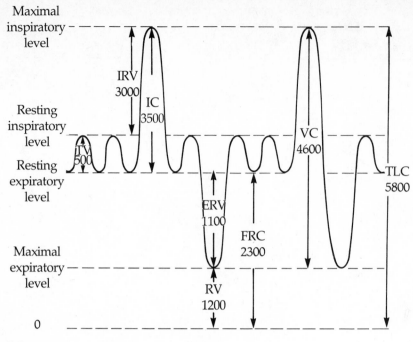

FIGURE 7–3

Lung volumes and capacities. *ERV,* expiratory reserve volume; *FRC,* functional residual capacity; *IC,* inspiratory capacity; *IRV,* inspiratory reserve volume; *RV,* residual volume; *TLC,* total lung capacity; *TV,* tidal volume; *VC,* vital capacity.

in emphysema. For such patients, a body plethysmograph ("body box") must be used to measure residual volume in the laboratory.

As mentioned above, two or more volumes combine to make a lung capacity. *Inspiratory capacity* is the maximum volume that can be inspired starting from a resting expiratory level, in other words, the tidal volume plus the inspiratory reserve volume. Inspiratory capacity measures about 3,500 ml and usually represents 75% of the vital capacity. *Functional residual capacity* (FRC) consists of the residual volume plus the expiratory reserve volume and represents the volume of air in the lungs at the end of a normal expiration. A usual value is 2,300 ml. The FRC functions to maintain a constant alveolar P_{CO_2}. It increases in hyperinflation, such as in emphysema or asthma. An increased FRC means an increased muscular effort of breathing, because thoracic size is increased. It also means impaired ability to increase ventilation and to alter quickly the composition of alveolar gas.

A decrease in FRC is seen in restrictive diseases that decrease the number of open alveoli, such as atelectasis, pulmonary edema, and pneumonia. A decrease

in FRC is the primary defect in the adult respiratory distress syndrome (ARDS) that causes hypoxemia due to severe atelectasis and alveolar edema. Positive end-expiratory pressure (PEEP) increases FRC by increasing alveolar surface area for gas exchange. (ARDS and PEEP are discussed in Chapters 8 and 9.) Deep inspiratory maneuvers also aid to reexpand alveoli and increase FRC.

The total amount of air in the lungs is called *total lung capacity* and measures about 5,800 ml. It consists of FRC and inspiratory capacity.

Vital Capacity *Vital capacity* (VC) is very important clinically. It equals the total lung capacity minus the residual volume and is a measure of the person's ability to take a deep breath. To measure it, the nurse should tell the patient to take a deep inspiration and then expel as much air as possible. The exhaled volume is measured with a spirometer. Normal vital capacity is about 4,600 ml. A decreased vital capacity is a helpful but nonspecific sign, since it may be caused by depression of the respiratory center, obstructive diseases, or restrictive conditions. It is important to recognize that a normal vital capacity does not rule out the presence of pulmonary disease, such as pulmonary embolism.

Maximum Inspiratory Force Although not a lung volume or capacity, *maximum inspiratory force* (MIF) measures the ability of the patient to move air and cough effectively. Bedside measurement of VC and MIF in the intubated patient can help predict the ability of that patient to cough and take deep breaths following extubation. MIF is measured by having the patient breathe in against a negative-pressure manometer while his or her airway is occluded. The normal MIF is about -60 to -100 cm H_2O pressure. If the MIF is less than -25 cm H_2O, the person probably cannot maintain a normal sigh volume or cough effectively.

Significance To interpret the patient's pulmonary volumes and capacities, group the data into the broad categories of obstructive and restrictive pulmonary diseases. *Obstructive* diseases are those associated with increased resistance to airflow, particularly during expiration, such as asthma and emphysema. Increased total lung capacity, increased functional residual capacity, and decreased expiratory flow rates characterize obstructive pulmonary diseases. *Restrictive* diseases are those that limit lung expansion. Decreased total lung capacity, vital capacity, and functional residual capacity characterize restrictive pulmonary diseases.

When interpreting lung measurements, remember that the trend of values is more important than one particular reading.

Airway Resistance

In order for air to move in and out of the lungs, the work of breathing must overcome a variety of resistances. These resistances can be subdivided into three categories: airway resistance, tissue resistance, and compliance (Guyton 1986).

Airway resistance to gas flow depends on the lumen size, velocity of air flow, and gas characteristics. In normal, quiet breathing, airway resistance is slight. Airway resistance can be evaluated by measuring the relationship between pressure and air flow. It is not feasible to measure airway resistance directly in the critically ill, but indirect measurements can be obtained by measuring expiratory flow rates. The patient is asked to breathe in as much air as possible and then to expel it as hard and fast as possible. This forced expiratory volume is recorded on a graph containing a time scale. The volume expired in one second is called FEV_1. The ratio

between it and vital capacity (FEV_1/VC) is an indicator of resistance in the larger airways. The normal person is able to expel about 80% of vital capacity in the first second. In the patient with obstructive airway disease (COPD) the FEV_1/VC may be as low as 45%.

The tissues of the lungs and thoracic cage exert tissue resistance; that is, they resist the molecular rearrangements necessary for lung expansion and contraction. Only a small amount of the work of breathing is necessary to overcome this nonelastic tissue resistance.

Compliance

The tissues of the lung and thorax also have elastic resistances that must be overcome during inspiration. The lung tissues resist inspiration because they contain elastic fibers and because the fluids lining the alveoli have surface tension, as explained below. These factors make the lungs tend to recoil (deflate). The thoracic muscles, tendons, and connective tissue also have elastic properties that make them resist expansion.

The expansibility of the lungs and chest wall is called *compliance*. It can be evaluated by measuring the relationship between pressure and volume and can be expressed as the change in volume (V) per unit of change in pressure (P): $C = \Delta V/\Delta P$. In the critically ill, effective dynamic compliance equals tidal volume (V_T) divided by inspiratory peak pressure; normal is about 45 ml/cm H_2O. Since peak pressure is affected by resistance in the airway and breathing circuit, a more accurate compliance measure may be effective static compliance. It equals V_T divided by inspiratory plateau pressure (end-inspiratory pressure); normal is about 70 ml/cm H_2O. (If PEEP is used, it is subtracted from the peak inspiratory pressure or the inspiratory plateau pressure, depending on whether dynamic or static compliance is being measured.) Compliance decreases in conditions that (a) increase the resistance of the chest wall, such as scoliosis, tight dressings, and musculoskeletal diseases such as polio, or that (b) reduce the distensibility of the lung, such as pulmonary congestion, atelectasis, restrictive diseases, and disorders characterized by decreased surfactant.

The surface between the alveolar gas and alveolar wall has the property of surface tension, that is, attraction between the surface molecules of the fluid. This property tends to make the alveoli collapse, thereby making expansion very difficult. Surfactant, a lipoprotein made by special alveolar cells, counters this tendency. It progressively decreases surface tension on expiration, thus helping to control alveolar volume and prevent alveolar collapse. When surfactant decreases (as in

ARDS), alveolar surface tension increases. Because of the resulting decrease in lung distensibility, compliance decreases.

Deadspace

The pulmonary symbol for a volume of gas is V. With a dot over it ($\dot{V}$), it means volume per unit time, assumed to be one minute unless stated otherwise.

The total volume of air that ventilates the lungs per minute is called the *minute ventilation* ($\dot{V}_E$). It is the product of tidal volume (V_T) and respiratory rate (f). Part of the minute ventilation merely fills the tracheobronchial tree and does not participate in gas exchange; this is called *deadspace* (V_D). The volume of gas per minute that actually reaches the alveoli and participates in gas exchange is called *alveolar ventilation* ($\dot{V}_A$).

There are two types of deadspace: anatomic deadspace and alveolar deadspace. *Anatomic deadspace* is the air in the tracheobronchial tree up to the terminal bronchioles. *Alveolar deadspace* is that air in the alveoli that does not participate in gas exchange, because the alveoli containing it are without adequate capillary blood flow. (In other words, ventilation exceeds perfusion, so the ventilation/perfusion ratio, or $\dot{V}/\dot{Q}$ ratio, is greater than normal.) The sum of anatomic deadspace and alveolar deadspace is called *physiologic deadspace*.

Alveolar ventilation equals tidal volume minus deadspace, times respiratory rate; that is $\dot{V}_A = (V_t - V_D)f$. A normal value is about 5,200 ml assuming $V_T = 500$, $V_D = 150$, and f = 15. Alveolar ventilation can be either estimated or measured. To estimate it, you must know the tidal volume, respiratory rate, and weight of your patient. Then assume that the anatomic deadspace equals 2 ml/kg (1 ml/lb) of body weight, subtract that value from the tidal volume, and multiply by the rate. Note that this formula does not take into account alveolar deadspace and will be inaccurate for patients with either increased alveolar deadspace (as in pulmonary embolism) or altered anatomic deadspace (as in a tracheostomy). Alveolar ventilation can be calculated more accurately by measuring physiologic deadspace. The patient's expired air is collected for several minutes and analyzed for expired Pco_2 ($P_{\overline{E}}co_2$). The arterial Pco_2 (P_aco_2*) is measured from an arterial blood sample. A modified Bohr equation is used:

$$V_D = V_T \times \frac{P_aco_2 - P_{\overline{E}}co_2}{P_aco_2}$$

The value obtained for deadspace then can be subtracted from tidal volume. The resulting number is multiplied by rate to calculate alveolar ventilation.

In the normal lung, deadspace is minimized by a protective reflex. When alveolar deadspace increases, the lack of matching perfusion causes local bronchoconstriction, which redirects ventilation to better-perfused areas.

V_D/V_T Ratio

More commonly in the clinical setting, we are less interested in the amount of alveolar ventilation per se than in the ratio between deadspace and tidal volume. This V_D/V_T ratio indicates what proportion of tidal volume is being wasted as deadspace. As explained later, the Pco_2 of arterial blood is a useful indicator of tidal volume. Comparing the Pco_2 of arterial blood and the Pco_2 of expired gas indicates the amount of wasted ventilation. Rearranging the terms of the modified Bohr equation gives the equation for the ratio:

$$\frac{V_D}{V_T} = \frac{P_aco_2 - P_{\overline{E}}co_2}{P_aco_2}$$

The usual V_D/V_T ratio is approximately 0.3; above 0.6, it is unlikely that the person can maintain spontaneous ventilation.

Blood Gas Values

The adequacy of gas exchange in the lungs can be evaluated by arterial blood gas analysis. The blood sample is withdrawn from an existing arterial line or by percutaneous puncture of an artery.

Interpreting Blood Gas Values

The laboratory report of arterial blood gases will state the Po_2, Pco_2, and a measure of bases in the body (either bicarbonate or base excess). A convenient progression in analyzing these values is first to analyze the partial pressures reported and then to analyze the acid–

*Note that P stands for *partial pressure*. A subscript written with a capital letter means the gas is in the gaseous phase; one written with a lowercase letter signifies the gas in a liquid phase. Thus, P_Aco_2 means alveolar Pco_2, whereas P_aco_2 means arterial Pco_2. A dash above a symbol signifies a mean value. See Table 7–3 for a complete list of abbreviations and their definitions.

TABLE 7–3 SYMBOLS RELATED TO PULMONARY FUNCTION

Elements, Chemicals

O_2	Oxygen	Cl^-	Chloride ion
CO_2	Carbon dioxide	HCO_3^-	Bicarbonate ion
N_2	Nitrogen	$NaHCO_3$	Sodium bicarbonate
He	Helium	H_2CO_3	Carbonic acid
H_2O	Water	CO	Carbon monoxide
Na^+	Sodium ion	CN	Cyanide
K^+	Potassium ion	CA	Carbonic anhydrase

Gas Fractions

F_{GAS}	Fraction of a gas	F_EO_2	Fraction of expired oxygen
F_IO_2	Fraction of inspired oxygen		

Gas Pressures

P_B	Barometric (atmospheric) pressure
P_{GAS}	Partial pressure of a gas
PO_2	Partial pressure of oxygen
P_IO_2	Partial pressure of oxygen in inspired gas
P_AO_2	Partial pressure of oxygen in alveolar gas
PaO_2	Partial pressure of oxygen in arterial blood
$P_{(A-a)}O_2$	Alveolar-arterial oxygen pressure difference
$P_{\bar{v}}O_2$	Partial pressure of oxygen in mixed venous blood
P_cO_2	Partial pressure of oxygen in capillary blood
PCO_2	Partial pressure of carbon dioxide
P_ICO_2	Partial pressure of carbon dioxide in inspired gas
P_ACO_2	Partial pressure of carbon dioxide in alveolar gas
P_aCO_2	Partial pressure of carbon dioxide in arterial blood
$P_{\bar{v}}CO_2$	Partial pressure of carbon dioxide in mixed venous blood
P_cCO_2	Partial pressure of carbon dioxide in capillary blood

Gas Saturations

S_aO_2	Saturation of oxygen in arterial blood
P_{50}	Partial pressure of oxygen at which one half of hemoglobin molecules are saturated
$S_{\bar{v}}O_2$	Saturation of oxygen in mixed venous blood

Gas Contents

C_aO_2	Content of oxygen in arterial blood
$C_{\bar{v}}O_2$	Content of oxygen in mixed venous blood
$C_{(a-\bar{v})}O_2$	Arterial-mixed venous oxygen content difference

Terms Describing Respiration

$\dot{V}O_2$	Oxygen consumption	RQ	Respiratory quotient
$\dot{V}CO_2$	Carbon dioxide production	R	Respiratory exchange ratio

Symbols for Perfusion

$\dot{Q}$	Blood perfusion (flow)	$\dot{Q}_s$	Shunt flow
$\dot{Q}_T$	Cardiac output	$\dot{Q}_s/\dot{Q}_T$	Shunt fraction

(Continues)

TABLE 7–3 SYMBOLS RELATED TO PULMONARY FUNCTION (Continued)

Symbols for Ventilation

$\dot{V}_E$	Minute ventilation	V_D/V_T	Dead space fraction
$\dot{V}_A$	Alveolar ventilation	$\dot{V}_A/\dot{Q}$	Ventilation-perfusion ratio
V_T	Tidal volume	$D_{L}CO$	Diffusion capacity for carbon monoxide
V_D	Dead space ventilation		

Terms Describing Compliance

P_{MAX}	Maximum (peak) pressure
P_{STAT}	Static (plateau) pressure
C_{DYN}	Dynamic compliance
C_{STAT}	Static compliance
C_{RS}	Respiratory system compliance

Terms Describing Pulmonary Function

FVC	Forced vital capacity
FEV_1	Forced expiratory volume in one second
FEF_{25-75}	Forced expiratory flow over .25 to .75 second
FRC	Functional residual capacity
TLC	Total lung capacity
RV	Residual volume
IC	Inspiratory capacity
IRV	Inspiratory reserve volume
ERV	Expiratory reserve volume
MVV	Maximum voluntary ventilation
MIF	Maximum inspiratory force
WOB	Work of breathing

Terms Describing Fluid and Acid–Base Balance

ECF	Extracellular fluid
ICF	Intracellular fluid
BE	Base excess

Terms Describing Diseases or Therapy

COPD	Chronic obstructive pulmonary disease
NRDS	Neonatal respiratory distress syndrome
ARDS	Adult respiratory distress syndrome
CF	Cystic fibrosis
PBL	Persistent bronchopleural gas leak
CPT	Chest physical therapy

Terms Describing Ventilation

SV	Spontaneous ventilation
IMV	Intermittent mechanical (mandatory) ventilation
AMV	Assisted mechanical ventilation
CMV	Controlled mechanical ventilation
PEEP	Positive end-expiratory pressure
CPAP	Continuous positive airway pressure
EPAP	Expiratory positive airway pressure
CPPV	Continuous positive pressure ventilation
IPPV	Intermittent positive pressure ventilation
IPPB	Intermittent positive pressure breathing

(Continues)

TABLE 7–3   SYMBOLS RELATED TO PULMONARY FUNCTION (Continued)

Terms Used in Hemodynamic Monitoring

HR	Heart rate
SV	Stroke volume
MAP	Mean arterial pressure
ICP	Intracranial pressure
SVR	Systemic vascular resistance
PVR	Pulmonary vascular resistance
P_{FAW}	Pulmonary arterial wedge pressure
EMD	Electromechanical dissociation

Source: Luce J et al.: *Intensive respiratory care.* Philadelphia: Saunders, 1984.

base values. Chapter 16 on metabolic imbalances presents the interpretation of acid–base values. This chapter will review the interpretation of partial pressures, which are reported in mm Hg, or torr (1 torr = 1 mm Hg at 0° C).

Diffusing Capacity   Before discussing factors related to interpretation of only P_{O_2} or only P_{CO_2}, it is helpful to review those factors affecting exchange of both gases. The ability of the alveolar-capillary membrane to exchange a gas is called its *diffusing capacity.* Guyton (1986) defines diffusing capacity as "the volume of a gas that diffuses through the membrane each minute for a pressure difference of 1 mm Hg." The diffusing capacity for a given gas is affected by the pressure gradient across the membrane, the area of the membrane, the thickness of the membrane, and the diffusion coefficient of the gas.

Pressure Gradients   The pressure gradients for O_2 and CO_2 are major determinants of gas exchange. In a mixture of gases, such as atmospheric or alveolar air, the pressure exerted by each gas is independent of the other gases and proportional to its percentage of the total gas (Dalton's law). The pressure exerted by each gas is called its *partial pressure*. The total pressure of the air inspired is the *barometric (atmospheric)* pressure, which varies in relation to distance above or below sea level; at sea level it is 760 mm Hg. The partial pressure of a gas is calculated by multiplying the total pressure by the percentage of the gas. Table 7–4 presents the approximate percentages and partial pressures for inspired (tracheal) air, which consists primarily of nitrogen, oxygen, carbon dioxide, and water vapor. (*Note:* To obtain the partial pressures of inspired gases, the pressure exerted by water vapor must be subtracted first. The reason for this subtraction is that gases in the airways are completely humidified; this means that at 37°C the other gases can exert a maximum partial pressure of 713 mm Hg.) The partial pressure of oxygen in inspired air is 150 mm Hg, while the partial pressure of CO_2 is 0.2 mm Hg.

Alveolar air differs somewhat from tracheal air. Nitrogen, which accounts for the greatest percentage,

TABLE 7–4   COMPOSITION OF INSPIRED (TRACHEAL) GAS AT SEA LEVEL

Total barometric pressure	760 mm Hg
−Water vapor at 37°C	47
Corrected barometric pressure	713 mm Hg

GAS	PERCENTAGE		PARTIAL PRESSURE
Nitrogen	79.03%	× 713 =	563.5 mm Hg
Oxygen	20.94%	× 713 =	149.3
Carbon dioxide	0.03%	× 713 =	0.2
Total	100%		713.0 mm Hg

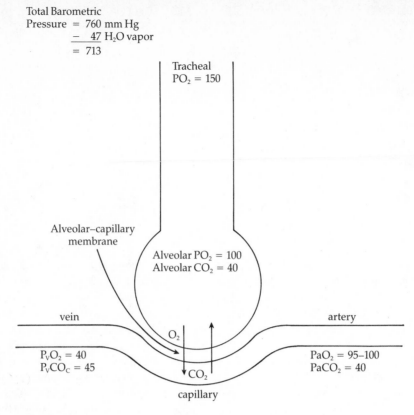

Total Barometric
Pressure = 760 mm Hg
       −   47 H$_2$O vapor
       = 713

Tracheal
PO$_2$ = 150

Alveolar–capillary
membrane

Alveolar PO$_2$ = 100
Alveolar CO$_2$ = 40

vein   artery

O$_2$

P$_V$O$_2$ = 40   PaO$_2$ = 95–100
P$_V$CO$_C$ = 45   PaCO$_2$ = 40

CO$_2$

capillary

FIGURE 7–4

Alveolar-capillary gas exchange.

readily establishes equilibrium across the alveolar-capillary membrane and therefore can be disregarded. The remaining gas consists of about 14% oxygen, 5% CO_2, and 6% water vapor. Thus, alveolar air contains less oxygen and more carbon dioxide than tracheal air.

The partial pressure of O_2 in alveolar air is about 100 mm Hg. The partial pressure of CO_2 in alveolar air is 40 mm Hg. Blood in the pulmonary capillaries has P_{O_2} of 40 mm Hg and P_{CO_2} of 45 mm Hg. The resulting pressure gradients cause oxygen to diffuse from the alveoli into the capillaries, and carbon dioxide to diffuse from the capillaries into the alveoli. Although the pressure gradient for CO_2 is small, carbon dioxide diffuses faster than oxygen because its solubility is much greater (Figure 7–4).

Surface Area and Thickness of Membrane In addition to the pressure gradients, factors affecting gas exchange in the alveoli are the alveolar surface area and the thickness of the alveolar-capillary membrane. The alveolar surface area varies with age, body size, lung volume, presence of surfactant, and other factors. It decreases with emphysema and pneumonectomy.

The thickness of the alveolar-capillary membrane occasionally becomes clinically important, because increased thickness reduces the diffusing capacity. The membrane's thickness increases with pulmonary edema and pulmonary fibrosis.

Diffusion Coefficient The diffusion coefficient expresses the rate of gas transfer across the membrane. According to Guyton (1986), the coefficient depends on both the gas's solubility and its molecular weight. The diffusion coefficient of carbon dioxide is approximately twenty times that of oxygen.

Ventilation/Perfusion Relationships Of the four factors affecting diffusing capacity, changes in pressure gradients are most important clinically. Pressure gradients depend on the relationship between ventilation and blood flow in alveolar-capillary units.

The relationship between ventilation ($\dot{V}$) and perfusion ($\dot{Q}$) has a critical influence on gas exchange. The lungs are perfused by two circulations: the bronchial and the pulmonary. The bronchial circulation provides oxygenated blood to supply the lung structures down to and

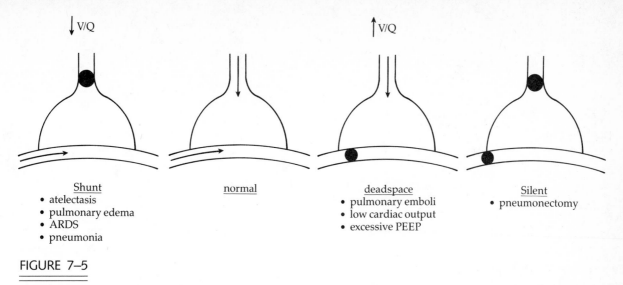

$\downarrow$ V/Q

$\uparrow$ V/Q

Shunt
- atelectasis
- pulmonary edema
- ARDS
- pneumonia

normal

deadspace
- pulmonary emboli
- low cardiac output
- excessive PEEP

Silent
- pneumonectomy

FIGURE 7–5

Types of ventilation-perfusion units.

including the terminal bronchioles (but not the alveoli). The pulmonary circulation provides deoxygenated blood to participate in gas exchange and incidentally nourishes the alveoli. After the pulmonary blood is oxygenated, it travels through pulmonary veins, which ultimately empty into the left atrium.

There is a continuum of relationships between ventilation and perfusion (Figure 7–5). At one end of the continuum is a unit that is perfused but not ventilated, the *shunt unit* discussed later in the chapter. In the middle of the continuum, the *normal unit* is both ventilated and perfused. At the other end of the continuum is a unit that is ventilated but not perfused, the *deadspace unit* already discussed. (If a unit is neither ventilated nor perfused, it is referred to as a *silent unit.*)

Even in the normal lung there is an uneven distribution of ventilation in relation to perfusion; in any given part of the lung, the ventilation and perfusion may not match. Some areas of the lung have too much ventilation in relation to perfusion, others too little. These regional $\dot{V}/\dot{Q}$ mismatches are unimportant in the healthy person.

The previous sections discuss factors common to exchange of both oxygen and carbon dioxide and therefore common to interpretation of P_aO_2 and P_aCO_2. The following sections discuss individual factors related to interpretation of P_aO_2 as an indicator of oxygenation and P_aCO_2 as an indicator of alveolar ventilation.

Po_2 and Other Indices of Oxygenation   In order to interpret Po_2 as an indicator of oxygenation, you need a clear understanding of the relationship between Po_2 and other indices of oxygenation. As the distinc-

tions among these measurements can be confusing, they are defined in the following sections.

Oxygen is carried in the blood in two ways: about 97% is bound to hemoglobin, and about 3% is dissolved in the blood. The total amount that can be dissolved in the blood is about 0.3 ml/100 ml blood. The amount that can be carried on fully saturated hemoglobin is 1.34 ml O_2/g hemoglobin. If you assume a normal hemoglobin level of 15 g/100 ml, the hemoglobin could carry 15 × 1.34 ml = 20.1 ml O_2 in each 100 ml of blood. The total amount Hgb *could* carry (20.1 ml) plus the dissolved amount (0.3 ml) is called the O_2 *carrying capacity.* The *actual* amount of oxygen the blood is carrying is the O_2 *content.*

A widely used index of oxygenation that affects O_2 content is the *partial pressure of oxygen (Po_2),* that is, the pressure of the O_2 dissolved in the blood. Po_2 is the major determinant of O_2 *saturation,* which in turn provides a close estimate of the O_2 content. O_2 saturation is a percentage expressing the relationship between the amount of O_2 the hemoglobin is carrying and the amount it could carry, that is, between the O_2 content and the O_2 carrying capacity.

Oxyhemoglobin Dissociation Curve   The relationship of Po_2 to O_2 saturation is expressed in the *oxyhemoglobin dissociation curve* (Figure 7–6). This relationship is not linear; a given amount of change in Po_2 may be associated with varying amounts of change in O_2 saturation.

In most cases, you do not need to know the precise O_2 saturation for nursing purposes. It is helpful, however, to realize the implications of the oxyhemoglobin

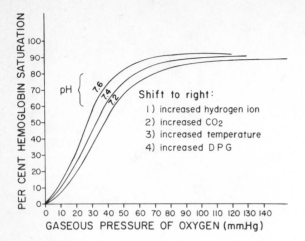

FIGURE 7–6

Shift of the oxygen-hemoglobin dissociation curve to the right by increases in *(1)* hydrogen ions, *(2)* CO_2, *(3)* temperature, or *(4)* DPG. (From Guyton A: *Textbook of medical physiology,* 7th ed. Philadelphia: Saunders, 1986.)

dissociation curve. A few examples will show its great clinical importance. At a high P_{O_2} (such as that in lung capillaries), hemoglobin becomes almost completely saturated with O_2, producing a normal O_2 saturation of 95–100% for arterial blood. This fact enables it to carry O_2 to areas of low P_{O_2} such as the tissue capillaries. There, P_{O_2} is about 40 mm Hg; as a result, hemoglobin becomes less saturated, giving up its O_2 to the tissues, which need it for cellular metabolism. The normal saturation for venous blood is about 70–75%.

You will notice that the upper portion of the curve is relatively flat while the middle and lower parts are steep. At the upper end of the curve, a large change in P_{O_2} is associated with only a small change in O_2 saturation. This fact is the reason we are not very alarmed when a patient's arterial P_{O_2} drops from 90 to 80; the hemoglobin still will be well saturated and therefore able to carry O_2 to the tissues. On the steep portion of the curve, however, a change in P_{O_2} is associated with a much greater effect on O_2 saturation. A drop in arterial P_{O_2} from 60 to 40, for instance, indicates a significant reduction in the amount of O_2 carried by hemoglobin to the tissues.

Another important implication of the curve is that an arterial P_{O_2} over 100 mm Hg does not really benefit a patient, because hemoglobin saturation cannot exceed 100%.

A number of conditions can alter the hemoglobin dissociation curve for the patient. Examples are fever and acidosis, which shift the curve to the right, indicating that hemoglobin has less affinity for O_2. As less oxygen

is picked up in the lungs, O_2 content decreases. Although oxygen is able to dissociate from hemoglobin more easily than normal at the tissue level, the decreased O_2 content limits the amount of oxygen that can be delivered to the tissues. A subnormal temperature or alkalosis will move the curve to the left, causing a higher than usual O_2 saturation, which indicates that hemoglobin has more affinity for O_2. Although the lungs pick up more oxygen than normal, so that O_2 content is increased, it is harder than normal for oxygen to dissociate from hemoglobin at the tissue level. As a result, the oxygen tension may be less effective in oxygenating the tissues.

A knowledge of what P_{O_2} and other indices of oxygenation represent will help you avoid erroneous conclusions based on them. For instance, you will recognize that P_{O_2} or O_2 saturation alone does not tell you how much oxygen actually is being carried in the blood. In order to calculate the amount of O_2 a given patient's blood is carrying, you must know both the O_2 saturation and the hemoglobin level; 95% saturation of 15 g is considerably different from the same saturation of 10 g. Similarly, even an adequate O_2 content in the blood does not mean the tissues are well oxygenated; the patient could be in shock and have a cardiac output too low to carry the O_2 to the peripheral areas of the body. In other words, *adequate tissue oxygenation depends on an adequate PO_2 for optimal hemoglobin saturation, a normal level of hemoglobin* to carry the oxygen, *and satisfactory circulation* to carry the oxygen to the tissues.

The previous sections discuss the significance of the P_aO_2. The following paragraphs describe the technique of interpreting the P_aO_2 and related measures.

P_aO_2 Interpretation When evaluating P_aO_2 data from the laboratory, make the following observations:

Note the measured P_aO_2 and the percentage of inspired oxygen at the time the sample was obtained. This percentage usually is expressed as the fractional inspired oxygen concentration, or F_IO_2; the value is given as a decimal. An F_IO_2 of 0.4, for instance, means 40% O_2 concentration. The F_IO_2 of room air is 0.21.

Compare the actual P_aO_2 and F_IO_2 to the desired P_aO_2 and F_IO_2 for that patient. Ideal values are P_aO_2 of 80–100 mm Hg on an F_IO_2 of 0.21 (room air). Also note O_2 saturation, which normally is 95% or higher.

Mixed Venous Blood Values So far, we have been discussing analysis of arterial blood samples. As arterial blood has not yet reached the systemic tissues, it does not give a full picture of what is happening on the cellular level. In some situations, it is helpful to analyze samples of mixed venous blood. Mixed venous blood cannot be obtained from peripheral veins. The P_{O_2} of peripheral venous blood represents the arterial-venous O_2 difference of only that area of tissue, and varies depending on the area sampled, its metabolic activity, and distance from the heart. Mixed venous blood is obtained from the distal port of a catheter in the pulmonary artery. By the time blood reaches the pulmonary artery, venous drainage from various peripheral areas, the coronary sinus, and Thebesian veins have become blended, so this blood reflects the state of overall tissue oxygenation. Current technology allows for continuous monitoring of mixed venous oxygen saturation ($S\overline{v}_{O_2}$) values from specially designed pulmonary artery catheters.

Normal values for mixed venous P_{O_2}, O_2 saturation, and O_2 content all are lower than for arterial blood. See Table 7–5.

If venous values are normal, it is possible to conclude that tissue oxygenation is adequate. Increases in these values imply that less O_2 than normal is being used by the tissues or that there is an abnormal source adding O_2 to venous blood (such as a left-to-right cardiac shunt). Decreases imply that there is a problem with the lungs and/or heart. If the lungs are oxygenating arterial blood inadequately, normal tissue oxygen extraction will result in an even lower venous P_{O_2} than normal. If the heart's CO is low, slowed circulation will allow more time for tissue oxygen extraction, again resulting in an abnormally low venous P_{O_2}.

Alveolar-Arterial O_2 Difference Often, a critically ill person will have a low $P_a{O_2}$. Identification of the cause is essential for optimal therapy.

A decreased $P_a{O_2}$ can occur in two general ways: First, the alveolar P_{O_2} may be low, as in hypoventilation or, rarely, decreased $F_I{O_2}$ in high altitudes. Second, alveolar P_{O_2} may be normal but diffusion into the capillaries may be impaired, as in ventilation/perfusion mismatch, increased shunting, or, rarely, a diffusion block at the alveolar-capillary membrane.

Because the diffusing capacity of carbon dioxide is about twenty times that of oxygen, damage to the alveolar-capillary membrane affects oxygen diffusion long before it affects carbon dioxide diffusion.

In the clinical setting, oxygen diffusing capacity cannot be measured directly. Instead, the adequacy of diffusing capacity can be inferred from the alveolar-arterial oxygen difference ($Aa_{D_{O_2}}$), sometimes called the *alveolar-arterial (A–a) gradient*. The $Aa_{D_{O_2}}$ can be calculated from a set of arterial blood gas values on a known oxygen percentage. A simplified version of the alveolar gas equation is used (Luce et al. 1984):

$$P_{A_{O_2}} = P_{I_{O_2}} - \frac{P_{A_{CO_2}}}{R}$$

In other words, the P_{O_2} of alveolar air equals the inspired P_{O_2}, minus the alveolar P_{CO_2} divided by the respiratory exchange ratio (R). The respiratory exchange ratio is the amount of CO_2 produced divided by the amount of oxygen consumed. The usual value on a mixed diet is 0.8. $P_{A_{CO_2}}$ is assumed equal to $P_a{CO_2}$, so the equation becomes:

$$P_{A_{O_2}} = P_{I_{O_2}} - \frac{P_a{CO_2}}{0.8}$$

To determine $P_{A_{O_2}}$, the appropriate values for $P_I{O_2}$ and $P_a{CO_2}$ are entered in the equation and the alveolar P_{O_2} is calculated. Finally, the difference between the alveolar and arterial P_{O_2} (the $Aa_{D_{O_2}}$) is determined, by subtracting the measured $P_a{O_2}$ from the calculated $P_{A_{O_2}}$. If the blood gases are drawn on room air, the normal $Aa_{D_{O_2}}$ is less than 15 mm Hg.

If the hypoxemic patient has a normal $Aa_{D_{O_2}}$, the cause of the hypoxemia probably is an inadequate alveolar P_{O_2}, that is, hypoventilation. If the patient has an increased $Aa_{D_{O_2}}$, the hypoxemia probably results from a problem at the alveolar-capillary level. Although theoretically such a problem could be due to uneven ventilation, alveolar-capillary block, or shunt, using 100% O_2 almost completely eliminates the first two causes. Therefore, an increased $Aa_{D_{O_2}}$ on 100% O_2 most likely is due to an increased shunt.

Shunt and Increased $Aa_{D_{O_2}}$ Physiologic shunt is the percentage of CO that is wasted perfusion because it does not exchange with gas in the alveoli. It is subdivided into: (a) anatomic shunt, (b) capillary shunt, and (c) $\dot{V}/\dot{Q}$ mismatch or venous admixture (Shapiro et al. 1985).

TABLE 7–5 MIXED VENOUS BLOOD VALUES AND ARTERIAL BLOOD VALUES COMPARED

	ARTERIAL BLOOD	MIXED VENOUS BLOOD
P_{O_2}	80–100 mm Hg	35–40 mm Hg
O_2 saturation	95% or above	70–75%
O_2 content	19.8 ml O_2/100 ml blood	15.5 ml O_2/100 ml blood

Anatomic shunt is that portion that anatomically bypasses the pulmonary capillaries and returns, unoxygenated, to the left atrium. Normally, it results from venous drainage from the bronchial, pleural, and Thebesian veins and represents 2–5% of CO. It accounts for the fact that arterial P_{O_2} normally is slightly lower (95 mm Hg) than alveolar P_{O_2} (100 mm Hg). Abnormal veno-arterial communications such as right-to-left cardiac shunts increase anatomic shunt.

Capillary shunt is that portion that goes through pulmonary capillaries in contact with completely unventilated alveoli. Because it does not exchange with alveolar gas, it also returns unoxygenated to the left atrium. The sum of anatomic and capillary shunt is referred to as *true shunt* or *absolute shunt*.

The third type of shunt, $\dot{V}/\dot{Q}$ *mismatch* or *venous admixture*, occurs in a unit that is well perfused but poorly ventilated. Blood returning to the heart from this unit has a lower P_{O_2} than blood returning from a normal unit. $\dot{V}/\dot{Q}$ mismatch is responsive to oxygen therapy.

Shunting is minimized in the normal lung by a protective reflex. When shunting increases, diminished or absent local ventilation causes a low $P_{A_{O_2}}$. The local blood vessels constrict, redirecting flow to better-ventilated areas. $\dot{V}/\dot{Q}$ mismatch may be due to failure of this protective reflex, or diffuse disease of the lung or vasculature, which prevents adequate matching or compensation.

It is helpful to estimate the degree of shunt both to follow changes in the patient's condition and to plan oxygen therapy. Shunt can be calculated using a complex shunt equation, or it can be estimated more simply by measuring the $P_{a_{O_2}}$ after the patient has received 100% oxygen for 15 minutes. In this situation, the normal alveolar P_{O_2} is about 670 mm Hg. When evaluating arterial P_{O_2}, the assumption is that every 20 mm Hg below 670 represents a 1% shunt. Normal subjects will have up to a 6% shunt by this method, so their normal arterial P_{O_2} will be approximately 550 mm Hg. Values below 550 mm Hg can be converted to percentages of shunt using the guideline of 20 mm Hg = 1% additional shunt. This method is accurate only for shunts up to 30% (Nadel 1981).

Evaluating $P_{a_{CO_2}}$ Carbon dioxide is produced by cellular metabolism and eliminated by the lungs. In the blood, it is carried in three forms (Guyton 1986). About 70% is converted to bicarbonate in this reaction:

$$CO_2 + H_2O \rightleftharpoons H_2CO_3 \rightleftharpoons H^+ + HCO_3^-$$

In other words, carbon dioxide combines with water to form carbonic acid, which then dissociates to a hydrogen ion and a bicarbonate ion. An enzyme called *carbonic anydrase* facilitates the formation of carbonic acid.

Because much more carbonic anhydrase is contained in red blood cells than in plasma, most of the body's bicarbonate is formed in the red blood cells. It then diffuses out of the cells into the plasma, where it is carried. About 20% of the CO_2 is carried in combination with hemoglobin and plasma proteins. The last 10% (approximately) is physically dissolved in the blood. It is the pressure of this dissolved CO_2 that is measured in $P_{a_{CO_2}}$.

Normal $P_{a_{CO_2}}$ is 35–45 mm Hg. $P_{a_{CO_2}}$ varies with both the production of carbon dioxide and its elimination by the lungs. Altered $P_{a_{CO_2}}$ levels reflect changes in alveolar ventilation. A decreased $P_{a_{CO_2}}$ indicates hyperventilation, as in hypoxia or compensation for metabolic acidosis. An increased $P_{a_{CO_2}}$ (hypercapnia or hypercarbia) indicates hypoventilation, as in respiratory center depression, increased V_D/V_T ratio, or compensation for metabolic alkalosis. The $P_{a_{CO_2}}$ is a better indicator of alveolar ventilation than is the patient's $P_{a_{O_2}}$. Abnormal CO_2 values are caused only by abnormal ventilation; abnormal O_2 values can be caused by many factors.

Diagnostic Procedures

Chest X-ray

Reading the chest x-ray report is another step in assessing a patient's aeration status. A basic understanding of chest x-ray interpretation is useful in reading x-ray reports and understanding medical discussions of your patient's condition. Occasionally, too, you may be the first person to see an abnormal film; your ability to spot abnormalities needing urgent attention may enable you to obtain medical therapy immediately for your patient. The following information is based on Cannobio (1984), Jacobs (1985), and Jacquith (1986).

Different substances allow varying amounts of x-ray energy to pass through them and strike the film, producing four x-ray densities. Because bone absorbs most of the energy and allows very little to strike the film, it produces a white color. Soft tissues and blood absorb less amount of energy and appear gray. Lungs appear black because they allow most of the energy to pass through. When the x-ray beam traverses several structures of different densities, it will produce an image combining their densities.

In examining a film, follow a logical sequence such as the one indicated here. The most significant principle to remember is that you can see a structure only if its edge is of a density that contrasts with the surrounding density.

Normal Characteristics   The normal chest film has the following pulmonary characteristics (Figure 7–7).

The ribs are intact and can be traced starting from their more superior attachment to the spine. The spine is straight and can be seen through the heart shadow in a film of good quality. The clavicles, visible in the upper thorax, are intact and equidistant, indicating the person was centered properly.

The hemidiaphragms appear rounded. The upper edge of each hemidiaphragm is visible (because of the contrast between air and water densities). The right hemidiaphragm usually is slightly higher than the left (because of the liver). On the left hemidiaphragm, the lower edge may be visible because the stomach often contains air. The lower edge of the right hemidiaphragm should not be visible. If it is, it signifies free air in the abdomen, such as from a perforated ulcer. The lateral angles between the diaphragm and ribs (the costo-phrenic angles) should be clear.

The pleura is not visible.

The trachea is midline, with the carina visible at the level of the aortic knob. The aortic knob, which is formed by the arch of the aorta, is seen as a knoblike water density to the left of the spine.

The heart appears solid, since the blood in it and its walls are the same density. The edges of the heart are clear because of the contrast with the surrounding air density of the lung.

Just above the heart, small bilateral water densities are visible. These densities mark the hila, where the pulmonary vessels and bronchi join the lungs. The left hilum usually is slightly higher than the right because the left main pulmonary artery is higher and more posterior than the right. The hilum consists primarily of the major pulmonary vessels. Lesser vascular markings (also called *lung markings*) are seen out to the edge of the lung fields; they are more prominent in the lower lungs when the person is upright. Because the vascular markings are water density, they cause the lung fields to look like a wispy air density. Beyond a small amount of mainstem bronchus visible to about one inch out from the hila, the bronchi usually cannot be seen. They have thin walls, and since they are filled with air, they do not contrast with the air density of the surrounding lung.

Individual lobes of the lung can be identified because the lobes are separated by *fissures* (also called *septa*). These interlobar septa are visible in different projections. Septa between *lobules (interlobular septa)* normally cannot be seen.

Abnormal Signs   Three important signs you may see or hear discussed are the silhouette sign, the air bronchogram, and Kerley's B lines.

Silhouette Sign   You will recall that in order for a structure to be visible, the density of its edge must contrast with the surrounding density. The loss of contrast is called the *silhouette sign;* it indicates that the densities of the two structures have become the same and are directly in contact with one another. This sign is useful in localizing processes that increase the water content of the lung, such as pneumonia and infiltrates. For instance, since the heart is an anterior organ, the complete loss of the right cardiac silhouette implies that the pathology lies in the anterior lobes (the upper or middle lobes) in an area in anatomic contact with the heart. A shadow overlapping a border without obliterating a silhouette implies that the process is located in the lower (posterior) lobes, the posterior mediastinum, or the posterior pleural cavity.

Air Bronchogram Sign   Another sign of a process that is making part of the lung a water density is the *air bronchogram sign.* You will remember that the bronchi normally cannot be seen because they and the surrounding lung are both of air density. When a process (such as pneumonia or pulmonary edema) makes the lung tissue a water density, the contrast makes the bronchi visible, unless the bronchi themselves are filled with secretions or destroyed. The appearance of the air bronchogram identifies the disorder as intrapulmonary.

Kerley's B Lines   Kerley's B lines are short linear shadows perpendicular to the pleural surface. They are thought to represent fluid in or thickening of the interlobular septae. They are seen frequently in pulmonary edema and mitral valve disease; pulmonary fibrosis or inflammatory exudate also may cause them.

Easily Identified Abnormalities   Differential diagnosis of chest x-ray finding is a complex science beyond the scope of this book. However, there are some abnormalities you will encounter so frequently they are worth reviewing here: collapse, pneumothorax, consolidation, and pleural effusion.

Collapse   Collapse of a part of the lung has many causes. It may be due to bronchial obstruction followed by absorption of the air remaining in the lung (atelectasis). Another cause may be compression, such as by air in the pleural space. A third cause is contraction, such as in pulmonary fibrosis.

Collapse is diagnosed by displacement of the septa, crowding of the vascular markings or air bronchograms, and increased radiopacity of the lung tissue. Other signs sometimes seen are shift of the trachea toward the area

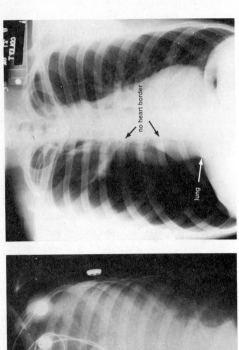

a

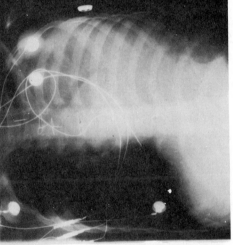

b

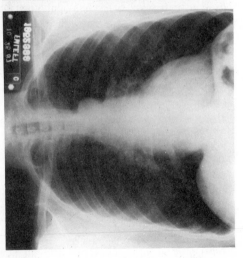

c

FIGURE 7–7

Chest x-rays. **a,** Normal posteroanterior (PA) chest film taken from 6 feet away, with the patient standing, and with as much of the anterior chest touching the plate as possible. Note that the normal heart is really quite small. **b,** a problem in the left lung is obvious in this x-ray; note the air bronchogram sign on the left indicating atelectasis. The air bronchogram clearly delineates the bronchus as it passes into the lower lobes of the left lung; left upper lobe bronchus is not visible indicating the probable presence of a mucus plug in that area. Vigorous endotracheal suctioning with ventilatory therapy produced significant clearing in 24 hours in this four-year-old girl. X-ray was taken two days post open heart surgery. Note endotracheal tube and wires used to close the sternum. **c,** The pneumothorax here is very extensive. Note that pressure in the right hemithorax must be greater than in the left, because the heart and other mediastinal structures are shifted away from the free air. This is a tension pneumothorax. Air entering the right pleural space is unable to escape because of a ball-valve effect, and each inspiration increases the intrapleural pressure. Prompt diagnosis and treatment, perhaps even with a large bore needle at first, are essential, often lifesaving. (From Tinker JH: Understanding chest x-rays. *American journal of nursing* 7:1:54–58. Courtesy, John H. Tinker MD, and American Journal of Nursing.)

of collapse (if the upper lobes are involved), displacement of the hilum, increased closeness of the ribs, elevation of the diaphragm on the affected side, and compensatory overexpansion of the adjacent parts of the lung causing increased radiolucency in those areas.

Pneumothorax   If you see an area of clear blackness (that is, no lung markings), it probably results from a pneumothorax. As air rises, look at the apices for this sign on an upright or semirecumbent film. Other signs you may see are increased radiopaqueness of the collapsed lung tissue, depression of the diaphragm, and tracheal and mediastinal shift away from the pneumothorax. The findings may be more apparent on an expiratory film, because the air-filled pleural space will contrast more with the more-solid compressed lung tissue during exhalation.

Consolidation   Areas of increased density (whiteness) are referred to as areas of consolidation. They can result from numerous causes. Broadly, causes of consolidation can be grouped into those that collapse the lung tissue, thereby making it more dense, and those that increase the fluid content of the lung. Increases in density due to fluid accumulation may be diffuse or localized. Diffuse increases are seen in pulmonary edema and pneumonia, as well as in other disorders. They can be differentiated on the basis of associated signs, such as air bronchograms, Kerley's lines, and the pattern of fluid distribution.

Pleural Effusion   Localized increases due to fluid are usually pleural (such as effusions or hemothorax). Fluid that causes partial or complete obliteration of the costophrenic angle on an upright film probably is *free pleural fluid*. When a film is taken with the patient on the side or back, this fluid will appear in the dependent part of the chest cavity. Fluid that does not shift with position is called *encapsulated* or *loculated*.

The above descriptions, although brief, will enable you to better interpret chest x-ray film reports and spot common abnormalities on chest films.

Lung Scans

Two types of lung scans can be performed: *perfusion scans* and *ventilation scans*. A *perfusion scan* is performed to evaluate arterial pulmonary blood flow and to detect pulmonary emboli. Patient preparation involves explanation of the purpose and technique of the test. It is unnecessary to withhold food or fluids. The scan takes approximately 30 minutes to perform. A radioactive contrast agent is injected via a peripheral vein in the arm. The agent used most often is human albumin tagged with technetium. After injection, a scintillation camera records distribution of the agent while the patient is in the supine position. The procedure then is repeated with the patient in a prone position. As with cardiac technetium scans, areas with normal perfusion show high uptake of the agent. The normal scan shows complete, even distribution. Areas of low uptake appear as "cold spots" and suggest the presence of an embolus.

A *ventilation scan* is performed to evaluate the distribution of ventilation after the patient inhales a radioactive gas, usually xenon. A nuclear scanner records gas distribution during the buildup phase, equilibrium phase, and washout phase (as the gas is removed from the lungs). A normal scan shows equal distribution during all phases. Uneven gas distribution or areas of slow washout indicate poor ventilation. The ventilation scan is particularly helpful when interpreted in conjunction with a perfusion scan. In diseases of the lung parenchyma, such as emphysema or pneumonia, ventilation is diminished. In pulmonary vascular conditions, ventilation is maintained but perfusion is decreased. Comparison of ventilation and perfusion scans thus is particularly helpful in the diagnosis of pulmonary embolism. Patient preparation is the same as that for perfusion scanning. You need provide no postprocedure care beyond continuing to provide emotional support while the patient waits for the diagnosis and therapeutic strategy recommendations.

Bronchoscopy

Bronchoscopy is a diagnostic procedure that utilizes a rigid metal bronchoscope or flexible fiberoptic bronchoscope to provide direct visualization of the tracheobronchial tree. The *rigid bronchoscope* is used to remove foreign objects and bronchial lesons. The *fiberoptic bronchoscope* is used more frequently because it is safer, more comfortable for the patient, and allows a greater viewing range because of its smaller size and flexibility. Fiberoptic bronchoscopy is used diagnostically, to examine possible sites of tumors, obstruction, cavitation, infection, or bleeding, and therapeutically, to remove mucus plugs, tenacious secretions, or sloughed mucosal eschar in inhalation injures. The fiberoptic bronchoscope is able to reach as far as the subsegmental bronchi.

Patient preparation includes a brief explanation of the purpose of the procedure, the steps involved, and the sensations to expect. Food and liquids usually are withheld for 6–8 hours preprocedure. Atropine may be administered prior to the procedure to reduce secretions and the danger of a vasovagal response. A sedative also may be given.

The patient is positioned in semi-Fowler's position or sits upright. A local anesthetic is sprayed into the nose and mouth to abolish the gag reflex. The anesthetic has a bitter taste and it is useful to alert the patient that the unpleasant taste is normal. When anesthesia occurs, the patient may have the sensation that there is something caught in the back of the throat that cannot be gotten out (Weaver 1982). This is an alarming sensation, and the person should be reassured that it is normal and that the airway will not be blocked during the procedure. Encourage the person to breathe through the nose, or pant, and to relax. If the patient is on a ventilator, a special adapter allows passage of the bronchoscope. The ventilator patient also should be reassured about the patency of the airway and encouraged to relax.

In the patient without an endotracheal tube, additional anesthetic usually is administered through one of the lumens of the bronchoscope when the bronchoscope is just above the vocal cords (Hollen et al. 1981). When the scope reaches the carina, anesthetic again is injected into the right and left mainstem bronchi to facilitate examination of deeper structures (Cameron 1981).

The physician examines the trachea and bronchi and performs additional procedures appropriate to the patient's clinical problems. These procedures may include suctioning of secretions and mucus plugs, bronchial brushings of lesions' surfaces, and biopsy. Bronchial wash specimens are taken for culture, sensitivity, and cytologic examination.

Nursing care during the procedure focuses on patient monitoring and emotional support. Complications can include laryngospasm, bronchospasm, hypoxemia, bleeding, and drug reactions (Weaver 1982). To minimize hypoxemia, supplemental oxygen is administered before, during and after the procedure. In a study of 67 bronchoscopic exams on surgical ICU patients, the most common complication was dysrhythmias related to a decrease in alveolar ventilation and oxygenation (Snow and Lucas 1984).

Postprocedure nursing care includes observation for the described complications, analysis of arterial blood gases 1–4 hours after the procedure, and withholding of food and fluids until the gag reflex returns, several hours postprocedure. Hoarseness, sore throat, and bloodstreaked sputum are common and subside spontaneously.

Pulmonary Angiography

Pulmonary angiography is an invasive diagnostic procedure in which the pulmonary vascular tree is visualized following injection of a contrast medium. It is used primarily to diagnose pulmonary embolism when scan results are equivocal.

Patient preparation includes a brief description of the technique and an explanation of its value in diagnosing disorders. Food and fluids are withheld for 6–8 hours prior to the test.

The procedure is performed in an angiography laboratory. The patient is placed supine, a cardiac monitor is attached, and an IV peripheral line is started if one is not already in place. Local anesthetic is injected into the antecubital space if the antecubital vein is to be used, or into the groin if the femoral vein is to be used. After a small incision is made, the catheter is introduced and passed antegrade through the right atrium and the right ventricle into the pulmonary artery. The contrast agent is injected and x-ray pictures taken for later examination. At the time of the injection, the patient may experience a flushed feeling or nausea, either of which usually passes rapidly.

The normal distribution of dye through the pulmonary vascular tree is unimpeded and symmetrical. Areas of narrowing may indicate stenosis, and areas of complete occlusion (cutoff) usually indicate emboli.

Complications of this procedure may include ventricular dysrhythmias from catheter stimulation of the myocardium, myocardial perforation, and allergic reaction to the dye. After the procedure, a pressure dressing is applied over the insertion site. Postprocedure complications and care are similar to those for cardiac catheterization and include monitoring for bleeding and hematoma formation, arterial occlusion, hypotension related to osmotic diureses, and delayed allergic reaction.

Thoracentesis

Thoracentesis is the procedure used to remove fluid from the pleural space. It can be done as either a diagnostic or a therapeutic modality. After receiving an explanation of the procedure, the patient is placed in the upright position and the lower posterior chest is prepared and anesthetized. A needle is introduced into the pleural space, and either a small amount of fluid is withdrawn for lab analysis or as much fluid as possible is withdrawn to evacuate the effusion. A biopsy of the pleura may also be obtained in this manner. The major complication is pneumothorax, and a postprocedure chest film should always be obtained. The patient should also be observed for any onset of respiratory distress.

Open Lung Biopsy

In the event that a diagnosis cannot be made using the previously described techniques, it may be necessary to surgically enter the chest via thoracotomy and obtain a biopsy specimen. Care of the thoracotomy patient is covered in Chapter 9.

REFERENCES

Bates B: *A guide to physical examination.* Philadelphia: Lippincott, 1983.

Benner P and Tanner C: Clinical judgment: How expert nurses use intuition. *Am J Nurs* 1987; 87:23–31.

Borg N et al. (eds): *Core curriculum for critical care nursing,* 2d ed. Philadelphia: Saunders, 1981.

Cameron T: Fiberoptic bronchoscopy. *Am J Nurs* 1981; 81:1462–1464.

Cannobio MM: Chest x-ray film interpretation. *Focus AACN* (Apr) 1984; 11:18–24.

Carrieri V et al.: The sensation of dyspnea: A review. *Heart Lung* 1984; 13:436–447.

Cherniack R, Cherniack L: *Respiration in health and disease.* Philadelphia: Saunders, 1983.

Grimes J, Iannopollo, E: *Health assessment in nursing practice,* 2d ed. Belmont, CA: Wadsworth, 1982.

Guyton A: *Textbook of medical physiology,* 7th ed. Philadelphia: Saunders, 1986.

Hollen E Sr et al.: Bronchoscopy. Pages 666–670 in *Diagnostics.* Horsham, PA: Intermed Communications, 1981.

Jacobs S: Radiographic and physical assessment of the chest. Chapter 4 in *Advances in cardiovascular nursing,* Douglas MK, Shinn JA (eds). Baltimore: Aspen, 1985.

Jacquith S: Chest x-ray interpretation: Implications for nursing intervention. *Dimen Crit Care Nurs* (Jan–Feb) 1986; 5:8–19.

Luce J et al.: *Intensive respiratory care.* Philadelphia: Saunders, 1984.

Murphey R, Holford S: Lung sounds. *Basics of RD* 1980; 8:1–6.

Nadel S: Adequate oxygenation. Pages 363–388 in *AACN's clinical reference for critical care nursing,* Kinney et al. (eds). New York: McGraw-Hill, 1981.

Shapiro B et al.: *Clinical application of respiratory care,* 3d ed. Chicago: Year Book Medical Pubs., 1985.

Snow N, Lucas AE: Bronchoscopy in the critically ill surgical patient. *Am. Surgeon* 1984; 50:441–445.

Weaver TE: Bronchoscopy, laryngography, and their potential complications. *RN* (Dec) 1982; 45:64–65.

West JB: *Respiratory physiology—The essentials,* 3d ed. Baltimore: Williams and Wilkins, 1984.

SUPPLEMENTAL READING

Blumsohn D: Clubbing of the fingers, with special reference to Schamroth's diagnostic method. *Heart Lung* 1981; 19:1069–1097.

Brandstetter R et al.: Hypoxemia following thoracentesis. *Heart Lung* 1982; 11:216–218.

Carrieri VK et al.: A framework for assessing pulmonary disease categories. *Focus AACN* (Apr) 1984; 10–16.

Celentano N, Conforti C: The effects of body position on oxygenation. *Heart Lung* 1985; 14:45–51.

Fuchs P: What you can learn from pulmonary function tests. *RN* (July) 1986; 49:24–27.

Harper R: Application of alveolar ventilation physiology. *Dimen Crit Care Nurs* (Mar–Apr) 1982; 80–86.

Husbey J: Radiographic evaluation of the chest. Ch. 16 in *Cardiac nursing,* Underhill S et al. (eds). Philadelphia: Lippincott, 1982.

Keely B: Ventilation-perfusion balance. *Dimen Crit Care Nurs* (May–June) 1984; 140–146.

Shapiro BA et al.: *Clinical application of blood gases,* 3d ed. Chicago: Year Book Medical Pubs., 1985.

Wade J: *Comprehensive respiratory care,* 3d ed. St Louis: Mosby, 1982.

Wimsatt R: Unlocking the mysteries behind the chest wall: Assessing the patient in respiratory distress. *Nurs* (Nov) 1985; 15:58–64.

8

Aeration Disorders

CLINICAL INSIGHT

Domain: Monitoring and ensuring the quality of health care practices

Competency: Getting appropriate and timely responses from physicians

The alliance between nursing and medicine in the critical-care unit can be an awkward one at times. A nurse who knows what she or he wants from a physician can be a sight to behold—resolute and determined. There's a fine line—some might say a tightrope—between being respectful of the physician's expertise and authority and being persistent in getting medical attention in a particular situation.

To present a convincing case to physicians, nurses learn to speak the language of medicine, to be conversant with the highly physiologically oriented knowledge base traditionally the purview only of physicians. Most physicians appreciate a nurse's alerting them to a problem, but an individual physician's receptivity to a nurse's approach may be less than ideal. Remaining persistent in the face of sometimes brusque or dismissive responses requires a solid experiential base and, at times, personal courage. Nurses also learn the value of timing, knowing a physician's idiosyncracies, and assertiveness in dealing

with touchy or inadequate responses, as the following exemplar shows (Benner 1984, pp. 142–143):

A patient was admitted with a diagnosis of thrombophlebitis. He had been on heparin therapy for about two days. . . . The report from the night shift said that he had had a difficult night. He had been having pain, more than usual. The intern on call was phoned, but did not come up to see the man. Instead Demerol was ordered I.M. Because the I.M. medication did not relieve the pain, the nurse phoned the intern again. By this time the nurse told the doctor that the patient was slightly short of breath. But the intern thought the nurse was being an alarmist and did not come up to see the man. The doctor then ordered Percodan. By 7 a.m. when I went in to see the patient, the man was clammy, cool, restless, and his vital signs were changing. He was more short of breath . . . , diaphoretic, had thready pulse, and was still in pain. I phoned the intern who regularly followed him and recounted the events of the night. He listened, paused, and then asked if I was calling to get more pain medication for the man. In a controlled manner I told him that something was going wrong with his patient and that giving him more narcotics would not solve the problem. I also said that I was calling because I wanted a doctor to see this man NOW. The intern came right up, and not a minute too soon. The man's level of consciousness was dramatically changing for the worse as were his vital signs. The patient had an infarction in his lung. Fortunately, swift action was taken and a specialist was called who, through surgery, was able to save the man's life and lung. The intern thanked me for my persistence in getting the patient seen promptly.

Persistence, like that demonstrated in the Clinical Insight exemplar, requires conviction in your understanding of the care a patient needs and confidence in your skills. This chapter is intended to help you provide nursing care that can anticipate, prevent, recognize, and alleviate various types of acute and chronic respiratory failure. *Respiratory failure* is defined as the inability of the cardiopulmonary system to provide adequate oxygenation and/or carbon dioxide removal to meet tissue metabolic needs. The diagnosis is based on laboratory data plus clinical assessment of the patient.

Respiratory disorders that affect lung parenchyma commonly are classified as restrictive, obstructive, or vascular. *Restrictive disorders* decrease lung compliance. Examples are pulmonary edema, adult respiratory distress syndrome (ARDS), and pneumonia. *Obstructive disorders* decrease air flow. Examples are bronchitis, emphysema, and asthma, collectively referred to as chronic obstructive pulmonary disease (COPD). *Vascular disorders* affect pulmonary blood flow and include pulmonary embolism and pulmonary hypertension.

Neuromuscular disorders do not affect lung tissue directly, but do affect movement of the chest wall. Neuromuscular causes of respiratory failure include central nervous system disorders, head trauma, spinal deformities such as kyphoscoliosis, neuronal diseases such as polio and myasthenia gravis, and chest wall trauma.

Restrictive disorders are the most common causes of acute respiratory failure in the critical-care unit, while obstructive disorders are the most common causes of chronic respiratory failure. The patient with stable COPD may be admitted to the critical-care unit for another disorder, e.g., hepatitis. The COPD patient also may develop an acute restrictive defect, such as pneumonia, which exacerbates chronic respiratory failure and may precipitate superimposed acute respiratory failure.

Pulmonary Edema

Pulmonary edema (excess fluid in the interstitial and/or alveolar spaces) results from two basic mechanisms. In the first, increased hydrostatic pressure in the pulmonary capillaries causes fluid to move across intact capillary membranes. This increased hydrostatic pressure can result from cardiac dysfunction and elevated left-heart pressures or from decreased pulmonary lymphatic drainage. This type of pulmonary edema sometimes is called *high-pressure pulmonary edema*. If it results from cardiac dysfunction, it may be termed *cardiogenic pulmonary edema*. In the second type of pulmonary edema, left-heart pressures are normal, but "leaky" capillary membranes (more permeable than normal) allow excessive fluid movement. This type is referred to as *normal-pressure or noncardiogenic pulmonary edema*. High-pressure pulmonary edema is discussed in the section that follows. Normal-pressure pulmonary edema is discussed in the next section (adult respiratory distress syndrome).

Assessment

Risk Conditions Recognize patients at risk for acute pulmonary edema; prevent it when possible. Conditions that increase risk include:

- Increased pulmonary capillary pressure: fluid overload, acute myocardial infarction, severe mitral stenosis, advanced aortic stenosis, severe hypertension, massive pulmonary embolism.
- Decreased lymphatic drainage: pneumonia, pulmonary contusion, microemboli, and increased central venous pressure (because lymphatics empty into systemic veins).

Prevention of Risk Consider ways to prevent the above conditions. Some examples follow. Closely monitor intake and output to avoid circulatory overload. If the patient has a pulmonary artery line, closely monitor hemodynamic readings for increased left ventricular end-diastolic pressure and increased pulmonary pressures. Minimize physical and emotional stress to decrease left ventricular workload. Teach the stable patient with chronic heart disease the importance of continuing medications at home, the symptoms of congestive heart failure, and the need for prompt medical attention if symp-

---

NURSING DIAGNOSES

The most important nursing diagnoses for the patient in pulmonary edema are:

• Impaired gas exchange
• Anxiety

---

toms occur. Prevent acute MI and shock as outlined in Chapter 13.

Signs and Symptoms The signs and symptoms of pulmonary edema are those of increased work of breathing, hypoxia, and fluid-filled alveoli.

Observe for signs of increased work of breathing due to decreased lung compliance, for example, use of accessory muscles, intercostal and supraclavicular retractions, expiratory wheeze, rapid, shallow respiratory pattern, and increased anxiety. Check for signs of hypoxia, such as tachypnea, tachycardia, hypertension, severe apprehension, diaphoresis, dysrhythmias, and peripheral vasoconstriction. Note signs of transudation of fluid into alveoli—profuse, frothy, pink sputum; cough; and rales. Monitor for increased PCWP and/or CVP.

Planning and Implementation of Care

Take measures described in the following paragraphs to relieve symptoms as promptly as possible.

Impaired Gas Exchange Related to Excess Lung Water Decrease lung water and improve gas exchange promptly by taking action as follows:

1. While summoning the physician, elevate the head of bed 45°–90°, and lower the legs to pool blood in the periphery if possible.

2. Give IV morphine sulfate as ordered by the physician to decrease apprehension and sympathetic stimulation (thereby decreasing peripheral arterial resistance and increasing venous capacitance). Anticipate a fall in pulmonary pressures and CVP. Assess systemic arterial pressure frequently. Morphine will decrease the circulating blood volume, so be alert for early signs of shock. It also decreases respiratory center sensitivity to P_aCO_2, so watch for respiratory depression and possible respiratory arrest.

3. Administer rapid-acting diuretics as ordered by the physican. Anticipate a drop in CVP and PCWP.

4. Apply rotating tourniquets, if ordered by the physician, to temporarily decrease the circulating volume while slower therapeutic measures take effect. When the treatment is discontinued, do *not* remove all the tourniquets at once, since the abrupt increase in venous return could again precipitate pulmonary edema.

5. Assist with a phlebotomy if the physician elects to perform such a procedure.

6. To improve oxygenation and ventilation, take these steps. Administer supplemental O_2 as described in Chapter 9. The patient will need particular emotional support to accept an oxygen mask, since it often reinforces the sensation of smothering. Also, administer intermittent positive pressure ventilation, as ordered by the physician. This treatment increases intrathoracic pressure, thereby decreasing venous return. Intubation and mechanical ventilation may be necessary if the work of breathing is excessive and exacerbates signs of myocardial ischemia and pump failure.

7. Work with the physician to alleviate the cause of the attack. For example, administer digitalis if the problem is poor myocardial contractility; assist with cardioversion if tachycardia precipitated the attack. For a more detailed description of pharmacological management, refer to Chapter 13 (Cardiovascular Disorders).

Anxiety Related to Difficulty Breathing and to the Unknown Take action to relieve the patient's anxiety. Stay with the patient, and try to provide a calm environment and brief, clear explanations. Also, administer morphine to relieve anxiety. For further interventions related to this diagnosis, see Chapter 13.

Outcome Evaluation

Evaluate the patient's progress according to these outcome criteria:

• Unlabored respirations 12–18 times per minute.
• BP and pulse WNL for patient.
• Lungs clear on auscultation.
• Skin warm and dry (and pink if the patient is Caucasian).
• No cough or sputum.
• Ability to tolerate level of anxiety or apprehension as indicated verbally or nonverbally (by facial expression and body posture).
• Arterial blood gases WNL for patient.

Adult Respiratory Distress Syndrome (ARDS)

Adult respiratory distress syndrome (ARDS) is a form of noncardiogenic pulmonary edema that occurs from diffuse injury to the alveolar-capillary membrane and results in stiff, wet lungs and refractory hypoxemia. This acute restrictive disorder is known by numerous other names, including *shock lung, wet lung, stiff lung, pump lung, congestive atelectasis, adult hyaline membrane disease, noncardiogenic pulmonary edema,* and *capillary leak syndrome.*

Assessment

Risk Conditions The clinical causes of ARDS are diverse; ARDS seems to be a final common pathway of lung injury as a result of a catastrophic event that results in increased permeability of the alveolar-capillary membrane. Incidence is approximately 150,000 per year, with a 50% mortality rate. Approximately one-third of survivors will have some permanent changes in pulmonary function (Brandstetter 1986; Stevens and Raffin 1984). Patients with two or more risk factors have a substantially higher chance of developing ARDS (Fowler 1983). Table 8–1 lists etiologies associated with ARDS.

Preventive Measures The critical-care nurse is in a key position to prevent or identify early this catastrophic syndrome. Knowing that the patient is at risk is the first step—the trauma patient who is now septic, for instance. Prevention lies in meticulous monitoring of fluid administration, filtering of blood products, maintaining strict asepsis, and preventing aspiration with the use of nasogastric drainage. Aggressive pulmonary care such as turning, suctioning, and hyperinflation may allow the use of lower oxygen concentrations (below 50%) to prevent oxygen toxicity, which can exacerbate the syndrome.

Pathophysiology ARDS is a syndrome characterized by: (1) a precipitating event, (2) pulmonary edema due to capillary injury and leak, (3) marked respiratory distress, (4) diffuse infiltrates on CXR, and (5) refractory hypoxemia. The injury to the pulmonary capillary is an integral factor in the development of the clinical presentation. Figure 8–1 illustrates the sequence of changes seen in ARDS.

Following the initial insult, there is a latent period of

TABLE 8–1 ETIOLOGIES ASSOCIATED WITH ARDS

Shock of any etiology
Trauma
  Fat embolism
  Lung contusion
  Nonthoracic trauma
  Head injury
  Burns
Aspiration
  Gastric contents
  Near drowning
Infections
  Gram negative sepsis
  Pneumonia (bacterial, viral, Legionnaire's, Pneumocystis-carinii)
  Radiation pneumonitis
Hematologic disorders
  Disseminated intravascular coagulation
  Massive transfusions
  Prolonged cardiopulmonary bypass
  Transfusion reactions
Inhaled toxic substances
  Oxygen
  Smoke
  Chemicals
Drug ingestion and overdose (heroin, barbiturates, methadone)
Metabolic
  Pancreatitis
  Uremia
Miscellaneous
  Paraquat ingestion
  Eclampsia
  Amniotic fluid embolism
  Fluid overload
  High altitude

about 12–24 hours after which vasoactive substances, such as complement, attract neutrophils to the pulmonary circulation. Other inflammatory substances, such as histamine, bradykinin, serotonin, platelets, and certain coagulation products (e.g., fibrin), serve to exacerbate damage to the capillary endothelium. These substances also cause bronchoconstriction and pulmonary vasoconstriction. This massive "capillary leak" promotes altered hydrostatic and oncotic pressure dynamics, with transudation of fluid and plasma proteins into the interstitium. Lymph flow also slows in its drainage of the interstitium. The result is frank pulmonary edema with progressive atelectasis due to surfactant dysfunction. Arterial hypoxemia and decreased compliance result.

In later stages, hyaline membranes line the alveolar ducts; and finally, fibrotic changes occur. This late stage is marked by decreased lung compliance, increased physiologic deadspace and pulmonary vascular resis-

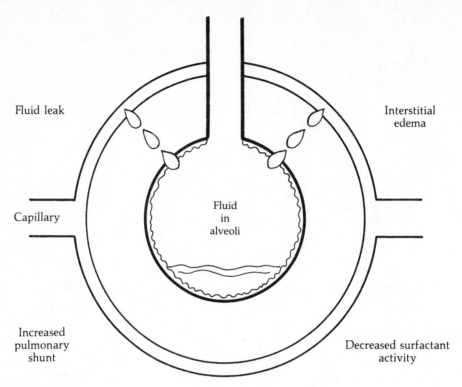

Fluid leak

Interstitial edema

Capillary

Fluid in alveoli

Increased pulmonary shunt

Decreased surfactant activity

Pathophysiologic sequence

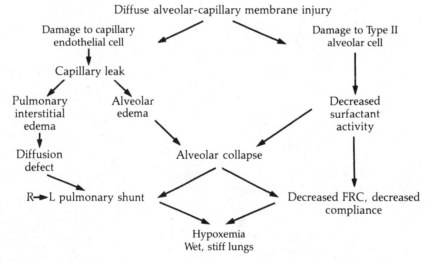

Diffuse alveolar-capillary membrane injury

Damage to capillary endothelial cell

Damage to Type II alveolar cell

Capillary leak

Pulmonary interstitial edema

Alveolar edema

Decreased surfactant activity

Diffusion defect

Alveolar collapse

R→L pulmonary shunt

Decreased FRC, decreased compliance

Hypoxemia
Wet, stiff lungs

FIGURE 8–1

Pathophysiologic sequence in ARDS: a pictorial presentation.

tance, and shunting unresponsive to PEEP. Intraalveolar septal thickening and the decreased surface area create a diffusion defect and increased deadspace hallmarked by an increased Pco_2 in addition to refractory hypoxemia.

Signs and Symptoms The clinical onset of respiratory distress typically lags behind the initial insult by 24–48 hours. The first sign you may notice at the bedside is visibly increased work of breathing, tachypnea, and patient complaints of breathlessness and air hunger.

Blood gas changes may or may not be present at this time; there may be only a respiratory alkalosis (Pco_2 25–35) without marked hypoxemia. Chest assessment findings are extremely variable and depend upon the underlying initiating insult; the same is true for the CXR.

As the syndrome progresses, respiratory distress becomes more marked with use of all accessory muscles and respiratory rates in the 40s. The P_aO_2 falls below 50 and does not respond to oxygen therapy. Your patient may exhibit new signs of being confused and agitated. The CXR, whose changes may lag 24 hours behind the clinical onset of respiratory distress, now shows increasing diffuse infiltrates. The patient requires intubation and mechanical ventilation. Increasing lung stiffness (altered lung compliance) is evidenced by high peak inspiratory pressures over 50 cm H_2O.

Hemodynamic instability increases, and its treatment depends on your patient's underlying problem. An important hemodynamic finding is that, despite pulmonary edema, your patient's pulmonary capillary wedge pressure may be normal. This finding confirms that the cause of your patient's pulmonary edema is a "leaky capillary" as opposed to left-ventricular failure. Some patients, however, may have a combination of a damaged capillary membrane and pump failure.

Other hemodynamic changes include elevated pulmonary artery systolic and diastolic pressures. Alveolar hypoxia and acidemia are both potent pulmonary artery vasoconstrictors. Other mechanisms contributing to pulmonary hypertension include the release of vasoactive substances like histamine, platelets, and bradykinin and accumulation of neutrophils and fibrin within the vessels (Stevens and Raffin 1984).

To maintain an adequate blood pressure and cardiac output, inotropic and vasopressor agents may be used, as opposed to fluid boluses, in order to maintain as dry a lung as possible.

The late stages of ARDS are reflective of the damage to the pulmonary capillaries preventing not only oxygenation of the blood but also removal of CO_2 from the blood. This is an important prognostic indicator because CO_2 diffuses much more easily than O_2, so if CO_2 diffusion is impaired, severe damage is present. In addition, the progressive hypoxemia is reflected by tissue hypoxia and a metabolic acidosis (decreased bicarbonate). This combination of metabolic and respiratory acidosis is a poor prognostic sign. The CXR usually has progressed to a "white-out," and sputum analysis shows that large amounts of albumin have leaked from the serum into the alveolus. Hypotension and bradycardia often follow, with death soon thereafter.

NURSING DIAGNOSES

A variety of nursing diagnoses can apply to the patient in ARDS, depending on the individual patient and the stage of development. The major diagnoses are:

- Impaired gas exchange
- Ineffective breathing pattern
- Ineffective airway clearance
- Anxiety

Care related to these diagnoses is discussed below.

Planning and Implementation of Care

Impaired Gas Exchange Related to Alveolar Edema and Alveolar Collapse Gas exchange is compromised in ARDS for a variety of reasons. Shunt increases because of fluid and cellular debris filling the alveoli and also due to alveolar collapse secondary to mechanical compression from interstitial edema and from decreased surfactant. Deadspace increases due to capillary compression and occlusion. The lung thus is characterized by mixed areas of shunt, deadspace, and silent (nonfunctional) and functional alveolar-capillary units. A diffusion defect also is present because of the presence of hyaline membranes, which probably are formed from transudated proteins.

Judicious fluid therapy is crucial to avoid further deleterious increases in lung water. The choice of intravenous fluids, a medical responsibility, is controversial. Colloids have been advocated on the theory that increasing the colloid osmotic pressure will mobilize water from the lungs—which may be true in the patient with intact alveolar-capillary function. In ARDS, however, most physicians prefer to avoid colloids, because capillary leak might allow colloids to migrate into the interstitial and alveolar spaces of the lung. Then the colloid particles in the lung would continue to attract water osmotically, increasing pulmonary edema.

Diuretics are administered cautiously to mobilize lung water. Furosemide and other rapid-acting diuretics are given in small doses, and fluid and electrolyte status and renal function are monitored closely.

Administration of steroids in ARDS is controversial. Although steroids possess theoretical advantage in stabilizing cell membranes and decreasing the release of lysosomal enzymes, their value remains to be proven. Side effects of increased susceptibility to infection, gastrointestinal bleeding, and diabetes mellitus may override their use on an empirical basis (Sladen 1986).

Attention to ventilation and oxygenation is of paramount importance. Because of the increased shunt, simple oxygen supplementation rarely is sufficient to achieve satisfactory P_aO_2 values. It usually is necessary to intubate and place the patient on mechanical ventilation with high tidal volumes to overcome the widespread alveolar collapse and decreased compliance. Oxygen is administered via the ventilatory circuit in an attempt to achieve normal P_aO_2 and oxygen saturation values. Because extremely high inspired oxygen fractions are necessary in ARDS, with the concomitant risk of oxygen toxicity, the patient is placed on positive end expiratory pressure (PEEP). By keeping alveoli constantly under positive pressure, PEEP increases functional residual capacity, allowing more surface area for gas exchange across the alveolar-capillary membrane. It thus allows the use of lower fractional inspired oxygen concentrations to achieve satisfactory levels of oxygenation.

When acceptable P_aO_2 values cannot be reached despite the use of PEEP, it may be necessary to use neuromuscular agents to paralyze and sedate the restless and hypoxic patient. This accomplishes two goals: First, the pressure needed to ventilate the patient is decreased by relaxing the chest wall, thus decreasing the risk of pneumothorax. Second, and more important, oxygen consumption by the respiratory muscles is decreased so that oxygen supply can better meet metabolic demand, thereby avoiding tissue hypoxia and resulting metabolic acidosis. It is **crucial to sedate** the patient, because paralytic agents do not change the patient's awareness of surroundings or discomfort.

Selected aspects of nursing care postintubation are presented in the nearby Nursing Care Plan.

Ineffective Airway Clearance Related to Depressed Ciliary Function, Increased Mucus Production, and Increased Airway Resistance In ARDS, the patient has difficulty clearing secretions for a number of reasons, including decreased ciliary transport and increased production of mucus. In addition, airway resistance increases because of early airway closure resulting from bronchoconstriction and mechanical compression from interstitial edema. To reduce retention of secretions, institute a program of vigorous pulmonary hygiene. This should include frequent turning, coughing and deep breathing, chest percussion and vibration, postural drainage, and suctioning. Some extremely hypoxic patients do not tolerate turning, postural drainage, or suctioning without hypotension and dysrhythmias. Close monitoring is essential. Humidification of oxygen and administration of bronchodilators

also enhance clearing of secretions. The patient should be protected against infection by meticulous attention to handwashing, care of invasive catheters, and decontamination of respiratory equipment. Nutritional needs should be closely met to assure an anabolic state and augmented defenses against infection.

Anxiety Related to Dyspnea and to the Unknown The patient with ARDS requires skillful, compassionate nursing care to reduce anxiety. Brief mention will be made here of effective measures, as they are discussed in detail in Chapter 3. Project a calm, competent air as you care for the patient. Encourage her or him to rest as much as possible; for example, group your nursing care activities to allow for uninterrupted periods of rest. Try to maintain normal day/night cycles. Ideally, assign a primary nurse to the patient, to facilitate a relationship of trust. Provide brief explanations of activities and procedures. Encourage family visits. Provide spiritual support if the patient wishes it by offering to contact a spiritual counselor. Use touch for reassurance if the patient is receptive.

Outcome Evaluation

The mortality rate in ARDS is high. For patients who survive, desirable outcome criteria are the following:

- Alert, oriented level of consciousness.
- Normal CO, as evidenced by arterial blood pressure WNL and normal thermodilution CO values.
- Good peripheral perfusion, as manifested by warm, dry skin, and bilaterally equal peripheral pulses of normal volume.
- PA, CVP, and PCWP readings WNL.
- Urinary output of 1 ml or more per minute.
- Arterial blood gases and serum electrolytes WNL.
- Normal respiratory pattern and rate.

Atelectasis

Atelectasis means collapsed alveoli in part or all of the lung. Although the term may be used to refer to collapse due to compression (as with a tumor), it commonly refers to collapse caused by (a) airway obstruction followed by absorption of gas in the alveoli, or (b) decreased surfactant production.

NURSING CARE PLAN

The Patient with ARDS (Postintubation)

NURSING DIAGNOSIS	SIGNS AND SYMPTOMS	NURSING ACTION	DESIRED OUTCOMES
Impaired gas exchange related to alveolar edema and alveolar collapse	• Reduced P_aO_2 • Restlessness, agitation • Confusion, disorientation • Dyspnea • Dysrhythmias • Tachycardia • Cyanosis (in severe hypoxemia) • Crackles, bronchial breath sounds • $S\bar{v}O_2 < 65\%$	1. Maintain airway for oxygen therapy; restrain patient PRN to prevent extubation. 2. Maintain PEEP at all times; use suction adapter, manual ventilation bag with PEEP valve. 3. Continuously monitor EKG. 4. Measure VS (BP, HR, PAD/PAW, CVP) q1hr. 5. Evaluate cardiac output q4hr. Monitor $S\bar{v}O_2$ (or S_aO_2) as ordered, preferably continuously. 6. Monitor ABGs as ordered. 7. Monitor fluid balance carefully; avoid fluid overload. 8. Weigh patient daily if tolerated. 9. Administer diuretics as ordered.	• $P_aO_2 > 60$ mm Hg on F_IO_2 < 0.60 • $S\bar{v}O_2 > 65\%$ • Patient is oriented • Clear CXR • Even fluid balance • No dysrhythmias
Ineffective breathing pattern related to patient breathing out of synchrony with ventilator	All the above plus: • Patient is "fighting" ventilator • Use of accessory muscles • Intercostal retractions	1. Verbally attempt to coach patient to breathe in phase with ventilator. 2. Sedate as ordered. 3. Frequently orient to time, place, and condition. 4. If coaching and sedation are unsuccessful with severe hypoxemia, consult with physician about paralyzing patient, **continuing sedation.** Explain to patient that he or she will be unable to move but you will keep him or her sedated and comfortable.	• $S\bar{v}O_2 > 65\%$ • Decreased work of breathing • Absence of inspiratory effort in the paralyzed patient
Ineffective breathing pattern related to decreased compliance	• Peak inspiratory pressures over 50 cm H_2O • Tachypnea • Elevated arterial carbon dioxide (P_aCO_2) • Dyspnea • Use of accessory muscles • Difficulty with manual ventilation	1. Check peak inspiratory pressures every 4 hours. 2. Decrease tidal volume and increase respiratory rate (RR) to decrease peak inspiratory pressures, as ordered. 3. Increase RR to decrease P_aCO_2 as ordered.	• Normal P_aCO_2 • PIPs < 40 cm H_2O • RR 8–18 • Normal CXR • Normal chest/diaphragm movement

(Continues)

NURSING CARE PLAN (Continued)

The Patient with ARDS (Postintubation) (Continued)

NURSING DIAGNOSIS	SIGNS AND SYMPTOMS	NURSING ACTION	DESIRED OUTCOMES
		4. Perform chest auscultation q1–2hr to detect pneumothorax due to high inspiratory pressures and damaged lung parenchyma. 5. Paralyze patient with severe decreased compliance to facilitate ventilation, as ordered. 6. In end-stage ARDS with uncorrectable CO_2 retention signifying irreversible lung damage, discuss prognosis/plan with physician and family.	
Decreased cardiac output related to high levels of PEEP	• Cool extremities • Decreased urine output • Decreased/loss of peripheral pulses • Decreased blood pressure • Tachycardia • $S\bar{v}o_2 < 65\%$	1. Measure cardiac output, ABG 30 min after each increase in PEEP. 2. Monitor $S\bar{v}o_2$ continuously, as ordered. 3. Monitor urine output. 4. Assess for signs of decreasing peripheral perfusion. 5. Use inotropes/vasopressors as ordered to maintain BP.	• Normal cardiac output • Normal renal function • Warm periphery

Assessment

Risk Conditions   Recognize the conditions that increase the risk of developing atelectasis: *shallow breathing* (as with pain), *dehydration, aspiration* of foreign objects, *retained secretions* (mucous plugs), *bronchospasm, ciliary depression,* and *decreased surfactant* (usually due to decreased alveolar expansion).

Preventive Measures   Take measures to prevent atelectasis:

1.   Auscultate the lungs to determine the need for, frequency of, and effectiveness of the interventions that follow.

2.   Establish rapport with the patient, and teach about deep breathing, coughing, turning, suctioning, chest physiotherapy, and intermittent positive pressure breathing. Emphasize the importance of these techniques in maintaining pulmonary function. Encourage the patient to practice breathing and coughing exercises several times a day. Observe that she or he performs them correctly. Praise the patient for participating in her or his own care, and inform the patient that during the stay in the critical-care unit you will assist with these measures. If the exercises cause pain, give adequate analgesics and wait long enough for them to take effect. Then capitalize on your relationship to motivate the patient to perform breathing exercises in spite of any remaining discomfort.

3.   Position the patient to facilitate lung expansion by elevating the head of the bed. Avoid pronounced compression of the diaphragm.

4.   Turn the patient every 1–2 hours to lessen pooling of secretions and prevent regional atelectasis.

5. Help the patient to deep breathe every 1–2 hours to reexpand closed alveoli. If she or he is unable to deep breathe, sigh the lungs with a hand ventilating bag a few times. Deliver a volume 2–3 times the patient's tidal volume. (Patients on continuous ventilation with high tidal volumes do not need to be sighed.)

6. Encourage oral fluids (if permitted) to reduce viscosity of secretions. If only intravenous fluids are allowed, maintain adequate hydration.

7. Mobilize secretions by performing chest physical therapy periodically, instilling saline before suctioning, and using mucolytic agents and bronchodilators as ordered.

8. Help the patient to cough effectively by splinting abdominal or thoracic incisions with a sheet. If necessary, stimulate the cough reflex by passing a nasal catheter down the trachea or by pressing over the trachea. If the patient has increased secretions and is unable to raise them, suction the trachea and bronchi.

9. Assist with intermittent positive pressure breathing or incentive spirometry if ordered by the physician.

Signs and Symptoms   Recognize the signs of developing atelectasis. If the airways to major atelectatic areas are open, bronchial breathing and increased tactile fremitus, voice sounds and whispered sounds may be present. If the airways are plugged, these signs will be absent. The chest x-ray may show patches or larger areas of consolidation, an elevated diaphragm, and a mediastinal shift, depending upon the site and extent of the collapse. Most postoperative atelectasis is microatelectasis (random alveolar collapse not detectable on chest x-ray). Signs and symptoms usually are subtle and may include restlessness, tachypnea, tachycardia, increased temperature, decreasing P_aO_2 or increasing $AaDo_2$, or dullness on percussion over areas that should be resonant.

NURSING DIAGNOSES

The nursing diagnoses most appropriate for the patient with atelectasis are:

- Impaired gas exchange
- Potential for infection

Planning and Implementation of Care

Atelectasis results in increased physiologic shunting (explained in Chapter 7) and often in stasis pneumonia as the retained secretions are an excellent medium for bacterial growth.

Impaired Gas Exchange Related to Alveolar Collapse   Relieve the hypoxia that results from increased physiologic shunting by taking these measures.

1. Implement steps 1–9 listed above under preventive measures.

2. Provide supplemental O_2 as ordered by the physician.

3. If the obstruction is massive, it may be necessary for the physician to bronchoscope the patient.

4. Maintain high tidal volumes or PEEP as ordered in the mechanically ventilated patient to promote alveolar expansion and surfactant production.

5. Assist with face-mask PEEP if prescribed for the spontaneously ventilating patient.

Potential for Infection Related to Decreased Host Defenses   Prevent or treat bacterial growth in the retained secretions and collapsed alveoli.

1. Monitor the patient's temperature every 4 hours.

2. Observe the quality of secretions. Send a daily specimen to the laboratory for examination.

3. Use scrupulous handwashing and sterile technique with suctioning, fluid lines, and incisions to avoid introducing bacteria into the patient's body.

4. Administer prophylactic or therapeutic antibiotics as ordered by the physician.

Outcome Evaluation

Use these outcome criteria to judge the patient's progress:

- Respiratory rate 12–18 times a minute.
- Pulse rate 60–100 times a minute.
- P_aO_2 80–100 mm Hg on room air.
- Lung physical examination normal (no bronchial breathing over lung fields; normal voice sounds and whispered sounds; resonance on percussion; normal tactile fremitus).
- Chest x-ray normal (no consolidation, diaphragmatic elevation, or mediastinal shift).

Pneumonia

It is estimated that 12–15% of all intensive care unit patients will acquire pneumonia (Podnos et al. 1985). The diagnosis is based on CXR, physical exam, and lab and bacteriological data. Infecting agents include bacteria, viruses, fungi, parasites, and others (such as *Legionella* and *Mycoplasma*). Mechanisms by which such organisms reach the lung include inhalation, aspiration, and hematogenous spread (bacteremia, septic emboli). In hospitalized patients, organisms are acquired almost exclusively by aspiration or direct inoculation of the lower respiratory tract (Kuhn 1985). The following section will focus on nosocomial (hospital-acquired) bacterial pneumonias.

Assessment

Risk Conditions Patients at greatest risk are those whose host defenses are compromised. Primarily this includes the elderly and chronically ill whose airway defenses such as mucociliary clearance mechanisms are damaged due to intubation and suctioning; or whose coughing and swallowing is neurologically dysfunctional, resulting in aspiration of oropharyngeal or gastric contents. Another group at great risk are those immunosuppressed patients with AIDS or cancer or those who have just undergone organ transplantation. Conditions such as pulmonary edema and previous lung infections also increase the likelihood of developing pneumonia. Abdominal and thoracic surgical procedures are associated with a high incidence of atelectasis and pneumonia due to decreased ventilatory muscle function (Kuhn 1985; Shapiro et al. 1985). Patients with COPD are at extremely high risk for pneumonias postoperatively due to poor diaphragmatic function, decreased cough, and impaired mucociliary clearance. Oxygen and cortico-steroids also depress alveolar macrophage function (Luce et al. 1984).

Preventive Measures Most all patients in critical-care units today fall under the category of high risk for the development of pneumonia. Specific measures by the nurse can help to decrease the incidence as well as to institute early treatment. In the surgical population, knowing the patient's preoperative pulmonary function will be key in identifying appropriate postoperative pulmonary care. Frequent repositioning and chest assessment are essential. Assessment of respiratory pattern with appropriate pain relief prevents hypoventilation and atelectasis; both are precursors of pneumonia. Mechanical support of ventilation is necessary until the patient demonstrates the ability to cough and deep breathe. Preoperative teaching of proper bronchial hygiene familiarizes the patient with equipment and routines and decreases pain and anxiety in the postoperative period.

Measures for the medical patient are similar. Prevention of aspiration is done by nasogastric drainage plus side positioning for neurologically impaired patients.

Vigorous mobilization of secretions, aseptic suctioning, handwashing, and careful fluid management are first-line management strategies in protecting your patient from contracting pneumonia. The use of disposable and closed-system ventilator tubing and humidifier has decreased this as a source of contamination.

Isolating patients with respiratory infections from other populations prevents cross-exposure to their bacterial flora.

Signs and Symptoms Bacterial pneumonias such as those caused by *Klebsiella* and *Pseudomonas* begin with a rapid onset of fever; in critically ill patients, however, fever may not be present. The patient with bacterial pneumonia appears more ill than patients with viral pneumonias. Bacterial pneumonias produce a localized infiltrate resulting in bronchial breath sounds, which contrasts with viral pneumonias that are more diffuse and produce chest findings of scattered rales and rhonchi. *Klebsiella* pneumonia may be multilobar; *Pseudomonas* pneumonia is also multilobar, but with a predisposition for the lower lobes. Atelectasis and small pleural effusions are common. Other gram negative bacterial pneumonias, such as *E coli, Enterobacter, Proteus,* and *Bacteroides,* appear similarly, though less in the lower lobes. These gram negative pneumonias are particularly severe due to their necrotizing effect on lung tissue.

Cough is a predominant symptom but may not be present in the critically ill. Sputum is purulent, although

---

NURSING DIAGNOSES

The nursing diagnoses most appropriate for the pneumonia patient are:

- Impaired gas exchange
- Ineffective airway clearance

it may be difficult to identify the responsible organism on gram stain. Tachypnea may be present due to fever plus consolidation.

Planning and Implementation of Care

Impaired Gas Exchange Related to Increased Shunting Oxygen therapy is instituted according to the degree of hypoxemia, and arterial blood gases are monitored. Chest x-rays are obtained daily and chest assessment findings correlated with chest x-ray reports. Turning and deep breathing (or manually sighing the ventilated patient) will enhance matching of ventilation and perfusion. Anticipate poorer oxygenation if your patient is positioned with the affected lung down, as blood flow will be greater to poorly ventilated areas.

Ineffective Airway Clearance Related to Secretions and Debilitation Humidify oxygen, and observe secretions for increased viscosity. Administer antibiotics as ordered, observing for side effects, particularly of aminoglycosides, as renal function may be affected. Avoid fluid overload. Use gentle and aseptic suctioning with chest percussion and postural drainage as tolerated by the patient. Observe sputum for changes that may indicate a superinfection, particularly in the patient on broad-spectrum antibiotics. Bronchodilators may be ordered to enhance mobilization of secretions; observe for side effects.

Outcome Evaluation

Evaluate the patient's progress according to the following desirable outcome criteria:

- Absence of fever.
- Arterial blood gas values WNL for the patient.
- Presence of normal breath sounds; absence of bronchial breath sounds.
- Absence of or normal-appearing sputum.

Pneumothorax

A *pneumothorax* is a collection of free air within the pleural space.

Assessment

Risk Conditions Anticipate and prevent a pneumothorax whenever possible, by first recognizing the patients at risk for developing a pneumothorax. Predisposing conditions are as follows:

1. Chest trauma, especially penetrating injuries or rib fractures.

2. Pneumonia, because it leads to lung abscesses.

3. Diseases causing degenerative changes in lungs, such as emphysema and bronchitis.

4. Airway obstruction due to bronchospasm, inflammation, or retained secretions.

5. Catheterization of subclavian vein, because it rests on the apical pleura.

6. Thoracentesis.

7. Pericardial tap.

8. Positive pressure ventilation. Risk of a pneumothorax from positive pressure ventilation increases if additional factors are present that increase intrathoracic pressure. If the patient has chronic obstructive lung disease or is fighting the ventilator, pressure inside the thorax may rise dangerously. The risk of pneumothorax also increases if the tidal volume is over 15 ml/kg, the peak inspiratory pressure is over 40–50 cm H_2O, or positive end expiratory pressure is applied.

The likelihood of pneumothorax escalates with increasing numbers of risk conditions. For example, the emphysematous patient on mechanical ventilation who develops retained secretions is more likely to develop a pneumothorax than the previously healthy person on mechanical ventilation whose nurses keep the airway clear. Pneumothorax also occurs in previously healthy people, for unknown reasons.

Preventive Measures Take whatever steps are possible to prevent the predisposing conditions. For example, encourage turning and deep breathing and coughing exercises to clear secretions. If the patient is unable to raise secretions through these methods, stimulate the cough reflex, perform chest physiotherapy, or suction the airway as a last resort.

Administer bronchodilators, steroids, and antibiotics prescribed by the physician to minimize airway obstruction, and antiemetics to control vomiting. Use Trendelenburg's position and have the patient perform a Valsalva maneuver during subclavian catheterization.

Signs and Symptoms Consistent and frequent chest assessment will ensure that you detect the pneumothorax promptly. Signs and symptoms will vary, depending on the size and type of pneumothorax. The types are: *open,* with a continued communication between the pleural space and the outside; *closed,* with closure of the pleural tear as the lung collapses; and *tension,* with the opening acting as a one-way valve to let air in but not out. The key signs and symptoms are pain, dyspnea, hypoxia, chest x-ray changes, and sometimes mediastinal shift. Signs of decreased cardiac output and shock may occur with tension pneumothorax due to compression of the heart and great vessels.

Watch for *chest pain* that is abrupt, sharp, and constant and usually appears unilaterally. Signs of *dyspnea* and *hypoxia* include tachypnea, nasal flaring, cyanosis, accessory muscle use, retractions, and decreased P_aO_2. On physical examination, the affected side may appear larger, with decreased movement, decreased tactile fremitus, hyperresonance or tympany, depressed diaphragm, and decreased breath sounds. The *chest x-ray* may show loss of lung markings peripherally, compression collapse centrally, or possible mediastinal shift.

Observe for signs of *mediastinal shift* away from the pneumothorax (if the pressure is great enough) as follows.

1. Check for tracheal deviation.

2. Monitor for signs of decreased venous return, such as jugular venous distention, increased central venous pressure readings, and liver tenderness.

3. Observe for signs of decreased CO, such as mental confusion, angina, oliguria, tachycardia, hypotension, and peripheral vasoconstriction.

4. Auscultate the precordium for deviation in heart sound locations. A crunching sound with the heartbeat (Hamman's sign, resulting from pneumomediastinum) may also be present.

NURSING DIAGNOSES

Among the possible nursing diagnoses for a patient with a pneumothorax are the following:

• Ineffective breathing pattern
• Chest pain
• Potential decreased CO

Planning and Implementation of Care

Ineffective Breathing Pattern Related to Restricted Lung Expansion The loss of pleural integ-rity causes lung collapse and interferes with lung reexpansion. Measures to alleviate the ineffective breathing pattern include stabilization of the thoracic cage, relief of positive intrapleural pressure, and compensation for altered lung volumes.

Stabilization of Thoracic Cage Stabilization of the thoracic cage is essential to minimize abnormal pulmonary dynamics. For an open pneumothorax *(sucking chest wound),* cover the wound with white Vaseline gauze until a chest tube can be inserted. If there is no sucking wound but there is an associated rib fracture or flail chest, paradoxical chest wall movement can be minimized initially by splinting the chest, for example, by placing your hands over the affected area. Obtain medical help for further stabilization, usually achieved with chest tube insertion and positive pressure ventilation.

Relief of Positive Intrapleural Pressure Reduce the positive intrapleural pressure that caused the lung collapse and interferes with its reexpansion. Methods of reducing the pressure vary with the type and size of pneumothorax.

1. For a small closed pneumothorax, the physician may prescribe bedrest and supplemental O_2. The air will be reabsorbed slowly, because of the pressure gradient between it and the surrounding blood and tissue.

2. For a tension or larger closed pneumothorax, assist with emergency decompression with a large-bore needle, stopcock, and syringe; Heimlich valve; or chest tube. (See Chapter 9 for information on the technique and nursing responsibilities related to chest tubes.)

3. Elevate the head of the bed 30° to facilitate expansion of the lung and evacuation of air via the chest tube. Use a footboard to keep the patient from slipping down in bed and restricting diaphragmatic movement.

4. For recurrent pneumothoraces, the physician may elect to create adhesions between the lung and chest wall via injection of an irritating substance into the pleural cavity under local anesthesia or via parietal pleurectomy under general anesthesia.

Chest Pain Related to Nerve Irritation To reduce the chest pain, consult with the physician about type, dosage, and frequency of analgesics. If the pain persists in spite of analgesics, consult with the physician about intercostal nerve blocks. As the pain usually is abrupt, sharp, constant, and unilateral, call to the attention of the physician any chest pain with different characteristics as a possible indicator of an additional disorder, such as acute MI.

Potential Decreased CO Related to Mediastinal Shift   Monitor the patient for signs of mediastinal shift as described earlier under signs and symptoms. If they occur in a patient without chest drainage, call them to the physician's attention immediately, as prompt decompression is mandatory. If they occur in a patient with chest drainage, immediately check the patency of the system and alert the physician.

Outcome Evaluation

Use these outcome criteria to evaluate the patient's progress:

- No chest pain.
- Unlabored spontaneous respirations 12–18 times per minute.
- Chest symmetrical in size and expansion.
- Normal tactile fremitus and breath sounds.
- Involved area of chest resonant on percussion.
- Trachea midline.
- Heart sounds in normal location; no Hamman's sign.
- Venous return normal (neck veins undistended, CVP readings normal, no liver tenderness or dependent edema).
- BP, pulse, and urinary output WNL for patient.
- Alert and oriented.
- Skin warm and dry (and pink if the patient is Caucasian).
- Chest x-ray—normal peripheral lung markings, no central compression collapse, no mediastinal shift.

Pleural Effusion

A *pleural effusion* is an accumulation of fluid in the pleural space. There are four main types of fluid found: exudative, transudative, hemorrhagic, and chylous. *Exudative* effusions have a pleural-to-serum-protein ratio greater than 0.5. *Transudative* effusions have a pleural-to-serum-protein ratio less than 0.5. *Hemorrhagic* effusions are bloody, and *chylous* effusions consist of lymph fluid (Luce et al. 1984). Because of the variety of etiologies resulting in fluid in the pleural space, effusions are common in the critical-care setting.

Assessment

Risk Conditions   Exudative effusions are seen in half of patients with pneumonia and have the potential of becoming infected. Grossly purulent pleural fluid is referred to as *empyema* or *pyothorax* if a large amount of pus is present. Empyemas may result as complications of respiratory infections, chest trauma, or chest surgery. Transudative effusions may be seen in patients with chronic left-sided heart failure and patients with low albumin due to cirrhosis and liver disease. Bloody effusions are seen following chest trauma and with some chest tumors. Serosanguinous effusions are seen after open heart surgery when the pleural space is entered. Chylous effusions are seen with obstruction to lymph flow, as in some malignancies. Malignant effusions tend to be large and to reoccur after drainage and are a poor prognostic sign.

Signs and Symptoms   The presence of symptoms depends on the size of the effusion and the rate at which it accumulated. Symptoms include complaints of dyspnea by the patient, decreased activity level, and decreased appetite. Signs include tachypnea, shallow respirations, tracheal deviation away from the side of the effusion, decreased breath sounds, and the absence of tactile and voice vibrations. A decubitus chest film helps identify free pleural fluid by a shift in the fluid level as the patient turns on his or her side. Percussion of the area results in a dull note.

Arterial blood gas analysis may show hypoxemia due to compression of lung tissue and shunting.

NURSING DIAGNOSES

Nursing diagnoses that may apply to the patient with a pleural effusion include:

- Impaired gas exchange
- Activity intolerance

Impaired Gas Exchange Related to Decreased Lung Expansion   Place the patient in a position to optimize lung expansion, and decrease patient feelings of breathlessness, usually by elevating the head of the bed. Avoid positions that restrict diaphragmatic movement. Assess the degree of effusion by frequent chest auscultation. Encourage deep breathing by use of incentive spirometry in the nonintubated patient. Follow blood gas analysis for hypoxemia, and observe the patient for signs of increasing hypoxia and/or hypercarbia.

Activity Intolerance Related to Inadequate Ventilation Space activities to avoid tiring the patient. Eating may be difficult due to extreme dyspnea, so encourage the patient to eat small amounts frequently. This will also avoid gastric distention and further lung restriction. Alert the physician of any decreasing activity tolerance and increasing dyspnea as most effusions are treated based on patient symptoms, not on the quantity of fluid estimated to be present in the pleural space.

Outcome Evaluation

Judge the patient's progress according to these desirable outcome criteria:

- Arterial blood gas WNL for patient.
- CXR WNL for patient.
- Normal breath and voice sounds.
- Normal percussion note.
- Decreased levels of dyspnea and energy as noted by the patient.

Pulmonary Embolus

An *embolus* is an undissolved mass that travels in the bloodstream and occludes a blood vessel. Emboli to the lungs include venous thromboemboli, air emboli, fat emboli, and catheter emboli. Incidence is 500,000 annually, with 50,000 deaths due to pulmonary embolus (Hayes and Bone 1983). Of patients who die due to pulmonary emboli, 40–60% are not diagnosed before death (Bell and Simon 1982).

Assessment

Risk Conditions Anticipate and prevent emboli whenever possible. Conditions increasing the likelihood of different types of emboli are stated in the next sections to enhance your ability to identify patients at risk.

1. *Thromboemboli* may result from blood stasis, venous wall abnormalities, clotting abnormalities, or irrigation of clotted catheter tips. In 1846, Virchow identified blood stasis, venous wall abnormalities, and clotting

abnormalities as factors promoting venous thrombosis. Remembering this triad can help you to recognize risk conditions for thromboemboli. For example, blood stasis may be caused by obesity, congestive heart failure, immobilization (bedrest), atrial fibrillation or standstill, or severely decreased myocardial contractility. Venous wall abnormalities can result from venous punctures or incisions, trauma, or atherosclerosis. Disorders causing abnormal blood clotting include thrombocytosis and dehydration.

The critical-care nurse also must be aware that forceful irrigation of clotted catheter tips can dislodge the clots, creating emboli.

2. *Air emboli* may result from surgery on the peritoneal cavity, air in intravenous lines, or breakage of a pulmonary artery catheter balloon.

3. *Fat emboli* can result from long-bone fractures (especially the femur and tibia), sternal splitting incisions, use of a pump oxygenator during cariopulmonary bypass, or trauma to subcutaneous fat. The exact mechanism of fat embolization is unclear; fat release from bones and tissues, alteration of circulating fats, and other causes have been implicated.

4. *Catheter emboli* may also occur. Many polyethylene intravenous catheters have a surrounding short steel needle to facilitate venipuncture. After venipuncture, the catheter is advanced through the needle, which is withdrawn and covered by a protective shield. If the catheter is advanced and then manipulated while the needle is unshielded, a portion of the catheter can be sliced off and embolize to the lung.

Preventive Measures Take measures to reduce the likelihood of embolization.

Virchow's triad of factors contributing to thromboemboli has numerous implications for nursing prevention. Follow the measures to reduce risk of *thromboemboli.*

1. Decrease *venous stasis* as follows:

    (a) Consult with the physician about the use of antiembolic stockings to maintain venous flow.

    (b) Ensure that active or passive exercises are performed, since muscular activity promotes venous flow by alternately compressing and releasing the veins. See Chapter 20 for recommended exercises.

    (c) Some physicians recommend elevating the supine patient's legs about 15° to aid venous flow without causing inguinal pooling. Avoid constant Fowler's position whenever not required by other conditions (such as acute pulmonary edema).

2. Reduce *venous wall trauma* as follows:

(a)   Avoid venous punctures on the legs whenever possible.

(b)   Observe vascular catheter insertion sites for inflammation and phlebitis. If they occur, discontinue the line (unless no other sites are available) and restart elsewhere.

3.   If you suspect a line has become clotted, first try to aspirate blood; reposition the tip; and then irrigate gently. Do *not* irrigate forcefully.

4.   Prevent dehydration to help maintain normal coagulability.

5.   Administer low-dose heparin if ordered by the physician. In a study of respiratory intensive care units, Pingleton (1981) found low-dose heparin both effective and safe in preventing pulmonary emboli. Research has also confirmed the effectiveness of mini-dose heparin in preventing fatal postoperative pulmonary emboli in major surgical procedures performed on patients over 40 years of age (Multicentre trial 1975).

Take preventive action against *air emboli*. The lethal dose of air is estimated to be 100 ml (Glennon et al. 1981). Although this is a sizeable amount, lesser amounts can occlude small vessels. Always remove air from vascular lines when assembling them. If you note a bubble once the line is in use, you can remove it with a needle and syringe without breaking continuity of the line. To prevent air embolization from breakage of a pulmonary artery catheter balloon, see Chapter 11, on cardiac assessment and hemodynamic monitoring lines.

Reduce the risk of *catheter emboli* by implementing the following measures. If it is necessary to reposition a catheter during insertion, withdraw the catheter and unshielded needle simultaneously. Once a catheter is positioned properly, withdraw the needle and cover it with the protective shield.

If a venous catheter is sliced off accidentally, it is imperative that you try to prevent it from reaching the heart. Immediately clamp your hands around the limb between the insertion site and the heart, and obtain immediate medical assistance to remove the catheter.

Signs and Symptoms   Detect the occurrence of pulmonary embolism promptly. Signs and symptoms vary, depending on the type, size, and hemodynamic consequences of the embolus.

Thromboembolism   A thromboembolus consists of fibrin, platelets, and red blood cells. When the platelets degranulate, they release substances that cause smooth muscle constriction in both the bronchi and the pulmonary arteries (Hamer and Lemberg 1982). Frequently,

chest pain, dyspnea, tachypnea, apprehension, and cough are present (Bell and Simon 1982).

Chest Pain   The cause of chest pain is unclear. Chest pain and tachypnea are the most common findings in pulmonary embolism.

Signs of Hypoxia   Watch for signs of hypoxia resulting from the increased alveolar deadspace. The signs include tachypnea, restlessness, and irritability. This wasted ventilation is reduced somewhat by the constriction of distal airways due to alveolar hypocapnia. This constriction is a protective measure, causing a redirection of ventilation to better perfused areas. Unfortunately, it also increases airway resistance and work of breathing.

Signs of Acute Right Ventricular Failure   Monitor for signs of possible acute right ventricular failure *(cor pulmonale)*. This condition results from a large embolus that occludes over 50% of the pulmonary vascular bed. An accentuated P_2 (pulmonic component of second heart sound), atrial dysrhythmias, increased CVP readings, distended neck veins, and liver engorgement all indicate right-heart failure. Mortality is 85–90% for this group. Pulmonary hypertension may also result from chronic multiple small emboli.

Signs of Decreased CO   Observe for indications of potential decreased CO. Signs resulting from decreased left ventricular filling are tachycardia, hypotension, dizziness or confusion, shock, or angina. The angina is a result of decreased coronary artery perfusion coupled with an increased right ventricular workload.

Air Embolism   A churning noise upon auscultation of the right ventricle is a sign of air embolism to the ventricle. It is accompanied by sudden dyspnea, shock, and cyanosis.

Fat Embolism   Suspect fat embolism if you see petechiae along with the signs and symptoms of increased deadspace, right ventricular failure, or decreased CO. Petechiae are most common on the anterior chest, neck, and axillary folds.

Pulmonary Infarction   Be alert for symptoms of a possible pulmonary infarction. The signs are those indicated above plus fever over 39°C; transient or persistent pleuritic pain and/or pleural friction rub; cough; and hemoptysis. A chest x-ray 12–24 hours postembolization frequently will show a localized density in the periphery with a rounded edge facing the hilum.

Infarction occurs in only about 10% of the known episodes of embolization. The probable reason is the dual blood supply to the lungs. There are numerous anastamoses between the bronchial and pulmonary capillaries and veins producing a network facilitating collateral flow in the event of an embolus.

Other Diagnostic Aids Keep abreast of the results of other diagnostic maneuvers. Additional tests may or may not be helpful in detecting an embolus. The ECG occasionally shows signs of right axis deviation and right ventricular strain. The routine chest x-ray may show nothing or may show an elevated diaphragm due to pneumoconstriction, decreased or absent vascular markings, or dilatation of the main pulmonary artery and right ventricle. Pulmonary angiography may show a filling defect due to an embolus or a cutoff due to a complete occlusion. Ventilation/perfusion scans usually show an area of normal ventilation with decreased or absent perfusion. Blood gases may be normal or show hypoxemia and an increased $AaDo_2$.

NURSING DIAGNOSES

Nursing diagnoses that may apply to the patient with a pulmonary embolus include:

- Chest pain
- Impaired gas exchange
- Potential decreased CO
- Potential knowledge deficit

Planning and Implementation of Care

If you suspect an air embolus in the right ventricle, immediately place the patient on the left side with the head dependent. This will prevent the air from obstructing the right ventricular outflow tract or migrating to the pulmonary artery. The air will be displaced to the apex, where a physician can aspirate it.

For any type of embolus reaching the pulmonary artery, the goals of care are to relieve the hypoxia resulting from the increased alveolar deadspace, combat any significant decrease in CO, and treat shock vigorously if present.

Chest Pain Possibly Related to Ischemia Relieve chest pain by administering analgesics as necessary, providing supplemental oxygenation, and encouraging relaxation.

Impaired Gas Exchange Related to Ventilation/ Perfusion Mismatch Observe for signs of progres-

sive hypoxemia and hypo/hypercapnia. Maintain bedrest, with the head of the bed elevated to promote respiratory excursion. Assist the person with bathing, eating, and other activities that increase dyspnea. Administer supplemental oxygen as ordered by the physician.

Potential Decreased CO Related to Increased Right Ventricular Afterload Decrease additional insults to the right ventricle by reducing its workload: provide physical rest; reduce emotional stress by providing as calm an atmosphere as possible, administering analgesics to control pain, and relieving anxiety as much as possible.

If shock occurs, follow measures outlined in the care plan for shock (Chapter 13). For persistent shock from a centrally located embolus, embolectomy may be attempted. After the patient is placed on cardiopulmonary bypass, the main pulmonary artery is incised and the embolus removed. Mortality is 40–60% (Hayes and Bone 1983).

Prevent recurrent embolization by administering anticoagulants and thrombolytic agents as ordered by the physician.

A mainstay of medical therapy for thromboembolism is anticoagulation. Heparin is the drug of choice in treating acute thromboembolism because it inactivates thrombin, thus blocking further clot formation, and also inhibits the degranulation of platelets surrounding the thrombus, thus limiting the release of substances causing smooth muscle constriction (Hamer and Lemberg 1982). It is administered intravenously. Controversy exists as to the best protocol for administration—intermittent high doses or continuous low doses. Therapy is monitored with Lee White clotting times or partial thromboplastin times kept at 2 to 2½ times normal. Heparin therapy is continued for several days or longer; a transition is made to oral anticoagulants as soon as the patient is ambulatory.

Because heparin does not directly affect fibrin, it has no fibrinolytic activity. Therefore, although it can prevent further clot formation, it cannot lyse already-formed clots. To achieve the latter therapeutic goal, thrombolytic agents such as intravenous streptokinase and urokinase also may be prescribed. A research study by Sharma et al. (1980) compared 40 pulmonary emboli patients randomly assigned to either heparin/oral anticoagulant therapy or urokinase or streptokinase/heparin/oral anticoagulant therapy. Measurements of pulmonary capillary blood volume and diffusing capacity at 2 weeks and 1 year showed that thrombolytic agents provided more complete resolution of thromboemboli than did heparin, and improved capillary perfusion and diffusion.

Potential Decreased CO Related to Bleeding Protect the patient from excessive anticoagulation and fibrinolysis by monitoring clotting and/or prothrombin times, observing for signs of internal or external bleeding, minimizing intramuscular injections, testing gastric contents and bowel movements for occult blood, and consulting with the clinical pharmacist on interactions between anticoagulants and the patient's other medications.

If anticoagulation is contraindicated or emboli persist despite anticoagulation, either the common femoral veins or the vena cava may be ligated; alternatively, an umbrella-shaped device may be inserted in the vena cava to trap further emboli.

Potential Knowledge Deficit When the patient's condition permits, teach him how to prevent, recognize, and respond to symptoms postdischarge. Emphasize the importance of exercise, hydration, measures to promote venous flow, and medical follow-up. Oral anticoagulants may be continued as long as the risk remains, permanently if necessary.

Outcome Evaluation

Judge the patient's progress according to these outcome criteria:

- Unlabored respirations 12–18 times a minute.
- Pulse, BP, and temperature WNL for patient.
- No signs of right ventricular failure (undistended neck veins, normal CVP readings, no liver engorgement).
- Alert and oriented.
- No churning noise when right ventricle is auscultated.
- No cough, hemoptysis, or pleural friction rub.

CHRONIC RESPIRATORY FAILURE

Chronic respiratory failure most commonly results from chronic obstructive pulmonary disease, those respiratory diseases associated with decreased expiratory flow rates (as evidenced by FEV_1). Bronchitis, emphysema, and asthma are chronic obstructive diseases whose sufferers live with a small respiratory reserve and easily develop acute respiratory failure. Asthma and bronchitis have reversible components, and those patients may be symptom-free between episodes, unlike patients with emphysema, which is irreversible. The American Lung Association estimates that over 450,000 new COPD patients are seen each year and that there may be as many as 15 million sufferers in the United States (Shapiro et al. 1985). In 1973, 70% of COPD patients survived their first episode of acute respiratory failure, whereas it is estimated that in 1986 95% would survive their first episode of respiratory failure (Bone 1986). COPD patients also are seen in increasing numbers in critical-care units for other procedures as well as for acute respiratory failure. The following sections focus on management of the COPD patient in the critical-care unit, including episodes of acute respiratory failure.

Bronchitis and Emphysema

Assessment

Risk Conditions Cigarette smoking remains the highest risk factor for developing bronchitis and emphysema, with an increase in female COPD patients as female smoking habits increase. Air pollution with noxious gases and particulate matter in urban areas also potentiates irritation to the lung and exacerbates COPD symptoms. Because COPD is more common in the elderly and because the geriatric population is growing, COPD is being seen with increasing frequency (Shapiro et al. 1985).

Preventive Measures Unfortunately, most of the time and money spent on COPD is during the acute phases of the illness. Measures to prevent acute exacerbations include smoking-cessation educational programs and pulmonary rehabilitation programs. Smoking-cessation education is appropriate for both the high school setting (to prevent development of COPD) and the adult public. Components of a successful pulmonary rehabilitation program include teaching bronchial hygiene measures, energy conservation techniques, dyspnea control, medication guidelines, and exercise programs to increase activity tolerance and independence.

The most common precipitating causes of acute respiratory failure in COPD patients are infection, left ventricular failure, myocardial infarction, pulmonary emboli, bronchospasm, sedative drugs, and removal of the hypoxic drive (Chin and Pesce 1983). Care of COPD patients who undergo other procedures, such as surgery, should reflect knowledge of these risk factors. Meticulous asepsis, fluid management, positioning, and drug (including oxygen) administration can help shorten their stay in the ICU and prevent precipitating acute respiratory failure.

During resolution of an episode of acute respiratory failure, the nurse and patient together can begin to identify areas of teaching needs. Some breathing retraining and dyspnea control techniques can be begun in the ICU postextubation in coordination with respiratory therapy personnel. Family should be included when possible. With physician guidance, referral to a pulmonary rehabilitation program may prevent future hospitalizations, increase exercise tolerance, and improve general feelings of well-being.

Signs and Symptoms *Chronic bronchitis* is characterized by inflammation of small airways and hypersecretion of mucus. It is defined as the presence of a recurrent, productive cough 3 months of the year for at least 2 successive years (American Thoracic Society 1982). Ciliary clearance is greatly impaired.

Emphysema is characterized by destructive changes of the alveoli, with resultant enlargement of the distal air spaces. The process is irreversible, causes lung tissue to lose its eleastic recoil, and results in increased lung compliance. The increase in air spaces results in a large increase in residual volume.

Bronchitis and emphysema are often overlapping so that many presenting signs and symptoms are common to both entities. Hyperinflation, or "barrel chest," is present due to air-trapping and increased residual volume, particularly in emphysema. This increased lung volume causes flattening of the diaphragm, decreasing inspiratory efficiency and increasing work of breathing, as noted by use of accessory muscles. Hyperresonance upon percussion and decreased chest excursion are also present. The respiratory rate may be reduced, with prolongation of the expiratory phase. Pursed-lip breathing may be present as the patient tries to reduce premature collapse of floppy airways and decrease air-trapping. Chest auscultation may reveal decreased breath sounds throughout in the pure emphysemic, or wheezing due to narrowing of airways on expiration, airway edema, and secretions in the bronchitic or mixed patient.

Cyanosis and hypoxemia are more common in the bronchitic patient due to secretions and shunting. When hypoventilation is present, CO_2 retention occurs. Chronic hypoventilation results in chronic CO_2 reten-

tion. These patients therefore depend on hypoxemia ($P_aO_2 < 60$ mm Hg) as their respiratory stimulus.

In the emphysemic, destruction of the alveolar-capillary membrane results in a diffusion defect that produces hypoxemia, particularly during exercise.

As hypoxemia and CO_2 retention progress, the patient may become agitated and combative, progressing to lethargy and confusion. Work of breathing becomes overwhelming due to increased air-trapping, secretions, and bronchospasm, and intubation and mechanical ventilation become necessary. With this chronically ill population the decision to intubate should ideally be discussed prior to its emergent need as some patients may not be able to be weaned from such support. Following previous intubations, some patients—along with family and physician support—may decide against reintubation should their condition deteriorate.

NURSING DIAGNOSES

The nursing diagnoses most applicable to the COPD patient are:

- Ineffective airway clearance
- Ineffective breathing pattern
- Impaired gas exchange
- Anxiety
- Hopelessness

Planning and Implementation of Care

Ineffective Airway Clearance Related to Ineffective Cough and Mucociliary Mechanisms Aggressive bronchial hygiene therapy is a necessity to clear secretions and decrease airway resistance as well as prevent infection. You should ensure that the patient is adequately hydrated, including having inhaled gases humidified. To ensure efficient coughing the patient should be assisted to a semi-Fowler's position. Drawing up the knees may help reduce pain of abdominal incisions (Luce et al. 1984). Patients unable to sit can be turned onto their sides with knees drawn upward. "Huff" coughing is a series of small coughs done with the glottis held open while saying "huff." In COPD patients this type of cough may produce higher flow rates despite airway collapse. Chest physical therapy and postural drainage are discussed in Chapter 9 and are appropriate to enhance secretion removal.

Ineffective Breathing Pattern Related to Decreased Diaphragmatic Function and Increased Lung Volumes Position your patient to augment diaphragmatic descent, i.e., high up in the bed and leaning over a bedside table if possible. Coordinate with the respiratory therapists the appropriateness of teaching diaphragmatic and pursed-lip breathing (see Chapter 9). Some COPD patients on ventilators increase air-trapping because they receive their next breath before they have finished exhaling the current one. To detect this problem, observe for increasing peak inspiratory pressures; lengthening the expiratory phase may prevent this. The use of expiratory retard may also be helpful.

Impaired Gas Exchange Related to Destroyed Alveolar-Capillary Membrane and Increased Secretions Perform maneuvers described under "Ineffective Airway Clearance." Monitor the patient for signs of hypoxia, and check arterial blood gases for degree of hypoxemia. Check the history and physical to ascertain what is normal for your patient.

Anxiety Due to Feelings of Breathlessness Establish a relationship of trust with the patient. Do not leave the bedside of a newly intubated or extremely dyspneic, panicked patient. Talk in a quiet, clear, concise manner. Many COPD patients do not like being hovered over or confined to a semisupine position. Explain in a concise manner exactly what you are doing or plan to do to help alleviate the feelings of breathlessness. Elicit the assistance of a respiratory therapist to "talk the patient through" dyspnea control maneuvers while you prepare an aminophylline infusion, send off lab work, etc. Broad statements such as "Just relax, Mrs. Jones" are ineffective and only serve to worsen the patient's panic.

Hopelessness Due to Irreversible Nature of Disease Dudley et al. (1980) has described the consequences of chronic dyspnea, anxiety, and depression as an "emotional straitjacket" because many patients use isolation, denial, and repression of emotions as defense mechanisms. Laughing, expressing anger, or crying all serve to increase their breathlessness. The resulting inactivity perpetuates lower levels of activity tolerance, and soon the patient is in a physically and emotionally confining world. Feelings of anger, despair, and hopelessness are common and may be taken out on caregivers. Pulmonary rehabilitation programs offer hope of increasing activity tolerance and independence. As the bedside nurse you can be instrumental in facilitating referral to such resources. In some cases psychiatric counseling may be helpful to treat severe depression.

Outcome Evaluation

Evaluate the patient's progress according to the following desirable outcome criteria:

- Arterial blood gases WNL for that patient.
- Absence of infection.
- Patient demonstration of bronchial hygiene maneuvers.
- Patient demonstration of diaphragmatic and pursed-lip breathing techniques.
- Patient able to describe signs and symptoms of infection.
- Patient report of decreased anxiety and hopelessness.

Status Asthmaticus

Asthma is a *chronic* disease characterized by recurrent attacks of reversible airway obstruction. *Status asthmaticus* is a *severe, unrelenting attack* unresponsive to the patient's usual forms of therapy. An acute asthmatic attack is a self-perpetuating complex characterized by three interrelated problems: spasm of bronchial smooth muscle, mucosal edema, and hypersecretion of mucus. The *smooth muscle spasm* is believed to be due to hyperreactivity of the bronchial smooth muscle caused by a variety of irritants. This hyperreactivity probably is due to an imbalance of both neurologic innervation and chemical mediators. Current research has implicated a group of vasoactive substances known as *leukotrienes* as being responsible for the acute airway narrowing, mucus production, and airway inflammation characteristic of acute asthma. These mediators may potentiate the effects of other substances on the airways (Gundel et al. 1986).

Neurological imbalance may also exist between the sympathetic and parasympathetic innervation of the bronchi. Normally, bronchi relax in response to sympathetic stimulation, specifically beta$_2$ receptor stimulation. This response is mediated by the production of cyclic 3'5' adenosine monophosphate (cyclic AMP), a chemical mediator that promotes relaxation of bronchial smooth muscle. In status asthmaticus, beta$_2$ stimulation is either abnormally low or blocked, so hyperreactivity and bronchoconstriction ensue.

Asthma is primarily a disease of the large airways,

but the widespread bronchoconstriction that occurs affects all exchange units. The constriction causes air-trapping, so that functional residual capacity increases and, as a result, vital capacity decreases. The overdistention of alveoli causes increased deadspace, which results in wasted ventilation. The overinflation of the lungs combined with the increased airway resistance markedly increases the work of breathing. Because of the reduced intake of air and of fatigue, hypoventilation occurs and leads eventually to hypercapnia.

Because asthma also is characterized by increased production of tenacious secretions, local areas of atelectasis occur. Continuing capillary flow past these areas of alveolar collapse results in increased shunting, which produces severe hypoxemia.

Assessment

Risk Conditions A number of risk conditions can precipitate an attack of status asthmaticus. Most common is respiratory infection, which typically is viral in nature. Other risk factors include failure to take prescribed medications or overuse of medications, particularly sympathomimetic agents. Weather changes, exposure to allergens, and emotional stress are other common precipitating factors.

Signs and Symptoms The clinical presentation of a patient in status asthmaticus is unforgettable. The patient presents with extreme dyspnea, exhaustion, and fear. Tachypnea, a compensatory response to the hypoxemia, is accompanied by accessory muscle use and often by cyanosis. Breath sounds are diminished. The patient may be wheezing markedly on inspiration and expiration. The absence of this sign is ominous, indicating that so little air is moving that a wheeze cannot occur. Coughing is almost impossible. The patient is tachycardic and diaphoretic. Clinical signs of dehydration usually are present. Most noticeable are the exhaustion and fear exhibited by the patient.

Planning and Implementation of Care

Impaired Gas Exchange Related to Increased Shunting Start the patient immediately on supplemental oxygen by Venturi mask at 24% F_IO_2. (Remember that a higher F_IO_2 may obliterate the hypoxic drive for ventilation on which this patient depends.) Draw arterial blood gases, on the physician's order, to determine the degree of hypoxemia; assist with arterial line placement if necessary for frequent blood gas assessments. Blood gases usually show severe hypoxemia, with P_aO_2 values of 50 mm Hg or less, and a normal pH and normal or low P_aCO_2 due to hyperventilation. A rising P_aCO_2 and falling pH are ominous signs, indicating that the patient is tiring in the effort to stave off impending respiratory failure. Unless checked, the continuing rise in P_aCO_2 will result in acute respiratory failure and apnea. Administer bicarbonate intravenously, as ordered by the physician, to combat the profound respiratory acidosis that results when compensation fails. Institute aggressive pulmonary care as described below.

Intubation and mechanical ventilation are used only as a last resort. The primary danger of mechanical ventilation for this patient is the increased risk of pneumothorax, due to the high inspiratory pressures necessary to overcome the increased airway resistance and the patient's tendency to breathe out-of-phase with the ventilator. Often, the mechanically ventilated asthmatic must be sedated and paralyzed to diminish the risk of fighting the ventilator. Expiratory retard may be used to maintain airway patency on expiration, thus allowing better emptying of lung volumes.

Ineffective Airway Clearance Related to Bronchospasm, Mucosal Edema, and Thick Secretions Humidify the oxygen administered to the patient. Start an IV line for administration of fluids and drugs, as ordered by the physician, because the patient usually cannot swallow safely due to gasping respirations. Obtain laboratory data to assess the degree of airway obstruction. Data collection usually includes a chest x-ray, which may be normal or show marked air trapping, and spirometry, which shows decreased vital capacity and decreased FEV_1. Administer sympathomimetic agents as prescribed. The patient may be given two doses of

---

NURSING DIAGNOSES

The nursing diagnoses applicable to the patient in status asthmaticus include:

- Impaired gas exchange
- Ineffective airway clearance
- Activity intolerance
- Actual fluid volume deficit
- Potential decreased CO
- Fear

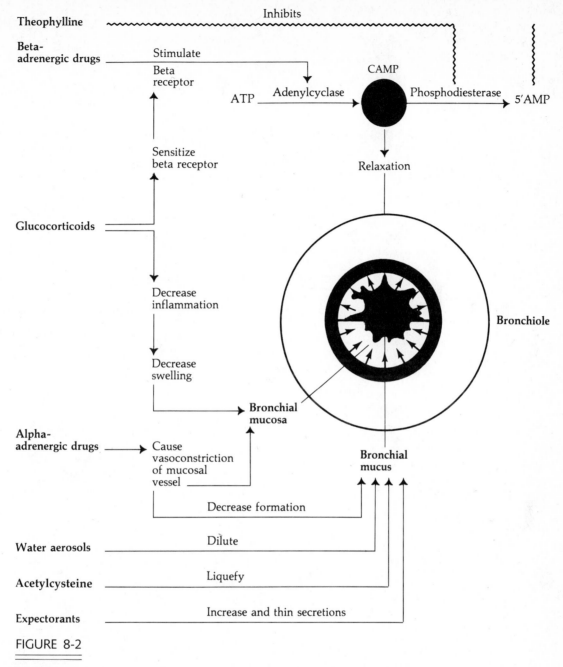

FIGURE 8-2

Possible benefits of various drugs in airway obstruction. (From Wilson R (editor-in-chief): *Principles and techniques of critical care.* Philadelphia: Davis, 1977.)

subcutaneous epinephrine or terbutaline as the initial pharmacologic maneuver. If this is unsuccessful, intravenous aminophylline may be prescribed. A theophylline derivative, aminophylline inhibits the activity of phosphodiesterase, thereby inhibiting the breakdown of cyclic AMP and promoting bronchial relaxation (Figure 8–2). Inhaled bronchodilators, such as albuterol, iso-

etharine and isoproterenol, also are used (Table 8–2). Steroids may be prescribed to diminish the nonspecific inflammatory reaction and inhibit the release of chemical mediators promoting bronchoconstriction, although the response is delayed in onset. Unless the patient is intubated, sedatives should not be administered, because they blunt the respiratory drive.

TABLE 8–2 NURSE'S GUIDE TO NEBULIZED MEDICATIONS

DRUG	DOSE	NURSING REMINDERS
Bronchodilators		

Albuterol (salbutamol)
  Proventil
  Ventolin
	0.5 ml of 0.5% in 2 ml normal saline every 4 hours	Monitor pulse and BP: may cause tachycardia and hypertension

Atropine (Atrovent)	1–2 mg in 2–3 ml normal saline, every 4–6 hours	Tachycardia, urine retention, blurred vision, dried secretions

Epinephrine
  Adrenaline
  Primatene Mist
  Vaponefrin
  Bronkaid
	0.2 ml of 2.25% racemic in normal saline every 2–4 hours	Monitor pulse and BP: may cause tachycardia and hypertension
		Also may cause excitement or shaking

Isoproterenol hydrochloride
  Isuprel
  Medi-haler-Iso
	0.5 ml of 1:200 in 2.5 ml normal saline every 4 hours	Monitor pulse and BP: may cause tachycardia and hypotension

Isoetharine Bronkosol	0.25–1.0 ml diluted with saline, via IPPB. Hand nebulizer: 3–6 undiluted inhalations	Monitor pulse and BP: may cause tachycardia and BP fluctuations

Metaproterenol sulfate
  Alupent
  Metaprel
	0.3 ml in 2 ml normal saline	Monitor pulse and BP: may cause tachycardia and hypertension
		Protect from light

Mucolytic		
Acetylcysteine Mucomyst	1–2 ml of 10–20% instilled into trachea; or 3–5 ml of 10%, or 6–10 ml of 20%, inhaled 3–4 times per day	After opening, store in refrigerator and use within 96 hours May cause nausea May cause bronchospasm: use very cautiously in asthmatics
Tyloxapol Alevaire	10–20 ml of 0.125% over 30–90 minutes, 3–4 times per day	May also be used to deliver epinephrine, isoproterenol, or other bronchodilator May produce nausea
Steroids		

Dexamethasone sodium phosphate
  Decadron Respihaler
 	
  Decadron Turbinaire
	2–3 inhalations, 3–4 times per day
	Two sprays per nostril, 2–3 times per day
		Antiinflammatory effect can cause infections of mouth: check for signs, and culture if necessary

Beclomethasone dipropionate
  Vanceril
  Beclovent
	100 micrograms in 2 inhalations, 3–4 times per day	As with Decadron

Antiasthmatic		

Cromolyn sodium
  Aarane
  Intal
	20 mg 4 times per day	Not used in emergency treatment of asthma, but for long-term prevention of attacks

Activity Intolerance Related to Hypoxemia Promote physical and emotional rest for the patient. Allow him or her to assume a position of comfort. The typical posture chosen by the acute asthmatic is sitting up, leaning forward, with arms supported and shoulders elevated. You can make this position more comfortable for the patient by providing an over-the-bed table or pillows on which to lean.

Actual Fluid Volume Deficit Related to Diaphoresis, Increased Lung Water Loss, and Diuresis Due to Aminophylline Administration Administer fluids as previously described. Assist with CVP line placement, if desired by the physician, to monitor fluid therapy. Monitor BP, pulse, level of consciousness, urinary output, breath sounds and peripheral perfusion closely. After the patient is stabilized and able to swallow safely, encourage the intake of oral fluids.

Potential Decreased CO Related to Right Heart Failure Monitor the patient for signs and symptoms of impending cardiac failure (see Chapter 13 for further details). Usually, the failure is right-heart failure precipitated by the high pulmonary vascular resistance (cor pulmonale).

Fear Related to Inability to Breathe Comfortably Provide emotional support by projecting a calm, competent air. If accepted by the patient, use touch to provide reassurance. Allow a loved one, if calm, to stay with the patient. For further suggestions on provision of emotional support, see Chapter 3.

Outcome Evaluation

Evaluate the patient's progress according to the following desirable outcome criteria:

- Vital signs WNL for patient.
- Arterial blood gas values WNL for patient.
- Presence of normal breath sounds.
- Absence of dyspnea and wheezing.
- Recovery of normal energy level.

REFERENCES

American Thoracic Society: Definition and classification of chronic bronchitis, asthma and pulmonary emphysema. *Am Rev Respir Dis* 1982; 85:762.

Bell W, Simon T: Current status of pulmonary thromboembolic disease: Pathophysiology, diagnosis, prevention and treatment. *Am Heart J* (Feb) 1982; 239–263.

Benner P: *From novice to expert.* Menlo Park, CA: Addison-Wesley, 1984.

Bone R: Acute respiratory failure in the setting of chronic obstructive lung disease. *Proceedings of the critical care medicine conference,* USC, Feb 27–Mar 2, 1986, Las Vegas, CA.

Brandstetter RD: The adult respiratory distress syndrome—1986. *Heart Lung* 1986; 15:155–164.

Chin R, Pesce R: Practical aspects in management of respiratory failure in chronic obstructive pulmonary disease. *Crit Care Quart* 1983; 6:1–19.

Dudley D et al.: Psychosocial concomitants to rehabilitation in chronic obstructive pulmonary disease. *Chest* 1980; 77:413–420.

Fowler A et al.: Adult respiratory distress syndrome: Risk with common predispositions. *Ann Intern Med* 1983; 98:593.

Glennon S et al.: Respiratory disorders. Pages 485–542 in *AACN's clinical reference for critical care nursing,* Kinney M et al. (eds). New York: McGraw Hill, 1981.

Gundel RH et al.: The leukotrienes: Pharmacologic and clinical implications for respiratory care. *Resp Care* (Feb) 1986; 31:137–145.

Hamer S, Lemberg L: A complication commonly overlooked. *Heart Lung* 1982; 11:588–592.

Hayes S, Bone R: Pulmonary emboli with respiratory failure. *Med Clin North Am* 1983; 67:1179–1190.

Kuhn M: Pneumonia: Pathogenesis, clinical and laboratory features. In *Comprehensive management of respiratory emergencies,* Brenner B (ed). Rockville, MD: Aspen, 1985, pp. 159–179.

Luce J et al.: *Intensive respiratory care.* Philadelphia: Saunders, 1984.

Multicentre trial: Prevention of fatal postoperative pulmonary embolism by low doses of heparin. *Lancet* 1975 (July); 45–51.

Pingleton S: Prevention of pulmonary emboli in an intensive care unit. *Chest* 1981; 79:647–650.

Podnos S et al.: Nosocomial pneumonia in patients in intensive care units. *West J Med* 1985; 143:622–627.

Sasahara AA et al.: Pulmonary embolism: Diagnosis and treatment. *JAMA* 1983; 249(21):2945–2950.

Schluttenhoffer N: The special challenge of empyemas. *Nurs 84* (Dec); 57–60.

Shapiro B. et al.: *Clinical Application of Respiratory Care,* 3rd ed. Chicago: Year Book, 1985.

Sharma G et al.: Effect of thrombolytic therapy on pulmonary-capillary blood volume in patients with pulmonary embolism. *N Engl J Med* 1980; 303:842–845.

Sladen J: Personal communication, 1986.

Stevens J, Raffin R: Adult respiratory distress syndrome—Etiology and mechanisms, management. *Postgrad Med J* 1984; 60:505–513, 573–576.

Virchow R: Weitere Untersuchungen uber die Verstopfung der Lungernareterie und Ihre Folgen. *Beit Exp Pathol Physiol* 1846; 2:21.

SUPPLEMENTAL READING

Ayres SM: Mechanisms and consequences of pulmonary edema: Cardiac lung, shock lung, and principles of ventilatory therapy in adult respiratory distress syndrome. *Am Heart J* (Jan) 1982; 103:97–111.

Bernard GR, Bradly RB. Adult respiratory distress syndrome: Diagnosis and management. *Heart Lung* 1986; 15:250–255.

Cherniack RM, Cherniack L: *Respiration in health and disease,* 3d ed. Philadelphia: Saunders, 1983.

Fahey AV: Life-threatening pulmonary embolism. *Crit Care Quart* (Sept) 1985; 8:81–88.

Fuchs, PC: Action STAT; Tension penumothorax. *Nurs* (Nov) 1985; 15:41.

Hanley ME, Bone RC: Acute respiratory failure. *Postgrad Med* (Jan) 1986; 79:166–176.

Jenkinson SG: Pneumothorax. *Clin Chest Med* (March) 1985; 6:153–161.

Shapiro BA et al.: Chronic obstructive pulmonary disease.

Chapter 30 in *Clinical application of respiratory care*. Chicago: Year Book, 1985.

Stratton CW: Bacterial pneumonias—An overview with emphasis on pathogenesis, diagnosis and treatment. *Heart Lung* 1986; 15:226–249.

Tafuro P et al.: Approach to hospital-acquired pneumonias. *Heart Lung* 1984; 13:482–485.

Woodruff ML: Pulmonary thromboembolism: Risk factors, pathophysiology and management. *Crit Care Nurse* (Jul/Aug) 1984; 4:52–63.

9

Aeration Treatment Techniques

CLINICAL INSIGHT

Domain: The helping role

Competency: The healing relationship: creating a climate for and establishing a commitment to healing

In the face of the devastation wrought by critical illness or injury, the nurse can help the patient maintain an awareness of the possibilities for recovery and a sense of optimism. Helping the patient this way requires a complex alloy of technical expertise, analytic skills, and intuition. Here, an expert nurse confidently builds on the trust established with physicians, and in doing so, achieves both an act of mercy and a victory, whose importance her patient well recognizes. The following exemplar comes from Benner (1984, pp. 52–53, 512).

The patient was a 17-year-old male admitted post c-spine fracture. The patient presented to the ICU awake, alert, and quadriplegic. Within 24 hours, due to poor ventilatory effort, significant lung consolidation developed. The doctors decided to intubate him in order to provide positive airway pressure from a ventilator. The patient was extremely apprehensive about his intubation. His respiratory rate increased dramatically after the tube was passed. His respiratory rate

increased into the 40s and his P_{CO_2} was dropping. The patient was unable to decrease his respiratory rate due to his high anxiety. The doctors were considering increasing his sedation enough to knock out his respiratory drive so that we could totally control his ventilation with this respirator. This increased his anxiety even more. This measure would have added to his already monumental problems with recovery and rehabilitation—something he didn't need. I just knew we could resolve this—his anxiety and thus rapid respiration rate—without using such drastic measures. I intervened in his behalf with his multiple physicians; I explained my "gut feeling," my concerns for his recovery, and negotiated for more time to attempt to resolve this problem. Then I began reassuring him, using my calmest voice. I spoke assuredly, honestly, professionally, and yet personally. He could not speak, as he was intubated. He could not write, as he was quadriplegic, and we didn't allow him to nod his head due to his unstable neck fracture. His only communication was with his eyes and his amazing ability to mouth words clearly and understandably. It took three and a half hours before he began to relax. He needed to know that we cared about him, as an individual, not just another helpless patient. He needed to be involved, not just prescribed to, and he felt so very helpless. This incident is critical to me because it was what nursing is all about for me. The

*point was made by one simple statement he mouthed
to me late in the day—when he had a respiration rate
in the 20s, and he was no longer threatened with
having the few remaining functional muscles chemi-
cally paralyzed. His words were: "Thank you. You've
really helped me a lot. I don't want to imagine what
would have happened to me if you weren't here and
hadn't cared."*

An arsenal of interventions to improve aeration lies at a
nurse's fingertips. Sometimes a given intervention
needs to be applied; at other times, as in the Clinical
Insight, it needs to be withheld and an alternate tried
instead. This chapter discusses oxygen therapy, chest
physiotherapy, artificial airways, tracheal suctioning,
mechanical ventilation, chest drainage, and thoracic surgery.

Oxygen Therapy

Specific signs indicating a possible need for supplemental oxygen are decreased mental status (confusion, impaired thought processes, drowsiness, or lethargy),
tachycardia, dysrhythmias, hypotension, pale cool extremities, dyspnea, fatigue, respiratory depression, cyanosis, and decreased P_aO_2. Oxygen therapy also is indicated for prevention of hypoxemia. The physician is
responsible for prescribing the type of therapy, its frequency and duration, F_IO_2 (fractional inspired oxygen),
and liter flow. In an emergency (such as shock, severe
respiratory depression, impending MI, or serious dysrhythmias), the nurse should be empowered to start oxygen therapy under standing unit guidelines.

Guidelines for Initial F_IO_2 Selection

The goals of oxygen therapy are to treat hypoxemia,
decrease work of breathing, and decrease myocardial
work using the lowest F_IO_2 possible (Shapiro et al.
1985). Selection of the appropriate F_IO_2 is based on the
medical history, clinical status, and probable baseline
blood gases. Tinits (1983) recommends the following
guidelines for selecting the initial F_IO_2.

For patients with no history of CO_2 retention and
mild-to-moderate respiratory distress, the exact F_IO_2 is
not critical. Because hemoglobin desaturation has been
mild, an intermediate O_2 concentration (approximately
40%) is appropriate.

Patients with no history of CO_2 retention and severe
respiratory distress have greater hemoglobin desaturation, and their initial F_IO_2 should be higher (50–100%).

Patients with chronic CO_2 retention and mild-to-moderate exacerbations of COPD often have a P_aCO_2
decreased from its normal level because of hyperventilation. If the resting P_aCO_2 is below 55 mm Hg, an initial
F_IO_2 of 28% may be selected. If the resting P_aCO_2 is
known to be above 55 mm Hg, the initial F_IO_2 should be
24%. The F_IO_2 can be titrated to higher levels if a lower
F_IO_2 is tolerated.

Patients with chronic CO_2 retention and severe exacerbations of COPD should receive 24% oxygen initially. The F_IO_2 may be increased incrementally. These
patients should be closely monitored because they may
require assisted ventilation because of deteriorating
status.

Intubated patients on positive pressure ventilation,
once stabilized, should receive the F_IO_2 that most nearly
reproduces their baseline arterial blood gases.

It should be emphasized that the above are guidelines for selection of initial F_IO_2 only, and should not
replace clinical judgment. Subsequent F_IO_2 adjustment is
based on arterial blood gas values and close monitoring
of the patient's clinical status.

Methods of Oxygen Therapy

The following information on methods of oxygen therapy is based primarily on Shapiro et al. (1985).

The ideal O_2 delivery system would deliver a consistent F_IO_2 that could be controlled easily, allow accurate
measurement of inspired F_IO_2, be comfortable for the
patient, be convenient for the therapist, and be inexpensive. Unfortunately, no current method meets all these
criteria. One must choose from a variety of devices the
one that will best meet the patient's needs. They may
be classified into low-flow and high-flow systems. Oxygen flow is *not* synonymous with oxygen concentration,
because concentration depends on the relationship between O_2 flow *and* total air flow.

Low-Flow Systems   A low-flow system is one in
which the gas flow is insufficient to meet all the requirements for inspiration; room air must also be inspired.
Table 9–1 describes low-flow devices that deliver oxygen concentrations from 21% to above 90%. (A low oxygen concentration is below 35%, a moderate concentration is 35–50%, and a high concentration is above
50%).

Low-flow systems have an oxygen reservoir that is
diluted with room air. The cannula, catheter, and simple

TABLE 9–1 SELECTED OPTIONS IN OXYGENATION (FOR SPONTANEOUSLY BREATHING PATIENTS)

	PATIENT CRITERIA	ADVANTAGES	DISADVANTAGES	NURSING PRECAUTIONS
Low-Flow Systems				
Nasal cannula 1–6 L 24–40%	Normal V_t Respiratory rate <25 Regular respiratory pattern	Comfortable No breathing of expired air Allows eating and talking Practical for long-term therapy Cost	Easily dislodged Cannot be used with nasal obstruction Straps irritate ears Nasal prongs irritate nose	Make sure the nares are patent. May use even with a mouth-breather, since oropharyngeal air flow creates Bernoulli effect, pulling in O_2 through nasopharynx. Do not increase L above 6 because it will not increase F_IO_2; switch to a mask.
Simple oxygen mask 5–8 L 40–60%	Same as above	Higher concentrations than cannula Cost	Tight seal may cause facial irritation, or increase anxiety in dyspneic patients Interferes with eating and talking	Do not run below 5 L, as exhaled CO_2 will not be washed out. To increase F_IO_2 above 0.60, do not increase liter flow; switch to a bag with reservoir.
Partial rebreathing mask with reservoir bag 6–15 L 35–60%	Same as above	Higher concentration because rebreathe from O_2 reservoir Cost	Tight seal, as above Interferes with eating and talking	Maintain flow rate sufficient to keep bag from completely collapsing on inspiration.
Nonrebreathing mask with reservoir 6–15 L 55–90%	Same as above	Highest concentration Cost	Seal may irritate skin Bag must be kept properly inflated Can lead to oxygen toxicity Valve can stick	Maintain flow rate sufficient to keep bag from completely collapsing on inspiration.
High-Flow Systems				
Venturi mask 4–8 L 24–40%	Patients relying on hyponic drive, needing constant precise F_IO_2	Delivers exact concentration despite variations in respiratory pattern F_IO_2 directly analyzed	May irritate facial skin Interferes with eating and talking Cost	To increase F_IO_2, switch to a higher-concentration mask/adapter.

mask use the nose, nasopharynx, and oropharynx as anatomical reservoir. The mask with reservoir bag adds an additional O_2 reservoir from which the patient inspires. Without a one-way valve between this bag and mask, the system is a partial rebreathing mask. If there is a one-way valve between the bag and mask, the system is a nonrebreathing mask.

The advantages and disadvantages of low-flow systems are summarized in Table 9–1. Variations in respiratory rate or tidal volume will affect the inspired oxygen concentration. The slower the rate or the lower the tidal volume, the higher the F_IO_2; the faster the rate or the higher the tidal volume, the lower the F_IO_2. This fact has great clinical significance. Consider the patient with chronic lung disease, started on a nasal cannula at 2 L/min. If tidal volume drops below 300 ml, the F_IO_2 may increase to the point where it suppresses the hypoxic ventilatory drive, and you may have an apneic patient on your hands!

For these reasons, monitor the respiratory rate, depth, and pattern every 2–4 hours. If the respiratory rate increases above 25, breathing becomes shallow, or the ventilatory pattern becomes irregular or inconsistent, alert the physician, who may want to switch to a high-flow system.

Another disadvantage is that since the patient is breathing air from outside as well as inside the system, the temperature and humidity cannot be controlled.

High-Flow Systems High-flow systems (described in Table 9–1) include Venturi masks and nebulizers using the Venturi device. This device is based on the Bernoulli principle, which states that as the velocity of gas flow increases, its lateral pressure decreases. In a device using this principle, the oxygen flows through a small orifice at a high velocity. Just after the oxygen leaves the orifice, the low lateral pressure pulls in, or "entrains," room air. By varying the size of the orifice and the flow of oxygen, one can provide a precise F_IO_2. The high-flow systems deliver a consistent, precise oxygen concentration. In addition, temperature and humidity are better controlled as the patient breathes only the system's air.

Complications

Prevent the complications of oxygen therapy: dehydration of mucosa, hypoventilation, absorption atelectasis, and acute oxygen toxicity. Preventive measures are described in the following paragraphs.

Dehydration of Mucosa Always humidify oxygen because it is a dry gas that can quickly dehydrate the mucosa. Humidification can be achieved with humidifiers or nebulizers. Heated humidifiers deliver fully saturated water vapor, while nebulizers deliver aerosols (tiny water particles).

Hypoventilation Avoid provoking hypoventilation in chronic lung disease patients. These patients depend upon the hypoxic stimulus to ventilation rather than the normal hypercapnic stimulus. Suppression of the drive to breathe may be due to removal of this hypoxic stimulus. It also may be due to further increases in P_aCO_2, secondary to: (a) depressed ventilation, (b) increased shunting, provoked by absorption atelectasis and vasodilatation in the lung, and (c) alteration in the CO_2 dissociation curve (Haldane effect) (Tinits 1983).

To prevent this problem, use low O_2 concentrations if the patient is not mechanically ventilated. Monitor the ventilatory pattern closely. Be especially alert if the patient is breathing slowly or shallowly, since as mentioned earlier these will increase the F_IO_2 in a low-flow system.

Absorption Atelectasis Prevent absorption atelectasis. This complication can occur because oxygen washes out nitrogen in the alveoli. Nitrogen normally maintains the residual volume that keeps the alveoli open because it is poorly absorbed, in equilibrium, and, at ambient pressures, metabolically inert. When it is replaced by oxygen, which is readily absorbed, the residual volume decreases and the alveoli collapse. This process occurs when the patient has a low tidal volume, a normal tidal volume without sighing, or early airway closure that traps alveolar gas, as in emphysema. Therefore, prevent this problem by limiting the duration of 100% inspired O_2, even at lower concentrations, maintaining a patent airway, mobilizing secretions, sighing the patient, or providing constantly high tidal volumes. The use of positive end expiratory pressure (described later in this chapter) may allow lower oxygen concentrations.

Acute Oxygen Toxicity Acute oxygen toxicity depends on both the alveolar oxygen pressure (not alveolar O_2 concentration or P_aO_2) and duration of exposure.

Oxygen toxicity presents a characteristic pathological picture (Tinits 1983). The earliest symptoms are those of tracheobronchitis—sharp pleuritic chest pain and dry cough—which occur after about 6 hours on 100% oxygen at 1 atm pressure. After 18 hours, pulmonary function tests become abnormal. The vital capacity decreases first; later, most lung volumes and capacities and compliance decrease. After 24–48 hours, ARDS may occur. This period corresponds with the early exudative phase of oxygen toxicity. This phase is marked by interstitial and alveolar edema and hemorrhage due to damage to the alveolar-capillary membrane. Alveolar cells become damaged after about 3 days, resulting in significant decreases in surfactant. After about 1 week, the second, proliferative phase begins, characterized by pulmonary fibrosis and hyperplasia of alveolar Type II cells and capillaries.

Guidelines for prevention of oxygen toxicity are somewhat uncertain. The following ones represent a reasonable consensus (Shapiro et al. 1985; Tinits 1983):

1. Limit the use of 100% oxygen to brief periods in emergency situations.

2. As early as possible, reduce the F_IO_2 to the lowest possible level that provides adequate oxygenation.

3. Up to 70% oxygen probably may be safely used for 24 hours.

4. Up to 50% oxygen probably may be safely used for 2 days.

5. After 2 days, an F_IO_2 above 40% is potentially toxic.

6. Prolonged use of F_IO_2s below 40% rarely causes acute oxygen toxicity.

These guidelines of course *must* be considered in light of the patient's need for relief of hypoxia. With many critically ill patients, the dangers of this therapy are outweighed by the need for high inspired oxygen concentrations over prolonged periods to maintain adequate tissue oxygenation. Above all, remember that ABG monitoring is critical for appropriate oxygen therapy.

Outcome Evaluation

Evaluate the effectiveness of O_2 therapy by using these outcome criteria:

- Improved level of consciousness, ideally alert, oriented, and relaxed.
- BP, pulse rate, and cardiac rhythm WNL for patient.
- Spontaneous, unlabored respirations 12–18 times per minute.
- Urinary output WNL for patient.

- Extremities warm and dry (and pink if the patient is Caucasian).
- ABGs WNL for patient.

Chest Physiotherapy

Used prophylactically, chest physiotherapy (PT) can benefit patients who have had a history of thoracic or abdominal surgery, smoking, coma, endotracheal or tracheostomy tube, or chest wall deformity. Therapeutic use of chest physiotherapy can benefit patients with respiratory depression, thoracic or abdominal incisions, atelectasis, copious or viscous secretions, pneumonia, bronchitis, or emphysema. Chest physiotherapy will provide no benefit for patients with pneumothorax, hemothorax, or pleural effusion (because the pleural space does not connect with bronchi); pulmonary edema; or congestive heart failure.

To assess the need for chest PT, examine a variety of indicators. Physical examination may reveal increased respiratory rate or effort, decreased chest excursion, decreased or bronchial breath sounds, rales or rhonchi. Arterial blood gases may show decreased P_aO_2 and/or increased P_aCO_2. Pulmonary function tests may reveal a decreased tidal volume or vital capacity. The chest x-ray may show consolidation, atelectasis, or infiltration.

Prevent patient apprehension and pain. Explain to the patient the benefits and techniques of chest PT. (Demonstrate them on yourself or gently on him or her.) Administer analgesics before starting, unless contraindicated by his or her pulmonary or systemic status.

Techniques of Chest PT

A repertoire of chest PT techniques includes: postural drainage, percussion, vibration, diaphragmatic breathing, and localized expansion.

Postural Drainage Use the diagrams in Figure 9–1 to position the patient to drain the desired segments. Patients in critical-care areas usually will only tolerate three or four position changes for postural drainage and chest percussion.

Percussion Use the postural drainage diagrams to position the patient according to the area you want to

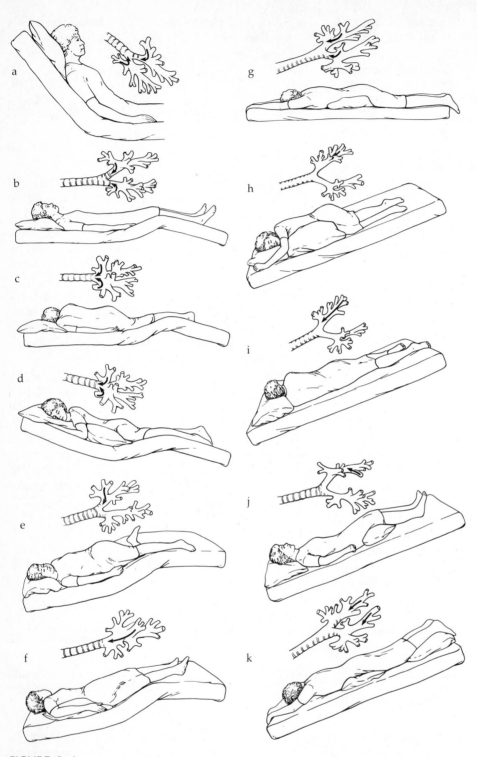

FIGURE 9–1

Postural drainage positions for specific pulmonary segments. **a,** Left and right upper lobes (apical segment). **b,** Left and right upper lobes (anterior segments). **c,** Right upper lobe (posterior segment). **d,** Left upper lobe (posterior segment). **e,** Left upper lobe (lingular segment). **f,** Middle lobe of right lung. **g,** Lower lobe (superior segment), patient lying prone with one pillow under abdomen. **h,** Left lower lobe (lateral basal segment). **i,** Left and right lower lobes (anterior basal segments). **j,** Left and right lower lobes (anterior basal segments). **k,** Left and right lower lobes (posterior basal segments). (Source: Kneisl C, Ames S: *Adult health nursing.* Menlo Park, CA: Addison-Wesley, 1986, p. 555.)

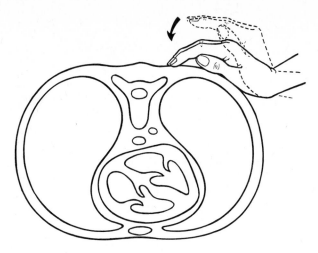

FIGURE 9–2

Chest percussion.

treat. Cover the skin with a thin towel. Do not percuss over bony prominences, female breasts, or bare skin.

Cup your hands. Relax your shoulders and elbows. Move your hands from the wrists (Figure 9–2) to produce a hollow percussion note rather than a slapping sound. The object is to trap and compress air between your hand and the chest wall, thus transmitting an energy wave to the lung tissue to loosen mucus.

Work with gravity; that is, percuss from the least dependent to the most dependent area. Do not percuss in the opposite direction, but instead return your hands to the starting position and repeat the movement.

Begin percussing slowly and gently to accustom the patient to the sensation. Increase the percussion until you are percussing vigorously about 200 times a minute. Percuss for 2–3 minutes in the same area to loosen secretions.

There now are available commercial devices for percussion and vibration that are quiet and comfortable for the patient.

Vibration Place one hand over the desired area. Place the other hand on top of and parallel to the first. Flex your elbows slightly. Using your shoulder muscles, vibrate your hands on the chest wall throughout exhalation. Repeat for at least five exhalations. Aim at delivering a vibration frequency of about 200 per minute.

Huffing Place the patient in a comfortable upright position. Tell the patient to take a deep breath, blow part of it out in a short huff by contracting the abdominal muscles, and continue huffing until he or she must inspire.

Diaphragmatic Breathing Place the patient in Fowler's position with slight knee flexion to facilitate diaphragmatic descent and relax the abdomen. Instruct the patient to use only the abdominal muscles, and reinforce the instruction by having the patient place his or her hands on the abdomen to obtain feedback. Have the patient breathe in by trying to push his or her hands apart and breathe out by letting them come back together.

Localized Expansion It is possible to improve the expansion of a general area of the lung, such as the apex, base, or lateral lung, with localized expansion techniques. Place one hand anteriorly and the other posteriorly over the area for treatment. Tell the patient to take a deep breath. As the patient inspires, compress the area with the anterior hand. At the height of inspiration, release the pressure suddenly.

Coordinating Techniques and Treatment Goals

From the preceding techniques, select those appropriate to the goal of treatment and your patient's condition.

1. To mobilize secretions, use percussion, vibration, or huffing, in conjunction with postural drainage. To improve tidal volume and exhalation, use diaphragmatic breathing, localized expansion, or huffing.

2. Do not use percussion at all if the patient has acute cardiac disease, thoracic inflammation, hemorrhage, or a very low platelet count. Percuss gently on patients who have or are prone to rib fractures, such as those with osteoporosis, bone cancer, or hypocalcemia. Do not percuss over an incision or area of pain, but percuss normally over the rest of the chest. Brace the incision or painful area with a sheet folded into a belt or with your hand.

3. Modify postural drainage for patients with increased intracranial pressure, orthopnea, or poor cardiovascular reserve.

If the problem is increased intracranial pressure, check with the physician as to acceptable positioning. If the patient has orthopnea or diminished cardiovascular reserve, lower the head as much as tolerable.

4. Coordinate the duration and frequency of the treatments to achieve the therapeutic goal without exhausting the patient. In general, perform chest PT every 2–4 hours, rotating treatment sites. Limit treatments to 10–20 minutes. Do not perform them within 30 minutes of oral feedings. Work together with respiratory therapists to time PT with bronchodilator therapy for optimal effect.

Outcome Evaluation

Evaluate the effectiveness of your treatments according to these outcome criteria:

- Lungs clear on auscultation.
- Arterial blood gases WNL for patient.
- Tidal volume and tidal capacity WNL for patient.
- Chest x-ray clear.

Artificial Airways

Patients who can benefit from an artificial airway are those with an upper airway obstruction, profuse secretions, a need for mechanical ventilation, or a likelihood of aspirating gastric secretions.

The most common upper airway obstruction in the nonalert patient is the tongue, which falls back and occludes the hypopharynx. For this reason, whenever possible place the nonalert patient on his or her side or prone. Do not leave such a patient unattended in the supine position, especially with a pillow under the head.

If the previously alert patient develops apnea or noisy breathing with diminished air movement, immediately open the airway, following current American Heart Association life support recommendations for initial airway establishment.

Types of Artificial Airways

For more secure maintenance, insert an artificial airway or assist a physician to do so. The three categories of artificial airways are the pharyngeal airway, the endotracheal tube, and the tracheostomy tube. Their advantages and disadvantages are summarized in Table 9–2.

Pharyngeal Airways   There are two types of pharyngeal airways: the oropharyngeal and the nasopharyngeal. Often, the nurse may insert these at her own discretion. The oropharyngeal or oral airway extends from the lips to the pharynx and therefore displaces the tongue anteriorly. It is made of curved, rigid plastic. To insert one, select a size suitable for the patient. Open the mouth with a tongue depressor or by inserting your crossed thumb and index finger into the corner of the mouth and crossing them further to force the mouth open. Turn the airway sideways and slide it along the buccal mucosa until the flange on the end touches the lips. Then turn it so the curve fits over the tongue. Tape it in position.

A nasopharyngeal airway is a soft rubber tube that extends from the nare to the pharynx. The end of the tube is funnel shaped to prevent it from entering the nostril. Select the largest-diameter tube that will fit the nostril. Choose the appropriate length by holding the tube against the patient's cheek, with the funnel-shaped end at the nostril and the other end pointing toward the back of the throat. The end of the tube should be about one inch beyond the earlobe. Lubricate the entire length with water soluble jelly and insert it gently. It should be changed every 8–12 hours to prevent occlusion with secretions.

Endotracheal Tube   An endotracheal tube extends from the nose or mouth into the trachea. An endotracheal tube may be inserted at the bedside by the physician or specially trained nurse or respiratory therapist. The orotracheal route is preferred in emergencies. Although the tube can be inserted rapidly by this route, it is more difficult to stabilize the tube and kinking develops more easily than with the nasotracheal route. The nasotracheal route of insertion is more difficult, and the diameter of the tube is limited by the size of the nares. To assist with orotracheal intubation:

1.   Bring the emergency cart equipped with the following to the bedside: laryngoscope with several sizes of curved and straight blades, extra bulb and battery; assorted sizes of endotracheal tubes; a stylet; topical anesthesia; Yankauer pharyngeal suction tip; suction apparatus; sterile catheters and gloves; syringes; needles; intravenous muscle relaxants (succinylcholine or pancuronium bromide); narcotics and sedatives such as morphine and diazepam; water-soluble lubricant; Magill forceps; benzoin; tape, a bite block or oral airway; and the ordered delivery system for oxygenation and/or ventilation.

2.   Snap the size and type of blade preferred by the physician onto the laryngoscope handle. Make sure the light works; if not, replace the bulb or the battery in the laryngoscope handle.

3.   Connect the Yankauer suction tip to the suction apparatus. Suction and preoxygenate the patient.

4.   Inflate the endotracheal tube cuff to test for symmetry of the cuff and any possible leak in the cuff. Then deflate it.

5.   Bend the stylet to a curve with a radius of about 30°. Insert it in the tube until it reaches half an inch proximal to the tube's end (if you protrude it past the tip, it may damage the trachea).

6.   Position the head in moderate dorsiflexion. If

TABLE 9–2 ARTIFICIAL AIRWAYS

TYPE	ADVANTAGES	DISADVANTAGES
Pharyngeal Airways		
Oral pharyngeal	Quick and easy to insert	May cause patient to gag
Nasopharyngeal	Quick and easy to insert	Clogs easily
		Kinks easily
		May cause pressure necrosis
Endotracheal		
Orotracheal	Rapid insertion	Special training needed for insertion
	Larger tube size possible than with nasotracheal	Can be bitten
	Less traumatic insertion than nasotracheal	Interferes with coughing
		Can cause pressure necrosis
		Possible tracheal damage from cuff or tube
		Kinks easily
		More difficult to stabilize position
		More uncomfortable for patient
Nasotracheal	Cannot be bitten	Special training needed for insertion
	Easier to stabilize position	Insertion more traumatic
	More comfortable for patient	Size of tube limited
		Can cause pressure necrosis of nose
		Possible tracheal damage from cuff or tube
		Interferes with coughing
		Kinks easily
Tracheostomy		
Uncuffed tube	Suitable for children due to small diameter of trachea	Danger of aspiration
	Decreased risk of tracheal damage	Cannot be used for mechanical ventilation in adults
Cuffed plastic (low pressure)	Large, low-pressure cuff reduces risk of tracheal damage	Expensive
	Cuff bonded to tube	
Cuffed plastic (high pressure)	Cuff bonded to tube	Increased risk of tracheal damage
Cuffed metal	Easy to clean because inner cannula removable	Cuff not bonded to tube; can slip off and occlude tube
		May need adapter for manual or mechanical ventilator
All	Decreased deadspace	Surgical insertion necessary, so is not suitable as method of emergency airway establishment
	Easier to suction	
	Patient can swallow	
Laryngectomy		
	Decreased deadspace	Permanent
	No risk of aspiration	Surgical procedure
		Patient unable to talk normally

the patient is conscious, the physician may apply topical anesthesia to the trachea and administer a muscle relaxant.

7. Lubricate only the tip of the tube; if you lubricate the whole tube, the physician will have difficulty handling it. Hand the tube to the physician.

8. The physician will insert the laryngoscope blade and visualize the vocal cords. Using the hand or the Magill forceps, the physician will pass the tube between the vocal cords, through the larynx, and into the trachea. When she or he indicates, quickly inflate the cuff. The physician will remove the stylet and laryngoscope and hold the tube in place. Observe the monitor closely for dysrhythmias, and check BP frequently.

9. Hand ventilate the patient until he or she is calm and tolerating the tube.

10. Connect the tube's opening to the ventilating device and begin ventilation. Auscultate the lung fields bilaterally to confirm tube placement in the trachea. Insert an oral airway or bite block, paint the skin with benzoin, and tape the tube securely. Mark the exit point of the endotracheal tube and/or chart the corresponding number of centimeters that are on the side of the tube.

11. Obtain an immediate chest x-ray to verify tube placement.

Tracheostomy Tube A tracheostomy tube must be inserted by a surgeon. A *tracheostomy* is an artificial opening into the trachea; *tracheotomy* is the operative procedure that creates it. A tracheostomy is indicated when the anticipated time interval for an artificial airway exceeds 2–3 weeks, when an upper airway obstruction prevents the use of an endotracheal tube, when radical neck surgery is performed, or as a measure to decrease anatomic deadspace.

Ideally, the tracheotomy rarely is performed in an emergency. For emergency airway establishment, the patient should be intubated at the bedside and transferred to the operating room, where the technically more difficult tracheotomy can be performed under calmer, sterile conditions. General anesthesia is administered and the head and neck extended. A horizontal incision is made between the second and third tracheal rings, and a window the size of the tracheostomy tube excised. The largest cannula that will fit the trachea is inserted. A fabric tape is placed around the neck and tied to the flange of the tube. The tube is not sutured to the skin.

If the patient has a severe upper airway obstruction precluding intubation before tracheotomy, an emergency cricothyrotomy may be performed at the bedside. The physician palpates the thyroid cartilage and cricoid ring. He or she then uses a scalpel or scissors to incise the cricothyroid membrane. A tracheostomy tube is inserted and the patient transported to the operating room for tracheotomy and closure of the cricothyrotomy.

Prevention of Complications

The critical-care nurse plays a crucial role in forestalling possible problems with an artificial airway. Such complications include: apprehension, malposition or loss of the airway, airway obstruction, infection, and tracheal damage.

Incorporate the following guidelines into your routine care of the person with an artificial airway. Many of them apply to any type of artificial airway. When one applies only to a specific type of airway, it is so stated.

Apprehension Relieve the patient's apprehension due to fear of the unknown, discomfort, or inability to talk. Whenever possible before insertion, prepare the patient psychologically. In many cases, you will have to delay this preparation until the airway has been established. Insertion of any of these airways is uncomfortable; the conscious patient will experience an unpleasant sensation of pressure or choking. The endotracheal tube is probably the most uncomfortable. The newly tracheotomized patient may require medication for the pain of the incision. Most patients learn to tolerate an artificial airway. The patient is justifiably anxious when he realizes the airway interferes with speech and he cannot call for help. Explain that he will be able to speak again when the airway is removed. In the meantime, establish a communication system (see Chapter 3) and call it to the attention of all staff caring for the patient.

Malposition or Loss of the Airway Prevent inadequate ventilation due to the malposition or loss of the airway. Take these preventive measures:

1. After an endotracheal or tracheostomy tube is inserted, obtain an x-ray to verify placement. Also, auscultate both lung fields at least every 2 hours. Sometimes the tube is placed improperly or migrates so that it enters the right mainstem bronchus rather than remaining above the carina as is necessary for bilateral ventilation. In this case, breath sounds will be present in only one lung.

If the tube slips forward to the hypopharynx, the patient may be able to vocalize. Mechanically ventilated patients will not receive their tidal volumes, and alarms should sound. Using a tongue blade and flashlight, you can check the back of the patient's throat for presence of the cuff. If the cuff is visualized, immediately notify the physician to advance the tube into the trachea or reintubate if necessary.

2.   Have readily accessible within the unit a largyngoscope, extra tubes, and tracheotomy tray. At the bedside, keep an airway mask and hand-ventilation bag; in addition, for a tracheostomy tube, keep the obturator (if one was used) and a tracheal dilator.

3.   Avoid accidental extubation. For a tracheostomy tube, be sure the tapes holding it in place are tied firmly. For an endotracheal tube, note the centimeter number on the tube at the point it enters the patient's nose or mouth and chart it, for reference in chest x-ray interpretation and repositioning. Restrain the hands of confused, agitated patients at risk for self-extubation, and sedate per orders.

Airway Obstruction   Forestall obstruction of the airway. Follow these steps to avoid obstruction:

1.   Eliminate airway obstruction due to kinking of the endotracheal tube. Position the patient's head normally; avoid flexing it. Support the ventilator tubing with a pillow or rolled towel. Some patients will bite an orotracheal tube, thereby occluding it. Prevent this by inserting an oral airway or bite block. If your unit does not stock commercial bite blocks, you can fashion a bite block yourself by wrapping adhesive tape into a rectangle that will fit comfortably between the patient's teeth. Be sure to leave a small tab protruding from the mouth so you can remove it for mouth care.

2.   Prevent obstruction due to herniation of the cuff over the tip of the tube. Avoid overdistending the cuff by checking cuff pressures whenever air is inserted.

3.   Prevent airway obstruction due to retained secretions. Because these tubes bypass the humidification provided normally by the upper airway, provide artificial humidification. Also maintain adequate systemic hydration. For a tracheostomy, remove the inner cannula (if there is one) at least every 8 hours, and rinse with normal saline. Tracheostomy tubes are now also available with disposable inner cannulas.

Institute a vigorous program of coughing, turning, and chest physiotherapy to mobilize secretions. A tube in the trachea, of course, prevents normal coughing, so meticulous attention to removal of secretions is vital. See other sections of this chapter on suctioning and chest physiotherapy for details.

4.   Inhibit the formation of tracheal granulation tissue. While this tissue will not cause obstruction during intubation, it may cause obstruction after extubation. To minimize the development of granulation tissue, reduce factors that irritate the trachea. Remove the secretions that accumulate above the cuff, causing chemical irrita-

tion of the trachea. Do not use aerosol sprays where the patient can inhale them. Keep cotton fibers from entering the airway by using noncotton gauze around a tracheostomy stoma. If your sterile gloves are powdered on the outside, rinse them with sterile solution before suctioning.

Infection   Because the upper airway defense mechanisms are bypassed, pulmonary infection frequently occurs. Sinusitis also is a problem with nasal intubation. Follow this procedure to prevent infection:

1.   Use meticulous sterile technique during suctioning and tracheostomy care. Keep the skin around a tracheostomy tube free of secretions by cleaning it with hydrogen peroxide and applying a dry sterile dressing around the stoma. Use sterile suctioning technique with a fresh sterile catheter for each episode of suctioning.

2.   Give thorough mouth care at least every 8 hours to reduce the potential of the oropharynx as a focus of infection.

3.   Drain the water that condenses in the ventilator tubing by disconnecting the tubing and letting it empty into a basin. Do *not* drain the condensed water back into the patient's lungs or the reservoir of the humidifier.

4.   Follow a prescribed schedule of changing ventilatory equipment. In most units, standard policy is to change the sterile water in the humidifier every 8 hours and to replace the humidifier or nebulizer and ventilatory tubing every 24 hours. Disposable tubing and humidifier units have decreased the risk of equipment-borne infections.

5.   Tie tracheostomy tapes snugly but not tight enough to irritate the skin. Reduce chafing by tying the tape so that there are no knots at the sides of the flange and by changing the tape when it becomes soiled. To eliminate knots at the sides of the flange, loop the tape through one side of the flange, pass both ends behind the patient's neck, and loop the bottom piece of tape through the other side of the flange. Then tie a knot several centimeters away from the flange so the knot is on top of the lower piece of tape. This method provides a smooth surface against the skin.

Upper Airway Damage   Avoid pressure necrosis of the nare by cleaning around a nasotracheal tube and observing for areas of pressure or necrosis that may necessitate changing nostrils. To prevent oral necrosis, reposition an orotracheal tube every 8 hours. Have one person hold the tube while you deflate the cuff and remove the tape securing the airway. Move the tube to the opposite side of the mouth, check that the same centimeter distance (as marked on the tube) has been maintained, tape it in position, and reinflate the cuff.

Also, forestall tracheal damage from cuffed tubes. Tracheal damage may consist of necrosis, stenosis, tracheoesophageal fistula, distension, or tracheomalacia (loss of cartilage). Numerous factors have been implicated in the genesis of tracheal damage. Among them are infection; the length of intubation; improper size or placement of the tube; cuff size, pliability and shape; intracuff pressure and hypotension (Shapiro et al. 1985). The following paragraphs describe measures that will reduce tracheal damage.

Minimize cuff pressure. Numerous studies have been reported on the relationship between cuff pressure and tracheal damage. Most have utilized animal models, and their conclusions are controversial and confusing. After surveying the available literature, Shapiro et al. (1985) conclude that, in the patient with a normal perfusion state and uninfected trachea, cuff pressure over 5 mm Hg obstructs lymphatic flow, producing edema; pressure over 18 mm Hg obstructs venous drainage, producing congestion; and pressure in excess of 30 mm Hg impedes arterial flow, causing ischemia. Cuff pressures over 50 mm Hg usually create ischemic and necrotic areas within 48 hours, but these areas are patchy. This tracheal mucosal damage is completely reversible unless necrosis and sloughing occur circumferentially (Shapiro et al. 1985). The potential for damage is increased with a small, rigid, unevenly inflating cuff; such a cuff may exert over 300 mm Hg pressure against the tracheal wall. Mucosal damage does not appear to be countered sufficiently by the ritual of deflating the cuff 5 minutes each hour.

The current literature has significant clinical implications. To minimize cuff pressure, take these steps:

1. Adjust cuff pressure according to the technique used in your unit: minimal occluding volume or minimal leak. In the *minimal occluding volume technique,* the cuff is inflated just until an inspiratory air leak (audible with your stethoscope) disappears. In the *minimal leak technique,* once the air leak has been obliterated, withdraw a small amount of air so that there is a slight leak present at peak inspiration. With either technique, once the desired point has been reached, note the pressure on the manometer and then close the cuff inflation line. Record the measured pressure.

2. Check cuff pressure every 8 hours, according to unit protocol. Call to the physician's attention pressures over 20 mm Hg, increases in cuff pressure or volume, or a leak (other than a deliberate minimal leak).

3. Tracheal necrosis is more common when both an endotracheal or tracheostomy tube and a large nasogastric tube are in place. If nasogastric drainage is necessary, use as small a size nasogastric tube as is effective.

Watch for other ways to reduce tracheal damage with a tracheostomy tube. Observe for bleeding around the tube or pulsations of the tube. Bleeding around the tube usually is minor and due to trauma. Pulsations of the tube when none were present previously may indicate imminent hemorrhage through the tube due to erosion of the tip into the innominate artery. This complication is rare but life threatening. If you spot new pulsations, obtain immediate medical evaluation. It may be necessary to reposition the tube or replace it with a shorter or narrower tube.

Observe for the appearance of oral feedings or tube feedings in the tracheal aspirate. Their presence suggests either a tracheoesophageal fistula or, more commonly, swallowing dysfunction resulting from the tube's interference with the normal swallowing mechanism. You cannot prevent this dysfunction but can minimize it by inflating the cuff and elevating the head of the bed during feedings and for 30 minutes afterward. Both swallowing dysfunction and a tracheoesophageal fistula will cause a positive methylene blue test. When this dye is added to the feeding, its appearance in tracheal secretions confirms the connection between the esophagus and trachea. Differentiating the two causes requires radiology or endoscopy. A fistula usually takes 2–4 weeks to develop, so a positive dye test before then probably indicates swallowing dysfunction. The dysfunction usually will disappear after the airway is removed.

Watch for puffed-up tissues that crackle when palpated, indicating subcutaneous emphysema. Possible causes include air escaping from the stoma into the tissues and a bronchopleural fistula. Call this finding to the physician's attention, as it will necessitate treatment if it continues and compresses the trachea. Once the source is controlled, the air is reabsorbed slowly. If the subcutaneous emphysema is severe, the physician may decompress the tissues by inserting several 18-gauge needles or making small incisions under local anesthesia. Stroking the skin towards the needles or incisions causes the air to escape.

Treatment of Complications

The previous section stressed the role you can play in preventing the complications of an artificial airway. If complications do occur, you must recognize them promptly and respond appropriately.

Relief of Airway Obstruction Retractions, increased inspiratory pressure on a ventilator, severe apprehension, and decreased or absent air movement signify acute airway obstruction. This life-threatening problem can be caused by kinking, placement of the end of the tube against the carina, tracheal wall, or bronchus, or by mucous plugs or herniation of the cuff over the tube's end if a cuff is overinflated.

If you suspect acute airway obstruction, (a) manipulate the head, neck, or tube slightly to eliminate kinking or reposition the tip; (b) suction the airway; and (c) deflate the cuff. If the airway is a tracheostomy with an inner cannula, remove the inner cannula. If the obstruction persists, summon medical help immediately.

Relief of Bleeding   Profuse frank bleeding from the endotracheal or tracheostomy tube indicates erosion of the tube into the innominate artery. Pulsation of the tube may precede this event. Summon medical assistance immediately. Hyperinflate the cuff to tamponade the bleeding. If the patient has a tracheostomy tube, inserting a finger into the stoma in front of the tube and applying upward pressure may slow bleeding (Luce et al. 1984). An immediate operation is necessary to suture the site of the erosion.

Response to Accidental Extubation   If accidental extubation occurs, *do not panic*. For a tracheostomy, use a tracheal dilator to maintain the stoma and attempt to reinsert the tube (using its obturator if it has one). For other airways, open the airway by hyperextending the head or using the jaw-thrust maneuver and manually ventilate the patient with a bag-valve-mask device. Call a physician immediately to reintubate the patient.

Treatment of Infection   Purulent or colored secretions or an elevated temperature may indicate a pulmonary infection. Culture the secretions to identify the specific organism, and consult with the physician about drug therapy.

Removal of Artificial Airways

When the airway is no longer needed, prepare the patient for its removal. Pharyngeal airways are removed in one step. An endotracheal or tracheostomy tube is removed in several steps. First, the patient must maintain spontaneous ventilation for several hours if he or she has been on a mechanical ventilator; this step is discussed in greater detail under the section on mechanical ventilation. The gag reflex and swallowing ability must be intact. When these criteria are met and it is time to remove the tracheostomy or endotracheal tube, first explain the extubation procedure to the patient. Preoxygenate the patient, suction the trachea, and then suction the pharynx. Ask the patient to take a deep breath, or inflate the lungs with a hand-ventilating bag. At the peak of inspiration, the physician or nurse will deflate the cuff and remove the tube. Immediately provide humidified supplemental oxygen. Observe the patient closely for signs of recurrent respiratory distress. A sore throat and hoarse voice are common after extubation and require no treatment other than an explanation to the patient and humidification. Inspiratory stridor occurring upon extubation or more commonly about 24 hours later indicates laryngeal edema. Alert the physician, who may reintubate the patient or order further observation, humidification, and local application of a steroid and vasoconstrictor (racemic epinephrine) to reduce the edema.

Outcome Evaluation

Evaluate the effectiveness of the artificial airway and your care according to these outcome criteria:

- Patient is able to communicate needs to staff.
- Calm, relaxed appearance.
- Unlabored respirations within limit desired for patient.
- Arterial blood gases WNL for patient.
- Lungs clear to auscultation.
- No signs of necrosis or bleeding around the airway.
- Tracheal cultures without pathologic flora.
- No oral feedings or tube feedings in tracheal aspirate.

Tracheal Suctioning

Be alert for patients who need tracheal suctioning. Conditions that indicate difficulty with spontaneous clearing of secretions include the following:

1. Increased viscosity of secretions.
2. Weak or paralyzed thoracic or abdominal muscles, for example, owing to thoracic surgery or paraplegia.
3. Depressed ciliary activity such as after general anesthesia.
4. Increased production of secretions.
5. Ineffective cough; a patient is unable to cough

effectively if he or she has an endotracheal or tracheostomy tube, or if vital capacity is less than 15 ml/kg or inspiratory capacity below 75% of normal (Shapiro et al. 1985).

Prevention of Complications

Suctioning is not a benign procedure. Potential complications include hypoxemia, dysrhythmias, sudden death, laryngospasm or bronchospasm, and infection.

Avoidance of Routine Suctioning Avoid routine suctioning by capitalizing whenever possible on the patient's ability to remove secretions.

1. Teach the cooperative and able patient how to cough effectively. Tell her or him to take in a deep breath and close the glottis on a count of "one," contract the thoracic and abdominal muscles on "two," and open the glottis on "three." Demonstrate the sound of an effective cough versus an ineffective one with the glottis open and no abdominal movement. An effective cough can generate an estimated velocity of 600 miles an hour.

2. Maintain adequate systemic hydration (and airway humidification if an artificial airway is in place).

3. Implement a program of chest PT and postural drainage to assist the patient to raise secretions.

4. If necessary, utilize cough stimulation techniques to enhance secretion removal by the patient. Following are some methods of cough stimulation. (a) Press firmly over the lower trachea until the patient coughs. (b) If recommended in your institution, instill 2–5 ml of sterile saline down the endotracheal or tracheostomy tube to loosen secretions and initiate a cough. This practice is controversial because, unless you take strict precautions to keep the bottle of fluid sterile, it rapidly becomes contaminated and you will introduce a source of infection. (c) Pass a suction catheter until it reaches the carina. In most patients, this contact will initiate a forceful cough.

Assess the effectiveness of these techniques by auscultating the lung fields every 1–4 hours for crackles and wheezes, examining serial lung x-ray reports (looking for infiltrates or atelectatic areas), and evaluating the blood gases.

Recommended Suctioning Technique Suction when secretions are retained in spite of the measures outlined above. Prevent or minimize complications by adhering closely to these recommendations:

1. Explain to the patient the purpose, technique, and sensations involved. Warn that she or he may feel out of breath or may feel like choking. Suctioning is not a pleasant experience; patients deserve to know this, as well as that the discomfort will be brief. The properly prepared patient is less likely to panic during the procedure. It helps for you to convey a positive rather than a punitive attitude. For example, say "I'm going to suction you so you can breathe more easily" rather than "I'm going to suction you because you just won't cough as I showed you before your surgery."

2. Do not suction if you note signs of laryngospasm (crowing respirations), bronchospasm (severe wheezing), or bradycardia.

3. Bring to the bedside single sterile gloves, sterile saline in a small cup, sterile suction cathers, sterile saline in a 10-cc syringe without a needle, sterile water-soluble lubricant, a hand ventilating bag connected to 100% oxygen and a mask or endotracheal/tracheostomy tube adaptor, and tissues. Turn the suction apparatus on to 80–120 mm Hg.

4. Wash your hands.

5. Preoxygenate the patient. (For options, see the discussion in the next section.)

6. Open the catheter package sterilely. Designate one hand as sterile, to handle the catheter only. Place a sterile glove on it. Designate the other hand as unsterile, to connect the suction and occlude the vent. To minimize resistance and trauma while passing the catheter, leave the vent open. Apply sterile water-soluble lubricant or sterile saline to the cather.

7. If the patient has an endotracheal or tracheostomy tube, disconnect the airway from the adapter on the hand ventilating bag with the unsterile hand. This is tricky; if you cannot do it rapidly, use an assistant to hand ventilate and to disconnect and reconnect the airway.

8. If the patient does not have an endotracheal or tracheostomy tube, facilitate catheter entry into the trachea by placing him or her in Fowler's position. Put a pillow behind the shoulders and tilt the head backward. Do not automatically turn the head to the right to enter the left bronchus or vice versa; these positions are not as effective as has been thought in the past, since it is difficult to enter the more sharply angled left bronchus without a curved-tip catheter. In a study reported by Kubota (1980), for example, the greatest success in suctioning the left mainstem bronchus was achieved with a curved-tip catheter, with the head in a midline position.

Grasp the tongue with a gauze square and pull it forward gently. To retract the epiglottis, have the patient cough or breathe deeply while you pass the catheter only on inhalation. When the catheter enters the trachea, the patient may become very restless and apprehensive. Talk soothingly, reminding him or her that the procedure will be over soon.

9. Advance the catheter gently and rapidly as far as it will go; then withdraw it 1–2 cm to avoid traumatizing the tracheal wall. Since the carina is very sensitive to mechanical stimulation, the patient may cough forcefully at this point.

10. Occlude the vent intermittently and suction no more than 10 seconds. Rotate the catheter gently as you withdraw it. Watch the cardiac monitor for the development of dysrhythmias.

11. Reoxygenate the patient. If secretions are thick, rinse the catheter with sterile solution.

12. Repeat the suctioning and oxygenating until the secretions are removed.

13. Next, suction the oropharynx using the same catheter. (Note: it is acceptable to use the same catheter to suction first the sterile trachea and then the oropharynx, but *not* the reverse.)

14. Discard the glove, catheter, and cup after *each* suctioning session.

Options for Preventing Hypoxemia The recommended techniques for preventing hypoxemia during suctioning are controversial, particularly for ventilator-dependent patients. Among the techniques that have been recommended are the following:

Ventilator Hyperoxygenation/Hyperinflation with Removal from the Ventilator During Suctioning Before suctioning, adjust the patient's ventilator to administer approximately 5 breaths of 100% oxygen, at a tidal volume 1.5 times larger than the maintenance volume being used to ventilate the patient. Disconnect the patient from the ventilator during suctioning. Then reconnect, maintain the increased tidal volume and 100% oxygen for another 5–8 breaths, and return the dials to their original settings.

The length of time required to reach the new F_IO_2 varies according to the ventilator type, baseline F_IO_2, and minute ventilation (Chulay 1987). In addition, in a busy critical-care unit the nurse may forget to return the dials to their previous setting, subjecting the patient to an increased risk of oxygen toxicity, barotrauma, and absorptive atelectasis.

Manual Hyperoxygenation/Hyperinflation with Removal from the Ventilator During Suctioning Before suctioning, disconnect the patient from the ventilator circuit; ventilate with a hand-held ventilating bag for approximately 5 breaths at 100% oxygen and a tidal volume 1.5 times larger than the patient's usual tidal volume. After suctioning, reoxygenate the same way and reconnect the patient to the ventilator.

Limited data are available on the effectiveness of these bags in providing the desired F_IO_2 and tidal volume (Chulay 1987). Most bags deliver an F_IO_2 below 1.0, even when an oxygen reservoir is used. Rates range from 0.7 to 1.0. Check with the manufacturer about the delivered F_IO_2 for the bags on your unit when used with an oxygen reservoir. Chulay (1987) recommends that a given bag should be used only when its F_IO_2 delivery capability exceeds the maintenance F_IO_2 level the patient is receiving.

Hyperoxygenation/Hyperinflation with Ventilator Maintenance During Suctioning Alternatively, to allow suctioning without disconnection from the ventilator circuit, use a special swivel adapter attached to the standard endotracheal tube adapter, or use a modification of the standard adapter itself. Jung and Newman (1982) have reported on a study utilizing a modified adapter with two accessory ports through which a patient can be lavaged and suctioned without disconnection from the ventilator circuit. They found that in patients with severe respiratory dysfunction, the fall in arterial O_2 saturation that accompanied the standard suctioning technique was lessened significantly by suctioning through the modified adapter. Bodai (1982) studied use of a valve that fits commercially available respiratory circuits and contains a diaphragm to allow catheter introduction. He found the drop in P_aO_2 was significantly less with the valve system than with the standard suction technique. Adapters and valves that allow suctioning without interrupting ventilation are particularly helpful for patients who are very sensitive to routine suctioning, such as those with severe pulmonary dysfunction and those on PEEP.

Oxygen Insufflation Without Ventilator Disconnect, Preoxygenation, or Hyperinflation Bodai et al. (1987) studied a new, commercially available double-lumen catheter that allows simultaneous oxygen insufflation into the trachea along with suctioning. After evaluating it with 24 ventilator-dependent patients in varying degrees of respiratory failure, with diverse medical diagnoses, and a variety of suctioning protocols, they concluded that oxygen insufflation alone was as effective as preoxygenation and hyperinflation in preventing suction-related hypoxemia. They recommend that oxygen insufflation replace bagging for most patients and that patients with severe pulmonary failure who are sensitive to suctioning be ventilated via a valve system that maintains ventilator connection and PEEP.

NURSING RESEARCH NOTE

Pierce B, Piazza D: Differences in post-suctioning arterial blood oxygenation values using two postoxygenation methods. *Heart Lung* 1987; 16:34–38.

Which method is better for oxygenating mechanically ventilated patients after suctioning: Ambu-bagging or mechanical sighing? Although both procedures are used in clinical practice, both have drawbacks, and there are no studies conclusively supporting the use of one and exclusion of the other.

To answer this question, this study compared postsuctioning arterial P_{O_2} after ventilatory sighing with arterial P_{O_2} after manual bagging, using a convenience sample of 30 cardiac surgery patients. All patients were preoxygenated with a hand ventilating bag, using 3 breaths of 100% oxygen and hyperinflation. Each subject was suctioned once

with each type of postoxygenation method. The order of the postoxygenation was randomized. The Ambu-bagging method used a PMR-2 self-inflating resuscitation bag with an O_2 reservoir connected to 100% oxygen. Ventilatory sighing meant the patient was connected to a Bear-2 ventilator after suctioning and 3 breaths of 100% oxygen were delivered by pushing the sigh control.

Four blood gas samples were collected from each subject's arterial line: one before and after each of the two postoxygenation methods. Duplicate readings were obtained, and the two means were compared by analysis of variance, with statistical significance level set at 0.05. (The reader interested in the details of the research methodology should consult the original source.)

The mean P_aO_2 showed highly

significant differences in relation to the type of treatment ($F = 14.67$, $p = 0.0007$). Compared to P_aO_2 before suctioning, mean P_aO_2 rose with ventilatory sighing but dropped with Ambu-bag postoxygenation. Arterial blood pH and O_2 saturation levels also showed significant differences. The pH and O_2 saturation remained relatively stable with ventilatory sighing but decreased with Ambu-bagging. For cardiac surgery patients in this hospital, the researchers therefore recommend that ventilatory sighing be used as a postoxygenation method whenever possible. They also recommend additional studies to evaluate the effectiveness of ventilatory sighing and Ambu-bagging with different patient populations, using various ventilators and/or transcutaneous or mixed venous oximetry.

Treatment of Complications

During and after suctioning, observe heart rate and rhythm, respiratory rate, blood pressure, and skin color and moisture in particular. Recognize and respond promptly to signs of complications. Restlessness, cyanosis, and sometimes worsened dysrhythmias usually indicate hypoxemia secondary to depletion of P_AO_2. Terminate the suctioning and oxygenate the patient. For future suctioning episodes, increase the duration of preoxygenation and decrease the duration of each suctioning episode.

Increased dysrhythmias may result from hypoxia, catecholamine release during anxiety, or mechanical stimulation of the vagal fibers innervating the trachea. Remove the suction catheter, oxygenate the patient, and calm him or her if apprehensive. If the dysrhythmia persists, notify the physician.

Crowing, wheezing, or resistance to catheter removal indicates laryngospasm or bronchospasm. If the catheter can move freely, remove it and do not attempt to suction again; otherwise, disconnect the suction and

leave the catheter in the trachea. Oxygenate the patient and summon a physician immediately.

Purulent or foul-smelling secretions suggest infection. Inform the physician and send a specimen for culture and sensitivity.

Outcome Evaluation

Evaluate the effectiveness of suctioning against these outcome criteria:

- Toleration of suctioning without panic.
- No restlessness, cyanosis, or more severe dysrhythmias during or after suctioning.
- No crowing, wheezing, or resistance to catheter removal.
- Tracheal cultures without pathologic flora.
- Improved breath sounds.
- Improved arterial blood gases.

Mechanical Ventilation

The physician's decision to institute mechanical ventilation is based not on the disease entity per se but rather on the physiologic stress it imposes on the patient. Objective signs that a person probably cannot maintain adequate ventilation for a prolonged period of time include a vital capacity of less than 15 ml/kg or twice a predicted tidal volume; a maximum inspiratory force of less than -20 cm of water within 20 seconds; arterial P_{CO_2} more than 10 mm Hg above the patient's normal value, a shunt of greater than 30%; and/or a deadspace/tidal volume (VD/VT) ratio greater than 60%. The broad indications for mechanical ventilation are apnea, impending or acutal acute ventilatory failure, and some cases of hypoxemia. Impending acute ventilatory failure is best documented by progressively increasing P_aCO_2 values and decreasing pH values. Mechanical ventilation may be indicated for hypoxemia without hypercapnea due to decreased functional residual capacity, severely increased work of breathing, or an inadequate pattern of breathing.

Procedure for Mechanical Ventilation

Prepare the patient psychologically. If time and the patient's condition permit, help the physician explain to both the patient and the family the purpose of mechanical assistance before it is instituted; otherwise, as soon afterward as feasible. Briefly, explain the equipment involved and the care the patient will receive, for example suctioning and blood gas checks. Emphasize the sensations the patient will experience—those of having something breathe for him or her and those related to the artificial airway. Establish a system by which the patient can summon help immediately. Assure the patient that the ventilator has mechanical alarms; demonstrate the noises the alarms make, and explain how the staff will respond. Also assure the patient that a nurse will always be at the bedside or within hearing distance. This psychologic preparation will not only reduce the patient's apprehension but also have physiologic benefits. The properly prepared patient is less likely to fight the ventilator. Fighting the ventilator is detrimental because it increases catecholamine release, oxygen consumption, and the need for paralyzing drugs.

Bring to the bedside the necessary equipment. From the respiratory therapy department, order the type of ventilator and the settings specified by the physician. Place at the bedside a hand ventilating bag, mask and oxygen tubing, and sterile suction supplies.

Types of Ventilators The ventilators most commonly used are those that produce IPPV (inspiratory [not "intermittent"] positive pressure ventilation). Positive pressure ventilators come in two basic types: pressure-limited and volume-limited. Pressure-limited ventilators include the Bird Mark 7 and Bennett PR II. Since the pressure is predetermined, the dependent variable is the volume of gas delivered. For example, when the airway is clear, the desired volume will be delivered; but if it becomes obstructed, the set pressure will be reached much earlier and only part of the volume will be delivered. Volume preset ventilators include the Bennett 7200, MA-1, and MA-2, Ohio 560, Bear, and Veolar ventilators; in these, the dependent variable is the pressure. The Servo ventilator is one that can be volume- or pressure-limited.

The type of ventilator chosen depends on the patient's need and in some cases the availability of the ventilator, since volume ventilators are considerably more expensive than pressure ventilators. The patient with normal compliance is a suitable candidate for the pressure ventilator, since one can be reasonably sure of the delivered volume for a given pressure. The patient with poor or variable compliance needs a volume ventilator, since it is more difficult to predict from a given pressure whether the patient will receive the desired volume. Because of their greater capabilities, volume ventilators are more popular than pressure ventilators in critical-care situations.

Ventilatory Modes When the decision is made to place the patient on a ventilator, the mode or pattern of ventilation must be chosen. Control, assist/control, and intermittent mandatory ventilation are the three most commonly used modes.

The *control* mode provides full ventilatory support and usually is used only in the apneic patient. The machine delivers a set number of ventilations per minute without regard to the patient's efforts.

The *assist/control* mode provides a minimum number of breaths per minute but allows the patient to initiate the breath and to breathe at a more rapid rate if desired. Whether the breath is initiated by the patient or by the machine (if the patient fails to breathe), each breath is of the same tidal volume and delivered under positive pressure.

Intermittent mandatory ventilation (IMV) is a mode capable of providing either full or partial ventilatory support (as may be desired during weaning). A preset number of breaths is delivered by the machine, and in between the patient may breathe spontaneously with no machine assistance and at his or her own varying tidal volumes. *Synchronized IMV* (SIMV) allows the predetermined breath to be delivered in phase with the patient's own efforts. If the IMV rate is set at 10, the machine is doing most of the ventilatory work; if the IMV rate is set at 4, the patient must assume part of the ventilatory work, as during the weaning process. Some of the purported advantages of IMV modes are active use of the respiratory muscles, less depression of venous return (fewer positive pressure breaths), and more flexibility for weaning (Weisman et al. 1982; Shapiro and Cane 1984).

Expiratory Maneuvers The most common expiratory adjustment or maneuver is the application of *positive end-expiratory pressure* (PEEP). PEEP can be applied to any of the above-described modes of ventilation. In addition, it can be applied to the spontaneously breathing patient via an endotracheal tube or by mask. When positive airway pressure is applied to the spontaneously breathing patient, it is called *continuous positive airway pressure* (CPAP). Figure 9–3 illustrates various ventilatory modes with PEEP and CPAP.

PEEP PEEP has several significant physiologic effects. Recall that critically ill patients often suffer alveolar collapse, due to the loss of surfactant, absorption atelectasis during the administration of oxygen, or early small airway closure.

When alveoli collapse during expiration, the continuing pulmonary capillary blood flow is not oxygenated; that is, increased shunting occurs. The alveolar collapse also causes a decreased residual volume and therefore a decreased *functional residual capacity* (FRC). In addition, alveolar collapse causes decreased lung compliance, because it takes a higher-than-normal airway pressure to reopen the alveoli. Thus, alveolar collapse causes both hypoxia and increased work of breathing. The application of PEEP causes airways to stay open longer, decreasing shunt, increasing FRC, and improving ventilation/perfusion match. As a result, the patient can oxygenate his blood more readily. PEEP often allows the use of a lower F_IO_2, an important consideration in preventing oxygen toxicity.

PEEP usually is instituted in any patient unable to maintain a P_aO_2 greater than 60 on less than 50% oxygen. There is a great deal of controversy regarding optimal levels of PEEP because of its potential detrimental effects, which include decreased venous return, increased risk of pneumothorax, and increased water retention due to stimulation of ADH production. For these reasons, PEEP is added in 2–3-cm H_2O increments with close surveillance of the patient's BP, pulse, car-

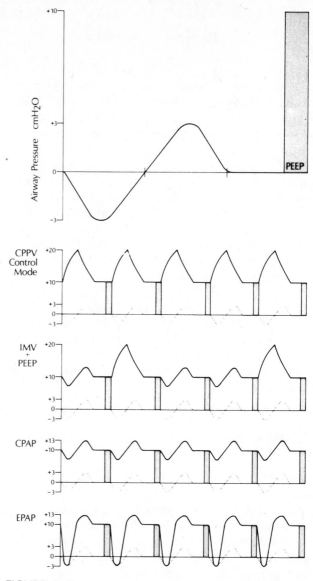

FIGURE 9–3

Airway pressure curves of various modes of positive end-expiratory pressure (PEEP). CPPV = continuous positive-pressure ventilation, sometimes referred to as "the ventilator with PEEP"; IMV = intermittent mandatory ventilation; CPAP = continuous positive airway pressure; EPAP = expiratory positive airway pressure. (Reproduced with permission from Shapiro, B.A., Harrison, R.A., Kacmarek, R.M., and Cane, R.D.: *Clinical application of respiratory care*, 3rd edition. Copyright © 1985 by Year Book Medical Publishers, Inc. Chicago.)

diac output, and ABGs. The usual therapeutic level of PEEP is 5–15 cm H_2O pressure (Katz 1984, Shapiro et al. 1984).

CPAP In the intubated patient who is weaning, oxygenation may be optimized by continuing some positive airway pressure (5 cm H_2O) during the trial of spontaneous breathing. The patient may then be extubated directly from the CPAP mode, or positive pressure may be removed and the patient placed on a T-piece or blow-by and then extubated.

In the unintubated hypoxemia patient, mask CPAP can help reopen and expand alveoli, correct hypoxemia, and possibly alleviate the need for intubation. Its use can also be applied to those patients deemed to be at high risk for developing an acute lung injury (Shapiro et al. 1984). The mask must be tight fitting, the patient alert and cooperative. A nasogastric tube is recommended to prevent aspiration from vomiting; otherwise, the patient's arms must be free to remove the mask should vomiting occur (Luce et al. 1984).

Expiratory Retard   One maneuver that may be used with positive pressure ventilation involves adding a resistance to the expiratory line. It does not disturb the baseline pressure, thus allowing the patient to reach atmospheric pressure at the end of exhalation. As all it does is retard the expiratory phase, it is analogous to the pursed-lip breathing used by patients with COPD, and allows better emptying of the lungs when FRC is increased.

Ventilator Settings   Initially, ventilator settings are approximate. Ideally, a slow ventilatory rate (10–14 per minute) and high tidal volume are chosen. The initial tidal volume setting usually is 10–15 ml/kg body weight. Other settings, such as F_IO_2, sensitivity, and PEEP, depend on the patient's condition. Patient observation and evaluation of blood gases must be used to refine these settings to the patient's need.

Large tidal volumes with slow rates have several physiologic advantages. The effects of deadspace are minimized. Mean airway pressure is lower with slow rates; as a result, venous return is not diminished as much as with faster rates. Ventilation with normal tidal volumes removes the normal sigh mechanism, which prevents collapsed alveoli and promotes surfactant production, so patients on normal tidal volumes need to be given periodic deep inflations. Large tidal volumes obviate the need for sighing and so are more effective in preventing microatelectasis.

Hemodynamic Monitoring and the Effects of Positive Pressure Ventilation   During normal respiration, pressure changes occur in the thoracic cavity that cause fluctuation in pulmonary artery waveforms. Patients receiving positive pressure ventilation will have additional variations in these pressure waveforms. Normal spontaneous breathing can be thought of as negative pressure breathing, since intrapleural pressures

drop during inspiration. On observing a pulmonary artery waveform readout on such a patient, you will note that the waveform dips during inspiration. The opposite effect is seen during positive pressure breaths given by a mechanical ventilator; the waveform will rise during inspiration.

In order to obtain standardized, accurate hemodynamic data readings it is recommended that values be obtained at end-expiration, or that period of the cycle preceding inspiration (Reidinger et al. 1981). The use of a graphic paper recording enables you to consistently identify end-expiration and its corresponding pulmonary artery pressure. Digital displays average consecutive waveforms over a set period of time. In the patient with marked fluctuation in waveforms, this averaging may lead to inaccurate pressures on which clinical interventions, such as fluid therapy, would be based (Dantzker 1986). Figure 9–4 shows examples of hemodynamic pressure interpretation in ventilated patients.

Prevention of Complications

Prevent the potential complications associated with mechanical ventilation. The primary complications are insufficient or excessive oxygenation and/or ventilation, water imbalances, decreased CO, pneumothorax, infection, atelectasis, and gastrointestinal hemorrhage or dilatation. Prevent them by incorporating the actions described in the following sections into your care of any ventilated patient.

Incorrect Ventilation   Monitor the ventilator settings and the delivered values at least hourly. (Ventilator settings often are slightly inaccurate; it is important to note *both* the machine settings and the delivered values.) Make the following checks or, if the respiratory therapist performs them, keep yourself informed of the values.

1.   Count the delivered respiratory rate by observing the patient's chest. Compare it to the set ventilator frequency.

2.   Monitor the exhaled tidal volume. The machine's gauge estimates only the set tidal volume. Delivered tidal volume is measured with a spirometer attached to the exhalation port.

3.   Read the peak inspiratory pressure (PIP) from a dial on the ventilator. Also note the maximum inspiratory pressure—the setting of the pressure pop-off valve. It usually is set about 10 cm above the pressure necessary to deliver the desired tidal volume. An increase in PIP signifies either an increase in lung stiff-

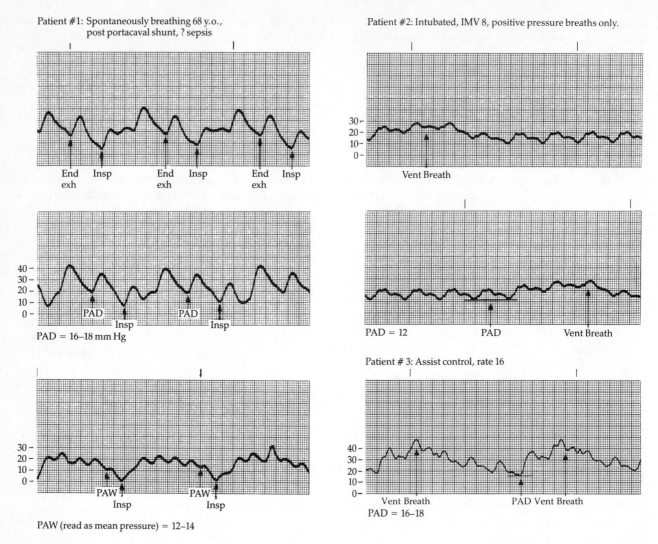

Patient #1: Spontaneously breathing 68 y.o., post portacaval shunt, ? sepsis

End exh — Insp — End exh — Insp — End exh — Insp

PAD — Insp — PAD — Insp
PAD = 16–18 mm Hg

PAW — Insp — PAW — Insp
PAW (read as mean pressure) = 12–14

Patient #2: Intubated, IMV 8, positive pressure breaths only.

Vent Breath

PAD = 12 — PAD — Vent Breath

Patient #3: Assist control, rate 16

Vent Breath — PAD Vent Breath
PAD = 16–18

FIGURE 9–4

Reading Hemodynamic Pressures in a mechanically ventilated patient. Insp = inspiration, End Exh = end-exhalation, PAD = pulmonary artery diastolic pressure, PAW = pulmonary artery wedge pressure, Vent Breath = ventilator breath continuous strip. Horizontal marks added to show where pressure is read.

ness (decreased compliance), secretions in the airway, patient biting the tube, or tube positioned low on the carina. A sudden increase in PIP may indicate pneumothorax.

4. Monitor the ratio between inspiration and expiration (I/E ratio), which usually is 1:2. Inspiration must be shorter than expiration to prevent trapping air in the chest.

5. Keep the alarms *on*. Most ventilators have a delay button you can press to prevent the alarm from sounding when you need to disconnect the patient temporarily—for example, to suction or to drain condensed

water from the tubing. Use this delay feature whenever possible. If you do turn the alarm off, be *absolutely* sure to turn it back on when you are finished.

6. Check the sigh settings. Most volume-cycled ventilators have an optional "sigh" mechanism to mimic the normal deep breaths we take unconsciously. These hyperinflations help to prevent atelectasis and promote surfactant production. The sigh mechanism usually is not used when the patient is on high tidal volumes or PEEP, since these maneuvers also help to prevent atelectasis. If the sigh mechanism is selected, check its rate (usually 6 sighs per hour), volume (usually 150% of tidal

volume), and pressure limit (usually the same or slightly higher than the maximum tidal volume inspiratory pressure).

Oxygen Toxicity As discussed earlier in this chapter, excessive amounts of oxygen can cause lung parenchymal damage (oxygen toxicity) and absorption atelectasis. For this reason periodically check the F_1O_2 setting and the delivered oxygen concentration. Note the machine setting, especially after the patient has been placed on an F_1O_2 of 1.0 prior to suctioning or blood gas sampling. If you fail to reset the F_1O_2 after these procedures, the person may develop nitrogen washout (absorption atelectasis) or oxygen toxicity. To determine the delivered oxygen concentration, use an oxygen analyzer and place its tip at the patient's airway.

Patients requiring more than 40% oxygen for several hours to maintain a normal P_aO_2 customarily are considered candidates for PEEP, which reduces the risk of oxygen toxicity by allowing the use of a lower F_1O_2.

Water Imbalances The patient may develop dehydration or a positive water balance. Dehydration may result from high temperature or low humidity of the inspired gas. To prevent dehydration, be sure there is a thermometer dial in the inspiratory tubing. Visually check it every 2 hours to maintain the temperature between 32° and 37°C. Also maintain the specified level of fluid in the humidifier. The etiology of positive water balance in mechanically ventilated patients is not clear; factors implicated include humidification of inspired air, reduced lymphatic flow, and inappropriate ADH (antidiuretic hormone). Nebulizers may add up to 500 ml fluid intake per 24 hours; in addition, nebulizers and humidifiers prevent the usual loss of water via the lungs (approximately 300–500 ml/24 hours). Place the patient on intake and output recording. When calculating water balance, consider both the retention of fluid normally lost and the addition of fluid from the equipment. Also monitor the patient's weight, compliance, hematocrit, serum sodium, and chest x-ray for signs of water retention.

Decreased Cardiac Output Positive pressure ventilation increases intrathoracic pressure and therefore decreases venous return to the heart. This effect is increased when PEEP is used. Most patients can tolerate this effect, increasing their peripheral venous tone to compensate. Patients with conditions that diminish sympathetic responses (for example, hypovolemia, drugs interfering with sympathetic tone, or old age) cannot compensate for increased intrathoracic pressure. Monitor the heart rate, arterial blood pressure, peripheral perfusion, and venous pressure to detect the patient's response to the increased intrathoracic pressure;

notify the physician promptly if you observe signs of falling cardiac output.

Pneumothorax Pneumothorax may occur due to rupture of a bleb in the lung, disruption of lung sutures, or procedures such as CVP line insertion while the patient is on the ventilator. Its incidence is increased in the patient with PEEP. See Chapter 8 for ways to prevent, recognize, and respond to this complication.

Infection Minimize the ventilator as a source of infection. Respiratory therapy should follow a regular program of decontaminating equipment. Change ventilator tubing once every 24 hours. When water condenses in the tubing, empty it externally rather than draining it back into the patient's lungs or into the humidifier reservoir.

Atelectasis Prevent atelectasis by following the measures outlined in Chapter 8. In addition, if normal tidal volumes are being used, periodically sigh the patient to prevent microatelectasis. If the ventilator does not have a sigh button, hand ventilate the patient with a tidal volume larger than the ventilator's. Once the patient has developed microatelectasis, the sigh will not reopen collapsed alveoli. To promote reexpansion, deliver a deep breath and hold the inflation momentarily, that is "yawn" the patient (Shapiro et al. 1985). Some ventilators have an end-inspiratory pause or "inflation hold" button; if yours does not, hand ventilate the patient and briefly hold inspiration to mimic a normal yawn.

Gastrointestinal Complications Prevent gastrointestinal complications. Hemorrhage occurs in about 25% of patients with prolonged mechanical ventilation. Consult with the physician about administering antacids, ranitidine, or cimetidine, which have been found effective in reducing the incidence of massive GI hemorrhage in intubated, mechanically ventilated patients in respiratory failure. Also, consult the physician about minimizing the use of steroids. Test gastric and fecal matter for occult blood, and notify the physician if present. Avoid gastric dilatation (caused by air swallowing) and aspiration by consulting with the physician about using nasogastric decompression.

Treatment of Complications

Recognize and respond promptly to the problems of loss of ventilation, cardiovascular deterioration, and/or a struggling patient.

Whenever adequate ventilation fails abruptly, immediately disconnect the ventilator and hand ventilate the patient while you evaluate the problem further. A sudden increase in inspiratory pressure often accompanied by release of the pop-off valve signifies obstruction. Check for kinks in the tubing, and suction the airway. A falling pressure in a volume-limited ventilator or a rapidly decreasing tidal volume in a pressure-limited ventilator indicates a leak in the system. Check the tubing connections. If these simple actions fail to correct the problem, summon the assistance of another nurse, respiratory therapist, or physician.

The cause of cardiovascular deterioration usually is increased intrathoracic pressure. Reversal of hypotension usually is accomplished by fluid and/or sympathomimetic drug administration. If the decompensation is acute, hand ventilate the patient. Obtain immediate medical reevaluation of the therapy.

A restless or struggling patient may indicate hypoxia or emotional panic. Bag breathe the patient while blood gases are checked; the ventilator settings may have been inadequate. If the gases are abnormal, inform the physician, who may want to alter the settings. If the gases are normal, the problem may be that the patient is terrified of the sensation of being unable to ventilate himself or herself. When this occurs, hand ventilate, starting at the person's spontaneous rate and slowly decreasing the frequency until the desired rate is reached. Then, reconnect the patient while you coach him or her to breathe in synchrony with the ventilator. The attitude you convey during this maneuver is very important. If your tone or actions are critical or demeaning, you will only increase patient anxiety. If you verbally acknowledge the fright and convey calmness, especially if the patient has developed trust in you before the episode, you will be considerably more effective in aiding adaptation to dependence on the ventilator. If the problem continues, consult with the physician about revising the ventilator settings. If all other measures fail, the physician may order the patient sedated with morphine or paralyzed with small doses of curare or pancuronium bromide along with the sedation.

Discontinuation of Mechanical Ventilation

Assist with discontinuation of mechanical ventilation as ordered by the physician. First, note how well the patient meets weaning criteria (Table 9–3). Shapiro et al. (1985) have identified guidelines for ventilator discontinuance. They point out that the primary criterion for ventilator discontinuance is improvement or reversal of the underlying disease process. Objective signs that the

TABLE 9–3   WEANING CHECKLIST

1. Clinical condition—Reversal of underlying process
2. Stable hemodynamics
3. Adequate muscle strength
4. Lungs optimally dry, compliant
5. Adequate nutrition
6. Normal acid–base, electrolytes, hematocrit
7. Oriented, able to follow commands
8. No respiratory depressants in system
9. Rested
10. No splinting due to pain of abdominal/thoracic incision
11. Trusting relationship with nurse, emotional support

PHYSIOLOGIC PARAMETERS TO ASSESS READINESS TO WEAN

1. Muscle mechanics
    Vital capacity > 10–15 ml/kg
    Inspiratory force > -20 cm H_2O
2. Oxygenation status
    A $-$ aDo_2 on 100% < 300–350 mm Hg
    Shunt fraction Q_s/Q_T < 10–20%
    Deadspace/tidal volume (V_D/V_T)< 0.6

---

ventilator probably may be discontinued safely include the following: vital capacity is greater than 10–15 ml/kg; respiratory rate is below 25; shunt is less than 20%; and arterial blood gas values and hemodynamic measurements are stable. Most patients do not need to be weaned from the ventilator gradually.

If the patient has been receiving PEEP, he must be weaned from PEEP before being weaned from the ventilator. Weaning from PEEP can begin when the P_aO_2 is acceptable on 40% oxygen. PEEP is decreased in small decrements, with arterial blood gases used to evaluate the effects of each reduction, until atmospheric pressure is tolerated or 5 cm CPAP is applied.

To discontinue the ventilator, first assist the physician in explaining the impending events to the patient: Let the patient know that there may be shortness of breath initially and that you will stay and monitor closely. Explain that if he or she has difficulty, mechanical ventilation will be resumed and discontinuation tried again later. Place the patient in high Fowler's position to promote optimal expansion of the lung, and suction the airway.

In previously healthy patients who have received short-term ventilation, connect the airway to a T-piece rather than the ventilator. In addition to the arm that connects to the patient, another arm of the T connects to wide-bore oxygen tubing; the third arm is an exhalation port. The patient usually receives 10–20% more oxygen when the ventilator is discontinued.

Monitor pulse, blood pressure, peripheral perfusion, level of consciousness, and rate and ease of breathing for the first 15 minutes. A mild increase in pulse, RR, and BP are normal. Suction as necessary, and coach the patient to breathe slowly and deeply along with you.

After 15 minutes, evaluate the blood gases, vital capacity, and cardiopulmonary status. If they are satisfactory, continue oxygen, deep breathing and coughing exercises, and chest PT. If the patient remains stable for several hours, the artificial airway then may be discontinued.

When the patient cannot maintain spontaneous breathing after the ventilator is discontinued, the cause may be physical or psychologic. The possible reasons require careful evaluation by you and the physician. The process of weaning often is facilitated by IMV and in some cases by CPAP.

Outcome Evaluation

Evaluate the effectiveness of mechanical ventilation according to these outcome criteria:

- Calm, relaxed, not struggling against ventilator.
- Arterial blood gases within desired limits for patient, usually P_aO_2 60–100 mm Hg and P_aCO_2 35–45 mm Hg.
- No signs of dehydration or fluid overload.
- BP, pulse rate, venous pressure, and peripheral perfusion WNL for patient.
- Tracheal aspirate without pathologic flora.
- No frank or occult blood in gastric or fecal matter; hemoglobin and hematocrit levels WNL for patient.

Chest Drainage

In order for the lungs to expand properly, the pleural space must remain a potential space, with a pressure more negative than the intrathoracic pressure. In addition, there must be no accumulation of fluid or air in the mediastinum, which could interfere with lung expansion or produce cardiac tamponade. When air and/or fluid accumulates in the pleural space or mediastinum, the increased pressure interferes with lung expansion. A

chest tube will relieve the pressure, drain the fluid, and thereby facilitate resumption of normal pulmonary dynamics.

Techniques of Chest Drainage

Recognize patients who could benefit from chest drainage, that is, those with pneumothorax causing respiratory embarrassment; hemothorax; pneumomediastinum; or hemomediastinum. Examples are the patient with a rib fracture and pleural tear and the thoracic surgical patient. Most hospitals use a disposable chest drainage system, such as the Pleurevac, because it is simpler to use, less cumbersome, and less prone to breakage than the older bottle system. The principles of chest drainage will be explained using the simplest type of Pleurevac; correlations with the three-bottle system will be included (Figure 9–5). The three-bottle system and the Pleurevac have three chambers: a collection chamber, a water seal chamber, and a suction control chamber. Depending on which chambers are used, you have the options of straight gravity drainage or drainage under low suction (from an external suction source). Fluid drainage accumulates in the *collection chamber*. The *water seal* allows displaced air from the collection chamber to escape but prevents atmospheric air from entering the pleural space. The *suction chamber* controls the amount of suction exerted on the chest. Displaced air leaves the system through a vent.

Assisting With Chest Tube Insertion Assist with bedside chest tube insertion by acting as the unsterile person and by monitoring the patient's condition. Before the tube is inserted, set up the drainage system according to the manufacturer's recommendations. Mark all fluid levels with the date and time. The physician will insert one or more tubes, depending on the problem. To evacuate air from the pleural space, the physician will insert the tube anteriorly at the second intercostal space. To remove fluid from the pleural space the physician will insert it in the eighth or ninth intercostal space in the midaxillary line.

(To evacuate air or fluid from the mediastinum, the tubes are inserted in the operating room. One tube is placed anteriorly at the base of the pericardium. The other is placed anteriorly just below the xiphoid process.)

When the tube is inserted and the obturator removed, connect the tube to the drainage system. The doctor will suture the tube to the chest wall and dress the site occlusively. If suction has been ordered, turn the suction source on until you see gentle bubbling in

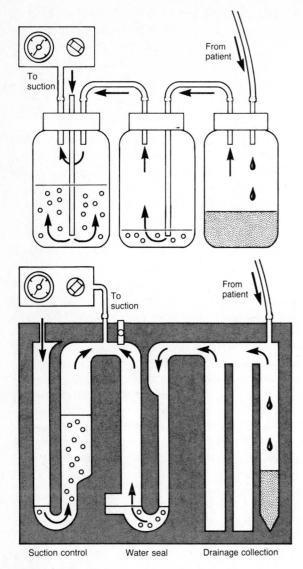

To suction

From patient

Suction control   Water seal   Drainage collection

FIGURE 9–5

Pleurevac pleural drainage system. Air vent is shown. (From Luce J et al.: *Intensive respiratory care.* Philadelphia: Saunders, 1983, p. 166.)

the suction chamber. Tape all connections securely. Tape in a circular fashion except at the connection between the chest tube and the connecting tubing. There, tape longitudinally, leaving a narrow space so you can observe the drainage.

Maintenance of Chest Drainage

Once the system is established, maintain its patency and effectiveness.

Amount, Rate, and Quality of Drainage Observe the collection chamber for the amount, rate, and quality of drainage. Mark the level of drainage each hour. Call a rate over 100 ml per hour or frank bleeding to the attention of the physician.

Decreased drainage may result from obstructions in the system, pooling of secretions, or reexpansion of the lung. Keep the tubing free of kinks by taping connections to tongue blades to stabilize them. Loosely coil the tubing flat on the bed; dependent loops cause increased pressure. Unless contraindicated, place the patient in Fowler's position to facilitate both air and fluid removal. Turn the patient regularly. In many units, the nurse is expected to strip routinely the tubes every 15 minutes to one hour if fluid is being evacuated. The usual stripping procedure is as follows. To strip the tube, lubricate about 12 inches at a time with hand cream, or use an alcohol swab. Pinch the tube shut proximal to the chest. Maintain the occlusion while you pinch the tube with your other thumb and forefinger and slide them away distally. Then, maintain the distal occlusion while you release the proximal one, creating suction. Finally, remove the distal pinch. Strip the tube down to the collection chamber, to suck fluid and clots into it. Hand-over-hand compression is another method to move fluid and clots. To strip the tube, start proximally. Squeeze it with one hand, place your other hand distally and squeeze it, and then release the proximal hand. Continue hand over hand to the collection chamber.

Alternate stripping methods include fan-folding several layers of tubing and squeezing them with both hands, and hand-over-hand stripping in which each hand's compression is released before the next one is applied.

Routine chest tube stripping has become controversial because there are so few objective data regarding its benefits and risks. An important nursing research project by Duncan and Erickson (1982) has demonstrated that, in human subjects, stripping can generate chest tube pressures far in excess of the amount of suction normally applied during drainage with suction. Stripping the entire length of the tube via the most common manual or roller method often generated pressures in excess of -400 cm H_2O! Hand-over-hand sustained compression generated up to -330 cm H_2O pressure. Fan-folding caused pressures of about -50 cm H_2O, and intermittent hand-over-hand compression created about -30 cm H_2O pressure. The length of tubing stripped was directly related to the amount of negative pressure generated.

As it is reasonable to assume that chest tube pressures are transmitted to the pleural space, these findings should give one pause and call into question the value and safety of routine stripping. A prudent course is to evaluate each clinical situation separately, use stripping only if fluid is not draining freely, and use whichever lowest-pressure stripping method is effective in that particular situation. Also, assess the patient's response to chest tube stripping, as the procedure can cause great discomfort.

Water Seal Fluid Level   Observe the water seal chamber for the level of fluid once every 8 hours. Too little fluid may allow air to enter the chest; too much means the intrapleural pressure will have to rise excessively before air or fluid can be expelled. Add or remove water as necessary.

Water Seal Fluctuations   Also observe the water seal chamber for fluctuations. The fluctuations ("tidaling") result from changes in intrapleural pressure with respiration. Normally, the Pleurevac's water seal will show fluid movement upward on inspiration and downward on expiration. In the bottle system, the fluid in the glass tube will move upward on inspiration and downward on expiration. (If the patient is on a positive pressure ventilator, the direction will be reversed.) Excessive fluctuations indicate coughing or respiratory distress. Decreased fluctuations may indicate an obstruction to drainage or reexpansion of the lung. Tidaling is less marked with mediastinal tubes.

Bubbles in Water Seal   Observe the water seal chamber for bubbles. Bubbles result from air leaking from the patient, into the collection chamber, and through the water seal before leaving the system. Thus, they reflect the amount of air leaking from the lung into the pleural space. You should see occasional bubbles in the seal if the patient has an air leak. You should not see continuous bubbles. Persistent continuous bubbling indicates an air leak in the system or a massive air leak from the patient. To identify which, briefly clamp the tube near the patient. If the bubbling stops, you know the leak is at the insertion site or inside the patient. (Palpate around the insertion site to see if the leak is there. If it is, notify the physician, who can put in a pursestring skin suture. If the leak is inside the patient, notify the physician; surgical repair may be necessary. Pleurevacs are available with an air-leak meter to help quantify changes in the size of an air leak.) On the other hand, if the bubbling does not stop when you clamp the tube, you know the leak is in the system itself. Continue clamping along the system to localize the leak. If it is in the tubing, replace it or tape the connections more firmly. If the leak is in the bottle or Pleurevac, replace it. The presence or absence of an air leak should be charted in your initial baseline assessment.

Fluid Level and Bubbling in Suction Control Chamber   Observe the suction control chamber for fluid level and bubbling. Note the level of fluid in the suction control chamber and the rate of bubbling, once every 8 hours. The amount of suction depends on the amount of fluid in the suction control chamber, not the setting on the external suction source or the rate of bubbling. Maintain a gentle, constant stream of bubbling; vigorous bubbling simply promotes evaporation of the fluid. Whenever the level of the water decreases, add more to maintain the desired suction. With a Pleurevac, minimize evaporation of fluid from the suction chamber by using the rubber cap with the small air vent to cover the large opening of the suction control chamber.

Placement of System   When using bottles, place them in holders and warn visitors and staff not to kick them accidentally. Pleurevacs may be hung from the bedside or placed in a holder on the floor. Keep the system below the patient's chest, even while transporting him or her. If necessary when turning the patient, the collection chamber may be lifted over the chest momentarily.

Prevention of Complications

Utilize preventive measures described in the following sections to avoid complications.

Pneumothorax   Prevent a tension pneumothorax by keeping the system vented and by clamping only when appropriate.

The drainage system must always be vented to air in order to prevent a dangerous buildup of pressure in the chest. When suction is applied with a Pleurevac, make sure the small hole in the rubber cap of the suction control chamber is not occluded. In the three-bottle system, be sure the upper end of the vent tube in the suction control chamber is not occluded. If it is necessary to interrupt the suction (to transport the patient or if the external source fails), be sure to vent the drainage system.

Keep two clamps at the bedside, and learn the principles underlying when to clamp and when not to clamp the chest tube. You may clamp the system briefly to locate the source of an air leak. You also may clamp the chest tube briefly near the thoracic wall when changing the collection chamber or when the chamber breaks, *unless* the patient has an air leak.

Ankylosis and Discomfort   Prevent shoulder ankylosis and discomfort. Assist the patient with range of motion exercises several times daily. Splint the insertion site while turning or coughing.

Removal of Chest Tubes

Assist with chest tube removal when the lung has expanded or drainage has become minimal. Signs of lung expansion are cessation of bubbling in water seal fluid, normal physical examination, and a chest x-ray showing fully aerated lungs. Explain the procedure to the patient, and premedicate if possible, since removal is moderately painful. Bring to the bedside a suture removal set, sterile Vaseline gauze, dressing supplies, and a towel. Spread the towel over the bed so the tube can be placed on it after removal. Remove the dressing. The physician will cut the suture and hold the Vaseline gauze over the insertion site. The doctor will tell the patient to take a deep breath and bear down while he or she quickly pulls out the tube and covers the site firmly with the gauze, to seal it off. Secure the Vaseline gauze with gauze squares and tape. (Some physicians prefer to place a suture around the tube on insertion and have you tighten it as the tube is removed. Also, some believe Vaseline gauze is unnecessary and instead use dry gauze squares to cover the site.) A small amount of serosanguinous drainage may occur after removal. If necessary, simply reinforce the dressing for the first 48–72 hours; then it can be changed.

Outcome Evaluation

Evaluate the effectiveness of chest drainage according to these outcome criteria:

- Calm, relaxed appearance.
- Unlabored respirations WNL for patient.
- Performs range of motion and breathing exercises and moves about willingly.
- Lungs fully aerated, as manifested by chest x-ray and physical examination.

Thoracic Surgery

Patients undergoing thoracic surgery are at 20–40% risk for pulmonary complications (O'Byrne 1985). Vital capacity is estimated to decrease 30–50% during the first 24 hours (Shapiro et al. 1985). The thoracic incision causes severe pain with resultant rapid and shallow respirations. These patients are typically middle-aged or older and frequently have significant smoking histories. The procedure itself usually involves manipulation or resection of lung tissue necessitating reexpansion of the lung during the postoperative period. All of these factors emphasize the role of the critical-care nurse in outlining a plan of aggressive, preventative pulmonary care beginning with preoperative teaching and continuing with vigilant postoperative assessment and interventions.

Preoperative Assessment

It is important for you to be able to identify the patient who is at high risk for postoperative complications such as ventilatory failure, pneumonia, and atelectasis. Even though you may not see the patient in the preoperative period, a quick review of the history and physical can provide two or three pieces of data that have been demonstrated to predict postoperative problems. A forced vital capacity less than 20 ml/kg (normal 55–85 ml/kg) and/or a FEV_1/FVC (see Chapter 7) less than 50% places the patient at greater risk for postoperative ventilatory failure (Shapiro et al. 1985). Other data, such as smoking history, nutrition, and activity level, are important to note.

Preoperative teaching of inspiratory maneuvers, splinting techniques, and, if appropriate, mechanical ventilation support should be reviewed by either the nurse or respiratory therapist.

Operative Procedures

For most procedures involving resection of lung tissue, the patient is intubated with a double-lumen endotracheal tube to allow independent ventilation of the unaffected lung while leaving the operative lung deflated for ease of manipulation. The operative lung is inflated occasionally during the procedure. Because the patient is placed in a side-lying position with the good lung dependent, the dual-lumen endotracheal tube prevents debris, blood, or infectious material from moving into that dependent lung. Stasis of secretions in the dependent lung and atelectasis in the operative lung are primary postoperative problems in addition to a large incision involving resection of ribs and separation of muscle. During chest closure, both lungs are maximally inflated and chest tubes are placed in positions to evacuate air and fluid and to reestablish normal negative intrapleural pressures.

Segmental Resection   The most common thoracic procedures are usually for removal of malignancies. *Seg-*

mental or wedge resections involve actual cutting into lung tissue and alveolar surfaces. Patients undergoing such procedures are more prone to air leaks of longer duration as well as atelectasis due to traumatized lung tissue. Chest tube drainage with applied negative suction is used to evacuate air and fluid. If lung expansion does not occur, a procedure to roughen up the visceral pleura is performed to make the lung adhere directly to the chest wall.

Lobectomy A *lobectomy* involves removal of an entire lobe; therefore, the surgical procedure involves closing of a bronchus or resectioning a bronchus to maintain ventilation of distal lung tissue. Following removal of such a volume of lung tissue, the remaining lung will eventually shift and fill the space, unless atelectasis and/or an air leak persists.

Pneumonectomy Removal of an entire lung *(pneumonectomy)* results in the closure of a mainstem bronchus. Rupture of such a bronchial stump results in a major and massive air leak due to its size. Following removal of the lung, the vacated hemithorax fills with serosanguinous fluid, which eventually solidifies to form a space-occupying mass. This process aids in preventing a shift of mediastinal contents. For this reason, chest tubes usually are not placed postoperatively. If they are placed, they may be clamped but are never applied to suction. If shifting of the mediastinum does occur, fluid can be intermittently drained. Bronchopleural fistula can be a serious complication following pneumonectomy, as fluid (blood or infectious fluid) can drain into the remaining lung, producing acute respiratory failure. Placing these patients on their back or operative side prevents pressure on the mediastinum and the remaining lung and prevents draining fluid via a fistula into the remaining lung (Finklemeier 1986).

Decortication *Decortication* is the surgical removal of the visceral pleura. This procedure is performed when other maneuvers, such as chest tube drainage, have failed to reexpand the lung, and air and/or fluid remains in the pleural space, placing the patient at risk for empyema or an infected pleural effusion.

Postoperative Complications

Hypoventilation Splinting due to pain and increased stiffness of the chest wall result in a pattern of rapid and shallow breathing. Subsequent atelectasis, secretion retention, shunting, and hypoxemia increase the risk for developing acute ventilatory failure. Careful pain control, combined with "stir-up" pulmonary regimes

every 1–2 hours, is directly coordinated by the ICU nurse and can prevent having to intubate and mechanically ventilate a patient. The advent of epidural narcotics now enables control of pain without oversedating the patient (Cousins 1984).

Hemorrhage Close monitoring of chest tube drainage in the first 8 hours is important to detect bleeding. In general, blood loss over 100 ml/hr or a sudden increase in blood loss should be reported to the surgeon. Keeping chest tubes in view, avoiding kinking, and turning the patient side to side will allow early detection of bleeding. In pneumonectomy patients without chest tube drainage, physical signs such as hypotension, tachycardia, and oliguria are used to monitor blood loss. Serial hematocrits are also followed.

Tension Pneumothorax The presence of an air leak is assessed in the immediate postoperative period by noting constant bubbling in the underwater seal of the chest drainage system. The absence of chest tubes in pneumonectomy patients places them at higher risk for the development of a tension pneumothorax. In that case, rupture of the bronchial stump allows air to pass into the chest, building up until pressure shifts the mediastinum (heart, trachea, and great vessels) towards the remaining lung. Cardiac output is impaired, and the patient presents in shock.

Cardiovascular Complications You should be aware of any pre-existing cardiac conditions that place your patient at risk for myocardial infarction. Most commonly, supraventricular dysrhythmias such as atrial flutter and atrial fibrillation may occur. Digitalis may be given prophylactically in the preoperative period (Finklemeier 1986). Fluid management is important to prevent overloading your patient with resultant congestive heart failure and/or respiratory failure.

Summary The thoracic surgical patient presents a great challenge to the ICU nurse, particularly when the patient has pre-existing pulmonary disease, as many do. Astute pulmonary care applied early and aggressively can forestall a prolonged ICU stay, with its many attendant complications.

REFERENCES

American Heart Association, Greater Los Angeles Affiliate and MICU Paramedic Training Institute, Department of Health Services, County of Los Angeles: *Pre-hospital care of cardio-vascular emergencies.* 1979.

Benner P: *From novice to expert.* Menlo Park, CA: Addison-Wesley, 1984.

Bodai B: A means of suctioning without cardiopulmonary depression. *Heart Lung* 1982; 11:172–176.

Bodai B et al.: A clinical evaluation of an oxygen insufflation/suction catheter. *Heart Lung* 1987; 16:39–46.

Brooks C: Endotracheal tube cuffs: Pressure is the answer. *Crit Care Nurse* (Feb) 1982; 66–68.

Chulay M: Hyperinflation/hyperoxygenation to prevent endotracheal suctioning complications. *Crit Care Nurse* 1987; 7:100–102.

Cousins M: Intrathecal and epidural narcotics. *Anaesthesiology* 1984; 61:276–310.

Dantzker DR: Diagnosis of secondary pulmonary hypertension: Invasive techniques. *Heart Lung* 1986; 15:423–429.

Duncan C, Erickson R: Pressures associated with chest tube stripping. *Heart Lung* 1982; 11:166–170.

Finklemeier BA: Difficult problems in postoperative management. *Crit Care Quart* (Dec) 1986; 9:59–70.

Jung R, Newman J: Minimizing hypoxia during endotracheal airway care. *Heart Lung* 1982; 11:208–212.

Katz J: PEEP and CPAP in perioperative respiratory care. *Resp Care* 1984; 29:614–629.

Khan F: Results of gastric neutralization with hourly antacids and cimetidine in 320 intubated patients with respiratory failure. *Chest* 1981; 79:409–412.

Kubota Y: Evaluation of selective bronchial suctioning in the adult. *Crit Care Med* 1980; 8:748–749.

Luce J et al.: *Intensive respiratory care.* Philadelphia: Saunders, 1984.

O'Byrne C: Postoperative care and complications in the thoracotomy patient. *Crit Care Quart* (Mar) 1985; 53–58.

Reidinger M et al.: Reading pulmonary artery and pulmonary capillary wedge pressure waveforms with respiratory variations. *Heart Lung* 1981; 10:675–678.

Samson L et al.: *Methods in critical care: The AACN manual.* Philadelphia: Saunders, 1980.

Shapiro B, Cane R: The IMV-AMV Controversy: A plea for clarification and redirection. *Crit Care Med* 1984; 12:472–473.

Shapiro B et al.: *Clinical application of respiratory care,* 3d ed. Chicago: Year Book, 1985.

Shapiro B et al.: Positive end-expiratory pressure therapy in adults with reference to acute lung injury: A review of the literature and suggested clinical correlations. *Crit Care Med* 1984; 12:127–141.

Skelly B et al.: The effectiveness of two preoxygenation methods to prevent endotracheal suction-induced hypoxemia. *Heart Lung* 1980; 9:316–323.

Tinits P: Oxygen therapy and oxygen toxicity. *Ann Emerg Med* 1983; 12:89–96.

Wagner R (ed): *Principles and techniques of critical care.* Kalamazoo, MI: The Upjohn Co, 1977.

Weisman A: Positive end-expiratory pressure in acute respiratory failure. *N Engl J Med* 1982; 1381–1384.

SUPPLEMENTAL READING

Brenner BE: *Comprehensive management of respiratory emergencies.* Rockville, MD: Aspen, 1985.

Chalikian J, Weaver T: Mechanical ventilation: Where it's at, where it's going. *Am J Nurs* (Nov) 1984; 1373–1379.

Darovic G: Ten perils of mechanical ventilation and how to hold them in check. *RN* 1983; 46:37–42.

Fromme LR, Kaplow R: High-frequency jet ventilation. *Am J Nurs* (Nov) 1984; 1380–1383.

Gershan J: Effect of PEEP on pulmonary artery wedge pressure. *Heart Lung* 1983; 12:143–148.

Grossbach-Landis I: Successful weaning of ventilator-dependent patients. *Top Clin Nurs* 1980; 2:45–65.

Janowski MJ: Accidental disconnections from breathing systems. *Am J Nurs* (Feb) 1984; 241–244.

Marini JJ: The physiologic determinants of ventilator dependence. *Resp Care* (Apr) 1986; 31:271–282.

Timms RM et al.: Hemodynamic response to oxygen therapy in chronic obstructive pulmonary disease. *Ann Intern Med* (Jan) 1985; 102:29–36.

Zori SJ: Mechanical ventilation: Bring the patient into focus. *Am J Nurs* (Nov) 1984; 1384–1388.

Unit 5

FLUID BALANCE

10

Cardiovascular
Physical Assessment

CLINICAL INSIGHT

Domain: Effective management of rapidly changing situations

Competency: Skilled performance in extreme, life-threatening emergencies: rapid grasp of a problem

In the ICU, life-threatening emergencies can occur with unnerving suddenness. The abilities to rapidly assess chaotic situations and quickly grasp life-threatening problems are hallmarks of skilled performance. In the following paradigm (Crabtree and Jorgenson 1986, p. 144), a nurse expertly orchestrates the care necessary to save a life in jeopardy.

Nurse: *I was in charge; it was a Sunday morning, and it was very quiet; we didn't have any beds open. The unit was full and we had no forewarning. All of a sudden one of the cardiac surgeons, with two residents, wheeled in this cart and said, have this patient.*

Interviewer: *They hadn't called?*

Nurse: *No, nothing. Absolutely nothing. Said, we need an ICU bed, or at least an ICU nurse. One or*

the other. *And I said, well, what is going on? They said, we just did a biopsy on this man, and he is in acute rejection. We believe he is acute rejection from a cardiac heart transplant a year and one-half ago. He needs an ICU bed. There was no time to argue with them about, why didn't you call first or do something, because this guy was obviously crashing. So, we had to move a patient out quickly, and I asked one of the nurses on the unit to go out and get a blood pressure on this guy and see if he needed to be bagged or needed to be intubated or needed anything. I said, keep him out in the hall, and watch him until we can move a patient out of the room. He was on a cart in the hall, so one of the nurses on the unit [who] wasn't busy at the time, but who had two of her own patients, went out there quickly while I wheeled a patient out bed 8. . . . That was a patient that was transferable, so we bumped that patient out to the floor. I was in charge and had to take this patient. I knew absolutely nothing about him except that he was desperately ill. The family was scared to death, and so was the patient. He had been, 24 hours earlier, in fine shape.*

Rapidly, the team springs into action: the patient is intubated, the pulmonary artery cannulated, and multiple vasopressors started. Then, since the patient must be transferred back to the state in which he received the transplant, the nurse not only manages this critically ill patient but also expertly coordinates the transfer.

So, for two hours I had to monitor this guy, knowing absolutely no medical history, and knowing that he was crashing. I was calling RT saying, I need this or I need that, setting up the lines I knew he would need. And, I was trying to deal with, over the phone—with an air ambulance company. It took a lot of coordination, a lot of work with the family, to try and alleviate their anxieties and patient's. And I think about 4 or so in the afternoon, we finally got him moved out. We took the patient on a ventilator over to the airport. When we left, when we were loading the patient up, the wife of the patient came up and told me—this was a very emotional moment, after trying so hard all day to deal with this—this woman came up and told me, it's so wonderful that there are people like you in nursing.

Astute practice of the competency illustrated in the Clinical Insight requires an extensive foundation of clinical experience built on a thorough understanding of normal and abnormal physiology. Chapters 10–18 provide a sound knowledge base related to fluid balance, a complex process regulated primarily by the interdependent functions of the cardiac, vascular, renal, endocrine/metabolic, and hematologic/immunologic systems. This chapter focuses on cardiovascular physical assessment. A convenient assessment format is shown in Table 10–1.

History

One of the most important steps in assessing a patient is rapid, accurate symptom evaluation. One simple, easily remembered method of evaluating cardiovascular complaints is to use the PQRST mnemonic, in which each initial identifies an important aspect of symptom analysis. The PQRST approach is presented in Table 10–2.

The cardiovascular symptoms that most often trouble patients are chest pain, shortness of breath, palpitations, syncope, intermittent claudication, and abnormal sensations or temperature of the extremities.

Chest pain is the most common cardiovascular complaint. Although it most often is due to myocardial ischemia, chest pain also can indicate a variety of other disorders. The differential diagnosis of chest pain is covered in Chapter 13. Chest pain due to cardiovascular disorders can radiate anywhere within the 6-dermatome region, which ranges from the jaw area to the epigastrium. This includes the back, neck, upper extremities, and so on.

Shortness of breath is the subjective sensation of being unable to draw in enough air to breathe. It most often is associated with congestive heart failure, but also may accompany other disorders, such as myocardial infarction. Related pulmonary variants include dyspnea on effort (DOE), orthopnea (the inability to breathe comfortably while lying flat), and paroxysmal

TABLE 10–1 CARDIOVASCULAR ASSESSMENT FORMAT

VITAL SIGNS

Temperature _____ Pulse _____ Respirations _____ BP _____

GENERAL APPEARANCE

Age _____ Sex _____ Race _____ Height _____ Weight _____
General:
   development _____ nourishment _____
   degree of distress _____

CARDIOVASCULAR SYSTEM

1. History _____

TABLE 10–1 CARDIOVASCULAR ASSESSMENT FORMAT (Continued)

2. Physical
  A. Inspection/palpation—Vasculature
    Skin: color _____ temperature _____
        trophic changes _____
        vascular lesions _____
        tenderness _____
        edema _____
  B. Auscultation—Vasculature
    BP _____
    Bruits _____
  C. Neck veins/jugular venous pressure _____ JV pulse _____
    Arterial pulses
        carotid _____ brachial _____ radial _____
        femoral _____ popliteal _____
        dorsalis pedis _____ posterior tibial _____
  D. Inspection/palpation
    PMI _____
    Precordial movements _____
  E. Auscultation—Heart
    Heart sounds
        S_1 _____ S_2 _____
        S_3 _____ S_4 _____
        Murmurs _____
        Rubs _____
  F. Auscultation—Lungs
        vesicular _____ adventitious _____
        bronchial _____ crackles _____
                        rhonchi _____
                        wheezes _____
  G. Activity level
    ADL _____
    Walking (approx. distance) _____
        symptoms _____
  H. Risk factors (please check)
        ___ smoking   ___ high-fat diet
        ___ hypertension   ___ sedentary lifestyle
        ___ hypercholesterolemia ___ stress
        ___ diabetes mellitus
3. Diagnostic procedures and laboratory tests
  A. CBC: RBC _____ Hgb _____ Hct _____
        WBC _____ Differential _____
  B. Clotting time _____ PT _____ PTT _____
  C. Cardiac enzymes _____
  D. ECG _____
  E. Chest x-ray _____
  F. Cardiac pressures CVP _____ RA _____ RV _____ LA _____
        LV _____ PA _____ PCWP _____ Aorta _____
  G. Cardiac cath _____
  H. Other (Echo/stress test) _____
4. Other relevant data _____

TABLE 10–2 PQRST MNEMONIC FOR SYMPTOM ASSESSMENT

LETTER	ASPECT	SAMPLE QUESTIONS
P	Precipitators	What were you doing when the _____ started? Have you ever had this before?
Q	Quality	What does it feel like? On a scale of 1 to 10, where would you rate this?
R	Region Radiation	Point to where it hurts. Does it move anywhere?
S	Signs and Symptoms	Have you had any other symptoms?
T	Time	When did it start? Is it constant or does it come and go? Did it come on suddenly or gradually?
	Treatment	What have you done to make it go away? Did it help?

nocturnal dyspnea (PND), in which the person has nighttime episodes of shortness of breath due to fluid movement into the lungs brought about by lying flat and thereby increasing venous return.

Palpitations are premature heartbeats or other cardiac rhythm abnormalities that the person experiences as skipping, pounding, or thumping sensations in the chest.

Syncope is a temporary loss of consciousness (fainting) from which the person recovers spontaneously. Cardiovascular causes include stenosis of the aortic valve, rhythm disturbances (most often heart block), abnormally sensitive carotid sinus, and pacemaker failure.

Intermittent claudication is leg pain on exertion due to arterial insufficiency. Decreased arterial perfusion also may cause severe pain, as in arterial thrombosis, or result in *prickling, numbness,* or *coolness of extremities.*

Physical Examination

Physical examination techniques elicit a significant portion of the database from which you generate nursing diagnoses. The usual four techniques of physical assessment are *inspection, palpation, percussion,* and *auscultation,* and they demand refinement of your senses of sight, touch, and hearing to detect subtle indicators of patient status. In addition, critical-care nurses often use

two less well-respected senses, those of smell and intuition.

This chapter presents cardiovascular assessment techniques in the order in which most nurses use them. This practical approach will enhance your ability to integrate these techniques comfortably in the daily care of your patients. The order is as follows:

- General inspection
- Examination of skin vital signs
- Palpation of arterial pulses
- Auscultation of blood pressure
- Inspection of neck veins
- Inspection and palpation of precordium
- Auscultation of heart sounds

Related anatomy and physiology are integrated in the following discussions to help you understand not only the *what* and *how* of assessment, but also the *why.*

General Inspection

Nurses sometimes hurry through the phase of general inspection in their eagerness to auscultate the heart and investigate data from mechanical equipment. Developing the skill of inspection, however, can provide you with a great deal of information about your patient.

For instance, does your patient look apprehensive? cyanotic? Is the patient gasping or doubled over in pain? diaphoretic? These signs suggest a serious illness, such as myocardial infarction or a large pulmonary embolus, and are hard to miss. Unless you look specifically for more subtle signs, however, you may not notice such clues as cyanosis of the tongue and clubbing of the fingers, both indicative of hypoxemia, or distended neck veins, indicative of right-sided heart failure.

Examination of the Skin

The skin reflects both systemic and local changes in cardiovascular status. Skin assessment can be grouped conveniently into three areas: for acutely decreased perfusion, for chronically decreased perfusion, and for edema.

Acute Decreases in Perfusion Acute decreases in perfusion can be detected by evaluation of "skin vital signs," that is, color, temperature, and moisture of the skin.

Inspect the skin for color. Color abnormalities may include pallor, mottling, cyanosis, or rubor (redness produced by reactive hyperemia when a severely ischemic limb is allowed to become dependent). Signs of bleeding include frank bleeding, hematomas, bruises, and petechiae (small, round red spots indicating an increased tendency to bleed). Also note the presence of varicose veins.

Inspect the nailbeds, too, for the presence of cyanosis or clubbing. Check capillary filling time by pressing the end of the nail and releasing it quickly. Normally, the nailbed blanches on pressure but quickly pinks up on release of pressure. A delay in return to the normal nailbed color indicates poor arterial perfusion.

Palpate the skin for temperature, and moisture. When checking for temperature changes, use the backs of your fingers, which are more temperature-sensitive than the palmar aspects. Coldness is a reliable sign of pathologic vasoconstriction only if you examine the patient in a warm environment and the patient normally does not suffer from cold extremities. Increased warmth is of less significance than coldness in evaluating the vascular system, although it often accompanies thrombophlebitis.

Skin moisture abnormalities can include diaphoresis, the clamminess of the patient in shock, or the excessively dry skin of the dehydrated patient.

Chronically Decreased Perfusion Chronically decreased perfusion causes trophic changes and clubbing. Trophic changes, which result from prolonged tissue malnourishment, include thickened nails, hairlessness, shiny taut skin, or skin ulcers.

Edema *Edema* is the accumulation of excessive fluid in the interstitial spaces of tissues. Normally, extracellular fluid and other substances move between the capillaries and interstitial spaces because of pressure gradients and capillary permeability. Movement is thought to occur primarily by diffusion, either through pores or the capillary membrane itself. *Diffusion* is the term that applies to the movement in one direction, *filtration* the term that describes the balance of outward and inward diffusion, that is, the net fluid movement.

Many years ago, Starling hypothesized that the direction and speed of fluid exchange across the capillary membrane depends on the interaction of pressures in the capillary fluid and interstitial fluid. The following descriptions of the mechanics of fluid exchange and edema formation are based upon Guyton (1986).

There are four pressures that affect filtration: two pressures exerted by fluid *(hydrostatic pressures)* and two by proteins *(colloid osmotic pressures)*. Hydrostatic pressure tends to "push" fluid out of a compartment, and colloid pressure tends to "pull" fluid into a compartment. The effective filtration pressure equals the sum of the forces tending to move fluid in one direction minus the sum of the forces tending to move fluid in the opposite direction.

At the arteriolar end of the capillary, the net force causes fluid movement out of the capillary and into the interstitial space. At the venular end, the net force causes diffusion of fluid back into the capillary. About 90% of the fluid that leaves the arteriolar end of the capillary is reabsorbed at the venular end. The remainder is reabsorbed by the lymphatic system, which also reabsorbs the small amounts of protein that leak continuously from the capillary. *Starling's law of the capillaries* states that the mean filtration forces at the capillary membrane exist in equilibrium, so that the amount of fluid that leaves the capillaries equals that returned to the capillaries and lymphatics.

The factors affecting capillary dynamics suggest the various causes of edema. Increased capillary hydrostatic pressure occurs with arteriolar dilatation (as in allergic reactions), venous obstruction (as with clots or congestive heart failure), or fluid retention (as in renal failure). Decreased plasma proteins can result from inadequate nutrition or accelerated protein loss, as in nephrosis. Increased capillary permeability occurs in capillary damage—for example, with burns or endotoxins. Finally, decreased lymphatic drainage can produce edema—for instance following surgical removal of diseased lymphatic glands.

There is a safety zone in which some of these causes can exist without producing clinically obvious edema (Guyton 1986). Interstitial hydrostatic pressure normally is negative. As it becomes more positive, it tends to produce increased lymphatic flow, which not only carries away some of the excess fluid but also some of the tissue proteins, thereby reducing their osmotic pull on capillary fluid. Edema usually is not detectable until the interstitial fluid volume is 30% above normal; it can reach several hundred percent above normal in severe cases.

Edema may be pitting or nonpitting. To determine the presence of peripheral edema, press with three fingers spread slightly apart for 10 seconds, and after release, feel for two "hills" between three "valleys" in the skin. A depression (pit) that slowly disappears following fingertip pressure indicates that edema fluid is soft enough to be displaced by outside pressure. Nonpitting edema usually indicates that protein has coagulated in the tissues.

Frequently, you can deduce the cause of edema from its characteristics. Edema that occurs bilaterally in dependent body parts (such as the sacrum in the bedridden patient or feet in the ambulatory patient), pits on pressure, and decreases with position changes is dependent (orthostatic) edema, caused by increased capillary hydrostatic pressure secondary to gravity. Unilateral or bilateral pitting or brawny edema, often associated with skin ulceration, is characteristic of increased hydrostatic pressure caused by venous obstruction or valvular insufficiency. Localized nonpitting swelling of the eyes, lips, tongue, hands, or genitals, or internal swelling (especially of the larynx), often associated with itching or burning sensations, typifies allergic (angioneurotic) edema. This type of edema results from increased hydrostatic pressure due to arteriolar dilatation following histamine release from damaged tissues.

Evaluation of Peripheral Arterial Pulses

A screening evaluation of peripheral pulses compares them bilaterally for volume, rhythm, and rate. The pulse volume depends on many of the same factors as arterial pressure (such as stroke volume and peripheral resistance) as well as characteristics of the vessel and its distance from the heart. Pulse volume may be described as absent, small (weak), normal or large (bounding).

Occasionally, you may find a decreased or absent pulse as a normal variant, particularly when checking the brachial, popliteal, and posterior tibial pulses. This finding is not a cause for alarm, providing that a more distal pulse is palpable or that other signs of adequate circulation (such as warm skin) are present.

The pulses of leg arteries sometimes can be difficult to locate. To find the popliteal artery, flex the patient's knee slightly and feel behind the knee with the fingertips of both hands. The dorsalis pedis pulse is congenitally absent or nonpalpable in about 10% of the population; however, when it is absent as a normal variant, the posterior tibial pulse usually is present. Abnormal pulses include the following:

- Loss of a previously present pulse
- Bilateral loss of radial or pedal pulses
- Unilateral pulse loss or inequality

Selected abnormalities of the arterial pulse are presented in Figure 10–1. Another abnormality that can be palpated is aortic stenosis, characterized by a slow rate of rise in the pulse fullness.

Blood Pressure Auscultation

Measurement of blood pressure (BP) is of vital importance in patient assessment because it is a prime indicator of the adequacy of organ perfusion.

Technique   When measuring BP noninvasively, it is essential to adhere to certain guidelines. These criteria often are overlooked in practice, resulting in the hasty recording of inaccurate pressures. The following are guidelines for accurate pressure measurement:

1.   Use a sphygmomanometer cuff with a bladder that is 20% wider than the limb diameter and long enough to go halfway around the limb. Too small a cuff produces a falsely high BP, and too large a cuff a falsely low one. Usually, a cuff 12–14 cm wide is appropriate for the arm and one 18–20 cm wide is appropriate for the thigh of an average adult.

2.   Identify the palpatory and auscultatory pressures. Place the limb so that the artery you will use is at the level of the heart, and palpate the arterial pulse. Center the bladder over the artery and wrap the cuff snugly. While palpating the pulse again, inflate the cuff to about 30 mm above the point at which the pulse disappears. Then lower the pressure 2–3 mm per second until you detect the pulse again. This point is the palpatory systolic pressure, and its importance will be explained shortly. Next, center the stethoscope over the artery and reinflate the cuff to about 30 mm above the palpatory systolic level. Auscultate the artery while you lower the pressure about 3 mm/second, noting the changes in arterial sounds (Korotkoff sounds).

The Korotkoff sounds are caused by the vibrations of turbulent flow in the partially compressed artery. The first ones occur when the cuff pressure

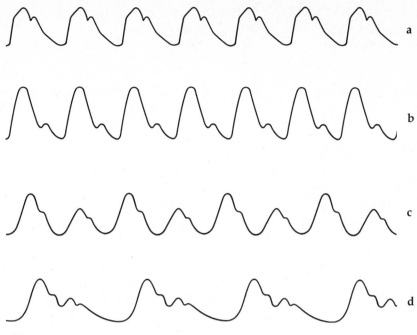

FIGURE 10–1

Abnormal arterial pulses. **a,** Normal. **b,** Large, bounding
(water hammer) pulse. Characterized by rapid rise, sharp
crest, rapid fall. Seen in hyperkinetic states (anxiety, fever,
anemia, exercise), rapid arterial runoff (aortic regurgitation),
sometimes in atherosclerosis and hypertension. **c,** Pulsus alternans. Regular alternation of pulse amplitude, due to alternation of left ventricular end-diastolic volume and contractility; seen in left ventricular failure. **d,** Bigeminal pulse.
Irregular alternation of pulse amplitude, most often due to
premature ventricular beats coupled to normal beats. Premature beats have small volume, normal beats larger volume
due to prolonged diastolic filling after premature beats.

reaches the peak systolic pressure in the artery and are
characterized by clear tapping sounds of increasing intensity. As the pressure is lowered, the sounds take on
a murmuring quality because of the increased volume of
blood flowing through the artery. When diastolic pressure is reached, the sounds muffle suddenly and take on
a blowing quality. They then gradually decrease in intensity until they disappear because the compression no
longer is sufficient to cause turbulent flow. The disappearance may never be reached in high-flow states such
as fever, anemia, and thyrotoxicosis.

The point at which the initial tapping sounds are
heard is recorded as the *systolic* level. The muffling
or disappearance of sounds represents the *diastolic*
pressure.

If you are unable to hear the pressure, deflate the
cuff completely and wait 2 minutes before rechecking.

Failure to observe this caveat causes venous congestion, which falsely elevates the diastolic BP.

Particularly on initial evaluation, check the pressure
in both arms. A difference of up to 10 mm Hg is normal.
An increased difference is seen in dissection of the aorta
and some congenital defects.

3. Mentally calculate the pulse pressure and mean
arterial pressure. The *pulse pressure* is the difference
between the systolic and diastolic readings. Pulse pressure depends primarily on stroke volume, peripheral resistance, and vessel distensibility. Increased pulse pressure is seen as a normal variant or in conditions that
increase stroke volume (for example, circulatory overload or anxiety.), decrease peripheral vascular resistance
(fever), or decrease arterial distensibility (aging, hypertension). Decreased pulse pressure is usually not seen
in normal subjects. Conditions that can cause it are de-

creased stroke volume (for example, shock, heart failure, hypovolemia), increased peripheral vascular resistance (shock, hypovolemia, vasoconstrictor drugs), and obstructions to ventricular ejection (mitral insufficiency, aortic stenosis).

The *mean arterial blood pressure* averages out cycle-to-cycle variations in BP and therefore is the average pressure under which blood flow to the tissues occurs. A true mean BP can be obtained electrically via an intraarterial line. To approximate the mean for patients without intraarterial lines, add one-third the pulse pressure to the diastolic pressure; for a pressure of 120/80, the mean BP is 93 mm Hg. (Note that this value is not an arithmetic mean, which would result from adding the systolic and diastolic values and dividing by 2. Because diastole is longer than systole, the mean BP is closer to the diastolic reading.)

Abnormal Findings

Auscultatory Gap In severely hypertensive patients, the sounds may completely disappear for an interval below the true systolic pressure. If you fail to establish the systolic pressure by palpation, and instead follow the common practice of inflating the cuff only a short interval above the disappearance of sounds, the point at which you stop inflation may well fall within this auscultatory gap. The first sounds you hear on deflation then will be the bottom of the auscultatory gap, rather than the true systolic pressure. Another source of error is to raise the cuff pressure high enough to hear the true systolic pressure but release the pressure when sounds disappear; in the person with an auscultatory gap, you will be misled into interpreting the point at which sounds disappear as the diastolic level. Obviously, hasty checking may underestimate seriously the true systolic reading or overestimate the real diastolic reading. For this reason, it is wise to develop the habits of checking the systolic level by palpation before auscultating the blood pressure and continuing to auscultate until the cuff pressure is 0, particularly in patients you suspect are hypertensive. Record an auscultatory gap in this manner: "280/140 with an auscultatory gap from 250 to 220."

Pulsus Paradoxus Inspiration normally makes intrathoracic pressure more negative, causing pulmonary vessels to expand and causing blood to pool in the vessels. The resulting decrease in venous return to the left side of the heart causes cardiac output to decrease. As a result, systolic arterial pressure normally may drop as much as 10 mm Hg on normal inspiration.

In conditions that restrict cardiac expansion, more blood pools in the pulmonary vessels and an exaggerated drop in systolic arterial pressure may occur. Ex-

amples are cardiac tamponade and constrictive pericarditis. Severe obstructive lung disease also causes an exaggerated response, because the increased fluctuations in pulmonary pressures are transmitted to the heart and great vessels. The exaggerated systolic arterial pressure response to inspiration is known as a *paradoxical pulse,* although the name is poor because the response is merely an accentuation of the normal response rather than a paradox (an apparently absurd but true situation). It often must be detected by auscultation rather than palpation.

To check for a paradoxical pulse, instruct the patient to breathe normally. Inflate the cuff above the known systolic level. Deflate the cuff during normal expiration and note the systolic pressure. Then wait, reinflate the cuff, and check the systolic BP when the patient inspires. A difference of less than 10 mm Hg between the two points indicates a normal BP response to inspiration. A greater difference indicates a paradoxical pulse. If its other causes are ruled out, this finding can be particularly valuable in confirming the presence of cardiac tamponade and the trend of readings useful in evaluating its progression.

Bruits Particularly on initial evaluation, it also is helpful to auscultate the major arteries. Auscultation normally reveals no bruits, although systolic abdominal bruits occur normally in about 25% of young people (Daily and Schroder 1985). In partially occluded vessels (primarily the carotid or femoral arteries), bruits indicate turbulent blood flow secondary to atherosclerosis or other pathology.

Interpretation To interpret the measurements you obtain, it is necessary to comprehend the factors that affect blood pressure and their interrelationships. These are presented graphically in Figure 10–2 and discussed in detail in the paragraphs that follow. The factors that affect blood pressure and their interrelationships are extremely complex and involve feedback mechanisms at many levels. The explanations presented here are simplified and are based primarily on the works of Guyton (1986) and Daily and Schroeder (1985).

Physics of Blood Flow Arterial pressure varies directly with cardiac output and peripheral resistance:

$$\underset{\text{(MAP)}}{\text{Mean arterial pressure}} = \underset{\text{(CO)}}{\text{Cardiac output}} \times \underset{\text{(SVR)}}{\text{Systemic vascular resistance}}$$

Cardiac output averages about 5 liters per minute. It equals the amount of blood the left ventricle ejects with each beat (the *stroke volume*) times the number of beats per minute (the *heart rate*). Both stroke volume and heart rate are related directly to arterial blood pressure.

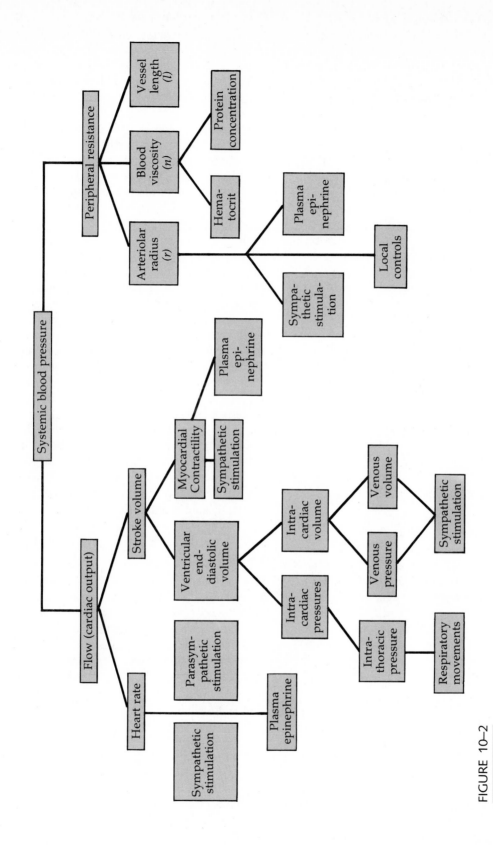

FIGURE 10–2

Multiplicity of factors affecting circulation.

The stroke volume is determined by the ventricular volume at the end of diastole and by the ventricular contractility. These factors in turn are influenced by the venous return to the heart and by nervous and hormonal stimulation. The heart rate, the other chief determinant of cardiac output, responds primarily to nervous and hormonal stimuli.

Peripheral resistance is affected chiefly by blood vessel radius, blood viscosity, and blood vessel length. Blood vessel radius and peripheral resistance are related inversely—as the radius increases, resistance decreases, and arterial pressure also may decrease. Even small changes in arteriolar radius can have a profound effect on arterial pressure. Changes in blood viscosity are much more important than changes in blood vessel length. As blood viscosity increases (for example, due to an increased hematocrit or serum protein level), peripheral resistance also tends to increase and so does arterial pressure.

Systemic vascular resistance (SVR) cannot be measured directly. It can be calculated, however, from mean arterial pressure (MAP), mean right atrial pressure $(\overline{RA})$, and cardiac output (CO), as follows:

$$\underset{\substack{\text{(expressed in} \\ \text{resistance units)}}}{\text{SVR}} = \frac{\text{MAP} - \overline{\text{RA}}}{\text{CO}}$$

$$\underset{\substack{\text{(expressed in} \\ \text{dynes/sec/cm}^{-5})}}{\text{SVR}} = \frac{\text{MAP} - \overline{\text{RA}}}{\text{CO}} \times 80$$

Normal values for SVR are 15–20 resistance units or 900–1600 dynes/sec/cm^{-5}.

Intrinsic Control of the Local Circulation   Blood flow is controlled both locally and systemically. The multiple factors controlling the circulation can be grouped into intrinsic, nervous, and humoral controls (Guyton 1986). To a large degree, the vascular system is capable of functioning without outside control. The inherent mechanisms that enable it to do so are termed *intrinsic controls*. The most important intrinsic control is local control of blood flow in response to tissue demands. The following description of local control is based upon Guyton (1986).

Local control of blood flow occurs in capillary beds. Blood flows into capillary beds through arterioles. From arterioles, blood flows next into metarterioles, courses through the capillaries, and exits through the venules.

Arterioles have a continuous muscular coat. Arterioles, and to a lesser extent venules, are innervated extensively by the sympathetic nervous system, so their constriction and dilatation are controlled by central nervous system stimulation.

In contrast, metarterioles are surrounded intermittently by smooth muscle fibers. At the point where metarterioles give rise to capillaries, smooth muscle fibers called *precapillary sphincters* surround the blood vessels. Metarterioles and precapillary sphincters are controlled not by nerves but instead almost completely by local factors.

There are two major theories for control of local blood flow: the vasodilator theory and the nutrient demand theory. According to the *vasodilator theory,* vasodilating substances may be released in response to increased tissue metabolism, decreased blood flow, or a shortage of oxygen or other nutrients. These substances may include carbon dioxide, lactic acid, hydrogen ions, histamine, adenosine, and other agents.

The *nutrient demand theory* presupposes that vessels dilate in response to a need for oxygen or other nutrients. Oxygen could control tissue flow, according to this theory, through its effect on precapillary sphincters. Normally, each individual sphincter either is completely open or closed at a given time and also displays intermittent contraction and relaxation, a phenomenon called *vasomotion*. Because of vasomotion, blood spurts intermittently into the capillaries. Each tissue can control its own blood flow by altering sphincter activity to influence the frequency and duration of the vasomotor cycle. In tissues that suffer a prolonged but moderate oxygen deficit, flow also is increased by dilatation of already existing bypass channels (collateral vessels) plus increases in the number and size of new blood vessels, which are laid down continuously in tissues.

It is thought that the tissues have an important role in regulating CO, since they control peripheral vascular resistance and venous return, both direct determinants of cardiac output.

Nervous Control of the Circulation   In addition to local controls, tissue blood flow is regulated by nervous and hormonal controls. Nervous control of the circulation is mediated via complex pathways, most of which are part of the autonomic nervous system. Parasympathetic control of the vascular system is relatively unimportant, affecting arterial pressure only through its ability to slow the heart rate.

In contrast, sympathetic stimuli are very important. The most important nervous regulator of the circulation is the sympathetic vasoconstrictor system, which operates through the vasomotor center. The "vasomotor center" is thought to be located in the lower pons and upper medulla. From this center, impulses pass through the spinal cord to vasoconstrictor fibers, which innervate arteries and veins. These fibers secrete norepinephrine, which acts directly on the smooth muscle of blood vessels to cause constriction.

The vasomotor center controls circulation chiefly by altering the degree of blood vessel constriction. The lateral parts of the center constantly discharge stimuli that keep the blood vessels partially contracted (vasomotor tone).

When stimulated to raise arterial pressure, the upper and lateral portions of the vasomotor center increase sympathetic stimuli. The stimulation can increase arterial pressure in a number of ways. It constricts the veins and venous reservoirs, diminishing their capacity and thereby increasing blood volume. It accelerates the heart rate. By increasing constriction of the arteries and arterioles, it raises peripheral resistance. The center can also send impulses to the adrenal medullae, provoking secretion of epinephrine and norepinephrine, which are carried in the bloodstream and reinforce vasoconstriction. All these mechanisms raise arterial pressure.

When stimulated to lower arterial pressure, the lower and medial portion of the vasomotor center inhibits the center's release of sympathetic stimuli, thereby inhibiting vasoconstriction and decreasing the effects described in the paragraph above. The medial portion of the center also sends parasympathetic impulses via the vagus nerve to the heart, slowing its rate.

Numerous stimuli affect the vasomotor center. Higher nervous centers located throughout the cerebral cortex, diencephalon, midbrain, and pons can produce excitation or inhibition of the vasomotor center. This fact explains why motor activity, emotional responses, and the "fight or flight" response to stress are accompanied by circulatory changes.

Humoral Control of the Circulation Humoral regulation of the circulation, the least significant of the three control types, is mediated through the actions of a number of substances in the body fluids, including both vasoconstricting and vasodilating agents. As mentioned earlier, norepinephrine release from sympathetic vasoconstrictor nerves plays an important role in nervous control of the circulation. Norepinephrine can also be secreted by the adrenal medullae in response to sympathetic stimuli from the vasomotor center, as can epinephrine. Norepinephrine causes vasoconstriction in almost all blood vessels. Epinephrine, however, causes some blood vessels to constrict and others to dilate. Angiotensin is produced by an interplay of several chemicals in the renin-angiotensin mechanism. When blood pressure drops below physiologic levels, the kidney secretes renin. Renin activates a series of reactions that finally produce angiotensin, a stimulator of aldosterone release and a powerful arteriolar vasoconstrictor. Histamine already has been mentioned as a controller of local arteriolar dilatation. The unclear roles of other chemicals, such as bradykinin, serotonin, and prostaglandins, remain a promising area for further investigation in the understanding of vascular dynamics.

Regulation of Mean Arterial Pressure Regulation of mean arterial pressure can be subdivided into two categories: short-term (rapid-acting) control mechanisms and long-term control mechanisms.

Rapid-acting controls include three major mechanisms that respond within seconds to blood pressure changes: baroreceptor reflexes, chemoreceptor reflexes, and the central nervous system ischemic response. The following information about these reflexes is derived from Guyton (1986). Within the physiologic range of blood pressure (approximately 60–180 mm Hg), baroreceptors are the major short-term regulators. *Baroreceptors* (pressoreceptors) sense changes in pressure. The most important ones are contained in the aortic arch and in the carotid sinuses, which are located in the internal carotid arteries just above the bifurcation of the internal and external carotid arteries. Baroreceptor response starts within seconds of a pressure change. When blood pressure drops, they transmit a decreased number of impulses to the vasomotor center. (Impulses from the aortic baroreceptors traverse the vagus nerve to the medulla. Those from the carotid baroreceptors travel along the carotid sinus nerve [Hering's nerve] to the glossopharyngeal nerve to the medulla.) The center responds by increasing vasoconstriction, increasing the heart rate, and increasing myocardial contractility.

If pressure falls below 80 mm Hg, *chemoreceptors* come into play. Chemoreceptors respond primarily to changes in O_2 concentration and, to a lesser extent, CO_2 concentration and pH of arterial blood. The most important are located in the aortic and carotid bodies (in the aortic arch and carotid bifurcations). They send impulses along the same paths as baroreceptors. An oxygen deficit causes increased chemoreceptor activity and excitation of the vasomotor center.

As pressure continues to fall below 50 mm Hg, the very powerful *CNS ischemic response* is triggered. Although the exact mechanism is uncertain, it is thought that the drop in pressure allows CO_2 to accumulate in the central nervous system, producing intense stimulation of the vasomotor center. An example of a CNS ischemic response is the Cushing reflex. It occurs when an extreme elevation in cerebrospinal fluid pressure cuts off the blood supply to the brain.

In addition to the three instantaneous control mechanisms mediated by the nervous system, several humoral and intrinsic control systems come into play within 20 minutes to several hours. As described above, the humoral or hormonal mechanisms include release of norepinephrine and epinephrine from the adrenal medullae, activation of the renin-angiotensin system, and secretion of antidiuretic hormone. These hormonal mechanisms result in vasoconstriction, cardiac stimulation, and retention of sodium and water to expand blood volume. In addition, a capillary fluid shift (intrinsic control mechanism) occurs. A decreased arterial pressure alters capillary dynamics in such a way that fluid shifts from the interstitial spaces into the capillaries to reestablish equilibrium. This fluid shift also helps to increase circulating blood volume.

These reflexes are effective only temporarily (hours to days), because baroreceptors adapt to the new pressure level, the circulatory system adapts to the sympathetic stimuli, and local controls override the sympathetic response. Longer-range restoration of blood pressure is provided by the kidneys, as discussed in Chapter 15.

Examination of Neck Veins

As part of the patient examination, you should examine the neck veins. There are two purposes for this procedure: to evaluate venous pressure noninvasively (a basic skill) and to study the waves of the venous pulse (an advanced skill).

The venous system is a low-pressure, low-resistance system. Because it is so distensible, it can easily accommodate an increase in blood volume. As it responds to a lesser degree of sympathetic stimulation than arteries and arterioles, the venous system easily shifts blood into the circulating blood volume when the need arises.

Venous reservoirs exist in all parts of the body except the heart, brain, and skeletal muscles. The most important are those in the abdominal organs, particularly the liver and spleen, and in the skin.

Among the factors affecting venous return to the heart are venous pressure (in turn affected by blood volume, venous distensibility, gravity, and right atrial pressure), venous valves, sympathetic stimulation, the contraction of skeletal and abdominal muscles, and intrathoracic pressure changes occurring during respiration.

Assessment of Venous Pressure   Although venous flow is nonpulsatile, pressure changes resulting from atrial and ventricular filling are transmitted to the neck veins and can be appreciated as pulsations. Following are procedures for evaluating venous pressure by examining the neck veins:

Estimate the venous pressure as normal or increased. To evaluate the venous pressure and pulse, first identify the neck veins, using the internal jugular

vein on the right. Elevate the head of the bed slightly if you anticipate a relatively normal venous pressure or approximately 45° if you suspect an elevated pressure, as in congestive heart failure. Place a small pillow under the neck to relax the neck muscles. Turn the head slightly away from you.

Shine a light tangentially across the neck. Identify the carotid artery, external jugular vein, and internal jugular vein. Because the external jugular vein is superficial and engorges easily, the internal jugular vein (especially the right one) is preferred for evaluation of venous dynamics. The inexperienced examiner easily may confuse the carotid artery with the jugular veins, particularly the internal jugular, which runs parallel to it. To distinguish them, keep these points in mind. The carotid pulse is palpable, with a single strong rapid upstroke. It is unaffected by respiration or position and cannot be obliterated easily by pressure. The internal jugular vein lies deep, under the sternocleidomastoid muscle, and runs parallel to the carotid artery. Its pulsations usually are not palpable, instead being seen in gentle movements of the overlying tissue.

Thompson (1981) suggests looking for the internal jugular pulse beginning at the base of the neck just lateral to the juncture of the sternum and clavicle and looking upward along the sternocleidomastoid muscle to the earlobe.

In contrast to the arterial pulse, the venous pulse consists of two or three slower, smaller upstrokes (the a, c, and v waves discussed in a later section). The level of pulsation descends with inspiration and rises with expiration. The pulsations are obliterated easily by pressure on the vessel just above the clavicle. The internal jugular pulse in a healthy person is visible only when the person is lying flat, and disappears as the head of the bed is elevated to 30–45°.

After you have identified the neck veins, use the following procedure. Vary the degree of elevation of the head of the bed until you can see the maximum pulsations of the upper level of the fluid column in the internal or external jugular veins. Then make the following observations:

1.   Note the degree of elevation of the head of the bed.

2.   Measure the level of the pulse. To do this, draw an imaginary horizontal line from the upper level of pulsation, and another imaginary horizontal line from the angle of Louis. Measure the vertical distance between these lines. The normal measurement is 3 cm or less. Adding 5–6 cm to the measurement will give you a rough estimate of the patient's central venous pressure.

3.   Note the relationship between the level of pulsation and the respiratory cycle. The normal respiratory variation is for the level to decrease on inspiration and increase on expiration. Severely increased pressure appears as a paradoxical rise in the level of distention during inspiration (*Kussmaul's sign*).

4. Perform a *hepatojugular reflux* (HJR) test. Ask the patient to breathe normally. Press the right upper quadrant of the abdomen firmly for 30 seconds while you observe the neck veins. This maneuver increases venous return from the abdomen to the heart. If this test increases venous distention 1 centimeter or less, venous pressure is normal. An increase of more than 1 cm (positive HJR) indicates increased venous pressure, such as in right heart failure or constrictive pericarditis. This test is invalid if the patient holds his or her breath or bears down during it.

If you are assessing the external jugular vein, one additional maneuver can be performed:

5. Apply pressure on the vein just above the clavicle. The vein will distend. Release the pressure suddenly and note how rapidly the vein empties. Normally, the vein immediately empties to less than 3 cm above the sternal angle (Nimoityn and Chung 1983).

Causes of increased venous pressure include right ventricular failure, fluid overload, high cardiac output states, pericardial constriction, and tricuspid valve disease.

Assessment of Venous Pulse Wave Contour The venous pulse consists of three positive waves and two descents, which are related to pressure changes during the cardiac cycle (Figure 10–3). When the right atrium contracts, forcing blood into the right ventricle during the end of diastole, the slight rise in atrial pressure produces the *a wave*. Atrial diastole causes a drop in pressure, known as the *x descent*. It is interrupted by the *c wave*, which occurs as a result of tricuspid valve closure, bulging of the tricuspid valve during ventricular systole, and/or a neck vein reflection of the nearby carotid pulse. During the last part of ventricular systole, venous return raises the atrial pressure and produces the *v wave*. The opening of the tricuspid valve and rush of blood into the ventricle create a drop in atrial pressure, the *y descent*. The cycle then repeats itself.

To identify the individual waves, look at the venous pulse while you either palpate the carotid artery on the other side of the neck or auscultate the heart. The a wave just precedes S_1 and the carotid upstroke. The c wave usually cannot be seen. The v wave coincides with S_2.

A variety of abnormal venous pulses may be seen and related logically to the conditions that produce them. In atrial fibrillation, for example, effective atrial contraction does not occur, and no a wave is seen. Large, regular a waves indicate resistance to atrial emptying into the right ventricle, as in tricuspid stenosis or pulmonary hypertension. Extremely large a waves (cannon waves) denote atrial contraction against a closed tricuspid valve. They may occur regularly, as in junctional rhythm, or irregularly as in AV dissociation.

Examination of the Heart

External Chest Landmarks External chest landmarks serve as reference points when reporting findings. The portion of the chest wall that overlies the heart is called the *precordium*. The heart itself sits in the mediastinum, between the lungs and above the diaphragm.

Findings commonly are described in relation to the nearest rib or intercostal space (ICS) and imaginary reference line. To locate the intercostal spaces, feel for a bony ridge across the sternum about 2 inches below the suprasternal notch. This ridge is called the *sternal angle* or *angle of Louis*. It marks the attachment of the second rib and is a handy reference point from which to count the ribs and intercostal spaces. Place your second and third fingers on either side of the ridge and slide them out past the sternal border until you feel a depression under your third finger. This depression is the second intercostal space. Continue numbering the ribs and spaces by palpating downward and laterally in an oblique line. Remember that the ribs slope down at about a 45°

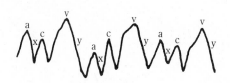

Key:	Atrial Stage	Ventricular Stage
	a wave—right atrial contraction	ventricular diastole
	x descent—atrial diastole	
	c wave—tricuspid bulging or impact of carotid arterial pulse; interrupts x descent	
	v wave—increased atrial pressure due to venous return	ventricular systole
	y descent—tricuspid valve opening, blood entering ventricle	ventricular diastole

FIGURE 10–3

Venous pulse waves.

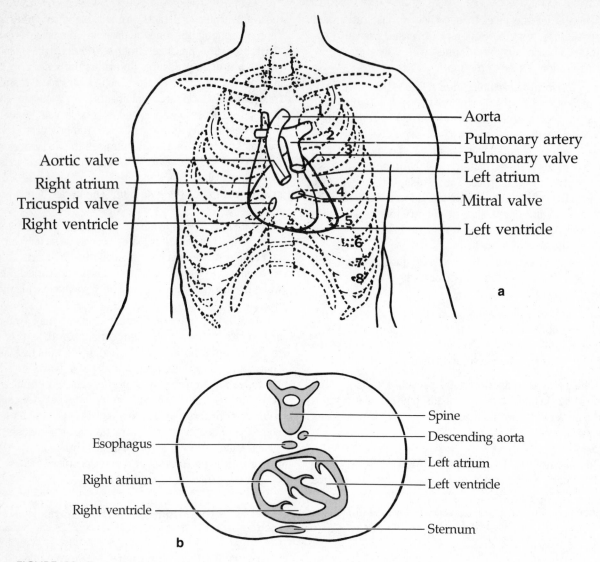

Aorta
Pulmonary artery
Pulmonary valve
Aortic valve
Right atrium
Left atrium
Tricuspid valve
Mitral valve
Right ventricle
Left ventricle

a

Spine
Descending aorta
Esophagus
Left atrium
Right atrium
Left ventricle
Right ventricle
Sternum

b

FIGURE 10–4

Position of cardiac structures. **a,** Frontal plane (numbers designate intercostal spaces);
b, horizontal plane.

angle from their attachment to the thoracic spine to their anterior attachment to the costal cartilages.

The imaginary reference lines on the anterior chest are the midsternal and the midclavicular. On the lateral chest, the lines are the anterior and posterior axillary lines—drawn downward from the axillary skin folds—and the midaxillary line.

The heart is a hollow muscular organ that lies obliquely in the anterior and inferior part of the chest. The sternum and ribs are anterior to the heart, and the esophagus, descending aorta, and the fifth through eighth thoracic vertebrae are posterior. The heart somewhat resembles an inverted triangle, with its narrow apex in the fifth intercostal space at approximately the left midclavicular line (MCL) and its broad base at the level of the attachments of the third ribs to the sternum. About two-thirds of the heart lies to the left of the midsternal line. The apex is more anterior than the base.

Because of the heart's oblique position in both the frontal and horizontal planes, each chamber is not equidistant from the chest walls (Figure 10–4). The right ventricle (RV) is most anterior, lying directly under the sternum. The left atrium (LA) is most posterior. The

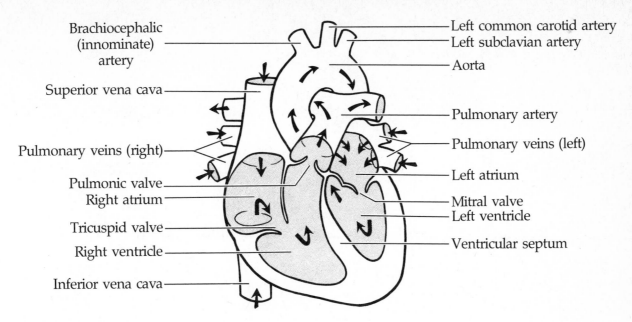

Brachiocephalic (innominate) artery

Superior vena cava

Pulmonary veins (right)

Pulmonic valve

Right atrium

Tricuspid valve

Right ventricle

Inferior vena cava

Left common carotid artery

Left subclavian artery

Aorta

Pulmonary artery

Pulmonary veins (left)

Left atrium

Mitral valve

Left ventricle

Ventricular septum

FIGURE 10–5

Cardiac structures. Arrows show direction of blood flow.

right atrium (RA) is closest to the right lateral chest wall, and the left ventricle (LV) is closest to the left lateral chest wall.

The major blood vessels enter and leave the heart at its base (Figure 10–5). The superior and inferior venae cavae (SVC and IVC) bring deoxygenated blood to the right atrium. The pulmonary artery (PA) arises from the right ventricle and slants off to the left. It carries deoxygenated blood from the right ventricle to the lungs, and the four pulmonary veins (PV) return oxygenated blood to the left atrium. The aorta (Ao) arises from the left ventricle and slants off to the right. It carries oxygenated blood from the left ventricle to the systemic circulation.

The cardiac valves help control blood flow through the chambers and great vessels. The tricuspid valve (TV) lies between the right atrium and right ventricle, at the attachment of the fifth rib to the right side of the sternum. The mitral valve (MV) lies between the left atrium and left ventricle, at the attachment of the fourth rib to the left side of the sternum. The mitral and tricuspid valves sometimes are called atrioventricular valves. Each is anchored by chordae tendinae to the papillary muscles on its ventricular floor.

The pulmonic valve (PV) lies between the right ventricle and the pulmonary artery. The aortic valve (AV) lies between the left ventricle and aorta. The pulmonic and aortic valves are located under the sternum at approximately the level of the attachments of the third

ribs to the sternum. They are not anchored by chordae tendinae, closing instead because blood presses against their cuplike cusps. Because of their shape, the aortic and pulmonic valves sometimes are called semilunar valves.

Because the valves are grouped so closely anatomically, it is not possible to differentiate them with a stethoscope applied directly over their actual locations. Instead, you must listen in the auscultatory areas to which the sounds produced by each valve are best transmitted. In general, these areas are "downstream" from the valve, along the path of blood flow through the heart; there are, however, some exceptions.

At present, there are several ways of labeling these favored sites (Figure 10–6). One way is to refer to the nearby valve; another is to refer to the nearby chamber; a third way is to give the general anatomical location; and a fourth is to give the specific anatomical location. Thus, *tricuspid area*, right ventricular area, and lower left sternal border all describe the same site on the chest wall, that is, the fourth and fifth intercostal spaces to the left of the sternum. *Mitral area*, left ventricular area, and apical area all describe the fifth intercostal space at the midclavicular line. *Pulmonic area* and upper left sternal border are synonymous with the region of the second intercostal space to the left of the sternum (remember that the pulmonary artery slants off to the left of the heart). *Aortic area* and upper right sternal border are synonymous with the second inter-

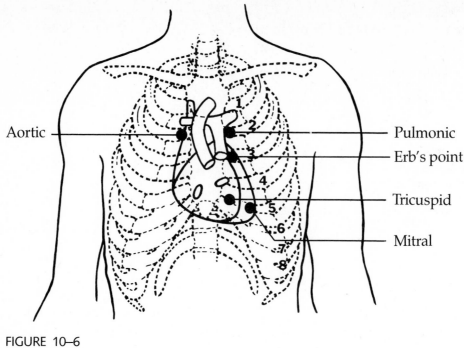

FIGURE 10–6

Auscultation sites. The second intercostal space at the right sternal border is referred to as the *aortic* area; the second intercostal space at the left sternal border is referred to as the *pulmonic* area; the third intercostal space at the left sternal border is *Erb's point;* the fifth intercostal space at the left sternal border is referred to as the *tricuspid* area or lower left sternal border; the fifth intercostal space at midclavicular line is referred to as the *mitral* area or apical area.

costal space to the right side of the sternum (the aorta slants off to the right of the heart). A secondary aortic area is *Erb's point,* located at the third intercostal space at the left sternal border.

There are several ways to fix the preceding information in your mind. One of the most helpful is to study anatomical specimens or a three-dimensional replica of the heart. Another is to use a mnemonic to remember the areas, as shown in Table 10–3. Comprehension of the relationships between the cardiac structures and the external chest landmarks is crucial to true understanding of the possible sources of phenomena detectable at a particular chest site.

Inspection and Palpation of the Precordial Pulsations Normally, the only pulsation detectable is the apical impulse, caused by forward rotation of the heart at the beginning of systole. Palpate with the palm of your hand to locate the point of maximal impulse (PMI). It usually is located at about the fifth intercostal space, in the left midclavicular line. The normal apical impulse is less than 2–3 cm in diameter and lasts for about a third of systole. In many patients, this impulse

is not detectable. If it is, note its location, size, and character. In left ventricular hypertrophy, the impulse is displaced to the left and is larger, longer, and more forceful than normal. Also note any other abnormal precordial movement, such as a systolic parasternal lift (indicative of right ventricular enlargement), extra impulses, or vibrations (thrills).

Percussion Percussion involves striking the chest and evaluating the resulting vibrations. It was once used to estimate heart size by percussing out cardiac borders. Today, x-ray is used as a more precise technique for estimating heart size. Being of limited value in examining the heart, percussion is not discussed here.

Auscultation

Cardiac Cycle and Normal Heart Sounds Auscultation allows you to assess the sounds generated by blood flow inside the heart. Before you can understand the data it provides, you must have a thorough understanding of the relationship of the cardiac cycle to the sounds generated by the heart.

TABLE 10–3 MNEMONICS TO HELP REMEMBER AUSCULTATION SITES

Aortic right, pulmonic left,

Tricuspid's at the sternum;

Mitral's at the apex beat—

This is how we learn 'em.*

Ape to Man:

A = aortic

P = pulmonic

E = Erb's point

To = tricuspid

Man = mitral**

---

*Sherman J, Fields S: *Guide to patient evaluation,* 2d ed. Garden City, NY: Medical Examination Publishing Company, 1974.
**Brykczynski K: Going ape over heart sounds. *Nursing 81* (September) 1981; 25.

The *cardiac cycle* is that series of events between one ejection of blood from the heart and the next. During the different phases of the cycle, blood rapidly accelerates or decelerates against myocardial structures. These rapid changes in blood flow cause tensing and vibration of valves and other cardiac structures. The vibrations are thought to generate sounds that can be assessed by auscultation. The events of the cardiac cycle are diagrammed in Figure 10–7.

The cycle begins with filling of the ventricles with blood. At this time, the atrioventricular valves are open, but the semilunar valves are shut. After about two-thirds of the atrial blood has entered the ventricles passively, the atria contract to actively fill the ventricles with the remaining third. At the end of this event, blood is decelerating very rapidly because it is entering against increasing pressure in the ventricles. This rapid deceleration causes the structures of the mitral and tricuspid valves to tense and vibrate just before the valves close. The closure of the valves signals the onset of ventricular systole.

The ventricles are now closed chambers, since both the atrioventricular and semilunar valves are shut. Ventricular contraction begins with a tremendous increase in ventricular pressure, because the blood has no place to go (ventricular isovolumetric contraction).

As ventricular pressure increases, it causes the pulmonic and aortic valves to open. Blood is ejected rapidly into the pulmonary artery and aorta. Toward the end of this phase, the blood decelerates very rapidly due to the increasing pulmonary arterial and aortic pressures. This deceleration causes the structures of the pulmonic and aortic valves to vibrate just before the valves close, ending ventricular systole.

The ventricles now are closed chambers again. As they relax, they cause a decrease in pressure without a change in volume (ventricular isovolumetric relaxation). When the pressure drops sufficiently, the tricuspid and mitral valves open, beginning the ventricular passive filling phase again. The cycle then repeats itself.

The rapid acceleration and deceleration of blood creates vibrations of the valves and surrounding structures. Authorities differ as to whether these vibrations or actual valve closure produce heart sounds. The first heart sound, S_1, occurs at the time the mitral and tricuspid valves close. The second heart sound, S_2, occurs at the time the aortic and pulmonic valves close. From this description, you can tell that S_1 marks the beginning of ventricular systole and S_2 its end. The time between S_2 and the next S_1 marks ventricular diastole. Because systole is usually shorter than diastole, the pause between S_1 and S_2 is shorter than that between S_2 and S_1.

Characteristics of S_1 and S_2 S_1, the sound associated with closure of the mitral and tricuspid valves, is heard best with the diaphragm at the apex. It forms the "lub" in the "lub-dub" sound of the normal heartbeat. Usually, S_1 is heard as one sound; however, a normal variant in adolescents and young adults is two closely associated sounds, a *split* S_1 caused by closure of the mitral valve slightly before the closure of the tricuspid valve. The split is heard best at the tricuspid area. Because S_1 signifies the onset of systole, it is heard just before the carotid arterial pulse is palpable.

S_2, the sound associated with closure of the aortic and pulmonic valves, is heard best with the diaphragm at the aortic area. S_2 is higher pitched and shorter than S_1, forming the "dub" in the normal "lub-dub" sound of the heartbeat.

Normally, the aortic valve closes slightly before the pulmonic, creating two components of S_2: the aortic sound (A_2), which is heard first, and the pulmonic sound (P_2). Usually, A_2 is louder and heard all over the precordium, while the softer P_2 is heard only in the pulmonic area. Therefore, a split S_2 is best heard at the pulmonic area. The reason for the split of S_2 is as follows.

As just mentioned, A_2 usually occurs before P_2. On inspiration, the split between these sounds widens. Although the exact cause is uncertain, many cardiologists believe that the increased negativity of chest pressure during inspiration causes different amounts of blood to be delivered to and therefore ejected from each ventricle. The negativity may cause pooling of blood in the pulmonary vasculature, so that less blood enters the left

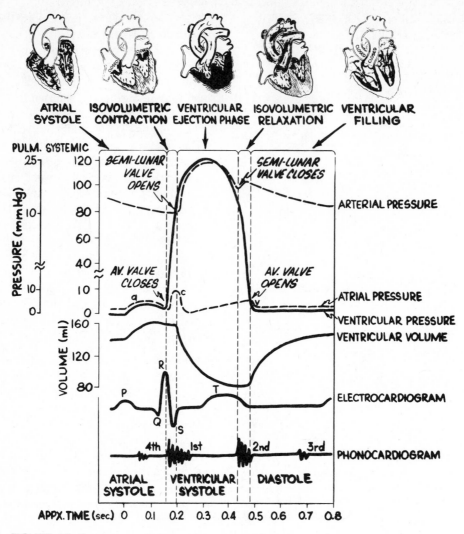

FIGURE 10-7

Hemodynamics of the cardiac cycle. From Rudd M: *Basic concepts of cardiovascular physiology.* Waltham, MA: Hewlett-Packard, 1973. Copyright (1973) Hewlett-Packard Company. Reproduced with permission.

ventricle. Because less blood is ejected, the aortic valve closes a little early. At the same time, the increased negativity produces a suction effect on the systemic veins, causing more blood to enter the right side of the heart. Because more blood is ejected from the right ventricle, the pulmonic valve closes a little later than on expiration. As a result of the early A_2 and late P_2 on inspiration, the split between the sounds widens. Physiologic split S_2's are heard most often in children and young adults.

Among the abnormalities of S_1 and S_2 that may be detected are increased, decreased, or varying intensity of either sound. It also is possible to detect an abnormal relationship between the components of the second heart sound.

A number of conditions may cause S_2 to have no variation (a *fixed split*) or reversed *(paradoxical)* split, in which P_2 occurs before A_2 and widens on expiration. Physiologic mechanisms and clinical examples of conditions characterized by abnormal S_1's and S_2's are shown in Table 10-4.

Characteristics of S_3 and S_4 Occasionally, as you auscultate the precordium, you will hear extra heart sounds. Often these are *gallop rhythms,* so called because they supposedly resemble the galloping of a horse. Gallop rhythms result from an extra ventricular sound during diastole, usually generated by the rapid deceleration of blood as it enters against elevated ventricular pressure. Some gallop rhythms result from an extra sound in early

TABLE 10–4 ABNORMAL HEART SOUNDS

SOUND	ABNORMALITY	MECHANISM	EXAMPLES
S_1	Louder than normal	1. Valve wide open	Short PR interval, premature beats, tachycardia, mitral or tricuspid stenosis
		2. Prolonged ventricular filling	Left to right shunts
	Softer than normal	1. Valve partly closed	First degree AV block
		2. Valve prematurely closed	Severe hypertension
		3. Normal tensing	Mitral or tricuspid insufficiency
		4. Damping of sound	Thick chest, pericardial effusion
S_2	Persistent or paradoxical split	1. Asynchronous ventricular activation	
		A. Block of bundle branch	RBBB (persistent split), LBBB (paradoxical split)
		B. Ectopy	Left ventricular (persistent), right ventricular (paradoxical)
		2. Prolonged ejection on one side of head A. Systolic overload	Pulmonary stenosis or hypertension (persistent), aortic stenosis or systemic hypertension (paradoxical)
		B. Diastolic overload	Pulmonary insufficiency (persistent), atrial septal defect (persistent), ventricular septal defect (persistent), aortic insufficiency (paradoxical), patent ductus arteriosus (paradoxical)
		C. Other	Right ventricular failure (persistent), left ventricular failure (paradoxical), myocardial infarction (paradoxical), angina (paradoxical)
		3. Two outlets for ventricular ejection	Mitral insufficiency (persistent), ventricular septal defect (persistent), tricuspid insufficiency (paradoxical)
S_2	Single sound	1. One component decreased	Severe aortic or pulmonic stenosis
		2. Aortic valve anterior	Tetralogy of Fallot
		3. Murmur obscuring A_2	Atrial septal defect, patent ductus arteriosus, pulmonic stenosis
S_3	Presence	1. Diastolic overloading of ventricles	Valvular insufficiency, atrial septal defect (RV), left-to-right shunts (LV), high output states†
		2. Decreased ventricular compliance and/or increased ventricular diastolic pressure	Ventricular failure, ischemic heart disease, constructive pericarditis, cardiomyopathies
S_4	Presence	1. Systolic overloading of ventricles	Aortic or pulmonic stenosis, hypertension (systemic or pulmonary)
		2. Systolic overloading of right atrium	Tricuspid stenosis
		3. Decreased ventricular compliance and/or increased ventricular diastolic pressure	Mitral insufficiency, ventricular failure, ischemic heart disease, cardiomyopathies
		4. Systemic diseases	Severe anemia, severe infections
		5. First degree AV block	

†RV = right ventricular overloading, LV = left ventricular overloading.

Source: Adapted from Marriott H: *Differential diagnosis of heart disease,* Oldmar, FL: Tampa Tracings, 1967.

diastole, during the phase of rapid passive ventricular filling. The sound is called S_3, and the rhythm is called a *ventricular gallop,* or *protodiastolic gallop.* An S_3 is normal in children and in adults under age 30 years. It is almost always pathologic in adults over 30 years of age. An S_3 usually signifies volume overload in the ventricle. It is heard in patients with CHF, valvular disease, and cardiomyopathy.

S_3 is low-pitched, so it is most audible with the bell of the stethoscope. Because it most often originates from the left ventricle, it is heard best in the mitral area, with the patient turned on the left side. It occurs so early in diastole that it immediately follows the end of systole. The pattern of S_1–S_2–S_3 sounds like "lub-*dub*-duh" or "Ken-*tuc*-ky."* Another helpful hint: S_3 is heard just after the carotid pulse wave disappears.

Another gallop rhythm results from an extra sound in late diastole, during the phase of active ventricular filling (which results from atrial contraction). The sound is called S_4, and the rhythm is called an *atrial gallop* or *presystolic gallop.* A physiologic S_4 may be heard in infants, small children, and healthy adults over 50 years of age (Thompson 1981). An abnormal S_4 is thought to result from increased resistance to ventricular filling during atrial contraction.

S_4 is heard best with the stethoscope bell at the mitral area. The sound occurs so late in diastole that it immediately precedes systole. The pattern of S_4–S_1–S_2 sounds somewhat like "de-lub-*dub*" or "Ten-nes-*see*."* S_4 is heard just before the carotid pulse wave is felt. S_4 occurs so close to S_1 that it may be hard at first to differentiate it from a split S_1. The key differentiating feature is the area in which the sounds are heard—a split S_1 is heard best at the tricuspid area, whereas a left-sided S_4 is heard best at the apex.

An S_4 implies decreased ventricular compliance or a "stiff" left ventricle. It is heard in hypertension, myocardial infarction, aortic or pulmonic stenosis, and cardiomyopathies, for example, and frequently is not accompanied by ventricular failure. It is a normal variant in people age 65 years or older.

In a patient with a severely failing heart, both an S_3 and an S_4 may be heard. Occasionally, during a run of tachycardia or in prolonged atrioventricular conduction, they may combine in a mid-diastolic sound called a *summation gallop.*

Physiologic mechanisms and clinical examples of disorders characterized by abnormal S_3's and S_4's are included in Table 10–4.

Other abnormal sounds are *snaps* and *clicks.* Opening *snaps* occur with movement of stenotic valves. Mitral

and tricuspid opening snaps are high-pitched diastolic sounds heard shortly after S_2 and often followed by rumbles. *Clicks* are systolic sounds. Systolic ejection clicks are high-pitched sounds heard in early systole, just after S_1. Systolic ejection clicks result from movement of stenotic valves or expansion of the great blood vessels. Thus, they may be heard with aortic or pulmonic stenosis and with systemic or pulmonary hypertension. Mid-systolic clocks usually are associated with mitral valve prolapse.

Murmurs   A *murmur* is a long series of audible vibrations generated by turbulent blood flow. A murmur usually results from an obstruction to blood flow, flow into a dilated vessel, a high rate of flow across a normal valve, forward or backward flow across an abnormal valve, or flow through an abnormal arteriovenous communication.

A murmur is identified on the basis of its timing, location, radiation, loudness, pitch, intensity (shape), quality, and response to respiration, position changes, and pharmacologic agents. *Timing* in the cardiac cycle may be systolic, diastolic, or continuous. A systolic murmur may be described further as holosystolic (lasting throughout systole) or systolic ejection (midsystolic) murmur. The chest site where the murmur is loudest is its *location,* while *radiation* describes its transmission to other chest sites, the neck, or extremities. *Loudness* is graded on a scale from 1 to 6. A grade 1 murmur can barely be heard; a 2 is faint, but detectable; 3, moderately loud; 4, loud; 5, louder; and 6 is so loud it can be heard with the stethoscope just above but not in contact with the chest wall. *Pitch* is produced by the number of vibrations per second; high-frequency sounds are high-pitched, low-frequency ones are low-pitched. The *shape* of a murmur is described as crescendo (increasing), decrescendo (decreasing), crescendo-decrescendo (diamond-shaped), or plateau (constant). The *quality* depends on the mixture of pitches creating the sound and usually is described as harsh, blowing, rumbling, or musical. The characteristics of murmurs vary considerably; only the most common are included here (Table 10–5).

The timing of murmurs is easier to understand if you recall the events of the cardiac cycle. For instance, S_1 occurs at the time of mitral and tricuspid valve closure and marks the onset of systole. At this time, the aortic and pulmonic valves still are closed. S_2 is heard at the time of aortic and pulmonic valve closure, marking the end of systole. A holosystolic murmur occurs when blood flows from a chamber with a continuously higher pressure during systole into one with a lower pressure; thus it logically may result from mitral or tricuspid insufficiency or a ventricular septal defect. It usually is high-pitched and blowing, harsh, or musical. The murmur of mitral insufficiency is best heard at the apex,

---

*The accented syllable in *Kentucky* and *Tennessee* corresponds with S_2.

TABLE 10–5 SIMPLIFIED CHARACTERISTICS OF MURMURS

TIMING	LOCATION	PITCH	QUALITY	TYPE
Holosystolic				
	Apex	High	Blowing	Mitral insufficiency
	LLSB	High	Blowing	Tricuspid insufficiency
	Left sternal border	High	Blowing	Ventricular septal defect
Systolic ejection				
	URSB	Medium	Harsh	Aortic stenosis
	ULSB	Medium	Harsh	Pulmonic stenosis
Early diastolic				
	URSB and Erb's point	High	Blowing	Aortic insufficiency
	ULSB	High	Blowing	Pulmonic insufficiency
Mid-to late diastolic				
	Apex	Low	Rumbling	Mitral stenosis
	LLSB	Low	Rumbling	Tricuspid stenosis

Key: LLSB = lower left sternal border; URSB = upper right sternal border; ULSB = upper left sternal border.

tricuspid insufficiency at the lower left sternal border, and ventricular septal defect at the left sternal border.

Systolic ejection murmurs occur after S_1, the phase of isovolumetric contraction, and the opening of the aortic and pulmonic valves. These murmurs, typical of aortic and pulmonic stenosis, have a crescendo-decrescendo shape due to the blood ejection increase and decrease. They end before their respective component of S_2 (A_2 or P_2) marks the closure of the valve. They usually are harsh and high-pitched. The murmur of aortic stenosis is heard best at the upper right sternal border; it often radiates to the apex and carotid arteries. The pulmonic stenosis murmur is loudest at the upper left sternal border. Systolic ejection murmurs also occur with flow into a dilated vessel (as in systemic or pulmonary hypertension) or increased flow across the valve (as in aortic or pulmonic insufficiency).

In diastole, the semilunar valves should be closed and the atrioventricular valves open. Early diastolic murmurs logically may result from aortic or pulmonic insufficiency (manifesting itself soon after closure of the valve, which is marked by S_2). They are soft, blowing,

high-pitched, decrescendo murmurs. The murmur of pulmonic insufficiency is heard best at the upper left sternal border, that of aortic insufficiency at the upper right sternal border or third left inter-space.

Mid- to late diastolic murmurs occur during the phase of rapid ventricular filling as blood rushes across the atrioventricular valves. They are heard in mitral and tricuspid stenosis. They cause low-pitched rumbles. A tricuspid stenosis murmur is appreciated best at the lower left sternal border, that of mitral stenosis at the apex.

Be particularly alert for the sudden appearance of the following murmurs. A new holosystolic murmur along the left sternal border may indicate rupture of the ventricular septum following myocardial infarction, while a new holosystolic murmur at the apex may result from rupture of the papillary muscles, which anchor the mitral valve. These murmurs are accompanied by sudden, severe left and right heart failure. In a patient with a suspected aneurysm or descending aortic dissection, the onset of a murmur of aortic insufficiency may herald additional proximal dissection.

Techniques of Auscultation There are many systems for listening to cardiac sounds; this is one useful method. Have the patient lie down. If the patient stands or sits, many low-frequency sounds, such as diastolic filling sounds or murmurs, will diminish or disappear because of orthostatic pooling.

First, create as quiet an environment as possible: turn off the television if one is present; ask visitors or staff to be quiet; and so on.

Start with the diaphragm. Press it against the chest firmly enough to leave a ring on the skin when you later remove it. Inch the diaphragm along the chest, progressing from the apex to the left lower sternal border, left upper sternal border, and finally the right upper sternal border. Repeat the process with the bell, but press it on the skin just enough to seal the edges. To keep both the diaphragm and bell from moving on the skin and creating distracting noises, keep the finger tips holding the chestpiece in contact with the chest.

Unless you use both chestpieces, you will miss some cardiac sounds. The diaphragm, best for detecting high-pitched sounds and murmurs, enables you to hear clearly S_1, S_2, and murmurs of valvular regurgitation. The bell, best for low-pitched sounds and murmurs, allows you to hear clearly S_3, S_4, and diastolic rumbles from the mitral and tricuspid valves.

As you auscultate the precordium, make the following observations:

1. What is the relationship between S_1 and S_2? Identify S_1 by listening to the heart while you palpate the carotid pulse. S_1 coincides with or slightly precedes the carotid pulse. To understand this fact, remember that S_1 represents the vibrations at the time of mitral and tricuspid closure. Closure of these valves is followed by ventricular systole, which causes the aortic (and therefore carotid) pulse. Although S_1 may be heard all over the precordium, normally it is louder than S_2 at the apex and softer than S_2 at the base. Try to identify whether S_1 is louder or softer than normal or is variable.

2. After you identify S_1 and S_2, listen at the left upper sternal area to hear the split of S_2. You can identify which component is A_2 by comparing the sounds you hear at the pulmonic area to the sound you hear at the aortic area. After you have identified the components, listen while observing the patient's respiration to identify whether the sounds widen normally, paradoxically, or not at all.

3. Next characterize any abnormal sounds. Do they occur during systole or diastole? In which areas do you hear them best? Can you hear them better with the bell or with the diaphragm? Are they continuous or dis-

crete? Do you hear them best with the patient supine or in another position?

Skill at auscultation takes considerable practice under the guidance of a knowledgeable practitioner. It helps to listen to audiotapes of heart sounds and to begin practicing with patients whose heart rates are under 70 beats per minute. Although you may be unable to diagnose abnormal sounds, your ability to identify their presence and to describe them will assist you in detecting changes in the patient's condition and in alerting a more experienced nurse or a physician to the need for further assessment.

REFERENCES

Brykczynski K: Going ape over heart sounds. *Nurs 81* (September) 1981; 25 (Innovations in nursing: personal communication).

Crabtree A, Jorgenson M: Exploring the practical knowledge in expert critical-care nursing practice. Unpublished master's thesis, University of Wisconsin, Madison, 1986.

Daily E, Schroeder J: *Techniques in bedside hemodynamic monitoring,* 3d ed. St Louis: Mosby, 1985.

Guyton A: *Textbook of medical physiology,* 7th ed. Philadelphia: Saunders, 1986.

Marriott H: *Differential diagnosis of heart disease.* Oldsmar, FL: Tampa Tracings, 1967.

Nimoityn P, Chung E: History taking and physical diagnosis of the cardiovascular system. In *Quick references for cardiovascular diseases,* 2d ed, (ed. Chung E). Philadelphia: Lippincott, 1983, pp. 1–19.

Thompson D: *Cardiovascular assessment: Guide for nurses and health professionals.* St Louis: Mosby, 1981.

SUPPLEMENTAL READING

Andreoli K et al.: *Comprehensive cardiac care,* 5th ed. St Louis: Mosby, 1983.

Bates B: *A guide to physical examination,* 3d ed. Philadelphia, Lippincott, 1983.

Guzzetta C, Dossey B: *Critical care nursing. Body-mind-spirit.* St Louis: Mosby, 1984.

Henderson B, Ferguson G: Concepts of physical assessment in critical care nursing. In *AACN's clinical reference for critical care nursing* (eds. Kinney M et al.), pp. 253–308. New York: McGraw-Hill, 1981.

Malasanos L et al.: *Health assessment,* 2d. ed St Louis: Mosby, 1981.

Newton K: Comparison of aortic and brachial cuff pressures in flat supine and lateral recumbent positions. *Heart Lung* 1981; 10:821–826.

Silverman ME: *Examination of the heart. I. The clinical history.* Dallas: American Heart Association, 1978.

Tilkian A, Conover M: *Understanding heart sounds and murmurs.* Philadelphia: Saunders, 1979.

11

Cardiovascular Diagnostic Procedures

CLINICAL INSIGHT

Domain: The diagnostic and monitoring function

Competency: Detection and documentation of significant changes in a patient's condition

The critical-care nurse functions with a constant, almost subconscious awareness of impending doom barely being held at bay by aggressively applied technologies. The expert nurse can provide care in the here and now despite this awareness; an important component of socialization into the role of critical-care nurse involves learning not to be paralyzed by this feeling or blinded to what is occurring moment to moment.

The nurse functions as the patient's first line of defense in the critical-care unit; when a harmful situation develops, it is the expert who first recognizes "something is wrong here." The ability to interpret a particular finding depends on a carefully crafted alloy of both nursing and medical knowledge, as well as recognition that the significance of a particular change is highly dependent on its context. It is only after considering multiple possibilities in the context of the moment that the nurse's knowledge, analytic thinking, and intuition coalesce into pattern recognition. The importance of honing perceptual abilities and staying attuned to the nuances in a given

situation is reinforced, sometimes painfully, in the crucible of clinical practice, as can be seen in the following words of a nurse with 9 years' critical-care experience (Benner and Tanner 1987, p. 28).

They tried to do a cardiac catheterization and were not successful. It was a clinical situation where I didn't look for certain things I should have looked for. I was more tuned to the fact that he was in pulmonary edema. I was treating that, giving a lot of drugs and a lot of different IV drips.

I completely forgot to look at the things you routinely look at after cardiac catheterizations, like pedal pulses. They had injured his artery when they attempted the cardiac catheterization, and he had clotted off the arteries in his feet. All through the night he had said to me that his feet were hurting and cold. My response was to get a warm blanket for his feet.

I was just so lost in the fact that he was in acute pulmonary edema. It was very apparent in the morning that there was something horribly wrong with his feet.

I can't believe that I overlooked this. When someone has a cardiac catheterization, you always check pulses. You always document them every 15 minutes, then every half hour and so on. But he hadn't had the bona fide catheterization done, and I wasn't thinking in terms of that.

237

This chapter presents the cardiac diagnostic techniques you are most likely to encounter in the bedside care of patients. At the end of this chapter, you will have the theoretical knowledge necessary for beginning skill in (1) interpretation of selected laboratory data, (2) nursing care related to selected diagnostic procedures, and (3) management of hemodynamic monitoring lines.

Laboratory Tests

Laboratory measures of serum enzymes can provide helpful assessment clues when used as adjuncts to the patient's history and physical examination.

Evaluation of Serum Enzymes

Organs contain enzymes, substances that accelerate metabolic reactions. When cells are damaged, they release enzymes into the interstitial fluid and thence into the serum. Serial determinations of serum levels of selected enzymes thus can be a valuable adjunct to the history and physical exam. Analysis of characteristic patterns of elevation can be of significant assistance in evaluating the presence and degree of organ damage. Both the trends of values and the amounts of increases are significant. As with other laboratory tests, the normal values vary among institutions and authorities. The values and time intervals included in Table 11–1 are

guidelines you should evaluate for applicability in your clinical setting.

In the setting of cardiac disease, the enzyme tests most frequently ordered are creatine phosphokinase (CPK), lactic dehydrogenase (LDH), and their isoenzymes. *Isoenzymes* are alternate molecular structures of an enzyme. Isoenzyme specificity is significantly greater than total enzyme specificity.

CPK is found in the brain, the myocardium, and skeletal muscle. A normal CPK level is less than 99 units per liter (U/L) for males and less than 57 U/L for females. In myocardial infarction, CPK begins to increase after 4–6 hours and peaks at 5–10 times normal by 24 hours. The elevation lasts 3–4 days. It is highly sensitive but relatively nonspecific. In addition to an elevated total CPK value, myocardial infarction causes significant changes in the levels of CPK isoenzymes.

Three CPK isoenzymes have been identified: the brain (CPK-BB or CPK_1), cardiac (CPK-MB or CPK_2), and skeletal muscle (CPK-MM or CPK_3) fractions. A normal CPK serum isoenzyme profile shows 100% of CPK from skeletal muscle and none from the heart or brain; that is, $CPK_3 = 100\%$. CPK elevations occur in cardiac disorders (cardioversion, angina, infarction), skeletal muscle injury (vigorous exercise, intramuscular injections, trauma, major surgery), and neurologic disorders (stroke, convulsions, head injuries). Being able to distinguish the source of CPK elevations as skeletal, cardiac, or cerebral obviously is of great diagnostic value. In the heart, most CPK is of the cardiac variety and the remainder is skeletal. In acute myocardial infarction, both the skeletal muscle and cardiac levels show increases.

Numerous studies have shown CPK-MB to be the

TABLE 11–1 CHARACTERISTIC SERUM ENZYME CHANGES IN ACUTE MYOCARDIAL INFARCTION

ENZYME	NORMAL VALUE*	ELEVATION†		
		Onset	Peak Time	Duration
CPK	<99 U/L (male)* <57 U/L (female)*	4–6 hrs	12–24 hrs	3–4 days
CPK_2(CPK-MB)	0–7 IU/L*	4–6 hrs	12–24 hrs	2–3 days
LDH	<115 IU/L	8–12 hrs	24–48 hrs	10–14 days
LDH_1: LDH_2	$LDH_1 < LDH_2$	$LDH_1 > LDH_2$: 12–24 hrs	48 hrs	Variable; for most patients, less than 7 days

Key: U/L = units per liter; CPK = creatine phosphokinase; CPK-MB = creatine phosphokinase, muscle-brain subunits; IU/L = international units per liter; LDH = lactic dehydrogenase

*Data from Kelber M Sr: Cardiac enzymes. In *Diagnostics*, pp. 103–107. Springhouse, PA: Intermed Communications, 1986.

†Data from Roberts R: 1981. Diagnostic assessment of myocardial infarction based on lactic dehydrogenase and creatine kinase iso-enzymes. *Heart Lung* 1981; 10:486–506.

most specific and sensitive enzyme indicator of myocardial damage. Utilization of CPK isoenzymes has provided a means for quickly determining myocardial damage. It has been extremely beneficial and cost effective because it permits more prompt implementation of appropriate therapy.

In assessing myocardial infarction with plasma CPK isoenzymes, it is important to sample blood on admission and every 8 hours $\times 3$. Cardiac function elevations occur in all myocardial infarction patients within the first 48 hours. The serum cardiac fraction begins to rise 4–6 hours after the onset of chest pain, peaks at 12–24 hours, and lasts up to 2–3 days. As a result, CPK isoenzyme levels are most useful in the early diagnosis of myocardial infarction. If the patient is admitted to the CCU more than 36 hours after onset of symptoms, analysis of CPK isoenzymes may not provide the necessary data; one should rely instead on LDH isoenzyme analysis.

LDH is present in almost all tissues. The normal serum level is less than 115 IU/L. LDH has five isoenzymes, labeled according to the speed with which they migrate toward the anode in an electrophoretic field. Each isoenzyme is found in a variety of tissues. The normal LDH isoenzyme values are: LDH_1, 18–29%; LDH_2, 29–37%; LDH_3, 18–26%; LDH_4, 9–16%; and LDH_5, 5–13% (Kelber 1986). The relationship between fractions is very important in evaluating LDH isoenzyme results. Normally, LDH_2 is the largest percentage, followed, in decreasing order, by LDH_1, LDH_3, LDH_4, and LDH_5. The heart contains primarily LDH_1, with a slightly lesser amount of LDH_2 and decreasing amounts of LDH_3, LDH_4, and LDH_5. Liver and skeletal muscle tissue have the opposite pattern, that is, no LDH_1 and increasing amounts of the isoenzymes up to LDH_5. Because LDH is so widely distributed in the body, LDH elevations occur in numerous conditions, including pulmonary embolism, liver disease, renal infarction, and neoplastic conditions. For this reason, an LDH elevation by itself would not necessarily indicate myocardial injury, but LDH isoenzymes would help to pinpoint the source. An elevated LDH_5, for instance, points to skeletal muscle or hepatic damage rather than cardiac damage.

Following an infarction, the LDH level begins to rise within 8–12 hours, peaks at 24–48 hours, and persists for up to 14 days. In addition to LDH elevation, the LDH isoenzyme profile often changes. As mentioned above, the serum normally contains slightly more LDH_2 than LDH_1. An LDH_1 greater than LDH_2 is called a "flipped LDH" pattern. Eighty percent of acute MI patients show this pattern within 48 hours post infarct. (Although other conditions [such as renal infarction] can cause the flipped LDH profile, they are rarer and readily differentiated from acute MI.) Therefore, when patients present longer than 24 hours after the onset of MI symptoms, LDH isoenzyme analysis is more revealing than CPK-MB analysis.

In the past, SGOT also was utilized in the diagnosis of myocardial infarction. However, it has been shown to be relatively insensitive and nonspecific. Therefore, SGOT should not be included in the diagnostic assessment of heart disease.

To summarize, the presence of myocardial infarction should be assessed with isoenzymes taken on admission and every 8 hours $\times 3$. CPK and LDH isoenzymes are highly sensitive. In conjunction with the clinical history and electrocardiogram, isoenzyme analysis provides a powerful tool for detecting myocardial infarction. If the CPK cardiac fraction is not elevated, no myocardial infarction has occurred. An elevated CPK cardiac fraction and flipped LDH indicate that a myocardial infarction definitely has occurred. An elevated CPK cardiac fraction without a flipped LDH may or may not indicate an MI.

In addition to acute myocardial infarction, isoenzyme analysis can provide clues that confirm the presence of other disorders common in acute MI patients. LDH_5 can be monitored to evaluate hepatic damage following infarction or congestive heart failure. LDH_2 and LDH_3 elevate with lung injury. The patient with acute chest pain, an elevated LDH_2 and LDH_3, normal $LDH_1 : LDH_2$ ratio, and normal CPK (MB) probably has suffered a pulmonary rather than myocardial infarction.

Because red blood cells contain LDH, hemolysis can significantly distort this test's value in diagnosing MI. When collecting blood samples for enzyme determination, perform the venipuncture as nontraumatically as possible, avoid shaking the container, and promptly send the specimen to the laboratory. Also, remember to draw the samples on time and note on the laboratory slip the date and time of drawing; when possible, also note the date and time of the suspected MI. These actions will help to ensure that results are arranged chronologically and peak elevations are detected.

Diagnostic Procedures

A wide variety of procedures is available to the physician in diagnosing cardiac disorders. Although you will not perform them yourself, you should read the reports and understand their significance. The diagnostic maneuvers reviewed here are chest roentgenology, echocardiography, Doppler ultrasonography, radionuclide studies, electrophysiologic studies, and cardiac catheterization.

Chest Roentgenology

This diagnostic technique utilizes an x-ray beam directed through the patient's chest to expose film placed against the opposite chest wall.

There are four basic roentgen densities. In order of increasing density they are gas, fat, water, and metal. The differing densities of chest structures allow differing amounts of radiation to pass through the thorax and strike the exposed film. As a result, it is possible to differentiate on the developed film the shadows cast by the various structures. Air, which is the most radiolucent, appears black. Fat appears dark gray. Water appears light gray. Bone, which is the most radiopaque, appears white. The following descriptions of radiographic findings are based on Strong (1986), Chen (1986), and Sanderson and Kurth (1983).

Because of the anatomic positions of the chambers, individual chambers are seen best on different projections. These projections are obtained by placing the chest in various positions in relation to the x-ray beam and film. In the preferred method, the patient is standing and takes and holds a deep breath while the film is taken with a beam 6 feet away.

In the *posteroanterior* (PA) view, the film is placed against the anterior chest so the beam travels from the back to the front of the thorax. The *lateral* view positions the film against the right or left lateral chest wall. The *right* or *left anterior oblique* (RAO or LAO) view positions the plate against the right or left chest so the beam traverses the thorax obliquely from the opposite portion of the posterolateral chest wall.

Since critically ill patients cannot tolerate being transported to the x-ray department or being positioned upright, the films most commonly seen in the critical-care unit are portable chest films. The patient is supine, or sometimes the thorax is elevated. The x-ray beam traverses the chest from about 2 feet away, in an *anteroposterior* (AP) projection. Although the AP view is more distorted than the PA view, it nonetheless provides useful information in patient care. For example, it can indicate whether an endotracheal tube is positioned properly and whether there is a collection of air or blood in the pleural space.

In analyzing the cardiac significance of chest films, the interpreter considers heart size, signs of chamber enlargement, calcifications of myocardial structures, and evidence of altered pulmonary blood flow.

Echocardiography

In this procedure, ultrasonic waves are beamed into the heart and their echoes recorded. It is a safe, noninvasive procedure for following the mechanical activity of intracardiac structures that can be repeated as often as needed. The procedure usually is performed by a physician or specially trained technician, either at the bedside or in a laboratory.

The patient is positioned supine or on the left side. A transducer is placed in various positions on the chest, avoiding the lungs and bones. Common locations are the left sternal border at the fourth intercostal space, the right sternal border, and the suprasternal notch. The transducer emits sound waves, which bounce back from the interfaces of dissimilar materials, such as blood and muscle. By aiming the transducer in different directions, the operator picks up echoes from different cardiac structures. Correct positioning of the transducer beam is difficult and time-consuming, so the procedure usually takes 30–60 minutes. Figure 11–1 shows an example of a position to record the mitral valve.

When the beam encounters a boundary between substances with different acoustic properties (such as cardiac muscle and blood), a portion of it is reflected. The returning sounds (echoes) are recorded as one-dimensional or two-dimensional views on a strip chart or on a videorecorder that is photographed. The acoustic characteristics of the substances determine the intensity of the echo. Blood is recorded as a black (echo-free) space, whereas tissue appears white. The length of time before the echo returns indicates the structure's distance from the transducer. By comparing the echocardiogram to a simultaneously recorded electrocardiogram, the physician can interpret the timing of various mechanical events.

Echocardiography has matured in the past 10 years. Initially, only M-mode (M for motion) echo techniques were available. Although these were extremely useful, several limitations became apparent, including the lack of spatial resolution and the inability to examine large areas of the ventricular myocardium. Thus, two-dimensional (2-D) echo has become the mainstay of ultrasound imaging. Today, the combination of M-mode and 2-D echo affords the best possible use of ultrasound. The strengths of 2-D echo are in terms of location and spatial orientation, while the strength of the M-mode is in allowing more precise measurement of wall thickness and valvular motion (Horowitz et al. 1980).

M-mode Echocardiography Among the conditions that can be diagnosed from an M-mode echocardiogram are disorders of mitral or aortic valve motion, left atrial

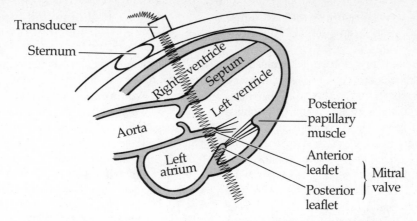

FIGURE 11–1

Echocardiography. With the transducer directed as shown, the echocardiogram will record echoes from the chest wall, right ventricular wall, ventricular septum, anterior and posterior leaflets of the mitral valve, and posterior left ventricular wall.

tumors, pericardial effusion, septal defects, and aortic aneurysms. In addition, it is possible to calculate chamber size and blood volumes, including cardiac output. In the setting of acute myocardial infarction, the M-mode can provide certain types of additional information, allowing the cardiologist to:

1. Estimate the extent of tissue damage due to the infarct.

2. Evaluate overall left ventricular function.

3. Assess for various complications of myocardial infarction, such as heart failure, papillary muscle dysfunction, myocardial rupture, thrombus formation, and pericarditis.

4. Provide prognostic information of value in planning overall approach to the patient.

Two-Dimensional Echocardiography Left ventricular function can be accurately and reproducibly estimated at the bedside in patients by using the 2-D echo. It is a more precise technique than M-mode for identifying, quantifying, and evaluating global and regional left ventricular wall motion abnormalities in patients with acute myocardial infarction. Abnormal wall motion occurs in infarcted as well as noninfarcted zones. Patients with large infarctions and individuals with left ventricular failure demonstrate reduced left ventricular function, compared with individuals with smaller infarcts or patients without heart failure. Using this technique it is possible to delineate alterations in right ventricular chamber size and wall motion abnormalities in cases of

right ventricular infarction. Of additional therapeutic importance is the ability to identify mural thrombi in all four chambers. Echocardiography can provide most of the information necessary for assessing congestive cardiomyopathy, including overall left ventricular function. It is also an extremely useful way to detect idiopathic hypertrophic cardiomyopathy and to assess the degree of outflow tract obstruction (Bommer 1985). Finally, two-dimensional echo is useful in detection and management of the serious and often catastrophic complications of acute infarction, which include:

1. Ventricular septal rupture and subsequent left-to-right shunting.

2. Mitral regurgitation due to papillary muscle dysfunction or rupture.

3. Flail mitral leaflets with subsequent severe acute mitral regurgitation.

There are no complications of echocardiography. Postprocedure nursing care involves resuming interventions, including providing emotional support as the patient tries to cope with concern about an impending or confirmed diagnosis.

Doppler Ultrasonography

Traditionally, a Doppler ultrasonic probe has been used to evaluate arterial flow when a patient's pulse is impalpable. In recent years, there has been much interest in the use of Doppler techniques to measure blood-flow velocity in the great vessels and through the heart valves.

In Doppler ultrasonography, a hand-held transducer is placed over the patient's artery after a small amount of conductive jelly has been put on the tip of the transducer. The transducer emits sound waves that bounce off moving red blood cells. These sound waves can be heard through the stethoscope attached to the transducer. Normally, you can hear phasic sounds with systolic and diastolic components. If blood flow in the vessel is decreased, the sounds will be decreased also. If partial obstruction is present, you will hear a high-pitched sound at the obstruction and weaker sounds distal to it. If complete obstruction is present without collateral flow, the sounds may be completely absent.

Blood pressure readings can be taken using the Doppler probe in patients in whom blood pressures are not audible using traditional auscultatory methods.

In addition to evaluation of arterial flow, the Doppler can be used to evaluate venous flow. Normal venous sounds are lower-pitched than arterial sounds, vary with respiration, and increase after the vessel is occluded proximally and the pressure then is released. If these normal signs are absent, venous thrombosis may have occurred.

According to Mauldin (1986), the Doppler is 95% accurate in detecting significant impairment of arteriovenous flow but may fail to detect small thrombi and plaques and usually fails to detect major thrombosis of the calf veins.

Doppler techniques have become part of the routine echo examination in many laboratories. Doppler *color-flow mapping* (CFM) is the newest and probably the most exciting addition to cardiac ultrasound. CFM is a type of *pulsed-wave* (PW) Doppler. In conventional pulse wave, a sample volume is positioned in a two-dimensional image to collect Doppler-shifted information from a small, discrete area. In contrast, the CFM instrument automatically gathers Doppler-shifted information from multiple sample volumes along the scan line. Mean velocities are calculated and blood flow is color coded for direction and velocity. The resulting colors are superimposed on the image of blood flow. These create a "noninvasive angiogram": a 2-D image of cardiac anatomy, with color representation of blood as it flows through the anatomy. Color-flow mapping is a combination of Doppler-flow information and 2-D imaging. It can simultaneously locate abnormal blood flow and identify the spatial extent and direction of the flow (DeMaria et al. 1985).

Radionuclide Studies

Radionuclide studies use radioisotopes to evaluate myocardial blood flow and to determine the location and extent of myocardial infarction. They are relatively safe, noninvasive procedures that can be repeated as often as necessary for serial evaluation. Several kinds of radionuclide studies are available: myocardial infarction imaging, myocardial perfusion imaging, cardiac blood pool imaging, computed tomography, nuclear magnetic resonance imaging, and positron-emitted tomography.

Myocardial Infarction Imaging In myocardial infarction imaging (technetium pyrophosphate or "hot spot" scan), the patient is given an intravenous injection of technetium-99 pyrophosphate and the chest is scanned with a special detector a few hours later. Pyrophosphate is taken up by bone and also selectively concentrated in recently infarcted tissue, probably because it is attracted to the calcium in destroyed mitochondria (Zeluff et al. 1980). The infarcted tissue appears as a "hot spot" on the scan due to the uptake of the radioisotope by dying cells. The infarct can be localized by comparing scans taken in various views and its size estimated by correlation with the area of uptake. Pyrophosphate scans can detect infarction as early as 12 hours after it occurs, although they are most sensitive 24–72 hours after, and likely to be negative by 4–7 days post infarction.

Myocardial Perfusion Imaging In contrast to myocardial infarction imaging studies, which can detect only acute infarctions, myocardial perfusion imaging (thallium or "cold spot" scans) can detect both acute and chronic infarctions. Thallium-201 chloride is a potassium analog that is actively transported into normal cells following injection (Pantaleo et al. 1981). In the normal scan, thallium is equally distributed throughout the myocardium because perfusion is equal. In ischemic, injured, or infarcted tissue, abnormal perfusion or abnormal uptake causes less thallium to be transported into cells, so the area appears as a "cold spot."

Thallium scans can be performed as resting or exercise scans. On a *resting scan,* a "cold spot" can result from a new infarct, an old infarct, or an area of ischemia. In an *exercise scan,* thallium is injected in the stress-testing laboratory while the patient exercises, and scans are taken immediately and 4 hours later. Comparison of the scans can help differentiate between an infarct, which shows up as a persistent "cold spot," and ischemia, in which the "cold spot" fills in on the later scans. Thallium scans thus are a powerful tool for evaluating regional myocardial perfusion.

Cardiac Blood Pool Imaging Cardiac blood pool imaging evaluates regional and global ventricular performance after IV injection of human serum albumin or red blood cells tagged with the isotope technetium-99m pertechnetate. A scintillation camera records the radioactivity emitted by the isotope. Blood pool imaging is more accurate and involves less risk to the patient than left ventriculography in assessing cardiac function. The purposes of this test are:

1. To evaluate left ventricular function.
2. To detect aneurysms of the left ventricle and other myocardial wall motion abnormalities (area of akinesis or dyskinesis).
3. To detect intracardiac shunting.
4. As a prognostic tool in evaluating left ventricular dysfunction post MI.
5. To follow patients with valvular disease and determine left ventricular deterioration.

Several imaging methods exist. In *first-pass imaging,* the camera records the isotope's radioactivity in its initial pass through the left ventricle. The ejection fraction is calculated by taking counts of radioactivity during end-diastole minus counts during systole, divided by counts at end-diastole. The portion of the isotope ejected during each heartbeat can then be calculated to determine the ejection fraction; the presence and size of intracardiac shunts can also be determined.

Gated cardiac blood pool imaging, performed after first-pass imaging or as a separate test, utilizes a signal from an electrocardiogram (EKG) to trigger the scintillation camera. In two-frame gated imaging, the camera records left ventricular end-systole and end-diastole for a total of 4 minutes and superimposes these gated images. Comparison of end-systolic and end-diastolic images allows assessment of left ventricular contraction in order to find areas of dyskinesia or akinesia.

In *multiple-gated acquisition (MUGA) scanning,* the camera usually records 16 frames (or 14–64 points) of a single cardiac cycle, yielding sequential images that can be studied like motion picture film to evaluate regional wall motion and determine the ejection fraction and other indices of cardiac function. In the stress MUGA test, the same test is performed at rest and after exercise to detect changes in ejection fraction and cardiac function. A bicycle is used to stress the myocardium. A normal response is for ventricular volume to decrease and ejection fraction to increase. If cardiac function is impaired, the ejection fraction will decrease during exercise. In the nitro MUGA test, the scintillation camera records points in the cardiac cycle after sublingual administration of nitroglycerin, to assess its effect on ventricular function (Forrester 1976).

Advanced Diagnostic Imaging Techniques
Computed tomography (CT), nuclear magnetic resonance (NMR) (also known as magnetic resonance imaging [MRI]), and positron-emitted tomography (PET) are three techniques of medical imaging that have revolutionized medical diagnosis. Each "scanning" technique presents information in the form of a "tomograph," which is simply the Greek word for cross-sectional slice (Oldendorf 1985). In CT, a narrow beam of x-rays is used to obtain information about the tissues. CT has been in clinical use for about a decade. Although it has been used primarily to evaluate brain tissue density, CT is gaining popularity in studies of cardiac evaluation. NMR scanners have also been used in the clinical setting. NMR is based on monitoring the concentration and location of hydrogen within the nuclei of the cells within the body. Studies are in progress that use NMR to assess a variety of cardiovascular disorders, such as atherosclerosis, MI, remote infarctions, and pericardial disease. PET scanners have been used in clinical research for several years and have proven useful in evaluating myocardial metabolism.

CT, NMR, and PET exploit different physical properties of the atoms and molecules making up the tissues of the human body. It is important to understand that the picture produced by each of these techniques represents some particular characteristic of the tissue density, water concentration, or metabolic rate (Oldendorf 1985). Consequently, each technique has its place in cardiac evaluation. For example, PET has been used to evaluate the metabolism of ischemic areas of the heart, while NMR has been used to evaluate the presence and extent of congenital abnormalities. The three procedures differ also in the form of radiation employed to provide the information about the tissue. CT uses conventional x-rays, which are emitted and recorded in a new and unique fashion. PET scanners measure isotopes, which are injected intravenously. In NMR, a magnetic field is applied and the response of nuclei against the magnetic field studied (Higgins 1985).

Details of physical preparation for radionuclide tests vary among institutions. In general, no physical preparation is needed, except for the exercise scans, for which the patient must fast for a few hours before the procedure. Emotional preparation involves explanations that the procedures are relatively safe and essentially painless, as well as specific details about when, where, and how the procedures will be performed. NMR is discussed in detail in Chapter 4.

Electrophysiologic Studies

During the past years much has been learned about cardiac dysrhythmias from clinical electrophysiologic studies (EPS) that use intracardiac recording and stimulation techniques. Recordings of local activity can be obtained from portions of the heart that are electrically silent on the body-surface electrocardiogram. It is possible to map the sequence and time of activation of the atria and ventricles and to separate atrioventricular conduction into the AV node and His-Purkinje system.

When recordings from selected sites are used in conjunction with pacing and programmed stimulation sequences, much can be learned about automaticity, conduction, refractoriness, and the origin of dysrhythmias. These techniques not only have enhanced our understanding of dysrhythmias and conduction defects but have also improved the ability to select and evaluate therapy for these disorders.

The clinical uses of electrophysiologic studies include:

1. Evaluting the mechanism, site, and extent of the ventricular or supraventricular dysrhythmia or conduction defect
2. Evaluating syncope: determining covert defects in impulse formation or conduction
3. Evaluating the efficacy of antidysrhythmic therapy (Wellens 1972).

Electrophysiologic studies are conducted in cardiac catheterization laboratories or a special procedure room. The equipment includes a fluoroscope, a magnetic tape recorder, a programmable stimulator, a multichannel recorder, and a defibrillator. Electrode catheters are introduced through the femoral and antecubital veins. The number and type of catheters depend on the conduction pathway being investigated. A recording is always taken from the bundle of His, along with other parts of the conduction system. In addition, intervals of activation time are recorded from each area. A catheter first is advanced to the right ventricle and then withdrawn to the area of the tricuspid valve, where the His bundle electrogram is recorded. A catheter with four electrodes then is introduced and placed against the lateral wall of the upper right atrium. The distal part of the electrode is used to stimulate the atrium. Additional electrode catheters are often placed in sites such as the coronary sinus and right ventricular apex.

Intracardiac electrograms are displayed on an oscilloscope along with tracings from several surface electrocardiographic leads and time markers. Recordings are made on a magnetic tape to insure that transient events do not escape detection. Spontaneous rhythms are recorded. In addition, programmed stimulation is applied with a timed pacing impulse so that patterns of either atrial or ventricular dysrhythmias can be recorded. After the dysrhythmia has been induced and recorded, programmed pacing is used to terminate it. If this is unsuccessful, defibrillation or cardioversion is applied. In addition, various antidysrhythmic drugs may be given during an EPS to evaluate their efficacy in dysrhythmia control.

Nursing care prior to the procedure includes an explanation of the events of the procedure and assurance that the patient will be given medication to relax. It is important that the patient know he or she will be awake during the procedure. Encourage the patient to verbalize fears and concerns regarding the procedure. Since these patients most often have a life-threatening dysrhythmia, they need a lot of nursing support and reassurance. Postprocedure care involves assessments similar to those after cardiac catheterization. The extremity involved should be checked for bleeding, pulses, temperature, and color. In addition, the patient's cardiac rhythm should be noted.

Cardiac Catheterization

Catheterization is an invasive diagnostic procedure designed to study anatomical and mechanical aspects of cardiac function. It is used to evaluate the patient with atypical chest pain or inadequate response to medical therapy, to identify anatomical lesions and associated conditions in order to plan drug or surgical therapy, and to evaluate postoperative hemodynamic status.

Patient Preparation Collaborate with the physician and catheterization laboratory staff in emotionally preparing the patient and the family. Before going to the procedure, the patient should have a clear idea of its benefits and risks, pre- and postprocedure care, and the steps of the procedure. In discussing the steps, focus on the sensations the patient may expect, and ways to interact effectively with the team.

Among the sensations the patient may experience are stinging as the local anesthetic is injected, the sense of pressure as the catheter is inserted or advanced, palpitations as the catheter is positioned in the heart, and intense warmth, a headache, and nausea as the dye is injected. These sensations are unpleasant but last only a minute or two. Let the patient know that in the room there will be many personnel in surgical dress. The patient should tell any of them if he or she experiences discomfort or does not understand what is being done.

Catheterization is a frightening experience to many patients. Assisting the patient to verbalize and cope with fears not only will contribute to equanimity during the procedure but also may reduce the likelihood of such complications as catecholamine-induced dysrhythmias and vasovagal reaction (hypotension and bradycardia resulting from massive discharge by the autonomic nervous system).

Physical preparation includes several steps. Blood is drawn for coagulation studies. If the patient is on anticoagulants, they may be discontinued several hours before the procedure. The patient usually is not permitted anything by mouth (except oral medications) for 8 hours prior to the procedure. Prophylactic antibiotics may be administered. Catheter insertion sites are scrubbed and shaved. The patient usually is premedicated with diazepam or another relaxation medication. Glasses or dentures may be worn to the laboratory.

In the laboratory, preparation consists of the application of ECG electrodes, insertion of an arterial line,

---

RESEARCH NOTE

Watkins LO et al.: **Preparation for cardiac catheterization: Tailoring the content of instruction to coping style.** *Heart Lung* 1986; 15:382–389.

In a study of 86 patients undergoing cardiac catheterization, the authors examined the effects of instructional content, coping style, and psychophysiologic response to heart catheterization. The two types of coping style studied were "blunting" and "monitoring." *Blunters* tend to diminish the psychologic impact of stressful events by denying or avoiding the threatening aspects; *monitors* tend to seek information about the stressful event. The sample consisted of consecutive patients admitted for first-time cardiac catheterization who could read and write and were not health professionals. Anxiety scores on admission were computed using both the state and trait forms of the Spielberger State-Trait Anxiety Inventory (SSTAI), and both the general and today forms of the Multiple Affect Adjective Check List (MAACL) completed by subjects.

Subjects were categorized as blunters or monitors according to their responses to stress-evoking scenarios on the Miller Behavioral Style Scale. Blunters and monitors were assigned randomly to a control group, a procedure-information group, or a sensation-information group. The control group derived any information they obtained from the cardiologist and other health care professionals. The procedure-information group watched an audio/slide presentation on catheterization procedures; the sensation-information group viewed the same program with integrated information about sensations frequently experienced during catheterization. The last two groups then retook the SSTAI State anxiety form and the MAACL today form.

After catheterization, the performing cardiologist assessed the patient's level of cooperation, using a previously validated scale. Within 2 hours after catheterization, all subjects completed the SSTAI state form and the MAACL today form, reporting how they felt during the procedure.

Blood pressure and pulse were measured after randomization and again prior to catheterization. Other data gathered included age, sex, race, years of education, diagnosis, length since diagnosis of cardiac disease, and length of catheterization.

Independent and interactive effects of information level and coping style were analyzed using a two-way analysis of variance of single and repeated measures. Two-way analysis of covariance was used for the SSTAI state anxiety and MAACL today anxiety measures after instruction and at catheterization (the SSTAI trait anxiety and MAACL general scores were the respective covariates.) Two-way analysis of covariance also was used for heart rate and blood pressure at catheterization (the postrandomization values were the respective covariates). Proportions were compared with chi-square tests.

The results demonstrated an interactive effect of information level and coping style on anxiety scores at catheterization ($p = 0.013$). Monitors who received sensation information were less anxious than monitors who had not, whereas blunters who received sensation information were more anxious than those who had not. A similar effect was found for heart rate at catheterization ($p = 0.01$), and there was no significant difference in blood pressure. The control group demonstrated the highest anxiety, mean heart rate, and systolic BP levels of all three groups.

This study supports the idea that a person's coping style determines whether teaching results in less emotional distress during a procedure. This research demonstrates the need for instruction to be individualized to differing styles of coping.

skin preparation, and draping with sterile sheets. The patient will be positioned supine on a narrow cradle that can be tilted sideways to facilitate various x-ray projections, since the procedure is performed under image-intensification fluoroscopy with television monitoring and videotape playback.

Catheterization Procedures The catheterization proceeds according to a protocol determined individually for each patient. The approach to the vascular system may be percutaneous (favored for femoral vessels) or by cutdown (favored for the brachial artery or basilic vein). Among the factors that influence the choice of site are the presence of obesity or peripheral vascular disease.

Catheterization of the right heart is achieved from the basilic or femoral vein most commonly. The left side of the heart may be catheterized via a retrograde arterial approach across the aortic valve, via a trans-septal puncture from the right atrium across the fossa ovalis, or via direct puncture through the chest wall.

Generally, the right heart is catheterized first. The catheter is left in place while the left heart is catheterized. Once that catheter is positioned, the peripheral arterial, left ventricular, and pulmonary capillary pressures are measured simultaneously.

Data Recorded During the catheterization the pressures are measured and the pressure waveforms are recorded for further study.

Oxygen contents and saturations are measured at several sites. These can be studied to determine the presence of shunts (abnormal blood flows within the heart). The usual oxygen saturation on the right side of the heart is 75%; on the left it is about 95%. Oxygen content varies from 14–15 volumes percent on the right side of the heart to 19 volumes percent on the left. An abnormal increase in oxygen content or saturation is called a *step-up* and is a clue to the presence of a shunt. For instance, an abnormally high oxygen content or saturation in the right atrium suggests that better-oxygenated blood is mixing with venous blood in the right atrium. Among the conditions that might cause this finding are a defect in the atrial septum and a pulmonary vein returning to the right atrium instead of the left.

Cardiac output (CO) also is calculated. CO is the amount of blood ejected by the heart each minute. It is a product of the heart rate and stroke volume, which is the amount of blood pumped out with each ventricular contraction. During catheterization, the CO usually is measured both at rest and after exercise with a hand-grip or bicycle wheel mounted at the end of the table.

CO can be calculated in several ways. The most common is the *Fick method*. It is based on the theory that the amount of oxygen the body consumes equals that used by the tissues times the blood flow to the lungs. Oxygen consumption is measured by occluding the nose, having the patient breathe in a known concentration of oxygen, and analyzing the concentration in the air expired. The amount of oxygen used by the tissues is measured by taking simultaneous arterial and mixed venous blood samples, and subtracting the venous oxygen content from the arterial. The values then can be entered into the Fick equation:

$$\frac{\text{Oxygen consumption (ml/min)} \times 100}{\substack{\text{Arteriovenous oxygen content difference} \\ \text{(ml/100 ml blood)}}}$$
$$= \text{Cardiac output (CO) (ml/min)}$$

CO also may be calculated by the indicator-dilution technique. In the catheterization laboratory, the indicator commonly used is a dye. A known amount of dye is injected centrally, and its concentration is measured continuously at a peripheral arterial site. A dye-dilution curve is recorded, and the cardiac output can be calculated by computing the area under the curve.

The value obtained for CO is more meaningful when related to the patient's size, specifically body surface area. The resulting value is the cardiac index; its normal range is 2.5–4.0 L per minute per square meter of body surface (2.5–4.0 L/min/m^2). Similarly, the volume pumped out with each stroke is more meaningful when related to the patient's size. The normal stroke index is 30–65 ml/beat/m^2.

The volume of blood in each chamber also can be measured. From the left ventricular volumes at end-systole and end-diastole, it is possible to calculate the ejection fraction. This value indicates the percentage of ventricular diastolic volume that the ventricle is able to eject. To maintain an effective cardiac output, the ejection fraction usually must be at least 0.60.

Myocardial metabolites such as lactate can be measured to evaluate oxygen supply to the myocardium. Valve orifice areas and gradients (pressure differentials) across the valves also can be determined.

Vascular resistance also can be calculated. Normal total systemic vascular resistance is 900–1600 dynes-sec-cm^{-5}; usual total pulmonary vascular resistance is 100–300 dynes-sec-cm^{-5}.

Contrast media may be injected to opacify various cardiac structures. The general term for this procedure is *angiography*. *Ventriculography* is the injection of dye into the left ventricle to assess its contractility. *Aortography* is the use of contrast media to examine the function of the aorta and aortic valve. *Coronary arteriography* is the injection of dye into the coronary arteries to assess their patency. These studies are filmed for further analysis.

At the completion of the catheterization (which may last 2–4 hours), the catheters are removed. The vessels may be stripped proximally and distally to remove clots. If a cutdown was performed, the vessel is sutured. If a percutaneous approach was used, pressure is applied at the site. The site then is covered with an antibiotic ointment and an occlusive dressing applied. As it is difficult to apply an occlusive dressing at the groin, a sandbag may be placed over the dressing at the femoral site.

Complications Among the complications that may occur during catheterization are cardiac arrest, acute myocardial infarction, dysrhythmias, vasovagal reaction, anaphylactic shock, dye injection into the myocardium or pericardium, emboli to the lungs or brain, and sudden fluid shift due to the hypertonicity of contrast media.

After the catheterization, potential complications include thromboemboli, hemorrhage or hematoma, renal failure, and hypotension because excretion of the hypertonic dye causes an osmotic diuresis. The patient usually is on bedrest until the next day and on intravenous fluids until oral intake equals fluid output. When the patient first returns from catheterization, check temperature, perfusion distal to the insertion sites, hemostasis at the sites, blood pressure, and intake and urine output. Usually, you should make these checks, excepting temperature, every 15 minutes until the patient is stabilized and then gradually decrease frequency of the checks for the first 24 hours. Transient diminution of the arterial pulse is common, but any pulse decrease should be reported promptly to the physician, because it may signal impending arterial occlusion. If you are unable to monitor the patient constantly at the bedside, be sure to teach the patient and family to alert you to any coolness, numbness, or paresthesias distal to the incision sites. Instruct the patient to keep the extremity straight and to rotate the ankle and flex and extend the foot while on bedrest.

A sound understanding of the above information will reinforce your comprehension of cardiac anatomy and physiology. In addition, your knowledge of the normal values will help you understand catheterization reports on your patients and use them to predict nursing problems. For instance, you might note that your patient had extremely high left atrial and pulmonary arterial pressures. This knowledge would alert you that your patient was at high risk for developing pulmonary edema; you then would know to monitor the patient closely for the onset of signs and symptoms, and take such preventive measures as close attention to fluid balance.

Arteriography

Arteriography is an invasive diagnostic procedure in which arterial systems are radiographically evaluated following injection of a contrast medium. Arteriography is performed to evaluate areas of hemorrhage, obstruction, aneurysm, or vascular abnormalities.

Preprocedure care is similar to that for cardiac catheterization. During the procedure itself, a catheter is placed in the femoral, brachial, or carotid artery and passed under fluoroscopic control to the desired vessel. The dye then is injected, the vessel visualized, and x-ray films taken for diagnostic evaluation.

Postprocedure care is analogous to that for cardiac catheterization.

Hemodynamic Monitoring

The Cardiac Cycle and Pressure Waves

As blood flows from chamber to chamber, as valves open and close, and as the myocardium contracts and relaxes, pressures are generated in various parts of the heart. These cardiovascular pressures can be measured and monitored through catheters whose tips are placed in the atria, pulmonary artery, or systemic arteries.

Uses of Hemodynamic Lines

Hemodynamic lines have several uses. They enable you to sample venous and arterial blood without repeated vascular punctures. They provide a way to monitor various waveforms, which can provide clues to patient status. The combination of pulmonary arterial and systemic arterial lines can be used to calculate cardiac output. Most important, these lines enable you to monitor directly various cardiac pressures. Interpretation of these pressures can guide you and the physician in planning and evaluating therapy in shock, fluid overload or deficit, cardiac failure, and other conditions.

Pressure Measurements

The most important cardiac pressure is that of the left ventricle, because it is a major determinant of systemic perfusion. The pressure in the left ventricle just before systole is called the *left ventricular end-diastolic pressure* (LVEDP). This pressure reflects the compliance of the left ventricle, that is, its ability to receive blood from the left atrium during diastole. When left ventricular compliance decreases, the LVEDP rises. Myocardial infarction and left ventricular failure are two examples of conditions in which left ventricular compliance decreases. Direct monitoring of LVEDP would be very helpful in detecting changes in the patient's condition and in guiding optimal fluid therapy in shock. Unfortunately, left ventricular pressure cannot be monitored at the bedside owing to the high potential for thromboembolization directly to the brain or other vital organs.

Correlation of Pressures There is a close correlation between LVEDP and other cardiac pressures.

In the presence of a normal mitral valve, LVEDP is reflected by *left atrial pressure* (LAP). In the person with a normal mitral valve and normal lungs, the LVEDP also is reflected by the pressure in the pulmonary capillary bed (*pulmonary capillary wedge pressure,* PCWP) and the pressure in the pulmonary artery at the end of diastole. This latter pressure sometimes is referred to as the *pulmonary artery end-diastolic pressure* (PAEDP).

This correlation is best understood if you visualize the left ventricle, left atrium, pulmonary capillary bed, and pulmonary artery as one chamber at certain points in the cardiac cycle (see Figure 11–2). When the left ventricle is filling, the mitral valve is open and the left ventricle and left atrium form a common chamber.

Therefore, LVEDP and mean LAP are similar. Moving backwards in the blood circuit, one realizes that since there are no valves between the left atrium and the pulmonary capillary bed, their pressures should be similar, too. Continuing backwards in the vascular circuit, one realizes that when the pulmonic valve is closed, pressures in the pulmonary capillary bed should approximate PAEDP; and in fact, they do, with PAEDP normally less than 5 mm Hg higher than wedge pressures (Kaye 1981). This "unichamber concept" is clinically useful, because it justifies the constant monitoring of PAEDP rather than frequent wedging of the balloon to obtain intermittent PCWPs, which increases the risk of balloon rupture and pulmonary artery trauma. Be aware, however, that this unichamber concept holds true only for patients with normal mitral valve function and no pulmonary disease.

Left atrial pressure can be monitored at the bedside, but a LAP line can be dangerous because it provides a direct path for air or clots to enter the left ventricle and become systemic emboli. The pulmonary capillary and pulmonary arterial pressures can be monitored at the bedside with a balloon-tipped catheter placed in the pulmonary artery. With the ballon deflated, one can measure pulmonary artery systolic, diastolic, and mean pressures with the catheter. When the balloon is inflated, it wedges the catheter in a small distal branch of the pulmonary artery. The pressure recorded is that reflected back from the left atrium through the pulmonary capillary bed. This pressure is the *pulmonary capillary wedge pressure* (PCWP).

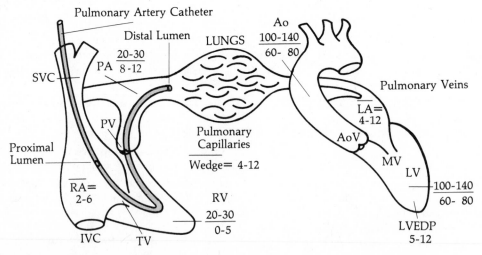

FIGURE 11–2

Normal cardiac pressures. Adapted with permission from unpublished figure, NSI Educational Systems, Inc., Beverly Hills, CA.

The least sensitive indicator of left ventricular pressure is the *central venous pressure* (CVP). It is monitored at the bedside through a catheter whose tip is located at the juncture of the superior vena cava and right atrium, or through one lumen of the balloon-tipped pulmonary artery catheter that opens in the same location. The CVP reflects the pressure in the right atrium and systemic veins. It is affected primarily by changes in right-sided heart pressures and only secondarily by changes in left-sided pressures, so the CVP may be the last cardiac pressure to reflect increased LVEDP. Moreover, because the CVP can be affected by pulmonary disease, pulmonic or tricuspid stenosis, and other right atrial or ventricular abnormalities, an elevated CVP is not necessarily an accurate indication of an elevated LVEDP. The CVP line is safer than the LAP and PA lines. It is used to measure venous pressure, estimate blood volume, obtain venous blood samples, and administer fluids and some medications. It may also be used to monitor the patient in heart failure when PA monitoring is unavailable.

Systemic arterial pressure can be monitored directly through a catheter (arterial line) placed into a major systemic artery.

Values for normal resting cardiac pressures vary somewhat from institution to institution. The following, slightly modified from Daily and Schroeder (1985), may be considered normal values, in millimeters of mercury (mm Hg), as shown in Figure 11–2:

- Superior vena caval or right atrial (RA) pressure: 2–6 mean
- Right ventricular (RV) pressure: 20–30 systolic and 0–5 diastolic
- Pulmonary artery (PA) pressure: 20–30 systolic, 8–12 diastolic, 10–20 mean
- Pulmonary capillary wedge pressure: 4–12 mean
- Left atrial (LA) pressure: 4–12 mean
- Left ventricular (LV) pressure: 100–140 systolic and 60–80 diastolic; left ventricular end-diastolic pressure (LVEDP): 5–12
- Aortic (Ao) pressure: 100–140 systolic, 60–80 diastolic, and 70–90 mean

Central Venous Pressure (CVP) Lines

Insertion The CVP line can be inserted at the bedside by a physician. It usually is inserted percutaneously in the antecubital, internal jugular, or subclavian vein.

The nurse has three primary responsibilities related to insertion of a CVP line: preparing the patient and family, preparing equipment, and assisting and observing.

Preparing the Patient and Family Prior to insertion, whenever possible, explain to the patient and immediate family how the procedure will help in the patient's care. Tell the patient what sensations to expect. Reassure the patient that you will be observing and that you should be told promptly of any discomfort. Consult with the physician before giving an analgesic or sedative, since such drugs can alter baseline pressure measurements. Obtain baseline vital signs. Mark on the patient's chest the reference point for measurements. This point usually is at the fourth intercostal space on the lateral chest wall, midway between the anterior and posterior chest. It is important to mark it so that readings are taken at a consistent level. If they are not, variations in readings may be attributed to changes in the patient's condition when they actually result from changes in the recording technique.

Preparing the Equipment Monitoring equipment usually consists of a specific type and size of catheter, a device to measure pressures, a flush solution and related tubing, and a carpenter's level. Insertion equipment includes local anesthetic, skin preparatory solution, sterile gloves, dressing supplies, and a cutdown tray if indicated.

The measuring device may be a water manometer or a pressure transducer and oscilloscope. The water manometer, commonly used for CVP measurement, is suitable for low pressures (under 40 cm of water), when it is not necessary to see the waveforms. A *transducer* (Figure 11–3) is an instrument that converts pressure waves to electrical energy, which then can be displayed on an oscilloscope. It usually is used for pressures too high for the water manometer or in situations where depiction of the waveform is useful, such as with pulmonary or systemic arterial pressures.

Flush systems consist of a solution (such as heparinized 5% dextrose in water) and a method of irrigating the line. The least desirable irrigation method is a syringe inserted in a stopcock port because of the potential for infection and excessively high flushing pressures. The most desirable method is a continuous low-flow flush device, which is a closed system that infuses solution at a constant slow rate. When you want a rapid flush, you can pull the "tail" on the device and flush the system without breaking sterility.

Details of the equipment and setup procedure vary from unit to unit. In general, before the procedure begins, connect the equipment (except for the catheter itself) together sterilely and securely. Flush air out of the system. If you are using a transducer, balance and

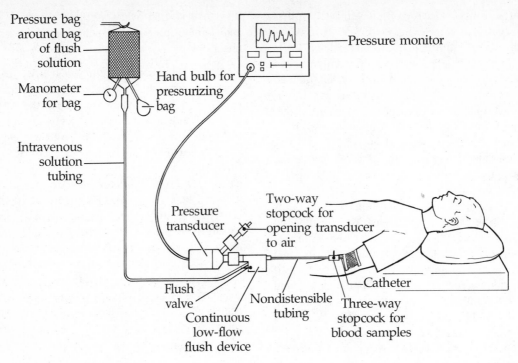

Pressure bag around bag of flush solution

Manometer for bag

Hand bulb for pressurizing bag

Pressure monitor

Intravenous solution tubing

Pressure transducer

Two-way stopcock for opening transducer to air

Flush valve

Continuous low-flow flush device

Nondistensible tubing

Catheter

Three-way stopcock for blood samples

FIGURE 11–3

Pressure monitoring with transducer. Pressure transducer and continuous flush device enlarged to show detail.

calibrate it according to the manufacturer's directions. Label the system with tags at several points: the solution bag or bottle, the tubing near the rate control clamp, and the tubing near stopcocks or medication ports. Critically ill patients often have several hemodynamic and fluid infusion lines. When they are unlabeled, it is easy to confuse them and accidently alter the flow rate or inject medication into the wrong line.

Assisting and Observing To assist the physician, first position the patient as necessary. If the subclavian or internal jugular vein is used, place the patient in reverse Trendelenburg with face turned away from the insertion site. Doing so maximizes ease of entry into the vein and minimizes the danger of air embolism. Also, act as the unsterile person to pour prep solution, hold the bottle of local anesthetic, and open the catheter package. As the line is inserted, observe the patient for pain and cardiopulmonary distress. As soon as blood drips out the end of the catheter, connect it to the system. The physician will dress the site of insertion while you obtain the initial measurement.

Obtaining Accurate Measurements Each time you measure the pressure, follow these steps:

1. Place the patient in the baseline position, that is, the position in which all readings are taken. The usual

position is supine with the bed flat. If necessary for a particular patient, the head of the bed may be elevated, but it should be placed at the same degree of elevation for each reading. If the patient is on a ventilator, you may leave it connected during the reading. Be sure to note "on ventilator" when you record the pressure.

2. Check the level of the measuring device. Use a carpenter's level to make sure the "O" on the manometer or the air–fluid interface of the transducer is level with the reference mark on the patient's chest.

3. Look for and remove any air bubbles in the line or transducer; they can cause a damped, distorted reading or failure to get any reading.

4. Check the patency of the line by observing on the oscilloscope the normal waveform transmitted by the transducer, observing fluctuations in the manometer when it is opened, or aspirating blood from the line.

5. Measure the pressures. Turn the stopcock on the manometer so that fluid flows from the fluid source into the manometer. Let the manometer fill several centimeters above the expected reading, but do not let the upper end of the manometer become contaminated with fluid.

Turn the stopcock to open the line between the manometer and the patient. The fluid level should fall and, after it stops falling, fluctuate with respirations. The average level of the fluid represents the reading. After noting the value, turn the stopcock so the fluid again can flow from the fluid source to the patient.

There are other nursing actions to maintain accurate pressure measurements:

6. To ensure that the catheter is positioned properly, immobilize the extremity.

7. Prevent kinking of the tubing. You will not only increase the accuracy of pressure readings but will also protect your patient from fluctuating dosages of any drugs being administered through the line.

8. To ascertain whether the tip is in the correct location, obtain a chest x-ray after insertion.

Analyzing the Pressures Critically The normal CVP when measured by the manometer method is 2–8 cm H_2O (Sedlock 1980).

As mentioned earlier, CVP also can be monitored by using a transducer connected to the proximal lumen of a flow-directed, balloon-tipped catheter in the pulmonary artery. In this situation, you will be able to record CVP by setting the pressure monitoring switch on mean pressure. When working with a transducer, the normal CVP is 2–6 mm Hg. (This value is equivalent to the normal CVP in cm H_2O, as 1 mm Hg equals 1.36 cm H_2O.)

The central venous pressure is affected by the amount of blood in the right ventricle just before systole *(preload)*, ventricular *contractility*, and the amount of resistance against which the right ventricle must eject blood *(afterload)*.

A low CVP indicates inadequate preload, that is, inadequate venous return, due either to true hypovolemia secondary to actual fluid deficit, or to relative hypovolemia due to excessive vasodilatation.

A high CVP can reflect one or more problems: increased preload, decreased contractility, or increased afterload.

Increased Preload When preload is increased, the ventricle may be unable to pump out the excess fluid efficiently. Preload can be increased by fluid overload, such as in excessive administration of IV fluids, fluid retention in cardiac or renal disease, valvular insufficiency, and left-to-right cardiac shunts—for example, a ventricular septal defect.

Decreased Contractility Contractile force can be diminished in right ventricular infarction, myocarditis, or restrictions to expansion such as cardiac tamponade.

Increased Afterload Right ventricular afterload increases whenever pulmonary vascular resistance increases due to obstruction or pulmonary vasoconstriction. Examples include chronic obstructive lung disease, pulmonary em-

bolism, and other pulmonary disorders. Right ventricular afterload also increases in the presence of mitral or pulmonic stenosis.

There are several principles to remember in interpreting pressure data:

1. Compare the values obtained at this time to the patient's normal values rather than an arbitrary standard. If the patient has undergone cardiac catheterization within the past few months, pressures obtained at that time may be used as baselines. If not, you must predict general values on the basis of your knowledge of the so-called normal values and your patient's pathology. For example, you would expect the patient with a narrowed tricuspid valve to have an elevated CVP. The patient with chronic obstructive lung disease probably would have both high PA pressures and CVP.

2. Single readings are not as significant as the trend of values.

3. Consider the pressures in relation to each other. If one pressure is measured with a manometer and another with a transducer, you may want to convert them to the same scale. To convert millimeters of mercury (Hg) to centimeters of water, multiply by 1.36. Remember that abnormal values are not always due to primary pathology of the monitored chamber. For example, an elevated CVP in association with normal or low PA pressures suggests that the cause lies between these two sites, that is, with the pulmonary valve, right ventricle, or tricuspid valve. In contrast, an elevated CVP in conjunction with elevated PA pressures suggests that the cause is pulmonary disease, left-sided heart disease, or fluid overload.

4. Remember that a normal value does not necessarily indicate an absence of pathology. For instance, a patient may have a normal CVP but be intensely vasoconstricted due to hypovolemia.

Observing the Waveforms Periodically If the patient is being monitored with a transducer, waveforms should be periodically observed. The CVP will display the characteristic atrial waveforms. The atrial curve consists of three ascending and two descending waves (Figure 11–4). The *a wave* is produced by atrial contraction. The *x descent* occurs as atrial pressure drops during atrial diastole. It is possible that the onset of ventricular contraction contributes to this descent by tugging downward on the atrioventricular valves. The *c wave* may result from bulging of the valves into the atria during ventricular contraction. The c wave may also result from the impact of the carotid arterial pulse on the nearby jugular vein. The *v wave* occurs as the atria fill and their pressure increases. The *y descent* shows the rapid drop in atrial pressure after the atrioventricular

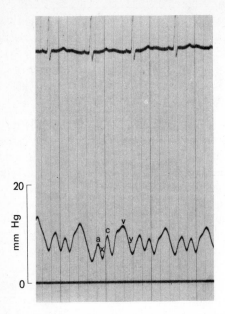

FIGURE 11–4

RA pressure waveform showing *a, c, and v waves* with *x and y descents*. Note that the recorded waveforms are delayed from the corresponding electrical event in the P-QRS-T. This delay occurs because of the delay in recording pressure events through a long catheter. (From Daily E, Schroeder J: *Techniques in bedside hemodynamic monitoring,* 3d ed. St Louis: Mosby, 1985.)

valves open and the rapid, passive ventricular filling phase ensues.

Changes in waveforms can be clues to malposition of the catheter tip, obstructions in the line, or changes in the patient's clinical state.

Prevention of Complications   Anticipate and prevent complications by taking the appropriate nursing measures. The most common complications associated with CVP catheters are pneumothorax, infection, fluid overload, and poor infusion of fluid.

Pneumothorax   Pneumothorax may occur during insertion of the CVP line into the subclavian or jugular vein. The reason for this complication is that the apex of the lung extends above the clavicle. Because it is in close proximity to these veins, it may be punctured accidentally during insertion. For information on the recognition and treatment of pneumothorax, see Chapter 8.

Infection   Maintain scrupulous sterile technique. Observe the insertion site every 8 hours for signs of inflammation. Clean the site and change the dressing at least daily. Check the patient's temperature at least once every 8 hours, and call unexplained elevations to the physician's attention.

Fluid Overload   Fluids commonly are administered only via the CVP or peripheral venous lines. To prevent accidental fluid overload via a CVP line, use measuring chambers and small-drop infusion sets.

Poor Infusion of Fluid   This problem occurs most commonly because of partial obstruction of the catheter tip due to fibrin deposition, but it may also occur due to kinking of the catheter. If the catheter is not kinked, try to aspirate fluid from the line or to irrigate it gently. Do not attempt to clear the line by a forceful manual flush, because you may cause a thrombus on the tip of the catheter to embolize to the pulmonary vessels.

Pulmonary Arterial (PA) Lines

PA and pulmonary capillary wedge (PCWP) pressures can be monitored at the bedside through a balloon-tipped, flow-directed catheter placed in the pulmonary artery. This type of catheter sometimes is referred to generically by the name of one specific brand of catheter, the *Swan-Ganz* pulmonary artery catheter.

A variety of catheters is available. The double-lumen catheter has two openings, one at the distal end and one for balloon inflation. With it, one can record PA pressures and PCWP only. The triple-lumen catheter has an additional lumen (proximal lumen) that opens in the right atrium, so it has the additional capability of recording CVP. The quadruple-lumen catheter has a fourth lumen, which connects with a temperature-sensitive thermistor on the end of the catheter. With this pulmonary artery catheter, one can record the pressures in the pulmonary artery, pulmonary capillaries, and right atrium, as well as calculate CO by the thermodilution method. Other catheters available include a multipurpose catheter, which enables not only pressure recordings but also electrical pacing of the right heart, and an $S\overline{V}O_2$ monitoring catheter, which allows continuous monitoring of venous oxygen saturation ($S\overline{V}O_2$), a sensitive indicator of tissue oxygen consumption.

Insertion   The catheter is inserted by a physician, percutaneously or via cutdown. The usual insertion site is the subclavian, internal jugular, brachial, or femoral vein. Preparation of the patient and family is similar to that for CVP line insertion. Preparation of the equipment is more elaborate, as each pressure-monitoring lumen must be attached to a heparinized, pressurized, calibrated monitoring system. Details of this setup vary, depending on how many pressures you plan to monitor with how many transducers and depending on the protocol for setup used in your unit. The general steps involved in setup include maintaining a sterile connection of the components of the monitoring system, flushing air from the tubing and transducers, balancing the system to zero, and calibrating it to a known calibration factor. (Opening the transducer to air and balancing to zero negates pressure contributions from the atmosphere so that only cardiovascular pressures will be measured. Calibration is accomplished by introducing a known pressure into the system and verifying that the readout is correct, to assure that the cardiovascular pressures will be recorded accurately.) Finally, the balloon on the catheter is submerged in sterile fluid in a basin and inflated to check for leaks, then deflated. The catheter is then filled with the heparinized solution and connected to the monitoring system. Most protocols call for lidocaine at the bedside because of the risk of ventricular irritability.

After the vessel is entered, the catheter is usually advanced under fluoroscopic and ECG observation, with the balloon deflated until it reaches the right atrium. At that point, the balloon is partially inflated, and blood flow inside the heart carries it though the tricuspid valve into the right ventricle, through the pulmonic valve into the pulmonary artery. The balloon is then inflated to enable floating the catheter through the pulmonary arterial tree until it wedges itself in a small pulmonary artery. The balloon then is allowed to deflate.

During insertion, the nurse's primary responsibility is to observe the patient for complications, which can include: ventricular dysrhythmias due to irritation of the heart by the catheter tip, especially when the tip is located in the right ventricle; hematoma at the insertion site; and pneumothorax if a subclavian approach is used and the lung is punctured. An additional responsibility is to observe the waveforms appearing on the monitor screen as the catheter passes through each chamber. Each chamber has a distinct waveform that indicates the catheter's exact location and progress.

Once the line is inserted, it is the nurse's responsibility to secure a portable chest x-ray to ensure correct placement of the catheter tip, to obtain accurate measurements, and to prevent or minimize complications.

Right Atrial (RA) Pressure The normal RA pressure is 2–6 mm Hg. The normal waveform includes *a, c,* and *v* waves (see Figure 11–4). Waveform interpretation and causes of abnormal pressure readings are reviewed in the previous section on CVP lines.

Right Ventricular (RV) Pressure RV pressure normally is monitored only during PA catheter insertion. Normal RV pressure is 20–30 mm Hg systolic, with an end-diastolic pressure of 2–6 mm Hg.

The RV waveform demonstrates a gradually increasing pressure during ventricular filling, with a small bulge at the time of atrial contraction (Figure 11–5). After the tricuspid valve closes, the pressure increases sharply

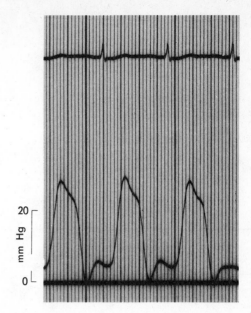

FIGURE 11–5

Normal right ventricular pressure tracing. (From Daily E, Schroeder J: *Techniques in bedside hemodynamic monitoring,* 3d ed. St Louis: Mosby, 1985.)

during systole until it causes the pulmonic valve to open. Then it peaks and drops rapidly, until the pulmonic valve closes and diastole begins.

There is one other situation in which you should be alert to the appearance of an RV waveform, and that is once the PA catheter has been placed in the pulmonary artery. In that situation, the appearance of an RV waveform signifies that the catheter has migrated backwards into the right ventricle and may precipitate the onset of possible ventricular ectopy resulting from irritation of the ventricular wall due to the catheter flipping around inside the ventricle. At times, in fact, the catheter may slip forward into the pulmonary artery and backward into the right ventricle, alternately producing PA and RV waveforms.

PA Pressures When the catheter is in the pulmonary artery with the balloon deflated, you can monitor systolic, diastolic, and mean PA pressures by placing the monitor switch on the appropriate setting. Normal PA pressures are: 20–30 systolic and 8–12 diastolic, both measured in mm Hg. It is important to realize that pulmonary artery pressures normally fluctuate in critically ill patients. According to research by Nemens and Woods (1982), defining a change of 5 mm Hg in PA systolic or mean pressure or a change of 4 mm Hg in PA diastolic pressure as clinically significant is likely to be valid for most patients.

The pulmonary arterial waveform has a characteristic

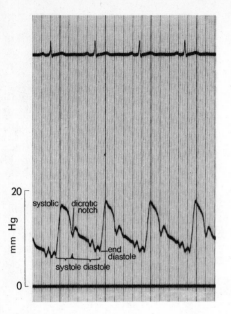

FIGURE 11–6

PA pressure waveform showing phases of systole, dicrotic notch (pulmonic valve closure), and diastole. Normally, PA end-diastole closely represents LVEDP. (From Daily E, Schroeder J: *Techniques in bedside hemodynamic monitoring,* 3d ed. St Louis: Mosby, 1985.)

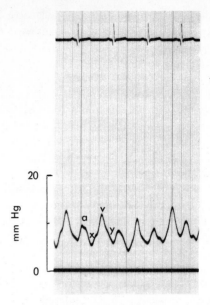

FIGURE 11–7

Normal pulmonary artery wedge pressure waveform showing *a* and *v* waves and *x* and *y* descents. (From Daily E, Schroeder J: *Techniques in bedside hemodynamic monitoring,* 3d ed. St Louis: Mosby, 1985.)

appearance (Figure 11–6). After the beginning of systole, the wave form shows a rapid upstroke during ventricular ejection, followed by a more gradual downstroke. The downstroke is interrupted by the dicrotic notch, signifying the closure of the pulmonic valve and the onset of diastole.

PA pressures reflect both pulmonary blood volume and pulmonary vascular resistance. Low PA pressures indicate hypovolemia due to either fluid loss or vasodilation. Elevated PA pressures can reflect increased pulmonary blood volume or increased pulmonary vascular resistance.

Increased Pulmonary Blood Volume This can occur in fluid overload, intracardiac shunts, mitral valve disease, left ventricular failure, or cardiac tamponade or constrictive pericarditis.

Increased Pulmonary Vascular Resistance This situation can occur when there is an obstruction to blood flow, such as in pulmonary embolism, when pulmonary hypertension is present in cardiac or pulmonary disease, or when pulmonary vessels vasoconstrict due to hypoxemia or hypercapnia.

PCWP When the balloon on the tip of the pulmonary artery catheter is inflated, the catheter tip is

moved along by blood flow until it wedges in a small pulmonary artery. The inflated balloon in effect "blocks" the recording of pressure behind it in the pulmonary artery and allows recording only of pressures forward from it, that is, the pressures in the pulmonary capillaries themselves. As there are no valves between the pulmonary capillaries and the left atrium, wedge pressure reflects mean LAP.

The normal PCWP is 4–12 mm Hg. A change of 4 mm Hg is likely to be clinically significant in most patients (Nemens and Woods 1982).

The wedge pressure waveform (Figure 11–7) is similar to the LA waveform (Figure 11–8) in that it displays the typical *a* and *v* waves of atrial contraction and ventricular systole. Normally, the *c* wave, which reflects bulging of the mitral valve during early ventricular systole, is so small it cannot be seen.

Decreased PCWP values are seen in hypovolemia, whether due to true fluid loss or to vasodilation. Increased PCWP values can indicate increased preload, decreased contractility, or increased afterload.

Increased Preload When more blood returns to the left ventricle than it can pump out, left ventricular end-diastolic volume and LVEDP increase. This increase is reflected in an elevated wedge pressure. This situation can occur in volume overload due to excessive intrave-

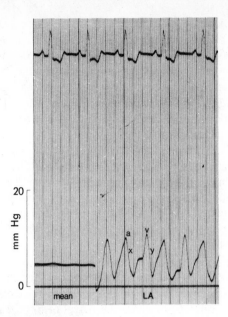

FIGURE 11–8

LA pressure waveform demonstrating similarity to PAW waveform. This pressure is normal. (From Daily E, Schroeder J: *Techniques in bedside hemodynamic monitoring,* 3d ed. St Louis: Mosby, 1985.)

nous solutions, fluid retention in cardiac or renal failure, aortic or mitral valvular disease, or intracardiac shunts.

Decreased Contractility Decreased left ventricular (LV) contractility can occur in myocardial ischemia or infarction, ventricular aneurysms, myocarditis, acid–base imbalances, cardiomyopathy, or restrictions to filling, such as cardiac tamponade.

Increased Afterload Resistance to LV ejection (increased systemic vascular resistance) will elevate wedge pressures. Situations in which this can occur include systemic hypertension and administration of vasoconstricting agents, and outlet obstructions such as coarctation of the aorta and aortic stenosis.

Measures to Obtain Accurate Pressures As with a CVP line, the nurse should ensure that the transducer is leveled and the line patent before attempting to record PA and wedge pressures. The reference point on the patient's chest (the phlebostatic axis, at the 4th intercostal space, mid-axillary line) should be leveled with the air–fluid interface in the transducer. Patency of the line can be checked by observing the normal waveform on the oscilloscope before recording the pressures.

If you are using a transducer, you will be able to measure systolic, diastolic, and mean pressures. You can obtain these pressures for the pulmonary artery by placing the switch on the pressure monitor on the appropriate settings. To measure pulmonary capillary pressure, place the switch on "mean." Inflate the balloon with no more than the specified amount of air for that size catheter. Insert the air until the characteristic PCWP wave form (containing *a* and *v* waves) appears on the oscilloscope. To keep the balloon inflated while you read the pressure from the monitor, hold the syringe in place or use the lever on the catheter's end to lock the air in place. After taking the reading, be sure to remove the syringe or release the lock so the balloon can deflate.

Numerous systems problems can occur to interfere with the recording of accurate pressures. Among the most common are damping, inappropriately high or low pressures, catheter whip artifact, and respiratory fluctuations. *Damping* results from poor transmission of the pressure wave to the oscilloscope and is recognized by decreased amplitude of the waveform. Possible causes include partial occlusion of the catheter tip by a clot, placement of the catheter tip against the vessel wall, and air bubbles in the line or transducer. To avoid damping, use a pressurized, heparinized, low-flow flush system, periodically rapid-flushing it. Close the line off to the patient and remove all air bubbles backwards through the system. If damping occurs, try aspirating the line for blood, having the patient cough, changing the patient's position, checking the system for air bubbles and removing them, and/or flushing the line. If none of those measures works, the line may need to be repositioned by the physician.

Inappropriately high or low pressures can be caused by improper leveling, loose connections, or migration of the catheter tip. To prevent them, always level the transducer before measuring pressures, and connect the system components securely. If inappropriate pressures occur, it helps to double-check the patient's position relative to the transducer, check the connections and tighten them if necessary, and alert the physician if inappropriate waveforms indicate the catheter tip has migrated from the pulmonary artery so it can be repositioned.

Catheter fling is an artifact of excessive movement of the catheter. To compensate for it, record only average (mean) pressures.

Respiratory variation in pressure recordings results from transmission of normal respiratory pressure fluctuations to the monitoring system. Record pressures at end-expiration (see Chapter 9 for details). Alternatively, if the patient is on a ventilator, try taking him or her off the ventilator to record the pressures, since the ventilator produces positive pressure. This latter measure should be done only if the patient can tolerate being off the ventilator, and only if it is acceptable to your colleagues, as the issue of whether to record pressures on or off the ventilator is controversial. Some professionals feel that the "true" pressures are those recorded off the ventilator, while others believe off-ventilator pressures are somewhat irrelevant, since the on-ventilator pressures represent the actual pressures under which the cardiovascular system is functioning the majority of the time. Until the issue is resolved, follow the prevailing practice in your unit, and remember that the consistency of measurement and trend of pressures are much more important than individual values in assessing the patient's clinical picture.

Cardiac Output (CO) Determinations   CO is the amount of blood ejected by the heart per minute. It is the product of heart rate times stroke volume. Stroke volume, the amount of blood ejected from the heart with each heartbeat, in turn depends on preload, contractility, and afterload. *Preload* is the volume of blood in the ventricles just prior to systole, that is, the end-diastolic volume. According to the Frank-Starling mechanism, an increased diastolic volume causes greater lengthening of the cardiac muscle fibers, which in turn provokes increased muscle shortening during contraction. Therefore, within a physiologic range of muscle stretching, an increased ventricular diastolic volume (increased preload) causes increased CO. *Contractility* is an inherent property of the ventricles that enables them to shorten muscle fibers independent of the Frank-Starling mechanism. *Afterload,* the third major determinant of stroke volume, is the impedance to ejection of blood from the ventricle. As afterload increases, resistance to ejection increases, and CO falls.

At the bedside, the most common method of measuring CO is the thermodilution method, using a balloon-tipped, flow-directed thermodilution catheter. A known amount of solution, at a known temperature, is injected into the right atrial port of the catheter. A thermistor in the pulmonary artery measures the resulting temperature change of the blood. A computer then calculates cardiac output.

To measure CO, a thermodilution output computer is attached to its connector on the end of the thermodilution catheter and is calibrated and checked. The injectate is prepared by drawing sterile solution, usually 5% dextrose in water, into plastic syringes. The best syringes to use are those that have finger rings on the barrel and a thumb ring on the plunger, because they allow you to hold the syringe without handling the barrel and therefore transmitting your body heat to the injectate. The injectate used may be either cold or at room temperature (Shellock and Riedinger 1983). The temperature of the injectate is fed into the computer.

To inject the solution, attach an injectate syringe to the three-way stopcock connected to the proximal (right atrial) port of the catheter. Turn the stopcock to shut off the routine drip to this port. Inject the solution evenly and as rapidly as possible. Then read the CO measurement off the computer. Usually, three CO determinations are made and the values averaged to obtain the measurement.

Normal cardiac output is 4–8 liters per minute. As these values do not take into account body size, however, a more meaningful measurement is cardiac index. The *cardiac index* equals the cardiac output divided by the body surface area, which can be determined using a Dubois body surface chart. The normal cardiac index is 2.5–4.0 liters/minute/meter^2.

If the individual measurements vary more than 25% from each other, suspect an error in measurements. Possible sources of error include varying injectate temperatures, due to touching the barrel of the syringe or injecting more slowly than 4 seconds; varying injectate amounts, due to inaccurate filling of the syringes; and catheter tip in the right ventricle or wedge position rather than in the pulmonary artery.

For discussion of the significance of changes in CO, please see Chapter 13.

Complications of PA Catheters   Complications of PA catheters include ventricular dysrhythmias, pulmonary infarction, thromboemboli, air emboli, and balloon rupture, as well as the problems of hemorrhage, infection, and patient discomfort common to any hemodynamic monitoring line.

Ventricular Dysrhythmias   Ventricular dysrhythmias can be caused by displacement of the PA catheter into the right ventricle. This displacement will cause a change in the contour of the waveform, from the typical PA tracing to an RV tracing. This problem again emphasizes the need to keep an eye on the waveforms displayed on the oscilloscope. Notify the physician, and inflate the balloon to see if it will float back up into the pulmonary artery. Repositioning the patient on the left side also may help the catheter float back into the pulmonary artery. If it does not, the physician will need to reposition the catheter. After repositioning, get a new chest x-ray to verify catheter placement.

Pulmonary Infarction   Pulmonary infarction may result if the PA catheter balloon is left inflated or if the deflated balloon spontaneously wedges itself in the capillary bed. Adhere to the safety precautions described below under the problem of balloon rupture. You may be able to dislodge a spontaneouly wedged catheter by having the patient cough or turn. If these measures are unsuccessful, notify the physician promptly.

Thromboemboli To minimize the risk of thromboemboli, utilize a continuous low-flow flush system whenever possible. Flush lines after blood samples are drawn, including flushing the stopcock port from which the sample was obtained. Also flush promptly if the tracing becomes damped (that is, the amplitude of the waveforms decreases). If you are unable to aspirate blood or infuse fluid, the line may be clotted. Do not attempt to clear the line by a forceful manual flush because you may cause a thrombus to embolize.

Air Emboli There are several ways to prevent air emboli. Be sure that air is flushed from the line before initial use. During insertion of the PA line in the subclavian vein or jugular vein, place the patient's head below the level of the thorax. If you spot air bubbles in the line, remove them with a needle and syringe or shut the line off to the patient and flush it. Whenever it is necessary to open the transducer to air (as in balancing it or removing blood that has leaked into the dome), first turn off the stopcock to the patient.

Ballooon Rupture The PA line presents another source of potential air emboli from breakage of the balloon used to obtain the PCWP. Minimize the risk of breakage by inserting no more air than appropriate for the specific size catheter, by releasing the air after the reading, and by aspirating before injecting air for subsequent readings. You should feel a slight resistance to inflation of the balloon. If the balloon breaks, you will know because the air will enter with minimal resistance, no wedge tracing will appear, and blood may leak out of the balloon lumen. If you suspect breakage, turn the lumen off to the patient and notify the physician. The small amount of air in the balloon is not dangerous, but repeated injections of air by well-meaning misinformed staff can be unsafe.

Arterial Lines

Arterial lines are catheters placed in systemic arteries to facilitate recording of continuous, accurate data about BP in the patient who has an unstable hemodynamic status, and to allow frequent sampling of arterial blood gases without the need for repeated arterial punctures. Arterial lines commonly are placed percutaneously in the radial, brachial, or femoral arteries.

To assist with insertion, prepare the patient as described in the section on CVP lines and set up a pressurized, heparinized pressure monitoring system. If the site chosen is the radial artery, either you or the physician should perform an *Allen's test* of the patency of the ulnar artery. To perform this test, have the patient make a fist, and then occlude both the radial and ulnar arteries. Have the patient open her or his hand, and release the pressure on the ulnar artery. If the hand pinks up quickly, you can assume that good collateral blood flow is available to the hand in the event the radial artery becomes occluded.

Once the line is inserted, recording of pressures and observation of the arterial waveform become nursing responsibilities. Normal arterial pressures vary widely; a general range of aortic systolic pressure is 100–140 mm Hg, with diastolic pressures of 60–80 mm Hg, and mean pressures of 70–90 mm Hg. Catheters terminating not in the central aorta but instead more distally will show higher systolic pressures. Systolic pressure in the femoral artery, for example, may be as much as 20 mm higher than aortic pressure, due to the amplification of the pulse pressure wave during systole (Daily and Schroeder 1985).

The normal arterial waveform has a sharp upstroke and a more gradual downstroke with an evident dicrotic notch, due to a small rise in pressure that occurs at the time of aortic valve closure (Figure 11–9). End-diastole should be clearly seen.

To ensure accurate recordings, balance and calibrate the transducer according to the manufacturer's recommended procedure at least every 8 hours. Also compare the recorded measurement to the blood pressure ob-

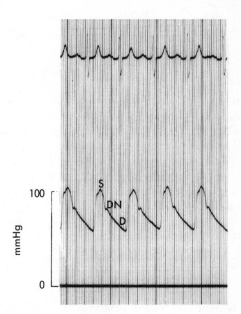

FIGURE 11–9

Normal arterial pressure tracing. S = systole, DN = dicrotic notch, D = diastole. (From Daily E, Schroeder J: *Techniques in bedside hemodynamic monitoring,* 3d ed. St Louis: Mosby, 1985.)

tained with a sphygmomanometer at least every 8 hours. Remember that many factors can give you discrepancies between the cuff BP and arterial line. Among the most common are wrong cuff size, dysrhythmias, peripheral vasoconstriction or vasospasm, and unbalanced or uncalibrated equipment.

Arterial lines share with PA lines the problems of damping, spurious readings, thrombosis, and infection. Exsanguination also can occur with arterial lines if a stopcock port is accidentally left open after an arterial blood sample is drawn. The blood in the artery is under such high pressure that a patient can lose a significant amount of blood if this occurs or if connections in the system are loose. For this reason, the limb with the arterial line should always remain uncovered and pressure alarms should be set to alert you if accidental disconnection occurs. In addition, when the line is removed, you should maintain firm pressure on the site for at least 5 minutes to prevent hematoma formation due to high intravascular pressure.

REFERENCES

Benner P and Tanner C: Clinical judgment: How expert nurses use intuition. *Am J Nurs* 1987; 87:23–31.

Bommer WJ: Analyzing blood flow with echocardiography. *Diagnostic Imaging* 1985a; 5:76–79.

Bommer WJ: Basic principles of flow imaging. *Echocardiography* 1985b; 11:501–509.

Byrne C et al.: *Laboratory tests: Implications for nurses and other allied health professionals.* Menlo Park, CA: Addison-Wesley, 1981.

Chen J: Chest roentgenography. In Hurst J et al.: *The Heart, arteries, and veins,* 6th ed. New York: McGraw-Hill, 1986.

Daily E, Schroeder J: *Techniques in bedside hemodynamic monitoring,* 3d ed. St Louis: Mosby, 1985.

DeMaria A et al.: Doppler flow imaging: Another step in the evolution of cardiac ultrasound. *Echocardiography* 1985; 2(6):495–500.

Forrester JS et al.: Functional significance of regional ischemic contraction abnormalities. *Circ* 1976; 54:64.

Galen R: The enzyme diagnosis of myocardial infarction. *Prog Human Pathol* 1975; 6:141–155.

Galen R: Enzymes in the diagnosis of myocardial infarction. *Heart Lung* 1981; 10:484–485.

Guyton A: *Textbook of medical physiology,* 7th ed. Philadelphia: Saunders, 1986.

Higgins CB et al.: Magnetic resonance imaging of the cardiovascular system. *Prog Cardiol* 1985; 109:136–151.

Horowitz SF et al.: Complementary roles of cardiac ultrasound and cardiovascular nuclear medicine. *Sem Nuclear Med* 1980; 10:94–105.

Kaye W: Invasive monitoring techniques. In *Textbook of advanced cardiac life support,* pp. XIII–1–32, eds McIntyre K, Lewis A. Dallas: American Heart Association, 1981.

Kelber M Sr: Cardiac enzymes. In *Diagnostics,* pp. 99–133. Springhouse, PA: Intermed Communications, 1986.

Mauldin N: Doppler ultrasonography. In *Diagnostics,* pp. 939–943. Springhouse, PA: Intermed Communications, 1986.

Nemens E, Woods S: Normal fluctuations in pulmonary artery and pulmonary capillary wedge pressures in acutely ill patients. *Heart Lung* 1982; 11:393–398.

Oldendorf WH, Oldendorf JR: CT, NMR and PET: Modern diagnostic imaging techniques in medicine. *Am J Cont Ed Nurs* 1985; 1:26–30.

Pantaleo N et al.: Thallium myocardial scintigraphy and its use in the assessment of coronary artery disease. *Heart Lung* 1981; 10:61–70.

Sanderson R, Kurth C (eds): *The cardiac patient,* 2d ed. Philadelphia: Saunders, 1983.

Sedlock S: Interpretation of hemodynamic pressures and recognition of complications. *Crit Care Nurse* (November/December) 1980; 39–54.

Shellock F, Riedinger M: Reproducibility and accuracy of using room-temperature vs. ice-temperature injectate for thermodilution cardiac output determination. *Heart Lung* 1983; 12:175–176.

Strong A: Cardiac radiography. In *Diagnostics,* pp. 900–902. Springhouse, PA: Intermed Communications, 1986.

Wellens HJ: Value and limitations of programmed electrical stimulation of the heart in patients with ventricular tachycardia. *Circ* 1972; 46:216.

Zeluff G et al.: Evaluation of the coronary arteries and myocardium by radionuclide imaging. *Heart Lung* 1980; 9:344–348.

SUPPLEMENTAL READING

Abbott N, Scanlon-Trump E: Infection related to physiologic monitoring: Venous and arterial catheters. *Heart Lung* 1983; 12:28–34.

Criss E: Digital subtraction angiography. *Am J Nurs* (Nov) 1982; 1706–1707.

Daily E, Schroeder J: *Hemodynamic waveforms: Exercises in identification and analysis.* St Louis: Mosby, 1983.

Gershan J: Effect of positive end-expiratory pressure on capillary wedge pressure. *Heart Lung* 1983; 12:143–147.

Grose B et al.: Effect of backrest position on cardiac output measurements by the thermodilution method in acutely ill patients. *Heart Lung* 1981; 10:661–665.

Kannell W, Dawber T: Contributors to coronary risk: Ten years later. *Heart Lung* 1982; 11:60–64.

Kaye W: Catheter- and infusion-related sepsis: The nature of the problem and its prevention. *Heart Lung* 1982; 11:221–228.

Laulive J: Pulmonary artery pressures and position changes in the critically ill adult. *Dimen Crit Care Nurs* 1982; 1:27–34.

Spaccavento L, Hawley H: Infections associated with intra-arterial lines. *Heart Lung* 1982; 11:118–122.

12

Dysrhythmias and Conduction Defects

CLINICAL INSIGHT

Domain: Administering and monitoring therapeutic interventions and regimens

Competency: Administering medications accurately and safely: Monitoring untoward effects, reactions, therapeutic responses, toxicities, and incompatibilities

With patients in precarious physiologic status, the ability to titrate multiple pharmacologic agents to maintain vital functions within normal limits often becomes a determining factor in patient survival. Often—but not always—medication administration falls within prescribed protocols; at other times, the nurse may be functioning in uncharted seas with new or experimental therapies.

Potent medications with a slim margin of safety are the rule rather than the exception in critical care, and a patient's life may depend on the nurse's knowledge of appropriate use of these powerful agents. In the following exemplar, from Crabtree and Jorgenson (1986, pp. 158–159), a nurse challenges a physician to expand his tunnel vision and reconsider an order for a medication, which, given the patient's history, could be lethal to her.

This lady came in with an MI, and this resident after

working with these people liked to push IV propranolol with anybody who has an acute cardiac event. He felt that the woman was having an acute MI, but he was not seeing the multiple problems associated with this. He was seeing an acute MI; he was really treating acute MI's, with this IV Inderal, which was contraindicated for various reasons. I think that it's a good drug in its right use. And I think that they've shown, . . . studies have shown propranolol in acute infarcts can limit the infarct size, but you can't use it on somebody that has severe COPD, who has heart block, and is in pulmonary edema. I think those are all strong contraindication to its use. He didn't look at the patient, because in this case, he was telling me to give this woman 1 mg of propranolol. The woman was bolt upright in bed and gasping. And she would just shake her head yes or no; she just didn't have enough air to say more than that. And I was trying to tell the resident, don't do that, because she was obviously in pulmonary edema. She was a terrible smoker. She had lung problems. And when she first came in, she had a prolonged PR interval, and as I was sitting there disagreeing with this doctor, she started going into a 2:1 and by the time I'm done giving my little dissertation . . . she's going into third-degree heart block. I said I could not do these things because—and I listed the reasons why I felt uncomfortable being forced to give this drug. And I said, le-

gally I am . . . responsible if I would inject this, and I had drawn up the medication and I said, if you feel strongly, you can do it.

Critically ill patients are subject to a wide variety of dysrhythmias, which range from inconsequential to lethal. Since the inception of ECG monitoring, nurses have assumed increasing responsibility for accurate recognition and rapid termination of life-threatening dysrhythmias. And, as illustrated in the Clinical Insight, nurses also play a key role in dysrhythmia prevention.

This chapter shows you the mechanics of analyzing the ECG. It also assists you in recognizing and responding appropriately to the dysrhythmias and conduction defects you are most likely to encounter in clinical practice. Remember that the monitor is but a tool in patient care. Focus on the patient, not just the monitor!

Dysrhythmia Diagnosis

ECG Recording

Contraction of the cardiac chambers is provoked by an electrical stimulus. The initiation and propagation of this stimulus can be recorded on an electrocardiogram (ECG).

12-Lead Electrocardiogram The standard electrocardiogram consists of six limb leads and six precordial leads, each of which has a slightly different orientation toward the heart. The limb leads are I, II, III, AVR, AVL, and AVF. They look at the heart in the frontal plane. The six precordial leads are V_1 through V_6. They give a transverse view of cardiac activity.

Leads I, II, and III, called *standard limb leads,* create Einthoven's triangle (Figure 12–1). In lead I, the machine reads the right arm (RA) electrode as negative and the left arm (LA) electrode as positive. In lead II, it reads the RA electrode as negative and the left leg (LL) as positive. In lead III, it reads the LA as negative and the LL as positive. Each of these leads measures the difference in potential between two electrodes. The standard limb leads therefore are called *bipolar* leads.

In contrast, the remaining limb leads and the precordial leads are *unipolar* leads, that is, they measure the actual potential under one electrode. If the electrodes from which these leads are recorded are connected to a

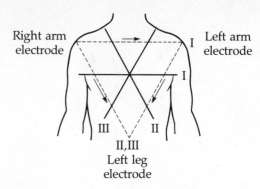

FIGURE 12–1

Standard limb leads, demonstrating Einthoven's triangle. The three dashed lines represent the leads as recorded and are labeled to show the direction of current, from negative to positive poles. The solid lines represent the shifting of these axes (without altering their direction) so that they intersect at the zero point, the heart. The lines are labeled at their positive poles.

common terminal, its potential is zero. This common electrode is called the *neutral* or *indifferent electrode*. If this electrode is connected to one pole of a galvanometer, an electrode connected to the galvanometer's other pole will record the true potential under itself. This electrode is called the *exploring electrode*.

Leads I, II, and III form an equilateral triangle whose apices are the right arm, left arm, and left leg electrodes. These electrodes are considered to be electrically equidistant from the heart, which is at zero potential. Because a unipolar lead records the difference between the common electrode at zero potential and the exploring electrode, it measures the difference between the center of the heart and the exploring electrode also.

For the augmented limb leads (AVR, AVL, and AVF) (Figure 12–2), the machine reads one electrode as pos-

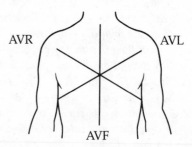

FIGURE 12–2

Augmented limb leads. Leads are labeled at their positive poles.

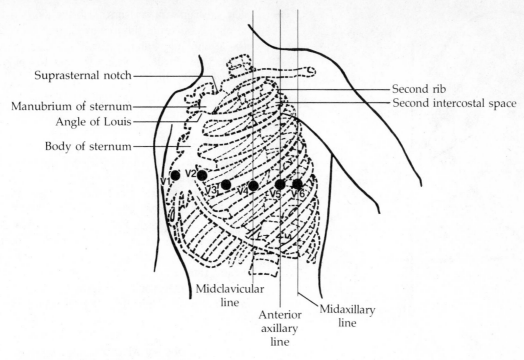

Suprasternal notch

Manubrium of sternum

Angle of Louis

Body of sternum

Second rib
Second intercostal space

V1 V2
V3 V4 V5 V6

Midclavicular
line

Anterior
axillary
line

Midaxillary
line

FIGURE 12–3

Placement of precordial (chest) leads. Positions of the precordial electrode: V_1, fourth intercostal space at right sternal border; V_2, fourth intercostal space at left sternal border; V_3, midway between V_2 and V_4; V_4, fifth intercostal space at midclavicular line; V_5, directly lateral to V_4 at anterior axillary line; V_6, directly lateral to V_5 at midaxillary line.

itive and combines the remaining two electrodes to create the neutral electrode. For example, to record AVR, the right arm electrode is read as positive and the left arm and left leg electrodes are joined to form the neutral electrode. Each augmented lead measures the difference in potential between the center of the heart and the limb wearing the positive electrode.

The remaining six leads (V_1 through V_6) also are unipolar leads (Figure 12–3). A separate exploring electrode is placed at different positions on the precordium, and the right arm, left arm, and left leg electrodes collectively serve to produce a zero potential reference point at the center of the heart.

The twelve leads intersect at the heart, thus providing 12 views of the heart, six frontal and six transverse (Figure 12–4). Occasionally the exploring electrode is moved to positions on the right chest for additional lead placements when a right ventricular infarction is suspected.

Bedside Cardiac Monitoring Modifications of the standard 12 leads are used for routine cardiac monitoring at the bedside. Specifics of monitors vary from man-

ufacturer to manufacturer. The following general guidelines will help you work with a variety of models.

The bedside monitor consists of a monitor console, a patient cable, and electrode wires that can be connected to disposable electrodes. The console contains an oscilloscope screen to display the tracing and various buttons and switches to obtain the tracing. In most units, the bedside monitors also are connected to displays at the nurses' station or central monitoring area.

When you are notified of an admission, turn the monitor on with the power switch to let it warm up. Connect electrodes to the electrode wires. Connect the electrode wires to the patient cable and plug the cable into the monitor itself. Check that the following switches are on their standard settings. The *sweep speed switch* controls the rate at which the beam traverses the screen; its usual setting is 25 mm per second. The *filter switch* controls the amount of external interference in the tracing. It has two settings, "diagnostic" and "monitor." The usual setting for routine monitoring is "monitor" because it filters out most of the muscle artifact.

a

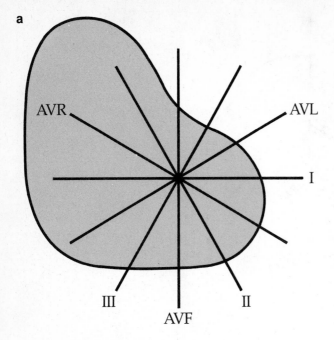

b

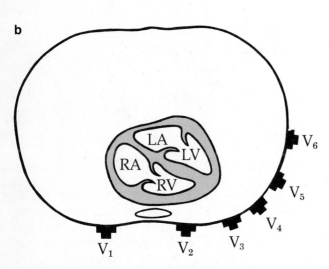

FIGURE 12–4

ECG views of the heart. **a,** Frontal plane (hexaxial reference system). Leads are labeled at their positive poles. **b,** Horizontal plane (precordial leads). *RA,* right atrium; *RV,* right ventricle; *LA,* left atrium; *LV,* left ventricle.

When the patient arrives, take these steps:

1. Explain to the patient why and how you will monitor cardiac rhythm. Depending on the patient's condition, you may need to modify or delay this explanation.

2. Prepare the electrode sites. If they are hairy,

clip the hair with scissors. Rub the skin briskly with an alcohol sponge (let the freshly clipped patient know that the alcohol may sting). Allow the sites to dry. Peel the electrodes off their backing without touching the gel or the adhesive surface.

3. Position the electrodes according to the lead you wish to monitor. The most common routine monitoring leads are lead 2 and MCL_1. Lead 2 provides the same view of cardiac activity as standard lead II; the difference is that lead 2 electrodes are placed on the chest, whereas lead II electrodes are placed on the limbs. Lead 2, however, is not the ideal lead for visualizing atrial activity or ventricular activity. A superior lead is the right chest lead, V_1, because it clearly records the sequence of ventricular depolarization. It thus facilitates differentiation of right from left premature ventricular beats; right from left bundle branch block; and premature left ventricular beats from premature right bundle aberrant beats. Unfortunately, routine monitoring in this lead is mechanically inconvenient, since it requires four limb electrodes plus a precordial electrode. MCL_1 is a lead developed by Marriott and Fogg (1970) to overcome the diagnostic disadvantages of lead 2 and the mechanical disadvantages of lead V_1. Placements of the electrodes will vary, depending on the lead you want to monitor (Figure 12–5) and the number of electrodes used.

4. After placing the electrodes and setting the selector knob, observe the ECG pattern on the screen. Adjust the position of the baseline with the position knob. If the complexes are not tall enough to be counted by the machine's rate meter, increase them with the sensitivity knob. (This knob sometimes is labeled "gain" or "size.")

5. Next note the rate being displayed on the rate meter. Set the rate alarms according to the limits at which you want to be alerted. For the patient with a satisfactory rate, these limits usually are ±20 beats from the patient's normal rate. For patients with abnormally slow or fast rates, you may wish to narrow the limits to deviations of 10 beats per minute in the abnormal direction. For example, for a patient with a heart rate of 60, you might place the low-rate alarm at 50 and the high-rate alarm at 90.

6. Trigger a printout of the rhythm by pressing the appropriate button or switch on the monitor. Analyze the rhythm and mount it in the patient's chart along with your admission nursing assessment.

Monitoring Problems Common monitoring problems include muscle artifact, 60-cycle interference, and wandering baseline (Figure 12–6). *Muscle artifact* appears as random, narrow deflections in the tracing. Make sure

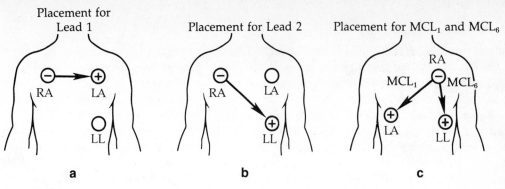

Placement for
Lead 1

Placement for Lead 2

Placement for MCL₁ and MCL₆

a

b

c

FIGURE 12–5

Placement of electrodes for routine monitoring. **a,** For lead 1, place electrode marked ⊖ or RA under right clavicle, electrode marked ⊕ or LA under left clavicle, and electrode marked ground or LL at sixth or seventh intercostal space in anterior axillary line. Place selector switch on lead 1. **b,** To monitor lead 2, place electrodes as in lead 1 and set switch on lead 2. The machine will read the RA electrode as negative and the LL electrode as positive. **c,** To monitor MCL₁ or MCL₆, place electrode marked ⊖ or RA under left clavicle, electrode marked ⊕ or LA in V₁ position, and electrode marked ground or LL in V₆ position. Then switch selector to lead 1 position to obtain MCL₁ and lead 2 position to obtain MCL₆.

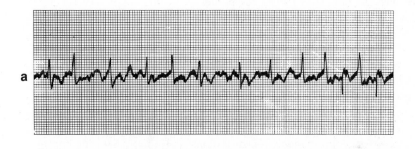

a

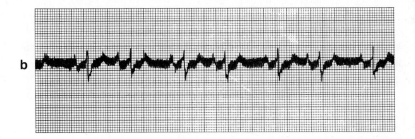

b

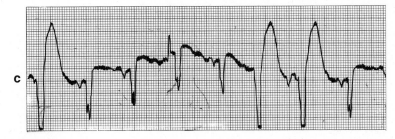

c

FIGURE 12–6

ECG artifacts. **a,** Muscle movement; **b,** 60-cycle interference; **c,** patient movement and wandering baseline.

the patient is in a comfortable position and is warm. Position the electrodes over less muscular areas.

The baseline may appear thickened due to poor electrode contact or electrical interference with the machine. Reposition the electrodes over more bony areas and make sure the straps are tight enough to hold them securely. With *60-cycle interference,* you actually may be able to see 60 tiny peaks per second in the baseline due to electrical interference. If the patient's bed is electric, unplug it. Also check for broken electrode wires or cable. Ground other electrical equipment in the immediate vicinity.

When the baseline does not remain centered on the paper but instead moves up and down, it is said to be wandering. *Wandering baseline* is due to respiratory or muscle movement. Reposition the electrodes.

ECG Analysis

ECG analysis is most meaningful when you comprehend the relationship between the electrical forces in the heart and the recording obtained at the chest surface.

Membrane Potentials and the ECG All heart cells have a membrane potential, which is simply a difference in electrical charge across a semipermeable cell membrane. There are two types of potentials: the *resting membrane potential* (RMP), and the *action potential,* which has two stages, depolarization and repolarization. These potentials and their relationship to ionic movement are depicted in Figure 12–7, which diagrams the potentials for a *ventricular* (nonpacemaker) cell.

Three channels allow ions to move across cell membranes: *fast* channels, *slow* channels, and *potassium* channels. Their characteristics are presented in Table 12–1.

Membrane potentials are affected by both the permeability of the cell membrane to sodium (Na^+) and potassium (K^+) ions and the rate at which these ions pass across the membrane. In the resting state, no electrical activity is occurring. This stage is represented by an isoelectric line. In the resting state, the cell membrane is less permeable to sodium than to potassium. Sodium and potassium each establishes its own equilibrium across the cell membrane. Relatively more sodium is outside than inside the cell. Relatively more potassium is inside than outside the cell. Although the cell contains many positively charged potassium ions and fewer positively charged sodium ions, these positive charges are exceeded by negatively charged ions, primarily proteins and phosphates. As a result, the cell is polarized with more negative charges inside and more positive charges outside.

When a sufficient stimulus occurs, membrane permeability changes. This stimulus may be electrical, chemical (as in hypoxia), or mechanical (as in chamber dilatation). If the stimulation is strong enough, the membrane will reach a certain point at which its potential changes significantly. This point is called the *threshold*. If the membrane reaches threshold, an action potential occurs on an all-or-none basis—that is, either the whole membrane changes its potential or none of it does. The action potential results from the movement of ions into and out of the cell according to the membrane's permeability for each ion and the gradient of each ion across the cell membrane.

When stimulation occurs and threshold potential is reached, the complex *fast-channel* gating mechanism opens, allowing the membrane to become much more permeable to sodium. It allows such a large amount of sodium ions to rush into the cell, carrying their positive charges with them, that the inside of the cell rapidly becomes positive. Because the cell now is more positive inside than outside (the reversal of the polarized state), this process is called *depolarization*. On the action potential diagram, it is seen as a rapid upstroke (phase 0), ending with a spike on the action potential diagram (phase 1).

TABLE 12–1 DEPOLARIZATION CHANNELS

CHANNEL	MEMBRANE POTENTIAL	IONIC MOVEMENT	RESULT
Fast	-90 mV	Sodium into cell	Rapid depolarization of muscle cells
Slow	-60 mV	Calcium-sodium into cell	Pacemaker activity of SA node, AV junction, and possibly ectopic sites Prolongation of phase 2 in nonpacemaker cells (follows fast-channel activity)
Potassium	————	Potassium out of cell	Speedy repolarization (follows slow-channel activity)

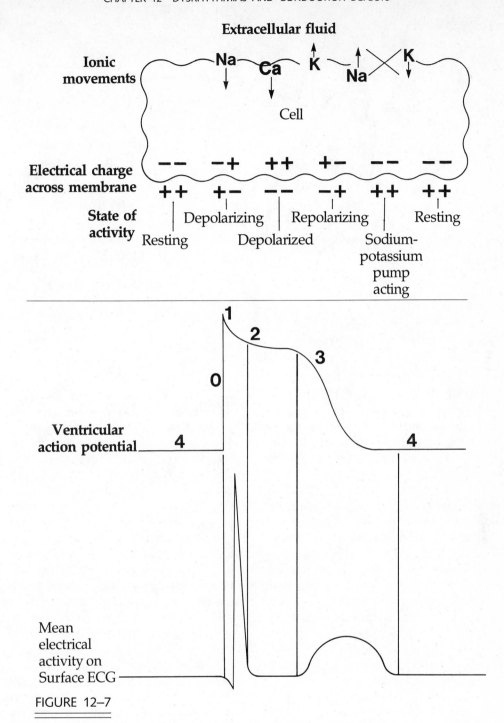

FIGURE 12–7

Ionic movements related to ventricular action potential.

The cell remains depolarized, with little or no voltage change, during a plateau period (phase 2) as the slow channels are activated and calcium leaks in. Because calcium ions are positive, they sustain the positivity inside the cell, which provides time for the release of intracellular calcium stores and contraction of the cardiac muscle cell. The fast channels are closed during this pe-

riod. The plateau ends abruptly with repolarization (phase 3) as the slow channels close and the potassium channels open (Guyton 1986). As potassium diffuses out of the cell, the potential becomes progressively more negative until it returns to resting potential (phase 4). Although the overall balance of positive versus negative charges is restored, the distribution of most of the so-

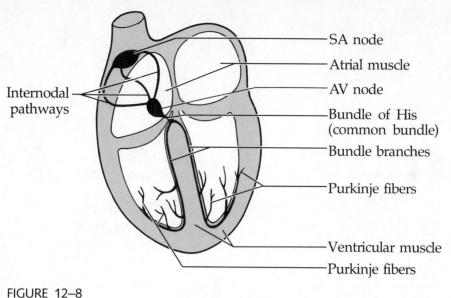

Internodal
pathways

SA node

Atrial muscle

AV node

Bundle of His
(common bundle)

Bundle branches

Purkinje fibers

Ventricular muscle

Purkinje fibers

FIGURE 12–8

Cardiac conduction system.

dium and potassium is the reverse of what it was in the original polarized state. Using energy, the sodium-potassium pump in the cell membrane transports sodium out of the cell and potassium back in to restore the correct balance. This restoration does not disrupt the phase 4 baseline.

Refractory Periods   During phases 0, 1, and 2, the myocardial cells cannot respond to another impulse. This time is called the *absolute refractory period*. During phase 3, repolarization, the cell may respond to an impulse. This period is called the *relative refractory period*. During the relative refractory period, a stimulus must be stronger than usual to evoke a response. At the end of phase 3, however, there is a temporary increase in excitability, during which a weaker than normal impulse can provoke repetitive depolarization; this time is called the *vulnerable period*. During phase 4, no refractoriness is present, so excitability is normal.

Conduction System   Changes in membrane potential spread more rapidly along the heart's conduction system than through other cardiac cells. Figure 12–8 shows the major components of the conduction system. They are not nerves but rather specialized muscle tissue. Normally, impulses arise in the SA node at the juncture of the right atrium and superior vena cava. From the sinus node, they spread across the atria and over preferential pathways to the atrioventricular (AV) node and left atrium. The preferential pathways to the AV node are the anterior, middle, and posterior inter-

nodal bundles. Bachmann's bundle, a branch of the anterior internodal bundle, is the preferential pathway to the left atrium. The AV node is located just to the right of the base of the interatrial septum and above the tricuspid valve. The impulses next travel to the bundle of His, which extends leftward from the AV node into the upper membranous part of the interventricular septum. (The AV node and bundle of His sometimes are referred to as the AV junction.) The bundle of His, also called the common bundle, splits into right and left bundle branches that travel down the muscular interventricular septum. The left bundle branch has two major divisions to the left ventricle, the anterior-superior branch and the posterior-inferior branch. The bundle branches split into the terminal part of the conduction system, the network of Purkinje fibers, which spreads the impulses from the endocardium to the epicardium.

Cells in the conduction system have different transmembrane potentials from cells outside the system (Figure 12–9). The most important difference relates to the resting phase. The phase 4 of cells outside the system is stable; they must wait for a stimulus to depolarize them. In contrast, the resting phase of cells inside the system shows a gentle positive slope. These cells are able to reach threshold potential spontaneously, thus depolarizing themselves. SA nodal fibers, for example, have a resting potential of approximately -60 mV. This level allows only slow calcium-sodium channels to be open, not the fast sodium channels, so the action potential develops and recovers more slowly than with ventricular cells; in addition, SA nodal fibers are

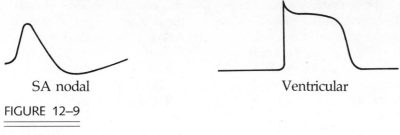

SA nodal   Ventricular

FIGURE 12–9

SA nodal versus ventricular action potentials.

"leaky" to sodium ions, which allows the resting potential to rise slowly until the calcium-sodium channels open and the action potential ensues (Guyton 1986). This property of spontaneous diastolic depolarization is called *automaticity*. These cells also have the property of *rhythmicity*; that is, they can depolarize themselves rhythmically.

Because cells in the conduction system can depolarize themselves, they can function as pacemakers to depolarize the rest of the heart. Pacemaker cells are of two types, dominant and latent. Although *latent* pacemakers exhibit diastolic depolarization, they usually become excited by an impulse transmitted from higher up in the system before they reach threshold spontaneously. A latent pacemaker may become a *dominant* pacemaker if it speeds up, a higher pacemaker slows down, or impulses from a higher pacemaker become blocked. Normally, the SA node is the dominant pacemaker because it can depolarize itself faster than the other potential pacemakers, 60–100 times a minute. If it slows down, fails, or becomes blocked, the next pacemaker to take over is the AV junction, at 40–60 beats per minute. If the Purkinje fibers are not depolarized by the SA node or AV junction, they will depolarize spontaneously at 20–40 beats per minute.

There are two major mechanisms of impulse formation: automaticity and re-entry. *Normal automaticity*, described earlier, is present in pacemaker cells. *Abnormal automaticity* may result from impulse formation related to abnormal slow-channel activity (Lewis 1981). The other mechanism of impulse formation is *re-entry*, which can occur inside or outside the conduction system. For re-entry to occur, there must be branching conduction pathways. One pathway must have a unidirectional *(antegrade)* block, or a longer refractory period than the other pathway.

Figure 12–10 diagrams one mechanism of re-entry. It shows a Purkinje fiber that branches in two and serves a ventricular muscle fiber. The impulse from the Purkinje fiber starts to travel down both branches but is blocked in one branch. It travels down the other branch, through the muscle fiber, and arrives at the bot-

RE–ENTRY

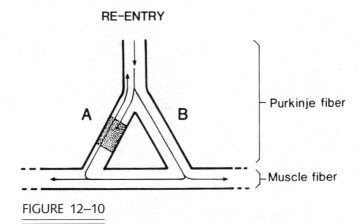

FIGURE 12–10

Re-entry mechanism. (From Lewis A: Monitoring and dysrhythmia recognition in advanced life support. In *Textbook of advanced life support*, eds. McIntyre K, Lewis A, pp. VI–1–28, Dallas: American Heart Association, 1981. Reproduced with permission. © American Heart Association.)

tom of the first branch. From there, it spreads retrograde (backward up the branch) to the original starting point, which by now has repolarized. From that point, it can travel through the rest of the conduction system, creating an isolated ectopic beat or a series of fast, repetitive beats, which appear as a tachycardia. In the atria, for example, this mechanism is thought to be responsible for producing atrial tachycardia.

Impulse formation and propagation are affected by many stimuli discussed elsewhere in the text. Briefly, sympathetic nerves (from the cervical and upper thoracic sympathetic ganglion chain) innervate the SA node, AV node, and ventricles. When sympathetic stimulation is increased, impulses are formed and conducted more quickly, and the ventricles contract more forcefully.

Parasympathetic control is provided by the vagus nerves from the medulla. Parasympathetic fibers innervate the SA and AV nodes. When parasympathetic stimulation is increased, impulses are formed and conducted more slowly.

Refer to Chapter 10 for detailed discussion of cardiovascular dynamics and hormonal and chemical influences on cardiac impulses. The blood supply to the conduction system is discussed in detail in the myocardial infarction section of Chapter 13.

Vectors and the ECG   To interpret an ECG, you must have a clear mental picture of the relationship between the 12 leads and the heart's position in the frontal and transverse planes. If you are unclear, review the previous sections of this chapter dealing with those topics before proceeding with the following sections on ECG analysis.

At a given point in time, numerous cardiac cells' individual membrane potential changes interact to form an electrical force. This force, called a *vector,* has both direction and magnitude. It can be recorded by an ECG electrode on the chest surface.

It is important to recognize that the ECG records only the heart's electrical activity, not its mechanical activity, which follows electrical activation. It thus can record depolarization and repolarization, but not chamber contraction and relaxation and not valvular motion.

The surface ECG is able to record the relatively large vectors of the atria and ventricles but not the smaller vectors of individual parts of the conduction system. Whenever it is unable to detect electrical activity, it records a straight line, called the *baseline* or *isoelectric line.* When it detects a vector, it records a deflection from the baseline.

The direction and magnitude of the deflection depend on (a) the distance between the force's starting point and the lead, and (b) the relation between the force's

direction and the lead's axis, the imaginary line between the poles of the lead (Figure 12–11). If the force's direction is toward the lead's positive pole, a positive deflection is recorded. If it is directed away from the positive pole, a negative deflection is recorded. The more parallel the force is to the lead, the larger the recorded deflection; the more perpendicular, the smaller the deflection. If the force and lead are completely perpendicular to each other, no deflection is recorded. When the positive and negative forces are equal, a diphasic deflection is recorded. In this case, the mean vector is perpendicular.

Labeling Deflections   By convention, the deflections are labeled with the letters P through U (Figure 12–12). Atrial depolarization (*not* atrial contraction) produces the P wave. Ventricular depolarization causes the QRS complex. Ventricular repolarization is seen as the T wave.

Intervals including or between these deflections are labeled as follows. The PR interval is from the start of atrial depolarization (the P wave) to start of ventricular depolarization (the QRS). It represents the length of time for an impulse to depolarize the atria and travel through the AV junction and bundle of His to the bundle branches. The ST segment is the interval between the end of ventricular depolarization (QRS) and the T wave. The end of the S wave and start of the ST segment sometimes is referred to as the J point. The QT interval is the duration of ventricular depolarization and repolarization. It is measured from the beginning of the QRS to the end of the T wave.

P and T waves are called those whether they are positive, negative, or diphasic (part positive, part negative). In contrast, the letters used to label the QRS complex vary with the polarity and sequence of the deflections. *QRS complex* is a generic term applied to any ventricular depolarization; combinations of these letters are used to designate specific ventricular configurations (Figure 12–13). The first negative deflection after the P wave is called a Q wave. The first positive deflection after the P wave is called an R wave. The first negative deflection after the R wave is called an S wave. If the QRS complex consists of only one negative wave, it is called a QS configuration. Other variations include the notched R, when the negative deflection after the R wave does not reach the baseline, and the RSR', when it does. The relative size of the ventricular deflections can be indicated by using small letters for small waves and capital letters for large ones.

Correlation with Action Potential   The QRST complex corresponds approximately to the phases of the ventricular action potential described earlier. The

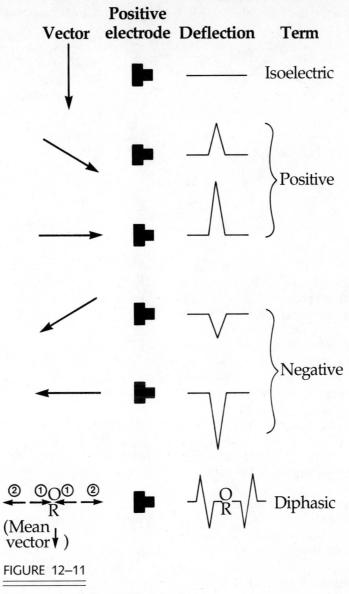

FIGURE 12–11

Vectors and associated ECG deflections.

QRS corresponds with ventricular depolarization and the rapid start of repolarization (phases 0 and 1). The ST segment represents phase 2, the plateau. (As mentioned earlier, during phases 0, 1, and 2 [QRS and ST segment], the cell is in its absolute refractory period.) The T wave corresponds with repolarization, and the relative refractory period. The T wave's downstroke corresponds with the vulnerable period during phase 3. The baseline between complexes corresponds with phase 4.

These facts are clinically significant. For example, a premature atrial beat falling during the ventricles' absolute refractory period cannot cause them to depolarize. A premature ventricular beat occurring during the vul-

nerable period of the T wave (R-on-T phenomenon), however, can provoke lethal ventricular tachycardia or ventricular fibrillation. For this reason, you should keep an eagle eye on the distance between T waves and premature ventricular beats!

Plotting Vectors Vectors can be plotted on reference systems to determine their normality. Although plotting is an advanced skill that you may not perform yourself, it is valuable to understand the vector concept for two reasons: axis normality or deviation is determined by vector analysis, and comprehension of normal vectors will help you spot whether a given deflection is normal for the lead in which it appears.

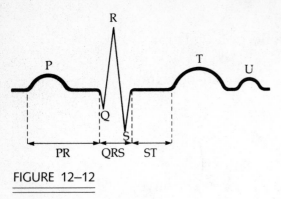

FIGURE 12–12

ECG deflections and intervals.

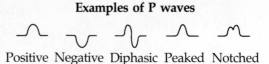

Examples of P waves

Positive   Negative   Diphasic   Peaked   Notched

Examples of QRS complexes

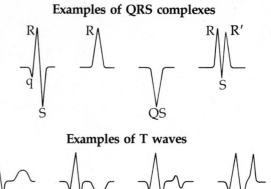

Examples of T waves

Positive   Inverted   Diphasic   Tall, peaked

FIGURE 12–13

Labeling ECG deflections.

Frontal plane vectors can be plotted on the hexaxial reference system (Figure 12–14). This reference system is formed by the intersection of the six frontal leads, which divide the frontal plane into 30° units. By convention, all degrees in the upper half of the figure are negative and all those in the lower half are positive. This convention is unrelated to the positive and negative poles of a lead. For example, AVL's positive pole is at −30°, while AVR's negative pole is at +30°.

The hexaxial reference system is divided into quadrants by leads I and AVF. Lead I divides the body into superior and inferior parts, and lead AVF, into right and left sides. By examining deflections in those leads, you can determine the quadrant of the reference figure into which the vector falls and the direction of the vector in the heart.

For instance, suppose you found a patient's QRS complex to be positive in both leads I and AVF. You could refer to Figure 12–14 and note that the quadrant in which both of these leads have positive QRS is the quadrant of normal axis. Alternatively, you could reason out the axis. If the QRS is positive in lead I, the electrical activity must be traveling toward the positive pole of lead I, that is, the left side of the body. If it is positive in lead AVF, it must also be traveling toward AVF's positive pole, that is, the foot. Thus, the vector is leftward and inferior.

It is possible to locate the vector more precisely. For details of the technique, consult a cardiology text. Horizontal plane vectors also can be plotted on a precordial reference figure formed by the six precordial leads.

Interpretation of Mean Vectors   The most important vectors are the mean frontal P, QRS, and T vectors and the initial QRS vector. The mean frontal P, QRS, and T vectors of the normal electrocardiogram lie within the quadrant bounded by the positive sides of leads I and AVF (0° to +90°). This signifies that the mean direction of atrial depolarization, ventricular depolarization, and ventricular repolarization is leftward and inferior. Since this is the normal direction, the person is said to have a normal axis. If the vectors fall outside the quadrant, axis deviation is present. Axis deviation can result from different positions of the heart within the chest cavity, cardiac disease (such as hypertrophy or conduction disturbances), or disease of other chest organs that alters their ability to conduct electrical impulses.

A mean QRS vector between +90° and −90° to the right of the axis of lead AVF indicates right axis deviation. That within the range of +90° to +110° may be normal. Right axis deviation from +110° to −90° is abnormal and usually results from right ventricular hypertrophy or right bundle branch block. A mean QRS vector between 0° and −90° represents left axis deviation. The range from 0° to −30° may be normal. Abnormal left axis deviation (−30° to −90°) suggests left ventricular hypertrophy or left anterior hemiblock.

Sequence of Depolarization and Related Vectors   The next section discusses the P, QRS, and T wave vectors and the ECG complexes they produce. The vectors are shown diagrammatically in Figure 12–15. Figure 12–16 is an example of a normal 12-lead ECG and associated patterns of depolarization.

The *P wave* represents right atrial depolarization followed by left atrial depolarization. Sinus P waves usually

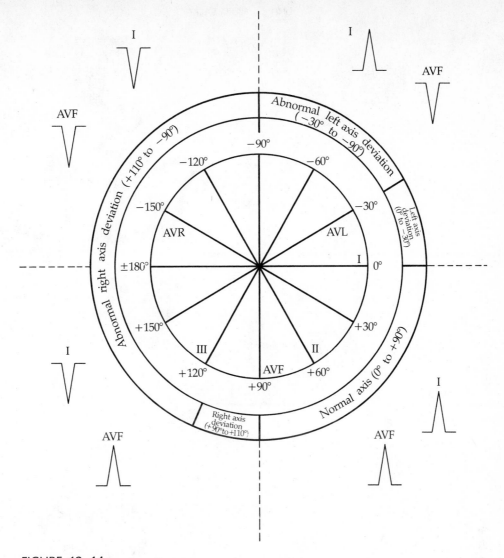

FIGURE 12–14

Hexaxial reference figure for determination of mean frontal QRS vector.

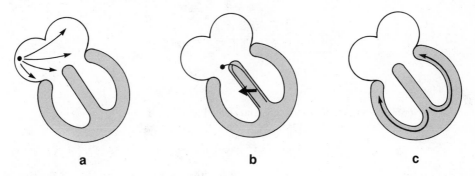

a   b   c

FIGURE 12–15

Sequence of depolarization. **a,** Atrial depolarization—P wave vector is anterior, inferior, and leftward; **b,** septal depolarization—initial QRS vector is anterior, either inferior or superior, and rightward; **c,** free ventricular wall depolarization—mean QRS vector is posterior, inferior, and leftward.

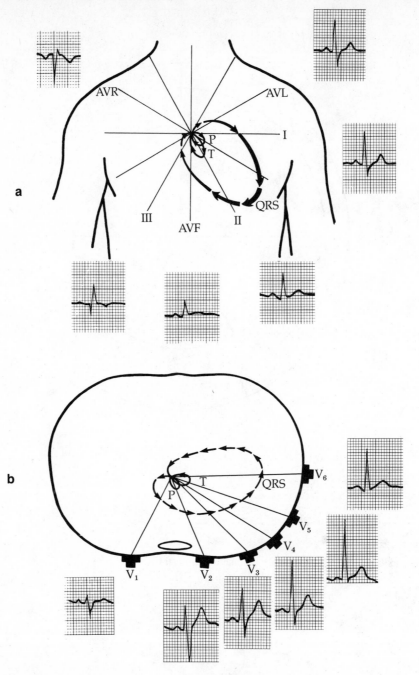

FIGURE 12–16

Normal patterns of depolarization and related deflections on
12-lead ECG. **a,** Frontal plane; **b,** transverse plane.

are rounded and symmetrical, with a maximum width of
0.12 seconds and maximum amplitude of 0.3 mV (Burrell and Burrell 1982). The normal mean frontal P wave
axis is about +60°. Looking on the hexaxial reference
figure, you can see that the leads closest to this vector
are II and AVR, with the vector moving toward the pos-

itive pole of lead II and away from the positive pole of
AVR. You can anticipate, then, that in normal sinus
rhythm, II and AVR are the leads which will best display
atrial activity, and the P wave will be positive in II and
negative in AVR. The P wave normally is positive in the
remaining limb and precordial leads. Occasionally, how-

ever, the normal P wave is negative, flat, or diphasic in III or AVL.

Following atrial depolarization, an isoelectric line is recorded as the impulse travels through the AV node, the bundle of His, and bundle branches. The interval from the start of the P wave to the end of this isoelectric line (that is, to the start of the QRS) is known as the *PR or PQ interval*. Its normal value is constant and within 0.12–0.20 seconds.

Atrial repolarization usually is not recorded because it is obscured by ventricular depolarization.

The *QRS complex* represents ventricular depolarization. The frontal plane QRS axis normally lies from 0° to +90° and varies with age. It is about +60° to +90° in the young adult and moves leftward (more horizontally) with increasing age. Ventricular depolarization normally starts on the left side of the interventricular septum and initially moves to the right across the septum and anteriorly to the tip of the right ventricle. This initial QRS vector also moves either inferiorly or superiorly. The inferior orientation is more common in the person with a more horizontal mean QRS vector. Small negative deflections *(normal Q waves)* may be present in some leads. These normal Q waves represent septal depolarization. In addition to the patient's axis and lead in which Q waves are seen, normal Q waves are defined by width and depth. These criteria vary with leads, but in general a Q wave is abnormal if it (1) appears in a lead where it was not present earlier, (2) is more than 0.04 seconds wide, (3) is greater than one-fourth the height of the R wave or (4) accompanies a left bundle branch block in leads I, AVL, AVF, V₄, V₅, or V₆. The reason for the latter criterion is that left bundle branch block usually causes the loss of normal Q waves in leads oriented toward the left ventricle; therefore, the appearance of even a small Q wave in these leads usually indicates an infarction in addition to the bundle branch block.

Depolarization next spreads through the right and left free ventricular walls, from endocardium to epicardium. Because the muscle mass of the left ventricle is larger than that of the right ventricle, the ECG reflects primarily left ventricular vectors, which are oriented leftward and inferiorly. They progress from the initial anterior orientation toward a strongly posterior orientation, because the bulk of the left ventricle is posterior.

The posterior base of the ventricles is the last area depolarized. This vector is posterior, superior, and rightward.

The changing QRS vectors are reflected in the ECG. They cause increasingly positive waves (R waves) in leads towards whose positive poles they are traveling and increasingly negative waves (S waves) in leads away from whose positive poles they are traveling.

Thus, lead II normally is characterized by a small Q wave (of septal depolarization) and large R wave. AVR displays a normal deep, wide QS wave, while V₁ normally is characterized by either a large wide Q wave or a small R wave and large S wave. The R wave becomes progressively larger and the S wave progressively smaller from V₁ to V₆. The normal duration of the QRS complex is 0.06–0.10 seconds. A QRS greater than 0.10 seconds is considered abnormal, and one that exceeds 0.12 seconds is usually caused by pathologic blocking (Guyton 1986).

The *ST segment* is isoelectric because early ventricular repolarization is very slow. The ST segment should be level with the PR interval line. Abnormal elevation is 1 mm or more above the line and abnormal depression 1 mm or more below it. ST segment deviations may indicate myocardial ischemia and injury. They are discussed in greater detail in Chapter 13.

The *T wave* represents ventricular repolarization and is evaluated by vector, size, and shape. Normally, the T wave is positive when the QRS is predominantly positive and negative when the QRS is negative. If the T wave's polarity is opposite to that of the QRS, the T wave is called *inverted*. The T wave usually is rounded and symmetrical. A T wave greater than 0.3 mV (3 mm) tall in a precordial lead is abnormally high or deep. Tall, narrow, peaked T waves are seen in hyperkalemia. Giant inverted T waves commonly appear with myocardial infarction and ventricular premature beats.

The *QT interval* represents the length of time for ventricular depolarization and repolarization. Measured from the beginning of the QRS to the end of the T wave, this interval varies with heart rate, and needs to be rate-corrected by calculating the QT_c ($QT_c = QT/\sqrt{RR \text{ interval}}$). The QT is lengthened by certain antidysrhythmics (e.g., quinidine, disopyramide, and procainamide), hypokalemia, and some psychoactive drugs. A lengthened QT may precipitate torsâdes de pointes.

Sometimes, a small wave is recorded after the T wave. This *U wave* is poorly understood but may represent the very end of ventricular repolarization.

Analyzing the ECG Train yourself to use a systematic approach to ECG analysis so that you do not overlook important data. The exact sequence is not as important as your consistency in using it. The following approach integrates analyses of vectors and the timing of cardiac events. It requires the use of a measuring device called *calipers*.

1. Note ventricular regularity and measure ventricular rate. The rate can be determined in relation to the measurements on the ECG paper (Figure 12–17). By convention, horizontal measurements represent time

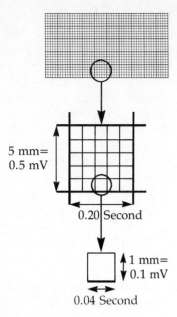

FIGURE 12–17

Time and voltage measurements on ECG paper (when recording speed is 25 mm/sec).

(vertical measurements represent electrical voltage). At the standard recording rate of 25 mm/sec, each small box measured horizontally equals 0.04 seconds. By remembering this value, you can figure out that each large box (five small boxes) equals 0.20 seconds, and 30 large boxes equal 6 seconds.

If the rhythm is regular, there are several ways to calculate rate. Since 300 boxes equal one minute, you can count the number of large boxes between the same point on two consecutive R waves and divide into 300. This method is accurate only if each of the R waves falls on the edge of a big box. Since 1500 small boxes also equal one minute, another way is to count the number of small boxes between two consecutive R waves and divide into 1500. A third method is that recommmended by Dubin (1974) (Figure 12–18):

A. *Find a deflection occurring on a heavy black line.* For instance, to calculate ventricular rate, look for a QRS on a heavy black line. Use the distance between it and the same point on the next QRS to calculate the rate. If there is no QRS falling exactly on a heavy line, measure the distance between two QRSs with your calipers by placing one caliper point on the first QRS and the other on the same point on the next QRS. Without changing the relative position of the points, lift the calipers to the edge of the strip and place the first point on a heavy line. Then

count to the second caliper point to determine the rate.

B. *Count out the rates represented by each heavy black line until you reach the ones closest to the second caliper point.* The rates represented by each heavy line are shown in the figure and may be memorized easily. You can see that the rate of the strip in the figure lies between 60 and 75. (A deflection occurring on each heavy line is occurring at a frequency of 1 per 0.2 seconds, or 300 per minute. One occurring every other black line equals a frequency of 1 per 0.4 seconds, or 150 per minute. The remaining rates were calculated in a similar fashion.)

C. *To pinpoint the rate, know the values represented by the small black lines.* Although they are not as easy to remember, frequent practice with them will make them second nature. The precise ventricular rate of the strip in the figure is 65. These smaller rate divisions also were determined logically, by dividing frequencies into 300. For example, the rate 125 was obtained by adding 0.4 seconds (the frequency of the next highest heavy line) to the 0.08 seconds (the frequency represented by two additional small boxes), and dividing the sum 0.48 into 60 to get 125 beats per minute.

If the rate is irregular, you can get an estimate by counting the number of R waves in a 6-second (30 large boxes) strip and multiplying it by 10.

2. Note atrial regularity and measure the atrial rate. Use the above methods, but calculate the distance between the same point on two consecutive P waves.

3. Examine the P waves to identify the source of atrial activity. What is their contour, width, and amplitude? Do all the P waves resemble each other? Do they occur before, during or after the QRS? Is their polarity normal for the lead you are examining?

4. Measure the PR interval to evaluate conduction through the atria, AV junction, and bundle of His. To do this, measure from the onset of the P wave to the onset of the first ventricular deflection (it may not always be an R wave). Multiply the number of small boxes between these points by 0.04 seconds to get the measurement. Is the measurement normal, shortened, or prolonged? Is the PR interval constant, irregular with a consistent pattern, or completely irregular?

5. Examine the QRS to analyze the length and sequence of ventricular depolarization. Measure from the onset of the first ventricular deflection from the baseline to the end of the last ventricular deflection, that is, the return to the baseline. (If the demarcation between the

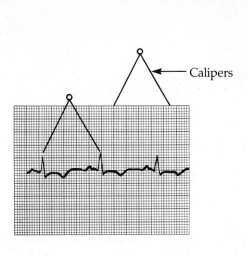

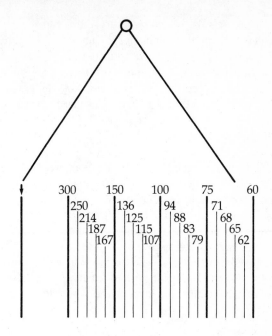

FIGURE 12–18

Rapid rate calculation for regular rhythms. (From Dubin D: *Rapid interpretation of EKGs,* 3d ed. Tampa, FL: COVER Publishing Company, 1974. Used with permission of Dale Dubin, M.D., and C.O.V.E.R. Publishing Company.)

baseline and the deflections is not clear, the onset and termination of the QRS may be difficult to detect. Sometimes, you will be able to see the change from a thick deflection, caused by slow electrical activity, to a thinner line resulting from the faster ventricular depolarization.) Multiply the number of small boxes by 0.04 seconds to get the measurement. Is the patient's value normal or prolonged? Is it constant, variable with a consistent pattern, or completely variable?

Examine the QRS deflections to assess the direction of ventricular depolarization. Are the deflections appropriate to the lead? If a Q wave is present, is its presence normal for that patient and lead? Is the appearance of the QRS similar for all complexes in a given lead?

6. Examine the ST segment and T wave to evaluate ventricular repolarization. Is the ST segment normal (isoelectric and level with the flat part of the PR interval), elevated above the baseline, or depressed? Is the T wave normal or abnormal?

7. Measure the QT interval, and rate-correct it using a nomogram. Is the QT_c normal, short, or prolonged?

In summary, the normal ECG has the following characteristics. The impulse originates in the SA node at a rate of 60–100 beats a minute. It produces a P wave that is symmetric and rounded and that precedes ven-

tricular activity. It travels across the atria, AV node, and the bundle of His in 0.12–0.20 seconds. It produces a QRS complex that lasts 0.06–0.10 seconds. The complex is followed by an isoelectric ST segment and a T wave that is symmetric, rounded, and of the same polarity as the QRS. The vectors of the P wave, QRS complex, and T wave are appropriate for the lead being examined. The rate-corrected QT interval is appropriate for the heart rate.

Common Dysrhythmias

Rhythms traditionally are classified on the basis of their origin and their underlying mechanisms. The origin of a dysrhythmia may be the sinus node, atria, AV junction, or ventricles. Mechanisms usually are grouped into disturbances of impulse formation and disturbances of impulse conduction (blocks). Definitions of disturbances of impulse formation follow.

A *bradycardia* is any rhythm with a regular ventricular rate under 60 beats per minute (bpm).

A *tachycardia* is any rhythm with a regular ventricular rate over 100 bpm. Not all interpreters use this terminology. For instance, a spontaneous ventricular rhythm usually has a rate between 20 and 40 bpm. If the rate exceeds 40, some interpreters call it ventricular tachycardia; similarly, a junctional rhythm over 60 bpm may be called a junctional tachycardia. You can see how confusing this usage is, since "tachycardia" used this way can refer to a ventricular rate above 40, 60, or 100 bpm. For clarity, restrict the term *tachycardia* to rates over 100. Rates less than 100 bpm, but above normal for their sources, are best called *accelerated*.

Flutter is a regular rhythm, more rapid than tachycardia, with a saw-toothed appearance. The term usually is applied only to an atrial dysrhythmia, although an occasional author calls ventricular tachycardia with this contour, ventricular flutter.

Fibrillation refers to chaotic depolarization. It produces an irregular, wavy baseline in which complexes cannot be distinguished clearly. Fibrillation may occur in either the atria or the ventricles.

The disturbances of impulse formation are named by combining their source with their mechanism—for example, *sinus bradycardia*. To enable you to compare and contrast the basic sinus, atrial, junctional, and ventricular rhythms, their characteristics are presented in tabular form and illustrated with ECG strips. Table 12–2 presents sinus rhythms; Table 12–3, paroxysmal supraventricular tachycardias; Table 12–4, atrial rhythms; Table 12–5, junctional rhythms; and Table 12–6, ventricular rhythms.

Conduction Defects

Disturbances of impulse conduction also may occur. These are called *blocks* and are subdivided into sinus, atrioventricular (AV), bundle branch, and hemiblocks (block of a subdivision of the left bundle branch). AV blocks, bundle branch blocks, and hemiblocks are the most common and are presented in this chapter.

A block may be superimposed on any disturbance of the cardiac rhythm; thus, a patient might have an atrial tachycardia with AV block or a normal sinus rhythm with bundle branch block. Labeling of atrioventricular blocks can be confusing. To label an AV block, count the number of P waves per QRS. For example, if a rhythm had two P waves for each QRS, it would be described as a 2:1 block. Occasionally, an atrial wave may be obscured by the QRS deflections. To detect a hidden wave, use your ECG calipers to measure the P–P interval on visible waves. If the distance between the P waves just before and just after a QRS is twice the measured P–P interval, you can deduce that a P wave is being obscured by the QRS. Atrioventricular blocks are shown in Table 12–7.

AV dissociation is a term that means the atria and ventricles are beating independently, that is, dissociated. Because AV dissociation can be associated with many different dysrhythmias, it is not a primary dysrhythmia. Whenever you use the term, you also must state the primary rhythms causing atrial and ventricular beating—for example, AV dissociation with sinus bradycardia and ventricular rhythm. AV dissociation may occur in three different ways. If the primary pacemaker slows, a rhythm may escape from a lower site. An example is the sinus bradycardia and ventricular rhythm mentioned above. AV dissociation also may occur if the primary pacemaker discharges at a normal rate but an ectopic pacemaker accelerates. An example of this category is sinus rhythm and ventricular tachycardia. The third way that AV dissociation may occur is if impulses from the primary pacemaker become completely blocked (third-degree AV block). This type of dissociation is detected easily if the atrial rate is greater than the ventricular. If the ventricular rate is greater than the atrial, however, you cannot say just from the ECG strip that a third-degree block is present, although it is possible that a third-degree block occurred and was followed by acceleration of a rhythm from a junctional or ventricular focus. In order to diagnose the cause of the dissociation in this case, the physician will attempt to accelerate the rhythm driving the atria to see whether a block is in fact present.

In the first two types of dissociation, AV conduction is normal. Occasionally, then, when a P wave is far enough away from a QRS, it may be conducted to the ventricles, thus capturing (depolarizing) them. Such a beat is called a *capture beat*. It occurs because the impulse reaches the ventricles at a time when they can respond, that is, when they are not already refractory from the impulses otherwise driving them.

Bundle branch blocks (BBB) are a type of conduction disturbance in which the right or left bundle branch fails to conduct impulses. To understand the ECG patterns that result from BBBs, it is helpful to understand the relationship between the sequence of ventricular activation and the corresponding ECG deflections (Table 12–8). Normally, ventricular depolarization occurs in two major steps. Septal depolarization proceeds from left to right, followed by free ventricular wall depolarization. The right ventricle depolarizes from left to right; simultaneously, the left ventricle depolarizes from right to left. Because left ventricular muscle mass exceeds that of the right ventricle, the ECG normally reflects primarily left ventricular depolarization. This normal sequence of ventricular depolarization can be seen clearly in ECG recordings from V_1, an electrode over the right ventricle, and V_6, an electrode over the left ventricle. The wave of septal depolarization travels toward V_1

TABLE 12–2 SINUS RHYTHMS

REGULARITY AND RATE			AV CONDUCTION		
Ventricular	**Atrial**	**P Waves**	**P:QRS Ratio**	**PR Interval**	**QRS**
Normal Sinus Rhythm (NSR)					
Regular, 60–100	Same as ventricular	Symmetrical, rounded	1:1	0.12–0.20 sec	0.06–0.10 sec

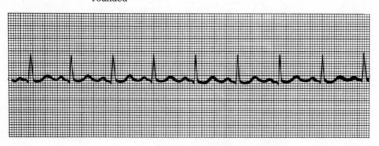

CAUSES Normal heart
SIGNIFICANCE Normal rhythm
TREATMENT None

REGULARITY AND RATE			AV CONDUCTION		
Ventricular	**Atrial**	**P Waves**	**P:QRS Ratio**	**PR Interval**	**QRS**
Sinus Bradycardia					
Regular, below 60	←————————————	Same as normal sinus rhythm		————————————→	

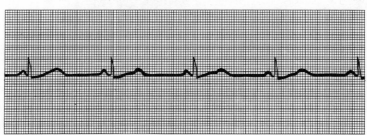

CAUSES Normal heart; athletic heart; sleep; vagal stimulation; myocardial infarction; increased
      intracranial pressure
SIGNIFICANCE Significance depends on rate. If moderate, allows for increased ventricular filling
      and decreased myocardial oxygen demand; if too slow, inadequate cardiac output
TREATMENT None if asymptomatic; if symptomatic, atropine, isoproterenol, or artificial pace-
      maker

(Continues)

TABLE 12–2   SINUS RHYTHMS (Continued)

REGULARITY AND RATE		AV CONDUCTION			
Ventricular	**Atrial**	**P Waves**	**P:QRS Ratio**	**PR Interval**	**QRS**

Sinus Tachycardia

Regular, above 100
(usually up to 180)   ←———————————————— Same as normal sinus rhythm ————————————————→

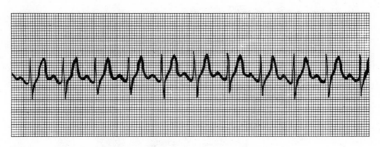

CAUSES   Normal heart: tea, coffee, tobacco, alcohol; physical or emotional stress; inflammatory
            heart disease; coronary artery disease
SIGNIFICANCE   Usually not significant except in patient with heart disease; then may cause an-
                  gina, infarction, congestive heart failure, shock
TREATMENT   If asymptomatic, none; if symptomatic, treat the cause

REGULARITY AND RATE		AV CONDUCTION			
Ventricular	**Atrial**	**P Waves**	**P:QRS Ratio**	**PR Interval**	**QRS**

Sinus Arrhythmia

| Irregular, 60–100 | Same as NSR | Same as NSR | Same as NSR | Same as NSR | Same as NSR |

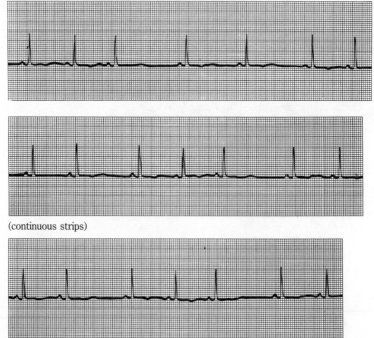

(continuous strips)

COMMENTS   Rate increases with inspiration, decreases with expiration, in cyclical fashion
CAUSES   Normal heart (variation in sympathetic and parasympathetic stimulation during respira-
            tion)
SIGNIFICANCE   Normal variant
TREATMENT   None

TABLE 12–2 SINUS RHYTHMS (Continued)

REGULARITY AND RATE			AV CONDUCTION		
Ventricular	**Atrial**	**P Waves**	**P:QRS Ratio**	**PR Interval**	**QRS**
Sinus Arrest					
Regular but with occasional absence of entire PQRST complex; any rate	←——————————————— Same as normal sinus rhythm ———————————————→				

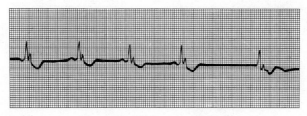

COMMENTS Cycle containing missed beat is not a multiple of the basic sinus cycle
CAUSES Failure of sinus node (owing to infarction), increased vagal tone, fibrosis, digitalis
         toxicity
SIGNIFICANCE May be transient or prolonged. If transient, no significance; if prolonged, patient
         develops asystole unless escape rhythm occurs.
TREATMENT If prolonged, atropine, isoproterenol, or artificial pacemaker

TABLE 12–3 PAROXYSMAL SUPRAVENTRICULAR TACHYCARDIAS

REGULARITY AND RATE			AV CONDUCTION		
Ventricular	**Atrial**	**P Waves**	**P:QRS Ratio**	**PR Interval**	**QRS**
Paroxysmal Atrial Tachycardia (PAT)					
Regular, 150–250	Same as ventricular	Contour slightly different from sinus P waves	1:1	Normal or prolonged or shortened	Normal

COMMENTS Onset and termination sudden
CAUSES Normal heart; stimulation from coffee, tea, tobacco; coronary artery disease; hyperthy-
         roidism; rheumatic heart disease
         Mechanism: re-entry at AV node
SIGNIFICANCE May produce heart failure, shock, angina, dizziness
TREATMENT Depends on patient's tolerance, cause, and history of previous attacks; vagal stim-
         ulation, verapamil, cardioversion, propranolol, procainamide, digitalization, sedation

(Continues)

TABLE 12–3 PAROXYSMAL SUPRAVENTRICULAR TACHYCARDIAS (Continued)

REGULARITY AND RATE			AV CONDUCTION		
Ventricular	**Atrial**	**P Waves**	**P:QRS Ratio**	**PR Interval**	**QRS**

Supraventricular Tachycardia

Regular, 150–250	←————————————— Not detectable —————————————→				Normal

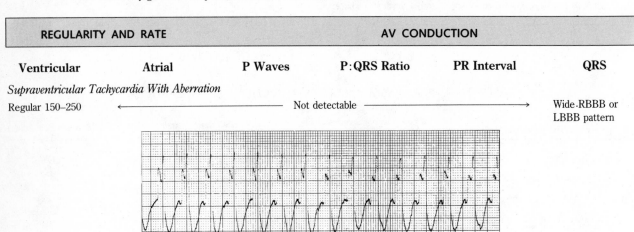

CAUSES See sinus, atrial and junctional tachycardia (Tables 12–2, 12–4, and 12–5, respectively)

SIGNIFICANCE Global term indicating rhythm originating above ventricles but whose source cannot be identified (because P waves are not clearly visible)

TREATMENT Differentiation requires additional maneuvers such as carotid sinus massage, study of a waves in jugular venous pulse, and assessment of S_1 intensity and S_2 splitting

REGULARITY AND RATE			AV CONDUCTION		
Ventricular	**Atrial**	**P Waves**	**P:QRS Ratio**	**PR Interval**	**QRS**

Supraventricular Tachycardia With Aberration

Regular 150–250	←————————————— Not detectable —————————————→				Wide·RBBB or LBBB pattern

SVT with RBBB aberration

CAUSES See sinus, atrial and junctional tachycardia (Tables 12–2, 12–4, and 12–5, respectively)

SIGNIFICANCE Same as in sinus, atrial and junctional tachycardia (Tables 12–2, 12–4, and 12–5, respectively); temporarily abnormal conduction through bundle branches because supraventricular impulses fall when one branch still refractory; easily confused with ventricular tachycardia

TREATMENT As for supraventricular tachycardia

TABLE 12–4   ATRIAL RHYTHMS

REGULARITY AND RATE			AV CONDUCTION		
Ventricular	**Atrial**	**P Waves**	**P:QRS Ratio**	**PR Interval**	**QRS**
Atrial tachycardia with block					
Regular if block is constant; irregular if block is variable; any rate	Regular, 150–250. If block is constant, atrial rate is multiple of ventricular rate	Contour slightly different from sinus P waves	More than 1:1	Normal or prolonged on conducted beats	Normal

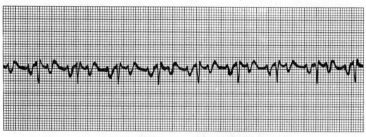

Atrial tachycardia with 2:1 block

COMMENTS   If atrial rate above 200, block usually is physiologic owing to arrival of some atrial
impulses at AV node during its refractory period
If atrial rate below 200, nonparoxysmal tachycardia, or block greater than 2:1,
block usually due to pathology
CAUSES   Coronary artery disease; digitalis intoxication
SIGNIFICANCE   Symptoms depend on ventricular rate
TREATMENT   If asymptomatic, observation; if digitalis is cause, discontinuation of drug, administration of potassium chloride; if digitalis not cause, digitalis to slow ventricular rate

REGULARITY AND RATE			AV CONDUCTION		
Ventricular	**Atrial**	**P Waves**	**P:QRS Ratio**	**PR Interval**	**QRS**
Atrial flutter					
Regular or irregular, depending on constancy of block; any rate	Regular, 200–350. If block is constant, atrial rate is multiple of ventricular rate	Sawtooth	More than 1:1. Usually constant, even block—2:1, 4:1, etc.	Normal on conducted beats	Normal

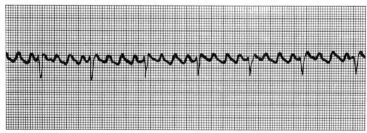

COMMENTS   Mechanism probably re-entry in atria
CAUSES   Coronary artery disease; mitral or tricuspid valvular disease; cor pulmonale
SIGNIFICANCE   Carotid sinus massage increases degree of block temporarily but does not terminate dysrhythmia
TREATMENT   Cardioversion; verapamil; digitalis; propranolol; quinidine; overdrive pacing

(Continues)

TABLE 12–4   ATRIAL RHYTHMS (Continued)

REGULARITY AND RATE		AV CONDUCTION			
Ventricular	**Atrial**	**P Waves**	**P:QRS Ratio**	**PR Interval**	**QRS**
Atrial fibrillation					
Irregular; rate varies, but averages 160–180	Unmeasurable	Chaotic (fine or coarse) fibrillatory (f) waves, seen as wavy baseline	Very variable; numerous f waves per QRS	Variable	Normal

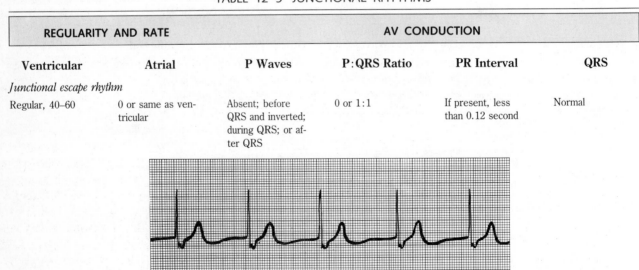

COMMENTS   If ventricular rate becomes regular in digitalized patient, clue to digitalis intoxication
           Chronic or paroxysmal
CAUSES   Normal heart; mitral stenosis; thyrotoxicosis; pericarditis; coronary artery disease; hypertensive heart disease
SIGNIFICANCE   No effective atrial contraction; predisposes to pulmonary or systemic thromboemboli (about one-third of patients develop). May precipitate or exacerbate congestive heart failure
TREATMENT   Cardioversion; digitalis; quinidine; verapamil; propranolol

TABLE 12–5   JUNCTIONAL RHYTHMS

REGULARITY AND RATE		AV CONDUCTION			
Ventricular	**Atrial**	**P Waves**	**P:QRS Ratio**	**PR Interval**	**QRS**
Junctional escape rhythm					
Regular, 40–60	0 or same as ventricular	Absent; before QRS and inverted; during QRS; or after QRS	0 or 1:1	If present, less than 0.12 second	Normal

COMMENTS   If P waves are present, junctional stimulus has been conducted retrograde to atria; usually seen best as negative P waves in leads II, III, and AVF
CAUSES   Failure of sinus node
SIGNIFICANCE   Protects patient from asystole
TREATMENT   Treatment of failure of sinus node; atropine, isoproterenol to increase junctional rate; or artificial pacemaker

TABLE 12–5 JUNCTIONAL RHYTHMS (Continued)

REGULARITY AND RATE		AV CONDUCTION			
Ventricular	**Atrial**	**P Waves**	**P:QRS Ratio**	**PR Interval**	**QRS**

Accelerated junctional rhythm

| Regular, 60–100 | 0 or same as ventricular | Same as junctional escape rhythm | Same as junctional escape rhythm | Same as junctional escape rhythm | Same as junctional escape rhythm |

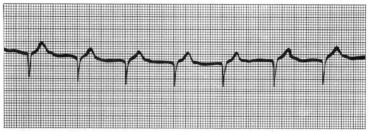

COMMENTS Also known as nonparoxysmal AV junctional tachycardia
CAUSES Digitalis intoxication, inferior infarction, myocarditis, postcardiotomy
SIGNIFICANCE Same as junctional escape rhythm; in addition, produces near-normal cardiac
output
TREATMENT Treatment of cause

REGULARITY AND RATE		AV CONDUCTION			
Ventricular	**Atrial**	**P Waves**	**P:QRS Ratio**	**PR Interval**	**QRS**

Junctional tachycardia

| Regular, over 100 | 0 or same as ventricular | Same as junctional escape rhythm | Same as junctional escape rhythm | Same as junctional escape rhythm | Same as junctional escape rhythm |

COMMENTS Same as junctional escape rhythm. Upright deflection in strip is standardization
mark.
CAUSES Digitalis intoxication, myocardial infarction, myocarditis, postcardiotomy
SIGNIFICANCE Depends on partient's tolerance; usually stops spontaneously if tolerated well
TREATMENT If asymptomatic, treatment of cause; if symptomatic, discontinuation of digitalis (if
cause); cardioversion, digitalis (if not cause)
Paroxysmal junctional tachycardia: see "Paroxysmal atrial tachycardia," Table 12–3

TABLE 12–6 VENTRICULAR RHYTHMS

REGULARITY AND RATE			AV CONDUCTION		
Ventricular	**Atrial**	**P Waves**	**P:QRS Ratio**	**PR Interval**	**QRS**

Ventricular rhythm

| Regular, 20–40 | Absent; or if present, unrelated to ventricular activity | | | | Greater than 0.12 second |

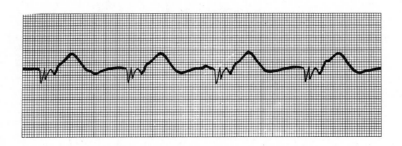

CAUSES Failure of higher pacemakers or complete AV block
SIGNIFICANCE Escape rhythm; if this rhythm occurs with no pulse or an insufficient pulse, treat
as electromechanical dissociation (EMD)
TREATMENT Atropine, isoproterenol, artificial pacemaker; if EMD, CPR and epinephrine

REGULARITY AND RATE			AV CONDUCTION		
Ventricular	**Atrial**	**P Waves**	**P:QRS Ratio**	**PR Interval**	**QRS**

Accelerated ventricular rhythm

| Regular, 40–100 | Absent; or if present, unrelated to ventricular activity | | | | Greater than 0.12 second |

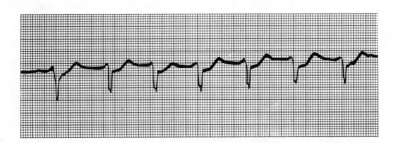

COMMENTS Transient episodes
CAUSES Acute myocardial infarction; digitalis intoxication
SIGNIFICANCE Ectopic ventricular pacemaker accelerates to rate approximating normal sinus
rhythm
TREATMENT Close observation; treatment of cause; rarely, atropine; lidocaine

TABLE 12–6 VENTRICULAR RHYTHMS (Continued)

REGULARITY AND RATE			AV CONDUCTION		
Ventricular	**Atrial**	**P Waves**	**P:QRS Ratio**	**PR Interval**	**QRS**

Ventricular tachycardia

Regular, 100–220   Absent; or if present, unrelated to ventricular activity   Greater than 0.12 second

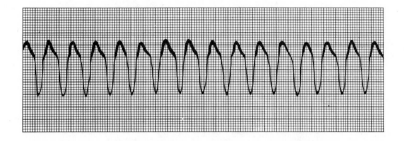

CAUSES   Acute myocardial infarction; coronary artery disease; premature ventricular beat (R on T phenomenon)

SIGNIFICANCE   Ominous as may progress to ventricular fibrillation; symptoms depend on underlying heart disease, rate, and duration of VT; may cause angina, cardiac failure, shock

TREATMENT   If pulseless, treat as ventricular fibrillation; if with pulse and hemodynamically stable, lidocaine, procainamide, cardioversion; if with pulse but hemodynamically unstable, cardioversion, lidocaine, procainamide, bretylium

REGULARITY AND RATE			AV CONDUCTION		
Ventricular	**Atrial**	**P Waves**	**P:QRS Ratio**	**PR Interval**	**QRS**

Ventricular fibrillation

400–600   Absent; or if present, unrelated to ventricular activity   None

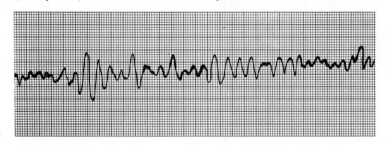

COMMENTS   Chaotic depolarization produces grossly irregular, bizarre ECG deflections

CAUSES   Acute myocardial infarction; coronary artery disease; electrical shock; premature ventricular beat (R on T phenomenon); dying heart

SIGNIFICANCE   Lethal within 4–6 minutes; symptoms include loss of consciousness, pulse, heart sounds and respirations; and absent blood pressure

TREATMENT   Precordial thump; immediate defibrillation; if ineffective, cardiopulmonary resuscitation; epinephrine, lidocaine, bretylium, sodium bicarbonate

(Continues)

TABLE 12–6 VENTRICULAR RHYTHMS (Continued)

REGULARITY AND RATE			AV CONDUCTION		
Ventricular	**Atrial**	**P Waves**	**P:QRS Ratio**	**PR Interval**	**QRS**

Torsâde de pointes (polymorphous ventricular tachycardia)

0	Absent				Greater than 0.12 second, varying morphology, twists around baseline

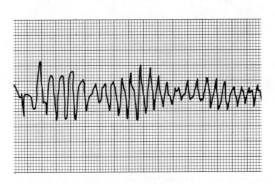

COMMENTS Frequently initiated with R-on-T phenomenon; associated with long QT interval
CAUSES Hypokalemia; quinidine-like drug toxicity; hypomagnesemia
SIGNIFICANCE May progress to ventricular fibrillation or spontaneously convert
TREATMENT Temporary pacing; lidocaine, magnesium sulfate

REGULARITY AND RATE			AV CONDUCTION		
Ventricular	**Atrial**	**P Waves**	**P:QRS Ratio**	**PR Interval**	**QRS**

Ventricular asystole

0	Absent, or if present, unrelated to ventricular activity		None

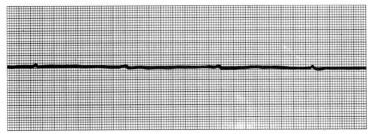

Ventricular standstill

COMMENTS In illustration, deflections are P waves
CAUSES Acute myocardial infarction; coronary artery disease; complete heart block; dying heart
SIGNIFICANCE Same as ventricular fibrillation
TREATMENT Immediate cardiopulmonary resuscitation; epinephrine, atropine, sodium bicarbon-
         ate, pacemaker

TABLE 12–7 ATRIOVENTRICULAR BLOCKS

REGULARITY AND RATE			AV CONDUCTION		
Ventricular	**Atrial**	**P Waves**	**P:QRS Ratio**	**PR Interval**	**QRS**
First degree AV block					
Regular, any rate	Same as ventricular	Sinus or atrial	1:1	Constant, but greater than 0.20 second	Normal

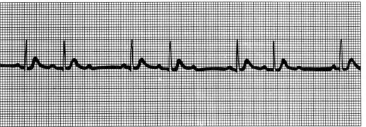

COMMENTS All impulses are conducted through AV node, but slower than usual
CAUSES Normal heart; coronary artery disease; digitalis intoxication; conduction system fibrosis; myocarditis; cardiac surgery
SIGNIFICANCE Relatively benign; may progress to second- or third-degree blocks
TREATMENT None necessary

REGULARITY AND RATE			AV CONDUCTION		
Ventricular	**Atrial**	**P Waves**	**P:QRS Ratio**	**PR Interval**	**QRS**
Second degree AV blocks: (1) Mobitz I (Wenckebach)					
Irregular but consistent pattern (group beating); any rate	Regular, faster than ventricular	Sinus or atrial	1:1 except for nonconducted P wave	Lengthens progressively until one P wave not conducted; cycle then repeats itself	Normal

Mobitz I second degree AV block

COMMENTS In second degree blocks, some impulses are not conducted; in Mobitz I, impulses are delayed progressively until one reaches AV node while it is absolutely refractory, so it cannot conduct that impulse
          Block usually at level of AV node
CAUSES Increased parasympathetic tone; digitalis intoxication; acute inferior myocardial infarction
SIGNIFICANCE Relatively benign: does not diminish cardiac output, usually transient, does not usually progress to greater degree of block
TREATMENT Usually, none necessary; if symptomatic, atropine; discontinue digitalis if cause

(Continues)

TABLE 12–7 ATRIOVENTRICULAR BLOCKS (Continued)

REGULARITY AND RATE			AV CONDUCTION		
Ventricular	Atrial	P Waves	P:QRS Ratio	PR Interval	QRS
(2) Mobitz II					
Irregular but with no consistent pattern, any rate	Regular, faster than ventricular	Sinus or atrial	1:1 except for non-conducted P wave	Constant on conducted beats, normal or prolonged	Wide with bundle branch block (if block infranodal) or normal (if block at AV node)

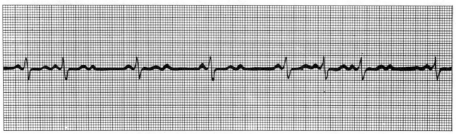

Mobitz II second degree AV block

COMMENTS   Impulses are conducted normally until one is suddenly blocked
            Block usually infranodal (below AV node), commonly at bundle branch level or
            uncommonly at bundle of His
CAUSES   Necrosis or fibrosis of conduction pathway; acute anterior myocardial infarction
SIGNIFICANCE   More ominous than Mobitz I; often precedes sudden complete heart block
TREATMENT   Atropine, isoproterenol, prophylactic artificial pacemaker

REGULARITY AND RATE			AV CONDUCTION		
Ventricular	Atrial	P Waves	P:QRS Ratio	PR Interval	QRS
Third degree (complete) AV block					
• with junctional escape rhythm					
Regular	Regular, faster than ventricular	Sinus or atrial	0; no relationship between Ps and QRSs	Appears variable, but P waves actually not conducted	Normal (due to junctional escape rhythm)

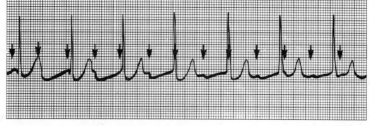

COMMENTS   In third degree blocks, no impulses are conducted through AV node
            Narrow QRS in this rhythm indicates block high in AV node (in illustration, arrows
            point to P waves)
CAUSES   Increased parasympathetic tone; drug effect; AV node damage; acute inferior MI
SIGNIFICANCE   Transient; favorable prognosis
TREATMENT   Atropine; temporary pacemaker

TABLE 12–7 ATRIOVENTRICULAR BLOCKS (Continued)

REGULARITY AND RATE		AV CONDUCTION			
Ventricular	**Atrial**	**P Waves**	**P:QRS Ratio**	**PR Interval**	**QRS**
• with ventricular escape rhythm					
Regular or absent	Regular, faster than ventricular	Sinus or atrial	0; no relationship between Ps and QRSs	Appears variable, but P waves actually not conducted	Wide (due to ventricular escape rhythm) or absent

COMMENTS Wide QRS indicates block at both bundle branches or bundle of His (infranodal block)
CAUSES Extensive conduction system disease; extensive anterior MI
SIGNIFICANCE Poor prognosis; likely to progress to asystole
TREATMENT Pacemaker

• with no escape rhythm:					
Absent	Regular	Sinus or atrial	None	None	None

COMMENTS Causes ventricular standstill
CAUSES Extensive conduction system disease; extensive anterior MI
SIGNIFICANCE Cardiac arrest
TREATMENT CPR; pacemaker

TABLE 12–8 BUNDLE BRANCH BLOCKS

REGULARITY AND RATE		AV CONDUCTION			
Ventricular	**Atrial**	**P Waves**	**P:QRS Ratio**	**PR Interval**	**QRS**
Normal conduction					
Regular or irregular, any rate, depending upon basic rhythm		Sinus or atrial	Normal or abnormal, depending on basic rhythm		0.06–0.12 second V$_1$: rS; V$_6$: qR

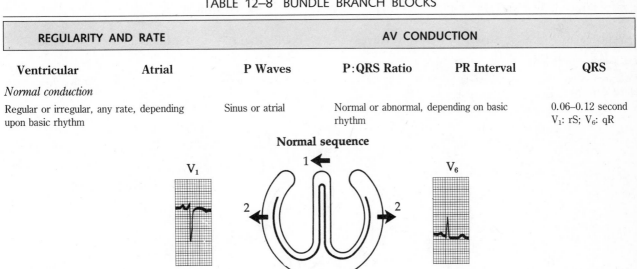

Normal sequence

COMMENTS Not a bundle branch block; included for comparison
CAUSES Normal heart
SIGNIFICANCE Normal conduction
TREATMENT None necessary

(Continues)

TABLE 12–8 BUNDLE BRANCH BLOCKS (Continued)

REGULARITY AND RATE		AV CONDUCTION			
Ventricular	**Atrial**	**P Waves**	**P:QRS Ratio**	**PR Interval**	**QRS**
Right bundle branch block					
Regular or irregular, any rate, depending on basic rhythm	Sinus or atrial	Normal or abnormal, depending on basic rhythm			Greater than 0.12 second; V_1: triphasic rSR'; V_6: triphasic QRS, with wide S wave

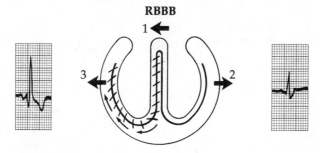

RBBB

COMMENTS   Does not affect recording of initial QRS waves; therefore, does not prevent ECG
                    signs of myocardial infarction
CAUSES   Normal heart; coronary artery disease; right ventricular hypertrophy; premature supra-
                    ventricular beats (aberration)
SIGNIFICANCE   Does not affect cardiac output
TREATMENT   None necessary, unless accompanied by block of one division of left bundle
                    branch; in that case, prophylactic artificial pacemaker

REGULARITY AND RATE		AV CONDUCTION			
Ventricular	**Atrial**	**P Waves**	**P:QRS Ratio**	**PR Interval**	**QRS**
Left bundle branch block					
Regular or irregular, any rate, depending on basic rhythm	Sinus or atrial	Normal or abnormal, depending on basic rhythm			Greater than 0.12 second; V_1: monophasic QS; V_6: monophasic wide R wave

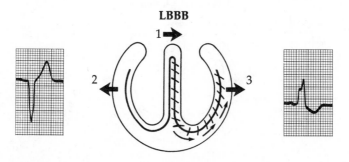

LBBB

COMMENTS   Block prevents recording of normal initial QRS waves, so can obscure ECG signs
                    of myocardial infarction
CAUSES   Normal heart; coronary artery disease; valvular heart disease; hypertension
SIGNIFICANCE   More serious than right bundle branch block because results from more serious
                    disorders and often accompanied by cardiomegaly
TREATMENT   None

(which records a small positive or R wave) and away from V_6 (which records a small negative or Q wave). The wave of free ventricular wall depolarization travels in the opposite direction—away from V_1 (which records a large negative or S wave) and toward V_6 (which records a large positive or R wave). As a result, normal bundle branch conduction produces an rS pattern in V_1 and a qR pattern in V_6.

When the right bundle branch is blocked, right ventricular stimulation is delayed. Septal depolarization proceeds normally, from left to right. The ventricles, however, no longer depolarize simultaneously; instead the left ventricle depolarizes before the right ventricle. Left ventricular depolarization proceeds normally, from right to left. Because the right bundle branch cannot conduct the impulse to the right ventricle, right ventricular depolarization occurs via spread of the impulse from the left ventricle. This spread occurs slowly because the impulse travels outside the conduction system; as a result, the QRS measures greater than 0.12 seconds. Although the length of right ventricular depolarization is prolonged, the direction remains the same, left to right. The three steps of ventricular depolarization are reflected in the ECG. Instead of the normal rS, a V_1 electrode records a triphasic (rSR′) deflection: a small positive wave of septal depolarization, a large negative wave of free left ventricular wall depolarization, and a large positive wave of free right ventricular wall depolarization. The V_6 electrode also records a triphasic deflection, but it is a qRS; the q wave reflects septal depolarization, the R wave reflects left free ventricular wall depolarization, and a wide S wave reflects the slow free right ventricular wall depolarization. Due to abnormal ventricular repolarization, the T wave that follows a right BBB is inverted.

When the left bundle branch is blocked, the pattern of depolarization is disrupted to a greater extent. Septal depolarization no longer proceeds from left to right; its direction is reversed. The right ventricle depolarizes next, in its normal direction (left to right). Left ventricular stimulation is delayed and occurs via spread of the impulse from the right ventricle, again outside the conduction system. The left ventricle therefore depolarizes last, but in the normal direction, right to left. The ECG patterns again reflect the ventricular activity clearly.

V_1 records a small negative wave of septal depolarization, sometimes a small positive wave of right ventricular depolarization, and a large negative wave of free left ventricular wall depolarization. These deflections usually are seen as a monophasic QS wave, sometimes with a small positive notch. The V_6 electrode records a small positive wave, sometimes a small negative wave, and a large positive wave, resulting in a wide, mono-

phasic R wave, occasionally with a small negative notch. The T wave usually is inverted, due to abnormal ventricular repolarization.

Because the initial forces in the right bundle branch block are not changed, ECG signs of myocardial infarction can be detected on the patient's ECG. In contrast, left BBB does alter the initial forces; when myocardial infarction occurs in the patient with left BBB, its characteristic ECG signs often are obscured.

Hemiblocks (a type of *fascicular block*) are blocks in one of the two divisions of the left bundle branch, which subdivides into an *anterior/superior fascicle* and an *inferior/posterior fascicle*. Hemiblocks are caused by the same factors that cause left BBB, which represents the block of both fascicles. The block of only one fascicle causes frontal axis deviation with a normal or slightly prolonged QRS duration.

Left anterior hemiblock (LAH) occurs more often than left posterior hemiblock (LPH). The anterior fascicle is more vulnerable to injury than the posterior fascicle, because it is thinner and supplied only by the left coronary artery. LAH thus is seen in anteroseptal and anterolateral myocardial infarctions, which result from blockage of the left coronary artery. The ECG signs of LAH include left axis deviation ($-45°$ or greater). Lead I will show an initial Q wave (qR configuration), while leads III and AVF will show predominantly negative complexes (rS configurations) rather than the predominantly positive complexes normally seen in those leads.

LPH is seen less often, probably because the posterior fascicle is less vulnerable to injury due to its thickness and its dual blood supply from both the right and left coronary arteries. When LPH is seen, it usually indicates a worse prognosis than LAH, because disease extensive enough to damage the posterior fascicle often damages the anterior fascicle and right bundle branch as well. ECG signs of LPH include an axis of $+120°$ or greater (right axis deviation). Leads I and AVL will show a negative (rS) complex instead of the positive complex usually seen, while leads III and AVF will have an initial Q wave (qR configuration).

No therapy is available for hemiblocks. Nursing care involves close monitoring for progression to more advanced degrees of block using a lead such as 1 or 3 to detect axis shifts. LPH is more likely to progress to more severe forms of block than is LAH. You should be particularly alert to the danger of progression to second- or third-degree heart block if the patient has right BBB with LAH or LPH, because only one unblocked fascicle remains to conduct impulses to the ventricles. Monitoring the patient in lead MCL_1 would be helpful in detecting the onset of right BBB. You should be especially alert to the development of Mobitz II block, which represents intermittent trifascicular block and heralds the development of constant trifascicular block (complete heart block). Because of the danger of progression, the patient with an acute myocardial infarction who develops a hemiblock usually will undergo prophylactic pacemaker insertion.

Funny-Looking Beats

Often when you examine an ECG strip you will notice "funny-looking" beats. These usually are *ectopic beats* (beats that arise outside the SA node). Because ectopic beats vary in significance, it is important to use a logical method to analyze a funny-looking beat. A good method of analysis is the following:

1. Determine whether a beat is early or late by comparing the interval between it and the preceding beat to an R–R interval of the dominant rhythm. If it is late, it is an escape beat. *Escape beats* occur when the dominant pacemaker fails to fire and depolarize slower sites of impulse formation. They appear "late," that is, after the next-expected dominant beat. If the funny looking beat is an escape beat, you can identify it further as an *escape junctional* or *escape ventricular* beat by looking for a P wave and measuring the QRS.

A beat that occurs early (before the next-expected dominant beat) is a *premature beat.* Supraventricular premature beats may be blocked, conducted normally, or conducted aberrantly. This last term means the beat is conducted down the bundle branches, although abnormally. *Aberration* is a transient conduction abnormality that occurs because the premature impulse reaches the bundle branches before they are fully repolarized. Since the bundle branches have unequal refractory periods, a premature impulse may find one branch still refractory (usually the right). The impulse still can travel the conduction pathway, but in a temporarily abnormal manner. At first glance, a premature supraventricular beat with aberration somewhat resembles a ventricular premature beat. It is important to differentiate them because their significance and treatment differ. Continue to follow a logical consistent approach to analyzing the beat.

2. Measure the QRS duration. A normal duration means the beat's origin is supraventricular. A wide QRS (when the dominant QRS is normal) can mean either a supraventricular beat with aberration or a ventricular beat.

3. Look for a P wave related to the premature beat. Its presence strongly suggests the beat is supraventricular.

4. Analyze the pause after the premature beat. To do this, compare the interval consisting of two dominant cycles to the interval between the two dominant beats surrounding the premature beat. (See Figure 12–19.) If the interval containing the premature beat is shorter than the interval containing two dominant cycles, the pause is called *noncompensatory.* It occurs because the premature impulse has depolarized the SA node, causing it, and therefore the ventricles, to pause. If the interval containing the premature beat is equal to or longer than twice the dominant cycle, the pause is called *compensatory.* It occurs because the impulse has not depolarized the SA node but instead has made the ventricles refractory to the next sinus impulse. That is, the SA node does not pause but the ventricles do—until the second sinus impulse after the premature beat, which arrives at a time when they can respond.

5. Compare the coupling intervals. The *couple* is the premature beat and the dominant beat immediately preceding it. Compare the interval between these R waves to that of other couples in the strip. Constant (fixed) coupling is a characteristic of ventricular premature beats.

6. Compare the R–R interval immediately preceding the premature beat to others in the dominant rhythm. A sudden lengthening just before the premature beat predisposes to aberration. The reason for this is that the refractory period of the bundle branches depends on the length of the preceding R–R interval—when the interval is long, the refractory period is long.

7. Examine the pattern of QRS deflections compared to the dominant QRS and to other premature beats:

A. Initial deflections similar to those of dominant beats suggest the impulse is traveling the usual conduction system; that is, it is supraventricular.

B. A pattern of deflections similar to that of other premature beats suggests that you probably are seeing a premature beat from the same source.

C. A BBB pattern may indicate supraventricular aberration or ventricular ectopy.

Abberation produces a BBB pattern when the early impulse reaches the ventricles while one bundle branch is still refractory. Since the refractory period of the right bundle branch usually is longer than that of the left bundle branch, aberration usually appears as a right BBB configuration.

Ventricular ectopy also may cause a BBB pattern. You will remember that in BBB, the impulse must spread cell to cell from the normally stimulated ventricle to the blocked one. As a ventricular premature beat arises outside the

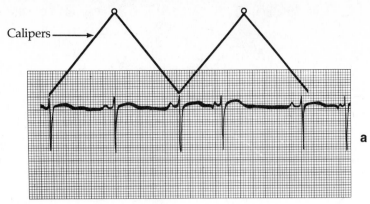

Noncompensatory pause

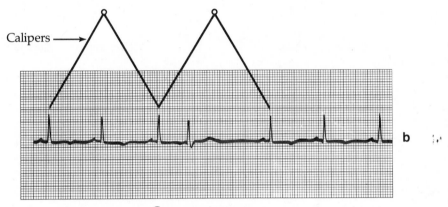

Compensatory pause

FIGURE 12–19

Noncompensatory versus compensatory pauses. To determine whether the pause following a premature beat is noncompensatory or compensatory, use your calipers to measure an interval consisting of two dominant cycles. Then,
without changing the relative position of the caliper points,
place the left point on the R wave preceding the premature
beat. **a,** If another dominant QRS falls *before* the right point,
the two cycles surrounding the premature beat are less than
two dominant cycles; that is, the pause is *noncompensatory.*
b, If the dominant QRS falls on or after the right caliper
point, the cycles surrounding the premature beat are equal to
or longer than the dominant cycles; that is, the pause is *compensatory.*

conduction system, it also spreads cell to cell to
the other ventricle. For this reason, a premature beat from the left ventricle may form the
same QRS configuration as a right BBB, while a
right ventricular premature beat may simulate a
left BBB.

Certain QRS configurations are more likely to represent ectopy than others. Clues to whether a QRS is

ectopic or aberrant are presented in Figure 12–20 and
Table 12–9.

Premature beats may be classified in many ways in
addition to the designations ectopic and aberrant. When
classified by site of origin, they are identified as atrial,
junctional, or ventricular. Another classification refers
to the number of foci (sites) from which they arise,
beats from one site with constant morphology being

Manifestation		Favors	Odds
RSR' variant in V_1 or MCL_1		Aberration	10:1
qRs in V_6 or MCL_6		Aberration	20:1
R or qR in V_1 or MCL, with taller left "rabbit ear"		LV ectopy	10:1
R or qR in V_1 or MCL_1 with taller left "rabbit ear"		Neither	—
QS in V_6 or MCL_6		LV ectopy	20:1
rS in V_6 or MCL_6(NO q)		LV ectopy	7:3
LBBB pattern with wide r in V_1 or MCL_1		RV ectopy	10:1

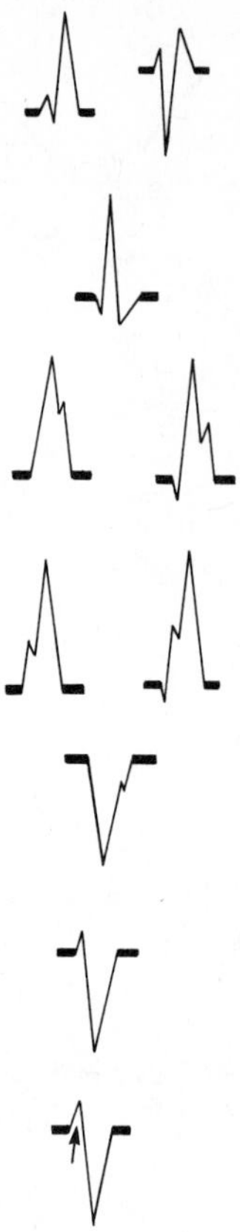

FIGURE 12–20

Ventricular aberration versus ectopy: morphologic clues.
(From Marriott H: *Workshop in electrocardiography.* Oldsmar, FL: Tampa Tracings, 1972.)

called *unifocal* and those from more than one site (or with different shapes) being called *multifocal* (or multiformed). These and other characteristics of premature beats are summarized and illustrated in Tables 12–10 and 12–11.

Differentiation of General ECG Patterns

So far, rhythms have been grouped primarily according to site of origin. You undoubtedly have noticed that different specific rhythms may have a similar general effect on the ECG. For instance, tachycardias from several sites have the same effect of a rapid, regular rhythm. When you first scan an ECG strip, it is the overall pattern that catches your eye, so your first impression is that of a tachycardia, bradycardia, or so on. Then, you proceed to differentiate the rhythms that

could cause that effect. Marriott (1972) has elaborated on this concept by originating an immensely useful list that identifies the specific rhythms that cause a similar general ECG pattern. Those causes discussed in this book are given in Table 12–12.

Nursing Care Related to Dysrhythmias

Assessment

To improve your ability to spot dysrhythmias promptly, develop good dysrhythmia detection habits. Auscultate the apical pulse for rate and regularity. Monitor the car-

TABLE 12–9   GUIDELINES FOR DISTINGUISHING VENTRICULAR DYSRHYTHMIAS FROM SUPRAVENTRICULAR ABERRATION.*

SUPRAVENTRICULAR TACHYCARDIA WITH ABERRANT VENTRICULAR CONDUCTION	VENTRICULAR TACHYCARDIA
1. Premature P wave of different morphology before the first beat of a run of tachycardia.	1. No P wave or a nonpremature P wave before the first beat of a run of tachycardia
2. QRS complex in an RBBB or LBBB pattern (triphasic)	2. QRS complex in a qS, rS, or R pattern (monophasic or biphasic)
3. Grossly irregular QRS pattern	3. Generally regular QRS pattern
4. Pattern changes in response to vagal stimulation (carotid pressure or Valsalva's maneuver)	4. Pattern does not change in response to vagal stimulation
5. Presence of P waves hidden in the T wave of the preceding beat	5. Signs of dissociated P wave within the pattern
6. Recent documented history of premature atrial beats	6. Recent documented history of ventricular ectopic beats
7. A rate greater than 170 bpm	7. A rate between 130 and 150 bpm
8. A taller right "rabbit ear" QRS complex MC_1	8. A taller left "rabbit ear" QRS complex in MCL_1
9. An incomplete compensatory pause after the last beat of the run of tachycardia	9. A full or complete compensatory pause after the last beat of the run of tachycardia
10. Patients with a history of atrial fibrillation or atrial flutter	10. Patients with a history of acute MI, especially anterioseptal MI
11. Central pulse should be present; may be weak; low BP	11. Generally absent central pulses; very low or no BP
12. Absence of hypoxic symptoms and no change in LOC	12. Unconscious; hypoxic seizures
13. Absence of capture or fusion beats	13. Captured or fusion beats during the tachycardia
14. Initial vector of the QRS complex identical with normal conducted beats	14. Initial vector of the QRS complex different from normally conducted beats

*Data from: Summerall CP: *Lessons in EKG interpretation.* New York: John Wiley & Sons, 1985, p. 81; Vinsant MO, Spence MI: *Coronary care.* St Louis: Mosby, 1985, pp 289–301; Conover MB: *Understanding electrocardiography.* St Louis: Mosby, 1984, pp 227–240.

Source: Catalano J: Arrhythmia quiz. *Crit Care Nurse* 1986; 6(4):18.

diac rhythm constantly with an oscilloscope. Observe the scope for changes in rate, rhythm, P wave, PR interval, QRS duration and configuration, ST segment, QT interval, and T wave. Analyze the rhythm strip, and mount it in the patient's record every 1–8 hours, depending on the stability of the patient's condition. When significant changes occur, document with a rhythm strip or 12-lead ECG. Read the 12-lead ECG reports (or the ECGs themselves) to keep informed about the progression of ECG changes.

Risk Conditions

Learn to anticipate and prevent dysrhythmias by recognizing the conditions that increase the patient's risk of developing a dysrhythmia. The risk conditions are numerous: major categories include myocardial hypoxia, electrolyte imbalances, catecholamine stimulation, vagal

stimulation, and trauma or structural interruption of the conduction system. Myocardial hypoxia can result from systemic hypoxia, inadequate coronary artery filling time (for example, in severe tachycardia), insufficient coronary artery perfusion pressure (for example, in shock), coronary artery disease, aortic valve disease, ventricular hypertrophy or dilatation, or anemia. In some cases, the patient with coronary artery disease may have an oxygen supply that is sufficient at rest or for minimal exertion, and may only develop myocardial hypoxia when myocardial workload increases (such as in tachycardia) because oxygen demand exceeds oxygen supply. Local areas of myocardial hypoxia may be present in myocardial infarction.

Electrolyte imbalances, particularly those of potassium and calcium, may contribute to dysrhythmias. These imbalances are discussed in Chapter 16.

Catecholamine stimulation, which predisposes toward tachydysrhythmias and premature beats, may occur in hypotension, hypertension, emotional excite-

TABLE 12–10   PREMATURE BEATS

QRS Duration	P Wave	PR Interval	Pause	Coupling	QRS Deflections
Atrial premature beat (APB)					
Normal	Atrial	Normal	Usually noncompensatory	Variable	Normal width; pattern same as dominant QRS

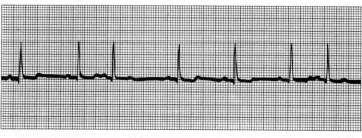

Atrial premature beat

COMMENTS   Wandering atrial pacemaker (WAP) might be mistaken for sinus rhythm with ABPs because of the varying shape and rate of P waves; but in WAP the ventricular rate remains essentially regular

CAUSE   Normal heart; caffeine, tobacco, alcohol stimulation; stress; myocarditis; myocardial ischemia; digitalis intoxication

SIGNIFICANCE   Ectopic atrial focus; usually benign but may precede atrial tachycardia, flutter or fibrillation

TREATMENT   Usually, none necessary; if very frequent, treat the cause; sedation; propranolol; digitalis (if not cause)

QRS Duration	P Wave	PR Interval	Pause	Coupling	QRS Deflections
Blocked or nonconducted APB					
Absent	Atrial	Absent	Usually noncompensatory	Variable	Absent

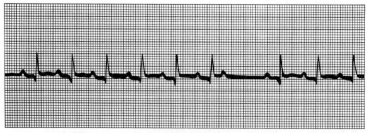

Blocked atrial premature beat

CAUSE   Same as APB
SIGNIFICANCE   Same as APB
TREATMENT   Same as APB

TABLE 12–10 PREMATURE BEATS (Continued)

QRS Duration	P Wave	PR Interval	Pause	Coupling	QRS Deflections
Aberrantly conducted APB					
Wide	Atrial	Normal	Usually noncompensatory	Variable	Wide QRS. Usually, initial deflection same as dominant QRS; usually, right bundle branch block pattern

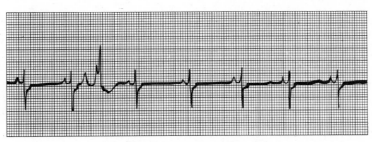

Aberrant atrial premature beat

COMMENTS Prolonged preceding R–R interval may be present
CAUSE Same as APB
SIGNIFICANCE Same as APB
TREATMENT Same as APB

QRS Duration	P Wave	PR Interval	Pause	Coupling	QRS Deflections
Junctional premature beat (JPB)					
Normal	Absent; before, during, or after QRS	Absent or less than 0.12 second	Usually noncompensatory	Variable	Normal width. Pattern same as dominant QRS

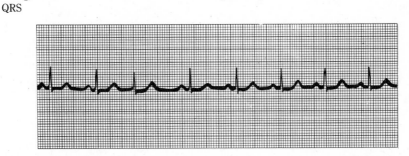

COMMENTS Retrograde atrial depolarization, so P wave negative in II, III, AVF
CAUSE Normal heart; caffeine, tobacco, alcohol stimulation; stress; myocarditis; myocardial ischemia; digitalis intoxication
SIGNIFICANCE Ectopic junctional focus; usually insignificant, but may precede junctional tachycardia
TREATMENT Usually, none necessary; if very frequent, treat the cause; sedation; propranolol; digitalis (if not cause)

(Continues)

TABLE 12–10 PREMATURE BEATS (Continued)

QRS Duration	P Wave	PR Interval	Pause	Coupling	QRS Deflections
Aberrantly conducted JPB					
Wide	Absent; before, during, or after QRS	Absent or less than 0.12 second	Usually noncompensatory	Variable	Wide QRS. Usually, initial deflection same as dominant; usually, right bundle branch block pattern

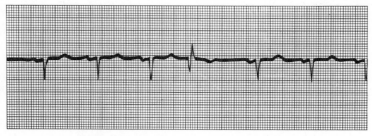

COMMENTS Prolonged preceding R–R interval may be present
CAUSE Same as JPB
SIGNIFICANCE Same as JPB
TREATMENT Same as JPB

QRS Duration	P Wave	PR Interval	Pause	Coupling	QRS Deflections
Ventricular premature beat (VPB)					
Wide	Unrelated	Absent	Usually compensatory	Depends on type	Wide QRS. Bizarre pattern; initial deflection usually opposite to dominant QRS

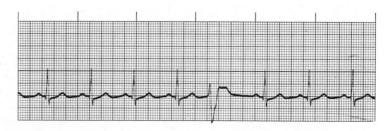

COMMENTS Followed by large inverted T wave; numerous subcategories shown in Table 12–11
CAUSE Normal heart; myocardial ischemia or infarction; electrolyte imbalances; others as in JPB
SIGNIFICANCE Ectopic ventricular focus; may progress to ventricular tachycardia or fibrillation, especially if more than 3 in a row, more than 6 per minute, multifocal, or falling on or near preceding T wave
TREATMENT None if infrequent; if frequent, lidocaine bolus IV followed by lidocaine infusion; tocainide; quinidine; procainamide; treat the cause

TABLE 12–10 PREMATURE BEATS (Continued)

QRS Duration	P Wave	PR Interval	Pause	Coupling	QRS Deflections
Fusion beat (shown by arrows)					
Intermediate between dominant and ectopic durations	Yes, but may be hidden in QRS	Normal or no more than 0.06–0.08 seconds less than dominant beat	Variable	Constant	Intermediate between dominant and ectopic contours

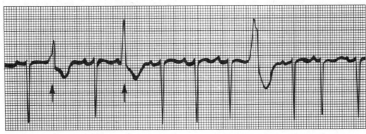

COMMENTS
CAUSE   As in other premature beats
SIGNIFICANCE   Simultaneous depolarization of atria or ventricles by one normal and one ectopic focus (normal sinus beat and artificial pacemaker; normal sinus beat and APB; or supraventricular beat and VPB)
TREATMENT   None necessary

TABLE 12–11 SUBCATEGORIES OF VPBs

CHARACTERISTICS	EXAMPLES

Unifocal VPB
Fixed coupling, constant QRS contour

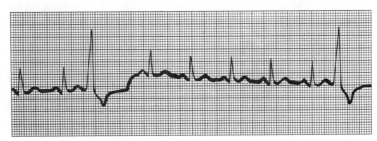

Multifocal (multiformed) VPB
Variable coupling, variable QRS contour

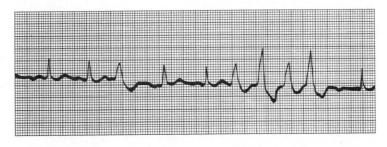

(Continues)

TABLE 12–11 SUBCATEGORIES OF VPBs (Continued)

CHARACTERISTICS	EXAMPLES

Interpolated VPB

No pause, "sandwiched" between dominant beats

Left ventricular VPB

Right bundle branch block pattern or primarily positive
deflection in leads oriented toward right ventricle (V_1, V_2)

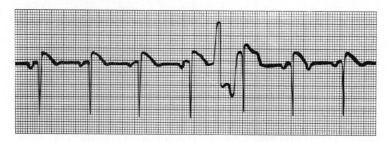

Right ventricular VPB

Left bundle branch block pattern or primarily positive
deflection in leads oriented toward left ventricle (V_5, V_6)

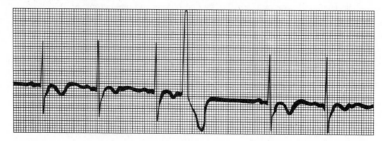

Isolated VPB

Occurring infrequently

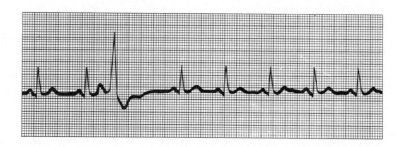

Bigeminy (ventricular)

VPB alternating with dominant beat

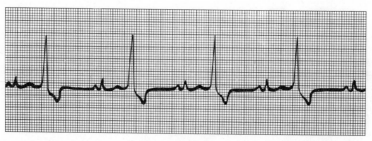

TABLE 12–12 SPECIFIC CAUSES OF GENERAL ECG PATTERNS*

GENERAL PATTERN	POSITIVE SPECIFIC CAUSES
Regular rhythm, normal rate	Normal sinus rhythm Accelerated junctional rhythm Accelerated ventricular rhythm Sinus tachycardia with 2:1 conduction Atrial flutter with 4:1 conduction AV dissociation: atrial fibrillation and accelerated escape rhythm
Bradycardia	Sinus bradycardia Junctional rhythm Ventricular rhythm Second-degree AV block with high-grade degree of block Third-degree AV block with escape rhythm
Tachycardia	Sinus tachycardia Atrial tachycardia Junctional tachycardia Ventricular tachycardia
Pauses	Nonconducted atrial premature beat Second-degree AV block (type I or II)
Premature beats	Atrial premature beat Junctional premature beat Ventricular premature beat Capture beat
Bigeminy	Premature beats coupled to a sinus, junctional, or ventricular beat Atrial flutter with alternating 4:1 and 2:1 conduction 3:2 AV block
Groups of beats	Premature beat occurring every third beat Two premature beats coupled to a sinus, atrial, or ventricular beat Premature beat in atrial fibrillation Grouping in atrial fibrillation Grouping in ventricular tachycardia 4:3 AV block
Chaos	Atrial fibrillation Atrial flutter with varying AV conduction Wandering pacemaker Multifocal atrial tachycardia Multifocal premature beats Mixed arrhythmias Ventricular fibrillation

*Table limited to those patterns and causes presented in this text.

Adapted from Marriott H: *Workshop in electrocardiography,* 1972; and *Differential diagnosis of heart disease.* Oldsmar, FL: Tampa Tracings, 1967.

ment, increased muscular work, and administration of certain drugs, such as vasoconstrictor agents. Vagal stimulation, which contributes to bradydysrhythmias and heart block, may occur with digitalis intoxication, Valsalva maneuvers, or tracheal stimulation. A *Valsalva maneuver* is a forced expiration against a closed glottis; it often occurs when a patient is moving about in bed or moving the bowels. Tracheal stimulation resulting in bradycardia or heart block may occur during tracheal suctioning, intubation, or vomiting.

Other factors that may provoke dysrhythmias are trauma to the conduction system (such as during cardiac surgery), structural defects (such as a ventricular septal defect), myocarditis, and stretching of myocardial fibers due to volume overload.

NURSING DIAGNOSES

The nursing diagnoses appropriate for a patient with a dysrhythmia may include one or more of the following:

- Decreased cardiac output
- Altered tissue perfusion
- Activity intolerance
- Anxiety

Planning and Implementation of Care

Prevention Whenever possible, plan to prevent dysrhythmias. One of the key goals of critical-care nursing is to develop the skill of taking preventive measures to avoid complications whenever possible. The following nursing measures are examples of planning to prevent dysrhythmias.

- Reduce catecholamine stimulation, which can produce tachycardias and premature beats. Minimize the patient's anxiety and pain and avoid hypotension. Promote physical and emotional rest.
- Avoid vagal stimulation, which can produce bradycardia and blocks. Take the following actions:
  1. Teach the patient to avoid Valsalva maneuvers. Also consult the physician about using stool softeners to reduce straining during bowel movements.
  2. When suctioning the trachea, watch the cardiac monitor for the onset of bradycardia and observe recommended time limits for suction-

ing. (The trachea is innervated with vagal fibers.)

- Monitor patients on digitalis, beta-blockers, or calcium-channel blockers to detect intoxication promptly.
- Avoid or alleviate fluid and electrolyte imbalances. Follow the care plans listed in Chapter 16.

Intervention

The actions the nurse takes when a dysrhythmia occurs depend on the nurse's judgment about its significance and on the nurse's authorized scope of practice.

Significance of the Dysrhythmia Once the rhythm has been identified, its significance must be evaluated in terms of both its etiology and its consequences. Consequences fall into two main categories: the rhythm's effect on cardiac output and its tendency to become more serious.

Effect on Cardiac Output (CO) CO equals heart rate times stroke volume. Normal sinus rhythm is the optimal rhythm because it provides enough time for atrial and ventricular filling, proper coordination of valve openings and closings, and coronary artery filling during diastole. The coordination of AV valve movements is important because it permits the active phase of ventricular filling. During this phase, atrial contraction contributes about 30% of ventricular filling volume. Patients with poor myocardial reserve are particularly dependent on this mechanism to maintain CO. When it is lost (as in sudden atrial fibrillation), the resulting drop in CO may produce signs of shock.

Bradycardia decreases CO if its onset is sudden. If its onset is gradual, a compensatory increase in stroke volume may occur to maintain a normal CO.

Tachycardia increases CO up to the point at which it infringes seriously on ventricular filling time. At that rate (which varies from patient to patient), cardiac output drops because of the limited filling time. The patient's ability to tolerate a tachycardia depends not on its source but on its rate, the heart size, and additional insults (such as systemic hypoxia).

Tendency to Become More Serious A dysrhythmia may progress to more serious dysrhythmias. It is good nursing practice to watch for such a tendency, and take appropriate measures when changes occur. Following are examples of some possible progressions to more serious problems.

Tachycardia predisposes to the development of faster rhythms by decreasing coronary artery filling time at the same time it increases myocardial oxygen demand. The resulting myocardial hypoxia alters the resting membrane potential of cardiac cells, enhancing the likelihood of spontaneous depolarization.

Premature beats indicate cellular irritability. They predispose toward rapid, repetitive depolarization, that is, tachycardia, flutter, and fibrillation.

Bradycardia encourages beats to escape from lower sites of impulse formation. It does so by failing to depolarize those sites and by decreasing coronary artery perfusion pressure. These escape beats may accelerate and become the dominant rhythm.

Lower degrees of block may progress to more complete blocks.

Treatment Treatment, in both emergency and nonemergency situations, depends on identification of the etiology of the dysrhythmia and selection of a therapeutic modality. The most frequently used options for treatment of each dysrhythmia are indicated in the tables throughout this chapter. The types of therapy are discussed in Chapter 14 and in Appendix 2.

Scope of Practice Selection of the treatment modality is the prerogative of the physician. As some dysrhythmias require immediate treatment and consultation with a physician may be delayed, many units have standing medical orders to guide the nurses and protect them legally in these situations.

General Principles Governing Treatment The general principles governing treatment instituted by the nurse under standing medical orders are as follows:

1. Do not initiate treatment of a dysrhythmia if the patient is stable hemodynamically and if the rhythm is unlikely to worsen.

2. Immediately treat life-threatening dysrhythmias causing pulselessness: ventricular asystole, ventricular fibrillation, and ventricular tachycardia.

3. Promptly terminate tachydysrhythmias that are causing hemodynamic deterioration or are likely to accelerate.

For monitored ventricular tachycardia causing pulselessness, a precordial thump may be done; if not effective, then countershock immediately. For monitored ventricular tachycardia not causing pulselessness, give a precordial thump, or lidocaine 1 mg/kg as an IV bolus. If unsuccessful, consult the physician about using procainamide or bretylium tosylate. Recurrent or persistent ventricular tachycardia may warrant amiodarone, atrial pacing, cardiac catheterization, myocardial revascularization, cardiac sympathectomy, or automatic implantable defibrillator.

4. Promptly relieve bradycardia causing hemodynamic deterioration. For sinus bradycardia and AV blocks, give 0.5 mg atropine as an IV bolus. If unsuccessful, this dose may be repeated to a total of 2 mg or contact the physician about the use of isoproterenol or artificial pacing.

5. Immediately suppress premature beats if they are dangerous. Supraventricular beats rarely are; keep the physician informed of their presence, and follow his or her therapeutic plan. If premature ventricular beats are more than six per minute, more than three in a row, multifocal, or falling on or near the T wave, administer an IV bolus of lidocaine 1 mg/kg.

Outcome Evaluation

Evaluate the patient's progress according to the following outcome criteria. Ideally, the dysrhythmic episode will be terminated and the patient will develop a normal sinus rhythm. The ideal may not occur, however, particularly in the critically ill patient with preexisting heart disease. Realistic outcome criteria in the absence of normal sinus rhythm are spontaneous, drug-controlled, or artificially paced rhythms with the following characteristics:

- Ventricular rate 60–100 beats per minute.
- Ventricular rate adequate to perfuse core organs and periphery, as manifested by alert mental state; absence of angina; urinary output WNL for patient; warm, dry skin; peripheral pulses bilaterally equal and of normal volume for patient.
- Infrequent atrial or junctional premature beats, if any.
- Six or fewer ventricular premature beats per minute.
- No more than three VPBs in a row.
- No multifocal VPBs.
- No VPBs falling on or near T waves.

REFERENCES

Andreoli K et al.: *Comprehensive cardiac care,* 5th ed. St Louis: Mosby, 1983.

Burrell L, Burrell Z: *Critical care,* 4th ed. St Louis: Mosby, 1982.

Crabtree A, Jorgenson M: Exploring the practical knowledge in expert nursing critical-care practice. Unpublished master's thesis, University of Wisconsin, Madison, 1986.

Dubin D: *Rapid interpretation of EKGs,* 3d ed. Tampa, FL: COVER Publishing Company, 1974.

Guyton A: *Textbook of medical physiology,* 7th ed. Philadelphia: Saunders, 1986.

Kenner et al.: *Critical care nursing: Body-mind-spirit,* 2d ed. Boston: Little, Brown, 1985.

Lewis A: Monitoring and dysrhythmia recognition in advanced life support. In McIntyre K, Lewis A (eds): *Textbook of advanced life support,* pp. VI-1–28. Dallas: American Heart Association, 1981.

Marriott H: *Workshop in electrocardiography.* Oldsmar, FL: Tampa Tracings, 1972.

Marriott H: *Practical electrocardiography,* 7th ed. Baltimore: Williams and Wilkins, 1983.

Marriott H, Fogg E: Constant monitoring for cardiac dysrhythmias and blocks. *Mod Concepts Cardiovasc Dis* 1970; 39:103–105.

Marriott H, Gozensky C: Arrhythmias in coronary care: A renewed plea. *Heart Lung* 1982; 11:33–39.

Scagliotti D et al.: Aprindine-induced polymorphous ventricular tachycardia. *Am J Cardiol* 1982; 49:1297–1300.

Standards and Guidelines for Cardiopulmonary Resuscitation (CPR) and Emergency Cardiac Care (ECC). *JAMA* (June 6) 1986; 255:2915–2954.

SUPPLEMENTAL READING

Duke D: Intraventricular conduction blocks. Part I: Introduction and electrocardiographic identification of right and left bundle branch block. *Crit Care Nurse* (May/June) 1982a; 30–39.

Duke D: Intraventricular conduction blocks. Part II: Axis calculation and electrocardiographic identification of left anterior fascicular block and left posterior fascicular block. *Crit Care Nurse* (July/Aug) 1982b; 58–70.

Hudak C et al.: *Critical Care Nursing,* 3d ed. Philadelphia: Lippincott, 1982.

Karnes J: Premature ventricular contractions: When to sound the alarm. *Nurs 84* (June) 1984; 14:34–39.

Kim HS, Chung EK: Torsade de pointes: Polymorphous ventricular tachycardia. *Heart Lung* (May) 1983: 12:269–273.

Kupper NS et al.: Tachycardia: Stay a step ahead of your patient's racing heart. *Nurs 84* (Aug) 1984; 14:34–41.

Marriott H, Conover M: *Advanced Concepts in Arrhythmias.* St Louis: Mosby, 1983.

Schultz D, Olivas G: The use of cough cardiopulmonary resuscitation in clinical practice. *Heart Lung* (May) 1986; 15:273–280.

Scordo KA: Skill booklet: Cardiac dysrhythmias—Recognizing the ones that matter. *Nurs Life* (Sept/Oct) 1984; 4:33–46.

Smith M: Rx for ECG monitoring artifact. *Crit Care Nurse* (Jan/Feb) 1984; 4:64–66.

Steger K et al.: Drug-induced Torsade des pointes: Case report and implications for the critical care staff. *Heart Lung* (March) 1986; 15:200–202.

Valladares BK, Lemberg L: Ventricular arrhythmias: A perspective on management. *Heart Lung* (July) 1985; 14:417–420.

13

Cardiovascular Disorders

CLINICAL INSIGHT

Domain: Effective management of rapidly changing situations

Competency: Contingency management: rapid matching of demands and resources in emergency situations

Rapidly changing situations are the norm in critical-care nursing, and coping with them can be both exhilarating and exhausting. Such situations demand an immediate response, and often it is the expert who steps forward to take charge, overtly or covertly. Acting with confidence in the midst of disaster requires extensive clinical experience. Managing life-threatening crises successfully also requires an intimate knowledge of how the system works, as shown in the following paradigm (Benner 1984, pp. 115–116). Finally, having others accept one's pronouncements in such catastrophes requires a known track record; precious minutes can be lost if others challenge one's leadership or argue with one's judgments. In the crucible of a crisis, however, role distinctions often fall away; others may recognize and respect the authority conferred by expertise. Here, Nurse Jolene talks about fighting to save the life of a patient with a carotid bleed, coping with the news that there is no blood in the blood bank for the patient, and directing the panicked ICU resident.

By this time the problem is blood, we need blood, and so I said, "OK, someone call the blood bank and get us some blood." And the nurse said, "We just called and there's none down there." No one had caught that the patient was sitting up there with no blood in the blood bank. So we took off a blood (sample) from the arterial line and sent it down for a type and cross-match. Meanwhile, I started plasmanate and lactated Ringers, because the mean pressure was dropping down to about 30 and the blood was just pumping out of his mouth. About this time the ICU resident came in. He said, "What shall I do?" And I said, "You need to go down to the blood bank and get some type-specific blood for this patient, because a nurse can't get that. You're the only person who can get type-specific blood." It was the best thing he could do under the circumstances. I said, "Bring two units, they will only give you two at a time, no matter how bad. But bring two and get back here as soon as you can." So he took off. (The patient's fluid resuscitation was successful and the bleeding was controlled enough to get the patient to surgery in time to repair the artery.)

The critically ill patient is at high risk for developing a number of cardiovascular disorders. Dysrhythmias are covered in Chapter 12. This chapter helps you recognize other cardiovascular disorders, identify appropriate nursing diagnoses, and understand the nursing and medical measures used to treat such problems. Such knowledge provides the foundation on which to build the clinical expertise illustrated in the Clinical Insight.

ACUTE CHEST PAIN

As a critical-care nurse, you often will be called on to perform a rapid, accurate assessment of a patient who has acute chest pain and to institute emergency stabilization of that patient. The patient's symptomatology can be assessed quickly yet thoroughly using the PQRST mnemonic. As explained in Chapter 10, each letter represents an area to be evaluated:

P   Precipitating factors
Q   Quality
R   Region and radiation
S   Associated symptoms and signs
T   Time and response to treatment

The most common causes of acute chest pain can be grouped into five categories: cardiac, pulmonary, mus-

culoskeletal, gastrointestinal, and psychosomatic. Table 13–1 presents the most common subcategories of acute chest pain, analyzing each according to the PQRST format.

In addition to assessing the patient's symptoms, you should perform a quick evaluation of blood pressure, pulse, monitor rhythm, respirations, level of consciousness, and peripheral perfusion.

NURSING DIAGNOSES

Nursing diagnoses for the patient who has acute chest pain include:

- Pain
- Anxiety
- Potential decreased cardiac output
- Potential altered tissue perfusion
- Potential disturbed self-concept: body image, role performance

Nursing measures for each of these diagnoses are discussed elsewhere in the text; this section focuses on emergency stabilization.

Emergency stabilization of the patient with acute chest pain is accomplished using the following measures.

1. Place the patient in high Fowler's position to facilitate diaphragmatic expansion.

TABLE 13–1   CHEST PAIN PROFILES

P PRECIPITATING FACTORS	Q QUALITY	R REGION AND RADIATION	S ASSOCIATED SYMPTOMS AND SIGNS	T TIME AND RESPONSE TO TREATMENT
Cardiac				
Angina				
Physical exertion	Pressure	Substernal	Diaphoresis	Gradual onset
Emotional stress	Tightness	Unable to pinpoint	Nausea, vomiting	Duration <30 min
Environmental factors	Squeezing	Radiates to arms, throat,	Dyspnea	Relief with rest or
Eating	Burning	jaw, back, upper abdomen	Syncope	nitroglycerin
	Mild to moderate pain		Uneasiness	

(Continues)

TABLE 13–1   CHEST PAIN PROFILES (Continued)

P PRECIPITATING FACTORS	Q QUALITY	R REGION AND RADIATION	S ASSOCIATED SYMPTOMS AND SIGNS	T TIME AND RESPONSE TO TREATMENT
Cardiac				
Acute Myocardial Infarction				
Same as angina; more likely to occur with no precipitators	Same as angina Severe pain Worsened by fear and movement	Same as angina	Same as angina plus: Apprehension more severe Extra heart sounds Pulmonary congestion	Sudden onset Duration >30 min No relief with rest, nitroglycerin, or change in posture Relief with narcotics
Dissecting Aortic Aneurysm				
Hypertension	Tearing sensation Excruciating pain worse at onset	Substernal Radiation to back and abdomen "Traveling" sensation	Dyspnea Apprehension Diaphoresis BP differences between arms Absence of pulse unilaterally Hemiplegia or paraplegia Murmur of aortic regurgitation	Sudden onset No relief with rest or nitroglycerin Relief with narcotics
Pericarditis				
Myocardial infarction Uremia Trauma Infections	Sharp Stabbing Knife-like Mild to severe Deep or superficial Worsened by inspiration, coughing, muscle movement, lying on left side	Precordial Retrosternal Radiation to neck, arms, or back	Dyspnea Friction rub	Sudden onset Continuous No relief with rest or nitroglycerin Relief with sitting forward or aspirin
Pulmonary				
Pulmonary Embolism				
Prolonged sitting or lying down Phlebitis Long-bone fracture	Crushing Deep ache Shooting Increased by deep inspiration or coughing	Lateral chest (over lung fields) Radiation to shoulder, neck	Dyspnea Pallor or cyanosis Syncope Cough with hemoptysis Apprehension Sinus tachycardia Pleural rub Fever	Sudden onset No relief with rest or nitroglycerin Relief with narcotics
Spontaneous Pneumothorax				
COPD None	Tearing Increased by breathing	Lateral chest	Dyspnea Decreased breath sounds Tachycardia Agitation	Sudden onset
Pneumonia				
Respiratory infection	Moderate ache Increased by coughing, inspiration, movement	Over lung fields Radiation to shoulder, neck	Dyspnea Tachycardia Pleural rub Fever Productive cough	Gradual onset Continuous duration Relief with sitting up

TABLE 13–1 CHEST PAIN PROFILES (Continued)

P PRECIPITATING FACTORS	Q QUALITY	R REGION AND RADIATION	S ASSOCIATED SYMPTOMS AND SIGNS	T TIME AND RESPONSE TO TREATMENT
Musculoskeletal (chest wall)				
Neck or arm stain Reproducible with movement	Soreness, tenderness Increased by movement	Localized to side of midline Able to pinpoint	None	Gradual or sudden onset Continuous or intermittent No relief with nitroglycerin Relief with rest, analgesic, heat
Gastrointestinal				
Food intake Alcohol	"Heartburn" Increased by eating or lying down	Lower substernal Upper abdominal Midline Radiation to upper abdomen, back, shoulder	Dysphagia Belching Vomiting Diaphoresis	Gradual or sudden onset Continuous or intermittent Relief with antacids or sitting up
Psychosomatic				
Emotional stress Fatigue	Dull ache to sharp stabbing Superficial	Precordium rather than center of chest Pinpoint localization No radiation	Palpitations Hyperventilation Dizziness Dyspnea Fatigue Frequent sighing	Gradual or sudden Variable duration Relief with rest or sedation

2. Start high-flow oxygen, usually 6 liters/minute via nasal cannula. If the patient has chronic lung disease, give oxygen via nasal cannula at 2–3 liters/minute.

3. Institute cardiac monitoring if not already in use.

4. Establish an intravenous (IV) lifeline, if one is not already in place. The usual fluid is 5% dextrose in water, administered at a "keep open" (very slow) rate via a microdrop infusion set.

5. Provide pain relief, per medical orders, with sublingual nitroglycerin or intravenous analgesics.

6. Obtain diagnostic studies, as ordered. They usually include a stat chest x-ray, 12-lead ECG, and cardiac isoenzymes (particularly CPK-MB), as well as a routine CBC and electrolyte panel.

These measures, particularly the first four, can be accomplished simultaneously with evaluation of the chest pain by the PQRST method. In addition, they can be accomplished simultaneously with nursing measures to relieve the patient's fear and anxiety, such as projection of a calm, competent persona, brief explanations of procedures, and therapeutic use of touch.

Definitive treatment of acute chest pain depends on its cause. For further details, consult other sections of this text that discuss cardiac and respiratory disorders, the most common causes of acute chest pain.

ACUTE MYOCARDIAL INFARCTION

Because of the prevalence of coronary atherosclerosis in the general population and because of the stresses imposed by being critically ill, your patients have a significant risk of developing an acute myocardial infarction (MI).

Assessment

Risk Conditions

Be alert for factors associated with an increased risk of MI. Among those implicated by epidemiologic studies are these:

- Middle or old age
- Male sex
- Female sex after menopause
- Elevated serum cholesterol or triglycerides
- Hypertension
- Manifestations of coronary atherosclerotic heart disease before the age of 50 in patient's parents or sibling
- Cigarette smoking
- Diet high in calories, sugar, salt, cholesterol, total fat, and/or saturated fat and low in fish
- Diabetes, fasting blood sugar over 120 mg/100 ml, abnormal glucose tolerance test
- Sedentary lifestyle
- Constant emotional tension
- Type A behavior

In the patient with suspected or confirmed coronary artery disease, the additional following factors are associated with an increased risk of MI:

- Previous MI
- Any factor reducing coronary artery perfusion or oxygenation (for example, systemic hypoxia, hypotension)
- Any factor increasing ventricular workload (for example, physical stress, emotional stress, hypertension, aortic stenosis)

Decrease the risk factors whenever possible. Following are some examples of ways to decrease coronary risk factors. Educate patients, their families, and the general public about the risk factors and ways to reduce them. (For specific recommendations, consult the most recent literature from the American Heart As-

sociation.) Administer antihypertensive or antilipidemic drugs if prescribed by the physician. Maintain adequate systemic oxygenation and coronary arterial perfusion. Reduce physical stress by limiting ambulation and self-care during acute ischemic attacks. Reduce emotional stress by the measures outlined in Chapter 3.

Signs and Symptoms

Be alert to the various signs and symptoms of acute myocardial infarction.

Note the *characteristics of pain.* Acute infarction pain is usually substernal. The patient may describe it as crushing, "like a weight on my chest," and when asked to localize it will place a clenched fist on the sternum. Frequently, the pain will radiate down the left arm, down both arms, or up into the neck. Less common sites of pain for which you should be alert are the jaw, back, and abdomen. Typically, the pain is constant and unrelieved by rest or by sublingual nitroglycerin (1 tablet q5min $\times$ 3).

Observe for *increased sympathetic stimulation.* Most patients develop increased sympathetic stimulation during an infarct. This stimulation produces tachycardia, slight hypertension, diaphoresis and clammy skin, and nausea or vomiting. Some patients suffer cardiovascular depression, possibly due to reflexes from the ischemic area. These people display bradycardia and hypotension.

Check for *additional findings:* On auscultation, you may hear an S_3, S_4, or paradoxically split S_2 due to decreased left ventricular compliance. The patient usually is short of breath. Blood gases show a metabolic acidosis (due to inadequate tissue perfusion) and respiratory alkalosis (due to hyperventilation). Severe apprehension is common.

Diagnostic Procedures

Causes of Infarctions Infarctions may occur for a variety of reasons; the exact cause may be difficult for the physician to diagnose. It is thought to occur most commonly as a result of occlusion of a coronary artery. In the past, thrombosis was believed to cause all infarctions. This concept has been proven erroneous. Although thrombosis precedes most infarctions, other causes have been identified. The occlusion may be due to atheromatous narrowing, spasm of the artery, or embolization of thrombi, fatty plaques, air or calcium. In some cases, the infarct may result not from occlusion but from a great disparity between myocardial oxygen demand and coronary arterial supply.

Types of Infarctions There may be two types of infarctions: subendocardial and transmural. The *transmural* infarction involves 50–75% or more of the total thickness of the ventricular wall and is characterized by abnormal Q waves and ST–T changes. It usually is due to atherosclerosis and arterial occlusion. The terms *subendocardial, nontransmural* and *non-Q-wave* have been used to describe infarcts with abnormal ST–T changes but no abnormal Q waves. Since these criteria also are consistent with small infarcts, the existence of subendocardial infarction is controversial. Infarcts limited to the subendocardium probably result not from arterial occlusion but rather from microemboli or a disparity between oxygen demand and supply. The subendocardium is particularly vulnerable to ischemia because of a combination of factors. Because it has the longest myofibrils in the heart, its O_2 need is greatest. Since coronary arteries lie on the epicardium, the epicardium is oxygenated better than the endocardium. As a result, at the same time the subendocardium needs more O_2 than other cardiac cells, the blood perfusing it has the lowest Po_2 in the heart. In addition, during systole the high pressure in the subendocardium and the wringing effect of contraction preclude perfusion of the subendocardium. Once subendocardial injury has occurred, it is particularly likely to progress to infarction and extension. The swelling of damaged cells and clotting combine to compress surrounding tissue. These factors also increase coronary arterial resistance, which creates a further decrease in flow both to the injured area and to the areas distal to it.

Coronary Blood Supply As many infarcts are due to arterial occlusion, it is helpful to understand the distribution of the coronary blood supply (Figure 13–1). The heart is supplied by three coronary arteries: the right and two branches of the left main coronary artery (the anterior descending and the circumflex coronary arteries). The right and left main coronary arteries arise from sinuses of Valsalva, recesses located on the aorta just above the aortic valve. The arteries lie on the epicardial surface and send small branches into the endocardium.

The right coronary artery courses along the anterior groove or sulcus between the right atrium and ventricle, giving off a branch (the marginal artery) to the apex. It continues along the posterior atrioventricular groove and in most cases descends along the posterior groove in between the ventricles, creating the posterior descending artery. In its course, the right coronary artery supplies the right atrium, right ventricle, posterior third of the septum, and the inferior (diaphragmatic) and posterior left ventricle.

The left main coronary artery splits into its two branches soon after arising from the aorta. The left anterior descending (LAD) coronary artery passes behind the pulmonary artery and travels down the anterior interventricular groove. In its course, it supplies the anterior two-thirds of the septum and the anterior and apical portions of the left ventricle, as well as portions of the right ventricle.

The left circumflex (LCX) coronary artery traverses the left atrioventricular groove from anterior to posterior. It sometimes ends as a descending artery along the posterior left ventricle. The LCX nourishes the left atrium, lateral left ventricle, and in some cases the posterior left ventricle and posterior ventricular septum.

All three coronary arteries supply parts of the conduction system. The SA node is nourished by the right coronary artery in about 60% of the population, and the circumflex artery in 40%. The internodal tracts are supplied by the right coronary artery. The AV node and bundle of His are supplied by the right coronary artery (90%) or circumflex artery (10%). The bundle branches are nourished primarily by the LAD and secondarily by the RCA.

Knowledge of the arterial blood supply will help you to understand the ECG signs of the infarction and predict specific patient problems that may occur.

ECG Indicators of Infarction If you suspect an infarct, obtain immediate medical help while you record a 12-lead ECG. If an infarct is diagnosed, obtain further recordings each of the next three days and thereafter as determined by the physician. Follow the serial 12-lead ECGs for the location and resolution of the infarct.

Myocardial ischemia, injury, and infarction usually produce characteristic changes on the ECG (Figure 13-2). These changes are detectable in leads whose positive poles overlie the involved area (indicative leads), as well as in leads whose positive poles overlie the opposite side of the heart (reciprocal leads). *Ischemia* impairs repolarization and therefore inverts the T wave. *Injury* to the myocardium prevents cells from becoming fully polarized; it therefore alters the ST segment. Indicative leads will show ST elevation, reciprocal leads ST depression. *Infarction* produces absence of electrical activity, creating in effect an "electrical window." Leads whose positive poles are closest to this window look "through" it, recording electrical activity on the other side of the heart. Consider a V_6 electrode, whose positive pole overlies the lateral left ventricle. You will recall that this lead normally displays a large R wave; it does not record right ventricular depolarization because that is obscured by the large positive wave of left ven-

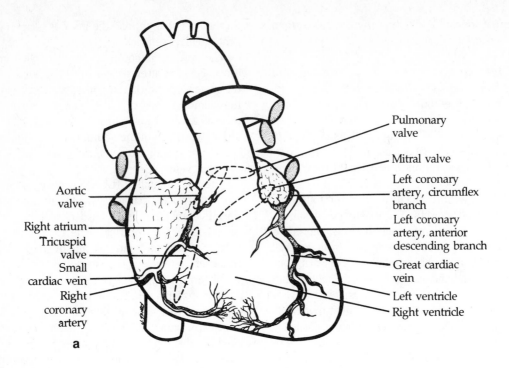

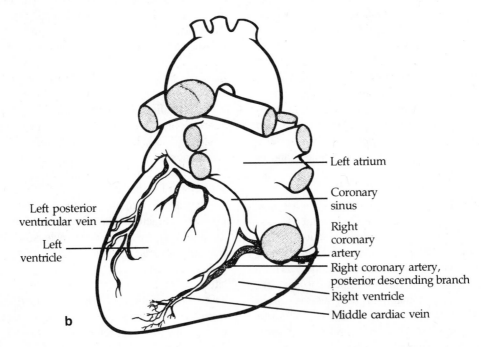

FIGURE 13–1

Coronary blood vessels. **a,** Anterior view; **b,** posterior view.

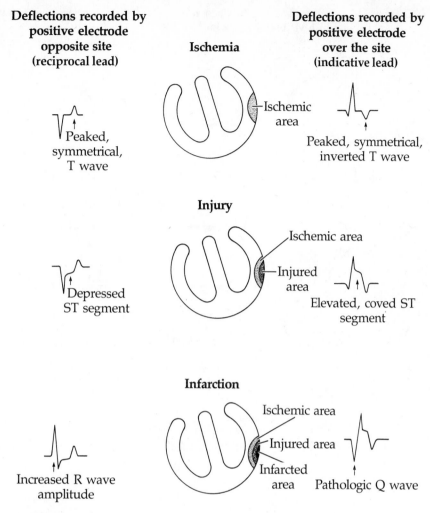

Deflections recorded by positive electrode opposite site (reciprocal lead)

Deflections recorded by positive electrode over the site (indicative lead)

Ischemia

Peaked, symmetrical, T wave

Ischemic area

Peaked, symmetrical, inverted T wave

Injury

Depressed ST segment

Ischemic area

Injured area

Elevated, coved ST segment

Infarction

Increased R wave amplitude

Ischemic area

Injured area

Infarcted area

Pathologic Q wave

FIGURE 13–2

ECG patterns of myocardial ischemia, injury, and infarction. Note that as damage progresses, signs are superimposed on earlier changes. For example, the pattern of infarction includes the pathologic Q wave (produced by the infarcted area), and elevated ST segment (from the surrounding injured area), and an inverted T wave (from the surrounding ischemic area).

tricular depolarization. When the lateral left ventricle infarcts, its cells no longer transmit current, so no R wave is recorded. Without the positive wave coming toward it, the electrode is free to record electrical activity on the other side of the heart. Because this current is moving away from it, the electrode records a significant negative deflection, that is, a Q wave. Now consider a V_1 electrode, whose positive pole is opposite the infarct. It normally records a small R wave of septal depolarization. Then it records a large S wave, because the combined effect of right and left ventricular depolar-

ization causes a current moving away from it. When the lateral left ventricle infarcts, V_1 will record an initial R wave as it usually does. Now, however, there are no negative left ventricular forces to oppose right ventricular depolarization. V_1 therefore continues to inscribe a positive wave, producing a large R wave.

Location and Evolution of Infarction The location of the infarct may be determined by noting in which leads the characteristic changes appear (Figure 13–3). The positive poles of leads I, AVL, and V_4–V_6 overlie

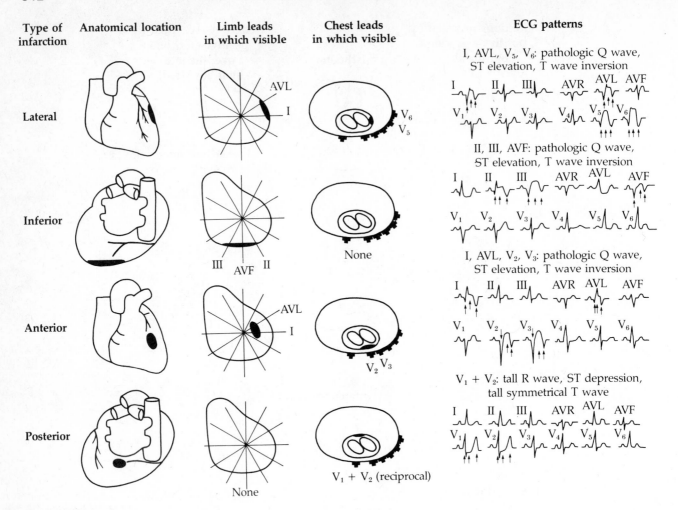

Type of infarction	Anatomical location	Limb leads in which visible	Chest leads in which visible	ECG patterns

Lateral

Inferior

Anterior

Posterior

AVL / I

III AVF II

None

AVL / I

V₂ V₃

None

V₆ V₅

V₁ + V₂ (reciprocal)

I, AVL, V₅, V₆: pathologic Q wave, ST elevation, T wave inversion

II, III, AVF: pathologic Q wave, ST elevation, T wave inversion

I, AVL, V₂, V₃: pathologic Q wave, ST elevation, T wave inversion

V₁ + V₂: tall R wave, ST depression, tall symmetrical T wave

FIGURE 13–3

Localization of infarcts. *Lateral infarct* usually results from occlusion of the left coronary artery, circumflex branch. *Inferior infarct* usually is due to occlusion of the right coronary artery, posterior descending branch. *Anterior infarct* usually results from occlusion of the left coronary artery, anterior descending branch. *Posterior infarct* usually is due to occlusion of the right coronary artery.

the lateral LV wall, and those of leads II, III, and AVF overlie the inferior LV wall. The lateral and inferior walls are opposite each other anatomically. When indicative changes occur in I, AVL, and V_4–V_6, reciprocal changes occur in II, III, and AVF, and vice versa.

The positive poles of chest leads V_1 through V_3 overlie, or "look at," the anterior left ventricular wall. Although the anterior and posterior LV walls are opposite anatomically, the 12-lead ECG contains no leads whose positive poles overlie the posterior wall. If an anterior infarction occurs, indicative changes are seen in leads V_2 and V_3, but there are no leads that display reciprocal changes. If a posterior infarction occurs, there are no leads that demonstrate indicative changes, but V_1 and V_2 may show reciprocal changes. For this reason, it is difficult to diagnose a posterior infarct from a 12-lead ECG; other techniques, such as vectorcardiography, are more informative.

These ECG changes can be used to identify the acuteness or evolution of an infarction (Figure 13–4). As the zone of infarction may be surrounded by a zone of injury, which in turn is enclosed by a zone of ischemia, signs of all three zones may be visible simultaneously on the ECG of a patient with a fully evolved fresh infarction. Alternatively, ECG changes may occur sequentially. In the earliest hours post-MI (the *hyperacute phase*), the ECG is characterized by ST elevation merging into giant, upright T waves. T wave inversion begins within 8–24 hours post-MI; abnormal Q waves develop within several days after MI.

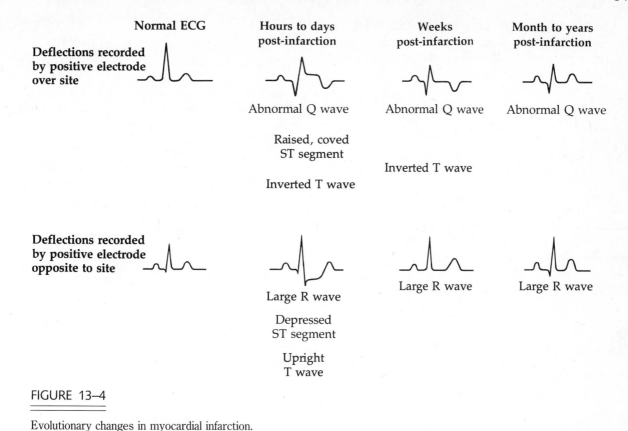

FIGURE 13–4

Evolutionary changes in myocardial infarction.

A few weeks post-MI, the ST segment becomes isoelectric. The T waves return to normal in anywhere from a few months to years post-MI. Typically, after 2–3 months the signs of a chronic or old infarction are apparent. The ST and T waves are normal, but the significant Q waves and the loss of R wave progression remain.

When examining the ECG for signs of ischemia, injury, and infarction, it is important to remember that changes in the T wave, ST segment, and QRS can be caused by conditions other than myocardial infarction. ST–T changes are nonspecific; tachycardia, hyperventilation, cerebral disorders, electrolyte imbalances, pericarditis, pulmonary embolism, and digitalis administration are common causes. QRS alterations also may result from left ventricular hypertrophy, pulmonary embolism, and complicated congenital heart defects, to name a few. These facts emphasize the importance of evaluating the ECG only in conjunction with other patient data.

Serum Enzymes and Radionuclide Imaging Additional measures used in the diagnosis of MI include evaluation of serum enzymes and radionuclide imaging. Serum enzymes show a pattern of characteristic changes, with elevations of CK-MB and the "flipped

LDH" pattern most diagnostic of acute MI. With Q-wave infarction CK-MB elevations are detected 4 hours post-MI and peak in 24 hours. In non-Q-wave infarction, there is more rapid release of CK-MB, peaking in 17 hours. For further details on normal values, onset and duration of elevations, and significance of abnormal values, please consult Chapter 11.

Radionuclide imaging enables imaging of the infarction and myocardial perfusion and provides indices of

---

NURSING DIAGNOSES

Nursing diagnoses that may apply to the patient suffering from an acute MI include:

- Anxiety
- Fear
- Chest pain
- Impaired gas exchange
- Potential decreased cardiac output
- Activity intolerance
- Constipation
- Ineffective coping

left ventricular function. Imaging is particularly valuable because it facilitates serial evaluation of infarction that can be repeated as often as necessary (see Chapter 11).

Planning and Implementation of Care

Nearby are presented plans of care, developed by the nursing staff of the University of Washington Critical Care Unit, for patients with uncomplicated MIs. They include specific problems and nursing actions for patients with particular types of infarcts.

Outcome Evaluation

Evaluate the patient's progress and the effects of your nursing interventions according to these outcome criteria:

- Heart rate and rhythm normal for patient.
- Cardiac output adequate, as manifested by: BP within patient's normal limits; alert, oriented state; absence of refractory angina or serious dysrhythmias; urinary output above 30–60 ml/hr; warm, dry skin; peripheral pulses WNL.
- Realistic plans made by patient and family for coping with changes in lifestyle and for return to a satisfying lifestyle after discharge.

NURSING CARE PLAN

Uncomplicated Myocardial Infarction

NURSING DIAGNOSIS	SIGNS AND SYMPTOMS	NURSING ACTIONS	DESIRED OUTCOMES
Behavioral responses observed in patients admitted to CCU to rule out MI: a. Anxiety/fear related to CCU admission	Appears restless Appears hostile, withdrawn Talks incessantly Has difficulty concentrating Muscular tenseness Watchful, frightened appearance	1. Introduce self to patient and family. 2. Limit nursing personnel caring for patient for continuity (Primary Care Nurse). 3. Stress that frequent assessments are part of the preventive purpose of unit and do not necessarily imply a deteriorating condition. 4. Inform patient/family of nurses' specialty training, if necessary. 5. Maintain a confident manner. 6. Repeat information PRN because of reduced attention span. 7. Judicious use of minor tranquilizers (e.g., Valium). 8. Educate patient about illness. 9. Encourage family visiting.	Decreased signs and symptoms of anxiety in patient/family.

NURSING CARE PLAN (Continued)

Uncomplicated Myocardial Infarction (Continued)

NURSING DIAGNOSIS	SIGNS AND SYMPTOMS	NURSING ACTIONS	DESIRED OUTCOMES
b. Fear of death, and anxiety over unfinished business	Verbalizes fatalism or acts extremely emotional, as if in grieving process. Verbalizes need to contact people, cancel appointments, "put affairs in order."	1. Allow patient/family to verbalize fears. 2. Answer questions when possible; don't avoid questions. 3. Facilitate the resolution of outside stressors by use of Social Services. Discuss alternatives.	Patient/family verbalize plans for activity progression upon discharge.
c. Fear of the unknown: medical/nursing procedures; changes in lifestyle; expectations of performance as a patient/family	Watches procedures with apprehension Asks questions about procedures Patient/family displays confusion/anxiety as to what actions are safe.	1. Provide brief and quiet explanation of admission procedure and rationale for: a. Placing in position of comfort (raise head of bed) and initially limiting activity to bedrest with commode privileges (activity plan). b. EKG monitor—purpose, alarm system, avoid tangling in wires, why continuous monitoring. c. Vital signs (BP, P, R, T) d. IV (meds, fluids) e. Labs (enzymes, electrolytes, UA, EKG, CXR). f. History-taking and cardiovascular assessment using CCC Admit Summary. 2. Orient family and patient to environment: a. How bed works, telephones, TVs b. How to call for RN c. Symptoms to notify RN of, including: chest pain, shortness of breath, palpitations, IV pain. d. Visiting hours	Patient/family verbalizes understanding of procedures.

(Continues)

NURSING CARE PLAN (Continued)

Uncomplicated Myocardial Infarction (Continued)

NURSING DIAGNOSIS	SIGNS AND SYMPTOMS	NURSING ACTIONS	DESIRED OUTCOMES

Alteration in comfort-chest pain related to myocardial ischemia/necrosis	Typically substernal, described as a heaviness, tightness, pressure, or aching. Radiation to arms (especially left) is common. May also c/o jaw, neck, throat, shoulder, back, or arm pain. Associated signs and symptoms:
	  nausea/vomiting
	  diaphoresis
	  weakness
	  anxiety
	  shortness of breath
	  dysrhythmias
	  palpitations
	  indigestion
		1. Chest vital signs.
		2. Note monitor rhythm.
		3. Administer medications to relieve pain:
		    nitroglycerin
		    MS (drug of choice)
		    or
		    Demerol IV
		4. Administer oxygen 3–8 L/min.
		5. Perform 12-lead EKG.
		6. Stay with patient until discomfort is relieved, offering reassurance and explanations of care.
		7. Prepare for IABP insertion, if unrelieved by drug therapy.
			Patient is free of pain
			Limitation of myocardial infarction size

Impaired gas exchange related to decreased cardiac output	Increased or decreased HR Decreased blood pressure Dusky color Decreased temperature Impaired capillary refill Restlessness Reduced arterial Po_2 Dyspnea	Administer oxygen at 3–8 liters per cannula for 24–48 hours	Normal vital signs Good skin color Absence of dyspnea $Po_2 \geq 100$ mm Hg
Potential for alteration in cardiac output: decreased, related to dysrhythmias	Dysrhythmias	1. Monitor EKG constantly (alarms on at all times). 2. Consider prophylactic use of antidysrhythmic drugs. 3. Monitor for side effects of antidysrhythmic drugs: hypotension, dizziness, nausea, vomiting.	Absence of life-threatening dysrhythmias
Decreased activity and exercise due to healing myocardium	See Cardiac Rehabilitation Manual		

Elevated enzymes confirming MI diagnosis	CPK >100 U/L*
	CPK_2 >6 U/L
	LDH >290 U/L
	LDH 1 > 82
	    2 > 119
	    3 > 87
	    4 > 68
	    5 > 85
	SGOT >25 U/L
		1. Ascertain approximate time of onset of pain.
		2. Draw enzymes as ordered. Ideally enzymes drawn 12 and 24 hours after onset of acute symptoms will confirm diagnosis. If not, draw again in 36 hours after acute MI symptoms.
			Enzymes within normal limits:*
			CPK_2 <6 U/L
			CPK <100 U/L
			LDH <290 U/L
			    1 $\leq$ 82
			    2 $\leq$ 119
			    3 $\leq$ 87
			    4 $\leq$ 68
			    5 $\leq$ 85

Alteration in bowel elimination: constipation related to bedrest	Straining at stool Subjective feeling of fullness	1. Ensure adequate bulk in diet and adequate fluid intake. 2. Prevent straining: administer stool softeners or laxatives PRN.	Elimination achieved without straining

*Values cited are those in use at University of Washington.

NURSING CARE PLAN (Continued)

Uncomplicated Myocardial Infarction (Continued)

NURSING DIAGNOSIS	SIGNS AND SYMPTOMS	NURSING ACTIONS	DESIRED OUTCOMES
		3. Give bedside commode privileges—ensure privacy. 4. Progress activity as tolerated.	
Ineffective individual coping related to behavioral responses commonly observed in patients who experience myocardial infarction: **a.** Acute anxiety	Decreased verbalization Inability to concentrate, understand, or retain information Restlessness or insomnia Muscular rigidity Palmar sweating Tremulousness Tachycardia	1. Maintain consistent, continuous nurse–patient contact. 2. Give repeated orientation to CCU routines, equipment, and procedures to patient and family. 3. Assess the patient's prior experience with illness, hospitalization, and severe stress and how it relates to current condition. 4. Solicit expressions of concern and questions from patient and family. 5. Prepare patient and family for each change or move in the patient's physical environment. 6. Allow at least 6 hours of uninterrupted sleep during night. 7. If not on a tranquilizer, assess need and discuss with physician. 8. Teach progressive relaxation. 9. Encourage patient to listen to soothing music.	Verbalizations and behaviors that demonstrate decreased emotional stress. Identifies primary nurse. Verbalizes "slept all night."
b. Denial	Avoids discussing the heart attack or its significance Minimizes the severity of the condition and its consequences Describes condition by quoting others (the doctor says . . .) May verbally acknowledge having had a heart attack, but disregards activity and diet restrictions	1. Assess whether denial is inhibiting the treatment plan: is it verbal or active denial? 2. If verbal, listen but do not reinforce the denial or force acceptance of a fact patient is not ready to cope with. 3. If active (i.e., disregards activity restrictions), assess consequences of pa-	Demonstrates adherence to activity and exercise program. Chooses foods based on restrictions. Verbalizes appropriate modifications in lifestyle.

(Continues)

NURSING CARE PLAN (Continued)

Uncomplicated Myocardial Infarction (Continued)

NURSING DIAGNOSIS	SIGNS AND SYMPTOMS	NURSING ACTIONS	DESIRED OUTCOMES
		tient's actions. Are they detrimental? Conveying concern and allowing more control of the environment are more successful than "threats." 4. If necessary, consult psychiatric clinical nurse specialist.	
c. Depression	Appearance, verbalizations, and behavior exhibiting depression	1. Verbally reflect your observations. 2. Solicit and listen to the patient's feelings; assess how he or she perceives the illness. 3. Allow and encourage tearfulness or crying. 4. Be "matter of fact" about patient's expressions of anger. 5. If patient becomes extremely hostile or angry, do not try to clarify or reason at that time. 6. Manipulate environment. 7. Educate patient about the illness.	Expresses feelings of anger.

Anterior Myocardial Infarction
See Uncomplicated MI, plus:

NURSING DIAGNOSIS	SIGNS AND SYMPTOMS	NURSING ACTIONS	DESIRED OUTCOMES
Anterior MI due to left anterior descending artery occlusion	ST segment elevation >1 mm T wave inversion Possible Q wave in leads I, AVL, V_1–V_4.	Obtain 12-lead EKG every morning for 3 days.	Return of the ST segment to baseline in leads 1, AVL, V_1–V_4 within 1–6 weeks.
Potential bundle branch block due to septal involvement	Widened QRS complex >0.12 sec. RBBB evidenced by: (1) rSR' in V_1; (2) Rs in V_6 (MCR_5) Complete LBBB evidenced by: (1) rS in V_1; (2) large monophasic R wave; no septal Q wave in V_6 (MCR_5) Left anterior divisional block (hemiblock) (1) Left axis deviation (axis $> -60°$) (2) negative QRS deflections in I, III, and MCR_5	1. Observe monitor closely, and document width of QRS. 2. Observe daily EKG closely for axis deviation. 3. Observe for development of biventricular block.	Sinus rhythm with QRS width within normal limits. Normal QRS axis on 12-lead EKG.

NURSING CARE PLAN (Continued)

Uncomplicated Myocardial Infarction (Continued)

NURSING DIAGNOSIS	SIGNS AND SYMPTOMS	NURSING ACTIONS	DESIRED OUTCOMES
Potential second degree AV block-Mobitz Type II with progression to complete heart block due to occlusion of left anterior descending coronary artery	Dizziness Syncope Alteration in LOC Mean arterial pressure (MAP) <80 mm Hg Second-degree AV block evidenced by: (1) nonconducted P waves; (2) constant PR interval of conducted beats Complete heart block evidenced by: (1) ventricular rate below 40/min; (2) atrial rate > ventricular rate; (3) QRS width >0.12 sec.	1. Observe monitor carefully for progression of heart block. 2. Notify physician of progressive block. 3. Observe: (1) vital signs; (2) skin for color, temperature, and moisture; (3) urinary output every 2 hours. 4. Correlate heart rate and rhythm with patient's clinical status. 5. See CCC Standing Orders re: Isuprel administration 6. Prepare equipment for possible pacemaker insertion.	HR > 50/min. MAP > 80 mm Hg. Clear mentation. Absence of dizziness and syncope. Urine output > 30 cc/hr.
Potential ventricular ectopy	Ventricular ectopy (PVBs, ventricular tachycardia, and ventricular fibrillation)	1. Observe monitor for ventricular ectopy. 2. Initiate therapy according to CCC Standing Orders. 3. Monitor for side effects of antidysrhythm drugs.	Absence of ventricular ectopy.
Potential interventricular septal rupture due to necrosis and scarring	Paradoxical pulse Distant heart sounds Holosystolic murmur at the apex and left sternal border MAP <80 mm Hg Significant HR change Decreased level of consciousness Sudden cardiac death	1. Observe and assess patient each hour: (1) vital signs; (2) breath sounds; (3) heart sounds (S_3, S_4 systolic murmur). 2. Initiate CPR if necessary. 3. Prepare patient for surgery.	Absence of paradoxical pulse. MAP >80 mm Hg. HR >50/min. Clear mentation. Skin warm and dry. Urinary output >30cc/hr. Absence of holosystolic murmur.
Potential ventricular aneurysm	Ventricular ectopy Paradoxical pulse Distant heart sounds MAP < 80 mm Hg Significant HR change Decreased level of consciousness Sudden cardiac death	1. Initiate activity progression and monitor patient's tolerance. 2. Observe monitor for ventricular ectopy. 3. Initiate therapy for ventricular ectopy according to CCC Standing Orders. 4. Initiate CPR if necessary.	Absence of ventricular ectopy. Absence of hemodynamic changes.
Potential dysfunction or rupture of papillary muscle	Abrupt onset of holosystolic murmur caused by mitral regurgitation Presence of S_3 and/or S_4 Mid-systolic ejection click Crackles in lung field	1. Assess heart sounds, lung sounds, and vital signs q2hrs. 2. Administer vasodilator drugs as ordered. 3. Prepare patient for IABP insertion. 4. Prepare patient for surgery.	Absence of holosystolic murmur. Absence of S_3, S_4, and mid-systolic ejection click. Absence of crackles. MAP >80 mm Hg.

(Continues)

NURSING CARE PLAN (Continued)

Uncomplicated Myocardial Infarction (Continued)

NURSING DIAGNOSIS	SIGNS AND SYMPTOMS	NURSING ACTIONS	DESIRED OUTCOMES
Potential acute congestive heart failure	See the nursing care plan for congestive heart failure, later in this chapter		
Potential cardiogenic shock.	See section on shock, later in this chapter		
Potential extension into lateral wall of myocardium.	See Lateral MI		

Diaphragmatic/Inferior MI
See Uncomplicated MI, plus:

NURSING DIAGNOSIS	SIGNS AND SYMPTOMS	NURSING ACTIONS	DESIRED OUTCOMES
Inferior MI due to occlusion of the right coronary artery	ST segment elevation >1 mm in leads II, III, and AVF T wave inversion in leads II, III, and AVF Q waves in leads II, III, and AVF	1. Obtain 12-lead EKG every morning for 3 days. 2. Observe for ST segment evolution in leads II, III, and AVF. 3. Observe for ST segment changes in other leads.	ST segment returns to baseline in leads II, III, and AVF.
Potential ischemia of SA node	Sinus bradycardia (<60 beats per minute)	1. Assess patient for hypotension, mentation changes, pallor, fatigue, and pain. 2. Observe for junctional or ventricular escape rhythms. 3. With significant hypotension, lower head of bed and elevate legs. 4. If symptomatic, give atropine 0.6 mg IV as per CCC Standing Orders (maximum of 2.0 mg over 2½ hrs).	Heart rate >60 beats per minute.
Potential ischemia of AV node resulting in second-degree AV heart block, Mobitz Type I (Wenckebach)	Second-degree AV block (Type I), evidenced by: (1) progressive lengthening of PR interval with each successive beat until a P wave appears without a QRS; (2) irregular R–R intervals	1. Observe rhythm carefully for progression of block. 2. If symptomatic, give atropine 0.6 mg IV as per CCC Standing Orders (maximum of 2.0 mg over 2½ hrs).	Absence of second-degree AV block, Mobitz Type I.
Potential pain related to extension to lateral or posterior myocardial wall	See Lateral MI Standard See Posterior MI Standard		
Pain related to inflammation of pericardium. a. Epistenocardia (focal pericarditis) within 4–5 days	Chest pain differs from myocardial pain in that it increases with deep inspiration or with movement	1. Reassure patient/family that disease is an inflammatory process rather than an MI.	Absence of chest pain. Absence of paradoxical pulse. Absence of pericardial friction rub.

NURSING CARE PLAN (Continued)

Uncomplicated Myocardial Infarction (Continued)

NURSING DIAGNOSIS	SIGNS AND SYMPTOMS	NURSING ACTIONS	DESIRED OUTCOMES
b. Dressler's syndrome (generalized pericarditis) within 10–14 days	Fever Tachycardia Paradoxical pulse Accentuated S_2 in pulmonic area Pericardial friction rub: (1) focal pericarditis shows ST segment elevation in II, III, and AVF; (2) generalized pericarditis shows ST segment elevation in limb and precordial leads ST segment elevation is concave in pericarditis versus convex in an infarction. Elevated sedimentation rate Leukocytosis	2. Administer steroids/antiinflammatory agents/salicylates as ordered. 3. Monitor for signs and symptoms of cardiac tamponade. 4. Monitor for potential arrhythmias. 5. Administer antipyretics for relief of fever. 6. Place in position of comfort. Usually if patient sits up and leans forward, pain may be somewhat relieved.	Return of ST segment to baseline
Potential right ventricular infarction	See Right Ventricular MI		

Lateral MI
See Uncomplicated MI Standard, plus:

NURSING DIAGNOSIS	SIGNS AND SYMPTOMS	NURSING ACTIONS	DESIRED OUTCOMES
Lateral MI due to occlusion of the left circumflex artery	ST segment elevation, T wave inversion, and possible Q wave in leads I, AVL, MCR_5, and V_6	Obtain a 12-lead EKG every morning for 3 days.	Return of ST segment to baseline in leads I, AVL, MCR_5, and V_6 within 1–6 weeks.
Potential acute congestive heart failure	See the nursing care plan for congestive heart failure, later in this chapter		
Potential ventricular ectopy			
Potential ventricular rupture	See Anterior MI		
Potential ventricular aneurysm			

Posterior MI
See Uncomplicated MI Standard, plus:

NURSING DIAGNOSIS	SIGNS AND SYMPTOMS	NURSING ACTIONS	DESIRED OUTCOMES
Posterior MI due to occlusion of circumflex branch of left coronary artery or occlusion of right coronary artery	Tall and slightly widened R wave in V_1 and V_2 Tall, upright symmetric T waves in V_1 and V_2 Depressed, concave, upward sloping ST segment or possibly isoelectric ST segment in V_1 and V_2	1. Refer to Diaphragmatic/Inferior MI Standard and Lateral MI Standard as posterior MI is usually an extension of either one and rarely stands alone.	Normal R wave progression in the precordial leads beginning in V_1 and V_2.

(Continues)

NURSING CARE PLAN (Continued)

Uncomplicated Myocardial Infarction (Continued)

Right Ventricular MI
See Uncomplicated MI Standard, plus:

NURSING DIAGNOSIS	SIGNS AND SYMPTOMS	NURSING ACTIONS	DESIRED OUTCOMES
Right ventricular infarction due to occlusion of the right coronary artery	Presence of inferior/diaphragmatic MI Elevated cardiac enzymes History of chest pain Pallor Possible hypotension Absence of pulmonary congestion Anxiety	1. Control pain with analgesics as per order. 2. Anticipate Swan Ganz catheter insertion.	Absence of chest pain. Uncomplicated inferior MI.
Right ventricular failure due to decreased contractility secondary to muscle damage	Elevated jugular venous pressure (neck vein distention) Elevated central venous pressure (CVP) with normal to low pulmonary capillary wedge (PCW) pressure Hypotension Pallor Lungs clear S_3 on inspiration	1. Administer fluid challenge to increase cardiac output by passive filling of left ventricle (as per order). 2. Avoid administering diuretics and nitrates, which decrease right ventricular filling volume and further decrease left ventricular filling. 3. Measure and record hemodynamic parameters.	Cardiac output 4–8 liters/min. Absence of neck vein distention. Normal CVP. Palpable peripheral pulses. MAP > 80 mm Hg.
Potential second-degree AV block, Mobitz Type I (Wenckebach)	See Inferior MI		

From University of Washington Critical Care Unit: Nursing care plan for MI patients. *Crit Care Nurse* (July/Aug) 1982; 79–84. Adapted with permission.

CARDIAC FAILURE

Cardiac failure may be defined as an inability of the heart to meet the body's metabolic demands. In cardiac failure, cardiac output per se may be low, normal, or high.

Cardiac output (CO) is the amount of blood ejected by the ventricle per minute. It is equal to the product of the heart rate and stroke volume. Therefore, abnormalities of the heart rate or stroke volume can result in a change in cardiac output. The heart rate can be assessed by the radial pulse or the apical pulse or evaluation of the EKG. When assessing heart rate, the cardiac response to varying stroke volumes should be evaluated. For example, the patient who is hypovolemic or in cardiac failure should develop a tachycardia. This normal response may be impaired by drug therapy, such as beta-blockers, or intrinsic atrial ventricular conduction defects. Other dysrhythmias that may contribute to altered cardiac output are junctional rhythm and atrial fibrillation, where the atrial component of cardiac output is lost.

Stroke volume in turn depends on myocardial preload, afterload, and contractility. *Preload* refers to the length of ventricular fibers at the end of diastole. It is directly dependent on the volume of blood in the ventricle; as the volume increases, preload—and therefore stroke volume—increases (Frank-Starling mechanism). This compensatory mechanism for regulating stroke volume will fail if the ventricular volume load becomes excessive. Because ventricular volume is in turn determined primarily by venous return to the heart, "preload" commonly is used as a synonym for "venous return." Preload is assessed from central venous or left atrial (pulmonary capillary wedge) pressure. An *elevated* preload may indicate cardiac failure or hypervolemia; a *decreased* preload may indicate hypovolemia (fluid volume deficit). Both problems can lead to an alteration in cardiac output.

Afterload refers to the tension and stress that develops in the wall of the ventricle during systole. It is determined by the peripheral resistence, the compliance of the arteries, the volume of the blood contained in the arterial system, and the status of the aortic valve. Since the major determinent of afterload is peripheral resistance, clinicians use peripheral resistance measurements as their guide for afterload.

Contractility is a complex process initiated by cellular depolarization. It cannot be measured directly, but changes can be demonstrated by the cardiac response to volume loading and by flattening of the arterial pressure waveform contour. Although the exact mechanism by which electrical energy is converted to mechanical energy awaits further study, one widely held theory follows, in simplified form (Guyton 1986).

The mechanical working cell of the heart is composed of bundles of very fine fibers called *myofibrils*. Each myofibril consists of small contractile units called *sarcomeres*. Each sarcomere in turn consists of two kinds of contractile proteins, actin and myosin. The thick myosin filaments partially overlap the thin filaments. The thin filaments consist of actin plus two regulatory proteins, tropomyosin and troponin.

The sarcomere is bounded at each end by a membrane to which the actin filaments are attached. The actin filaments extend partway in toward the center of the sarcomere. The myosin filaments alternate with the actin filaments but are not attached to the membrane.

Myosin filaments contain projections, called *cross-bridges*, that jut out toward the actin filaments, which contain binding sites. When the muscle is relaxed, the myosin and actin do not form cross-bridges because the tropomyosin/troponin complex covers actin's binding sites.

The last important component of the myocardial fiber is the sarcoplasmic reticulum, a complex network of tubules and sacs that surround the myofibrils. This system plays an important role in electrical impulse conduction and excitation-contraction coupling. In between sarcomeres in the transverse direction is a system of transverse tubules (T tubules). A T tubule is an invagination of the cell membrane (sarcolemma); therefore, it communicates with the extracellular fluid. In between myofibrils in the longitudinal direction is another system of longitudinal tubules (L tubules). The L tubules end in chambers (cisterns) where calcium is stored.

When an electrical impulse occurs, it is spread from the outer membrane of the fiber into the fibril along the T tubules. The spread of the impulse into the L tubules causes the release of calcium ions from the cisterns. Calcium also diffuses into the myofibrils from the T tubules. Because troponin has a strong affinity for calcium, they bind together, thereby uncovering actin's binding sites. Myosin's cross-bridges then can link up with the actin. This interaction pulls the actin in toward the center, so the filaments slide along each other. Using the energy source adenosine triphosphate (ATP), the bridges break and reform several times, each time pulling the actin in closer. When this process occurs in many fibers, it causes the muscle to contract. The efficiency of this mechanism is optimal within only a narrow range of myofibril stretch. When the ventricles are distended excessively, the fibers are pulled too far apart to permit effective coupling of the cross-bridges, and failure ensues.

The right or left ventricle may fail independently, or left ventricular failure may lead to right ventricular failure. At times, the left ventricle may fail so severely that the patient goes into shock. Shock is such an important consideration in the critically ill that it is discussed separately later in this chapter.

Assessment

Risk Conditions

Risk conditions for cardiac failure can be grouped conveniently into those that affect blood volume, those that affect the heart, and those that affect the periphery.

Risk conditions affecting blood volume alter the *preload*. With increased preload, the ventricles are unable to contract with maximum efficiency because the excessive end-diastolic volume disrupts the optimal relationship between cardiac fiber length and force of contraction. Valvular regurgitation, intracardiac shunts, severe bradycardia, fluid overload, and dysfunction or rupture of chordae tendinae are examples of conditions that cause increased preload.

Risk conditions directly affecting the heart are those that alter the heart's *contractility*. Contractility may be impaired by depressant drugs (such as propranolol), myocardial ischemia, acidosis, electrolyte abnormalities, decreased area of functional myocardium (as in myocardial infarction, ventricular aneurysm, or ventricular dyskinesis), myocarditis or cardiomyopathy, and ventricular fibrillation or asystole. In addition, because of the Frank-Starling relationship, contractility is decreased when the ventricles are not sufficiently distended due to obstructions to filling. Examples of filling impediments are cardiac tamponade, tricuspid or mitral stenosis, and restrictive cardiac diseases. Severe tachycardia, although not an actual physical obstruction, also limits CO by sharply decreasing ventricular filling time.

Risk conditions affecting periphery are primarily those that increase *afterload*. Increased afterload can precipitate failure when the heart becomes unable to expel blood efficiently against the increased resistance. Increased right ventricular afterload occurs with pulmonary hypertension and massive pulmonary embolism; increased left ventricular afterload occurs with systemic hypertension and intense vasoconstriction.

In addition to increased afterload, the periphery can cause the heart to fail because of *increased metabolic demand*. When metabolic demand is increased, cardiac output is high but is still insufficient for the body's needs. This high-output failure may be seen in fever, anemia, hyperthyroidism, or severe physical or emotional stress.

When you can identify risk factors, you can take steps to reduce them. For example, follow the measures to prevent and/or relieve dysrhythmias (Chapter 12), myocardial infarction, and cardiac tamponade. Also observe the patient for other risk states, and call them to the physician's attention.

Signs and Symptoms

Signs and symptoms of cardiac failure vary with the ventricle involved and the acuteness of the process. When the heart starts to fail, numerous compensatory mechanisms are called into play. Recall the CO equals heart rate times stroke volume. Increases in heart rate are an immediate compensatory response, but, particularly in the patient with decreased myocardial reserve, they are a costly way to increase CO. Because coronary artery perfusion occurs primarily during diastole, the shortened perfusion time can seriously compromise coronary artery blood flow. In addition, with tachycardia, ventricular diastolic filling time decreases, so that at high heart rates ventricular filling volume actually can be decreased. Finally, tachycardia increases myocardial oxygen demand. These three factors—decreased coronary artery perfusion time, decreased ventricular filling time, and increased myocardial oxygen demand—can interact in an already weakened heart to provoke myocardial ischemia or even MI.

Stroke volume can be increased by altering preload, increasing contractility, or decreasing afterload. A normal acute compensatory mechanism to increase preload is accomplished by vasoconstriction resulting from increased sympathetic nervous system stimulation. Longer-range compensatory mechanisms to increase preload include sodium and water retention by the kidneys.

Sympathetic nervous system stimulation also increases myocardial contractility, as does ventricular dilatation resulting from the increased preload, via the Frank-Starling mechanism. Ventricular dilatation is limited as a compensatory mechanism, however; when myocardial fibers are stretched too far apart, they are no longer able to contract as forcefully as when the ends of the actin and myosin myofibrils overlap sufficiently. A final mechanism by which contractility can increase is muscular hypertrophy. This compensation can occur only if cardiac failure develops slowly—for example, in systemic hypertension. Hypertrophy increases contractility, unless it becomes so severe that the increased muscle mass outstrips coronary artery perfusion capability, in which case ischemia will decrease contractile force.

Changes in afterload also occur in response to decreased CO. The normal physiologic response when cardiac failure begins is vasoconstriction, which increases afterload. While vasoconstriction helps to maintain blood pressure, it also increases the resistance against which the ventricle must pump to eject blood. Therefore, excessive vasoconstriction, or lesser degrees of vasoconstriciton confronting an already weakened ventricle, can actually worsen cardiac failure. Afterload reduction does not occur naturally in response to decreased cardiac output but instead is a therapeutic manuever used in refractory heart failure. By capitalizing on the interrelationships between CO and afterload, afterload reduction therapy enhances CO by decreasing the resistance to ventricular ejection.

Right Ventricular Failure When the right ventricle is unable to pump out blood adequately, blood inexorably backs up into the right atrium and then into the systemic veins. Right ventricular failure thus produces increases in right ventricular pressure, right atrial pressure, and systemic venous pressure. The elevated right ventricular pressure causes the following manifestations:

- S_3 due to filling against an already distended ventricle. The appearance of an S_3 is an important early sign of ventricular failure. An S_4 also may be present.

- Increased myocardial oxygen consumption.
- Pansystolic murmur at the lower left sternal border owing to stretching of the tricuspid ring (relative tricuspid insufficiency).

The increased right atrial pressure may produce atrial fibrillation or other atrial dysrhythmias. Elevated venous pressure causes the following signs and symptoms:

- Increased CVP reading
- Distended jugular veins
- Prominent jugular venous pulsations
- Liver engorgement and tenderness
- Positive hepatojugular reflux (momentary pressure over the liver produces increased jugular venous distention)
- Dependent edema
- Ascites due to fluid accumulation in the peritoneal space
- Decreased appetite, nausea, or vomiting due to pressure on the stomach and bowel from venous engorgement of abdominal vessels
- Increased arterial-venous O_2 difference

Because right ventricular output is decreased, the patient may also show nonspecific weakness or easy fatiguability.

Left Ventricular Failure In left ventricular failure, the left ventricle is unable to pump out blood into the systemic circulation efficiently. Initially, the right ventricle is unaffected and continues to pump blood into the pulmonary circuit. Left ventricular failure thus causes increases in left ventricular pressure, left atrial pressure, and pulmonary pressures. The left ventricular pressure elevation produces the following manifestations:

- S_3 and sometimes S_4, due to filling against an already distended ventricle. The appearance of an S_3 is an important early sign of ventricular failure.
- Increased myocardial oxygen consumption.
- Pansystolic murmur at the apex caused by relative mitral insufficiency.

Atrial fibrillation or other atrial dysrhythmias may result from left atrial distention.

Elevated pulmonary pressures cause transudation of fluid into the pulmonary interstitium and alveoli, reflected by the following signs and symptoms:

- Crackles or wheezing

- Dyspnea (This may appear as dyspnea on exertion, dyspnea at rest, orthopnea, or paroxysmal nocturnal dyspnea.)
- Frequent cough
- Hyperventilation and respiratory alkalosis
- Frank pulmonary edema

Because left ventricular output is decreased, the patient may also manifest:

- Dizziness or syncope, because of decreased CO to the brain
- Fatigue, because of diminished oxygenation of skeletal muscles and loss of cardiac reserve
- Metabolic (lactic) acidosis, because of insufficient oxygen for normal cellular aerobic metabolism
- Generalized edema
- Pulsus alternans (alternating volume of arterial pulse), for which the exact cause is unknown. One explanation is that the ventricle does not empty fully with the first contraction. The resulting increase in volume provokes a stronger contraction for the next beat (according to the Frank-Starling mechanism), emptying the ventricle more completely. As a result, the end-diastolic volume for the third beat resembles that for the first, and the cycle repeats itself.

If the ventricular failure is severe enough, blood will back up from the pulmonary vessels into the right side of the heart. In that case, signs and symptoms of right heart failure also will be present.

NURSING DIAGNOSES

Nursing diagnoses that may apply to the patient with congestive heart failure include:

- Alteration in cardiac output: decreased
- Impaired gas exchange
- Potential for fluid volume deficit
- Potential for injury: dysrhythmias
- Activity intolerance

Planning and Implementation of Care

Nearby is presented a plan of care for the patient with congestive heart failure. This plan utilizes the nursing

NURSING CARE PLAN

Congestive Heart Failure, Acute Phase

NURSING DIAGNOSIS	SIGNS ·AND SYMPTOMS	NURSING ACTIONS	DESIRED OUTCOMES
Alteration in cardiac output: decreased, related to decreased myocardial contractility	Decreased measured cardiac output Hypotension Increased systemic vascular resistance (>1400 dynes/sec/cm^{-5}) Decreased urine output Cool, clammy skin Decreased mental alertness Metabolic acidosis Increased arterial-venous oxygen saturation difference Diminished peripheral pulses Fatigue Decreased exercise tolerance Restlessness Anxiety *With left ventricular failure:* crackles orthopnea elevated pulmonary capillary wedge pressure (PCWP) *With right ventricular failure:* elevated right atrial pressure (RAP)	1. Administer supplemental oxygen. 2. Position patient with head of bed elevated if BP stable. 3. Administer positive inotropic agents *intravenously* as ordered: dopamine dobutamine amrinone calcium chloride *When taking p.o.:* digitalis milrinone 4. Monitor BP, heart rate, and hemodynamic measures every 15 minutes until stable, then every hour. 5. Monitor urine output every hour. 6. If patient is normovolemic, administer vasodilators as ordered: nitroprusside nitroglycerin captopril hydralazine isordil 7. Administer diuretics as ordered. 8. Monitor electrolytes, arterial blood gases every 6 hours until stable. 9. Administer volume, as ordered, for right ventricular failure. 10. Provide for a quiet environment. 11. Provide for periods of uninterrupted sleep. 12. Instruct patient in relaxation techniques. 13. Avoid the use of myocardial-depressing drugs, such as propranolol.	Cardiac output within normal limits. Absence of the signs and symptoms of decreased cardiac output.
Alteration in cardiac output: decreased, related to increased afterload	Decreased measured cardiac output Hypotension Increased systemic vascular resistance	1. Administer vasodilators as ordered: nitroprusside nitroglycerin captopril	Afterload within normal limits.

NURSING CARE PLAN (Continued)

Congestive Heart Failure, Acute Phase (Continued)

NURSING DIAGNOSIS	SIGNS AND SYMPTOMS	NURSING ACTIONS	DESIRED OUTCOMES
	Decreased urine output Cool, clammy skin Decreased mental alertness Metabolic acidosis Increased arterial-venous oxygen saturation difference Diminished peripheral pulses Fatigue Decreased peripheral pulses Fatigue Decreased exercise tolerance Restlessness Anxiety Normal or elevated PCWP, RAP Normal heart rate	hydralazine Isordil 2. Monitor BP every 15 minutes until stable; monitor SVR every hour, CO every hour. 3. Administer pain medication as needed. 4. Instruct patient in relaxation techniques. 5. Provide for a quiet environment. 6. Encourage patient to listen to soothing music. 7. Provide sedation as needed.	
Impaired gas exchange related to ventilation-perfusion imbalance	Confusion Somnolence Restlessness Irritability Inability to move secretions Hypercapnea Hypoxia	1. Administer supplemental oxygen as ordered. 2. Position patient with head of bed elevated if BP stable. 3. Monitor arterial blood gases every 4 hours until stable. 4. Assess breath sounds every 2 hours. 5. Instruct patient in relaxation techniques that utilize deep breathing. 6. Monitor fluid balance to maintain normovolemic—i.e., daily weights, hourly I & O. 7. Monitor hemoglobin and hematocrit daily for anemia. 8. Treat fever as ordered. 9. Provide for adequate rest and periods of uninterrupted sleep.	Normal arterial blood gases. Absence of respiratory distress.

Potential for fluid volume deficit related to excessive diuresis	*Early:*
	    precipitous weight loss
	    output greater than intake
	Late:
	    tachycardia
	    hypotension
	    thready pulse
	    confusion
	    weakness
	    oliguria
	    decreased RAP, PCWP
		1. Monitor urinary output every hour.
		2. Monitor response to diuretic.
		3. Monitor hourly I & O.
		4. Monitor daily weights.
		5. Instruct patient on importance of measuring all fluids and urine.
		6. Instruct patient on rationale for fluid restrictions/fluid encouragement.
			Patient will be normovolemic and will not develop a fluid volume deficit.

(Continues)

NURSING CARE PLAN (Continued)

Congestive Heart Failure, Acute Phase (Continued)

NURSING DIAGNOSIS	SIGNS AND SYMPTOMS	NURSING ACTIONS	DESIRED OUTCOMES
		7. In late phase, terminate diuretic therapy, give volume, and administer vasopressor agents, as ordered.	
Potential for injury: dysrhythmias, related to electrolyte imbalance	Hypokalemia Hyperkalemia Hyponatremia Metabolic alkalosis Metabolic acidosis ST segment depression T wave tenting U wave prominence U wave/T wave flattening Ventricular extrasystoles Complete heartblock Junctional rhythm Atrial tachycardia with block	1. Monitor electrolyte/acid–base balance. 2. Administer potassium as ordered while patient on diuretic therapy. 3. Monitor I & O. 4. Monitor EKG for signs of hypo/hyperkalemia and digitalis toxicity. 5. If suspected dysrhythmias occur, check electrolytes, arterial blood gases and digitalis level. Consult with physician regarding treatment.	Absence of dysrhythmias
Activity intolerance related to generalized weakness and imbalance between oxygen supply and demand	Increased heartrate (over 20 beats/min above resting) with activity Increased BP with activity Verbal reports of fatigue or weakness Exertional discomfort or dyspnea EKG changes with activity, reflecting dysrhythmias or ischemia	1. Maintain supplemental oxygen during activities. 2. Space out activities and encourage rest periods. 3. Instruct patient in energy conservation methods. 4. Encourage patient to use assistive devices with activities, e.g., walker. 5. Monitor patient response to exercise, and gradually increase activities according to response. 6. Instruct patient in relaxation techniques to be used during exercise. 7. Assist patient with activity as needed.	Increased level of activity without fatigue, weakness, discomfort, or other abnormal response.

diagnoses identified above and addresses the nursing interventions to be used in the acute phase.

Pharmacologic Therapy

A wide variety of pharmacologic agents can be used to promote cardiac output in patients in severe failure. To understand the rationale for use of various agents, it is helpful to recall related physiologic concepts.

Physiologic Concepts The key determinants of left ventricular performance are heart rate and stroke volume. Increasing the heart rate is a physiologically costly way to increase cardiac output because of tachycardia's effects on myocardial oxygen consumption and coronary artery filling time. To date, therefore, our major therapeutic efforts have been directed toward improvement of stroke volume.

Preload, contractility, and afterload all are affected by sympathetic nervous system stimuli, as well as other factors. Within the cardiovascular nervous system,

---

NURSING RESEARCH NOTE

Kadota L: Systematic overestimation of sequential thermodilution cardiac output measurements in coronary care patients. *Circulation* 1985; 72(supp III): III-24.

When nurses measure thermodilution cardiac outputs (CO), they commonly take the average of three sequential measurements. Is that really necessary? Furthermore, with iced injectate, does initial catheter cooldown result in a falsely elevated CO?

This study was designed to answer these questions.

Triplicate measurements were obtained from 61 patients, using a commercial CO computer, strip chart recorder, and 10 ml of iced 5% dextrose as injectate. Data were examined with a repeated-measures analysis of variance. The mean CO for the first measurement was 4.91 (SD = 1.71); the mean for both the second and third measurements was 4.65 (SD = 1.49). This difference was significant at p = .00001 (F 2,120 = 12.20).

The researcher concluded that when 10 ml of iced 5% dextrose is used as injectate, the first of three CO measurements is falsely high and should be discarded, and the second and third measurements should be averaged to calculate CO. The researcher also recommended replication of this study.

---

there are three major types of sympathetic receptors: alpha, beta, and dopaminergic. *Alpha receptors* are located primarily in vascular smooth muscle. When stimulated, they produce vasoconstriction. *Beta receptors* are located primarily in the heart, vascular smooth muscle, and bronchi. Stimulation of beta$_1$ receptors, found in the heart, causes increased heart rate and contractility. Stimulation of beta$_2$ receptors, found mostly in vascular smooth muscle and bronchi, causes vasodilatation and bronchial dilatation. The third type of receptors, *dopaminergic receptors,* are found in renal and mesenteric blood vessels. When stimulated, they increase blood flow to the kidneys and mesentery.

Vasoconstrictors The major pharmacologic agents used in pump failure can be classed broadly into vasoconstrictors, positive inotropes, and vasodilators. Vasoconstrictors are primarily alpha stimulators, such as norepinephrine (Levophed). Although widely used in the past, they are used less frequently now because of their troublesome side effects and the availability of other agents. Their major disadvantage is an extension of their therapeutic action: in addition to causing peripheral vasoconstriction, they cause renal vasoconstriction. The resulting decrease in blood flow to the kidneys contributes to the very real risk of acute renal failure (specifically acute tubular necrosis) in patients on these drugs. In addition, alpha stimulators used in a patient who already is vasoconstricted (as most shock patients are) can significantly decrease tissue perfusion.

Inotropes Inotropes are drugs that alter cardiac contractility; positive inotropes improve contractility. In the sections that follow, "inotrope" is assumed to be positive. Digitalis, a well-known inotrope, now is used less often in severe failure than in the past because of

the sensitivity of ischemic myocardium to it. Currently, the inotropes most commonly used in pump failure are dopamine and dobutamine.

Dopamine is a drug used in cardiogenic shock, hemodynamically significant hypotension, and refractory severe congestive heart failure. Its complex pharmacologic actions are dose-related. In the low-dose range (1–2 mcg/kg/min), its major action is dopaminergic receptor stimulation. As its major effect is on the kidney, increased urinary output results. The resulting diuresis lowers preload, thus decreasing the workload of the heart. In the mid-dose range (2–10 mcg/kg/min), dopamine's major action is beta stimulation in addition to the dopaminergic stimulation. The target organ most affected is the heart; contractility increases significantly, with relatively little increase in heart rate. In the high-dose range (above 10 mcg/kg/min), dopamine's major effect is alpha receptor stimulation. Because the drug is a precursor of norepinephrine, administration in this range causes peripheral vasoconstriction. The vasoconstriction produced can become so intense that it can counteract the dopaminergic effect of increased renal blood flow and increase afterload. Side effects that may occur with dopamine include hypotension, especially in hypovolemic patients; tachydysrhythmias or ectopic beats; excessive vasoconstriction; and tissue necrosis and sloughing, similar to that seen with Levophed, if the infusion infiltrates.

Dobutamine (Dobutrex) is a synthetic catecholamine that is a direct beta$_1$ stimulator. It is indicated in refractory congestive heart failure, cardiogenic shock, and significant hypotension. It has a stronger inotropic effect than chronotropic effect, so it causes a marked increase in contractility with relatively little increase in heart rate. Renal and mesenteric blood flow increase indirectly, due to the improved cardiac output. Its most significant side effects are tachycardia and dysrhythmias. The usual dose range is 2.5–10 mcg/kg/min, as an IV infusion.

Amrinone (Incor) is a new inotropic agent that acts directly on the contractile fibers of the myocardium, unlike Digitalis or the catecholamines. It also has vasodilator properties, decreasing afterload and preload. Hemodynamically it produces an increased CO, decreased left-ventricular end-diastolic pressure (LVEDP), decreased PCWP, and a slight decrease or no change in MAP. It is administered 400 mg/250 ml of normal saline, at a rate of 5–10 mcg/kg/min. Possible side effects include: dysrhythmias, thrombocytopenia, GI effects (nausea, vomiting, abdominal pain, anorexia), and hypotension.

Vasodilators Vasodilators are drugs that can improve cardiac output by reducing resistance to ventricular ejection. Their use in shock may seem paradoxical at first but is based on a sound physiologic rationale. Recall that blood pressure equals the cardiac output times systemic vascular resistance (BP = CO × SVR). Dilating peripheral vascular vessels reduces their resistance to flow. By reducing resistance to flow, these drugs reduce impedance to left ventricular ejection. Afterload reduction thus increases cardiac output, ultimately improving tissue perfusion.

The vasodilators most often used in shock are sodium nitroprusside and intravenous nitroglycerin. Sodium nitroprusside (Nipride) is indicated in pump failure, as well as in hypertensive crisis. It is a direct peripheral vasodilator with no direct inotropic or chronotropic activity. It acts on both the arterial and venous circuits, thus reducing both afterload and preload. As a result, systolic emptying increases, pulmonary congestion lessens, myocardial oxygen consumption decreases, and cardiac output increases. The most significant side effects are hypotension, altered ventilation-perfusion relationships due to reversal of compensatory pulmonary vasoconstriction in areas of local hypoxemia, thiocyanate toxicity, and inhibited platelet aggregation. The drug is photosensitive, so solutions must be protected from light. The usual dose range is 0.5–8.0 mcg/kg/min, as an IV infusion.

Intravenous nitroglycerin (Tridil, Nitrostat) is used in unstable angina; congestive heart failure complicating myocardial infarction; perioperative hypertensive episodes; and induced hypotension during surgery. It appears to be particularly helpful in management of angina due to vasospasm and may help to preserve ischemic myocardium in acute myocardial infarction. It affects both the arterial and venous circuits, thus reducing both afterload and preload, but its greater effect is on the venous side. It thus lessens venous return, pulmonary congestion, myocardial workload, and oxygen consumption. The mechanism by which it relieves angina is controversial, and probably includes a combination of its effects on the peripheral vascular system, redistribution of myocardial blood flow, and relief of coronary vasospasm. The most significant side effect is hypotension, especially in patients with borderline hypovolemia. Because the drug is absorbed by the plastic used in usual intravenous solution bags and tubing, it must be administered using glass bottles and special plastic tubing. The initial IV infusion dose is 0.5 mcg/min, with subsequent increments titrated to the patient's clinical response.

Captopril is an oral vasodilatating agent that may be used to decrease preload and afterload. It has been found to reduce postinfarction ventricular dilatation and it improves exercise tolerance in chronic congestive heart failure. Major side effects include hypotension and bradycardia, which may occur with the first dose.

Inotrope/Vasodilator Combination Therapy When caring for patients in severe heart failure, you may at times find yourself nursing a patient receiving both an inotrope and a vasodilator, typically dopamine and sodium nitroprusside. Managing a patient on such combination therapy can be confusing, because these drugs have synergistic effects on some determinants of cardiac output and opposing effects on other determinants. The following information to guide you is abstracted from Dracup et al. (1981). The goals of combination therapy are to increase cardiac output, lessen pulmonary congestion, and improve myocardial oxygen supply/demand balance. It is easiest to comprehend the effects of combination therapy by grouping them according to preload, contractility, afterload, and oxygen balance.

Nitroprusside and dopamine both decrease preload. Nitroprusside reduces preload by two mechanisms: increasing venous capacitance and improving ejection fraction. Dopamine reduces preload indirectly, by increasing urinary output and increasing ejection fraction (percentage of ventricular volume ejected during systole). Together, these agents provide greater reduction in LVEDP (leading to lessened metabolic demand) and lower wedge pressure (leading to lessened pulmonary congestion) than either drug does alone.

Nitroprusside has no direct effect on contractility but can improve it indirectly by reducing myocardial ischemia. Dopamine improves contractility directly through beta receptor stimulation. Together, the agents provide better augmentation of ejection fraction than nitroprusside alone, with less demand on the left ventricle than if dopamine were used alone.

Nitroprusside directly reduces afterload. If the reduction in afterload does not cause a sufficient compensatory increase in cardiac output, however, blood pressure will fall and tissue perfusion will suffer. Dopamine has no effect on afterload in low- to mid-dose ranges but will increase cardiac output, so its addition to nitroprusside is distinctly advantageous. In high-dose ranges, dopamine can counteract nitroprusside's afterload reduction and thus defeat its use. As long as high-dose dopamine is not used, the combined use of the two drugs can cause reduced afterload, improved cardiac output, and better maintenance of blood pressure and tissue perfusion than if the agents were used separately.

Nitroprusside may decrease oxygen supply if it causes a marked decrease in diastolic pressure and therefore in coronary perfusion pressure. Adding dopamine can overcome this problem by increasing cardiac output and therefore coronary arterial perfusion. On the other hand, dopamine may decrease oxygen supply it if increases vascular resistance or causes tachycardia. As each drug may cause decreased oxygen supply, the nurse should be especially alert for signs of increased ischemia when combination therapy is used.

Nitroprusside probably reduces oxygen demand by decreasing LV end-diastolic volume and vascular resistance. Dopamine, on the other hand, can increase oxygen consumption by increasing heart rate and contractility. The advantage of using the two agents together, therefore, is that their effects on oxygen demand can cancel each other out. As a result, dopamine can be used more safely in the setting of myocardial ischemia than it could by itself.

In summary, simultaneous use of these agents reduces preload, reduces afterload, increases contractility, and may improve myocardial oxygen supply/demand balance. They thus can increase cardiac output, improve systemic perfusion, and may preserve ischemic myocardium.

Outcome Evaluation

Evaluate the patient's progress and the effect of therapeutic measures according to these outcome criteria:

- Arterial pressure, pulmonary artery, and wedge pressures WNL for the patient.
- When thorax elevated 45°, jugular venous distention and hepatojugular reflux absent; normal jugular venous pulsations.
- Heart rate and rhythm normal for the patient; preferably normal sinus rhythm.
- No edema, ascites, or liver enlargement or tenderness.
- Lungs clear to auscultation.
- Blood gases within normal limits for patient.
- No dyspnea, orthopnea, or cyanosis.

ACUTE CARDIAC TAMPONADE

The heart is surrounded by the pericardial sac, which fits loosely around it and protects it against friction. The sac attaches to the great vessels, diaphragm, sternum, and posterior mediastinal structures. The inner layer of the sac (the part in direct contact with the heart) is the visceral pericardium or epicardium. The outer layer, the parietal pericardium, is fibrous. Both layers are lined with serous tissue. The space between the layers, the pericardial space, normally contains only 10–20 ml of pericardial fluid but can accommodate up to 2 liters of fluid without hemodynamic changes.

Cardiac tamponade results when increased intrapericardial pressure interferes with diastolic filling of the heart. The pressure may rise because of a space-occupying lesion, such as a tumor, or more commonly because of bleeding into the pericardial sac. Etiologies for cardiac tamponade are listed in Table 13-2.

Assessment

Risk Conditions

Certain conditions increase the likelihood of tamponade. Be on the alert for these conditions.

- Pericarditis, especially in an anticoagulated patient
- Cardiac trauma, penetrating or nonpenetrating, such as: cardiac surgery, cardiac biopsy, perforation by a transvenous pacing wire, myocardial infarction, stabbing or impalement
- Rupture of heart or great vessels

TABLE 13–2 ETIOLOGIES OF CARDIAC TAMPONADE

Cardiovascular causes:
   chest trauma
   heart surgery
   aneurysm
   coronary angiography
   insertion and removal of pacing wires
   insertion of central venous catheter

Neoplasms

Purulent pericarditis:
   bacterial
   viral
   tubercular

Myxedema

Collagen diseases
   rheumatoid arthritis
   systemic lupus erythematosus

Uremic pericarditis

Radiation pericarditis

Hypersensitivity states

Anticoagulants

Source: Estes ME: Management of the cardiac tamponade patient: A nursing framework. *Crit Care Nurse* 1985; 5:17.

Prevent or alleviate high-risk conditions whenever possible. For instance: consult with the physician about discontinuing anticoagulants when a patient develops pericarditis; maintain the patency of mediastinal chest tubes postcardiotomy and decrease cardiac workload for the patient with a recent myocardial infarction.

Signs and Symptoms

Recognize the signs of developing tamponade. They vary with the amount of fluid and the rapidity of its accumulation.

Precordial chest pain can vary from mild to severe. The pain is stabbing and knifelike, and is worsened by breathing, coughing, swallowing, moving, or lying supine. A pericardial friction rub is present in pericarditis, due to the movement of the two inflamed pericardial surfaces rubbing against each other.

Observe for signs of *systemic venous congestion* due to restricted venous return to the heart. These include distended neck veins, liver enlargement, elevated CVP or right atrial pressure readings, and/or dyspnea. A paradoxical arterial pulse (pulsus paradoxus) is an important finding in tamponade as well as in certain other cardiac disorders. Its etiology and assessment technique are presented in Chapter 10.

Observe for signs of *decreased CO*. Especially watch for a falling systolic blood pressure. Other signs include agitation, cyanosis, poorly palpable apical pulses, tachycardia, and sometimes muffled heart sounds.

Follow the results of diagnostic procedures. The ECG may be normal or show nonspecific signs of pericarditis. Alternating voltage (electrical alternans) of all P, QRS, and T deflections is thought to be diagnostic of tamponade; however, it is an infrequent finding. The echocardiogram will show an echo-free zone. The chest x-ray usually shows a widened mediastinum.

NURSING DIAGNOSES

Nursing diagnoses for a patient suffering from cardiac tamponade include:

- Pain
- Fear
- Decreased cardiac output
- Altered tissue perfusion

Planning and Implementation of Care

Relieve the *pain related to pericardial inflammation* by allowing the patient to assume the most comfortable position; preferably sitting up or leaning forward. Administer salicylates, analgesics, and/or steroids as ordered by the physician.

Relieve the *fear related to the unknown*. Using language appropriate to the patient's condition, explain that the symptoms are temporary and will be relieved by treatment. Inform the patient about the diagnostic and therapeutic procedures used to help her.

Relieve the *decreased CO* and *altered tissue perfusion related to impaired ventricular filling*. As a temporary measure, the physician may want you to infuse intravenous fluids rapidly to raise ventricular filling pressure above pericardial pressure. Definitive treatment for acute cardiac tamponade is removal of the pericardial fluid, as explained below. A rule of thumb used to determine when fluid removal is indicated is the "rule of 20": a CVP greater than 20 cm H_2O, a paradoxical pulse greater than 20 mm Hg, and a pulse pressure of less than 20 mm Hg (Guzzetta and Dossey 1984).

Assisting with Pericardiocentesis

If the symptoms are progressing rapidly, obtain *immediate* medical help and prepare for a pericardial tap *(pericardiocentesis)*. Following are the steps to take in assisting with pericardiocentesis:

1. Elevate the head of the bed about 60°.

2. Monitor the cardiac rhythm, CVP, and BP before and during the procedure. Have an emergency cart and defibrillator nearby. Ventricular fibrillation or accidental laceration of a coronary artery or the myocardium can cause shock and death.

3. Obtain a pericardiocentesis tray, sterile gloves, prep solution, and ECG machine and sterile "alligator" clips and wires. Act as the unsterile person to unwrap the tray and add to it the alligator clips and wire. The physician will connect the clips to the sterile needle and pass you the end of the wire. Connect it to the precordial lead wire of the ECG machine.

4. The physician will insert the needle at the cardiac apex or in the angle between the left costal margin and the xiphoid. As he or she does so, watch the pattern on the ECG machine and say immediately when the PR segment or ST segment elevates. These elevations indicate the needle has reached the myocardium, producing a local current of injury. They therefore warn the physician to withdraw the needle a few millimeters to avoid myocardial laceration.

5. After the fluid is aspirated, the physician will withdraw the needle and apply pressure on the site.

6. Send the aspirated fluid for diagnostic studies ordered by the physician.

Aspiration usually will cause dramatic hemodynamic improvement, with stabilization of the BP and pulse and disappearance of the paradoxical pulse. Continue monitoring the patient for recurrent tamponade. Repeated tamponade may necessitate surgical creation of a "pericardial window" to allow continuous fluid drainage.

Outcome Evaluation

Use these outcome criteria to evaluate the patient's progress:

- Heart rate and rhythm normal for patient.
- CO sufficient, as evidenced by arterial blood pressure, mental status, urinary output, peripheral pulses, skin temperature and color normal for patient.
- Heart sounds as loud as before the tamponade.

SHOCK

Cardiovascular health is maintained by the interaction of three elements: the heart pump; the blood vessels; and their contents, the blood volume. Shock is an acute process of hemodynamic and metabolic derangements resulting from disruption of one or more factors in this triad. It is an ever-present specter in the care of the critically ill.

Assessment

Risk Conditions

Conceptualizing three major types of shock, based on the triad components of the cardiovascular system, can assist you in determining which patients are at risk of shock. Major categories of shock (which often overlap) follow.

Hypovolemic Shock Fluid volume deficit may lead to hypovolemic shock—for example, following profound hemorrhage, excessive diuresis, or severe dehydration.

Cardiogenic Shock Cardiogenic shock results from failure of the heart to pump adequately. It can be subdivided into two types: *coronary cardiogenic shock,* in which pump failure results from ischemia or infarction due to compromised coronary arterial circulation, and *noncoronary cardiogenic shock,* in which pump failure results from abnormalities of the cardiac muscle or heart valves.

Distributive Shock Distributive shock results from abnormal distribution of blood volume due to altered vessel resistance. It can be subdivided into neurogenic shock and vasogenic shock. Neurogenic shock results from loss of normal sympathetic vasoconstrictor stimuli, which leads to vasodilatation. Because the capacity of the blood vessels expands in relation to the normal blood volume, a relative hypovolemia is present. Possible causes are spinal cord injury, severe pain, and vasomotor center depression due to drug overdose. Vasogenic shock results from diminished arterial resistance and increased venous capacitance, due to the release of vasodilating substances. Clinical examples are anaphylactic shock and septic shock.

Pathophysiologic Changes

For information on pathophysiologic changes leading to cardiogenic shock, please consult the section of this chapter on decreased cardiac output. The following pathophysiologic discussion focuses on hypovolemic and septic shock.

Hypovolemic Shock   *Hypovolemic shock* is primarily a defect in the microcirculation. In the compensated stage, sympathetic stimulation causes constriction of both the precapillary sphincter and the venule. As a result, fluid flow through the capillary decreases and pressure inside the capillary drops. The disparity in pressure between the outside and inside of the capillary promotes the movement of fluid from the interstitium into the blood vessels, thus helping to increase circulating blood volume. If shock persists and there is a pro-

longed decrease in capillary flow, decompensation occurs and a vicious circle of events develops. The long period of diminished flow results in microcirculatory hypoxia and acidosis, which increase capillary permeability. The acidosis also promotes relaxation of the capillary sphincters, allowing more blood to enter the capillary. As venule constriction continues, the net result is an increase in capillary pressure. Combined with the increased capillary permeability, the increased pressure results in the flow of the fluid out of the capillaries into the tissues, worsening the drop in circulating blood volume and creating a self-perpetuating cycle.

On the cellular level, shock disrupts vital cellular activities. Sodium/potassium transport mechanisms falter with the accumulation of excess sodium inside the cell and excess potassium outside it. Altered cellular permeability allows proteins to enter the cell, pulling water along with them and causing intracellular swelling. Mitochondria become depressed. Oxygen metabolism suffers.

Normally cells receive energy from a highly complex series of chemical reactions, briefly summarized here (Guyton 1986). These steps are diagrammed in Figure 13-5. During glycolysis, glucose is split to form pyruvic acid. This step does not require oxygen. In addition to the pyruvic acid, it produces a small number of hydrogen atoms and a small amount of energy, which is used in the synthesis of the high-energy bonds of *adenosine triphosphate* (ATP). These phosphate bonds store energy until the cell needs it. The pyruvic acid is con-

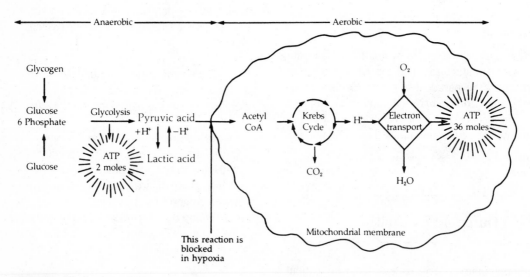

FIGURE 13–5

Cellular aerobic and anaerobic energy production. The conversion of pyruvate to acetyl coenzyme A (CoA) is blocked if not enough oxygen is available to combine with the hydrogen released during the Krebs cycle.

verted to acetyl coenzyme A and enters the Krebs (citric acid) cycle, during which the acetyl portion is broken down into carbon dioxide and hydrogen atoms. These hydrogen atoms plus those released during glycolysis undergo oxidative phosphorylation, in which huge amounts of energy are released and again stored as ATP.

Cellular hypoxia has drastic effects on energy availability. It is unclear at present whether the energy deficit results from decreased energy production or from adequate energy production accompanied by insufficient formation of ATP causing energy to be lost as heat rather than stored as ATP.

Because glycolysis does not require oxygen, it continues to provide a small amount of energy, as well as pyruvic acid and hydrogen atoms. These cannot be metabolized in the Krebs cycle or undergo oxidative phosphorylation in the absence of oxygen. Instead, the excessive amounts of pyruvic acid and hydrogen atoms combine with each other and produce lactic acid. The lactic acid diffuses out of the cell into the extracellular fluid, thus allowing glycolysis to continue providing energy for a few minutes. This shift from aerobic to anaerobic metabolism has three important consequences (a) cellular activities are hampered severely due to lack of available energy; (b) the increased demand for glucose causes rapid depletion of glycogen stores; and (c) lactic acidosis deranges the body's acid–base and electrolyte balances. By the time metabolic acidosis is detectable in arterial blood gas values, significant physiologic derangement has occurred.

If the person resumes adequate oxygenation, the lactic acid can be reconverted to pyruvic acid and utilized in the Krebs cycle. If not, the worsening metabolic acidosis and loss of energy result in cellular destruction.

As cells are damaged, disruption of their lysosomes frees proteases and other enzymes, which may hasten cellular destruction. These enzymes also are believed to provoke the release or activation of bradykinin, histamine, and other substances which cause severe vasodilatation and depress the heart.

Septic (Endotoxin) Shock   The pathophysiology of septic shock deserves special recognition due to the increasing importance of sepsis in mortality among the critically ill. The major pathogens responsible for septic shock are the aerobic, gram-negative organisms, particularly *E. coli,* the *Klebsiella-Enterobacter-Serratia* group, *Proteus,* and *Pseudomonas aeruginosa* (Root and Merle 1985).

The cell wall of gram-negative bacilli contains lipopolysaccharides, which are released as endotoxin when the bacteria die. This endotoxin is a principal cause of the pathogenicity of these organisms, which produce a type of septic shock called *endotoxin shock.*

Endotoxin stimulates the immunologic system, causing complement activation. The complement cascade produces these important effects:

1.   Attraction of leukocytes to the injured area. These leukocytes increase bacterial destruction and therefore cause further release of endotoxin.

2.   Production of inflammatory chemical mediators. Cells damaged by infection release powerful chemical substances. The most important of these substances are histamine and lysosomal enzymes, which cause severe inflammatory injury.

3.   Release of histamine from mast cells, causing vasodilatation, increased capillary permeability, and decreased peripheral resistance.

Lysosomal enzyme release not only damages surrounding tissue but, in conjunction with endotoxin, also activates vasoactive polypeptides (Proctor 1986). One of the most significant vasoactive polypeptides is bradykinin, a powerful vasodilator that markedly increases capillary permeability.

Sepsis is a powerful stimulator of the sympathetic nervous system, resulting in greatly increased catecholamine release. Heart rate and cardiac contractility increase due to beta stimulation. Because of the resulting increase in cardiac output, a hyperdynamic state ensues. The patient feels warm due to vasodilatation. Because vasodilatation increases the capacity of the vascular bed, blood pressure is low despite the increased cardiac output—hence the term "warm shock" for this phase. The increased capillary permeability causes marked extravasation of fluid from the vascular space, further worsening the disparity between the capacity of the vascular bed and the volume available to fill it.

As septic shock evolves, the hemodynamic picture changes from one of vasodilatation to vasoconstriction. The change is provoked by the marked constrictive effects of catecholamines and of prostaglandins released from damaged tissue. Perfusion of organs slows because of hypotension and vasoconstriction. Ischemia of the splanchnic bed triggers the release of myocardial depressant factor (MDF). As venous return decreases and MDF depresses contractility, cardiac output drops. In this hypodynamic state, the patient is in "cold shock." From this point on, the pathophysiologic events are similar to those of hypovolemic shock.

Blood gas values may vary, depending on the progression of septic shock. Initially, respiratory alkalosis is present due to hyperventilation induced by endotoxin. As septic shock progresses, metabolic alkalosis may develop. The cause of the metabolic alkalosis is unclear and may be related to impaired anaerobic metabolism, so that not as much lactate is produced as one would expect given the degree of hypoxemia. Metabolic (lactic) acidosis is a late development due to profoundly disrupted cellular metabolism. It may be combined with respiratory acidosis, if pulmonary deterioration becomes so severe that carbon dioxide elimination is impaired.

The septic shock patient is particularly at risk for developing adult respiratory distress syndrome (ARDS) and disseminated intravascular coagulation (DIC). Endotoxin directly damages pulmonary vascular endothelium (Proctor 1986). Disruption of capillary endothelium and increased permeability result in platelet aggregation, pulmonary vasoconstriction, pulmonary interstitial edema, leakage of fluid and protein into alveoli, and surfactant reduction. Because of alveolar collapse, diminished pulmonary perfusion, and impaired oxygenation, the patient develops widespread atelectasis, profound ventilation/perfusion imbalances, severe hypoxemia, pulmonary edema, and finally respiratory failure—the hallmarks of ARDS.

In addition to the effects of complement activation mentioned earlier, the complement sequence also triggers both the intrinsic and extrinsic coagulation pathways. The accelerated coagulation in turn triggers accelerated fibrinolysis—the classic "setup" for DIC.

Signs and Symptoms

The traditional criteria for shock are a systolic BP below 70 mm Hg; confusion or other signs of diminished cerebral perfusion; pale, cool, clammy skin; a urinary output below 30 ml per hour; and metabolic acidosis. Dependence on these classic signs, however, will cause you to deprive many of your patients of prompt assistance in the early stages of shock. These signs are late, may not occur in some shock states (especially septic shock); and/or may be inappropriate for a given patient, such as the hypertensive, in whom shock can occur within the range of so-called normal systolic pressures.

Because of the importance of early detection and aggressive management of shock, it is vital that you be alert to the early signs of shock. Hemodynamic responses to the different types of shock are presented in Table 13-3.

Hypovolemic Shock In early hypovolemic shock, powerful compensatory mechanisms are called into play when the blood pressure starts to drop. Baroreceptor stimulation excites the vasomotor center in the medulla, leading to tachycardia, increased peripheral resistance due to arteriolar constriction, and increased circulating blood volume due to venoconstriction. The kidneys also attempt to restore blood volume via ADH- and aldosterone-mediated sodium and water retention. As a result, CO is increased to near-normal levels. The blood flow is redistributed away from the skin and kidneys to preserve the vital heart and brain.

The signs and symptoms of this compensated stage of shock correlate with its pathophysiology. Pulse rate is slightly increased. BP is normal or slightly decreased. However, positive postural vital signs may be present at this stage of hypovolemic shock; that is, systolic BP drops 10 mm Hg or more and pulse increases 20 beats per minute or more when supine and sitting vital signs

TABLE 13–3 HEMODYNAMIC RESPONSES IN DIFFERENT TYPES OF SHOCK

Type	HYPOVOLEMIC	CARDIOGENIC	SEPTIC EARLY	SEPTIC LATE	NEUROGENIC
Cause	DECREASED CIRCULATING BLOOD VOLUME	DEPRESSED CARDIAC CONTRACTILITY	VASODILATATION DUE TO ENDOTOXINS		PERIPHERAL VASODILATATION DUE TO LOSS OF NERVOUS STIMULATION
Filling pressures	↓	↑	↓	↑	↓
Cardiac output	↓	↓	↑	↓	normal or ↑
Systemic vascular resistance	↑	↑	↓	↑	↓
Pulmonary vascular resistance	normal	normal	↑	normal	normal

From Bodai B, Holcroft J: Use of the pulmonary artery catheter in the critically ill patient. *Heart Lung* 1982; 11:406–416. Reprinted by permission of the C.V. Mosby Company.

are compared. Positive postural vital signs indicate the presence of orthostatic hypotension, due to the body's inability to compensate for the challenge of a sudden change in position in addition to compensating for the challenge of the developing shock. The skin of the periphery is cool and pale, with poor capillary filling evident in the nailbeds. Urinary output is slightly decreased. The person is alert and oriented.

As shock deepens to the level of approximately 25% loss of circulating blood volume, the pulse becomes rapid and thready. Frank hypotension becomes evident. The skin of the trunk becomes cool. Oliguria (urinary output below 30 cc per hour) is present and the person is markedly thirsty. Restlessness, confusion, or agitation develops. The respiratory rate increases in response to the continuing biochemical abnormalities.

In late shock, with loss of 40% or more of circulating blood volume, the pulse becomes very rapid and weak. BP drops below 80 mm Hg systolic. The skin appears mottled or cyanotic and feels cold. Urinary output drops below 20 cc per hour, and the person becomes disoriented. Finally, with just a few minutes of life remaining, the skin becomes deeply pale or cyanotic, sensation decreases, and unconsciousness intervenes.

Cardiogenic Shock Similar events occur in cardiogenic shock, but one area of difference exists. In hypovolemic shock, cardiac filling pressures are normal or slightly low in the compensated stage and definitely low in the decompensated stage, because of the actual loss of blood volume. In cardiogenic shock, filling pressures are elevated, because of the vascular congestion that results from the heart's inability to pump effectively.

Neurogenic Shock In neurogenic shock, the normal sympathetic responses to hypotension are disrupted. As a result of vasodilatation, vascular resistance decreases and filling pressures drop. CO may actually increase, however, due to the reduction in afterload.

Septic Shock Hemodynamic parameters in septic shock are markedly different from those in other types of shock. In *early sepsis,* beta stimulation causes increased CO, but vasodilatation causes filling pressures and systemic vascular resistance to fall. Pulmonary vascular resistance increases due to the release of prostaglandins from injured vascular endothelium and platelets (Proctor 1986). In *late septic shock,* when the heart is failing, cardiac output falls and filling pressures rise. Catecholamine and prostaglandin releases result in generalized vasoconstriction, so systemic vascular resistance increases.

The signs and symptoms of septic shock correlate with its pathophysiology. The signs of sepsis prior to the onset of shock are subtle. They include restlessness, confusion, tachycardia, and increased respiratory rate. In the *hyperdynamic "warm shock"* state, the patient becomes hypotensive. Nevertheless, the skin is warm and dry or flushed. Confusion, restlessness, and hyperventilation increase. In the *hypodynamic "cold shock"* state, the patient resembles one in late hypovolemic shock. The skin is cold and clammy, and severe oliguria is present. Due to the huge interstitial fluid accumulation and increased capillary permeability, the patient appears to be fluid-overloaded and to have pulmonary congestion. This appearance is deceptive, however, because the effective circulating volume is severely reduced.

Temperature changes may be confusing due to endotoxin's effect on the temperature-regulating center of the hypothalamus. Initially, the patient may be hypothermic due to depression of the center. Later, the patient may become hyperthermic as a result of the temperature-stimulating effects of the endotoxin and of pyrogen release from leukocytosis (Proctor 1986).

Laboratory Data

Laboratory data can provide valuable assistance in assessing the degree and type of shock. The most common laboratory parameters followed in shock, their normal values, changes in shock, and the mechanisms of abnormalities are presented in Table 13–4.

Prevention

The nurse plays a critical role in prevention of shock. Now that you are familiar with the types of shock and their pathophysiologies, take measures to prevent or ameliorate risk conditions. For example, to prevent hypovolemic shock: (a) closely monitor the intake and output of traumatized patients, patients on diuretics, and

---

NURSING DIAGNOSES

Because of the rich complexity and diverse causality of shock, many nursing diagnoses may be applicable. Examples include:

- Alteration in tissue perfusion
- Impaired gas exchange
- Alteration in urinary elimination
- Alteration in nutrition: less than body requirements

TABLE 13-4 COMMON LABORATORY DATA IN SHOCK*

TEST	NORMAL	IN SHOCK	MECHANISM
Blood Chemistries			
NUTRITIONAL SUBSTANCES			
Glucose	70–100 mg/100 ml	↑ Early	Sympathetic stimulation
		↓ Late	Depletion of body glycogen stores; decreased liver function
Total serum proteins			
Total	6.0–7.8 g/100 ml	↓	Leakage from capillary and decreased synthesis in liver cells
Albumin	3.2–4.5 g/100 ml	↓	
Globulin	2.3–3.5 g/100 ml	Normal or ↓	Larger particle size, less leaks from capillary
EXCRETORY SUBSTANCES			
Urea nitrogen	5.0–20.0 mg/100 ml	↑	Decreased renal excretion
Creatinine	0.6–1.2 mg/100 ml	↑	Decreased renal excretion
Bilirubin			
Total	0.5–1.2 mg/100 ml	↑	
Direct (conjugated)	up to 0.2 mg/100 ml	↑	Liver cell damage
Indirect (unconjugated)	0.1–1.0 mg/100 ml	↑	
FUNCTIONAL SUBSTANCES			
Sodium	136–142 mEq/L	↑ Early	↑ aldosterone causing renal retention of sodium
		↑ or ↓ Late	Altered renal function (ATN)
Potassium	3.8–5.0 mEq/L	↓ Early	↑ aldosterone causing renal excretion of potassium
		↑ Late	Acidosis, cell necrosis, and decreased renal function
Chloride	95–103 mEq/L	↓ Early	Alkalotic state and bicarbonate excess
		↑ Late	Acidotic state and bicarbonate deficiency
Carbon dioxide (carbonate)	21–28 mEq/L	↑ Early	Alkalotic state
		↓ ↓ Late	Severe metabolic and respiratory acidosis
SERUM ENZYMES			
Creatinine phosphokinase (CPK)	5–35 U/ml	↑	Necrosis of muscle cells and/or heart cells
Serum glutamic oxaloacetic transaminase (SGOT)	15–40 U/ml	↑	Necrosis of heart cells and/or liver cells
Serum glutamic pyruvic transaminase (SGPT)	15–35 U/ml	↑	Necrosis of liver cells
Lactic dehydrogenase (LDH)	150–450 Wroblewski U/ml	↑	Necrosis of liver and/or heart cells
Amylase	60–160 somogyl U/100 ml	↑	Necrosis of pancreatic cells
Lipase	0–1.5 Cherry-Crandall U/ml	↑	Necrosis of pancreatic cells
BLOOD CULTURES	No growth	Positive	Variety of causative microbes
Hematology			
Hemoglobin	male 14.0–16.5 g/100 ml female 12.6–14.2 g/100 ml	↓	Hemorrhage (if present)
Hematocrit (packed cell volume = PCV)	male 42–52% female 37–47%	↑ or ↓	Fluid leakage from the capillary Loss of blood (Note: does not occur until 6 hrs after blood loss)
Red blood cell count	male 4.6–6.2 million/ml female 4.5–5.4 million/ml	↓	Hemorrhage (if present)
White blood cell count	4,500–11,000/ml	↑	Body's response to infection (if present)
Platelet count	150,000–400,000/ml	↓	Platelet aggregation and microemboli

*Normal values cited from: Halstead JA: *The laboratory in clinical medicine,* 1976.

TABLE 13-4 COMMON LABORATORY DATA IN SHOCK* (Continued)

TEST	NORMAL	IN SHOCK	MECHANISM
Coagulation test:			
Prothrombin time (PT)	12–14 sec	Prolonged	Hypercoagulable state (if present)
Partial thromboplastin time (PTT)	45–65 sec	Prolonged	Hypercoagulable state (if present)
Arterial Blood Gases			
pH	7.38–7.42	↑ Early	Hyperventilation and carbon dioxide exhalation
		↓ Late	Carbon dioxide retention and lactic acid production
P_{CO_2}	35–45 mm Hg	↓ Early	Hyperventilation
		↑ Late	Hypoventilation
P_{O_2}	80–100 mm Hg	↓	Hypoventilation and hypoperfusion (ventilation/perfusion imbalances)
Bicarbonate	22–28 mEq/L	↓ Late	Severe acidotic state
Urine Measurements			
Creatine clearance	male 1.0–2.0 g/24 hr female 0.8–1.8 g/24 hr	↓	Impaired renal excretion
Osmolality	500–800 mOsm/L	↑ Early	Water retention, secondary to ADH
		↓ Late	Inability of the kidney to concentrate urine
Specific gravity	1.001–1.035	↑ Early	Same as for osmolality (influenced by administration of Dextran)
		↓ Late	
Sodium	80–180 mEq/24 hr	↓ Early	Sodium reabsorption secondary to aldosterone
		↓ or ↑ Late	Abnormal renal function
Potassium	40–80 mEq/24 hr	↑ Early	Potassium excretion secondary to aldosterone
		↓ or ↑ Late	Abnormal renal function

Source: Rice V: Shock, a clinical syndrome. Part III: The nursing care: Prevention and patient assessment. *Crit Care Nurse* (July/August) 1981; 38–39.

those unable to satisfy their thirst, such as unconscious patients; (b) promptly control frank bleeding; and (c) securely fasten arterial line connections to avoid accidental disconnection and hemorrhage. To prevent cardiogenic shock, take the measures outlined in the sections on MI to reduce myocardial workload and the risk of infarction extension, and those outlined in the sections on altered cardiac output and cardiac tamponade. Prevention of septic shock can be accomplished by removing sources of infection, such as contaminated IV lines and infected or necrotic tissue, and enhancing host defenses, for example, by maintaining adequate nutrition.

Planning and Implementation of Care

Alteration in Tissue Perfusion Related to Loss of Circulating Blood Volume

If you detect signs of rapidly developing shock, act promptly to identify the type of shock and take appropriate emergency measures:

1. Mentally review the patient's history, and quickly do a physical assessment, looking for clues to the cause of shock, such as a site of active bleeding.

2. While summoning medical assistance, take these emergency measures:

A. For hemorrhagic shock, control bleeding if possible. For frank bleeding from hemodynamic lines, reconnect the line or shut it off between the break and the patient. For blood vessel ruptures, apply direct pressure and elevate the site.

B. For hypovolemic shock, elevate the person's legs, which increases circulating blood volume 400–800 ml by promoting venous drainage from the legs. Do not use this measure for patients with cardiogenic shock, increased intracranial pressure, or active bleeding from the head and neck. Increasing the circulating blood volume can actively worsen these conditions. Trendelenburg's position, popular in the past in the treatment of shock, is used less often now because of its detrimental effects on diaphragmatic excursion and therefore ventilation, as well as its ability to further lower BP by reflex depression of baroreceptor activity.

C. Adminsiter supplemental oxygen so that the blood that does reach the tissues is optimally oxygenated.

D. If no IV lines are in place, establish two large-bore IV lines to facilitate rapid administration of fluid.

E. In selected instances, you may care for a patient in whom a *Medical Antishock Trousers* (MAST) suit is being used to control internal bleeding and shock. The MAST suit is a vinyl garment that fits over the patient's legs and abdomen and can be inflated to promote internal autotransfusion of blood from the legs and abdomen to the central circulation. You are most likely to encounter the use of the MAST suit in trauma patients preoperatively or in patients with neurogenic shock. It is crucial that you *not* deflate the garment in an attempt to examine the underlying areas; sudden removal of the suit can cause the BP to drop precipitously (Millar et al. 1985).

3. Establish baseline values and initial diagnostic data by recording a 12-lead ECG and by obtaining routine laboratory studies, such as a complete blood count; type and cross-match; serum electrolytes; arterial blood gases; and urinalysis. Additional specimens such as blood cultures should be obtained as indicated.

4. Assist the doctor in inserting an arterial line and a central venous or PA line to monitor hemodynamic pressures. Insert a Foley catheter to monitor urinary output. Monitor these parameters every 15 minutes to 1 hour, depending on the severity of shock and the rapidity of its progression.

5. Administer a fluid challenge if the physician orders one. Evaluation of the preceding data frequently identifies the type(s) of shock present. For instance, a history of angina coupled with ECG signs of a recent infarct strongly suggest cardiogenic shock. In many cases, however, the data are equivocal. For example,

low blood pressure, CVP, and urinary output could be present in any type of shock. In such a case, the physician may want you to administer a fluid challenge to evaluate the hemodynamic response to an increased blood volume. The appropriate amount of fluid challenge can be titrated by judicious use of hemodynamic data. Although the details vary among physicians, one common protocol is presented in Table 13–5.

Depending on the patient's condition and the physician's preference, crystalloids, colloids, and/or blood

TABLE 13-5 FLUID CHALLENGE PROTOCOL ACCORDING TO WEIL AND RACKOW

1. Obtain baseline measurements of either the central venous pressure (CVP) or the PCWP or pulmonary artery diastolic (PAD) pressure for an initial 10-minute observation period prior to beginning fluid administration.

2. Determine the infusion rate based on the filling pressure: When PCWP is used:

PCWP	Fluid Infusion Rate
<12 mm Hg	20 cc/min
12–18 mm Hg	10 cc/min
>18 mm Hg	5 cc/min

When CVP is used:

CVP	Fluid Infusion Rate
<12 cm H_2O	20 cc/min
12–18 cm H_2O	10 cc/min
>18 cm H_2O	5 cc/min

3. Infuse the appropriate amount of fluid for 10 minutes via an infusion pump. If at any time during the infusion, the PCWP increases by more than 7 mm Hg, or if the CVP increases by more than 5 cm H_2O, *discontinue the infusion.*

4. At the end of the 10-minute infusion period, measure the PCWP or CVP. If the PCWP has increased by 3 mm Hg or less, or if the CVP has increased by 2 cm H_2O or less, repeat the fluid challenge.

    If the PCWP has increased more than 3 mm Hg but less than 7 mm Hg, or if the CVP has increased more than 2 cm H_2O but less than 5 cm H_2O:
    a. Discontinue the infusion, and observe the patient for 10 minutes
    b. During this 10-minute observation period, if the PCWP falls to within 3 mm Hg of the initial PCWP or if the CVP falls to within 2 cm H_2O of the initial CVP, administer another fluid challenge over another 10-minute period.
    c. During this 10-minute observation period, if the PCWP does not fall to within 3 mm Hg of the initial PCWP, or if the CVP does not fall to within 2 cm H_2O of the initial CVP, discontinue the fluid challenge.

Source: Adapted from Rice V: Shock management, Part I: Fluid volume replacement. *Crit Care Nurse* 1984; 4:80–81. Based on data from Weil MH, Rackow EC: A guide to volume repletion. *Emerg Med* 1984; 16:101–110.

may be given to restore volume. The characteristics of the most commonly used solutions are presented in Table 13–6. The relative merits and drawbacks of each remain the subject of considerable debate. The amount used depends on the volume lost and on the degree of vascular capacitance.

Whatever fluids are used, remember to closely monitor intake and output, follow the trend of vascular pressures, and watch for the signs of fluid depletion and overload, discussed in Chapter 16.

Alteration in Tissue Perfusion Related to Diminished Myocardial Contractility

Administer inotropes—pharmacologic agents ordered by the physician to improve myocardial contractility. *Digoxin* may be given as a loading dose of 0.5 mg IV followed by additional 0.25 mg doses every hour until an optimum therapeutic effect is achieved. The actions of

TABLE 13-6 GUIDE TO PARENTERAL FLUID REPLACEMENT

TYPE	DESCRIPTION	USES	SPECIAL CONSIDERATIONS
Whole Blood and Blood Products			
Whole blood	Complete blood	To replace volume and maintain Hgb at 12–14 g/100 ml. Given in slow or rapid hemorrhage and hypovolemic shock	Best replacement for loss of whole blood is whole blood.
Red blood cells (packed, fresh or frozen)	Whole blood with 80% of plasma removed	To correct RBC deficiency and improve oxygen-carrying capacity of the blood. Given in anemia, slow hemorrhage, with PCV ↓ 25–30%. Frozen (thawed) RBCs given to organ transplant patients (because freezing destroys leukocytes). Used in cardiogenic shock (avoids fluid overload)	Frozen (thawed) RBCs—very expensive. Washed RBCs (suspended in saline) may be given in progressive shock to ↓ red cell adhesiveness (↓ fibrinogen coating).
Plasma (fresh or frozen)	Uncoagulated plasma separated from whole blood	To restore plasma volume in hypovolemic shock without ↑ PCV. To restore clotting factors (except platelets)	Used effectively for immediate volume replacement.
Platelets	Platelet sediment from platelet-rich plasma, resuspended in 30–50 cc of plasma	To restore platelets (in thrombocytopenia) and to maintain normal blood coagulability	
Plasma protein fraction (Plasmanate) (Plasma-plex)	5% solution of selected proteins from pooled plasma in buffered stabilized saline diluent (0.9% NaCl). Contains albumin, alpha and beta globulins	To expand plasma volume (while cross-matching is being completed) in hypovolemic shock. To correct hypoproteinemia and increase serum colloid osmotic pressure	Use cautiously in patients with CHF (due to added fluid) and in patients with renal failure (due to added proteins). Is osmotically equivalent to plasma. Does not carry danger of hepatitis (heat-treated).
Albumin 5% (buffered saline) 25% (salt-poor) (Albuminate)	Aqueous fraction of pooled plasma	To increase serum colloid osmotic pressure and expand plasma volume in shock (while cross-matching is being completed)	Does not carry danger of hepatitis (heat-treated). Use cautiously in patients with CHF. In shock, leaky capillaries may ↑ tissue proteins and augment interstitial and intracellular edema (may remain in circulation longer than crystalloid solutions). 5% albumin is osmotically equivalent to plasma.

(Continues)

TABLE 13-6 GUIDE TO PARENTERAL FLUID REPLACEMENT (Continued)

TYPE	DESCRIPTION	USES	SPECIAL CONSIDERATIONS
Plasma Substitutes (pharmaceutical plasma expanders)-Hypertonic Solutions			
Dextran	Large polysaccharide polymer of glucose		
LMWD (Dextran 40) (Rheoma-crodex) (Gentran 40)	Solution that contains 10% dextran (average molecular weight = 40,000) in 0.9% NaCl or in 5% dextrose in water	To rapidly expand plasma volume	Used if PCV ↑ 30%. Lasts about 12 hours. ↓ platelet adhesiveness, so may ↑ bleeding from raw surfaces (avoid in hemorrhage). May ↓ capillary sludging in progressive shock. Alters urine specific gravity.
HMWD (Dextran 70) (Macrodex) (Gentran 70)	Solution that contains 6% dextran (average molecular weight = 70,000) in 0.9% NaCl or 5% dextrose in water	To effectively expand plasma volume for up to 24 hours	May leak from capillary less readily than LMWD. ↑ platelet adhesiveness. Alters urine specific gravity. Same molecular weight as human plasma albumin.
Hetastarch (Hespan) (Volex)	500 ml unit of a 6% solution containing a synthetic polymer of hydroxethyl starch in normal saline	To expand plasma volume	Potential dilution of clotting factors with resultant coagulation changes. Potential circulatory overload in patients with severe CHF and compromised renal function. Increased serum amylase level, peaking within one hour of IV administration and persisting for 3–4 days. Do not use if solution is cloudy or deep brown. Monitor clotting studies and platelet counts. Compatibility with other substances is not established; infuse through separate line. Maximum infusion rate in hemorrhagic shock is 20 ml/kg/hr. Monitor serum albumin.
Crystalloid Solutions (contain electrolytes and water)			
Isotonic Solutions: Normal Saline	0.9% NaCl in water	To ↑ plasma volume when RBC mass is adequate	Contains 154 mEq/L sodium. Replaces losses without altering normal fluid concentrations.
Lactated Ringer's (Hartmann's)	Normal saline to which K^+ and Ca^+ have been added; also contains buffers	To replace fluid and to buffer pH (contains lactate, which is quickly converted to bicarbonate to buffer acidosis)	Contains 130 mEq/L sodium, 3 mEq/L calcium, 4 mEq/L potassium, 28 mEq/L lactate, 109 mEq/L chloride.
Ringer's	Normal saline to which K^+ and Ca^+ have been added	To replace fluid and to give additional K^+ and Ca^+. Contains high concentration of chloride and may increase plasma chloride level	Contains 147 mEq/L sodium, 4 mEq/L potassium, 5 mEq/L calcium, 156 mEq/L chloride.
Hypotonic Solutions: ½ normal saline	0.45% NaCl in water	To raise total fluid volume	Contains 77 mEq/L sodium and 77 mEq/L chloride. Rapidly leaves vascular space; may potentiate intersitial and intracellular edema. Dilutes plasma proteins and electrolytes.
D_5W (physiologically hypotonic)	5% dextrose in water	To raise total fluid volume and to provide calories for energy (200 calories/1000 cc)	Glucose is metabolized rapidly so that water remains in vascular space (hypotonic). Dilutes plasma proteins and electrolytes.

Source: Rice V: Shock management, Part I. Fluid volume replacement. *Crit Care Nurse* 1984; 4:71–73.

digitalis and related nursing responsibilities are discussed in Appendix 2. Other agents that may improve contractility are *dopamine* and *isoproterenol,* discussed on pages 329 and 348.

Alteration in Tissue Perfusion Related to Excessive Vasoconstriction

A wide variety of inotropes, vasoconstrictors, and vasodilators can be used to treat patients with hemodynamically significant hypotension due to decreased myocardial contractility or increased vasoconstriction. They include dopamine, dobutamine, amrinone, norepinephrine, sodium nitroprusside, and intravenous nitroglycerin. The rationale for use, actions, and side effects were presented earlier in this chapter, under treatment of severe heart failure.

If the above measures are ineffective, the physician may resort to more aggressive or experimental forms of therapy. Devices to implement mechanical support of the cardiovascular system include a pneumatic suit on the lower extremities (medical antishock trousers [MAST], sometimes called a pneumatic antishock garment [PASG]), an intra-aortic balloon pump, and prolonged cardiopulmonary bypass. Another controversial area is the use of steroids, particularly in massive doses. Some physicians believe steroids may minimize cell damage by stabilizing lysosomes and may improve myocardial contractility. Others believe they are useless in shock or may promote gastric bleeding and ulceration. Often, physicians will try steroids when standard therapy fails to produce improvement, on the theory that the patient's adrenal glands may be unable to secrete adequate levels of steroids due to prolonged or severe stress.

Impaired Gas Exchange Related to Ventilation-Perfusion Imbalance

Impaired gas exchange can result from microatelectasis, microemboli, increased shunting, increased pulmonary congestion, and worsening acidosis. It is particularly troublesome because it superimposes respiratory acidosis on metabolic acidosis, and the combination often is lethal.

Maintain a patent airway by using the head-tilt maneuver, inserting a pharyngeal airway, or assisting with endotracheal intubation. Keep the airway clear of secretions by suctioning as necessary.

Administer supplemental oxygen via the method appropriate for the patient's needs. Initially, patients in relatively light degrees of shock may be managed with a nasal cannula, oxygen mask, or Venturi mask. As shock becomes more profound and the patient is intubated, oxygen may be administered via a mechanical ventilator.

Assess respiratory rate and rhythm, chest excursion, and lung sounds at least every hour. Monitor arterial blood gas values at least every 4 hours for trends, watching especially for hypoxemia, hypercapnia, and acidosis.

Provide aggressive pulmonary hygiene measures to prevent the development of atelectasis and pneumonia.

Administer sodium bicarbonate intravenously as ordered, to buffer acidosis. The need for and appropriate dose of bicarbonate should be titrated according to arterial blood gas values. Preferably administer the drug as a bolus rather than continuous infusion, as the solution frequently precipitates if other drugs are added to it.

Altered Urinary Elimination Related to Decreased Renal Perfusion

Acute renal failure is discussed in detail in Chapter 15. Briefly, monitor urinary volume and maintain output above 30 ml/hr. Monitor BUN, creatinine, and urine electrolytes as ordered. In addition to fluid administration, the physician may prescribe diuretics, usually mannitol or furosemide (Lasix). Monitor patients carefully during diuresis; fluid overload and congestive heart failure may occur with osmotic diuretics, rapid diuresis may provoke cardiovascular collapse, and a variety of electrolyte imbalances may develop during diuresis.

Altered Nutrition (Less Than Body Requirements) Related to Diminished GI Perfusion

Paralytic ileus may result from autonomic hyperactivity. Even if it does not, it is unwise to create an increased need for blood flow to the digestive organs at the very time blood is shunted preferentially away from them. For the duration of the shock episode, give the patient nothing by mouth, and insert a nasogastric catheter to drain the stomach. Provide nutritional supplementation as ordered. Before resuming oral feedings, be sure bowel sounds are present.

Definitive Care

Often, specific correction of the cause of shock is not the first line of defense but rather must wait until the patient's hemodynamic status is stabilized. Once the patient has been stabilized, assist the physician in treating the underlying cause of shock. Such treatment may include sending the patient to surgery to ligate bleeding vessels *(hemorrhagic shock)* or repair a post-myocardial infarction septal rupture *(cardiogenic shock)*, administering antihistamines *(anaphylactic shock)*, or starting intravenous antibiotics *(septic shock)*.

Complications of shock may include MI, adult respiratory distress syndrome *(shock lung)*, acute renal failure, disseminated intravascular coagulation, and cardiopulmonary arrest.

Outcome Evaluation

Evaluate the patient's progress toward health. Without vasopressor or vasodilator support, the patient ideally should maintain these outcome criteria:

- Arterial blood pressure within ± 10 mm Hg of preshock levels.
- Adequate perfusion of vital organs, as manifested by a return to preshock level of consciousness, cardiac status, and renal function.
- Adequate peripheral perfusion, as manifested by warm, dry skin, and by peripheral pulse volume WNL for patient.
- Arterial blood gases and serum electrolytes WNL for patient.

REFERENCES

Benner P: *From novice to expert.* Menlo Park, CA: Addison-Wesley, 1984.

Bodai B, Holcroft J: Use of the pulmonary artery catheter in the critically ill patient. *Heart Lung* 1982; 11:406–416.

Brewer CC, Markis JE: Streptokinase and tissue plasminogen activator in acute myocardial infarction. *Heart Lung* 1986; 15:552–558.

Catalano JT: Antiarrhythmic medications classified by their autonomic properties. *Crit Care Nurse* 1986; 6:44–49.

Chesney M, Rosenman R: Type A behavior: Observations on the past decade. *Heart Lung* 1982; 11:12–19.

Chyun D: Intravenous nitroglycerin in ischemic heart disease. *Dimen Crit Care Nurs* 1983; 2:10–21.

Dracup K et al.: The physiologic basis for combined nitroprusside-dopamine therapy in post-myocardial infarction heart failure. *Heart Lung* 1981; 10:114–120.

Estes ME: Management of the cardiac tamponade patient: A nursing framework. *Crit Care Nurse* 1985; 5:17–26.

Guyton A: *Textbook of Medical Physiology,* 7th ed. Philadelphia: Saunders, 1986.

Guzzetta CE, Dossey BM: *Cardiovascular nursing: Bodymind tapestry.* St Louis: Mosby, 1984.

Hoaglund PA: Right ventricular infarction. *Crit Care Quart* 1985; 7:19–26.

Keck S et al.: Cardiac tamponade: An initial study in the development of a predictive tool. *Heart Lung* 1983; 12:505–509.

Lamb IH: The angina that kills. *RN* 1985; 48:28–34.

Mathewson M: Current vasodilator therapy. *Focus Crit Care* 1983; 10:49–53.

Millar S et al.: *AACN procedure manual for critical care.* Philadelphia: Saunders, 1985.

Packer M et al.: Comparison of captopril and enalapril in patients with severe chronic heart failure. *N Engl J Med* 1986; 315:847–853.

Partridge S: The nurse's role in percutaneous transluminal coronary angioplasty. *Heart Lung* 1982; 11:505–511.

Perry A, Potter P: *Shock: Comprehensive nursing management.* St Louis: Mosby, 1983.

Proctor RH: *Clinical aspects of endotoxin shock.* New York: Elsevier Science Publishers, 1986.

Rice V: Shock management, part I. Fluid volume replacement. *Crit Care Nurse* 1984; 4:69–82.

Rice V: Shock management, part II. Pharmacologic intervention. *Crit Care Nurse* 1985; 5:42–57.

Root RK, Merle AS: *Septic shock.* New York: Churchill Livingston, 1985.

Sarkar A, Krupadev H: Myocardial rupture in acute myocardial infarction: Case report and review of the literature. *Heart Lung* 1983; 12:88–91.

Sipperly ME: Thrombolytic therapy update. *Crit Care Nurse* 1985; 5:30–34.

Weil MH, Rackow EC: A guide to volume repletion. *Emerg Med* 1984; 16:101–110.

SUPPLEMENTAL READINGS

Bourdarias JP et al.: Inotropic agents in the treatment of cardiogenic shock. *Pharm Ther* 1983; 22:53–79.

Douglas MK, Shinn JA: *Advances in cardiovascular nursing.* Rockville, MD: Aspen Publishers, 1985.

Keely BR: Septic shock. *Crit Care Quart* 1985; 7:59–86.

McCarthy C: Percutaneous transluminal coronary angioplasty: Therapeutic intervention in the cardiac catheterization laboratory. *Heart Lung* 1982; 11:499–504.

Michaelson C: *Congestive heart failure.* St Louis: Mosby, 1983.

Srebro J, Karliner JS: Congestive heart failure. *Curr Prob Cardiol* 1986; 23:302–365.

14

Cardiovascular Interventions

CLINICAL INSIGHT

Domain: The teaching-coaching function

Competency: Providing an interpretation of the patient's condition and giving a rationale for procedures

Patients in the surreal world of the intensive care unit, their minds blurred by medications, physiologic imbalances, and psychologic stress, may interpret their ordeals in bizarre ways. Often, these are recollections of profoundly disturbing episodes. Nurses can help such distraught patients make sense of their memories, thus eliminating the power of those memories to haunt them. In the following exemplar, from Benner (1984, pp. 88–89), a physician gives an account of his experience as a patient in an ICU.

All nurses coming on duty tried to make their own assessments of their patients' emotional level as well as their physical status. At times I would try to be falsely cheerful, and they would see through it. On one memorable Monday, I was obviously depressed, and my nurse, coming on duty, asked me gently what was wrong. I didn't have a clue. I wept buckets, something I don't usually do. I felt unashamed but puzzled. She said with some confidence: "We'll figure

this out," and then went on to ask a few questions. She wanted to know, "Is the sound outside disturbing you?" I realized that it was. After a little further thought she said: "You didn't hear this noise Saturday and Sunday, but you did hear it Friday when your aortic balloon came out. That was a bad time. You remember not only how painful that was but you also remember how the balloon sounded inside you during all those rough days. I bet you are remembering all that pain." My distress disappeared.

An understanding of the treatment techniques commonly used for patients with cardiovascular disorders will enhance your ability to implement a treatment plan, evaluate its effectiveness, and protect the patient from harmful side effects. In addition, such an understanding will enable you to interpret these treatments to the patient and family, as demonstrated in the Clinical Insight. This chapter presents information on common treatments for cardiac ischemia, rhythm disturbances, and cardiac failure. Included are emergency cardiac drug therapy, cardiac pacemakers, percutaneous transluminal coronary angioplasty (PTCA), the effects of cardiopulmonary bypass following surgical treatment of cardiac disorders, and intra-aortic balloon pump (IABP) therapy.

Emergency Cardiac Drug Therapy

Sudden Death

Sudden death is defined as death within one hour of the onset of symptoms. It is one of the three major syndromes of coronary heart disease (the other two being angina pectoris and acute MI). There is a high incidence of coronary heart disease, but not necessarily of acute MI, in patients who undergo sudden death. In a 4-year study of resuscitation following ventricular fibrillation outside the hospital setting, Cobb et al. (1975) found that acute MI was not common in the people who died, and was present in only about one half of those who survived. In contrast, diffuse coronary atherosclerosis and previous MI were common. Other cardiovascular conditions associated with sudden death were massive pulmonary thromboembolism, intracerebral hemorrhage, mitral valve prolapse, aortic aneurysm, and hypertrophic cardiomyopathy.

Studies have shown that ventricular fibrillation is very common in the early hours post-infarct. It also is important to realize that ventricular fibrillation can occur with no warning signs at all. These facts emphasize the importance of responding promptly to symptoms suggesting myocardial ischemia. When prodromal symptoms *are* present, the most common is chest pain.

There are certain possible indications for risk of sudden cardiac death (Chiang et al. 1970; Friedman et al. 1979). Among the risk factors are symptomatic heart disease, hypertension, diabetes, smoking, sedentary lifestyle, Type A personality, and premature ventricular beats post-infarction. On the resting ECG, findings that correlate with an increased incidence of sudden death include abnormal Q waves, ST segment depression, left BBB, bifascicular block, and premature ventricular beats in patients with known coronary artery disease.

Sudden death can occur through tachyfibrillatory mechanisms or bradysystolic mechanisms. About 60% of patients who arrest do so in ventricular fibrillation, about 10% in pulseless ventricular tachycardia, and about 30% in asystole or electromechanical dissociation. (Electromechanical dissociation is present when there is an electrical rhythm but no associated cardiac contractions.)

Initial approaches to the patient in cardiac arrest include cardiopulmonary resuscitation (CPR); general advanced cardiac life support measures such as intubation, oxygenation, and establishment of an IV line; and management of specific dysrhythmias. The following section discusses emergency antidysrhythmic agents, based on resuscitation standards developed by the 1985 National Conference on Cardiopulmonary Resuscitation (CPR) and Emergency Cardiac Care (ECC) (1986).

Emergency Cardiac Drugs

Key points for the most commonly used emergency drugs are presented here and in Table 14–1. Appendix 2 also contains information on numerous antidysrhythmic agents that are not considered emergency drugs.

Epinephrine   Epinephrine is an endogenous catecholamine with both alpha and beta adrenergic stimulating properties. Its complex pharmacologic actions depend in part on dose and in part on the body's reflex circulatory adjustments to this drug. In cardiac emergencies, epinephrine can be expected to increase heart rate, improve myocardial contractility, and increase systemic vascular resistance. As a result of these actions, blood pressure increases. In asystole, epinephrine can generate a spontaneous contraction. Epinephrine also can convert fine (low-amplitude) ventricular fibrillation into coarse (high-amplitude) ventricular fibrillation, which is easier to defibrillate.

Epinephrine is indicated in asystole, electromechanical dissociation, and ventricular fibrillation. The usual dose is 0.5–1.0 mg (5–10 ml of the 1:10,000 solution) every 5 minutes as needed. The drug usually is given intravenously but also can be given into the tracheobronchial tree via an endotracheal tube, where it can be absorbed via the pulmonary vascular bed. If neither route is feasible, it may be given as an intracardiac injection; however, this route is hazardous due to the risks of cardiac tamponade, myocardial or coronary artery laceration, and pneumothorax.

The major side effects of epinephrine are exaggerations of its therapeutic properties. The expected increase in heart rate can accelerate into a dangerous tachycardia. Increased automaticity can produce premature ventricular beats and ventricular fibrillation. Increased heart rate, contractility, and vascular resistance increase myocardial work and therefore myocardial oxygen consumption. As a result, epinephrine can increase myocardial ischemia or precipitate myocardial infarction.

Sodium Bicarbonate   Bicarbonate is no longer recommended for routine use in cardiac arrest, because of the dangers of extracellular alkalosis, shift of the hemoglobin dissociation curve, impairing; oxygen release;

TABLE 14-1 DRUGS USED IN CARDIAC ARREST: ADULT DOSES

DRUG	INDICATIONS	AVAILABILITY	MIXING DIRECTIONS	FINAL CONCENTRATION	USUAL DOSE	ADMINISTRATION
Epinephrine (adrenalin)	Asystole Electromechanical dissociation Ventricular fibrillation	10 ml preloaded syringe = 1 mg 1 ml ampule = 1 mg	As is = 1:10,000 dilution Dilute 1 ampule with 9 ml saline = 10 ml of 1:10,000	0.1 mg/ml	0.5–1 mg Always use as 1:10,000 solution	IV bolus or endotracheally every 5 minutes as needed
Sodium bicarbonate	Acidosis	50 ml preloaded syringe = 50 mEq	None	1 mEq/ml	1 mEq/kg initially, then 0.5 mEq/kg	IV bolus, according to arterial blood gases or every 10 minutes as needed
Calcium chloride	Hyperkalemia Hypocalcemia Calcium channel blocker toxicity	10 ml ampule = 1 g	None	100 mg/ml (10%)	2 ml	IV bolus every 10 minutes as needed
Atropine	Bradycardia AV block Asystole	10 ml preloaded syringe = 1 mg	None	1 mg/ml	0.5 mg–1.0 mg, to total of 2.0 mg	IV bolus or endotracheally every 5 minutes as needed
Lidocaine	Ventricular tachycardia Premature ventricular beats Ventricular fibrillation	5 ml preloaded syringe = 100 mg	None	20 mg/ml	1 mg/kg initially Additional 0.5 mg bolus every 8–10 minutes as needed, to total of 3 mg/kg	IV bolus
Bretylium	Ventricular tachycardia Ventricular fibrillation	10 ml ampule = 500 mg	Dilute to 50 ml Do not dilute		5–10 mg/kg 5 mg/kg initially, then 10 mg/kg, to total of 30 mg/kg	IV infusion over 10 minutes IV bolus every 15–30 minutes as needed
Procainamide (Pronestyl)	Ventricular ectopy Ventricular tachycardia	10 ml vial = 1000 mg	None	100 mg/ml	50 mg every 5 minutes, to total of 1 g, 50% QRS widening, or hypotension	IV bolus (up to 20 mg/min)

Important: Preparations differ among manufacturers. Always check the drug's label for specific information.

hypernatremia; hyperosmolality; production of (para-doxical) intracellular acidosis; and inactivation of cate-cholamines administered simultaneously. In addition, its use has not been found to improve survival. Its use should be considered only after initiation of better-proven interventions (such as defibrillation and antidys-rhythmics), typically about 10 minutes into the resuscitation. Thereafter, it may be used at the team leader's discretion. Earlier use is appropriate only for clearly defined situations, such as preexisting acidosis. The initial dose is 1 mEq/kg. Subsequent doses may be up to half that amount every 10 minutes.

Calcium Chloride With cardiac arrest, calcium administration does not improve survival, and excess calcium may be detrimental. It is indicated only for hyperkalemia, hypocalcemia, and calcium-channel-blocker toxicity. The customary dose is 2 ml of 10% calcium chloride, IV bolus every 10 minutes as necessary.

Atropine Atropine blocks the transmission of parasympathetic impulses from the vagus nerve. It does so by competing with acetylcholine (the usual parasympathetic chemical mediator) for receptor sites. Because stimulation of the vagus nerve inhibits impulse initiation by the SA or AV node and impulse conduction through the AV junction, blocking the vagus causes improved impulse initiation and conduction. Atropine is indicated for symptomatic sinus bradycardia, AV block, and asystole. The usual dose is 0.5 mg IV bolus every 5 minutes until a total of 2.0 mg is reached. It may also be administered endotracheally. Possible side effects include tachydysrhythmias, increased ischemia due to increased myocardial workload, and paradoxical bradycardia with doses less than 0.5 mg.

Isoproterenol (Isuprel) Isoproterenol is a synthetic sympathomimetic. Because it is almost a pure beta stimulator, it causes increased heart rate and increased contractility, accompanied by peripheral arterial dilatation. Because of its potent chronotropic and inotropic effects, cardiac output usually increases. Systolic blood pressure usually remains the same or increases due to the increased cardiac output, whereas diastolic pressure may fall due to the decreased peripheral vascular resistance. As a result, mean perfusion pressure may fall. Isoproterenol is used primarily to treat symptomatic bradycardias unresponsive to atropine in the patient with a pulse. It is not appropriate in cardiac arrest. It is administered as an IV infusion, at a rate of 2–10 μg/min, titrated to the desired blood pressure and heart rate. Side effects include increased automaticity leading to tachycardias and ventricular irritability, and increased oxygen consumption leading to increased myocardial ischemia.

Lidocaine (Xylocaine) Lidocaine is particularly useful in suppressing ventricular dysrhythmias. It apparently has different actions in normal and ischemic tissue. In animal experiments, lidocaine has been found to slow the rate of spontaneous phase 4 depolarization and depress conduction in reentrant pathways. It also has been found to reduce the difference in action potential duration between normal and ischemic myocardium, prolong the effective refractory time, and slow conduction in ischemic tissue, further suppressing reentrant activity. Lidocaine also raises the fibrillation threshold, especially in ischemic tissue.

Lidocaine is the first-line agent for ventricular tachycardia and ventricular fibrillation. Other indications for use include ventricular premature beats (VPBs) more frequent than 6 per minute; multiformed VPBs; R-on-T phenomenon, in which a VPB occurs close to the preceding T wave; and bursts of two or more VPBs. In addition, many physicians use lidocaine prophylactically in suspected myocardial ischemia.

The appropriate route and dose depends on the setting. In cardiac arrest, only bolus therapy should be used. An initial bolus of 1 mg/kg may be followed by 0.5 mg/kg boluses every 8–10 minutes, to a total of 3 mg/kg. Once resuscitated, the patient should receive an infusion of 2–4 mg/min. In the nonarrest situation, boluses may be given every 2–4 minutes. An infusion also should be started, beginning at 2 mg/min. It should be increased by 1 mg/min after each additional bolus, to a maximum of 4 mg/min.

Toxic effects of lidocaine are related primarily to the central nervous system and include drowsiness, confusion, tinnitus, slurred speech, muscle twitching, and seizures.

Because lidocaine is metabolized in the liver, it should be given cautiously to patients with impaired hepatic function, such as in chronic alcoholism or hepatitis, or decreased hepatic blood flow, such as in congestive heart failure or shock.

Bretylium Tosylate (Bretylol) Bretylium has complex electrophysiologic and hemodynamic properties. It increases the threshold for ventricular fibrillation and also facilitates defibrillation. It has dual effects on hemodynamics. Initially, it causes catecholamine release from adrenergic nerve endings, producing a transient increase in heart rate and blood pressure. Then, it produces an adrenergic blockade, resulting in decreased arterial pressure.

Bretylium is useful in treatment of ventricular tachycardia and ventricular fibrillation, but is no better than lidocaine. It is recommended for (1) ventricular fibrillation refractory to defibrillation and lidocaine, (2) recurrent fibrillation, and (3) ventricular tachycardia (with pulse) refractory to lidocaine and procainamide.

The dose depends on the clinical setting. In refractory or recurrent ventricular tachycardia, bretylium is given as an infusion of 5–10 mg/kg, diluted to 50 ml with 5% dextrose in water and administered over 10 minutes. After the loading dose, the drug may be given as a continuous infusion of 1–2 mg/min. In ventricular fibrillation, the initial dose is 5 mg/kg undiluted rapid IV bolus, followed by defibrillation. If fibrillation persists, the dose is increased to 10 mg/kg and repeated every 15–30 minutes as necessary during the resuscitation to a total of 30 mg/kg. Doses are interspersed with attempts at defibrillation.

Bretylium's major side effect is supine hypotension, which occurs in at least one-half the patients who receive it. This hypotension responds to leg raising and volume administration. Because the initial catecholamine release may cause increased dysrhythmias or hypertension, bretylium is not the drug of choice in treating digitalis-induced dysrhythmias. If other treatments are ineffective, however, bretylium may be tried even in the presence of digitalis toxicity.

Verapamil Hydrochloride (Isoptin, Calan) Verapamil is a slow-channel conduction blocker, which functions by inhibiting calcium ion influx into cardiac and smooth muscle. As slow-channel conduction plays a significant role in the electrical activity of the AV node, verapamil is useful in prolonging AV conduction. Its ability to interrupt reentrant AV nodal mechanisms makes it particularly useful in terminating paroxysmal supraventricular tachycardias. Verapamil also depresses myocardial contractility by blocking the role of calcium in the contractile mechanism. Finally, verapamil decreases contractile tone in vascular smooth muscle, thus interrupting coronary vasospasm and producing peripheral vasodilatation. The combination of decreased contractility and decreased afterload reduces myocardial oxygen requirements.

Verapamil is indicated for paroxysmal supraventricular tachycardia, atrial flutter, and atrial fibrillation. It terminates AV nodal reentrant tachycardias in almost 90% of patients, and slows ventricular response in atrial flutter and fibrillation. Verapamil is contraindicated in patients with impaired atrioventricular conduction; severe bradycardia may occur. Other detrimental effects include hypotension, precipitation of congestive heart failure, and exacerbated accessory conduction in Wolf-Parkinson-White syndrome. Because both beta-blocking agents and verapamil reduce contractility and AV conduction, verapamil should not be used concomitantly with intravenous beta-blockers.

The recommended initial dose is 5 mg IV bolus over 1–2 minutes. The repeat dose is 10 mg 30 minutes later if needed.

Procainamide (Pronestyl) Procainamide, an agent that suppresses ventricular ectopy, is recommended for PVCs and ventricular tachycardia when lidocaine is ineffective or contraindicated. The dose is 50 mg every 5 minutes until one of the following endpoints is reached: (1) rhythm termination, (2) hypotension, (3) increase of 50% in QRS width, or (4) total of 1 g administered. In the urgent situation, a slow IV bolus of up to 20 mg/min is administered; a faster rate may cause precipitous hypotension.

Defibrillation and Cardioversion

A direct-current electrical countershock may be successful in terminating both atrial and ventricular tachydysrhythmias. Cardioversion and defibrillation are similar in that each involves a countershock that depolarizes all the cells simultaneously, thereby allowing the sinus node to resume its dominance. They differ in that cardioversion uses a lower wattage and requires synchronization of the shock with the R wave. (Synchronization is necessary so that the shock will not fall during the vulnerable period of repolarization and therefore cause repetitive depolarization.) Cardioversion usually is not an emergency procedure; defibrillation is. Cardioversion usually is performed by a physician, defibrillation by the nurse if no physician is immediately available.

Defibrillation Defibrillation is the definitive treatment for ventricular fibrillation. It is critically important, since it is the major determinant of survival.

The optimal energy dose for defibrillation is not yet established. There is no clear-cut relationship between the size of the patient and the amount of energy necessary for defibrillation. The ideal dose probably varies considerably, depending on the length of fibrillation, previous electrical shocks, the functional state of the myocardium, and other factors.

Current American Heart Association standards recommend three rapid, consecutive shocks. The initial attempt at defibrillation should be made with 200 joules of delivered energy. If unsuccessful, defibrillation should be repeated at 200–300 joules immediately. If still unsuccessful, third and subsequent attempts should be made at 360 joules.

Cardioversion Prior to cardioversion, prophylactic quinidine and/or atropine may be administered, food and fluids restricted for 6 hours, and administration of digitalis stopped for up to 24 hours before the procedure. (Both cardioversion and defibrillation are contraindicated in the digitalized patient, because they may provoke refractory ventricular tachycardia.) The patient is anes-

NURSING RESEARCH NOTE

Kolar J, Dracup K: Survival from sudden cardiac death: The emotional aftermath. *Heart Lung* 1987; 16:326–327.

As burgeoning technology enables us to resuscitate more patients from episodes of sudden death, nurses increasingly wonder about the emotional impact of surviving such a traumatic experience. This study compared the emotional adjustment of survivors of sudden cardiac death and people who experienced recent episodes of recurrent ventricular tachycardia without sudden death. It also identified high-risk factors for severe psychosocial distress after sudden death survival.

Forty electrophysiology service patients who had neither a myocardial infarction nor a chronic medical illness were studied. Nineteen had survived sudden cardiac death, and 21 had experienced recurrent ventricular tachycardia. Seven measures of adjustment to illness were studied via patients' self-reports on the Psychosocial Adjustment to Illness Scale (PAIS), which has construct and convergent validity and internal consistency reliability coefficients of 0.47–0.85 for its seven subscales. The means of the two groups for each subscale and the total score were compared using a Hotelling's T square; no significant differences were found. Nonstepwise multiple linear regression analysis revealed three statistically significant variables ($p < 0.05$) predicting psychosocial adjustment: (1) marriage, which helped it, and (2) the number of dysrhythmias and (3) heart failure history, both of which hindered adjustment.

The results indicate that the sudden-death patient or ventricular tachycardia patient at greatest risk for psychosocial distress is single, has experienced several dysrhythmic episodes, and has had one or more congestive heart failure episodes. The research was based on psychologic control theory, *control* being defined as the belief that one can influence an event's unpleasantness. The researchers hypothesized that ventricular tachycardia patients would report less distress than sudden death survivors. The study results suggest that both sudden death and recurrent ventricular tachycardia cause an equally decreased sense of control and that both types of patients can benefit from similar nursing interventions that decrease psychologic distress.

thetized with diazepam or thiopental sodium and a synchronized countershock delivered.

Postcardioversion or postdefibrillation, monitor the ECG, blood pressure, and neuromuscular activity. Transient dysrhythmias such as premature beats and sinus bradycardia are common; so is transient hypotension. Neurologic assessment is particularly important in patients who have been in atrial fibrillation prior to cardioversion. During fibrillation, thrombus can form along the wall of the atria. With restoration of synchronized depolarization and regular atrial contractions, thrombus may break free and embolize. Potential complications from emboli are not limited to the cerebrovascular bed. Thrombus can also embolize to the coronary arteries, renal vascular beds, and splanchnic vascular beds, causing serious ischemia from occlusion of smaller vessels. Patients need to be elevated for this potential alteration in tissue perfusion.

Pacemakers

Patients who require pacemaker support are experiencing dysrhythmias that have resulted in alterations in cardiac output and possibly tissue perfusion. The goal of cardiac pacing is to restore regular rhythm and/or increase heart rate to optimize cardiac output and tissue perfusion. To effectively evaluate a patient with a pacemaker, the nurse needs to understand the reason for insertion, the characteristics of the pacemaker, placement of the electrodes, and the method of placement. Effective evaluation of pacemaker function requires an ability to distinguish pacemaker rhythm from spontaneous rhythm. Also, the nurse should be able to determine the effectiveness of the pacemaker's sensing mechanism and the ability of the pacemaker stimulus to initiate depolarization of cardiac muscle cells.

Indications

An artificial pacemaker may be inserted prophylactically or therapeutically. The indications for temporary pacing that are generally accepted by most professionals are shown in Table 14–2.

Approaches

A pacemaker may be temporary or permanent. Temporary pacemaker electrodes can be inserted through a

TABLE 14-2 INDICATIONS FOR TEMPORARY PACEMAKER

Bradydysrhythmias

Symptomatic sinus bradycardia

Sinus arrest

Slow ventricular rhythm

Asystole

Heart Blocks

Second-degree AV block with slow ventricular response

Third-degree AV block with slow ventricular response

Mobitz II second-degree AV block in anterior myocardial infarction

Right bundle branch block with left anterior or posterior fascicular block in anterior myocardial infarction

Alternating bundle branch block

Recurrent Ventricular Tachycardia

Sick Sinus Syndrome (bradycardia-tachycardia syndrome)

---

transvenous, transthoracic, or direct epicardial approach.

The *transthoracic* approach is used as a "last ditch" effort in CPR. The physician inserts an intracardiac needle into the right ventricle, through a subxiphoid approach or the left parasternal area. The pacing catheter is inserted, and the electrode is connected to the external power source. This method is rapid but not suitable for prophylactic use or long-term pacing. Complications include possible pneumothorax, cardiac tamponade, and myocardial or coronary artery laceration.

Epicardial pacing requires a thoracotomy and is often used temporarily during and after cardiac surgery. The temporary electrodes are sutured directly to the epicardium and brought out through the chest wall. If pacing becomes necessary, the terminals can be connected quickly to the power source. When pacing is no longer necessary, a pull on the wire will break the epicardial sutures so the electrodes can be pulled out.

The most common method of pacing is *endocardial (transvenous)* pacing. The system consists of a transvenous catheter electrode and a pulse generator. This method can be used for permanent or temporary pacing.

Permanent pacemakers are implanted in the patient's chest or abdomen. Most are powered by batteries that last 8–10 years. Many of the newer ones can be externally programmed with signals from a special programming unit. Programmable pacemakers allow noninvasive adjustment of settings to better meet the needs of an individual patient. *Temporary* pacemakers have external pulse generators with easily accessible controls to allow individual adjustment.

Modes of Pacing

The mode of pacing may be asynchronous or synchronous. The *asynchronous (fixed-rate)* pacemaker delivers a stimulus regardless of the patient's spontaneous cardiac activity. This mode is used only for the patient with no spontaneous beats—for example, in asystole. The *synchronous (demand)* pacemaker senses spontaneous activity and either inhibits the artificial stimulus or triggers its delivery while the ventricles are refractory. Therefore, this pacemaker mode allows spontaneous beats to occur without competition from the pacemaker. The pacemaker initiates a beat only when a preset interval has passed with no spontaneous activity. This preset interval (the *escape interval*) is the same as the interval between paced beats on most pacemakers. Some pacemakers have a longer escape interval, called *rate hysteresis,* to allow for a delay before the pacemaker fires and so allow for more opportunity for spontaneous impulse generation.

A three-letter pacemaker identification code has been developed by the Inter-Society Commission for Heart Disease Resources (ICHD); this has become the standard language to describe pacemaker function. Table 14–3 outlines the code and what each of the three letters describes about the function of any pacemaker. The ICHD code immediately tells the nurse which chambers the pacemaker paces, in which chambers the pacemaker senses electrical activity, and how the pacemaker is programmed to respond to what is sensed.

The most popular external pulse generator is the *ventricular QRS-inhibited (VVI) pacemaker,* which both senses and paces the right ventricle. Because it does not pace the atrium, synchronized atrial filling is lost, and patients with poor cardiac reserve may develop heart failure or hypotension without this "atrial kick." The *A-V sequential (DVI) pacemaker* can overcome this disadvantage. It senses ventricular activity and paces

TABLE 14-3 INTER-SOCIETY COMMISSION FOR HEART DISEASE RESOURCES (ICHD) PACEMAKER CODES

1st LETTER	2nd LETTER	3rd LETTER
Chamber Paced	**Chamber Sensed**	**Mode of Response**
A = atrial	**A** = atrial	**O** = not applicable
V = ventricular	**V** = ventricular	**I** = inhibited
D = dual chamber	**D** = dual chamber	**T** = triggered
		D = inhibited and triggered

TABLE 14-4 PACEMAKER TYPES BY ICHD CODE AND FUNCTION

ICHD CODE	FUNCTION	COMMENT
Single Chamber		
AOO	Atrial fixed rate	Asynchronous
AAI	Atrial demand	Inhibited by atrial impulse
AAT	Atrial demand	Triggered by atrial impulse
VOO	Ventricular fixed rate	Asynchronous
VVI	Ventricular demand	Inhibited by ventricular impulse
VVT	Ventricular demand	Triggered by ventricular impulse
Dual Chamber		
VAT	Atrial-triggered, ventricular-paced	Committed to pace by atrial impulse
VDD	Atrial-triggered, ventricular-demand	Inhibited by ventricular impulse
DVI	A-V sequential	Inhibited by ventricular impulse
DDD	Fully automatic	Inhibited by atrial and/or ventricular impulses

both the atria and ventricles in the proper sequence and with enough delay between atrial and ventricular stimulation to allow synchronized filling of the chambers. Table 14–4 lists the major pacemakers in use today by their ICHD code and describes their method of function.

Pacing Catheters

A wide variety of pacing catheters is available. The *transthoracic lead* is a straight wire with a J-shaped tip that resumes its shape inside the ventricle after insertion. *Screw-in electrodes* are available for permanent epicardial pacing. *Transvenous catheters* come as stiff pacing leads, which are inserted under fluoroscopic control, and flexible, soft leads on balloon-tipped, flow-directed catheters better suited for emergency insertion at the bedside (Morrelli 1983).

The pacing catheter is either unipolar or bipolar, depending on whether there are one or two electrodes inside the catheter itself. The *unipolar* catheter has a negative electrode at its tip. The positive pole, necessary to complete the electrical circuit, is either the gen-

erator case (in permanent pacing) or a skin electrode (in temporary pacing) (Hoffman 1982). The *bipolar* catheter has both poles at the internal tip of the catheter and two wires at the external end that fit into the matching terminals on the generator. Most temporary pacing leads are bipolar.

Bedside Insertion

In an elective situation, the catheter usually is inserted in a cardiac catheterization laboratory under fluoroscopy. In an emergency, a physician may perform a bedside catheter insertion into the femoral, external jugular, subclavian, or brachial vein. If the jugular or subclavian site is to be used, position the patient flat or lower the head to minimize the risk of air embolism by creating positive venous pressure so air will not be sucked into the vein.

The procedure for electrode catheter insertion varies with the type of catheter selected. The balloon-tipped, flow-directed catheter is inserted without fluoroscopic guidance and placed in position by balloon inflation in the vena cava. Blood flow then carries the catheter into the right ventricle.

If a stiff lead is selected, the physician ideally will position the catheter under fluoroscopy. If a portable unit is unavailable, he or she will attach a sterile alligator clamp to the negative electrode on the catheter and pass you the end of the wire. Attach it to the precordial ("V" or exploring) lead of the ECG machine. While the catheter is advanced, keep the physician informed of changes in the P wave, QRS, and ST segment. When the catheter reaches the right atrium, the P and QRS will be about the same height. As the catheter enters the right ventricle, the QRS amplitude will increase significantly. When the tip touches the endocardium, the ST segment will elevate. The physician will try to wedge the tip in the trabeculae of the right ventricle. He or she will then suture the catheter to the skin and dress the site.

Attach the negative distal electrode to the negative terminal of the pulse generator and the positive proximal electrode to the positive terminal.

The external pulse generator (see Figure 14–1) contains an on/off switch, a sensitivity setting to indicate what voltage the generator should interpret as a spontaneous QRS, a milliamperage (MA) dial to determine how much voltage the pacemaker discharges, a rate setting, a pacing indicator such as a light or moving line, and, in some cases, a test indicator for battery function. Turn the pacemaker on and set the dials as ordered by the physician. Start with the MA dial at its lowest set-

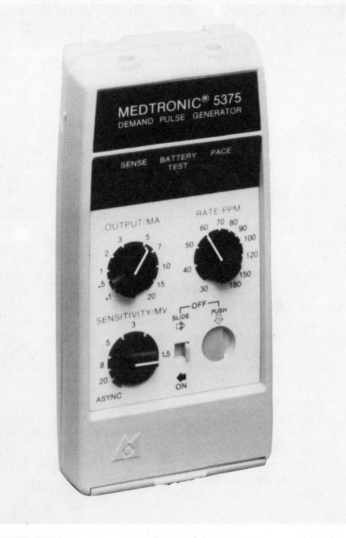

FIGURE 14–1

External pacemaker. (Courtesy Medtronic, Inc., Minneapolis, Minnesota.)

ting. Increase it until the ECG shows that each pacing spike is capturing (being followed by a QRS). The level at which this occurs is the *pacing threshold*. Increase the MA setting to twice threshold to allow for variations in discharge voltage and for fibrosis around the catheter tip.

The sensitivity dial determines the pacemaker's response to spontaneous cardiac activity. At greatest sensitivity, it may interpret any amount of voltage as a ventricular depolarization. At least sensitivity, it will ignore all cardiac voltage and will pace at a fixed rate. The usual setting is at a 12 o'clock position, where only a fairly large voltage will be read as a ventricular depolarization.

Insertion-related complications are most significant with a subclavian insertion site; pneumothorax, hemothorax, air embolism, and injury to the brachial plexus may occur. Following insertion, obtain chest x-ray films to verify position of the pacing wire and to detect any pneumothorax. Also obtain a 12-lead ECG to verify the position of the pacing wire.

Local hematoma and infection are possible with all methods of insertion. Check the insertion site for inflammation and the patient's temperature for elevation at least once every 8 hours. Clean the skin and apply a dry sterile dressing daily.

Postinsertion Nursing Care

After pacemaker insertion, the nursing goals are maintenance of electrical safety, maintenance of pacemaker effectiveness, prevention and treatment of complications, and education of the patient.

Electrical Safety Elimination of electrical hazards is essential because the pacing catheter provides a direct pathway for electricity to reach the heart and induce ventricular fibrillation. All electrical equipment should have three-prong plugs; the third prong connects the instrument to the hospital ground. Never use "cheater" adaptors to connect a three-prong plug and a two-hole electrical outlet. Disconnect from the patient any electrical equipment not currently in use. Connect all other electrical equipment in contact with the patient to a common receptacle. Avoid touching the patient and electrical equipment simultaneously. Use battery-operated razors and radios.

Newer-model pacemakers have insulated catheter tips and terminals. If you are using an older model with exposed tips or terminals, insulate the pacemaker terminals and exposed electrodes with a rubber glove. Wear rubber gloves whenever you work with the terminals or handle pacemaker wires or catheters.

Maintenance of Pacemaker Effectiveness The patient with a temporary or new permanent pacemaker should receive continuous ECG monitoring. Periodically, analyze a rhythm strip, noting in particular these characteristics:

- The appearance of the spike in relation to the P wave and QRS. In atrial pacing, it should be before the P wave; in ventricular, before the QRS, that is, after the P wave (if one is present). In a QRS-inhibited pacemaker, no spike should be visible during a spontaneous beat.
- The polarity and amplitude of the spike.
- The appearance of the paced QRS. The appearance will depend on the type of pacemaker. With a right ventricular pacemaker, the paced QRS should be wide, have a left BBB appearance in V_1 and V_6, and a deep S wave in II, III, and AVF.
- Whether the pacemaker rate calculated from the ECG matches the set rate.
- Whether the paced beats are synchronized with spontaneous beats. If a demand pacemaker is used, a paced beat should occur only when a spontaneous beat fails to appear on time. Fusion beats are common (Figure 14–2).

Also check the pacemaker threshold at least once every 8 hours. To do this, turn the MA dial down just to the point at which each spike is capturing. Note the reading and reset the dial at the previous setting.

Complications Use the aforementioned observations to detect problems promptly and take appropriate action. Some possible problems are described in the following paragraphs and shown in Figure 14–2.

Failure to Pace Failure to pace is indicated by absent pacemaker spikes, bradycardia or asystole, and signs of decreased cardiac output. There are numerous possible causes. Check the generator to make sure it is on and the dials are on the correct settings. Make sure the sensitivity dial is on the correct setting; it may have been dislodged to the position where it reads P waves as QRSs. Check the rate setting. Make certain connections are secure. The pacemaker components may have failed. If the patient's pacemaker is not pacing, change the battery or whole generator. If none of these interventions works, the cause may be a fractured electrode. You can prevent this by limiting tension on the pacing wire or catheter. If you suspect a fractured electrode, notify the physician. If a bipolar electrode has been used and only one wire is fractured, the unit can be converted to a unipolar system. Attach the intact electrode to the negative terminal and a skin electrode to the positive terminal. This serves as a temporary solution until the catheter is replaced.

Failure to Capture Failure to capture the ventricles is shown by spikes not followed closely by paced ventricular complexes; bradycardia or asystole; and decreased cardiac output. This problem usually is caused by catheter displacement. To prevent displacement, minimize movement at the insertion site. Should the pacemaker fail to capture, the catheter may be floating free in the right ventricle; if so, you may see ECG signs of ventricular irritability. Attempt to reposition it by moving the patient's arm or turning him on his side. The catheter may have moved into the right atrium; in this case, the spike will be followed by a P wave instead of a QRS. The catheter may have perforated the septum; the QRS then will manifest a RBBB pattern, being primarily positive in the right chest leads and negative in the left, and ventricular irritability may occur. If you are unable to reposition a floating catheter or if you suspect migration to the atrium or left ventricle, notify the physician to reposition the catheter.

Another possibility is that the MA setting may be inadequate due to fibrosis at the tip, infection, or potassium imbalance. Increase the MA until a new threshold is reached; then again set the MA dial at two to three

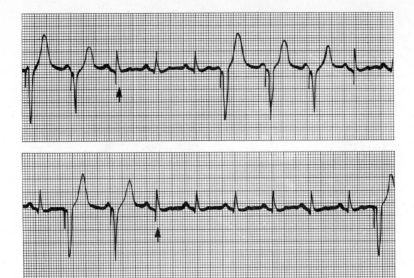

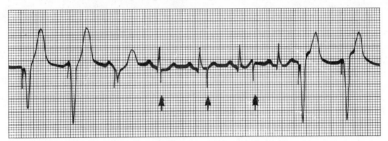

Demand ventricular pacemaker
(Continuous strip; arrows point to fusion beats)

Failure to sense

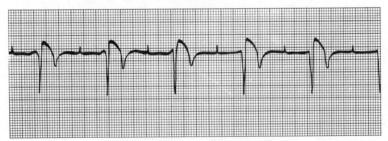

Failure to capture

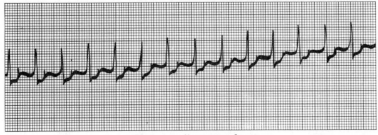

"Runaway" pacemaker
(rate is 150)

FIGURE 14–2

Pacemaker rhythms.

times threshold. Notify the physician of the increase in threshold.

Failure to Sense (Competition)   Failure to sense is indicated by pacemaker spikes occurring when they should not. This problem may be due to catheter malposition; try the measures suggested above. It also may result from too low a sensitivity setting; try adjusting the setting. If failure to sense continues and if the spontaneous rhythm is adequate, turn the pacemaker off. If not, leave it on. In either case, notify the physician. Competition rarely causes ventricular fibrillation, but be prepared in case it does occur.

A pacing rate change of more than 10 beats from the set rate indicates failure of the pacemaker components. Change the battery or the whole pulse generator.

Other, rarer problems include hiccoughs due to phrenic stimulation by the pacing stimulus, pericardial tamponade due to myocardial perforation, and thromboemboli from the catheter tip.

Patient Education   Teach the patient and family about the pacemaker. If the patient has a temporary pacemaker, briefly explain to patient and family how it works to aid the heart. Assess their current knowledge and clarify misconceptions. Review cardiac anatomy and emphasize how the pacemaker will relieve the symptoms that led to hospitalization. If the patient has a permanent pacemaker, teach patient and family more extensively about it. Teach the patient and a family member how to check the pulse daily. Stress the need for medical follow-up and the signs of pacemaker failure (rate change greater than ±10 beats, dyspnea, persistent dizziness, and fluid retention). Explain the need for a periodic battery change. Although permanent pacemaker generators are shielded from external electrical interference, the patient still should be aware of possible electrical hazards of high-voltage areas. The patient may use electrical devices providing he or she does not become dizzy. Encourage specific physical activities, but not to the point of fatigue. Make sure the patient has a pacemaker warranty card and knows to carry it at all times.

Percutaneous Transluminal Coronary Angioplasty (PTCA)

Angina that becomes poorly controlled by conventional medical therapy can be quite debilitating to patients. For some, percutaneous transluminal coronary angioplasty

(PTCA) may be an option. The technique of transluminal angioplasty first was used clinically by Dotter and Judkins in 1964 when they dilated a stenotic femoral artery in a woman threatened with limb loss from ischemia (Dotter and Judkins 1964). The procedure first was used in a patient with coronary artery obstruction by Grüntzig in 1977. (Grüntzig et al. 1979). The procedure, which has become common, is performed in institutions that have an active cardiac surgery program as an alternative to coronary artery bypass surgery for certain patients with coronary artery occlusive disease. The goal of PTCA is to dilate stenotic coronary arteries and increase flow using a double-lumen catheter with an expandable dilatation balloon.

Candidates for PTCA

Not all patients with coronary artery disease are suitable candidates for PTCA. First, patients must have angina that has become intolerable and is poorly controlled or refractory to medical therapy. There should also be objective evidence of ischemia documented by ST segment depression or other tests such as a defect in thallium uptake with thallium scanning (Shillinger 1983). It also is important that the patient have good left ventricular function, as little would be gained by restoring blood flow to myocardium that has already been damaged. If the patient's clinical condition is not improved by the procedure, the risk-to-benefit ratio for the procedure is increased (Killpack 1983). Any patient undergoing PTCA also must be a candidate for coronary artery bypass surgery and must understand that surgery is a possibility if complications occur. Approximately 6% of patients undergoing PTCA will require emergency bypass surgery (Kent 1982). This surgery is required due to sudden occlusion of the artery, rupture of the coronary artery, dissection of the atheroma, or persistent, irreversible coronary spasm. All of these conditions could precipitate myocardial infarction. In addition, coronary artery rupture may precipitate life-threatening cardiac tamponade.

Patients also must have coronary artery lesions that are amenable to the procedure. Initially, patients were required to have lesions of a single vessel. However, some experts in the field of PTCA now perform PTCA in patients with lesions in more than one vessel. The lesion must be accessible to the catheter, so patients with distal lesions are not candidates. Lesions must also be discrete, concentric, and noncalcified (Killpack 1983). Calcified lesions cannot be compressed by PTCA.

Patient Preparation for PTCA

The PTCA procedure itself lasts approximately 2–3 hours and is done in the cardiac catheterization laboratory. Patients may be admitted the evening before or the morning of the procedure and are generally discharged within 24 hours following the procedure. Even though patients are seen for only a few hours before the procedure, they may have significant deficits in knowledge about the procedure and possibility of surgery. Needed teaching includes information about basic anatomy and physiology, their disease process, and the procedure.

Nurses can help to minimize patient anxiety during the procedure by preparing them for what they will see and hear and by describing other sensations they will experience (Shillinger 1983). The cardiac catheterization laboratory is a rather foreign environment to most patients. They can be told to expect to see large numbers of people in surgical gowns, extensive monitoring equipment, and drapes covering themselves. They will also experience the room being darkened several times during the procedure. They need to know they likely will hear loud noises and alarms. They will feel sensations associated with catheter advancement and injection of contrast medium and may even experience angina as the dilatation is done. Adequate preparation for these events can help to minimize anxiety during the procedure and potentially abate physiologic responses to anxiety such as tachycardia and hypertension; both of these conditions increase oxygen demand, a situation to avoid in a patient with myocardial ischemia.

It also is important to prepare the patient and family for the possibility of coronary bypass surgery. The uncertainty of the outcome of PTCA likely will provoke a lot of anxiety for both patient and family. It can be emphasized that, though preparatory teaching is standard, only a small percentage of patients actually go to surgery. Instruction should include information about the intensive care unit routines, the noise level, the endotracheal tube, chest tubes, the incision, expected chest discomfort, and the use of pain medication. Families will need to know where the patient will go after surgery and how they can be kept informed of the patient's progress. Available information booklets about the intensive care unit might be given to them at that time.

PTCA Procedure

Prior to beginning the PTCA procedure, baseline data are obtained. These include a 12-lead electrocardiogram and assessment of lower-extremity pulses. Patients also

TABLE 14-5 MEDICATIONS USED FOR PTCA

MEDICATION	FUNCTIONS
Analgesics	Control of pain Sedation
Nitroglycerin	Minimize or prevent coronary artery spasm Relieve angina
Lidocaine	Control dysrhythmias
Heparin	Anticoagulation during procedure Maintain partial thromboplastin time (PTT) at 2–2½ times normal
Coumadin	Anticoagulation postprocedure for up to 3 months Maintain PTT at 2 times normal
Dipyridamole	Antiplatelet agent for up to 3 months Decrease platelet adhesion over injured vessel wall
Aspirin	Antiplatelet agent Decrease platelet adhesion (may take life-long)

will be typed and cross-matched so blood can be prepared if surgery becomes necessary. Coronary arteriography usually is performed to compare the exact location and size of the lesion with previous films. Temporary pacemaker wires are inserted in the event that transient heart block occurs during the procedure. Anticoagulation with heparin is achieved prior to insertion of the dilatation catheter. Table 14–5 outlines medications used for PTCA and their functions.

The double-lumen catheter is designed to allow for injection of contrast medium and recording of vessel pressures through one lumen and inflation of a sausage-shaped balloon accessible via a second lumen. The catheter is inserted via the femoral artery and advanced to the coronary ostia with fluoroscopic guidance. The catheter is advanced over a soft guidewire that directs the catheter to the coronary artery lesion and minimizes vessel wall damage from the stiffer dilatation catheter. Vessel pressures are recorded both proximal and distal to the obstruction. This recording helps localize the obstruction and also provides information about the degree of relief of obstruction achieved. Pressures distal to the obstruction will be lower than pressures proximal to the obstruction prior to the procedure. In addition to recording pressures, the balloon itself has radiopaque markers that assist in proper positioning. During this time, intravenous nitroglycerin is infused to minimize or prevent coronary artery spasm. The incidence of spasm is approximately 2% (Kent 1982).

Once the balloon is properly positioned, it is rapidly

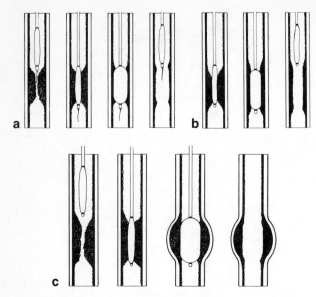

FIGURE 14–3

Theories of vessel expansion: **a,** compression with rupture of atheroma; **b,** compression with redistribution of atheroma; **c,** compression with tearing and stretching of the media. (From Killpack A: 1983. The use of intracoronary streptokinase and percutaneous transluminal angioplasty. In *Cardiovascular critical care nursing,* Woods S (ed). New York: Churchill-Livingstone Inc. 1983, p. 23. Used with permission.)

inflated with a combination of normal saline and contrast medium. The balloon is inflated to a pressure of up to 6 atmospheres and is kept inflated for up to 15 seconds (Shillinger 1983). During this time, the coronary artery is totally obstructed and the patient may experience angina. One inflation may only partially increase the diameter of the vessel lumen, so subsequent inflations might be considered. Inflations may be repeated to (1) increase distal vessel pressures, (2) improve washout of the contrast medium, and (3) improve the angiographic appearance of the stenosis (McCarthy 1982; Shillinger 1983). Failure of PTCA may result from an inability to maneuver the balloon over the lesion because of anatomic factors. This accounts for approximately one-fourth of PTCA failures. Failure also may occur because the lesion is too rigid to dilate or because of previously described complications.

Mechanism of Dilatation

The actual mechanism by which the coronary artery lesion is dilated is still under debate and may differ according to the developmental stage of the lesion (Bou-

man 1984). Figure 14–3 illustrates three possible mechanisms. Some researchers feel inflation compresses and possibly tears or ruptures the atheroma (Essed et al. 1983). Compression also may redistribute the atheroma within the vessel wall as water is expressed (Dotter and Judkins 1964). A third explanation is that compression results in tearing and stretching of the media, resulting in an increased coronary artery vessel diameter (Castaneda-Zuniga et al. 1980).

Care Following PTCA

Patients will require monitored care following PTCA in either a coronary care unit or intermediate intensive care unit. Complete bedrest will be required for 8 hours, with immobilization of the leg where the catheter was inserted. The following nursing diagnoses may be applicable to any patient following PTCA.

Potential for Fluid Volume Deficit The contrast medium acts as an osmotic diuretic and significant diuresis may occur. The patient likely will be thirsty and should be encouraged to drink freely. Serum potassium levels should be monitored closely as supplemental potassium may be required. Intravenous fluids will be used initially to supplement oral intake. Assessment of the patient for orthostatic hypotension is important before the patient is allowed out of bed.

Potential for Injury Myocardial ischemia, bleeding, and femoral artery occlusion are all potential complications of PTCA. Following PTCA, patients are monitored for dysrhythmias, ST segment changes, and cardiac enzyme elevation, all of which might indicate myocardial ischemia or injury. Intravenous nitroglycerin usually is maintained following the procedure, to promote coronary artery dilatation and to prevent coronary artery spasm. Any reports of chest pain by the patient should be documented and reported to the physician. Obtaining an electrocardiogram during the episode of chest pain may aid in identifying the origin of ischemia.

Following PTCA, heparin is not reversed. This increases the risk of bleeding at the femoral artery insertion site. Immediately after the catheter is removed, manual pressure is applied over the insertion site for at least 10 minutes. This is followed by placement of a pressure dressing. A sandbag should be placed over the pressure dressing. Bedrest and avoidance of hip flexion also help the femoral artery to seal off. The pressure dressing should be checked frequently for signs of bleeding. Any color change or evidence of hematoma at the insertion site should alert the nurse to the possibility of internal bleeding. Hematocrit levels also are evaluated to detect internal bleeding. It is important to remember that the patient is anticoagulated and internal bleeding could occur from other sources.

The presence of the catheter in the femoral artery may precipitate thrombus formation, which could embolize to the distal extremity. Evaluation following PTCA includes assessment of peripheral pulses in both legs, along with assessment of color, temperature, and capillary filling. Recording of data will assist others in determining if changes have occurred.

Knowledge Deficit A knowledge deficit related to the long-term anticoagulant and antiplatelet medication may exist. Patients will require instruction on action, dosage, and side effects of therapy. They will need to be able to recognize signs of bleeding and actions to take should bleeding occur. The nurse should inform patients of precautions to take to prevent uncontrolled bleeding while on anticoagulant therapy, e.g., no contact sports, no dental surgery. It also will be important that the patient understand the need for regular laboratory appointments to evaluate coagulation status.

Alterations in Self-Concept PTCA can have dramatic results for some patients, who may be able to leave the hospital after a 48-hour stay and be free of angina. Patients may view the procedure as a cure of their problem. They need to understand that the atherosclerotic disease process can still progress and risk factor modification is important. Successful PTCA may cause an abrupt change in lifestyle, which may require role adjustments at home, at work, or socially (Shillinger 1983). The nurse may be able to assist patients in preparing for this change and in developing strategies to facilitate transition. For some patients, PTCA will be unsuccessful, and they may have considerable anger about the outcome (Shillinger 1983). The nurse can help the patient express that anger, identify ways to work through the anger, and develop constructive plans to adjust to the outcome or select alternative options.

Cardiopulmonary Bypass

For some patients, coronary artery bypass surgery will be the intervention of choice to relieve myocardial ischemia. Some patients with coronary heart disease also may have concomitant valve disease. It is beyond the scope of this chapter to review the many cardiac lesions that might require the support of cardiopulmonary by-

pass (CPB) during surgery. Cardiopulmonary bypass results in some predictable alterations in hemodynamics and physiologic function that will persist in the early postoperative period. Nursing care of patients following cardiac surgery is focused on anticipating these expected hemodynamic and physiologic effects of CPB.

Principles of Cardiopulmonary Bypass

In order to perform surgery on the heart, it is necessary that the heart be in an arrested state, with rare exceptions. It also is desirable to collapse the lungs so they are not inflating over the surgical field. The role of CPB is to support blood pressure, systemic perfusion, oxygenation, and carbon dioxide removal during the time the heart is arrested and the lungs are not ventilated, thus preserving tissue perfusion and tissue viability.

One or two cannulas are placed in the right atrium or vena cavae, which bring venous blood to the CPB apparatus. Blood is then filtered and oxygenated. Temperature of the blood is also adjusted during this time. Once oxygenated, it passes through a pump and a filter to remove air and debris and is then pumped back to the body via a cannula placed in the ascending aorta. The three basic components of CPB are the plastic circuitry carrying the blood, the pump, and the oxygenator. During the surgical procedure, blood is continuously circulated between the patient and CPB system. Three principles that allow for effective CPB are hemodilution, hypothermia, and anticoagulation (Weiland and Walker 1986).

The CPB circuit can be thought of as additional vascular space that has to be primed with fluid. This is achieved with a lactated Ringer's solution. Hemodilution with a crystalloid solution decreases blood viscosity and peripheral vascular resistance. Hematocrits after hemodilution typically drop to around 25%. Hemodilution and subsequent decreased blood viscosity protect the patient from impaired flow from CPB due to peripheral resistance and sludging of blood that might result in poor capillary perfusion and microthrombus. Microthrombi could also form in the CPB unit itself. Hemodilution also lowers the plasma oncotic pressure, which results in fluid shifts and accumulation of interstitial fluid (Weiland and Walker 1986; Ream 1982). It is not unusual for a patient on CPB to gain 1–8 kilograms of weight from fluid accumulation.

Hypothermia is necessary to decrease metabolic demand, consumption of oxygen, and production of carbon dioxide. Patients typically are cooled on CPB to a temperature of 28°C. This provides major organs with protection against ischemia during surgery. This protection also allows for lower flow rates through CPB, which protects red blood cells from trauma and hemolysis (Weiland and Walker 1986). Hemodilution prevents the increase in blood viscosity that would normally occur with hypothermia. Patients are rewarmed to 36°C prior to the termination of CPB but will lose heat from the open chest and cold operating room suite. It is not uncommon to have a patient return from the operating room with a temperature below 36°C. Hypothermia will contribute to vasoconstriction and increased systemic vascular resistance, which contributes to the potential for postoperative hypertension.

Anticoagulation is required to prevent clotting of blood in the CPB system. Heparin is used to achieve an activated partial thromboplastin time (PTT) that is five to six times normal. At the conclusion of CPB, heparinization is reversed with protamine sulfate, a heparin antagonist. Inadequate heparin reversal may be one origin of postoperative bleeding, and careful monitoring of the PTT will reflect inadequate reversal. Heparin may also be sequestered in tissues and later released into the bloodstream, causing a heparin rebound effect. This may also be the cause of an abnormal PTT and bleeding in the postoperative period. It is corrected by additional protamine.

Postoperative Implications of CPB

Potential for Fluid Volume Deficit Following CPB, patients have the potential for fluid volume deficit due to blood loss, fluid shifts, osmotic diuresis, or inadequate replacement secondary to increased systemic vascular resistance.

Postoperative blood loss may be due to surgery-related problems such as oozing from small vessels that were not cauterized or from disruption of a suture line. Although philosophies vary from institution to institution, persistent mediastinal tube bleeding over 300–400 ml/hr for more than 3 hours usually warrants a return to the operating room for reexploration. This assumes that coagulation studies are normal. A patient who is bleeding excessively should also be monitored closely for an *alteration in cardiac output* as the result of cardiac tamponade. Blood can accumulate behind the heart, clot, and impair filling of the heart. This may be true even when mediastinal tubes are patent if they are not draining the area of accumulation.

Bleeding also may be due to inadequate reversal of heparin, which is discussed previously. Another origin of bleeding is consumption of clotting factors and injury or destruction of platelets during CPB. The roller pump

and filtration unit are particularly damaging aspects of CPB. The longer the patient has been supported with CPB, the more likely bleeding of this nature will occur. Abnormal PTTs and prothrombin times (PTs) indicate abnormal coagulation requiring treatment with fresh-frozen plasma. Platelet counts will guide platelet replacement. Platelets also may be given to bleeding patients with low-normal counts if there is suspicion of platelet dysfunction from injury.

Fluid volume deficit also may occur as a result of fluid shifts from hemodilution. This may persist for up to 6 hours postoperatively (Weiland and Walker 1986). Patients may require large amounts of volume replacement during this time to maintain optimal preload and to compensate for losses into the interstitial space. Another contributing factor is the activation of the complement and kinin systems by CPB, which induces a capillary leak syndrome, further increasing the tendency for interstitial fluid accumulation (Sladen 1982).

Osmotic diuresis is another contributing factor to fluid volume deficit. Mannitol is given on CPB to preserve renal tubular flow and to reduce myocardial edema. This osmotic diuresis caused by mannitol can result in a urine output of up to 3 liters in the first 4 hours after CPB (Sladen 1982). Many patients also will develop hyperglycemia (300–600 mg/dL) following CPB (Weiland and Walker 1986). This contributes to the osmotic diuresis. CPB is a physiologic stress that results in release of epinephrine and produces a catabolic state. Thus, insulin secretion is diminished and glycogenolysis is stimulated. Hypothermia also impairs the release of insulin by the pancreas (Weiland and Walker 1986). Serum glucose levels normalize as diuresis progresses, and insulin administration is not indicated. Diuresis also will occur as a result of the hemodilution itself as the body attempts to normalize fluid balance.

Great care must be taken to monitor serum electrolytes during diuresis. Of particular importance is potassium. Potassium is lost in large amounts during this time. Hypokalemia is the most common cause of myocardial irritability and dysrhythmias in the early postoperative period. Almost all patients will require potassium replacement.

Adequate replacement of volume during the early postoperative period may be hampered by the vasoconstriction associated with hypothermia. This increased systemic vascular resistance may cause hypertension and mask the true intravascular volume deficit. Other contributing factors are circulating catecholamines, vasopressin, and renin-angiotensin release as a result of low flows and pressure on CPB. Controlled vasodilation is the goal of treatment. Eventual rewarming will cause vasodilatation, but it may be rapid and result in hypotension as a result of inadequate fluid volume. Con-

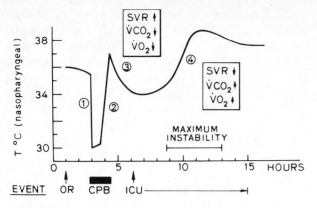

FIGURE 14–4

Temperature changes that occur during and after cardiac surgery. **1** and **2** demonstrate the cooling and rewarming that occur on CPB. **3,** Heat is lost to the periphery and ambient air after CPB. **4,** Rewarming occurs. Systemic vascular resistance (SVR), CO_2 production ($\dot{V}CO_2$) and oxygen consumption ($\dot{V}O_2$) change dramatically with rewarming. (From Sladen R: Management of the adult cardiac patient in the intensive care unit. Page 495 in *Acute cardiovascular management: Anesthesia and intensive care,* Ream A, Fogdall R (eds). Philadelphia: Lippincott/Harper & Row, 1982. Used with permission.)

trolled vasodilatation is achieved with vasodilators. Hypertension can then be controlled and fluid can be appropriately administered. Figure 14–4 illustrates the fluctuations of temperature and systemic vascular resistance that occur during the early postoperative period.

Potential for Alteration in Cardiac Output Hypothermia may depress cardiac performance in the early postoperative period. Cardiac output may be mildly depressed, and there is a tendency towards sinus bradycardia (Weiland and Walker 1986). Bradycardia is treated with chronotropic drugs or temporary epicardial pacing. Myocardial edema, as a result of CPB, also will contribute to low cardiac output as a result of the subsequent decreased compliance. This depression is transient and may not require further treatment. In many patients, however, transient depression of contractility is treated with positive inotropic drugs, particularly dopamine hydrochloride. This may be maintained for the first 12–24 hours. The exception to that is in patients who have incurred myocardial injury during surgery or who have had preoperative myocardial dysfunction. Those patients may require prolonged inotropic support and afterload reduction for greater than 24 hours after surgery.

Any depression of cardiac output should alert the nurse to assess patients for *alterations in tissue perfu-*

sion. Alterations in tissue perfusion also may occur during CPB. As a result, assessment will reveal impaired organ dysfunction. Renal and cerebrovascular function will be particularly affected by long periods of poor perfusion. Evaluation of tissue perfusion should include acid–base status, skin temperature, skin color, peripheral pulses, urine quantity and quality, and sensorium.

Alterations in tissue perfusion also may result from emboli during CPB. Sources of emboli may be thrombus in the heart, atherosclerotic plaque, calcium or vegetations on abnormal valves, or air. Any of these can seriously alter organ function, causing stroke or renal failure from thromboemboli.

Potential for Ineffective Airway Clearance or Impaired Gas Exchange As mentioned before, the lungs are collapsed while the patient is on CPB. As a result, some alveolar collapse occurs, secretions accumulate and poor lung perfusion may result in microthrombus formation (Sladen 1982; Weiland and Walker 1986). Therefore, all patients will have some degree of atelectasis and pulmonary shunting. This usually is not a major problem unless the patient has a history of lung disease. Care is directed at increasing ventilation of alveoli with mechanical ventilation and positive end-expiratory pressure. Nursing care focuses on techniques to enhance the ventilation-to-perfusion ratio. This includes frequent turning and suctioning. Following extubation, patients are mobilized as soon as possible. Coughing and deep breathing are encouraged and supported with adequate administration of pain medication.

For some patients who develop significant depression of cardiac output, the routine care described will not be adequate. Intra-aortic balloon counterpulsation may be one treatment of choice for this group of patients.

Intra-aortic Balloon Counterpulsation

Intra-aortic balloon counterpulsation (IABP) is a method of augmenting a patient's CO and increasing coronary artery perfusion during periods of transient myocardial depression. It is achieved through the placement of a balloon device in the aorta. Because the balloon deflates when the heart is in systole and inflates when it is in diastole, its pumping action is counter to that of the heart—thus the term *counterpulsation.*

Physiologic Effects

Normal coronary blood flow occurs during diastole. The coronary arteries are compressed during systole, so little blood flow occurs then. During diastole, when the heart is relaxing, there is little resistance to blood flow. When the balloon inflates during diastole, it increases intra-aortic volume, thereby increasing intra-aortic pressure. The increase in intra-aortic pressure is called *diastolic augmentation*. The elevated aortic pressure increases coronary artery perfusion pressure, thereby improving oxygen supply to the myocardium.

Normal ventricular ejection depends on preload, contractility, afterload, and heart rate. *Afterload* is the resistance to ejection against which the heart must work, created by the blood pressure and the vascular system. Resistance to ejection *(impedance)* often is increased in patients in shock, because of vasoconstriction. When the intra-aortic balloon is deflated during systole, it rapidly drops pressure in the aorta (Bitran et al. 1981). It thus lowers aortic end-diastolic pressure and resistance to ventricular ejection. Because it lowers afterload, it decreases left ventricular work and thus lowers myocardial oxygen demand. Because more oxygen is supplied to the ventricle, contractility improves. As blood is pumped out of the heart more efficiently, *preload* (the volume in the ventricle just prior to systole) decreases. This reduction in preload also improves contractility. The improved contractility indirectly causes heart rate to slow toward normal, because as perfusion improves, there is less sympathetic stimulation.

Indications

Indications for IABP include post-infarction cardiogenic shock, pre-infarction angina, and high-risk surgical patients. Post-infarction cardiogenic shock can follow extensive left ventricular damage, ventricular septal rupture, or acute mitral regurgitation from capillary muscle rupture or dysfunction. In pre-infarction angina, the pump allows safer cardiac catheterization and prompt cardiovascular surgery. In high-risk patients, preoperative pumping allows safer induction of anesthesia. The balloon also can be used to wean patients who have undergone open heart surgery off cardiopulmonary bypass. The IABP allows time for them to recover from the temporary myocardial depression produced by ischemia resulting from low perioperative blood flow or prolonged aortic cross-clamping. It also allows time for recovery if there is severe compromise from the surgery itself, as may occur, for example, with aneurysmectomy, in which a large portion of the heart muscle is removed.

IABP requires a competent aortic valve and ideally a healthy aortic wall. Contraindications include: (a) aortic valve insufficiency, which would allow blood to flow backward into the ventricle during diastolic augmentation; (b) aortic aneurysm, which could rupture during augmentation; (c) aortic dissection, because of the danger of rupture; and (d) severe peripheral vascular disease, which may prevent passage of or cause damage to the balloon.

Equipment

The balloon pump consists of two components: the balloon itself and the console that drives it. Balloons are available with one, two, or three pumping chambers (Daily and Schroeder 1985). Inflation of the single-chambered balloon displaces blood both retrograde toward the aortic arch and anterograde toward the periphery. The double-chambered balloon has a small distal balloon that inflates first, with a larger proximal balloon that inflates next. The distal balloon inflation adds a downstream resistance to flow, so that when the proximal balloon is inflated, a greater amount of retrograde flow occurs. The triple-chambered balloon has a middle section that inflates first, with sections on the distal and proximal ends that inflate next; flow occurs in both anterograde and retrograde directions.

The size of the balloon is important. Balloon capacities vary from 10–40 ml. A size is selected to occlude approximately 80% of the aortic diameter. Occlusion of a greater area can result in aortic damage and red blood cell hemolysis.

Insertion

The balloon usually is inserted in the critical-care unit, cardiac catheterization laboratory, or operating room. Prior to insertion, the patient must be placed on a cardiac monitor, and have in place an arterial line, balloon-tipped PA line, central IV line, and peripheral IV line.

The usual insertion site is the common femoral artery. Typically, the balloon is inserted percutaneously. The balloon catheter is advanced to the thoracic aorta, where it is positioned so that it lies distal to the left subclavian artery and proximal to the renal arteries (Figure 14–5). This position is crucial to maintain flow to the left arm and the kidneys. To secure the catheter, it is sutured to the skin.

With the percutanous method, local anesthesia is infiltrated and the artery punctured with a needle through which a guidewire is passed. The needle is removed and the puncture wound enlarged with a dilator, followed by

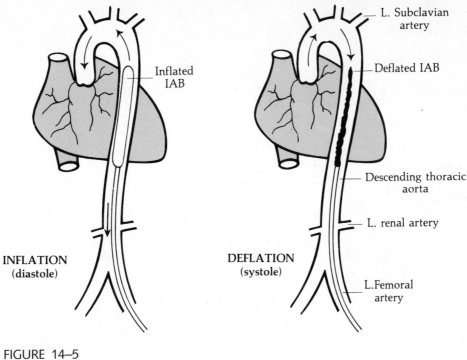

L. Subclavian artery

Inflated IAB

Deflated IAB

Descending thoracic aorta

L. renal artery

L. Femoral artery

INFLATION
(diastole)

DEFLATION
(systole)

FIGURE 14–5

Position of the IAB catheter in the aorta. (From Bullas J: Percutaneous intra-aortic counterpulsation balloon. *Crit Care Nurse* (July/August) 1982; 41.)

insertion of a dilator sheath. To make the balloon small enough to fit through the dilator sheath, the balloon is wrapped around the catheter using a special wrap control handle on the end of the catheter (Bullas 1982). After the balloon is inserted, the balloon is unwrapped by turning the handle counterclockwise. Correct balloon placement is verified by x-ray or fluoroscopy.

Once balloon position has been confirmed, the console is set to begin pumping. The balloon usually is filled with helium.

Nursing Care

Nursing care of the patient on IABP is much like that of any extremely ill patient. Most IABP patients, for instance, require intubation and mechanical ventilation. Because it is assumed that the nurse is familiar with general care of an unstable patient, this section will address only those aspects of care specific to IABP.

Timing Optimal timing of inflation and deflation requires console adjustment by a balloon console technician or specially trained nurse. The skill of the console operator is paramount to establishment and maintenance of optimal counterpulsation. To best coordinate

cardiac and balloon pumping, the ECG is used as the trigger for balloon activity (Figure 14–6). The lead best displaying R wave amplitude should be selected because the R wave is the usual trigger for inflation of the balloon. The balloon will deflate prior to the onset of the QRS complex so that it is deflated by the time ventricular contraction occurs. It will inflate shortly after the peak of the T wave.

Balloon timing is adjusted from the arterial waveform. The dicrotic notch is identified on the unassisted arterial tracing; this notch corresponds with closure of the aortic valve. Balloon inflation is adjusted so that pressure elevation from the balloon begins at the dicrotic notch, that is, so that balloon inflation begins just as the aortic valve is closing after ventricular ejection. The balloon remains inflated during diastole. Deflation is set to occur just prior to systole, producing an end-diastolic pressure dip just before the next cardiac systole. If balloon inflation is too early (and depending on the position of the valve leaflets), the aortic valve may close early (thus limiting stroke volume and increasing afterload). If balloon inflation is too late, diastolic augmentation decreases because of the rapidity of arterial runoff. If balloon deflation is too early, blood may flow retrograde from the carotid and coronary arteries into the aorta, and decrease coronary perfusion. More likely, early deflation will allow pressure in the aorta to rise to

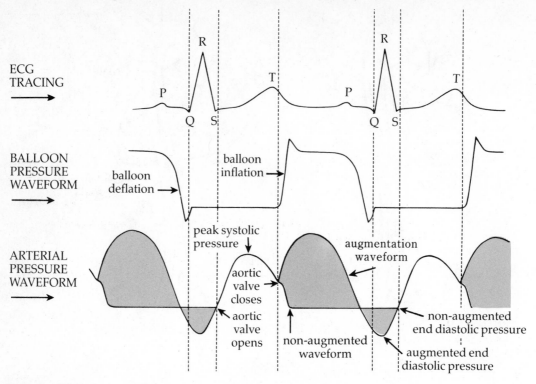

ECG TRACING →

BALLOON PRESSURE WAVEFORM →

ARTERIAL PRESSURE WAVEFORM →

FIGURE 14–6

Schematic relationship of balloon pressure waveform, ECG tracing, and arterial pressure. (Adapted from Bullas J: Percutaneous intra-aortic counterpulsation balloon. *Crit Care Nurse* (July/August) 1982; 44. Used with permission.

unassisted end-diastolic levels so that there is no drop in pressure just before the next systole. Therefore, there will be no decrease in the resistance to ventricular ejection. If it is too late, it will increase resistance to left ventricular ejection.

Interpretation of waveforms requires you to be extremely familiar with cardiovascular dynamics. During pumping, diastolic pressure is elevated and systolic pressure is reduced, when compared to unassisted tracings. For this reason, peak diastolic pressure may be higher than peak systolic pressure.

Weaning

Most patients show improvement in cardiovascular parameters within an hour of the onset of pumping, with peak improvement at approximately 24 hours post-IABP insertion (Shinn 1986). Patients then fall into three subsets: those who fail to respond to pumping and die; those who become pump-dependent and die; and those who, with or without surgery while on the pump, survive to be weaned.

The patient is weaned from the balloon when the hemodynamic condition is stable, often after 24–48 hours. Weaning can be achieved by decreasing the assist ratio and/or the balloon volume. Although the process varies, weaning typically is achieved by decreasing the frequency of balloon inflation from every beat to every second beat, and so on until the patient is receiving minimal support. The balloon then is removed under local anesthesia and a Fogarty catheter passed proximally and distally to remove any clots.

Complications   Complications associated with pumping fall into two categories: patient complications and technical complications.

Patient Complications   The patient complications specific to balloon counterpulsation are arterial occlusion, thromboemboli, platelet aggregation, and infection. *Arterial occlusion* can result from impaired circulation to the catheterized extremity or to displacement of the balloon. Compare peripheral pulses, color, temperature, and sensation hourly. Alert the physician immediately to any signs of decreased perfusion. Pay particular attention to the pulse in the left radial artery. If it diminishes or disappears, the balloon may have moved and occluded the left subclavian artery. Also monitor urinary output. A sudden drop may indicate that the balloon has moved distally and is occluding the renal arteries. To minimize the risk of displacing or kinking and cracking the catheter, elevate the head of the bed no more than 20° and avoid flexing the catheterized leg at the hip. Patients can be turned safely from side to side.

Thromboemboli can result from dislodgement of plaque during insertion or clotting around the catheter or balloon itself. Although the balloon surface is antithrombogenic, the surface can be damaged if it comes in contact with instruments during the insertion. Even if the balloon is undamaged, clot formation still can be a danger. To minimize the danger of thromboembolism with an undamaged balloon, do not allow the balloon to remain deflated longer than a few minutes; instead, you can turn the balloon volume way down to make it quiver so that thrombi will not form.

The physician may order anticoagulation during IABP after careful consideration of benefits versus risks for a particular patient (Ford and Buckley 1981; Bullas 1982; Bitran et al. 1981). If anticoagulation is employed, be alert for overt signs of bleeding and test nasogastric drainage and stools for occult blood.

The balloon may trigger *platelet aggregation*. To reduce this risk, the physician occasionally may order the administration of low-molecular-weight dextran, which "coats" the platelets to decrease clumping (Ford and Buckley 1981).

Infection is a serious potential complication. The balloon acts as a conduit for infection. To minimize the risks of infection, use meticulous aseptic technique not only at the insertion site but with all invasive procedures. An occlusive dressing usually is maintained over the insertion site. If the patient develops a fever, blood cultures should be drawn promptly. Opinion about the value of prophylactic antibiotics is divided. Some physicians advocate antibiotic use only if signs of infection appear. The majority, however, place the patient on antibiotics prior to catheter insertion and maintain prophylaxis until after catheter removal.

Technical Complications Technical complications that may occur include *balloon leak, balloon rupture,* and *inadequate pumping* because of dysrhythmias. Normally, a small amount of gas diffuses out of the balloon, so it must be periodically purged and refilled, usually every 2–4 hours. Some consoles do this automatically; others require manual filling. The nurse should be aware of the frequency and volume of balloon filling. Any increase in frequency or volume suggests that the balloon is leaking and will need to be replaced. Balloon rupture is unlikely unless the balloon was damaged during insertion. Careful handling of the balloon decreases the risk of balloon rupture.

Dysrhythmias will affect the efficiency of pumping, since the balloon timing is set from the regular R–R interval on the ECG. They should be treated promptly. If dysrhythmias are persistent, the balloon inflation can be set to trigger from the peak of the systolic arterial waveform. Most pumps also have a pacing mode, which will trigger off a pacer spike.

Conclusions

Although the overall death rate associated with IABP may seem high because of the underlying disease state, balloon counterpulsation offers the physician and nurse a powerful therapeutic tool for helping the gravely ill cardiovascular patient.

Outcome Evaluation

Evaluate the patient's response to cardiovascular interventions according to the following outcome criteria. Ideally, the patient will develop a normal sinus rhythm and adequate cardiac output. The ideal may not occur, however, particularly in the critically ill patient with preexisting heart disease. Realistic outcome criteria in the absence of normal sinus rhythm are spontaneous, drug-controlled, or artificially paced rhythms with the following characteristics:

- Ventricular rate 60–100 beats per minute.
- Ventricular rate and contractility adequate to perfuse core organs and periphery, as manifested by alert mental state; absence of angina; urinary output WNL for patient; warm, dry skin; peripheral pulses bilaterally equal and of normal volume for patient.
- Infrequent atrial or junctional premature beats, if any.
- Six or fewer ventricular premature beats (VPBs) per minute (unless the patient has a history of frequent VPBs).
- No more than three VPBs in a row.
- No multifocal VPBs.
- No VPBs falling on or near T waves.

- If on maintenance antidysrhythmic medication or permanent pacing, the patient should show no major toxic effects or complications from the therapy.

REFERENCES

Benner P: *From novice to expert.* Menlo Park, CA: Addison-Wesley, 1984.

Bitran D et al.: Intra-aortic balloon counterpulsation in acute myocardial infarction. *Heart Lung* 1981; 10:1021–1027.

Bouman C: Intracoronary thrombolysis and percutaneous transluminal angioplasty. *Nurs Clin North Am* 1984; 19:397–409.

Brown B et al.: Asystole and its treatment: The possible role of the parasympathetic nervous system in cardiac arrest. *J Am Coll Emerg Physicians* 8:448.

Bullas J: Percutaneous intra-aortic counterpulsation balloon. *Crit Care Nurse* (Jul/Aug) 1982; 40–49.

Castaneda-Zuniga W et al.: The mechanism of balloon angioplasty. *Diag Radiol* 1980; 135:565–571.

Chiang B et al.: Predisposing factors in sudden cardiac death in Tecumseh, Michigan: A prospective study. *Circulation* 1970; 41:31–37.

Cobb L et al.: Resuscitation from out-of-hospital ventricular fibrillation: Four years followup. *Circulation* 1975; 52:223–235.

Daily E, Schroeder J: *Bedside hemodynamic monitoring.* St Louis: Mosby, 1985.

Detre K et al.: Collaborative randomized study of cardiopulmonary-cerebral resuscitation. *Crit Care Med* 1981; 9:395–402.

Dotter C, Judkins M: Transluminal treatment of atherosclerotic obstruction. *Circulation* 1964; 30:654–670.

Essed C et al.: Transluminal coronary angioplasty and early restenosis: Fibrocellular occlusion after wall laceration. *Brit Heart J* 1983; 49:393–397.

Ford P, Buckley M: Circulatory assistance. Pages 933–943 in *AACN's clinical reference for critical care nursing.* Kinney M et al. (eds). New York: McGraw-Hill, 1981.

Ford P, Preston R: Circulatory assist devices. Pages 126–128 in *Methods in critical care: The AACN manual.* Sampson L et al. (eds). Philadelphia: Saunders, 1980.

Friedman G et al.: Mortality in middle-aged smokers and nonsmokers. *N Engl J Med* 1979; 300:213–217.

Grüntzig A et al.: Nonoperative dilatation of coronary artery stenosis. *N Engl J Med* 1979; 301:61–68.

Hoffman S: Artificial cardiac pacing. Pages 30–93 in *Critical care nursing.* Hudak C et al. (eds). Philadelphia: Lippincott, 1982.

Jouve R et al.: Bretylium tosylate-induced stabilization of electrical systole duration in patients with acute myocardial infarction. *Heart Lung* 1982; 11:399–404.

Kent K et al.: Report from the registry of the national heart, lung and blood institute. *Am J Cardiol* 1982; 49:2011–2117.

Killpack A: The use of intracoronary streptokinase and percutaneous transluminal angioplasty. Pages 15–29 in *Car-

diovascular critical care nursing.* Woods S (ed). New York: Churchhill Livingston, 1983.

Lambrew T et al.: Adjuncts for artificial circulation. Pages V1–5 in *Textbook of advanced cardiac life support.* McIntyre K, Lewis A (eds). New York: American Heart Association, 1981.

McCabe J et al.: Preliminary experience with percutaneous intraortic balloon pumping. *Circulation* 1980; 62:I–123.

McCarthy C: Percutaneous transluminal coronary angioplasty: Therapeutic intervention in the cardiac catheterization laboratory. *Heart Lung* 1982; 11:499–504.

Morelli R: The temporary cardiac pacemaker. Pages 77–117 in *Cardiac arrest and CPR.* Auerbach P, Budassi S (eds). Rockville, MD: Aspen Systems Corporation, 1983.

National Conference on Cardiopulmonary Resuscitation (CPR) and Emergency Cardiac Care (ECC): Standards and guidelines for cardiopulmonary resuscitation (CPR) and emergency cardiac care (ECC). *JAMA* 1986; 255:1:2905–2984.

Pantridge J, Geddes J: A mobile intensive care unit in the management of myocardial infarction. *Lancet* 1967; 2:271–273.

Ream A: Cardiopulmonary bypass. Pages 420–455 in *Acute cardiovascular management: Anesthesia and intensive care.* Ream A, Fogdall R (eds). Philadelphia: Lippincott, 1982.

Redding J (ed): 2nd Wolf Creek Conference on CPR. *Crit Care Med* 1981; 9:357–362.

Rich S: Percutaneous transluminal angioplasty: Nonsurgical therapy of occlusive arterial disease. *Postgrad Med J* 1980; 68:217–220.

Shillinger F: Percutaneous transluminal coronary angioplasty. *Heart Lung* 1983; 12:45–50.

Shinn J: Intra-aortic balloon counterpulsation. Pages 189–201 in *Crit Care Nurse* 3d ed. Hudak et al. (eds). Philadelphia: Lippincott, 1986.

Sladen R: Management of the adult cardiac patient in the intensive care unit. Pages 481–548 in *Acute cardiovascular management: Anesthesia and intensive care.* Ream A, Fogdall R (eds). Philadelphia: Lippincott, 1982.

Weaver W et al.: Ventricular fibrillation: A comparative trial using 175-J and 320-J shocks. *N Engl J Med* 1982; 307:18–23.

Weiland A, Walker W: Physiologic principles and clinical sequelae of cardiopulmonary bypass. *Heart Lung* 1986; 15:34–39.

White R: Cardiovascular pharmacology: Part I. Pages VIII 1–16 in *Textbook of advanced cardiac life support.* McIntyre K, Lewis A (eds). New York: American Heart Association, 1981.

SUPPLEMENTAL READING

Abello J, Lemberg L: Coronary artery thrombolysis in acute myocardial infarction. *Heart Lung* 1983; 12:100–103.

Arcebal A, Lemberg L: The diagnosis of myocardial infarction in patients with permanent pacemakers. Part I. *Heart Lung* 1981; 19:1111–1116.

Beeler B: Infections of permanent transvenous and epicardial pacemakers in adults. *Heart Lung* 1981; 11:152–156.

Bergin K: Counterpulsation: External or intra-aortic. *Crit Care Nurse* (Nov/Dec) 1981; 29–33.

Bicking M: Nursing care plan: The patient on the intra-aortic balloon pump. *Crit Care Nurse* (Jul/Aug) 1982; 50–53.

Birkholz G: IABP: Legal and ethical issues. *Dimen Crit Care Nurs* 1985; 5:285–287.

Brundage B et al.: The role of aortic balloon pumping and postinfarction angina. *Circulation* 1980; 62:220–226.

Cantwell R et al.: Think fast: What do you know about cardiac drugs for a code? *Nurs 82* (Oct) 1981; 99–103.

Carlson R, Weil M: Axioms on critical care of shock. *Hosp Med* (Oct) 1981; 99–102.

Conry K, Bies C: Compartment syndrome: A complication of IABP. *Dimen Crit Care Nurs* 1984; 4:247–284.

Cooper K: Electrical safety: The electrically sensitive ICU patient. *Focus* (Dec/Jan) 1982; 27–29.

Cowley, M, Gold H: Use of intracoronary streptokinase in acute myocardial infarction. *Mod Concepts Cardiovasc Dis* 51:97–102.

Cronin K et al.: Defibrillation. *Crit Care Nurse* (Nov/Dec) 1981; 32–35.

Crumpley L: Drug Corner: Aprindine (Fibocil). *Crit Care Nurse* (Sep/Oct) 1982; 20–23.

Doran K: PCTA: Patient education. *Dimen Crit Care Nurs* 1983; 2:55–64.

Downing T: Therapeutic efficacy of intraaortic balloon counterpulsation. *Circulation* 1982; 64:110–116.

Dreifus L et al.: Long-term monitoring of patients with implanted pacemakers. *Heart Lung* 1982; 11:417–420.

E.P.S.I.M. Research Group: A controlled comparison of aspirin and oral anticoagulants in prevention of death after myocardial infarction. *N Engl J Med* 1982; 307:702–708.

Ewy G: Defibrillating cardiac arrest victims. *Cardiovasc Med* 1982; 7:28–49.

Gever L: Streptokinase and urokinase. *Nurs 83* (Jan) 1982; 76–80.

Gurevich I: Infectious complications after open heart surgery. *Heart Lung* 1984; 13:472–480.

Halpern J, Davis J: Beta-adrenergic blocking agents. *JEN* 1982; 8:204–207.

Harvey J: Complications of percutaneous intra-aortic balloon pumping. *Circulation* 1981; 64:111–116.

Hazard P et al.: Transvenous cardiac pacing in cardiopulmonary resuscitation. *Crit Care Med* 1981; 9:666–668.

Isaacson J et al.: Post pump psychosis. *Crit Care Nurse* (Jan/Feb) 1982; 14–16.

Kaye W: Invasive therapeutic techniques: Emergency cardiac pacing, pericardiocentesis, intracardiac injections, and emergency treatment of tension pneumothorax. *Heart Lung* 1982; 12:300–319.

Kluge R: Infections of prosthetic cardiac valves and arterial grafts. *Heart Lung* 1982; 11:146–150.

Kowey P et al.: Pacemaker therapy. *Surg Clin North Am* 1985; 595–611.

Landymore R et al: Importance of topical hypothermia to ensure uniform myocardial cooling during coronary artery bypass. *J Thoracic Cardiovasc Surg* 1983; 82:832–836.

Lapinski M: Cardiovascular drugs and the elderly population. *Heart Lung* 1982; 11:430–434.

Lasche P: Permanent cardiac pacing: technology and follow-up. *Focus Crit Care* 1983; 10:28–36.

Lazar H, Roberts A: Recent advances in cardiopulmonary bypass and the clinical application of myocardial protection. *Surg Clin North Am* 1985; 65(3):455–476.

O'Brien E: Environmental dangers for the patient with a pacemaker. *Brit Med J* 1982; 285:6356–6358.

Ott B: Percutaneous transluminal coronary angioplasty and nursing implications. *Heart Lung* 1982; 11:294–298.

Parsonnet V: Indications for dual-chamber pacing. *PACE* 1984; 7:318–319.

Partridge S: The nurse's role in percutaneous transluminal coronary angioplasty. *Heart Lung* 1982; 11:505–511.

Patacky M et al.: Intra-aortic balloon pumping and stress in the coronary care unit. *Heart Lung* 1985; 14:142–148.

Patros R. Goren C: The precordial thump: An adjunct to emergency medicine. *Heart Lung* 1983; 12:61–64.

Quaal S: *Comprehensive intra-aortic balloon pumping*. St Louis: Mosby, 1984.

Roach A: Atenolol (Tenormin). *Crit Care Nurse* (Nov/Dec) 1981; 21–22.

Rossi L, Antman E: Calcium channel blockers. *Am J Nurs* 1983; 83:382–387.

Rutman R, Miller W: *Transfusion therapy: Principles and procedures*. Rockville, MD: Aspen Systems Corp, 1982.

Shively M: The physiologic principles of intra-aortic balloon counterpulsation. *Crit Care Quart* (Sept) 1981; 83–88.

Slusarczyk S, Hicks F: Helping your patient to live with a permanent pacemaker. *Nurs 83* (Apr) 1983; 58–63.

Stack J et al.: Automatic implantable defibrillator for the patient with recurrent refractory malignant ventricular arrhythmias: Case report. *Heart Lung* 1982; 11:512–515.

Stanford J: Who profits from coronary artery bypass surgery? *Am J Nurs* (Jul) 1982; 1068–1072.

Sturm J et al.: Combined use of dopamine and nitroprusside therapy in conjunction with intra-aortic balloon pumping for the treatment of post-cardiotomy low output syndrome. *J Thoracic Cardiovasc Surg* 1981; 82:415–420.

Thorpe C: A nursing care plan—The adult cardiac surgery patient. *Heart Lung* 1979; 8:690–698.

Werner W, Chrzanowski A: Streptokinase intracoronary thrombolysis in acute myocardial infarction. *JEN* 1982; 8:277–284.

Wold B: Advances in pacemaker therapy. Pages 1–16 in *Advances in Cardiovascular Nursing*. Douglas M, Shinn J (eds). Rockville, MD: Aspen Systems Corp, 1985.

Wulff K: Use of temporary epicardial electrodes for atrial pacing and monitoring. *Cardiovasc Nurs* 1982; 18:1–5.

15

Renal Assessment and Acute Renal Failure

CLINICAL INSIGHT

Domain: Organizational and work-role competencies

Competency: Building and maintaining a therapeutic team to provide optimum therapy

The multiple specialty services in a critical-care unit present a complex web of interrelationships within which the nurse sometimes must negotiate to meet patients' needs. Even though specialty teams may have little contact with each other and may have conflicting goals, the nurse knows they must work well together for the patient to benefit. Often, the nurse assumes a primary role in coordinating care. In the following paradigm, from Crabtree and Jorgenson (1986, pp. 168–169), Tracy, the nurse, intervenes in a situation in which care is poorly coordinated for a dialysis patient whose only kidney recently has been removed for a cancerous tumor. Although the patient has two medical teams—nephrology and surgical transplant—no one really is in charge. The patient is threatening to leave because she has been denied satisfaction of the most basic of human needs—food and water.

She was getting no fluids, nothing, no diet, no fluids. And there was nobody to really go to. This was

through the time when all the fellows, the nephrology fellows, were gone. And so there was one staff person on and they came in once, early in the morning, and nobody would really make a decision as to what to do with her. And her reaction was, if they don't give me anything to drink, I'm leaving, you know. And somebody would say, well, you know, you need to have a dialysis. And she'd say, I don't care, you know, I can't live like this. And you know, it makes sense, she's right. So she was in limbo between the two teams. And so I guess I had talked to her a little bit. I felt really frustrated because I thought, she's right, I mean I would be angry too, to go two days without anything at all. And you know, even dialysis patients get stuff to drink and they don't have kidneys that work, you know. She went down to dialysis and I talked to the nurse that was taking care of her and said, you know, I would call somebody and tell them how she feels and what her feelings are and that really there was no reason she shouldn't be able to have a diet. And that it would be important for her to have a diet. So, anyway, she did call and finally they came over and talked to her a little bit and she said, you know, she'd leave. I think she would have. And, they said she could have a little bit of ice chips.

Ice chips may not seem like much, but for this patient, caught in a frustrating no-man's-land between

368

the teams, the nurse's obtaining them was an act of mercy.

Caring for the renal failure patient poses unique nursing challenges. The chronic form of renal failure is well known to most nurses and may be reviewed in any medical-surgical nursing text. This chapter focuses on the acute form.

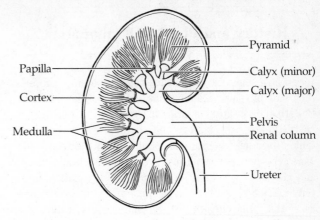

FIGURE 15–1

Gross renal anatomy.

ASSESSMENT

The kidneys, which measure about 6 by 12 cm, lie retroperitoneally on either side of the vertebral column. The left kidney is slightly higher than the right. The upper border of the left kidney is protected by the eleventh and twelfth ribs and that of the right kidney by the twelfth rib. Their lower borders are at the level of the third lumbar vertebra.

The kidney's gross structures consist of the cortex, medulla, pyramids, papillae, calyxes, and pelvis (Figure 15–1). The cortex, the outermost layer, contains glomeruli arranged like bunches of grapes, proximal and distal tubules, and first parts of the loops of Henle and collecting ducts. The medulla, the middle layer, contains 10–15 wedge-shaped pyramids formed by the loops of Henle and collecting ducts. The apices (papillae) of these pyramids empty into cup-shaped structures called calyxes, which in turn empty into the hollow inner section of the kidney, the pelvis. From the pelvis, urine travels down the ureter into the bladder and is excreted.

The kidneys have excretory, regulatory, and secretory (endocrine) functions. In addition to their well-known role in excretion of metabolic wastes, the kidneys function in regulation of extracellular fluid volume and osmolality, electrolyte balance, and partial control of acid–base balance. Endocrine functions are the secretion of both renin, which affects blood pressure, and erythropoeitin, which influences production of red blood cells.

Because of the diversity of renal functions, you must evaluate several parameters in order to judge the health of the kidneys. A convenient assessment format is shown in Table 15–1.

TABLE 15–1   RENAL ASSESSMENT FORMAT

1. History _____

2. Physical _____

3. Diagnostic procedures and laboratory tests

   Urine: volume _____

       sp. gr. _____ osmolality _____

       color _____ clarity _____

       pH _____ sediment _____

   BUN _____ Creatinine _____ Creatinine clearance _____

   Other _____

4. Other relevant data _____

History and Physical Examination

When assessing the patient for renal problems, the history and physical examinations often are less informative than laboratory tests, discussed in detail below. Nevertheless, the history and physical are very important, so do ask the patient about a history of renal disease; the presence of renal symptoms such as dysuria and changes in volume or frequency of urination; systemic diseases such as hypertension and diabetes mellitus; the family health history; and the medication history. Usually, physical signs and symptoms of renal disease are nonspecific. Often, they are those of fluid, electrolyte, or acid–base imbalances, presented in Chapter 16. When checking vital signs, particularly note the presence of hypertension and Kussmaul's respirations, which represent the body's attempt to compensate via the pulmonary system for the metabolic acidosis present in renal dysfunction.

The kidneys generally are not palpable, but they may be palpable normally in the thin person or abnormally in renal disease. Palpate both anteriorly, over the lower halves of the upper abdominal quadrants, and posteriorly, over the flanks. In the normal person, the lower poles of the kidneys, particularly the right kidney, may be felt in the upper abdominal quadrant(s).

If pain is present, evaluate its characteristics. Pain associated with kidney inflammation, such as with glomerulonephritis, may be constant, dull, and located over the flanks. The pain of pyelonephritis is sharp and severe. That associated with renal calculi may radiate toward the bladder or scrotum. If the stone becomes lodged in the ureter, severe spasmodic pain *(ureteral colic)* may occur.

If the patient is unable or unwilling to talk about the pain, you may be able to detect it by noting any attempts to guard the area when he or she moves or by other signs of pain such as a drawn facial expression. Sometimes, too, blunt percussion over the lower back will elicit pain. Remember, however, that many renal disorders are not characterized by pain, so its absence is not necessarily indicative of a healthy kidney.

Laboratory Tests

The most commonly monitored parameters of renal function are urinary output, urine solute concentration, and ability to excrete nitrogenous waste products. This section describes common tests of renal function and their significance.

Related Anatomy and Physiology

To accurately interpret these tests, you must have a clear understanding of urine formation. The following paragraphs review the anatomy and physiology of urine formation.

Urine is an ultrafiltrate of blood, formed by the kidney's microscopic structures. Urinary output depends on a multiplicity of factors, including integrity of the structures in the nephron, renal blood flow, adequacy of the countercurrent mechanisms, and hormonal influences.

The Nephron   The functional unit for urine formation is called the *nephron;* there are about a million in each kidney. Each nephron contains basically two sets of microscopic structures, one for blood flow and one for urine flow (Figure 15–2). As much as 75% of the nephrons can be destroyed before laboratory tests of renal function show significant abnormalities, and up to 90% can be destroyed before renal failure develops.

The renal artery carries blood to the kidney. Blood then flows through increasingly smaller arteries, the interlobar, arcuate, and interlobular arteries. After passing through the renal capillaries, blood returns via the corresponding veins to the renal vein.

The nephron's structures for blood flow arise from the interlobular artery. Blood travels through the *afferent arteriole* to a tuft of capillaries called the *glomerulus.* The glomerular capillaries recombine to create the *efferent arteriole,* which carries away from the glomerulus arterial fluid that was not filtered. Because the glomerular capillary bed is surrounded on both ends by arterioles, it is a high-pressure system. (The clinical significance of this fact will be elaborated on later.) From the efferent arteriole, blood enters a second capillary bed, the *peritubular system,* and then empties into venules. As its name implies, the peritubular system surrounds the renal tubules. Because it lies between an arteriole and a venule, the peritubular system is a lower-pressure capillary bed.

Vasa recta are straight capillary loops that arise from the peritubular capillary network of the juxtamedullary nephrons. They descend around the lower parts of the loops of Henle, loop into the medulla, and then return to the cortex. Their role in forming concentrated urine is discussed later.

Urine is filtered from the glomerulus into a surround-

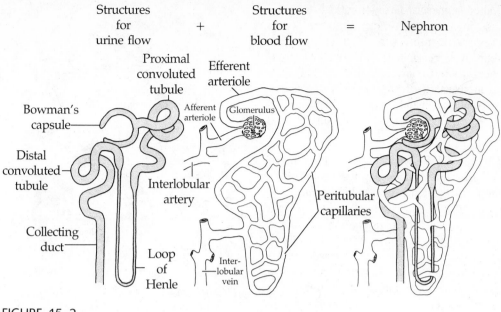

FIGURE 15–2

Nephron structures.

ing structure called *Bowman's capsule*. From there it travels through the *renal tubule*. The tubule consists of a proximal convoluted section, a U-shaped turn called *Henle's loop,* and a distal convoluted portion. From the tubule, urine passes through a collecting duct (or collecting tubule); then this duct joins other collecting ducts to empty into the calyx. Several calyces empty into the renal pelvis, from which urine flows down the ureter into the bladder.

There are two types of nephrons, *superficial cortical* and *juxtamedullary*. Both have glomeruli and proximal and distal tubules in the cortex, with part of the collecting ducts and loops of Henle in the medulla. The superficial cortical nephrons (about seven-eighths of the total) lie in the outer cortex, so their loops of Henle extend only a short distance into the medulla. The juxtamedullary nephrons lie in the inner cortex, near the medulla, so their loops of Henle extend much deeper into the medulla. The juxtamedullary nephrons are more active in urinary concentration than the cortical nephrons.

Glomerular Filtration   Tracing the formation of urine will help you to better understand the interrelationships of these structures. The first step in urine formation is filtration from the glomerulus to Bowman's capsule.

About 20% of the cardiac output, or 1200 ml/min, flows through both kidneys. Of this renal blood flow, 650 ml is the normal renal plasma flow. From the plasma, the kidneys form about 125 ml/min of glomerular filtrate. The portion of the plasma that becomes filtrate is called the *filtration fraction;* it also averages 20%.

Filtration occurs both because the glomerulus is a high-pressure capillary bed and because its membrane is very permeable. As with other capillaries, glomerular filtration depends on the balance between hydrostatic and osmotic pressures on each side of the membrane. All substances except protein and blood cells are filtered, so the filtrate is similar to plasma.

Autoregulation   Renal blood flow (RBF) and glomerular filtration rate (GFR) remain relatively constant in spite of wide fluctuations in mean arterial pressure, all the way from 80 mm Hg to 180 mm Hg. This regulation appears to be relatively independent of outside nervous control, blood-borne hormones, and systemic arterial pressure. Because control appears to reside within the kidney itself, this phenomenon is called *autoregulation.*

Factors controlling autoregulation are not completely understood. Two major hypotheses have been advanced to explain autoregulation: intramural pressures and juxtaglomerular feedback.

Intrarenal Pressure Theory   The first theory, based on *intrarenal pressures,* holds that changes in afferent arteriolar blood pressure cause changes in glomerular pressure and alter glomerular filtration rate. For example, a decrease in afferent arteriolar pressure would tend to lower glomerular pressure, thus slowing glomerular filtration. A decrease in afferent arteriolar pressure also would tend to lower peritubular capillary pressure, thus increasing reabsorption from the tubule. The retention of fluid resulting from both mechanisms would help to return afferent arteriolar pressure toward normal.

Juxtaglomerular Feedback Theory   The second and more complex hypothesis—juxtaglomerular feedback—maintains that a feedback system exists within the nephron itself to adjust blood flow and glomerular filtration rate to their optimal levels. The following explanation is based on Guyton (1986). The intranephronal feedback mechanism probably occurs at the *juxtaglomerular complex,* so called because it is near the glomerulus (Figure 15–3). The distal tubule passes in the angle formed by the afferent arteriole, leading into the glomerulus, and the efferent arteriole, leaving the glomerulus. It thus is in anatomic contact with both arterioles. The cells of the distal tubule that come in contact with the arterioles are more dense than other tubular cells and are called the *macula densa.* The smooth muscle cells in the corresponding portions of the arterioles are called *juxtaglomerular cells.* They contain granules of inactive renin. The macula densa and the juxtaglomerular cells together comprise the *juxtaglomerular apparatus.* The anatomical arrangement of the juxtaglomerular apparatus thus strongly implies that fluid in the distal tubule helps control nephron function by supplying feedback to both the afferent and efferent arterioles.

The feedback mechanism at the *afferent* arteriole probably depends directly on sodium and chloride ion concentration in the distal tubule. Inadequate flow of glomerular filtrate into the tubules causes excess tubular reabsorption of sodium and chloride, thereby lowering their concentration in the tubular fluid. The decreased sodium and chloride ion concentration at the macula densa causes dilatation of the afferent arteriole. This dilatation increases glomerular blood flow and glomerular pressure, which increase glomerular filtration rate back toward normal.

The feedback mechanism at the *efferent* arteriole probably depends primarily on renin release. When sodium and chloride ion concentration at the macula densa drops, the juxtaglomerular cells release renin. Renin causes formation of angiotensin II, a powerful vasoconstrictor. Angiotensin II constricts both the afferent and efferent arterioles, although the efferent arteriole is more sensitive to it. The greater constriction of the efferent arteriole causes glomerular pressure to rise. In

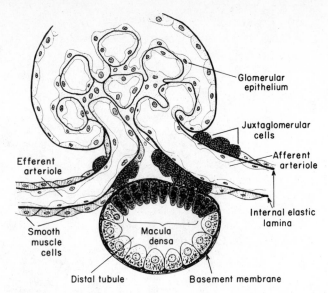

FIGURE 15–3

Structure of the juxtaglomerular apparatus, illustrating its possible feedback role in the control of nephron function. (From Guyton A: *Textbook of medical physiology,* 7th ed. Philadelphia: Saunders, 1986, p. 411. As modified from Ham: *Histology.* Philadelphia: Lippincott.)

turn, the increased pressure returns glomerular filtration rate to normal.

When arterial pressure drops for a few minutes, renal blood flow and glomerular filtration rate are autoregulated simultaneously: the dilatation of the afferent arteriole improves both renal blood flow and glomerular filtration. Within 10–20 minutes, however, renal blood flow autoregulation disappears as the powerful efferent arteriolar vasoconstrictor mechanism takes over and renal blood flow decreases. Glomerular filtration rate autoregulation persists, however; the greater constriction of the efferent arteriole over that of the afferent arteriole helps to maintain glomerular filtration pressure and therefore kidney function.

Formation and Effects of Angiotensin II   As mentioned previously, renin release causes formation of angiotensin II. This section explains in detail how the renin–angiotensin system functions. *Renin* is an enzyme that converts angiotensinogen, a circulating inactive substance formed by the liver, into angiotensin I, an inert substance. A converting enzyme, released primarily in lung capillaries but possibly also in the kidney itself, then converts angiotensin I to angiotensin II.

Angiotensin II has multiple roles in elevating arterial perfusion pressure. It intensely stimulates the adrenal glands to release aldosterone, promoting sodium reabsorption and thus water reabsorption. It is a powerful vasoconstrictor, acting directly on arteriolar smooth muscle to cause contraction. In the kidney, the vasoconstriction of the efferent arterioles reduces sharply the excretion of both salt and water. Angiotensin II also is believed to act on the brain to stimulate thirst. The resulting rise in blood volume and pressure returns afferent arteriolar pressure toward normal.

Autonomic Nervous Control The kidneys (especially the afferent arteriole) are supplied with autonomic nerve fibers. Sympathetic stimulation constricts the afferent and efferent arterioles. Because it reduces renal plasma flow (RPF) more than glomerular filtration rate (GFR), it usually increases the filtration fraction (GFR/RPF), the portion of renal plasma flow that becomes glomerular filtrate. Sympathetic stimulation also may lead indirectly to renin secretion, by constricting the afferent arteriole, thus reducing glomerular filtration rate and altering the ion load in the distal tubule. Strong sympathetic stimulation causes such great arteriolar constriction that glomerular blood flow drops severely. The autonomic nerve fibers appear to play little role in the autoregulation of the kidney, since a transplanted kidney is able to function without a nerve supply.

Tubular Reabsorption and Secretion From Bowman's capsule, the filtrate enters the tubules, where the processes of reabsorption and secretion separate substances to be conserved from those to be excreted. *Reabsorption* is the movement of solutes and water from the tubule into the peritubular network, that is, from the filtrate back into the bloodsteam. *Secretion* is the movement of substances in the opposite direction—from the peritubular network into the tubule.

Reabsorption can occur passively or actively. Passive movement, *diffusion,* results from concentration or electrical gradients. Among substances reabsorbed this way are water, urea, and negative ions such as chloride. Active movement occurs against gradients and requires both chemical carriers and energy. Numerous substances are reabsorbed this way, including sodium, potassium, calcium, and glucose.

There is a maximum rate of reabsorption for some solutes, called the *transport maximum.* When it is exceeded by the amount filtered, the remaining solute is excreted in the urine.

Secretion of substances also can be active or passive and is determined by hormones and the concentration of the substance in the extracellular fluid. Substances that may be secreted include hydrogen ion, potassium, penicillin, and x-ray contrast dye.

Countercurrent Mechanisms As the glomerular filtrate passes through the proximal convoluted tubule, loop of Henle, and distal convoluted tubule, its osmolality varies. In the proximal tubule, about 65% of the filtered sodium is reabsorbed actively. Water is reabsorbed because of the osmotic gradient established by the reabsorption of sodium. Other substances reabsorbed in the proximal tubule include all of the glucose, nearly all the amino acids, potassium, bicarbonate, and urea.

As the tubular fluid passes through Henle's loop, it is exposed to increasingly hypertonic interstitial fluid in the medulla, which results from complex countercurrent mechanisms in the loops of Henle and vasa recta (Figure 15–4). Because of these mechanisms, tubular fluid flowing down the loop becomes very hypertonic; the fluid flowing up and out of the loop becomes hypotonic.

Excretion of Dilute or Concentrated Urine Final adjustment of urine concentration takes place in the distal tubule and collecting duct. If the body does not need to retain water, no adjustment is necessary. Usually, the distal tubule and collecting duct are impermeable to water. As fluid passes through them, sodium and other substances are actively transported out but water is not reabsorbed. The already hypotonic urine becomes even more hypotonic, and a dilute urine is excreted.

Sometimes, however, the body needs to retain water to offset an increased osmolality of the extracellular fluid, such as occurs in dehydration. When this happens, the hypertonicity of the medullary interstitial fluid enables the kidney to concentrate urine as it passes through the distal tubule and collecting duct. The increased extracellular fluid osmolality is sensed by osmoreceptors in the hypothalamus. These stimulate the release of *antidiuretic hormone* from the posterior pituitary. ADH travels to the kidneys, where it increases the permeability of the distal tubule and the collecting duct to water. Because the surrounding interstitial fluid is so hypertonic due to the countercurrent mechanisms, a *concentration gradient* is created. This gradient makes water diffuse from the tubule into the interstitial fluid. This mechanism, if necessary, can make the urine in the collecting duct isotonic with the medullary interstitial fluid (up to 1200 mOsm/L). As a result, highly concentrated urine can be excreted. The water reabsorbed from the collecting duct re-enters the bloodstream to return serum osmolality to normal. This delicate mechanism fails early in kidney disease, and its loss is the reason renal patients often have dilute urine with a fixed osmolality or specific gravity.

In addition to urine concentration being adjusted in the distal tubule and collecting duct, reabsorption and

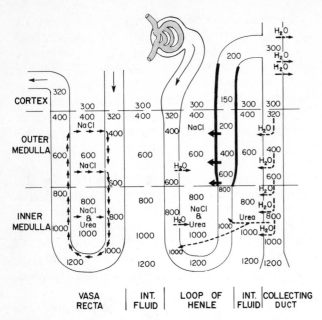

FIGURE 15–4

Countercurrent mechanism for concentration of urine. Values in mOsm/L. (From Guyton A: *Textbook of medical physiology,* 7th ed., p. 415. Philadelphia: Saunders, 1986.)

secretion of solutes may occur. Selective reabsorption of sodium will occur in the presence of *aldosterone,* a hormone secreted by the adrenal cortex in response to decreased serum sodium concentration, increased renin secretion, and other stimuli. Bicarbonate may be reabsorbed and hydrogen, ammonia, and potassium secreted by the distal tubule and collecting duct.

Urine Volume   As mentioned earlier, blood flow to the kidneys approximates 1200 ml/min. About 125 ml/min becomes glomerular filtrate. During its journey through the nephron, nearly all of this volume is reabsorbed, producing a urine output of 1 ml/min in the healthy adult.

Simply measuring the volume of urine can indicate the presence of a problem with urine formation but gives very limited information about its cause or about the adequacy of other kidney functions. For these items, you must rely on the results of more definitive tests of renal function.

Tests of Renal Function

Most of the following measures of renal function are done routinely on admission to the hospital as a screen-

ing device. Some, such as creatinine clearance, the physician will order only if renal damage is suspected.

Urine Osmolality and Specific Gravity   Evaluate the kidney's ability to concentrate or dilute urine by interpreting the serum and urine osmolalities or the specific gravity of urine. *Osmolality* is a measure of the number of osmotically active particles in solution. It is a laboratory determination reported as milliosmols (mOsm) of solute per kilogram of solvent. Normal serum osmolality is about 285–295 mOsm/kg. Maximal dilution can make urine osmolality as low as one-sixth of serum osmolality (down to 50 mOsm/kg), and maximal concentration can raise urine osmolality to four times serum values (up to 1200 mOsm/kg). Although the absolute values for each are important, the relationship between them is more significant. Urine osmolality should vary in the same direction as the serum value. When serum osmolality is increased, indicating an elevated concentration, urine osmolality also should increase, because the kidneys should conserve water to return the serum value to normal.

A cruder bedside measurement of the ability to alter urine concentration is the *specific gravity* of urine, which compares the concentration of urine to that of water. There are two bedside instruments for measuring specific gravity: the hydrometer and the refractometer. In the first method, you place urine in a small cylinder and float a *hydrometer* in it. The specific gravity is read in thousandths according to the level of the bottom of the fluid meniscus. In the second method, you place a drop of urine in a measuring device called a *refractometer* and read the value off a scale. Normal specific gravity of urine is 1.010–1.025.

Hydrometer readings reflect not only the concentration of particles but also their size and molecular weight. Falsely high readings occur when protein, glucose, radiographic contrast medium, and other high-molecular-weight substances are in the urine. In contrast, the refractometer, also known as the *total solids meter,* provides an accurate measurement of the total solids in a drop of urine. With both measures, serial determinations are more significant than single ones.

The healthy kidney is able to vary urine osmolality and specific gravity according to the concentration of serum. It does this through the countercurrent mechanism and under the influence of ADH. When kidneys are damaged, the ability to concentrate urine is one of the first functions lost. Urine osmolality becomes fixed within 50 mOsm of the serum value. Specific gravity readings also become fixed, near 1.010.

Routine Urinalysis   Routine urinalysis evaluates urine color, clarity, pH, and sediment. Urine usually is yellow or amber, due to the presence of urobilin. When red blood cells are destroyed or die, their hemoglobin is split and the heme portion is converted by reticuloendothelial cells into bilirubin. The bilirubin circulates to the liver, where it is conjugated and excreted into bile. It empties into the intestine, where it is modified into urobilinogen. Some of the urobilinogen is reabsorbed into the blood and is excreted into the urine, where it becomes oxidized into urobilin, producing the characteristic color of urine. Abnormal urine colors may be due to the presence of blood, diagnostic media, or therapeutic drugs, or to disease.

Normal urine is clear. Cloudy urine may indicate the precipitation of urates or phosphates on standing or the presence of blood, bacteria, or pus. The pH of urine ranges from 4.5–8.0. Although usually acid, it rapidly becomes alkaline on standing due to bacteria decomposing its urea into ammonia. More acid urine is seen commonly in acidosis and sodium depletion, alkaline urine in alkalosis and infections.

The mechanisms by which the kidneys alter urinary pH include hydrogen ion secretion/bicarbonate retention, secretion of ammonia, and acidification of phosphate salts. They are explained and diagrammed in the section on acid–base balance (Chapter 16).

Routine urinalysis includes a microscopic examination for blood cells, crystals, casts, and bacteria. Red blood cells are a sign of pathology or menstruation, while a few scattered white cells are common. A variety of crystals may be included, especially when the urine is concentrated; most are of no significance. Casts are abnormal and are often diagnostic of the location of renal damage. They are formed when the lumen of the tubules becomes filled with a material that then hardens, forming a cast of the lumen. Bacteria may not be significant except in "clean catch" or catheterized urine samples. If present in those samples, they must be identified further through cultures. The urine normally contains no detectable protein, glucose, or ketones. Proteinuria is common in renal disease, and may occur in diabetes, pregnancy, and marked athletic exertion; glycosuria in diabetes mellitus; and ketonuria in diabetic ketoacidosis and starvation.

BUN Urea is an end product of protein metabolism, both endogenous protein (muscle) and exogenous protein (dietary intake). According to Guyton (1986), amino acid degradation forms large amounts of ammonia, and bacteria in the gut constantly form additional ammonia, which is absorbed into the bloodstream. The ammonia molecules are converted to urea and excreted in the urine. The normal *blood urea nitrogen* (BUN) value is 8–20%. Because the level of urea nitrogen in the blood varies with urine output, the BUN level can be a useful indicator of renal function. Its value is limited, however, because factors other than renal function also may affect it: intake of urea precursors, the body's metabolic state, and blood volume. The level decreases in malnutrition or severe liver failure. It increases in conditions with increased urea formation (such as ingestion of protein-rich meals, gastrointestinal bleeding, infection, or administration of glucocorticoids), decreased urea excretion (such as renal disease), or altered relative concentration in the blood (such as dehydration).

Creatinine Creatinine is an end product of muscle metabolism. As its production is endogenous, the serum creatinine level is relatively independent of protein intake and metabolic state and therefore is a better guide to renal function than the BUN. Because serum creatinine concentration depends on lean body mass, the value varies from person to person; the normal range is 0.7–1.25 mg/100 ml for women and 0.85–1.5 mg/100 ml for men (Lancaster 1982). Within one person, the value normally is constant, so serial determinations are a useful way to follow the patient's progress.

Normal urine creatinine production is 1–1.8 g/24 hr. The relationship between plasma and urine creatinine concentrations can be helpful in differentiating two common causes of acute oliguria, as explained later.

Creatinine Clearance One of the kidney's functions is to clear the extracellular fluid of waste products. *Clearance* may be defined as the volume of plasma per minute that the kidneys completely clear of a substance. The clearance of a given substance can be a clinically useful indicator of glomerular filtration rate if the substance is freely filtered at the glomerulus but neither reabsorbed nor secreted.

Clearance is determined by measuring the plasma concentration of a substance, the urine concentration of the same substance, and the urine flow rate. Logically, the plasma concentration times the glomerular filtration rate equals the urine concentration times the urine flow rate. This relationship can be expressed mathematically as follows, where P_x = plasma concentration, U_x = urine concentration, GFR = glomerular filtration rate, and V = urine flow rate:

$$P_x \times GFR = U_x \times V$$

Rearranging the terms of the equation yields:

$$GFR = \frac{U_x V}{P_x}$$

Creatinine clearance is the most precise test of renal clearance that is commonly available. Creatinine is a normal by-product of muscle metabolism. It is excreted in the urine primarily by glomerular filtration, with a small amount contributed by tubular secretion. When creatinine is used to measure glomerular filtration rate, the following formula, derived from the general formula given above, applies. Here, C = creatinine clearance, U = urine creatinine concentration, V = urine flow rate, and P = plasma creatinine concentration:

$$C = \frac{U \times V}{P}$$

To determine creatinine clearance, a 24-hour urine specimen must be collected carefully. Have the person empty the bladder; record the time as the onset of the collection period but do not save that first specimen. Collect *all* urine voided during the *next* 24 hours. At the end of the collection period, obtain the final specimen. Add it to the volume and record the exact time. Obtain a blood sample for serum creatinine. The laboratory will measure the plasma and urine creatinine concentrations and calculate urine flow by dividing the total volume by the duration of the collection. By entering these figures in the clearance equation, the laboratory will determine the value for creatinine clearance.

Lancaster (1984) reports normal creatinine clearance as 100–150 ml per min for men and 85–125 ml per min for women.

Hemoglobin and Hematocrit When oxygen tension decreases, the healthy kidney secretes erythropoietin, which stimulates the bone marrow to produce red blood cells. Patients with kidney disease may not secrete erythropoietin adequately and therefore rapidly become anemic.

ACUTE RENAL FAILURE

Although a variety of renal disorders may afflict the critically ill, the one seen most frequently and the one you can play the greatest role in preventing is acute renal failure. *Acute renal failure* is the abrupt diminution of renal function, with a progressive retention of nitrogenous compounds such as urea and creatinine. It usually, but not always, is accompanied by oliguria.

Nursing care in acute renal failure begins with assessment of the patient for risk conditions and signs and symptoms.

Assessment

Risk Conditions

Conditions predisposing to acute renal failure can be divided into three categories: prerenal, renal, and postrenal causes. *Prerenal causes* are those that diminish renal perfusion without causing tubular damage. They are divided into two main categories:

a. Decreased circulating blood volume as in:
   - Hypovolemia due to severe hemorrhage, burns, or dehydration
   - Diminished cardiac output due to severe ventricular failure or cardiogenic shock
   - Septic shock
b. Obstructed renal perfusion due to renal arterial thrombosis or stenosis

In prerenal conditions, the kidney itself is normal. However, prolonged severe hypoperfusion can lead to ischemia and actual damage to the nephrons.

Renal causes are characterized by interstitial, glomerular, and/or tubular damage. The major categories are:

a. Acute tubular necrosis from:
   - Severe prolonged ischemia
   - Nephrotoxic substances such as insecticides, heavy metals, sulfonamides, and some antibiotics (most often streptomycin, gentamycin, kanamycin, neomycin, cephaloride, tetracycline, and penicillin)
   - Crush syndrome
b. Acute glomerulonephritis

Advanced age, diabetes mellitus, and chronic hypertension result in renal impairment. Patients with these preexisting conditions are at greater risk of developing acute renal failure from ischemia or exposure to nephrotoxins (Whittaker 1985).

Postrenal causes are urinary tract obstructions. Examples are: bilateral ureteral stones, benign prostatic hypertrophy, carcinoma of the bladder, and congenital malformations. Although the postrenal kidney itself is normal, uncorrected obstructions can lead to chronic, irreversible renal damage.

Acute tubular necrosis represents about 75% of the cases of acute renal failure (Richard 1981). Several pathophysiologic mechanisms have been proposed to explain acute tubular necrosis. The most likely are "tubular backleak" (in which epithelial disruption causes increased permeability, allowing backflow of filtrate out of the tubule) and obstruction by edematous tubular cells, casts, and cellular debris. In addition, there is evidence to suggest that intrarenal vasoconstriction occurs in response to tubular damage (Schrier and Conger 1986).

Prevention To prevent acute renal failure, eliminate as many causes as possible. For instance, check for a history of allergic reactions before administering drugs. Follow the measures outlined in other chapters to prevent or treat dysrhythmias, ventricular failure, cardiac tamponade, shock, acidosis, and extracellular fluid deficit. Maintain strict aseptic technique during urethral catheterization.

The most important prevention measure is to maintain adequate blood flow through the kidneys. If a patient develops hypotension, promptly restore blood volume. Administer vasoactive agents, such as dopamine (at 2–5 µg/kg/min), as ordered, which promote rather than deprive renal blood flow. Increased urine flow through the tubules decreases the nephrotoxic agent's ability to bind to the tubular cells. Force diuresis by administering mannitol, furosemide, or ethacrynic acid, as ordered by the physician. Monitor and prevent hypokalemia, which may increase the nephrotoxicity of aminoglycoside antibiotics.

Signs and Symptoms

Because the kidneys do not function normally in acute renal failure, they are unable to excrete waste products or regulate fluid, electrolyte, and acid–base balances.

The signs and symptoms of acute renal failure vary somewhat in intensity from those of chronic renal failure. For example, hyperkalemia is a major problem in acute failure but usually is relatively less severe in chronic failure. Signs and symptoms also vary with the cause. In the clinical setting, the most common causes of acute failure are decreased perfusion and acute tubular insufficiency (with or without necrosis). The latter is caused by severe ischemia or nephrotoxic agents. Differentiation of the two most common causes of acute renal failure is essential, because the treatments for prerenal hypoperfusion and for acute tubular necrosis differ significantly. Table 15–2 presents the key differentiating features of the two conditions.

Urine Volume Urinary output may vary with both the cause and the duration of failure. Anuria indicates complete obstruction or total renal shutdown. Oliguria (less than 400 ml/24 hr) is most common in the early stage of failure, the first 2 weeks. It occurs both in reduced perfusion and in acute tubular insufficiency. Nonoliguric failure (>400 ml/24 hr) occurs in 20–50% of all cases of acute tubular insufficiency. The increased incidence of nonoliguric failure seen in the past 5 years is thought to be due to early detection and treatment with fluids and diuretics.

Urine Osmolality and Specific Gravity If the cause of failure is diminished perfusion, then the urine osmolality will be greater than the plasma osmolality and the specific gravity will be elevated. This results from the kidney's attempts to conserve sodium and water. If the cause is tubular damage, then urine osmolality will be within 50 mOsm/kg of serum osmolality and the specific gravity of the urine will be low. The reason for this is that the ability to concentrate urine is one of the first functions lost when nephrons are damaged.

Urinary Sodium Levels Urinary sodium levels usually are decreased in prerenal causes of failure because the healthy tubules' normal response to stimuli is avid sodium retention. In acute tubular insufficiency, urinary sodium is increased because the damaged tubules fail to reabsorb sodium.

BUN and Creatinine The BUN and plasma creatinine will be elevated in both prerenal hypoperfusion and acute tubular insufficiency. In tubular insufficiency, BUN and creatinine values vary with the stage of failure. BUN and creatinine rise during the oliguric phase of failure due to diminished glomerular filtration. During the early diuretic phase, although urinary output increases due to the gradual return of renal function, the BUN and creatinine continue to rise because of diminished glomerular function. During the late diuretic phase, the BUN and creatinine fall and stabilize.

BUN/Creatinine Ratio In prerenal hypoperfusion, the BUN rises more rapidly than the plasma creatinine. In the hypoperfused kidney, urine flows slowly through the tubule, allowing a greater proportion of filtered urea to be reabsorbed into the circulatory system. Creatinine excretion is not appreciably affected by urine flow; therefore the ratio between BUN and creatinine is high, almost always over 20:1. In acute tubular insufficiency, the damaged tubules allow reabsorption of both urea and creatinine. The BUN and creatinine rise proportionately, maintaining a ratio of approximately 10:1.

TABLE 15–2 DIFFERENTIAL DIAGNOSIS OF OLIGURIA

	PRERENAL HYPOPERFUSION	ACUTE TUBULAR NECROSIS
Blood Values		
BUN	Increased	Increased
Creatinine	Normal or slightly increased	Increased
BUN:creatinine ratio	20:1 or greater (increased)	10:1 or less (not increased because both values elevated)
Urine Values		
Urine sodium	15 mEq/L or less (decreased)	40 mEq/L or more (normal or increased)
Specific gravity	1.020 or more (increased)	1.010 (not increased)
Osmolality	400 mOsm or more (increased)	250–350 mOsm (not increased)
Urine Plasma Comparisons (Ratios)		
Urine/plasma urea	Greater than 14:1	Less than 14:1
Urine/plasma creatinine	Greater than 20:1	Less than 20:1
Response to Fluids and Diuretics	Increased urinary output	None, or increased urinary output

Potassium Imbalances Evaluation of the ECG and the patient's muscles and reflexes may point to potassium imbalances. Peaked T waves, prolonged PR intervals or QRS durations, twitching, cramps, or hyperactive reflexes suggest hyperkalemia. This condition is a common, major problem in acute failure. In addition to impaired potassium excretion, hyperkalemia may result from acidosis, increased cellular breakdown, or excessive potassium intake in diet, medications, or intravenous solutions.

Flattened T waves, muscle weakness, nausea or vomiting, and hypoactive reflexes implicate hypokalemia. Although this condition is less common than hyperkalemia during renal failure, it can result from vomiting, diarrhea, some diuretics, decreased intake, or increased renal exchange of potassium for sodium.

Other Signs and Symptoms Drowsiness, weakness, twitching, convulsions, itchy skin, confusion, mental irritability, slowed thinking, and altered thought processes may result from uremia.

Anorexia, nausea, vomiting, and diarrhea or constipation may indicate metabolic acidosis. This acid–base imbalance may result from decreased reabsorption of bicarbonate and diminished excretion of ammonia, phosphates, and hydrogen ions.

Hypertension, rales, and signs of congestive heart failure or pulmonary edema may result from fluid overload.

Bruising, oozing of blood or frank bleeding, and decreased hemoglobin and hematocrit values may indicate anemia, increased capillary fragility, and/or decreased platelet adhesiveness. Anemia may appear within a few days of renal shutdown due to the diminished synthesis of erythropoietin.

Phases

There are three phases of acute oliguric renal failure: oliguric, diuretic, and recovery. The *oliguric phase* is the period of time in which urinary output is less than 400 cc per day. It begins within 48 hours of the renal insult and lasts 1–2 weeks. During this time, plasma creatinine increases approximately 1 mg/100 ml/day and BUN increases approximately 20 mg/100ml/day. The *diuretic phase* is the period of time in which the urinary output increases above 400 cc per day but BUN and creatinine continue rising. It marks the time during which tubular regeneration is occurring and lasts about 2 weeks. The *recovery phase* is characterized by stabilization of laboratory values followed by their return to normal values. It marks the time in which tubular function is returning, and lasts from 3–12 months.

Nursing diagnoses for the oliguric and diuretic phases are discussed in the following sections. In addition, selected diagnoses for the oliguric phase and diuretic phase are shown in the nearby nursing care plan.

NURSING CARE PLAN

Acute Renal Failure, Oliguric Phase

NURSING DIAGNOSIS	SIGNS AND SYMPTOMS	NURSING ACTIONS	DESIRED OUTCOMES
Excess fluid volume related to fluid retention	Oliguria Elevated CVP Peripheral edema Pulmonary edema Hypertension	1. Monitor and record intake and output. 2. Maintain fluid restriction. 3. Observe for increase in body weight. 4. Observe for peripheral edema, tachycardia, hypertension, elevated CVP, and distended neck veins. 5. Perform dialysis to remove excess fluid as prescribed.	Patient does not exhibit signs of fluid volume overload.
Potential for injury related to electrolyte imbalance, uremia, and metabolic acidosis	Hyperkalemia Acidemia Dysrhythmias Lethargy Nausea/vomiting Hypocalcemia	1. Restrict potassium intake in food/fluids. 2. Monitor electrolytes, BUN, and creatinine. 3. Monitor ECG for peaked T waves and other dysrhythmias. 4. Administer phosphate binders as prescribed. 5. Monitor for mental status changes. 6. Perform dialysis to correct uremia and electrolyte imbalance.	Patient exhibits normal electrolyte levels and does not have signs or symptoms of uremia.
Activity intolerance related to anemia/uremia	Decreased hemoglobin level Complaints of fatigue/weakness Dyspnea with activity	1. Minimize blood loss. 2. Administer blood as directed. 3. Assist patient with ADL. 4. Encourage self-care activities as tolerated. 5. Space activities to allow for rest periods.	Patient exhibits decreased fatigue/weakness.
Alteration in nutrition: less than body requirements related to dietary restrictions and uremia	Loss of appetite Nausea/vomiting Decreased lean body mass	1. Provide adequate protein, high-calorie diet. 2. Monitor BUN and electrolytes to evaluate response to diet. 3. Offer small, frequent meals. 4. Help patient to maintain good oral hygiene. 5. Administer antiemetics as prescribed. 6. Monitor for hyperglycemia if patient is receiving total parenteral nutrition.	Patient maintains adequate nutritional intake.

(Continues)

NURSING CARE PLAN (Continued)

Acute Renal Failure, Oliguric Phase (Continued)

NURSING DIAGNOSIS	SIGNS AND SYMPTOMS	NURSING ACTIONS	DESIRED OUTCOMES
Potential for infection	Temperature elevation Purulent sputum/drainage	1. Monitor temperature for elevations. 2. Provide frequent pulmonary care. 3. Assess pulmonary secretions, wound drainage, and urine for indications of infection. 4. Use aseptic technique during dressing changes, insertion of lines, and catheterization. 5. Minimize use of in-dwelling catheters. 6. Perform skin care and oral care on a regular basis.	Patient remains free of infection.

NURSING DIAGNOSES

In the oliguric phase, nursing diagnoses are numerous. They include:

- Excess fluid volume
- Potential for injury
- Activity intolerance
- Potential for infection
- Altered nutrition (less than body requirements)
- Potential pain
- Fear

In the diuretic phase, the primary nursing diagnoses are:

- Potential fluid volume deficit
- Potential activity intolerance

Planning and Implementation of Care: Oliguric Phase

Patient assessment serves as the basis for planning and implementing care to relieve the effects of acute renal failure and to prevent its complications. In addition to taking the following measures, it is of course essential to assist the physician in identifying and treating the cause of the failure.

Excess Fluid Volume Related to Inability to Excrete Water and Waste Products

Weigh the patient daily, under the same baseline conditions. A change in weight of 1 kg corresponds to a change in fluid volume of 1 L. Maintain strict intake and output records. Remember to include in these records insensible losses from pulmonary and integumentary excretion of water; these usually average 500 ml per day. Adhere to the fluid restrictions prescribed for the patient. Usually, the patient will be allowed an amount equal to urinary output plus 500 ml. This amount should be divided over a 24-hour period and provided in ways that help to satisfy the patient's thirst—for instance, in ice chips. Encourage patients to drink some water during the night to prevent the urea-induced nausea that often occurs. Monitor BP carefully, especially noting hypertension, which could signal excess fluid retention. Examine the patient for peripheral edema, congestive heart failure, and pulmonary edema. Assist with preparation for dialysis, as explained later in the chapter.

Potential for Injury Related to Hyperkalemia-Induced Dysrhythmias

Hyperkalemia is associated with both decreased renal potassium excretion and increased release of potassium from cells due to acidosis. Monitor the serum potassium daily. Observe the patient for signs and symptoms of hyperkalemia.

Monitor the ECG for the development of tall, peaked T waves, absent P waves, and broad, slurred QRS complexes, as well as abnormal cardiac rhythms. Limit potassium intake from IVs, food, and medications. Assess the patient for other possible causes of hyperkalemia—for example, GI bleeding. When transfusions are necessary, use fresh blood to help avoid the potassium released from cell deterioration in stored blood. If the patient develops hyperkalemia, assist with treatment as outlined in Chapter 16. Among the methods that may be used are administration of calcium chloride, ion exchange resins, insulin/bicarbonate/glucose infusions, and dialysis.

Activity Intolerance Related to Anemia

Because of the anemia that afflicts renal patients due to inadequate synthesis of erythropoietin, it is essential to monitor hemoglobin and hematocrit daily and to minimize blood loss. Draw minimal amounts of blood for laboratory specimens. Handle the patient gently to avoid bruising due to the increased capillary fragility. Minimize irritation from nasogastric tubes to prevent nosebleeds. Avoid hypodermic injections. Prevent or promptly treat stress ulcers. Use stool softeners to avoid constipation and prevent bleeding from hemorrhoids. Watch carefully for signs of anemia, hemorrhage, or occult bleeding, and alert the physician to them. Administer packed cells when ordered by the physician.

Potential for Infection Related to Decreased Immunologic Defenses

Give meticulous attention to asepsis for wounds and invasive catheters. Maintain a vigorous regimen of pulmonary hygiene to prevent pooling of secretions and bacterial growth. Avoid skin breakdown through well-aligned body positioning and frequent turning.

Potential for Injury Related to Diminished Drug Excretion

Avoid or give reduced dosages of nephrotoxic drugs or those that depend on the kidneys for excretion. For example, give reduced doses of antibiotics dependent on renal excretion. Even though digitalis is prescribed in reduced dosages, monitor closely for signs of digitalis toxicity. Avoid antacids containing magnesium (such as Maalox). Instead, use antacids containing phosphate binders, such as Amphogel. In addition to being excreted more easily, they help to prevent bone disease, as explained later.

Altered Nutrition (Less Than Body Requirements) Related to GI Distress and Decreased Mental Alertness

Maintain adequate nutrition with enough calories, carbohydrates, and protein to prevent negative nitrogen balance. Carbohydrates also forestall the production of ketones from fat metabolism and prevent gluconeogenesis from body protein.

Nutrition is a real challenge in the face of the gastrointestinal symptoms and decreased mental alertness. Maintaining mouth care, giving small portions, and providing social interaction during meals may encourage the oral intake of a high-calorie diet. If oral intake is insufficient to prevent protein catabolism (worsening the uremia) or fat metabolism (worsening the acidosis), the physician may prescribe hyperalimentation. See Chapter 19 for the care related to this type of nutrition.

Potential Pain Related to Uremic Pericarditis

Uremic pericarditis is a common complication of acute and chronic renal failure. Avoid predisposing factors. The most common ones are bacterial infection (shunt, respiratory, wound, or other) and poor dietary control. Watch for fever, chills, chest pain, a pericardial friction rub, and gallop rhythm. The pericarditis frequently is fibrinous. The most serious acute complications of pericarditis are cardiac failure, from myocarditis, and cardiac tamponade. (See Chapter 13 for discussions of prevention, recognition, and treatment of failure and tamponade.) Treatment of uremic pericarditis includes treatment of infection, good dietary control, and increased frequency of dialysis (with regional heparinization). If pericarditis is severe or persistent, pericardiocentesis, creation of a pericardial "window," or pericardiectomy may be necessary.

Potential Pain Related to Bone Disease

A troublesome complication of prolonged renal failure is defective bone metabolism. In renal failure, bone disease may occur because of calcium depletion. Because kidney failure impairs tubular excretion of phosphate, the serum phosphorous level rises. Since serum phosphorous and serum calcium maintain an inverse relationship, elevation of phosphorous results in a decrease in the serum calcium level. The serum calcium level also decreases because the kidney is unable to convert vitamin D to its active form. The low serum calcium stimulates parathyroid hormone secretion. An excess of this hormone leaches calcium from the bones into the serum, and in time the patient may develop osteodystrophy and secondary or tertiary hyperparathyroidism. Administration of phosphate binders can help to prevent this cycle by increasing excretion of phosphorous from the G.I. tract. Phosphate binders combine with dietary phosphorous in the intestine, thereby reducing absorption and preventing hyperphosphatemia.

Fear Related to Seriousness of Illness

Encourage the patient and family to discuss their concerns with you and the physician. Allow frequent family visits if the patient wants them. Promote the patient's participation in activities of daily living to the extent of his or her energy. For further supportive measures, please see Chapter 3.

Planning and Implementation of Care: Diuretic Phase

Potential Fluid Volume Deficit Related to Excessive Diuresis

Continue to monitor the fluid volume through daily weights and intake and output records. Observe for signs and symptoms of dehydration. Provide fluid intake to compensate for losses, remembering to include replacement for insensible fluid losses.

Potential Injury Related to Hypokalemia

Continue to monitor serum potassium levels. Observe the patient for muscle weakness, nausea and vomiting, personality changes, and other signs and symptoms of hypokalemia. Observe the ECG for flattening and broadening of the T wave, prominence of the U wave, and merging of the T and U waves. Provide oral and parenteral potassium to balance losses, as ordered.

Dialysis

Dialysis is the process by which dissolved particles diffuse from a fluid compartment across a semipermeable membrane into another fluid compartment. The purposes of dialysis are: removal of waste products of protein metabolism, removal of excess water, and reestablishment of electrolyte and acid–base balance. In the past, dialysis was prescribed only when more conservative management failed to control uremia, hyperkalemia, acidosis, or other effects of failure. Now, physicians are prescribing it early in the course of failure as part of an aggressive attempt to forestall the more severe manifestations and complications of failure.

There are three types of dialysis in use: hemodialysis, peritoneal dialysis, and continuous ultrafiltration/hemofiltration. In hemodialysis and continuous ultrafiltration, the blood is one fluid compartment, the membrane is an artificial one in the dialysis filter, and the dialysate is the second fluid compartment. In peritoneal dialysis, the semipermeable membrane is the peritoneum. The first compartment is the peritoneal capillary network, and the dialysate infused into the peritoneal cavity is the second compartment. Each type of dialysis has advantages and disadvantages. They are summarized in Table 15–3.

Hemodialysis

Nursing care for the hemodialysis patient includes maintaining circulatory access, initiating dialysis, attending to patient status and technical aspects of dialysis, discontinuing dialysis, promoting patient health between dia-

TABLE 15–3 COMPARISON OF HEMODIALYSIS, PERITONEAL DIALYSIS,
AND CONTINUOUS ULTRAFILTRATION

	HEMODIALYSIS	PERITONEAL DIALYSIS	CONTINUOUS ULTRAFILTRATION
Speed	Rapid—up to 8 hours per treatment	Slow—up to 72 hours initially, up to 12 hours per treatment thereafter. Can be advantage in patients who cannot tolerate rapid fluid and electrolyte changes.	Slow—treatment is continuous during oliguric phase. Continuous slow removal of fluid and electrolytes is an advantage in patients who cannot tolerate rapid changes.
Cost	Expensive	Manual—relatively inexpensive; automated—expensive	Relatively inexpensive. One-to-one nursing care may be required.
Equipment	Complex	Manual—simple and readily available; automated—complex	Manual—simple and readily available
Vascular access	Required	Not necessary, so suitable for patients with vascular problems	Arterial and venous access required
Heparinization	Required; systemic or regional	Little or no heparin necessary, so suitable for patients with bleeding problems	Heparinization of filter/tubing required; minimal systemic heparinization
Technical nursing skill necessary	High degree	Manual—moderate degree; automated—high degree	Moderate degree
Complications (other than fluid and electrolyte imbalances common to all)	Dialysis disequilibrium syndrome (preventable) Mechanical dysfunctions of dialyzer	Peritonitis Protein loss (0.5 g/L of dialysate) Bowel or bladder perforation	Blood loss—filter rupture/disconnection; system clotting

lyses, and coordinating other aspects of care as well as providing standard nursing care.

Dialyzers and Dialysate Solutions There are numerous models of dialyzers on the market, generally grouped into *coil, parallel plate,* and *hollow fiber* types. Within the parallel plate and hollow fiber dialyzers are two hydrostatic pressures: the positive pressure in the blood compartment, and the negative pressure in the dialysate compartment. The balance of these two pressures controls the rate and amount of fluid removal. Only a positive pressure is utilized with the coil.

The dialysate consists of specially formulated water, electrolytes, sodium acetate, and other substances, depending on the patient's needs. The solution usually is not sterile, because bacteria and viruses are too large to pass across the dialysis membrane. The concentration of waste products such as urea is zero; they diffuse out because of the concentration gradient between the blood and dialysate. Glucose may be added to the dialysate to create an osmotic gradient enhancing water removal. The concentration of electrolytes depends on the individual patient's needs. To prevent diffusion of substances for which the patient has desirable serum concentrations, an equivalent concentration is added to

the dialysate. For example, a higher-than-usual potassium concentraton will be used in the dialysate of a patient on digitalis, to prevent hypokalemia and precipitation of digitalis toxicity. In some cases, it may be advisable to add substances to the dialysate that will diffuse into the bloodstream. Sodium acetate, for example, will be metabolized by the body to bicarbonate ions, which then can buffer the metabolic acids the kidneys are unable to excrete

There are two types of dialysate delivery systems: the *batch system* and the *proportioning system.* Either type can be utilized in the portable dialysis machines used in the ICU. Where many patients are being dialyzed, as in chronic outpatient units, a central dialysate delivery system can be used. This is a proportioning system, and all patients receive the same dialysate composition.

Hemodialysis is a highly complex technical procedure. In order to implement it and respond rapidly and effectively to complications, the nurse needs specialized training and practice under the guidance of an experienced practitioner. Although you may not perform the dialysis, being knowledgeable about the process will help you support the patient and family and enhance your awareness of potential problems.

Circulatory Access   There are many routes of circulatory access for hemodialysis. In the patient with acute failure, the most common ones are the arteriovenous (AV) cannula, or shunt, and the femoral and subclavian catheters.

Catheters and Shunts   Percutaneous femoral catheterization using Shaldon catheters can be accomplished quickly but is suitable for only short-term use (24–48 hours). One catheter may be inserted low in the femoral vein for blood removal and a second one higher in the vein for blood return. Alternatively, a special catheter with a double lumen *(Mackintosh catheter)* may be used. Infection, clotting, and hemorrhage are potential complications of femoral catheterization. *Quenton double-lumen subclavian catheters* are commonly used for temporary access (days to months). Complications are similar to those of any subclavian line.

The AV *cannula,* or *shunt,* is used for patients needing short-term, repeated hemodialysis. The average life expectancy is 8–10 months, although some last for longer periods of time. It is inserted under local anesthetic in the operating room or occasionally at the bedside. Common sites of insertion are the radial artery and cephalic vein in the forearm and the posterior tibial artery and saphenous vein in the leg. Hard Teflon vessel tips are placed in an artery and vein. Soft cannulae made of Silastic are attached to these tips and tunneled subcutaneously to skin exit sites 2–4 cm from the vessel tips. Between dialyses, the cannulae are connected with a Teflon connector and blood flow is maintained

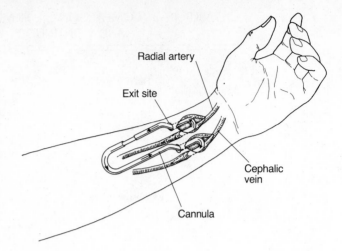

FIGURE 15–5

Standard AV shunt (cannula).

directly from the artery to the vein. Two kinds of shunts are in common use: the Scribner shunt and the Ramirez shunt. The *standard,* or *Scribner, shunt* (Figure 15–5) has curved U-shaped ends near the cannula tips, whereas the *straight,* or *Ramirez, shunt* (Figure 15–6) has suturable wings near the cannula tips.

Common problems with an AV shunt include thrombosis, hemorrhage, ischemia of the extremity, and infection. Forestall them with the measures described in the following sections.

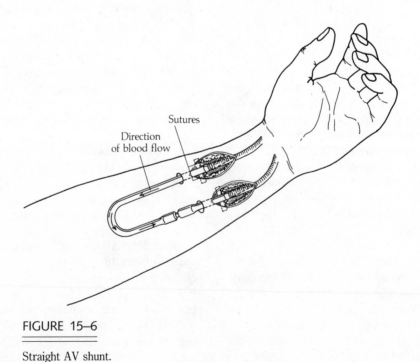

FIGURE 15–6

Straight AV shunt.

Thrombosis Thrombosis (clotting) is a serious complication that frequently can be prevented by meticulous nursing care. The following measures will assist in prevention of clots:

1. Inspect, palpate, and auscultate the shunt at least every 2 hours, more often if the shunt is new or there are problems with flow. Blood in the shunt should be uniformly red, warm, and pulsatile to the touch. Distal to the shunt (on the venous side), you should hear a bruit (murmur) and feel a thrill, caused by the turbulence resulting from the transmission of arterial pressure to the vein.

2. Prevent thrombosis by maintaining arterial blood pressure and avoiding trauma and infection at the shunt site. Elevate the extremity for the first 2–3 days, and handle it and the tubing gently. Limit activity on the extremity. Avoid taking blood pressures on or drawing blood samples from that limb. Warn the patient not to fall asleep with the limb bent. Do not apply constrictive dressings. Be careful to maintain cannulae alignment when you manipulate the cannulae or change the dressing. Misalignment can cause kinks or epithelial damage, which enhance clotting and infection.

3. The decrease of a bruit, thrill, or pulse in the shunt may indicate clotting; notify the physician. Very dark blood or blood that has separated into serum and red blood cells indicates thrombosis of the shunt. Notify the physician or hemodialysis nurse promptly, as the success of declotting attempts depends on how rapidly they are instituted. The physician or nurse will try to aspirate the clot, irrigate both cannulae tips with a heparinized solution, or strip the vessel with a special tube or a Fogarty catheter. Even if declotting is successful, thrombosis may recur unless the precipitating factor is corrected.

4. Minimize trauma to other vessels, which may be needed later for placement of another shunt, a graft, or arteriovenous fistula. For example, whenever possible, draw blood samples from the shunt rather than piercing another potential access site.

Hemorrhage Hemorrhage can be lethal within a matter of minutes. Make sure cannulae connections are secure. Keep bulldog clamps instantly available. If the cannulae separate, immediately clamp first the arterial cannula and then the venous cannula to prevent massive blood loss. After reconnecting them, remove the venous clamp and finally the arterial clamp. If a cannula or the whole shunt falls out, you may need to control bleeding with a tourniquet. Emergency surgery will be necessary to ligate the vessels.

Ischemia Ischemia to the extremity may occur if collateral supply is inadequate. Periodically, palpate the limb's pulses and observe skin color and temperature. (In the artery containing the cannula, the pulse distal to the cannula will be absent.) Alert the physician if ischemia develops; it may be necessary to reposition the shunt.

Infection Prevent infection by scrupulous attention to sterile technique. Shunt care should be given by nurses specially trained in the cleaning, positioning, and dressing of shunts, to prevent accidental damage. The following measures are especially important in shunt care.

1. Keep the dressing dry, and check periodically for drainage. Inspect the exit sites for erythema, edema, or tenderness whenever the dressing is changed or dialysis is performed.

2. When cleaning the sites, use separate sterile supplies for each site. Start the cleaning at the exit site and move outward to avoid contaminating the site with organisms from the distal epithelium. Apply an antibiotic ointment if the physician or unit procedure calls for it.

3. If you observe signs of infection, culture each site, draw blood cultures, and notify the physician or hemodialysis nurse. An infected site is a serious problem, because it predisposes toward thrombosis, embolism, systemic spread of the infection during hemodialysis, bacterial endocarditis, and septic shock. The infection is treated with appropriate antibiotics. Sometimes the shunt is removed, although maintenance of dialysis may be more important than infection at the access site.

Fistulas and Grafts If chronic hemodialysis is necessary, the surgeon may create an arteriovenous fistula or implant a graft. A *fistula* (Figure 15–7) is formed by a subcutaneous anastomosis of an artery and vein, most often the radial artery and cephalic vein. The pressure from the artery causes the vein to dilate. After 4–6 weeks, the vein can be used for dialysis. A *graft* is a vessel or synthetic implant anastamosed between an artery and vein. A fistula or graft can be used for hemodialysis by inserting large-gauge needles for blood flow into and out of the patient. Potential problems include thrombosis, hemorrhage, infection, ischemia of the extremity, aneurysm formation, and *arterial-steal syndrome*, in which arterial perfusion suffers because too much blood is diverted into the vein.

Preparation for Hemodialysis Specific procedures for initiating dialysis vary but include the steps discussed below.

1. Assess the patient emotionally, and assist the patient and family to approach the dialysis calmly. Reinforce the physician's explanation of the procedure. Ex-

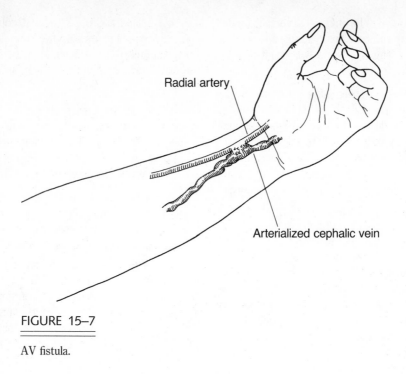

Radial artery

Arterialized cephalic vein

FIGURE 15–7

AV fistula.

plain the upcoming sequence of events to the patient and family, and answer their questions about it.

2. Assess the patient physically, and review the clinical record and laboratory reports. Particularly assess the fluid and electrolyte imbalances present. Record baseline values for the patient's weight, blood pressure, pulse, respirations, temperature, emotional state, and any other indicated parameters.

3. Draw blood samples for serum electrolytes, BUN, hematocrit, and clotting time.

4. Begin heparinization. Heparin is used to prevent clotting in the extracorporeal circuit. There are two techniques of heparinization: systemic and regional. In *systemic heparinization,* the clotting times of both the dialyzer and the patient are increased to the values appropriate for the dialyzer model in use. The heparin may be administered intermittently or continuously in the arterial line. *Regional heparinization* is preferred if the patient is bleeding already (such as in gastrointestinal bleeding) or is at high risk for bleeding (such as with recent surgery, pericarditis, or intracranial hematoma). In this method, the clotting time of the dialyzer, but not that of the patient, is increased by adding heparin to the dialyzer but neutralizing it with protamine sulfate before blood returns to the patient.

Heparin doses are individualized by body weight. Clotting times are monitored if the patient is acutely ill or has a potential bleeding problem. If an infusion is used, check its rate frequently.

Observe the patient closely for gastric bleeding, cardiac tamponade, and other signs of bleeding. These observations are particularly important if the patient has been on heparin before dialysis—for example, for a myocardial infarct. If bleeding occurs, protamine sulfate usually is administered to return the clotting time to the desired range. Dialysis may be discontinued if bleeding is severe.

5. Connect the patient to the dialyzer. For an AV shunt, clamp the arterial and venous cannulae and disconnect them. Connect the arterial line to the dialyzer, discard the saline in the dialyzer as it fills with blood, and then connect the venous line.

For an AV fistula or internal graft, you may want to infiltrate the puncture sites with xylocaine to reduce patient discomfort. For the arterial line, insert a large-gauge needle or catheter close to and directed toward the fistula or graft. The tip should be at least 3–4 cm away from the fistula or graft (Figure 15–7). For the venous line, insert a second needle further away and directed away from the fistula or graft in the direction of venous flow. Anchor the lines so there is no tension on them or kinking.

6. Begin blood flow to the dialyzer slowly to avoid precipitating hypotension. Monitor the blood pressure every 2–5 minutes while the dialyzer fills and the flow rate is increased.

7. Set alarm limits for blood flow rate, and dialysate concentration, flow rate, and temperature. Also activate the monitors for air bubble and blood leak detection.

Monitoring Hemodialysis Monitor the patient closely during the dialysis, and respond promptly to problems. The major potential problems during dialysis are fluid volume deficit, decreased CO, fluid overload, altered level of consciousness, and impaired physical mobility. In addition, a number of mechanical problems may occur. These problems are described in the following sections.

Potential Fluid Volume Deficit Related to Medications, Large-Volume Dialysis, or Ultrafiltration Hypotension, tachycardia, falling CVP, and/or thirst indicate volume depletion. The most common causes are antihypertensive or diuretic drugs, excessive volume removal for dialysis, and excessive ultrafiltration (water removal). (Accidental disconnection of the lines will not cause these signs; the alarms go off early enough to prevent the amount of blood loss which would produce them.) Before the dialysis, check with the physician about omitting any diuretic agents and antihypertensives (unless the patient is in hypertensive crisis). If sudden hypotension occurs anyway, immediately give normal saline intravenously in 50-ml doses through the extracorporeal circuit. Excessive volume removal for dialysis is a problem particularly with smaller patients and those who are hypovolemic before dialyses. To forestall this problem, a small-volume dialyzer may be employed, little pressure may be used to enhance fluid removal, and normal saline may be given intermittently or continually via the venous line to replace excess fluid loss. *Ultrafiltration* is the process of removing water from the circulation by manipulating pressure in the blood compartment and/or the dialysate compartment to increase the blood-to-dialysate pressure gradient. Ultrafiltration pressure is individualized according to the weight loss desired during dialysis. If the patient on ultrafiltration becomes hypotensive secondary to hypovolemia, the pressure gradient can be reduced. Fluid removal during dialysis can be monitored easily if bed scales are used.

Potential Decreased CO Related to Bleeding Observe the patient continuously for signs and symptoms of frank or occult bleeding. Monitor the clotting time, and maintain it within the limits appropriate for the patient. If the clotting time exceeds those limits, infuse protamine sulfate as necessary. If the patient has other risk conditions for bleeding, use regional rather than systemic heparinization. If the patient has a severe bleeding problem, use peritoneal dialysis rather than hemodialysis.

Potential Fluid Volume Excess and Electrolyte Imbalances Hypertension; weight increase; headache; ankle, sacral, and/or periorbital edema; crackles in lungs; or symptoms of pulmonary edema suggest fluid overload. They can be corrected by increasing the pressure gradient and thus increasing ultrafiltration.

Dysrhythmias, muscle weakness or cramps, hypoactive or hyperactive reflexes, or other signs of electrolyte imbalances call for a prompt check of serum electrolytes and consultation with the physician for possible orders regarding changes in the dialysate solution.

Potential Altered Level of Consciousness Related to Dialysis Disequilibrium Syndrome Headache, nausea, vomiting, hypertension, confusion, and/or seizures may indicate the dialysis disequilibrium syndrome. This syndrome, seen primarily at the completion of dialysis or occasionally with 1–2 hours of the start, may be due to too-rapid removal of urea from the bloodstream or to ultrafiltration. One explanation of the syndrome holds that because of the blood-brain barrier, rapid removal of urea from the bloodstream is not accompanied by equivalent removal from brain tissue. The hypertonic cerebrospinal fluid may cause water to shift from the plasma into brain tissue until equilibration occurs, and this cerebral edema may produce the signs of the syndrome. The syndrome may be prevented by early dialysis (before the BUN becomes excessively high), by dialyzing the acutely uremic patient gradually over 2–3 days, or by using the less efficient peritoneal dialysis. If the symptoms appear during hemodialysis, the blood flow rate may be reduced, medications may be administered to control seizures, or dialysis may be discontinued.

Impaired Physical Mobility Related to Danger of Dislodging Dialysis Lines The reduced mobility necessitated by dialysis contributes to discomfort, boredom, thrombosis, and atelectasis. Change the patient's position and give back rubs and range of motion exercises. Establish with the patient a schedule of deep breathing and coughing exercises. Provide diversion with books, television, crafts, or visits from family or friends. Remember to continue other regular treatments such as intermittent positive pressure breathing.

Mechanical Problems Mechanical problems include changes in dialysate concentration, flow, or temperature; blood flow or pressure; and many others. Although these items usually are monitored mechanically, the availability of such aids should not replace astute nursing observation and intervention. Follow these measures:

1. Maintain dialysate flow within the optimal range by checking the flowmeter and making necessary adjustments hourly. Excess flow rate will waste dialysate fluid, while insufficient flow will cause inefficient dialysis.

2. Maintain the dialysate temperature near body temperature. Too high a temperature causes hemolysis, fever, and pain; too low, chills and vessel spasm.

3. Maintain dialysate concentration. Changes in dialysate concentration can cause neurologic symptoms or red blood cell destruction. Most dialysate delivery systems have, in addition to a concentrate alarm, a bypass mode in which overly-concentrated dialysate automatically bypasses the dialyzer and is dumped. Problems with concentration are corrected by checking the water inflow lines (if the concentration is too high) or adding dialysate concentrate (if the concentration is too low). Use a chloride meter or chloride test before each dialysis to measure the number of chloride ions present in the solution. As most positive ions are combined with chloride when added to the mixture, this check is an indicator of the correct dialysate mixture. This is the only specific dialysate electrolyte test that can be performed at the bedside.

4. Quickly investigate when alarms are triggered. Pressure alarms on the extracorporeal circuit's arterial and venous blood lines monitor changes in blood flow into and out of the dialyzer. High-pressure alarms may indicate obstructions in the venous line, clots, or vessel spasm. Low-pressure alarms may indicate a problem with arterial flow from the patient and may reflect hypotension, clotting in the arterial line, or displacement of the shunt or cannula needle.

5. If a blood leak alarm occurs, look at the dialysate and check it with a blood indicator dipstick, since air bubbles can cause false alarms. A small blood leak may seal over and allow continuation of dialysis. A large blood leak usually calls for immediate cessation of dialysis. The return of contaminated blood to the patient depends on her or his condition and the physician's judgment of the risk/benefit ratio between the augmentation of blood volume and the risk of septicemia.

Discontinuing Dialysis When dialysis is completed, discontinue it in the following manner.

Discontinue heparinization (if not already done). When needles are used with internal access routes, heparin may be discontinued 1–2 hours before the dialysis is stopped so that puncture sites can clot more readily.

Clamp the arterial line but leave the venous line open for blood return to the patient. Rinse the venous line with saline and discontinue it.

For an AV shunt, reconnect the cannulae and dress the sites as described earlier. For an AV fistula, use a gloved finger and folded 4 × 4 gauze to apply direct pressure as the needles are removed and maintain it until bleeding stops. Use just enough pressure to prevent bleeding but not enough to occlude flow.

Problems Between Dialyses Be alert for problems between dialyses. Post-dialysis, anticipate that the patient's weight, blood pressure, and urinary output (if any) will be decreased. Since serum potassium will have been returned to normal, be alert for conditions that could provoke hypokalemia, such as diarrhea, persistent vomiting, and nasogastric drainage. Also observe for the dialysis disequilibrium syndrome, as outlined above. As the length of time since the last dialysis increases, be alert for problems with hyperkalemia and fluid overload. An acceptable weight gain between dialysis is 0.5 kg (1 lb) per 24 hours.

Peritoneal Dialysis

Peritoneal dialysis uses the peritoneum as the dialyzing membrane. One surface of the peritoneum lines the abdominal cavity; the other covers the abdominal viscera. The space between is the peritoneal cavity into which the dialyzing fluid is instilled. On the other side of the membrane is extracellular fluid. From it, the dialysate removes fluid through osmosis and metabolic wastes through diffusion and filtration. Peritoneal dialysis is contraindicated in adhesions of the peritoneal cavity. Unless it is being used to treat peritonitis, it is contraindicated in that condition also.

Access Several types of peritoneal catheters exist. A temporary catheter is used when dialysis is needed immediately or infrequently. Other types of catheters remain in place for repeated use.

Dialysis Systems Several types of dialysis systems are available. The *manual* method relies on manual infusion, monitoring, and drainage of fluid. It is easily learned and inexpensive, but its disadvantages include the amount of nursing time consumed and the danger of infection due to the breaks in sterility necessary in order to hang and discard fluids. *Automated* units cycle infusion, equilibration, and drainage mechanically. Although more convenient, they still require nursing attention to monitor their functioning, empty the drainage bag, and troubleshoot problems.

Continuous ambulatory peritoneal dialysis (CAPD) is a variation on the manual method, suitable for use with stable chronic renal failure patients. The dialysis is performed continuously, with fluid remaining in the peritoneal cavity for several hours at a time during the day and night.

Preparation for Peritoneal Dialysis To prepare the patient for peritoneal dialysis, follow these steps.

1. Assist the physician in explaining the necessity of dialysis and the technique involved. Inform the patient of common sensations associated with dialysis, such as pressure during catheter insertion and fluid instillation.

2. Record baseline vital signs and weight.

3. Assist the physician to insert the peritoneal catheter. Bring to the bedside skin prep supplies, dressing supplies, the size and type of catheter the physician prefers, its trocar, and the dialysis delivery system. Peritoneal dialysis may be done either with bottles of solution run in via gravity or by a machine that mixes the dialysate and delivers it via a pump. The dialysate should be at body temperature to minimize discomfort and optimize clearance of waste products. Add to the solution any prescribed medications such as potassium or heparin.

Immediately prior to catheter insertion, have the patient empty his or her bladder to minimize the risk of bladder perforation. Clean and shave the abdomen. Drape it with sterile towels. The physician will anesthetize the area just below the umbilicus and make a small incision. Through this, he or she will insert the trocar into the peritoneal cavity. After the catheter is passed through the trocar, the trocar is removed and the catheter is sutured in place. Urine, feces, or blood dripping out of the catheter indicate perforation of the bladder, intestine, or abdominal blood vessels. If no such catastrophe occurs, connect the administration set to the catheter.

4. Begin dialysis. The physician will specify the type and amount of fluid to be instilled and the length of the infusion, equilibrium, and drainage periods. One common order is 2 liters of fluid per cycle with an inflow time of 10 minutes, equilibrium time of 30 minutes, and outflow period of 20 minutes. If you are using an automated delivery unit, it will cycle by itself. If you are not, clamp the outflow tubing and infuse the dialysate over a 10-minute period. When it has run in, clamp the tubing before air can enter the peritoneal cavity. The equilibration period (dwell time) may last 15–45 minutes. At the end of the period, unclamp the outflow tubing to permit the dialysate to drain by gravity into the closed drainage system. During this time, turning the patient from side to side may help to facilitate drainage. Fluid drained from the first few cycles after catheter insertion may be slightly bloody. The cycles usually are repeated over 12–48 hours.

Monitoring Peritoneal Dialysis During and after the dialysis respond promptly to problems. The poten-

tial complications of peritoneal dialysis are fluid retention, pain, peritonitis, dyspnea and/or atelectasis, hyperglycemia, bladder or bowel perforation, and protein loss. These complications are described in the following sections.

Potential Excess Fluid Volume Related to Incomplete Drainage Inadequate fluid drainage, hypertension, and signs and symptoms of fluid overload or congestive heart failure indicate fluid retention. Be sure that the bottles of dialysate contain exactly the amount ordered for infusion; some manufacturers add an extra small amount, which you should pour off or include in your calculations of intake and output.

Keep a running record of inflow, dwell, and outflow times; volume instilled; volume drained; and the cumulative fluid balance. The amount drained should equal or exceed the amount instilled. Frequently, the patient may retain some of the dialysate, running a positive fluid balance. The amount of positive fluid balance allowable varies with the patient and should be specified in the doctor's orders for the procedure. In some cases, as in the patient with congestive heart failure, it may be as low as a few hundred milliliters. Incomplete drainage can result from pooling of fluid due to body position, obstruction to the catheter if it is buried in the omentum or clogged with fibrin clots, or escape of the fluid via a bowel or bladder perforation. When drainage is less than expected, try these measures: Turn the patient from side to side, elevate the head of the bed, and/or massage the abdomen gently. Should the problem continue and the patient continually retain fluid on each exchange, consult with the physician before initiating another cycle. He or she may attempt to clear the catheter by rotating it or probing it to dislodge any fibrin clots.

Pain Related to Peritoneal Distention or Irritation Prevent the common occurrence of mild pain by making sure the dialysate is at body temperature and by promoting effective drainage of fluid. If pain persists, notify the physician, as it may indicate peritonitis. Once peritonitis has been ruled out, the doctor may prescribe the instillation of a local anesthetic at the start of each cycle, decrease the volume instilled, or have you administer analgesics. Serving meals in small portions and providing diversion through family visits, television, and radio may also help reduce the discomfort.

Potential Pain Related to Peritonitis Abdominal pain, fever, rebound tenderness, and/or cloudy return fluid suggest peritoneal infection. Prevent peritonitis by scrupulous attention to sterile technique. Observe the outflow fluid; it should be pale yellow and clear. Routinely culture fluid drained from the first cycle and one cycle daily thereafter. If you note signs of infection, alert the physician. Antibiotics will be given in the dialysate and/or systematically in the hope of maintaining use of the catheter.

Impaired Gas Exchange Related to Interference with Diaphragmatic Motion   Dyspnea or atelectasis may result from restricted diaphragmatic descent due to the pressure of the fluid. Elevate the head of the bed. Prevent atelectasis by promoting deep breathing and coughing. If the patient develops acute dyspnea, drain the dialysate immediately and summon medical assistance.

Potential Altered Level of Consciousness Related to Hyperglycemia   Confusion and lethargy may result from fluid overload or hyperglycemia. Measures to prevent fluid overload are discussed above. When the dialysate fluid has a high glucose concentration, hyperglycemia may occur if glucose crosses the peritoneal membrane. To forestall hyperglycemia, make sure that the dialysate fluid has the ordered dextrose concentration (1.5%, 2.5%, or 4.25%) and drain dialysate promptly at the end of the specified equilibration period. Place diabetics on routine urine and/or blood tests for sugar and acetone.

Potential Altered Bowel and Urinary Elimination Related to Bowel or Bladder Perforation   Diarrhea and diminished or fecal-colored peritoneal drainage imply bowel perforation. Notify the physician, because laparotomy may be necessary to repair the perforation and minimize peritonitis. Bladder fullness, increased urinary output, and decreased peritoneal drainage suggest bladder perforation. Confirm your suspicion by testing both the drainage fluid and the urine for sugar; in perforation, they will have the same concentration. Alert the physician, who will repair the bladder surgically.

Altered Nutrition (Less than Body Requirements) Related to Protein Loss   Protein loss has been estimated at 0.2–0.5 g/L of drained fluid. Since dialysis often includes 24–48 cycles initially, this loss can be significant. High-protein meals and intravenous protein infusions may be contraindicated because of the diminished urea excretion. Because patients with low protein intake will develop edema, poor resistance to infection, and wasting after several months of peritoneal dialysis, some physicians prefer a high-protein diet, to minimize catabolism.

With proper management, patients may be sustained on intermittent or continuous home peritoneal dialysis for years.

Continuous Ultrafiltration/ Hemofiltration

Continuous ultrafiltration is a relatively new method of controlling fluid and electrolyte balance in critically ill patients who cannot tolerate hemodialysis or peritoneal di-

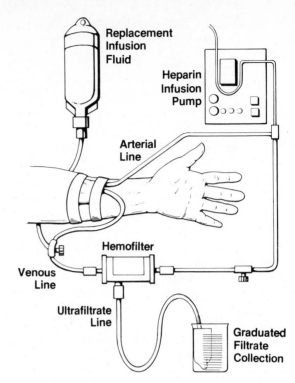

FIGURE 15–8

AV hemofiltration. (From Whittaker A et al.: Preventing complications in continuous arteriovenous hemofiltration. *Dimen Crit Care Nurs* 1986; 5:74, Philadelphia: Lippincott/Harper & Row.)

alysis. Water, electrolytes, and metabolic waste products are gradually removed as the patient's blood passes through a small-volume, low-resistance hemofilter (Figure 15–8). The procedure is powered by the patient's own arterial blood pressure. The system is maintained by the critical-care nurse and does not require hemodialysis machinery.

Access   The continuous ultrafiltration procedure requires access to both the arterial and the venous circulations. The femoral artery is frequently utilized, because it is easily accessed and provides adequate blood flow. Any large-bore venous access can be used to return blood to the patient. If continuous ultrafiltration will be required for more than a few days, an external arteriovenous shunt is preferred. The shunt can be placed in the patient's arm or leg. It provides high blood flow and access to both the arterial and the venous systems.

Continuous Ultrafiltration Systems   Continuous ultrafiltration is a continuous extracorporeal blood treatment in which plasma water, electrolytes, and nonprotein-bound solutes are removed from the blood. The ultrafiltrate produced is a protein-free fluid whose electrolyte concentration is similar to that of plasma. The cellular elements of the blood remain in the blood circuit. The principal use of continuous ultrafiltration is in the treatment of acute oliguric renal failure. There are three variations of ultrafiltration therapy: continuous arteriovenous hemofiltration, slow continuous ultrafiltration, and continuous arteriovenous hemofiltration dialysis. The purpose and mechanism of each of these therapies will be discussed in the following sections.

Continuous Arteriovenous Hemofiltration   Continuous arteriovenous hemofiltration (CAVH) is a renal replacement therapy for patients with uncomplicated acute oliguric renal failure. Plasma water and electrolytes usually are removed at rates of 400–800 ml/hr. Usually, one-half to three-fourths of the ultrafiltrate removed is replaced during the next hour with intravenous fluid such as normal saline. The ultrafiltrate contains the same level of solutes (e.g., potassium and urea) as the patient's plasma. Replacing it with solute-free intravenous solution dilutes the plasma solute level. The slow, continuous removal of fluid and solutes is closer to the kidney's normal functioning than is hemodialysis. Therefore, it is ideal for hemodynamically unstable patients or those with cerebral edema. If the patient's BUN, serum creatinine, and potassium are not rapidly rising, CAVH may be the only dialysis therapy required for fluid and electrolyte control.

Slow Continuous Ultrafiltration   Slow continuous ultrafiltration (SCUF) differs from CAVH in that a much smaller volume of plasma water is removed during each hour of treatment. When using SCUF, 150–300 ml of ultrafiltrate is removed each hour. In most patients, the replacement fluid will consist of only the patient's normal infusions, such as vasoactive drips and total parenteral nutrition. SCUF can be used to control fluid balance between hemodialysis treatments in patients requiring large volumes of total parenteral nutrition. It may also be used to control fluid volume overload in patients with congestive heart failure who do not respond to diuretic therapy.

Continuous Arteriovenous Hemofiltration Dialysis   Continuous arteriovenous hemofiltration dialysis (CAVHD) combines the convective transport of CAVH with the diffusive transport of hemodialysis. Sterile dialysate is infused into the ultrafiltration compartment of the hemofilter. The dialysate runs countercurrent to blood flow, enhancing electrolyte, urea, and creatinine clearance (Geronemus 1985). Fluid removal usually is less than 100 ml/hr; therefore, less fluid replacement is required. Since both fluid and electrolyte balance are controlled, CAVHD can be used to treat patients with severe hyperkalemia and azotemia.

Preparation for Continuous Ultrafiltration   Initiation of continuous ultrafiltration is not technically complex, and includes the following steps.

1. Prime the arterial tubing, hemofilter, and venous tubing with heparinized saline. Normally, 2 liters will be required.

2. Remove all air bubbles from tubing and hemofilter. Tap gently and rotate the hemofilter to expel stubborn bubbles.

3. Connect the heparin infusion and the arterial and venous replacement infusion lines to the hemofilter tubing.

4. Assess the patient's hemodynamic function. Record baseline values for heart rate, blood pressure, central venous pressure, cardiac output, and pulmonary artery wedge pressure.

5. Draw blood samples for baseline serum electrolytes, BUN, creatinine, plasma proteins, and hematocrit. Obtain a PTT or ACT for baseline coagulation status.

6. Administer the intravenous loading dose of heparin as directed by the physician.

7. Connect the patient to the ultrafiltration system as described in Preparation for hemodialysis on p. 386.

8. Begin the heparin infusion. In the majority of patients, hourly heparin requirements vary from 10–20 U/kg.

9. Monitor the ultrafiltration rate by collecting ultrafiltrate for one minute. Adjust the ultrafiltration rate to that prescribed by the physician.

Monitoring Continuous Ultrafiltration   Observe the patient closely during continuous ultrafiltration therapy. Monitor for problems related to fluid volume depletion, clotting of the filter, and bleeding. These problems are discussed in the following sections.

Potential for Fluid Volume Deficit   The primary determinant of ultrafiltration is the hydrostatic pressure exerted by the patient's blood pressure. Monitor the patient's blood pressure hourly. Administer intravenous fluids and vasopressors to maintain the mean arterial blood pressure above 60 mm Hg. Negative pressure, created by the distance between the hemofilter and the collection bag, pulls fluid through the filter membrane. Decrease the ultrafiltration rate by raising the collection bag toward the level of the hemofilter. Place a C-clamp on the ultrafiltrate line if further decreases in ultrafiltration rate are necessary. Measure ultrafiltrate output hourly. Observe for decreased ultrafiltrate, hypotension, tachycardia, and other signs of fluid volume depletion. Since ultrafiltration is opposed by the oncotic pressure exerted by the plasma protein level, monitor for elevations in hematocrit and plasma protein levels, which would indicate that the patient is becoming hemoconcentrated. Adjust intravenous fluid and electrolyte replacement to maintain balance.

Alteration in Tissue Perfusion Related to Clotting Clotting in the hemofilter and tubing results from inadequate heparinization or stasis of blood within the extracorporeal circuit (Whittaker et al. 1986). Draw blood, from the venous port, for PTT or ACT every 4 hours. Adjust the heparin infusion to maintain the PTT/ACT within the prescribed range. Observe the hemofilter and tubing for darkening or separation of the blood. If this occurs, flush the hemofilter with heparinized saline. Replace the hemofilter if a large portion of the fibers are clotted. Draw blood for clotting studies, and recalculate the patient's heparin requirements. Prevent stasis of blood by maintaining the patient's blood pressure and cardiac output. Promote optimal blood flow through the system. Place the hemofilter at the level of the right atrium. Position the tubing to avoid compression or kinking.

Decreased Cardiac Output Related to Bleeding Although only a low level of heparinization is required for continuous ultrafiltration, blood loss during the procedure is a major nursing concern. Observe and test the ultrafiltrate for occult blood; replace the hemofilter if blood is present. Stabilize all lines to prevent stress on the insertion sites. Bridge-tape tubing connections to prevent accidental disconnection. Monitor for occult blood in the urine and feces. Avoid tissue trauma during routine patient care.

Discontinuing Continuous Ultrafiltration Once the continuous ultrafiltration therapy is completed, discontinue it using the following procedure.

1. Turn off the heparin and replacement infusions.
2. Clamp the arterial tubing on the patient side of the arterial infusion port. Return the blood in the hemofilter and venous tubing by flushing saline through the arterial port.
3. Clamp the arterial tubing on the hemofilter side of the arterial infusion port. Use a pressure bag on the saline flush to clear blood from the arterial tubing.
4. Clamp the arterial and venous cannulae, and disconnect the hemofilter and tubing.

If using an AV shunt, reconnect the cannulae and dress the insertion sites. Maintain pressure over the femoral insertion site following removal of a femoral artery catheter. Monitor the patient closely after termination of the continuous ultrafiltration procedure. Observe for signs and symptoms of recurrent fluid volume excess or electrolyte imbalance.

Renal Transplantation

Although renal transplantation is not a treatment modality for acute renal failure, the critical-care nurse may care for patients immediately following transplant surgery. The early postoperative nursing care of the renal transplant recipient is directed toward maintaining fluid and electrolyte balance, monitoring for graft rejection, and prevention of infection.

Potential Fluid Volume Deficit

Most patients receiving a functional graft will have a high urine output during the first 24 hours following transplantation. Monitor intake and output closely. Replace urinary losses with intravenous fluids as directed. Consult with the physician to calculate the replacement fluid volume based on a percentage of the previous hour's urinary output. Evaluate the patient's response to fluid loss and replacement by observing for tachycardia and changes in blood pressure. Obtain a preoperative or admission weight, and weigh the patient daily. Expect a decrease in body weight due to fluid loss.

Be particularly alert for fluid volume depletion in patients with diabetes mellitus. Administration of corticosteroid drugs during or immediately after surgery frequently results in hyperglycemia and glucosuria. Observe the patient for signs of a developing osmotic diuresis. Test the urine for glucose, and monitor the serum glucose closely. Administer insulin as prescribed. Infuse glucose-free intravenous fluids until the serum glucose level is below 300 mg/dl.

Alteration in Tissue Perfusion Related to Graft Rejection

In order to prevent rejection of the transplanted kidney, the patient must be immunosuppressed. Immunosuppression therapy consists of a combination of prednisone with either azathioprine or cyclosporine (Strom and Carpenter 1984). The nurse is responsible for administering these medications and assessing for signs and symptoms of early graft rejection. Monitor the urine output, and report any significant decrease. Draw daily BUN and serum creatinine levels, and note any upward trends. Take the patient's temperature every 4 hours, and evaluate for elevations. Check for tenderness or swelling of the graft site.

Potential for Infection

Infection is an ever-present danger to the immunosuppressed kidney transplant recipient. Follow the infection control practices described in this and other chapters relating to catheter care, IV sites, wound care, and so on. Be aware that corticosteroid medications may change the patient's fever response to infection. Report any elevations in temperature. Consult with the physician before administering any medications with antipyretic properties. Monitor the white blood cell count daily for any downward trend. Also observe for any upward trend, which may indicate bacterial infection. Initiate protective precautions for significant leukopenia. Teach the patient health practices that decrease the risk of infection.

Outcome Evaluation

To evaluate the patient's progress, use these outcome criteria:

- Urine output WNL for patient, ideally 600–1600 ml/24 hr.
- Urine osmolality WNL for patient, ideally 500–800 mOsm/kg.
- Serum osmolality WNL for patient, ideally 285–295 mOsm/kg.
- Plasma and urine electrolytes WNL for patient.
- BUN WNL for patient, ideally 8–20 mg%.
- Creatinine concentrations WNL for patient, ideally 0.5–1.2 mg% for plasma and 1–1.8 g/24-hr urine.
- Level of consciousness unchanged or improved from that before onset of acute renal failure.
- Nutrition and elimination WNL for patient.
- Vital signs, ECG, and arterial blood gases WNL for patient.
- No signs or symptoms of fluid overload/deficit, anemia, infection, malnutrition, or uremic pericarditis.

REFERENCES

American Association of Critical Care Nurses: *Core curriculum for critical care nursing.* Philadelphia: Saunders, 1985.

Crabtree A, Jorgenson M: Exploring the practical knowledge in expert critical-care nursing practice. Unpublished master's thesis, University of Wisconsin, Madison, 1986.

Geronemus R: Continuous arteriovenous hemodialysis. *The first international symposium on acute continuous renal replacement therapy.* Cleveland, OH: Cleveland Clinic Foundation, 1985.

Guyton A: *Textbook of medical physiology,* 7th ed. Philadelphia: Saunders, 1986.

Lancaster L: Renal failure: Pathophysiology, assessment, and intervention. *Crit Care Nurse* (January/February) 1982; 40–63.

Lancaster L: *The patient with end-stage renal disease,* 2d ed. New York: Wiley, 1984.

Richard C: Management of patients with critical renal and gerintourinary disorders. Pages 657–696 in AACN's *Clinical reference for critical care nursing,* Kinney et al. (eds). New York: McGraw-Hill, 1981.

Schrier R, Conger J: Acute renal failure: Pathogenesis, diagnosis and management. Pages 423–460 in *Renal and electrolyte disorders,* 3d ed., Schrier R (ed). Boston: Little, Brown, 1986.

Stark J: How to succeed against acute renal failure. *Nurs 82* (July) 1982; 26–33.

Strom T, Carpenter C: Prophylaxis of allograft rejection. Pages 376–380 in *Current therapy in nephrology and hypertension, 1984–1985,* Glassock R (ed). Ontario: Decker, 1984.

Whittaker A: Acute renal dysfunction: Assessment of patients at risk. *Focus Crit Care,* 1985; 12:12–17.

Whittaker A et al.: Preventing complications in continuous arteriovenous hemofiltration. *Dimen Crit Care Nurs* 1986; 5:72–79.

SUPPLEMENTAL READING

Arenz R: Do-it-yourself. *RN* (July) 1981; 57–60.

Atkins C: Renal transplantation. Pages 851–889 in *Critical care nursing: Body-mind-spirit,* Kenner C et al. (eds). Boston: Little, Brown, 1985.

Crespo J: Dialysis-related infections. *Heart Lung* 1982; 11:111–117.

Doyle J: Treating renovascular hypertension: Bypass graft surgery. *Am J Nurs* 1982; 82:1559–1562.

Doyle J, Sequeira J: Treating renovascular hypertension: Renal artery dilatation. *Am J Nurs* 1982; 82:1563–1564.

Felsenfeld A: Dialysis, osteomalacia and aluminum toxicity: A form of renal osteodystrophy. *ANNA J* 1985; 12:189–191.

Flood S: Pericardial effusion in the uremic patient: Nursing considerations and management. *ANNA J* 1985; 12:294–298.

Irwin B: Using cyclosporine: Results of planned conversion to azathioprine after transplantation. *ANNA J* 1986; 13:14–28.

Johnson D: The dialysis disequilibrium syndrome. *Nephrol Nurse* 1980; 2:27–41.

Kidd P: Trauma of the genitourinary system. *J Emerg Nurs* 1982; 8:232–238.

Killion A: Reducing the risk of infection from indwelling urethal catheters. *Nurs 82* (May) 1982; 84–88.

King G: Continuous arterio-venous hemofiltration: A nursing perspective. *ANNA J* 1986; 13:151–154.

Lancaster L: Kidney transplant rejection: Pathophysiology, recognition, and treatment. *Crit Care Nurse* (September/October) 1982; 50–53.

Locke et al.: Continuous arteriovenous hemofiltration: An alternative to standard hemodialysis in unstable patients. *ANNA J* 1985; 12:127–131.

Mars D, Treloar D: Acute tubular necrosis—Pathophysiology and treatment. *Heart Lung* 1984; 12:194–201.

Metheny N: Renal stones and urinary pH. *Am J Nurs* 1982; 82:1372–1375.

Millar et al. (eds): Methods in Critical Care, *AACN manual.* Philadelphia: Saunders, 1985.

Norris M: Dialysis disequilibrium syndrome: A critical care nursing challenge. *Dimen Crit Care Nurs* 1982; 1:17–21.

Orr M: Drugs and renal disease. *Am J Nurs* 1981; 81:969–971.

Schrier R: Acute renal failure: Pathogenesis, diagnosis, and management. *Hosp Prac* (March) 1981; 93–112.

Stark J: BUN/creatinine: Your keys to kidney function. *Nurs 80* (May) 1980; 33–38.

Stark J: Acute poststreptococcal glomerulonephritis. *Nurs 82* (May) 1982; 114–115.

Toner M: Urinary tract obstruction: The hidden threats in treatment. *RN* (May) 1982; 58–63.

Valtin H: *Renal dysfunction: Mechanisms involved in fluid and solute imbalance.* Boston: Little, Brown, 1979.

Williams J: Hypotensive crises: Identifying the high-risk patient on hemodialysis. *Heart Lung* 1981; 10:309–316.

Winkelman C: *Hemofiltration: A new technique in critical care nursing. Heart Lung* 1985; 14:265–271.

16

Fluid, Electrolyte, and Acid–Base Imbalances

CLINICAL INSIGHT

Domain: The diagnostic and monitoring function

Competency: Detection and documentation of significant changes in a patient's condition

Becoming an expert critical-care nurse demands not only finely honing skills at detecting subtle physiologic changes but also developing the ability to present to the physician a convincing case for why this change is significant in this patient at this time. In the following examplar, from Crabtree and Jorgenson (1986, p. 133), Jill, a nurse, speaks eloquently of how she developed this skill, describing an incident that occurred early in her career, while caring for a freshly postoperative patient who had undergone an abdominal aortic aneurysm repair.

My cardinal rule in nursing is, look at your patient. I don't care what any of the monitors say, what the papers say—look at your patient. So, I always looked at the patient and the patient looked like hell. And, I looked down, and the first thing I noticed was his Foley bag was totally full, and I said to this physician, I wonder what his K^+ is, and he said, don't worry about the potassium; don't worry about his I & O; you nurses get so hung up in this. And, he really verbally *castrated me, and, well, I was worried about the potassium because I felt totally responsible. The surgeon would walk in and then would leave, and I had already learned that I really had to do my own thinking. So, I had a potassium drawn and, again—some people say this is very gutsy—who's going to pay for it? all these different things. I didn't worry about any of it. I worried about the patient. So, I had a potassium drawn, and it came back 2.8, and what I had never thought through was, now what am I going to do with this information? Because this surgeon that I had to call was, in my opinion, very difficult to deal with. So, now I'm in the position of, my God, Jill, you didn't think this through. You've got to call him with this information. So, I called him at home. And I told him what the patient's potassium was, and we did rectify the situation. But, the point that I'm making is, how much energy, how much time I used up just taking care of one small detail. Where, now, today, I would never concern myself with this. I would follow through; none of my energy would be worrying about what the interaction was going to be with me. I would not hesitate to call him at home, and I wouldn't worry about it. But, it was I was so new in dealing with surgeons. I was the new kid on the block; what did I know? and I had to prove myself. And, I was very concerned with what the surgeons thought of me—their interactions with me—be-*

cause to me the bottom line was, you had to get the order for the patient. And, there is a certain protocol that the nurse learns very early on: that she likes this relationship with the physician, or she's not going to get what the patient needs.

Fluid, electrolyte, and acid–base disorders are common in the critically ill. The risk factors and signs and symptoms may be so subtle, however, that at times it takes special alertness to detect them and assertiveness to ensure appropriate treatment for them, as illustrated in the Clinical Insight. This chapter discusses the pathophysiology of each disorder and presents measures to assist you in nursing your patients more effectively.

FLUID AND ELECTROLYTE IMBALANCES

Assessment

As a critical-care nurse, you should develop skill at effective intervention to protect the critically ill from the ravages of fluid and electrolyte imbalances. Such intervention requires you to maintain a high index of suspicion in conditions that increase the patient's vulnerability to such imbalances. You should anticipate and forestall the development of these disorders whenever possible. If they do occur, you should recognize their signs and symptoms, alert the physician, and help him or her institute treatment early.

Table 16–1 presents a useful format for assessing the patient's fluid and electrolyte status. Assessment includes evaluation of serial body weights, fluid intake and output, serum and urine osmolalities, serum and urine electrolytes, and signs and symptoms.

Serial Body Weights

Monitor serial body weights daily in patients susceptible to fluid imbalances.

The proportion of body weight that is body fluid varies with the patient's sex and fat content. In average-sized males, approximately 60% (40 L) of body weight is water. Women have more fat and less water than men: In the average-sized female, body water averages 50% (35 L).

Body fluid is divided into two main compartments: *intracellular* and *extracellular*. For a 70-kg man, about 25 L represents intracellular water, whereas about 15 L represents extracellular water. (Estimates of the volumes of fluid compartments vary considerably with the test substance used. The percentages given here are approximate and represent averages of those reported by various authors.) The extracellular compartment is subdivided into *functional* extracellular spaces, into and out of which fluid exchange can occur freely, and *non-*

TABLE 16–1   FLUID AND ELECTROLYTE ASSESSMENT FORMAT

1. History _____
2. Physical _____

   Admission weight _____ date _____

   Yesterday's weight _____ date _____

   Today's weight _____ date _____

   Signs and symptoms _____
   _____

3. Diagnostic procedures and laboratory tests

   Intake and output (24 hr) _____

   Osmolality: serum _____ urine _____

   Electrolytes: serum Na^+ _____ K^+ _____ Cl^- _____

   Ca^{2+} _____ Mg^{2+} _____

   urine Na^+ _____ K^+ _____ Cl^- _____

   Other _____

4. Other relevant data _____

functional spaces, from which fluid is not readily accessible to the circulation. The small nonfunctional fluid spaces include the peritoneal, pleural, cerebrospinal, bone, joint, and connective tissue fluids. The functional spaces consist of fluid outside the cells in the vascular system (plasma) and that outside the cells in body tissues and cavities (interstitial fluid). Plasma equals about 3 L and interstitial fluid about 12 L. Dynamic fluid exchange occurs continuously among the intracellular, plasma, and interstitial compartments. Of these three, only the plasma can be influenced directly by the intake of fluid from outside the body or by the elimination of fluid from the body. For instance, when you drink water, the first fluid compartment that is affected is the plasma. The intracellular and interstitial compartments then respond to changes in the volume or concentration of the plasma.

A rapid weight change (over 0.5 kg/day) suggests a fluid imbalance and often appears before other, more subtle signs and symptoms. Since a kilogram equals 2.2 lb and a liter of body fluid equals 2.2 lb, a general guideline is that each liter of fluid retained is reflected by a rapid weight gain of 1 kg; and each liter lost, by a loss of 1 kg. A patient's weight therefore can serve as a valuable guide to estimating fluid deficit or excess.

Fluid Intake and Output

For the internal environment to remain in a steady state from day to day, the intake and output of fluids must be equal. In the healthy adult, intake or output varies between 1500 and 3000 ml daily. The major routes of water intake are ingestion of liquids (500–1700 ml), the ingestion of water in foods (800–1000 ml), and the oxidation of food and body tissues (200–300 ml). The primary normal routes of water output are urine (800–1600 ml), water vapor excreted through the lungs and skin (600–1200 ml), and feces (50–200 ml). There is an obligatory loss of approximately 600–800 ml daily of water vapor from the lungs and skin (insensible water loss). Vaporization from the lungs and skin occurs even when water intake is zero. It is important to note that the amount of water vapor lost from the lungs and skin may greatly increase with critically ill patients.

The osmolality of body fluids is determined almost solely by sodium concentration. In turn, sodium concentration is controlled by two separate but closely associated systems: *antidiuretic hormone* (ADH) and *thirst* (Guyton 1986). Oral intake is regulated by the thirst center, believed to be located in the anterolateral hypothalamus. When plasma osmolality increases or blood volume decreases, the neurons in the thirst center become stimulated by intracellular dehydration, and the person becomes thirsty and increases water intake.

Water output is under multiple controls, the most significant of which are antidiuretic hormone (ADH), aldosterone, and barorerceptors. ADH is a hormone made in the supraoptic nuclei and stored in the posterior pituitary gland. On the surface of the anterior hypothalamus are cells, called *osmoreceptors,* that sense changes in the sodium concentration of the extracellular fluid that bathes them. When osmotic pressure increases, the supraoptic neurons become dehydrated and discharge impulses to the posterior pituitary at a faster rate, so there is an increased release of ADH. Conversely, when osmotic pressure decreases, ADH release falls. ADH travels in the bloodstream to the kidneys. There it alters tubular permeability to water, creating increased reabsorption of water (and therefore decreased urinary output). The retained water dilutes the extracellular fluid, reducing its concentration toward normal. The restoration of normal osmotic pressure then feeds back to the osmoreceptors to inhibit their discharge. The thirst center and supraoptic nuclei are close together and appear to respond to the same stimuli.

Another substance that plays an important role in the control of extracellular volume is aldosterone. *Aldosterone* is a hormone secreted by the adrenal cortex in response to many stimuli. In probable order of decreasing importance, the four most potent stimuli are: (a) increased potassium ion concentration in extracellular fluid; (b) increased angiotensin level (resulting from increased renin secretion by the juxtaglomerular apparatus in the kidneys); (c) decreased quantity of total body sodium; and (d) increased adrenocorticotropic hormone (ACTH) (Guyton 1986).

Aldosterone travels in the bloodstream to the kidneys, where it is believed to cause the formation of carrier proteins or enzymes necessary for active sodium transport through the tubular epithelium of the distal tubule and collecting duct (Guyton 1986). An increased level of aldosterone therefore causes increased sodium retention and an obligatory increase in water retention, thus reducing the urinary output. The retained sodium and water serve to increase the volume of extracellular fluid and feed back to inhibit aldosterone secretion.

Baroreceptors that sense high-pressure (arterial) changes are located in the arch of the aorta and in each carotid sinus, just above the bifurcation of the internal and external carotid arteries. When arterial pressure drops, these receptors transmit fewer impulses from the carotid sinuses (via the Hering and glossopharyngeal nerves) and from the aortic arch (via the vagus nerves) to the vasomotor center. The decrease in impulses excites the sympathetic (cardioaccelerator and vasoconstrictor) center and inhibits the parasympathetic (cardioinhibitor) center. As a result, heart rate accelerates and the peripheral vasculature constricts, increasing the central blood volume. At the same time, sympathetic stimulation constricts the renal afferent and efferent arterioles. This constriction reduces glomerular filtration, so less water is excreted.

Body Fluid Osmolality

When you consider the concentration of body fluids, it is important to realize that concentration may be expressed in several different ways. The term *concentration* in itself expresses the ratio between dissolved substances *(solutes)* and dissolving fluid *(solvent).*

Concentration expressed as weight is equal to the grams of solute per 100 ml of fluid; an example is a serum albumin value of 5 g/100 ml, also reported sometimes as 5 g/dl or 5 g%. An *equivalent weight* equals the molecular weight of a substance divided by its valence. In clinical situations, the value is given as milliequivalents per liter of fluid (mEq/L). This method is often used for reporting serum electrolyte values, for example, a serum sodium level of 140 mEq/L.

Osmosis is the movement of water from a solution with fewer solute particles across a semipermeable membrane into a solution with more solute particles. An *osmol,* a unit for measuring osmotic pressure, is the gram molecular weight of a substance multiplied by the number of dissociating ions. Because of the small concentrations with which we work in clinical situations, values are expressed in thousandths of an osmol, that is, milliosmols (mOsm).

The *osmolarity* of a solution is the solute concentration per volume of solution, or mOsm/L. The *osmolality* is the solute concentration per weight of solvent, or mOsm/kg of solvent. In clinical practice, osmolarity and osmolality often are preferred to other measures of concentration, because they express the number of osmotically active particles without regard to their size, electrical charge, or molecular weight. Normally in the body, the difference between osmolarity and osmolality is slight, and the terms often are used interchangably. The normal serum osmolality is 285–295 mOsm/kg.

Normal serum osmolality consists primarily of sodium, its anions, glucose, and urea. Osmolality can be measured in the laboratory; or it can be estimated at the bedside by using the following formula (sodium = Na):

$$\text{Osmolality} = (\text{Na} \times 2) + \frac{\text{BUN}}{3} + \frac{\text{Glucose}}{18}$$
$$(\text{mOsm/L})$$

The rationale for this formula makes it easier to remember. The value for sodium is multiplied by 2 to account for its accompanying anions. BUN and glucose values are divided by their approximate molecular weights to convert them from mg/100 ml (the units in which they are reported) to mOsm/L (Abels 1986). The calculated value usually is within 10 mOsm of the measured osmolality.

Urine osmolality is discussed in detail in Chapter 15.

Electrolytes

An *electrolyte* is a substance that will carry an electrical current when it is dissolved. The electrically charged particles into which it dissolves are called *ions.* Negatively charged ions are *anions,* and positively charged ones are *cations.* The number of ionic bonds per liter is expressed as milliequivalents per liter of fluid (mEq/L). For example, sodium chloride dissolves into a cation, sodium (Na^+), and an anion, chloride (Cl^-). Each ion has one ionic bond. The normal serum concentration for sodium is 135–144 mEq/L and for chloride 96–106 mEq/L. (The reason sodium concentration is higher than chloride concentration is that additional sodium exists in the serum in forms other than NaCl—for instance, as sodium bicarbonate.)

Often you will hear an electrolyte solution described in terms of its *tonicity,* that is, its osmotic pressure as compared to that of another solution, such as plasma. The tonicity of plasma is about 310 mEq/L. Tonicity is determined by adding the mEq of particles that cannot be ionized (such as urea), the mEq of those that can be but are not (such as undissolved sodium bicarbonate), and the mEq of ionized particles (anions plus cations). If the sum is within the range of 250–375 mEq/L, the solution is said to be *isotonic with plasma.* A *hypotonic* solution is less than 250 mEq/L, and a *hypertonic* one is over 375 mEq/L. The method of calculating tonicity explains why normal saline is isotonic with plasma in spite of the fact that normal saline contains more sodium and more chloride than plasma. (Isotonic saline contains 154 mEq/L each of sodium and chloride. Plasma has about 142 mEq/L of sodium and 102 mEq/L of chloride. Although plasma contains less sodium and chloride, it includes protein, urea, and other substances that add to its tonicity.)

Electrolytes are taken into the body in food and fluids. They are lost normally through sweat and urine. They also may be lost through hemorrhage, vomiting, and diarrhea.

The distribution of electrolytes varies considerably within fluid compartments and body fluids. Intracellular fluid consists primarily of potassium, phosphate, proteins, and magnesium. Extracellular fluid consists primarily of sodium, chloride, and bicarbonate.

The signs and symptoms of fluid and electrolyte imbalances also vary considerably. They are discussed under individual disorders below.

Fluid Imbalances

In attempting to understand fluid imbalances, it is important to remember the relationship between the intracellular and extracellular compartments. As mentioned earlier, the normal ratio is for one-third of total body water to be in the extracellular space and two-thirds to be in the intracellular space. Although fluid intakes or losses initially affect the extracellular space, fluid readily moves across the cell membrane.

The two primary fluid imbalances that occur are *fluid volume deficit* and *fluid volume excess*.

Fluid Volume Deficit

Information on fluid volume deficit is summarized in Table 16–2.

Signs and Symptoms An acute weight loss; decreased pulse volume, pulse pressure, and blood pressure; decreased urinary output; tachycardia; and dry skin and mucous membranes indicate the patient has a fluid volume deficit. Infants and the elderly are particularly susceptible to this condition.

If the serum sodium concentration is normal (135–144 mEq/L), isotonic fluid must have been lost from the extracellular space *(hypovolemia)*. This loss causes fluid and electrolytes to move out of the cell, so that both the extracellular and the intracellular compartments end up with volume deficits. When this occurs, the osmoreceptors in the hypothalamus stimulate ADH release and thirst, to attempt to return body fluids to normal. If water intake remains inadequate, however, this mechanism will be unable to restore normal fluid balance. Conditions that predispose to fluid volume deficit include decreased intake (anorexia, lethargy, unconsciousness); loss of electrolyte-rich secretions through blood loss, vomiting, diarrhea, fistulas, and nasogastric suction; and *third-spacing,* in which extracellular fluid moves to spaces where it is functionally inaccessible. As with any fluid or electrolyte disorder, clues from the patient's history can be invaluable in identifying the imbalance present.

TABLE 16–2   EXTRACELLULAR VOLUME DEFICIT

PREDISPOSING CONDITIONS	SIGNS AND SYMPTOMS	TREATMENT

Loss of Fluid and Electrolytes
Gastrointestinal secretion loss:
  vomiting
  diarrhea
  nasogastric suction
  fistulas
Blood loss
Burns
Profuse diaphoresis
Diuretic abuse
 	
Decreased Intake
Anorexia
Lethargy
Unconsciousness
Unavailability
 	
Third Spacing
Burns
Intestinal obstruction
Ascites
Peritoneal inflammation:
  peritonitis
  pancreatitis
	Acute weight loss
	Dry skin and mucous membrane
	Capillary filling time prolonged
	Positive postural vital signs
	Hypotension
	Skin turgor poor
	Thirst
	Laboratory data:
	  Hemoglobin
	  Hematocrit } ↑ due to hemoconcentration
	  BUN
	
	Serum osmolality ↑
	Urine specific gravity and osmolality ↑
	Urinary sodium level ↓
		Rehydration solutions
		Balanced salt solutions
		Replacement of specific losses

TABLE 16–3 EXTRACELLULAR VOLUME EXCESS

PREDISPOSING CONDITIONS	SIGNS AND SYMPTOMS	TREATMENT
Increased Ingestion or Retention of Isotonic Fluid	Acute weight gain	Restricted intake of fluid and electrolytes
Excessive infusion of intravenous fluid, especially sodium chloride	Bounding pulse	Diuretics
	Hypertension	Dialysis
Prolonged steroid therapy	Pitting edema	
Hyperaldosteronism	Jugular venous distention	
Severe congestive heart failure	Puffy face and eyelids	
Decreased Renal Excretion	Pulmonary congestion:	
Chronic renal failure	shortness of breath	
Severe stress (such as trauma, surgery)	cough	
	crackles	
	pulmonary edema	
	Laboratory data:	
	Hemoglobin and hematocrit ↓ due to hemodilution	
	Serum osmolality ↓	
	Urinary specific gravity and osmolality ↓	
	Urinary sodium ↓	

NURSING DIAGNOSIS

• Fluid volume deficit

Treatment The treatment for hypovolemia requires replacement of both fluid and electrolytes with an isotonic solution. (Of course, one must treat the cause, too. This is an obvious point and will not be belabored in the remaining discussions.)

Fluid Volume Excess

Information on this disorder is given in Table 16–3.

Signs and Symptoms Acutely increased weight; increased pulse volume, pulse pressure, and blood pressure; increased urinary output; and edema suggest that the patient has a fluid volume excess. A combination of intracellular and extracellular excesses can occur as a result of the intake of isotonic fluid.

Normal serum and urinary sodium concentrations confirm an isotonic imbalance. In this state, an increased volume of isotonic fluid in the extracellular space causes both fluid and electrolytes to move into the cell. The result is both an extracellular and an intra-

cellular volume excess. Pathologic conditions that can produce this imbalance include increased ingestion or retention of isotonic fluid (steroid therapy, severe congestive heart failure, or hyperaldosteronism), and decreased renal excretion (chronic renal failure or severe stress).

NURSING DIAGNOSIS

• Fluid volume excess

Treatment The treatment of isotonic excess is to remove both fluid and electrolytes by limiting their intake and utilizing diuretics, salt-poor albumin, or dialysis. Intravenous fluids usually are not indicated when isotonic excess is present.

Outcome Evaluation

Evaluate the patient's progress toward healthy water balance according to these outcome criteria:

• Weight WNL for patient.

• Blood pressure and pulse volume normal for patient.

- Level of consciousness and respiratory rate normal for patient.
- Skin warm, dry, and with normal turgor.
- Moist mucous membranes.
- Urinary volume WNL for patient, ideally 800–1600 ml/24 hr.
- Serum sodium normal for patient, ideally 135–145 mEq/L.
- Urinary sodium WNL for patient, ideally 50–130 mEq/L.
- Serum osmolality WNL for patient, ideally 285–295 mOsm/kg.
- Urinary osmolality WNL for patient, ideally 500–800 mOsm/kg.

Sodium Imbalances

Roles of Sodium

Sodium is the major cation of the extracellular fluid. It plays a crucial role in many body processes. Sodium has major responsibility for maintenance of normal osmolality (concentration) of body fluids. Many metabolic processes depend on sodium. It is a part of many energy-dependent cell membrane transport mechanisms (e.g., the sodium-potassium pump). Because of its function in the maintenance of transmembrane cellular potential, it also plays a major role in the transmission of electrochemical impulses and in neuromuscular conduction. Finally, through its combination with anions during sodium reabsorption in the renal tubules and through its role in the sodium/potassium/hydrogen ion exchange mechanism in the kidney, it participates in consistency of acid–base balance in the body.

The normal serum sodium level is 135–145 mEq/L. Serum sodium concentration is controlled primarily by the renal system, under the major influence of the ADH–thirst mechanism. Aldosterone has a mild effect on sodium ion concentration (Guyton 1986). Although aldosterone is a potent stimulus for sodium reabsorption, the accompanying obligatory reabsorption of water means that extracellular volume increases but relatively little change in sodium concentration occurs.

The two primary imbalances of sodium that occur are *hyponatremia* and *hypernatremia*. Differential diagnosis of sodium imbalances depends on the patient's history, the serum sodium concentration, and the urine sodium concentration. The serum sodium concentration expresses the relationship between the amount of sodium in the serum and the volume of plasma. If more water is lost than sodium, the sodium concentration rises. If more sodium is lost than water, the serum sodium concentration decreases.

Hyponatremia

Hyponatremia is defined as a serum sodium concentration of less than 135 mEq/L. There are two ways in which a patient may become hyponatremic: ingestion or retention of excess water (water intoxication), and actual loss of sodium (Table 16–4). In *water intoxication,* also known as *dilutional hyponatremia,* the patient's serum sodium has been diluted by an increase in the ratio of water to sodium. The increased proportion of water causes water to move into the cell, so the patient develops not only an *extracellular* fluid volume *excess* but also an *intracellular* fluid volume *excess*. Situations that may produce this state are: (a) excessive water ingestion, through administration of electrolyte-poor intravenous fluids, tap water enemas, or irrigation of gastric tubes with water instead of saline; (b) congestive heart failure; and (c) the syndrome of inappropriate secretion of antidiuretic hormone (SIADH).

SIADH occurs when there is uncontrolled production of ADH; that is, ADH release is not triggered by decreases in blood volume but instead occurs ectopically. SIADH may occur in a number of disorders. The most common include neurologic disease (head trauma, cranial surgery, and tumors) and pulmonary disease (tumors, severe pneumonia, and mechanical ventilation). SIADH causes dilution of blood volume due to water retention by the kidneys; however, the feedback mechanism that normally would limit ADH production does not operate, and water retention continues. Urine volume usually is concentrated due to water retention, and urine sodium is elevated, because the increased blood flow through the kidneys causes a sodium diuresis. SIADH is confirmed by comparison of serum and urine osmolalities; the serum osmolality will be considerably lower than the urine osmolality.

The other key mechanism by which hyponatremia can occur is true *loss of sodium.* A history of a low-sodium diet, diuretic use, gastrointestinal fluid losses, renal disease, or adrenal insufficiency usually is present. Because the patient has lost sodium and water, an extracellular fluid volume deficit exists. However, since the sodium loss exceeds the water loss, water tends to move into the cells. True sodium deficit thus produces an *extracellular deficit* and an *intracellular* fluid volume *excess.*

TABLE 16–4 HYPONATREMIA

PREDISPOSING CONDITIONS	SIGNS AND SYMPTOMS	MECHANISM	TREATMENT
Water Excess			
Excessive water ingestion	Fluid overload, *plus*:	Extracellular fluid excess, *plus*:	Fluid restriction
Excessive electrolyte-free IV solutions	Central nervous system:	Intracellular fluid excess (dilutional hyponatremia)	Diuretics
Excessive tap water enemas	Headache		Demeclocyline (for SIADH)
Irrigation of gastric tubes with water	Lethargy, confusion, delirium		
Congestive heart failure	Convulsions, coma		
Inappropriate ADH (SIADH)	Gastrointestinal system:		
Hyperglycemia	Nausea, vomiting, diarrhea, cramps		
	Laboratory data:		
	Serum sodium ↓		
	Urine sodium ↓ *		
	Urine specific gravity and osmolality ↓ *		
Sodium Deficit			
Low-sodium diet		Extracellular fluid deficit, *plus*:	Replacement of sodium:
Diuretics		Intracellular fluid excess	normal saline solution; hypertonic (3%) sodium chloride solution
Gastrointestinal losses:	Dehydration, *plus*:		
Severe vomiting	Central nervous and gastrointestinal systems: as above		
Diarrhea			
Nasogastric suction			
Renal disease	Laboratory data: as above		
Adrenal insufficiency			

*except SIADH

Signs and Symptoms The signs and symptoms of hyponatremia vary somewhat with the mechanism causing it. In both water intoxication and sodium loss, the patient will have signs and symptoms of cerebral edema—for instance, headache, lethargy, and confusion—and gastrointestinal symptoms. In true sodium deficit, however, signs and symptoms of dehydration also may be present.

Laboratory values include a decreased serum sodium concentration, decreased urine sodium level (except in SIADH), and decreased urine specific gravity and osmolality (except in SIADH).

Treatment The treatment of hyponatremia varies with its mechanism. Dilutional hyponatremia usually responds well to fluid restriction and diuretics. Demeclocycline (Declomycin) may be prescribed for the SIADH patient also, to block the action of ADH (Zucker and Chernow 1983). In true sodium loss, the appropriate treatment is sodium replacement, with either normal saline or, in severe depletion, hypertonic sodium chloride.

Hypernatremia

Hypernatremia, a serum sodium concentration in excess of 145 mEq/L, can occur in two ways: a *disproportionate water loss,* or a sodium excess (Table 16–5). In the first situation, the patient loses more water than sodium; as a result, serum sodium concentration increases, and the increased concentration "pulls" fluid out of the cells. This type of hypernatremia is characterized by *both extracellular and intracellular* fluid volume *deficits.* Causes

NURSING DIAGNOSES

Nursing diagnoses that may apply to the hyponatremic patient include:

- Alteration in comfort: pain
- Sensory-perceptual alteration
- Altered thought processes
- Altered bowel elimination
- Fluid volume deficit (with true sodium loss)

TABLE 16–5 HYPERNATREMIA

PREDISPOSING CONDITIONS	SIGNS AND SYMPTOMS	MECHANISM	TREATMENT

Water Loss Exceeding Sodium Loss
 Watery diarrhea
 Excessive osmotic diuresis
 Diabetes insipidus
 Fever
 Excessive dialysis
	Dehydration, *plus*:
	 Central nervous system irritability:
	   Restlessness, confusion, lethargy, stupor
	   Tremors
	   Seizures (if >160 mEq/L)
	   Coma (if >160 mEq/L)
		Extracellular fluid deficit, *plus*:
		 Intracellular fluid deficit
			Isotonic or hypotonic fluid replacement

Decreased Water Intake
 Coma
 Unavailability of water
	Laboratory data:
	   Serum sodium concentration ↑
	   Urine sodium concentration ↓
	   Urine specific gravity and osmolality ↑		

Sodium Excess Salt craving Excessive sodium bicarbonate administration Excessive steroid administration Hyperaldosteronism Renal failure Excessive sodium chloride administration	Fluid overload, *plus*: Central nervous system irritability: as above Laboratory data: as above	Extracellular fluid excess, *plus*: Intracellular fluid deficit	Restricted sodium intake Diuretics Hypotonic intravenous solutions

include water loss—for example, watery diarrhea, osmotic diuresis, and diabetes insipidus—and decreased water intake—for instance, in coma. In *sodium excess,* the patient ingests or retains more sodium than water. Examples are salt craving and excessive sodium bicarbonate administration. As the serum sodium concentration rises, water again is "pulled" out of the cells. This shift causes an *extracellular* volume *excess* in combination with an *intracellular* volume *deficit.*

Signs and Symptoms Signs and symptoms again vary somewhat with the mechanism of the hypernatremia. In both types, central nervous system irritability will be present, because the extra sodium concentration alters transmembrane electrical potential in such a way that cells become more easily excited. In addition, in water deficit, signs and symptoms of dehydration usually are present, whereas in sodium excess, signs and symptoms of fluid overload are observed.

Treatment Hypernatremia due to water loss responds to isotonic or hypotonic fluid replacement. In contrast, hypernatremia due to sodium excess is managed with restricted sodium intake, hypotonic intravenous fluids, and diuretics.

NURSING DIAGNOSES

The nursing diagnoses that may apply to patients with hypernatremia include:

- Sensory-perceptual alteration
- Altered thought processes
- Either fluid volume deficit or fluid volume excess, depending on the cause

Outcome Evaluation

Outcome criteria appropriate for the patient with a sodium imbalance include the following:

- Level of consciousness WNL for patient.
- Skin warm, dry, and with normal tugor.
- Blood pressure, pulse volume, and pulse rate WNL for patient.
- Serum sodium concentration 135–145 mEq/L.

- Serum osmolality 285–295 mOsm/kg.
- Urine sodium WNL for patient, ideally 50–130 mEq/L.
- Urine osmolality WNL for patient, ideally 500–800 mOsm/kg.

Potassium Imbalances

Roles of Potassium

Potassium is the major intracellular cation; nearly 98% of total body potassium is found inside the cells. The extracellular concentration of potassium is 3.5–5.5 mEq/L, and it is important to remember that this small extracellular concentration is not an accurate reflection of the amount of total body potassium. Although large fluctuations in *intracellular* potassium can be tolerated by the body, even small fluctuations in *serum* potassium can be toxic.

Potassium plays a number of important roles in the body. It is one of the ions responsible for maintenance of cellular transmembrane electrical balance and therefore is instrumental in normal neuromuscular transmission. It also contributes to maintenance of normal cellular osmotic pressure and to normal acid–base balance. Finally, it participates in numerous intracellular processes, including enzyme systems involved in the production of energy, synthesis of protein and glycogen, and metabolism of carbohydrates.

Potassium is absorbed from the GI tract and freely filtered at the glomerulus. Most of it is reabsorbed in the proximal tubule, with the distal tubule primarily responsible for secretion of potassium. Potassium excretion is under multiple controls, the most important of which are the sodium load delivered to the tubules, acid–base status of the body, potassium intake, and aldosterone level. The kidney does not conserve potassium effectively and urinary losses will continue even in the face of a potassium deficit.

Two imbalances of potassium exist: *hyperkalemia*, in which the serum potassium level exceeds 5.5 mEq/L, and *hypokalemia*, in which the serum potassium level is less than 3.5 mEq/L.

Hypokalemia

Conditions that increase susceptibility to hypokalemia are numerous in the critically ill. As indicated in Table 16–6, general causes are: (a) inadequate dietary intake; (b) loss of gastrointestinal secretions; (c) increased urinary loss; (d) aldosterone excess; and (e) intracellular potassium shift in alkalosis. (The interrelationships between potassium balance and acid–base balance are explained in the section of this chapter on acid–base abnormalities.)

An important role of the critical-care nurse is to prevent the development of hypokalemia. For example, consult the physician about adding potassium to the intravenous fluids of patients fasting postoperatively, particularly if they have GI suction or diarrhea. Monitor serum potassium levels of patients on potassium-wasting diuretics, especially furosemide and ethacrynic acid. Be particularly alert with patients receiving both digitalis and diuretics, since hypokalemia potentiates digitalis toxicity.

Signs and Symptoms   The signs and symptoms of potassium imbalances are easier to understand and remember if you recall the effect of potassium on the resting membrane potential. During hypokalemia, the serum deficit allows potassium to move out of the cell more easily than is normal. Since potassium has a positive charge, its loss results in increased negativity inside the cell, a condition known as *hyperpolarization*. Hyperpolarization reduces membrane excitability, making depolarization more difficult and prolonging repolarization.

On the ECG, the decreased responsiveness to stimuli may be seen as flattened T waves, prominent U waves, and prolonged PR intervals (Figure 16–1). However, these signs correlate poorly with the degree of hypokalemia. Because hypokalemia potentiates digitalis toxicity, you may see rhythms common in digitalis toxicity, such as ectopic beats and tachycardias. Ventricular asystole and fibrillation also may occur.

NURSING DIAGNOSES

Depending on the degree and effects of hypokalemia, a number of nursing diagnoses may apply. These include:

- Decreased CO
- Altered tissue perfusion
- Altered urinary elimination
- Ineffective breathing pattern
- Altered bowel elimination
- Impaired verbal communication
- Activity intolerance
- Self-care deficits
- Sensory-perceptual alteration

TABLE 16–6 POTASSIUM IMBALANCES

PREDISPOSING CONDITIONS	SIGNS AND SYMPTOMS	TREATMENT
Hypokalemia		
Inadequate dietary intake: Lethargy, anorexia, coma, postoperative fasting *Loss of gastrointestinal secretions:* Persistent vomiting, diarrhea, gastrointestinal drainage, fistulas *Increased urine output:* Diuretics, diabetic acidosis, diuretic phase of renal failure, burn diuresis *Aldosterone excess:* Severe prolonged stress, corticosteroid therapy, adrenal tumor, Cushing's disease *Intracellular shift:* Alkalosis *Hemodilution*	Flattened T waves Prominent U waves ST depression Prolonged PR interval Ventricular asystole or fibrillation Digitalis toxicity Hypoactive reflexes Paresthesias Weakness, ascending flaccid paralysis Hypotension Respiratory arrest Abdominal distention, ileus, anorexia, nausea, vomiting	Treatment of cause Increased potassium intake: foods, oral supplements, intravenous solutions Correction of alkalosis Potassium-sparing diuretics
Hyperkalemia		

Excessive intake:
Rapid IV potassium administration
 	
Cellular breakdown:
Crush injury, burns, stored bank blood transfusions
 	
Decreased urine output:
Oliguric phase of renal failure
 	
Aldosterone deficiency:
Addison's disease
 	
Extracellular shift:
Acidosis
 	
Hemoconcentration
	Tall, peaked T waves
	Decreased height of R wave
	Prolonged PR interval
	Absent P waves
	Prolonged QRS duration
	Sine waves
	Weakness
	Cramps
	Twitching
	Abdominal cramps, diarrhea
	  Later:
	Bradycardia, escape rhythms
	Ventricular asystole or fibrillation
	Paresthesias, paralysis
	Intestinal ileus
		Treatment of cause
		Limited potassium intake
		Emergency measures:
		  Sodium bicarbonate
		  Calcium chloride
		  Hypertonic glucose and insulin
		  Hemodialysis
		Nonemergency measures:
		  Ion exchange resins (e.g., Kayexalate/
		  sorbitol)
		  Peritoneal dialysis

Skeletal muscle depression appears as progressive weakness, hypoactive reflexes, paresthesias, and paralysis. Smooth muscle hypoactivity causes the gastrointestinal symptoms of distention, paralytic ileus, anorexia, nausea, and vomiting. Central nervous system signs are uncommon but may appear as drowsiness or lethargy. In the kidney, the ability to concentrate urine is lost, so polyuria, nocturia, and thirst may be present. Hypotension, due to impaired vasoconstriction, and respiratory arrest may be late findings.

Treatment Minimize the effects of hypokalemia while you assist the physician to treat the disorder. Implement the following measures:

1. Conserve the patient's energy to lessen weakness and fatigue.

2. Relieve gastrointestinal discomfort symptomatically.

3. Be prepared for emergency defibrillation, cardiac massage, and artificial respiration if the person arrests.

4. Correct alkalosis if present. Treatment may include acetazolamide. By blocking the action of carbonic anhydrase, acetazolamide increases excretion of bicarbonate and decreases the excretion of hydrogen ions. This action helps to correct the alkalosis (Gilman et al. 1985).

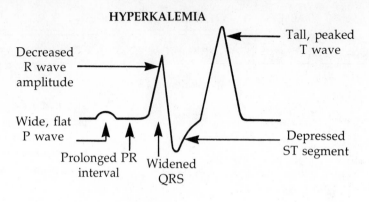

HYPERKALEMIA

Decreased R wave amplitude

Tall, peaked T wave

Wide, flat P wave

Prolonged PR interval

Widened QRS

Depressed ST segment

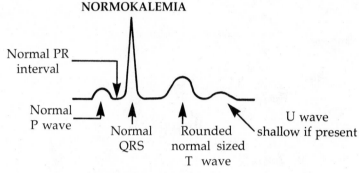

NORMOKALEMIA

Normal PR interval

Normal P wave

Normal QRS

Rounded normal sized T wave

U wave shallow if present

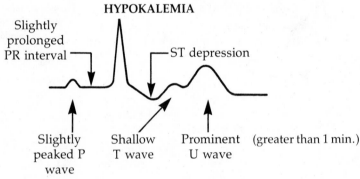

HYPOKALEMIA

Slightly prolonged PR interval

ST depression

Slightly peaked P wave

Shallow T wave

Prominent U wave

(greater than 1 min.)

FIGURE 16–1

Effects of potassium levels on ECG.

5. Increase the oral intake of potassium by giving potassium-rich foods, such as oranges, bananas, dried figs, and peaches, or oral potassium supplements if ordered. Oral potassium can produce small-bowel lesions, so alert the physician if the patient develops abdominal distention, pain, or gastrointestinal bleeding.

6. Administer intravenous potassium as ordered by the physician. Be sure that the patient has an adequate urinary output before giving increased oral or intravenous potassium; decreased renal excretion can quickly convert therapy for hypokalemia into precipitation of hyperkalemia. Dilute intravenous potassium and adminis-

ter it slowly. Rapid intravenous administration of potassium can exceed the kidney's ability to excrete a surplus, and create hyperkalemia. For this reason, do not exceed a rate of 20 mEq/hr unless the patient is on a cardiac monitor and the physician specifically orders a faster rate.

7. Teach patients, especially those to be discharged on digitalis or diuretics, the importance of eating potassium-rich foods at home, the signs and symptoms of hypokalemia, and the necessity of prompt medical attention if they appear.

Hyperkalemia

Conditions predisposing to hyperkalemia include excessive potassium intake, cellular breakdown, decreased renal excretion, aldosterone deficiency, and extracellular shift in acidosis (Table 16–6). Preventive measures that can help protect patients from hyperkalemia include assurance of adequate urinary output prior to administration of supplemental potassium and prompt treatment of acidosis. For patients with renal failure, transfusions should be performed with fresh blood; as stored blood ages, its cells break down and release potassium.

Signs and Symptoms In hyperkalemia, the excess serum potassium opposes the normal potassium leak from the cell in its resting state. As a result, the inside of the cell becomes less negative (more positive) than usual, a condition known as *hypopolarization*. Because fewer positive ions must flow in to initiate depolarization, the cell fires more easily. Action potential amplitude decreases, and repolarization is shortened. As the degree of hyperkalemia increases, however, the cell eventually has too many positive charges inside it to respond to all stimuli. Impulse formation and transmission slow and eventually cease.

Progression of hyperkalemia often is associated with specific ECG signs that correlate with serum potassium levels (Rice 1982). The earliest sign, which appears at a serum potassium level of about 6.5 mEq/L, is shortened repolarization, seen as tall, symmetrical, peaked T waves. R wave amplitude decreases and ST depression develops. Above 8 mEq/L, atrial conduction slows, producing flattened P waves and prolonged PR intervals. As hyperkalemia worsens, atrial excitability ceases and P waves disappear, although QRS complexes remain. At 10 mEq/L, the QRS complexes widen. Eventually, at 11 mEq/L, they widen so much that they merge with T waves to form sine wave configurations. This abnormality occurs because some areas of the myocardium still are undergoing depolarization while others are being repolarized. Among the dysrhythmias that may appear are blocks, bradycardia, escape rhythms, and sinus arrest. Ventricular fibrillation or asystole may occur as terminal events.

In the earlier stages of hyperkalemia, skeletal muscle excitability is manifested by weakness, cramps, and twitching. During the later stages, when cellular excitability diminishes, skeletal muscle depression produces paresthesias and ascending flaccid paralysis, and smooth muscle hypotonicity causes intestinal ileus.

Treatment Severe hyperkalemia is present when the serum potassium level exceeds 7.0 mEq/L or the

NURSING DIAGNOSES

The nursing diagnoses that may apply to a patient with hyperkalemia include:

- Decreased CO
- Altered urinary elimination pattern
- Activity intolerance
- Ineffective breathing pattern
- Altered bowel elimination
- Self-care deficits

ECG shows absent P waves, widened QRS complexes, or ventricular dysrhythmias. To relieve cardiac toxicity, potassium can be antagonized by IV administration of calcium gluconate or chloride. This treatment does not lower serum potassium, and its effects are transient, so it must be followed by sodium bicarbonate and hypertonic glucose and insulin therapy. The bicarbonate helps to correct acidosis, encouraging the return of potassium to the intracellular space. The hypertonic glucose and insulin infusion also helps move potassium intracellularly. The insulin facilitates the movement of glucose into the cell, which carries potassium along with it. Details of the measures used in emergency treatment of hyperkalemia are summarized in Table 16–7.

Lesser degrees of hyperkalemia may be treated by administration of diuretics, dialysis, or cation-exchange resins. The most commonly used resin is sodium polystyrene sulfonate (Kayexalate) given orally or by retention enema.

Outcome Evaluation

Use the following outcome criteria to gauge the patient's progress toward a healthy potassium balance:

- Serum potassium WNL for patient, ideally 3.5—5.3 mEq/L.
- Arterial blood gases WNL for patient, ideally pH 7.35–7.45, Po_2 80–100 mm Hg, Pco_2 35–45 mm Hg, and HCO_3 23–28 mEq/L.
- ECG WNL for patient, ideally with normal sinus rhythm, rounded P waves, PR interval 0.12–0.20 seconds, QRS duration of 0.06–0.10 seconds, isoelectric ST segments, and rounded T waves.
- Deep tendon reflexes, neuromuscular irritability, and muscular strength WNL for patient.
- Gastrointestinal function WNL for patient.

TABLE 16–7 EMERGENCY TREATMENT OF SEVERE HYPERKALEMIA (SERUM K$^+$ ABOVE 7.0 mEq/L AND/OR ECG SIGNS)

AGENT	ONSET	DURATION	DOSE	MECHANISM	PROBLEMS AND IMPLICATIONS
Sodium bicarbonate	5 min	1–2 hrs	1–2 amps	Promotes intracellular shift of K$^+$	Sodium intake ↑ Metabolic alkalosis Serum K$^+$ ↓ but not total body K$^+$ ↓
Calcium chloride	1–5 min	1–2 hrs	2.5–5.0 ml of 10% solution	Antagonizes effects on heart by raising threshold potential	Cardiac arrest in patients with digitalis toxicity No change in serum or total body potassium
Hypertonic glucose and insulin infusion	15 min	4–6 hrs	250–500 ml of 10% dextrose with 10–15 units of regular insulin, over 30–60 minutes	Promotes intracellular shift of K$^+$	Rebound hypoglycemia Serum K$^+$ ↓ but not total body K$^+$ ↓ Rebound hyperkalemia

Calcium Imbalances

Roles of Calcium

Calcium (Ca^{++}) is important in cellular excitability, excitation–contraction coupling, smooth muscular contractility, bone and tooth formation, blood clotting, and intracellular energy storage and use. Calcium is believed to bind with the protein linings of the sodium channels. Its positive charges theoretically block the entrance of sodium. It thus helps to establish the normal resting membrane potential, in which the cell is more negative on the inside than on the outside of the membrane. When a sufficient stimulus occurs, the calcium ions are displaced from the sarcoplasmic reticulum, and sodium enters the cell, initiating depolarization. In addition, calcium participates in both slow-channel and fast-channel depolarization of cardiac cells (Porth 1986).

Calcium also plays an important role in muscle contractility. Skeletal, cardiac, and smooth muscle all contain myofibrils of protein called actin and myosin. One current theory of contractility postulates that the actin and the myosin are inhibited from interacting in the resting state. When a stimulus causes depolarization, calcium ions are released from their storage sites (cisternae, or sacs abutting the longitudinal tubules of the sarcoplasmic reticulum). Large amounts also diffuse from the transverse tubules into the sarcoplasm. The calcium allows actin and myosin to link up in cross-bridges. The subsequent breaking and reforming of the cross-bridges pulls the actin and myosin filaments closer together, producing the muscle contraction.

In blood coagulation, calcium is thought to be essential in the formation of prothrombin activator by the intrinsic and extrinsic pathways, the conversion of prothrombin to thrombin, and the stabilization of fibrin threads. Calcium also is important for activation of the complement system, circulating proteins that augment the clotting process.

Calcium exists in several forms in the body. Most calcium (approximately 99%) is found in the bone. Because of this large reservoir, it is usually unnecessary to add calcium to routine IV solutions. The other 1% is located in tissue spaces and extracellular fluid. Extracellular calcium exists in three forms. About 45% of the total calcium is ionized. Ionized calcium is the form that is important physiologically because it can leave the capillaries and enter the cells. Approximately 50% of total calcium is nonionized and bound to plasma proteins. The remaining 5%, also nonionized, is combined with substances such as citrate, phosphate, and sulfate. Calcium can be released from the bound form and converted to the ionized form. This occurs during acidosis. Conversely, during alkalosis the binding of calcium increases and may cause a decrease in measured serum calcium. The ionized portion also varies with the level of plasma proteins. That is, as plasma proteins decrease, there usually will be a decrease in serum calcium. It is important to note, therefore, that a serum calcium of 10 mg% in the presence of a low level of serum proteins may actually indicate hypercalcemia (McFadden and Zaloga 1983).

Calcium is absorbed from foods in the presence of normal gastric acidity and vitamin D. About 87% of calcium excretion is via the feces and the remainder is in the urine. The serum calcium is controlled by two feedback loops, one involving parathyroid hormone and the other involving calcitonin. (The parathyroid glands also control the serum phosphorous level inversely with calcium.) When ionized serum calcium drops, the glands secrete increased parathyroid hormone. This hormone causes increased calcium absorption from the gastrointestinal tract, increased calcium reabsorption from the renal tubule, and resorption (release) from bone. The

resulting rise in calcium ion concentration feeds back to lower parathyroid hormone secretion. This control mechanism is slow, taking hours to days to function. When ionized calcium rises excessively, the thyroid gland secretes calcitonin. This substance acts quickly and briefly to inhibit calcium reabsorption from bone. Acute changes in serum calcium also are buffered by the easily exchangeable calcium in the bones and some mitochondria.

Hypocalcemia

The normal total serum calcium level is 8.5–10.8 mg%. A deficit of calcium is called *hypocalcemia*. Information on this condition is summarized in Table 16–8.

Be alert for conditions that can lead to hypocalcemia.

TABLE 16–8 CALCIUM IMBALANCES

PREDISPOSING CONDITIONS	SIGNS AND SYMPTOMS	TREATMENT
Hypocalcemia		
Decreased calcium absorption: Vitamin D deficit, hypoparathyroidism	Irritability	Seizure precautions
Decreased ionization of calcium: Alkalosis	Convulsions	CO_2 rebreathing
Immobilization of calcium in inflamed tissues: Massive subcutaneous infection, generalized peritonitis	Numbness and tingling of the extremities	Possible emergency tracheotomy
Increased gastrointestinal loss: Diarrhea, acute pancreatitis	Circumoral tingling	Calcium administration: intravenous, oral, dietary
Increased urinary loss: Diuretic phase of renal failure	Hyperactive deep tendon reflexes	Treatment of cause
Increased calcium binding: Massive transfusions of citrated blood	Twitching	
	Muscular cramps	
	Diarrhea, nausea, vomiting	
	Positive Chvostek's sign	
	Positive Trousseau's sign	
	Carpopedal spasms	
	Generalized tetany	
	Prolonged QT interval	
	Bronchospasm	
Hypercalcemia		
Increased calcium intake: Vitamin D excess, hyperparathyroidism	Lethargy	Saline solutions
Decreased urinary loss: Oliguric phase of renal failure	Coma	Diuretics
Increased ionization: Acidosis	Constipation, nausea, vomiting	Sodium bicarbonate
Increased reabsorption from bone: Prolonged immobilization	Hypoactive deep tendon reflexes	Phosphate administration
Malignant tumors (with or without metastasis to bone)	Weakness	Mithramycin
	Shortened QT interval	Dialysis
	Bradycardia, heart blocks	Reduced digitalis doses
	Digitalis toxicity	Acidification of urine
	Polyuria, thirst, dehydration	Treatment of cause
	Renal calculi, flank pain	
	Deep bone pain, pathologic fractures	

It occurs in conditions characterized by decreased calcium absorption, decreased calcium ionization, or increased calcium losses.

Signs and Symptoms Watch for the signs and symptoms of hypocalcemia. As with potassium imbalances, these are easier to remember if you understand the roles calcium plays in the body.

A calcium deficit (hypocalcemia) increases neuronal membrane permeability and allows sodium to enter the cell more easily than usual, facilitating spontaneous depolarization. Although this effect occurs in both the central and peripheral nervous systems, most manifestations appear peripherally. Central nervous system manifestations include irritability and convulsions. Early peripheral nervous system signs are numbness and tingling of the extremities, circumoral tingling, hyperactive reflexes, twitching, and muscular cramps. Smooth muscle hyperactivity may cause diarrhea, nausea, and vomiting.

Spasmodic muscular contractions (tetany) also may occur. At first, tetany may not be apparent unless you add another stimulus to depolarization, such as tapping the nerve or causing ischemia, or unless hyperventilation worsens the hypocalcemia by reducing calcium ionization. If you tap the facial nerve just below the temporal bone anterior to the ear, the facial muscles on that side of the head may twitch. This result is called a *positive Chvostek's sign*. Similarly, you can apply a blood pressure cuff to the arm and raise its pressure slightly above the patient's systolic level. If the hand folds in, *carpal spasm* (tetany of the hand) is present. This spasm following pressure on the nerves and vessels of the upper arm is known as a *positive Trousseau's sign* and is indicative of latent tetany. As hypocalcemia progresses to approximately 6 mg%, tetany will appear even without added stimuli. Tetany usually is fatal at about 4 mg% (Guyton 1986).

Prolonged ventricular systole is seen on the ECG as a prolonged QT interval. Hypocalcemia theoretically causes dysrhythmias, diminished cardiac contractility, and bleeding due to inadequate clotting. In reality, however, death from tetany usually occurs first.

Treatment Prevent complications of hypocalcemia while you assist the physician in treating it. Implement these measures:

1. Minimize the likelihood and effects of seizures by reducing environmental stimuli and placing the patient on seizure precautions.

2. Be prepared to assist with an emergency tracheotomy if laryngospasm occurs.

3. Administer calcium chloride, gluconate, or gluceptate as ordered by the physician. Do not add calcium to intravenous solutions containing bicarbonate or phosphate; it will precipitate. 5% dextrose is a better diluent than normal saline, because saline can further calcium loss (McFadden and Zaloga 1983).

4. Implement medical orders aimed at removing the cause of the calcium deficit.

Hypercalcemia

A calcium excess is called *hypercalcemia*. Information on this disorder is presented in Table 16–8. Conditions that predispose to hypercalcemia include increased calcium intake, acidosis, increased bone reabsorption, and malignant tumors.

Signs and Symptoms A calcium excess diminishes neuromuscular excitability theoretically because the extra calcium in the cellular pores repels sodium. Decreased excitability of the central nervous system is seen as lethargy or coma. Gastrointestinal signs include constipation, nausea, and vomiting. The skeletal muscles display hypoactive deep tendon reflexes and weakness. The ECG shows a shortened QT interval, indicative of a shortened ventricular systole. Decreased impulse formation and conduction may appear as bradycardia or heart blocks. Since hypercalcemia potentiates the effects of digitalis, rhythms of digitalis toxicity may occur. Because hypercalcemia impairs glomerular filtration and the kidneys' ability to concentrate urine, polyuria occurs and leads to thirst and dehydration. Renal calculi and flank pain also may appear. In hyperparathyroidism, increased parathyroid hormone causes excessive calcium resorption from the bones, and deep bone pain and pathologic fractures may occur. The effects of hypercalcemia begin at approximately 12 mg% and worsen as the level rises. Near 17 mg%, calcium precipitates in the body tissues themselves (McFadden and Zaloga 1983).

NURSING DIAGNOSES

Nursing diagnoses that may apply to the patient with hypocalcemia include:

- Alterations in comfort: pain
- Altered thought processes
- Sensory-perceptual alterations
- Altered bowel elimination

Treatment For hypercalcemia, include these interventions:

1. Maintain ambulation or active or passive exercises to minimize bone cavitation. Avoid rough handling or trauma, which increase bone pain and can induce pathologic fractures.

2. Record intake and output. Because hypercalcemia impairs the kidney's ability to concentrate urine, urinary output will be high. Be sure intake is at least 1000 ml over output to prevent dehydration.

3. Encourage a fluid intake of at least 4000 ml daily to minimize possible precipitation of calcium as renal calculi. Maintain an acid urine by encouraging the intake of foods that acidify urine (such as cranberry juice) and by preventing urinary infections, which alkalinize the urine.

4. Strain all urine for renal calculi.

5. For patients on digitalis preparations, observe closely for signs of digitalis intoxication. Ask the physician about reducing digitalis doses.

6. Restrict dietary calcium.

7. Administer pharmacologic agents as ordered. These may include calcitonin and mithramycin if the cause is bone resorption.

8. Administer intravenous or oral phosphate if ordered by the physician to increase calcium excretion.

9. Administer sodium chloride and furosemide as ordered to cause diuresis and calciuresis.

Outcome Evaluation

Evaluate the patient's progress toward restoration of normal calcium balance according to the following outcome criteria.

- Serum calcium level 8.5–10.8 mg%.

- Normal deep tendon reflexes, muscular strength, and irritability (for example, negative Chvostek's sign and Trousseau's sign; no carpopedal spasms or other signs of tetany).

- Gastrointestinal function and urinary output normal for patient.

- Signs or symptoms of deep bone pain, renal calculi, or pathologic fractures absent or controlled by therapy

Magnesium Imbalances

Roles of Magnesium

Magnesium is an essential catalyst for many important enzyme systems, especially those involved with carbohydrate metabolism and protein synthesis. It also is instrumental in the maintenance of normal ionic balance, osmotic pressure, neuromuscular transmission, and bone metabolism.

Magnesium is primarily an intracellular cation; a small amount (1.5–2 mEq/L) is found extracellularly. About half of the body's total is found in bones, with the remainder in muscles, soft tissues, and body fluids. Magnesium must be ingested daily. The body's requirement usually is met through eating chlorophyll-containing vegetables, meat, milk, and fruits. Extracellular magnesium concentration is regulated by the kidneys, though the mechanism is unclear.

Hypomagnesemia and Hypermagnesemia

Information on these conditions is summarized in Table 16–9. Be aware of conditions that increase the patient's susceptibility to these disorders. Conditions disposing to magnesium depletion are those characterized by decreased intake or absorption and those resulting from increased urinary excretion. States predisposing to magnesium intoxication are less frequent: excessive parenteral administration and oliguric renal failure.

Take measures to prevent magnesium imbalances. To avoid hypomagnesemia, encourage patients on oral intake to eat magnesium-containing foods. Ask the physician about magnesium supplements for alcoholic or malnourished patients, those suffering from excessive

TABLE 16–9 MAGNESIUM IMBALANCES

PREDISPOSING CONDITIONS	SIGNS AND SYMPTOMS	TREATMENT
Hypomagnesemia		
Decreased intake or absorption: malnutrition, severe diarrhea, alcoholism	Twitches	Increased intake of magnesium-rich foods (chlorophyll-containing vegetables, meat, milk, fruits)
Increased urinary loss: diuretic phase of renal failure, diuretics, alcoholism	Muscle cramps	Magnesium supplementation (oral or intravenous)
	Positive Chvostek's and Trousseau's signs	Treatment of cause
Hyperaldosteronism	Convulsions	
Hyperparathyroidism	Tetany	
Hypermagnesemia		
Decreased urinary excretion: oliguric phase of renal failure	Flushing	Decreased intake of magnesium-rich foods
Excessive parenteral administration	Tachycardia leading to bradycardia	Use of nonmagnesium antacids
	Prolonged PR interval	Slowing or discontinuation of parenteral magnesium
	Prolonged QRS	Intravenous calcium
	Drowsiness	Diuretics
	Loss of deep tendon reflexes	Dialysis
	Weakness	
	Coma	
	Cardiorespiratory arrest	

diarrhea or diuresis, and those receiving total parenteral nutrition.

To forestall hypermagnesemia, do not give drugs containing magnesium (such as antacids containing magnesium hydroxide) to patients in oliguric renal failure. When administering magnesium sulfate intravenously, do not exceed the rate recommended by the physician and watch for the signs of magnesium intoxication.

Signs and Symptoms Recognize the signs of magnesium disorders. Magnesium depletion causes increased neuronal excitability and neuromuscular conduction, and produces signs and symptoms similar to those of hypocalcemia. At a serum concentration of 1 mEq/L or less, you may see twitches, muscle cramps, convulsions, or tetany. There are no diagnostic ECG signs.

Magnesium intoxication is rare and usually related to a decrease in renal function or abuse of magnesium sulfate as a cathartic. Excess will depress neuronal excitability and neuromuscular transmission. During hypermagnesemia, peripheral vasodilatation produces flushing. Tachycardia appears initially due to hypotension, and later changes to bradycardia. Although ECG signs are not diagnostic of this disorder, you may observe certain changes including prolonged PR intervals and longer QRS durations. Drowsiness, loss of deep tendon reflexes, and weakness occur between 5–10

mEq/L; above 10 mEq/L, coma and finally cardiorespiratory arrest ensue (Porth 1986).

Treatment If signs of magnesium imbalances appear, notify the physician. Magnesium depletion is treated by correcting the underlying disorder and/or administering magnesium supplements. Magnesium intoxication is treated by slowing or discontinuing the administration of magnesium-containing drugs, by diuretics, and by dialysis. When appropriate to the patient's condition, teach ways to prevent the reoccurrence of magnesium depletion or intoxication. For instance, provide the renal failure patient with the names of antacids that do not contain magnesium.

Outcome Evaluation

Use these outcome criteria to evaluate the patient's progress.

- Serum magnesium level 1.5–2 mEq/L.
- Normal neuromuscular excitability and deep tendon reflexes.
- Spontaneous respirations, at rate normal for patient.

- ECG within patient's normal limits.
- Magnesium-depleted patient verbalizes knowledge of foods containing magnesium, awareness of importance of eating such, and ability to purchase them at home.
- Magnesium-intoxicated (oliguric renal failure) patient states intention to avoid magnesium hydroxide and names acceptable alternative antacids.

ACID–BASE IMBALANCES

Assessment

Acid–base imbalances are ubiquitous in the critically ill. Their causes, signs, and symptoms can be subtle and confusing. A hasty or simplistic interpretation of arterial blood gas values can cause you to identify acid–base disorders incorrectly. It is essential that you develop a systematic method to detect these imbalances and that you interpret blood gas values only in the context of the clinical situation.

The approach recommended in this chapter is a clinically useful one. This approach consists of the following steps:

1. Consider the patient's history, noting conditions that predispose to imbalances.
2. Next, note signs and symptoms suggesting acid–base imbalances.
3. Then, interpret the blood gases.

In order to utilize this approach, you must have a sound understanding of normal acid–base physiology as well as acid–base pathophysiology. Accordingly, the first portion of this assessment section is devoted to a review of key concepts in acid–base physiology.

Key Physiologic Concepts

Acids, Bases, and pH An *acid* is a substance that can release a hydrogen ion (H^+) when it dissociates; a *base* is a substance that can accept a hydrogen ion. Clinically, the H^+ concentration is expressed as pH. Since pH is the negative logarithm of the H^+ concentration, pH and H^+ concentration are related inversely. In other words, as H^+ concentration rises, pH falls; a low pH thus indicates the blood is more acid than normal. Similarly, a high pH indicates the blood is less acid (more alkaline) than normal.

Human metabolic processes produce several acids. The Krebs cycle, the major source of cellular energy, forms carbon dioxide and water as end products. Carbon dioxide and water combine to form carbonic acid (H_2CO_3), which is the most plentiful body acid. Because carbon dioxide can be excreted as a gas, it is sometimes referred to as a *volatile,* or respiratory, acid. Other less plentiful body acids, such as sulfuric acid and phosphoric acid, are breakdown products released by the metabolism of proteins or fats for energy or by other body processes. Because they cannot be excreted as a gas but instead must be excreted in water, they are called *nonvolatile, fixed,* or *metabolic* acids. Other metabolic acids are lactic acid, formed by anaerobic metabolism when tissues are hypoxic, and keto acids, commonly the result of metabolic pathways used when insulin is lacking.

The primary base in our bodies is bicarbonate. Lesser bases include forms of hemoglobin, protein, and phosphate.

To maintain the various life processes, human cells can tolerate only minor deviations in the concentration of hydrogen ions. Three primary systems interact to maintain the pH range most suitable for cellular processes. These systems are the chemical buffers in body fluids; the lungs; and the kidneys.

Chemical Buffers A chemical buffer consists of a weak acid and its salt. Chemical buffers are important because they are the body's first line of defense against an acid–base imbalance. When excessive acid or base is present, the chemical buffer system combines with it immediately, thus preventing pronounced changes in H^+ concentration.

There are four major chemical buffers in the body fluids, of which the most important are the bicarbonate/carbonic acid system in plasma and red blood cells. Other important buffers include the oxyhemoglobin/reduced oxyhemoglobin system (in red blood cells), the plasma protein system, and the phosphate system.

A variety of bicarbonate salts participates in the carbonic acid/bicarbonate system. Extracellularly, sodium bicarbonate is most important. Lesser salts in the extracellular fluid and those present in the intracellular fluid are potassium bicarbonate, calcium bicarbonate, and magnesium bicarbonate.

Carbonic Acid/Bicarbonate Buffer System As mentioned previously, carbonic acid is formed from carbon dioxide and water. It tends to dissociate into its ions: hydrogen and bicarbonate. This system can be expressed as follows:

$$H^+ + HCO_3^- \rightleftharpoons H_2CO_3 \rightleftharpoons CO_2 + H_2O$$

An important expression of this balance is the Henderson-Hasselbach equation. This equation states that the pH equals the sum of a constant value (pK) plus the logarithm of the ratio of bicarbonate to carbonic acid:

$$pH = pK + \log \frac{HCO_3^- \text{ (mEq/L)}}{H_2CO_3 \text{ (mEq/L)}}$$

Carbonic acid is a weak acid and dissociates readily. Since carbonic acid exists in the body mostly as CO_2 gas, you can substitute a P_{CO_2} value in the denominator of the equation. Clinically, P_{CO_2} is measured in mm Hg; to convert that value to mEq/L, multiply by 0.03.

$$pH = pK + \log \frac{HCO_3^- \text{ (mEq/L)}}{P_{CO_2} \text{ (mm Hg)} \times 0.03}$$

The normal ratio between bicarbonate and carbonic acid is 20:1. Since the log of this value is 1.3 and the pK equals 6.1, their sum gives the value of 7.4 as the normal pH. The normal range is considered to be 7.35–7.45. It is essential to remember that the pH is determined by the *ratio* between the two values rather than the absolute amount of HCO_3^- or carbonic acid. This fact has great clinical importance as shown later.

Respiratory Buffer System When the chemical buffers are unable to maintain balance, the respiratory and renal buffer systems come into play to control the concentrations of CO_2 and HCO_3^-, respectively.

The respiratory buffer system responds to an imbalance within minutes to hours. This system controls the level of CO_2 in the blood, and therefore the level of carbonic acid. When carbonic acid increases, the lungs increase their excretion of CO_2 gas by increasing the rate and depth of ventilation. If the body needs more acid, the lungs can decrease ventilation, thereby retaining CO_2 and increasing the amount of carbonic acid.

Renal Buffer System The renal buffer system responds slowly (within hours to days) but powerfully to an acid–base imbalance. It affects pH primarily by controlling the concentration of bicarbonate ion in the extracellular fluid. It also excretes fixed acids (which the lungs cannot eliminate).

Bicarbonate is filtered freely at the glomerulus and "reabsorbed" in the proximal and distal tubules, collecting ducts, and thick part of the loops of Henle; in addition, the kidney has two important systems for creating new bicarbonate and at the same time excreting hydrogen ions: the ammonia buffer system and the phosphate buffer system (Figure 16–2).

Classification of Acid–Base Imbalances

Acidosis and Alkalosis The classification of acid–base abnormalities can be confusing, so the basic terms will be reviewed. Two general processes can cause the pH to deviate from normal: an acidosis or alkalosis. An *acidosis* is a process that causes *acidemia,* a state in which the blood is more acid than normal. An *alkalosis* is a process that causes *alkalemia,* a state in which the blood is more alkaline (less acidic) than normal. Information about acidoses and alkaloses is shown in Tables 16–10, 16–11, and 16–12 and discussed in the remainder of the chapter.

Overview of Imbalances

The patient's history can provide valuable information in identifying acid–base disorders. Tables 16–10, 16–11, and 16–12 give examples of significant conditions to note when reviewing the patient's history. The following paragraphs relate the types of acid–base disorders to predisposing conditions.

Single Disorders An *acidosis* is present when there is an *acid excess or a base deficit* in the body, causing the blood's pH to be below 7.35. The acid excess can be a carbonic acid excess (in which case the condition is called *respiratory acidosis*) or a metabolic acid excess *(metabolic acidosis).* A base deficit can occur only from metabolic causes, such as the loss of alkaline fluids via a fistula of the lower gastrointestinal tract.

An *alkalosis* is present when there is either an *acid deficit or a base excess* in the body, causing the pH to be above 7.45. The acid deficit can be a carbonic acid deficit *(respiratory alkalosis)* or a metabolic acid deficit *(metaolic alkalosis).* A base excess can occur only from metabolic causes (such as increased bicarbonate retention because of a chloride deficit) or from an exogenous source—for example, excessive infusion of sodium bicarbonate.

Respiratory acidosis, metabolic acidosis, respiratory alkalosis, and metabolic alkalosis are the four single acid–base disorders.

Compensation When a single disorder first occurs, it will cause an abnormal pH and also an abnormal value

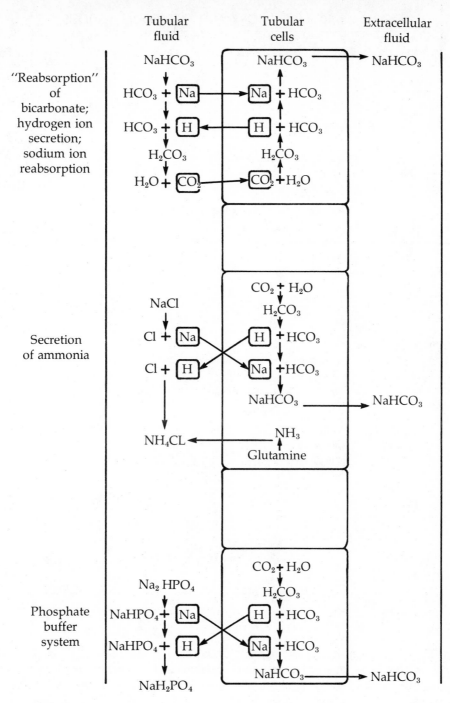

FIGURE 16–2

Renal mechanisms for reabsorbing and creating bicarbonate.

for the parameter associated with the system causing the imbalance. For instance, a respiratory acidosis causes an abnormal increase in P_{CO_2} and a resultant decrease in pH. The other value (in this case, HCO_3^-) will be normal initially. At this point, the disorder is called

acute or *uncompensated*. As time goes on, the system not causing the problem will try to compensate for it by altering its parameter to return the ratio of bicarbonate/carbonic acid to the normal 20:1; in this example, the kidney will retain bicarbonate. If the alteration *is not*

TABLE 16–10 RESPIRATORY AND METABOLIC ACIDOSIS

PREDISPOSING CONDITIONS	SIGNS AND SYMPTOMS	TREATMENT
Respiratory Acidosis		
Carbon Dioxide Retention		
Bronchial obstruction, chronic obstructive pulmonary disease	Hypoventilation (primary)	None (if compensated in chronic pulmonary disease)
Inadequate mechanical ventilation	Headache	Treatment of cause
Central nervous system depression (example: narcotic poisoning)	Restlessness, apprehension	Increased CO_2 elimination (by suctioning, aggressive pulmonary hygiene, or mechanical ventilation [cautiously to avoid alkalosis])
Neuromuscular disorders affecting respiration (example: poliomyelitis)	Drowsiness, confusion, coma	
	Acute respiratory failure	
	Hyperkalemia (peaked T waves, twitching, etc.)	Bicarbonate replacement
	Hypercalcemia (weakness, lethargy, flapping tremors, etc.)	Treatment of electrolyte imbalances
	Blood gas changes: pH ↓ P_{CO_2} ↑ HCO_3 normal or ↑	
Metabolic Acidosis		
Excessive Metabolic Acids		
Starvation	Hyperventilation (compensatory)	Treatment of cause
Diabetic ketoacidosis	Headache	Bicarbonate replacement
Lactic acidosis	Drowsiness, confusion, coma	Treatment of electrolyte imbalances
Renal failure	Nausea, vomiting	
Hyperkalemia	Hyperkalemia	
	Hypercalcemia	
	Blood gas changes: pH ↓ HCO_3 ↓ P_{CO_2} normal or ↓	
Loss of Alkali		
Diarrhea		
Fistulas of lower gastrointestinal tract		
Chloride excess		

sufficient to return the pH to normal, the disorder is *partially compensated*. At this point, the pH, P_{CO_2} and HCO_3^- all will be abnormal. If the alteration *is* sufficient to restore a more normal ratio and hence a normal pH, the condition is called *chronic* or *fully compensated*. In this stage, the pH will be normal but both the P_{CO_2} and HCO_3^- values still will be abnormal. Although their ratio will cause the pH to be within the normal range, the pH usually will tend more toward the acidic or alkaline end of the range, depending on the primary process.

In general, the pulmonary and renal systems compensate for each other. The renal system compensates for respiratory disorders by altering bicarbonate retention and hydrogen ion secretion. In respiratory acidosis,

the kidneys compensate by increasing bicarbonate retention and accelerating hydrogen secretion. In respiratory alkalosis, the kidneys decrease bicarbonate retention and hydrogen secretion.

The lungs compensate for metabolic acid–base imbalances by varying CO_2 excretion. In metabolic acidosis, stimulation of the respiratory center increases the rate and depth of ventilation, so increased CO_2 is blown off. This compensation is limited, however: a falling P_{CO_2} eventually causes respiratory depression, returning P_{CO_2} toward normal. In metabolic alkalosis, the lungs decrease ventilation and therefore retain CO_2. Respiratory compensation for metabolic alkalosis also is limited, however. At a P_{CO_2} of about 60 mm Hg in most

TABLE 16–11 RESPIRATORY AND METABOLIC ALKALOSIS

PREDISPOSING CONDITIONS	SIGNS AND SYMPTOMS	TREATMENT
Respiratory Alkalosis		
Increased CO₂ Excretion		
Hypoxia	Hyperventilation (primary)	Treatment of cause
Excessive mechanical ventilation	Giddiness, dizziness, syncope, convulsions, coma	Increased CO_2 retention (by decreased mechanical ventilation, breathing into paper bag, sedation, or 3–5% CO_2 administration)
Central nervous system stimulation (examples: pain, anxiety, hysteria, brainstem damage)	Hypokalemia (weakness, paresthesias, etc.)	Treatment of electrolyte imbalances
	Hypocalcemia (tingling, numbness, twitching, carpopedal spasms, tetany, convulsions, etc.)	
	Cardiac dysrhythmias	

	Blood gas changes:
	    pH ↑
	    P_{CO_2} ↓
	    HCO_3 normal or ↓	

Metabolic Alkalosis		
Loss of Metabolic Acids		
Nasogastric drainage	Hypoventilation (compensatory)	Treatment of cause
Vomiting	Hypokalemia	Increased H^+ retention (by administration of KCl)
Hypokalemia	Hypocalcemia	Increased bicarbonate excretion (by administration of acetazolamide (Diamox), ammonium chloride, or arginine hydrochloride)
Steroid administration	Cardiac dysrhythmias	

	Blood gas changes:
	    pH ↑
	    HCO_3 ↑
	    P_{CO_2} normal or ↑
		Dialysis

		Treatment of electrolyte imbalances
Excessive Intake or Retention of Alkali		
Excessive sodium bicarbonate administration		

Chloride depletion:
    Diuretics
    Low-salt diet without chloride supplementation		

people, the hypoxic stimulus to respiration becomes dominant. This stimulus causes ventilation to increase toward normal.

As mentioned earlier, the lungs respond to acid–base imbalances within minutes, while the kidneys take hours. As a result, compensation for metabolic imbalances occurs faster than compensation for respiratory imbalances.

Mixed Disorders   If two single disorders occur simultaneously, the patient suffers from a *mixed disorder (mixed disturbance)*. There are four mixed disturbances (Table 16–12). Mixed disturbances result from either two processes with similar effects on the pH (such as respiratory and metabolic acidosis in cardiac arrest) or

two processes with opposite effects on the pH (such as respiratory acidosis and metabolic alkalosis in the patient with chronic lung disease who is on diuretics).

Signs and Symptoms

Assess the patient for the clinical signs and symptoms of acid–base imbalances as described in the following sections.

Altered Level of Consciousness   Cerebral status changes result from alterations in cerebrospinal fluid pH. Confusion and coma often are present in acidosis, while dizziness and giddiness are more characteristic of

TABLE 16–12 MIXED DISORDERS

COMBINATION	EXAMPLES	MECHANISMS
Mixed acidoses	Cardiac arrest Severe hypoventilation	Absent ventilation or hypoventilation → respiratory acidosis Hypoxemia → anaerobic metabolism → metabolic (lactic) acidosis
Mixed alkaloses	Patient with compensated respiratory acidosis rapidly and excessively mechanically ventilated	Elevated bicarbonate level → metabolic alkalosis Hyperventilation → respiratory alkalosis
Respiratory acidosis and metabolic alkalosis	Chronic obstructive pulmonary disease plus diuretics or low-salt diet without chloride replacement	COPD → respiratory acidosis Chloride depletion → obligatory bicarbonate retention → metabolic alkalosis
Respiratory alkalosis and metabolic acidosis	Hepatic and renal failure	Liver failure → toxic metabolites → hyperventilation → respiratory alkalosis Kidney failure → ↓ H^+ excretion and ↓ bicarbonate production → metabolic acidosis

alkalosis. Because CO_2 crosses the blood-brain barrier more quickly than HCO_3^- ions, these symptoms occur sooner in respiratory disorders than metabolic ones.

Assess cerebral status by checking orientation to day, time, and location; ability to follow simple commands; and presence of dizziness or lightheadedness.

Ineffective Breathing Pattern Evaluation of ventilatory changes can be confusing, since they may either cause or compensate for acid–base imbalances. Hyperventilation can cause respiratory alkalosis or compensate for metabolic acidosis, in each case by increasing CO_2 elimination. Hypoventilation can cause respiratory acidosis or compensate for metabolic alkalosis, in each case by increasing CO_2 retention. Acid–base imbalances affect the respiratory center by altering the pH of arterial blood and cerebrospinal fluid. Acidosis lowers the pH, stimulates the respiratory center, and produces hyperventilation. Alkalosis raises cerebrospinal fluid pH and produces hypoventilation. To detect hypoventilation or hyperventilation, evaluate the rate and depth of respiration. Because only gross changes in depth of respiration are detectable on physical examination, use a spirometer to check the tidal volume.

Respiratory failure may occur in acute respiratory acidosis when the P_{CO_2} reaches 60 mm Hg. A patient with chronic hypercapnia, however, may tolerate a P_{CO_2} above 60 mm Hg without developing acute respiratory failure. Because the slow development of hypercapnia has allowed time for the kidneys to increase the serum bicarbonate level in compensation, the chronic patient can maintain a more normal pH than an acutely afflicted person.

Impaired Gas Exchange or Tissue Perfusion Dysrhythmias, angina, or shock may result from hypoxia or from the electrolyte imbalances discussed later. Both acidosis and alkalosis cause shifts of the oxyhemoglobin dissociation curve. In alkalosis, the curve shifts to the left, causing decreased dissociation of oxygen from hemoglobin. This effect contributes to tissue hypoxia. Acidosis causes the curve to shift to the right, so that oxygen is released more readily from hemoglobin. However, acidosis also causes decreased responsiveness to catecholamines, which in turn can cause decreased myocardial contractility and arteriolar dilatation. As a result, less efficient circulation of the blood may counterbalance the increased availability of oxygen in the blood.

To detect dysrhythmias, angina, or shock, implement the following measures. Auscultate the apical pulse for irregularities and the presence of gallops or murmurs. Monitor the electrocardiogram for signs of new or increasing atrial or ventricular dysrhythmias. Also monitor perfusion to the brain, heart, kidneys, and extremities.

Arterial Blood Gas Analysis

Definitive diagnosis of acid–base imbalances depends on arterial blood gas values. The values important in acid–base interpretation are the pH, P_{CO_2}, and a measure of base (HCO_3^- or base excess). Base excess is the preferred measure of base, because it measures both bicarbonate and other buffer anions of whole blood, such as those of hemoglobin and plasma proteins. Base excess reflects only metabolic activity. (It is reported as base mEq/L above or below the normal range of buffer base. Thus, a negative base excess actually means a base deficit.) When evaluating a patient's blood gases, always compare the reported values to the normals for your institution. Also compare them to the actual or expected normal values for your patient, as indicated by previous measurements or pre-existing conditions such as chronic obstructive pulmonary disease.

pH   First evaluate the general acid–base status by examining the pH. The normal range is 7.35–7.45. If the value is lower than normal (below 7.35), an acidosis is present. If the value is elevated (above 7.45), an alkalosis is present. If the value is within the normal range, there are two possibilities: The patient could have a normal balance or an abnormal process that is compensated. Since you cannot tell which situation exists from examining the pH alone, just note at this point whether the value is normal and, if so, whether it falls more toward the acid side of the normal range or more toward the alkaline side.

Pco_2   Evaluate the respiratory parameter by examining the Pco_2. The normal range is 35–45 mm Hg. Decide whether the value is normal, elevated above 45 and therefore tending to make the blood acidic, or decreased below 35 and therefore tending to make the blood alkaline.

HCO_3^- or Base Excess   Evaluate the renal parameter by examining the HCO_3^- or base excess. Normal ranges are 23–28 mEq/L for HCO_3^- and $+2.5$ to -2.5 for base excess. Decide whether the value is normal, elevated and therefore tending to make blood alkaline, or decreased and therefore tending to make the blood acidic. (For the sake of simplicity, only one measure of base is given in the following examples.)

Next, compare the pH, Pco_2, and base value to each other. Since blood gas values can indicate a variety of disorders and stages of compensation, a given set of numbers may be compatible with more than one interpretation. Explain *each* value, considering *all* the possible interpretations.

After considering the possible interpretations of the values, choose the most probable one for your patient, based on the clues from the other patient data and the likelihood of a given disorder.

Following are principles and examples illustrating interpretation of acid–base values.

Abnormal pH and Abnormal Pco_2 or HCO_3^-   If only the pH and one other value are abnormal, the blood

gases indicate a single uncompensated disorder. You can identify the disorder by deciding which process the pH represents and which other value (the Pco_2 or HCO_3^-) is abnormal. For example:

pH   7.32
Pco_2 50 mm Hg
HCO_3^- 24 mEq/L

The pH is decreased, so it tells you that an acidosis is present. The HCO_3^- is normal, so a metabolic problem cannot be the cause. The Pco_2 is elevated, making the blood more acidic. The values thus indicate an acute respiratory acidosis.

Note that in this example that the pH and Pco_2 are changing in *opposite* directions. This example thus illustrates one of two *rules of thumb* that can help you to identify quickly the type of disturbance present:

1. *If the pH and Pco_2 are changing in opposite directions, a respiratory disorder is present.*

2. *If the pH and HCO_3^- are changing in the same direction, a metabolic disorder is present.*

Abnormal pH, Abnormal Pco_2, and Abnormal HCO_3^-   If all three values are abnormal, they often indicate a single disorder with incomplete compensation. For example:

pH   7.30
Pco_2 25 mm Hg
HCO_3^- 12 mEq/L

The pH is decreased, again telling you that an acidosis is present. The Pco_2 is decreased, tending to make the blood alkaline. The HCO_3^- is decreased, tending to make the blood acidic. As the pH and HCO_3^- are changing in the *same* direction, a metabolic disorder is present (second *rule of thumb*). The Pco_2 is decreased because the body is attempting to compensate for the disorder, but as the pH is still abnormal, only partial compensation is present. The values thus indicate partially compensated metabolic acidosis.

Note that in this example, the Pco_2 and HCO_3 are changing in the *same* direction. This example illustrates a third *rule of thumb*.

3. *If the Pco_2 and HCO_3^- are changing in the same direction, the body is compensating for an imbalance.* (In this case, as the pH still is abnormal, the imbalance is only partially compensated.)

Normal pH, Abnormal Pco_2, and Abnormal HCO_3^-   If the pH is normal but both the Pco_2 and HCO_3^- are not, the values usually indicate a fully compensated single disturbance. Determining whether the pH lies more toward the acid or alkaline end of the normal range will help you decide whether the imbalance is an acidosis or alkalosis. For example:

pH   7.42
P_{CO_2} 50 mm Hg
HCO_3^- 32 mm Eq/L

The pH is normal, but more toward the alkaline end of the range. The P_{CO_2} is elevated, tending to make the blood acidic. The HCO_3^- is elevated, tending to make the blood alkaline. The values represent a metabolic alkalosis compensated by increased CO_2 retention.

This example also illustrates the third rule of thumb: If the P_{CO_2} and HCO_3^- are changing in the same direction, the body is compensating for an imbalance. In this case, however, as the pH is normal, the imbalance is fully compensated.

Mixed Disorders   At times, a patient will have both a respiratory and metabolic imbalance present. Depending on the clinical circumstances, a combined or mixed disorder may consist of two acidoses, two alkaloses, or an acidosis plus an alkalosis. For example:

pH   7.20
P_{CO_2} 55 mm Hg
HCO_3^- 20   mEq/L

The pH identifies the presence of a severe acidosis. The *pH* and *P_{CO_2}* are changing in *opposite* directions, so a respiratory disorder is present (first rule). However, the *pH* and *HCO_3^-* are changing in the *same* direction, so a metabolic disorder also is present (second rule). The values therefore indicate a mixed respiratory and metabolic acidosis. Such a combination may be seen in cardiac arrest, where respiratory acidosis may be present due to inadequate ventilation, and metabolic acidosis may be present due to inadequate tissue oxygenation. This example illustrates a fourth *rule of thumb*:

    4.   *If the P_{CO_2} and the HCO_3^- are changing in opposite directions, a mixed imbalance is present.*

To further help you differentiate simple imbalances from mixed imbalances, Sladen (1981) has identified two *golden rules*, presented in the American Heart Association's *Textbook of Advanced Cardiac Life Support*.

Golden **1.** *If an uncomplicated respiratory disorder is*
Rule   *present, a change in P_{CO_2} of 10 mm Hg will cause a change in pH of 0.08.*

To utilize this guideline, first examine the measured pH and P_{CO_2}. Calculate the difference between the measured P_{CO_2} and the "normal" P_{CO_2} of 40 mm Hg. Then calculate the pH that would be expected by using

this rule. Finally, compare the measured and calculated pHs. If they are reasonably close, only a respiratory disorder is present. If they differ significantly, a metabolic disorder also is present.

Examples from Sladen (1981) will demonstrate these concepts. Suppose a patient's blood gas values were pH 7.30 and P_{CO_2} 52 mm Hg. The difference between the measured P_{CO_2} and the exact "normal" of 40 mm Hg is 12 mm Hg. Use a simple algebraic equation:

$$\frac{\text{Rule}}{\text{expected } P_{CO_2} \text{ difference (10)}}{\text{expected pH change (0.08)}}$$

$$= \frac{\text{Patient}}{\text{measured } P_{CO_2} \text{ difference (12)}}{\text{calculated pH change } (x)}$$

Then

$$10x = 12\,(0.08)$$

so

$$x = \frac{12\,(0.08)}{10}$$

and therefore

$$x = 0.096 \quad \text{rounded off to } 0.10$$

The calculated pH change of 0.10 gives a calculated pH of 7.3. As this is identical to the measured pH, only a respiratory disorder is present.

Using a more complicated example, suppose the pH were 7.26 and the P_{CO_2} were 50 mm Hg.

$$\frac{\text{Rule}}{\text{expected } P_{CO_2} \text{ difference (10)}}{\text{expected pH change (0.08)}}$$

$$= \frac{\text{Patient}}{\text{measured } P_{CO_2} \text{ difference (10)}}{\text{calculated pH change } (x)}$$

Then

$$10x = 10(0.08)$$

so

$$x = 0.08$$

Therefore, the calculated pH is $7.40 - 0.08$, or 7.32. As the measured pH is 7.26, a considerable difference exists between the calculated and measured pHs, and so both a respiratory acidosis and a metabolic acidosis are present.

The amount of base deficit present due to the metabolic acidosis can be figured using the second golden rule:

Golden   **2.**   *A change in pH of 0.15 equals a change*
Rule   *in base of 10 mEq/L.*

In the example just given, the change in pH is represented by the calculated pH minus the measured pH: $7.32 - 7.26$, or 0.06. Again use a simple algebraic equation:

Rule

$$\frac{\text{expected pH change (0.15)}}{\text{expected base deficit (10)}}$$

Patient

$$= \frac{\text{measured pH change (0.06)}}{\text{calculated base deficit } (x)}$$

Therefore

$$0.15\,x = 0.06\,(10)$$

so

$$x = 4$$

There is a base deficit of 4 mEq/L.

For further examples of the application of these golden rules, consult Sladen (1981).

Venous Acid–Base Values Thus far, we have been discussing arterial values. In some cases, an arterial blood sample may be unavailable and values may be determined instead on a mixed venous sample. Normally, the venous P_{CO_2} is slightly higher (40–50 venous versus 35–45 arterial), and the pH slightly lower (7.31–7.41 versus 7.35–7.45) than arterial blood. Venous bicarbonate and base excess values are about the same as arterial values.

Electrolyte Imbalances

Accurate diagnosis of acid–base imbalances requires arterial blood gas values, as already explained. However, a certain amount of information about acid–base imbalances can be gleaned from signs and symptoms of electrolyte imbalances and from the serum electrolyte panel routinely obtained on patients. This panel typically includes values for serum sodium, potassium, chloride, and CO_2 content. The following sections describe the complex interrelationships between acid–base balance and electrolyte balance.

Sodium (Na^+) Because there is so much sodium in the extracellular space, shifts in acid–base balance do not affect sodium balance significantly. An increased serum sodium level also does not affect acid–base balance much. A decreased serum sodium level, however, can be associated with great derangements in acid–base

balance. The sodium deficit does not cause the derangements directly; the culprit is the accompanying chloride deficit. You may remember that the kidney can reabsorb sodium in three ways: with the negative chloride ion, with the negative bicarbonate ion, or in exchange for the positive potassium or hydrogen ion. In the presence of a depletion of both sodium chloride and water (such as in hypovolemic shock), the kidney will have a potent stimulus for sodium reabsorption. As relatively little chloride will be available in this situation, the kidney will reabsorb an increased percentage of the sodium with bicarbonate and an increased percentage in exchange for H^+ or potassium. Thus, hyponatremia, through its relationship to hypochloremia, may be associated with alkalosis and hypokalemia.

Potassium (K^+) Acid–base and potassium balance profoundly affect each other. Acidosis often is accompanied by hyperkalemia and alkalosis by hypokalemia. These associations are due to two mechanisms: exchange of potassium and hydrogen ions across the cell membrane, and altered renal excretion of potassium and hydrogen.

The body's cells contain buffer systems that can either accept or donate H^+ ions. H^+ ions and potassium ions (K^+) freely exchange across the cell membrane. Because the amount of extracellular K^+ is quite small compared to the intracellular amount, even small shifts of K^+ across the cell membrane cause significant changes in the serum level. In acidosis, excess H^+ ions in the serum migrate into the cell, where their buffering displaces K^+ ions. To maintain intracellular electrical balance, the K^+ ions diffuse out into the serum. As a result, acidosis can cause hyperkalemia. The $Na^+/K^+/H^+$ ion exchange mechanism in the kidney also plays a role in the interrelationships of K^+ imbalances and acid–base imbalances. In the kidney, Na^+ ions normally are retained in exchange for K^+ or H^+ ions. In acidosis, because H^+ ions are more abundant, the kidney tends to excrete H^+ ions rather than K^+ ions in exchange for sodium. As the excess H^+ ions block the secretion of K^+, hyperkalemia develops.

In alkalosis, the opposite situation exists. The intracellular buffers dissociate to release H^+ ions. As they move out of the cell, K^+ ions move in. Thus, alkalosis can cause hypokalemia. In addition, the kidney tends to retain H^+ ions, instead excreting K^+ in exchange for Na^+. This preferential retention of H^+ ions helps to compensate for the alkalosis, but at the expense of further contributing to hypokalemia.

In contrast to the above situations, in which acid–base imbalances cause K^+ imbalances, the converse can also exist; that is, K^+ imbalances can cause acid–base imbalances. Hyperkalemia causes more K^+ ions to move intracellularly, displacing H^+ ions into the serum and producing acidosis. In the kidney, more K^+ ions are exchanged for Na^+, and the retention of H^+ ions increases the acidosis. Hypokalemia favors the transmembrane shift of K^+ ions in the opposite direction from hyperkalemia—that is, from the cell into the serum. To maintain intracellular electrical balance, more H^+ ions then move into the cell, leaving the serum alkalotic. In the kidney, fewer K^+ ions are available for exchange, so more H^+ ions are excreted, and the alkalosis deepens.

The signs, symptoms, and treatment of potassium imbalances are discussed in detail earlier in this chapter.

Calcium (Ca^{++}) Serum calcium exists in both ionized and nonionized forms. The ionized form is the physiologically active one. Calcium ionization increases in acidosis and decreases in alkalosis. As a result, an acidotic patient may have signs of hypercalcemia, while an alkalotic person often shows signs of hypocalcemia. Acidosis can mask hypocalcemia because of its ability to increase calcium ionization. When the acidosis is treated and pH returns to normal, twitching, convulsions, paresthesias, carpopedal spasms, tetany, and other signs of hypocalcemia may become evident.

For a complete discussion of signs, symptoms, and treatment of calcium imbalances, refer to this chapter's section on electrolyte imbalances.

Chloride (Cl^-) Chloride is primarily an extracellular anion. Its serum concentration varies inversely with bicarbonate for two reasons: (a) it shifts across the cell membrane during buffering in exchange for bicarbonate (the chloride shift); and (b) renal absorption of chloride varies inversely with reabsorption of bicarbonate. For these reasons, hypochloremia can cause metabolic alkalosis, and vice versa; hyperchloremia can cause metabolic acidosis, and vice versa. The interrelationship of hypochloremia and metabolic alkalosis is particularly important clinically. As mentioned in the section on sodium, if insufficient chloride is present in the renal tubules, the kidney will reabsorb an increased proportion of sodium with bicarbonate, causing a metabolic alkalosis.

If the hypochloremic, alkalotic patient also has a stimulus for avid sodium retention, a vicious cycle may develop in which the electrolyte and acid–base imbalances feed on each other. A clinical example is the person with chronic congestive heart failure who is on a low-salt diet without adequate chloride replacement. The abnormal volume regulation causes an intense stimulus for sodium reabsorption. Because of chloride depletion, an increased percentage of sodium will be reabsorbed with bicarbonate; the stimulus for sodium

retention overrides the body's need to reduce alkali, and alkalemia worsens. As there also may be an increased renal exchange of potassium for sodium, hypokalemia may worsen also.

Serum Electrolyte Summary Because the changes in electrolyte balance are difficult to remember, they are summarized here.

The normal serum sodium level is 135–145 mEq/L. Hyponatremia, through its relation to hypochloremia, often is associated with alkalosis.

The usual serum potassium concentration is 3.5–5.5 mEq/L. Hyperkalemia often is present in acidosis or recovery from alkalosis. Hypokalemia may be associated with alkalosis or recovery from acidosis. A normal serum potassium may be present in the previously hypokalemic patient who has become acidotic.

The normal serum calcium level is 8.5–10.8 mg/100ml. Hypercalcemia may be present in acidosis and hypocalcemia in alkalosis.

The normal serum chloride concentration is 96–106 mEq/L. Hyperchloremia may be present in acidosis; hypochloremia frequently is associated with alkalosis.

CO_2 Content As mentioned earlier, the serum electrolyte panel usually includes a measurement of CO_2 content. CO_2 content consists of about 95% bicarbonate and 5% carbonic acid. It thus can reflect metabolic and/or respiratory activity. The normal CO_2 content is 24–30 mEq/L. CO_2 content is increased in respiratory acidosis and metabolic alkalosis. It is decreased in metabolic acidosis and respiratory alkalosis. Because of its relatively nonspecific nature, the CO_2 content value can indicate only that an acid–base abnormality is present. It cannot indicate whether that abnormality is an acidosis or alkalosis, nor can it pinpoint whether respiratory or metabolic dysfunction is at fault. To identify the type of imbalance, arterial blood gas values should be analyzed.

Anion Gap The serum electrolyte report can provide you with another useful clue to acid–base imbalance, called the *anion gap*, or delta, that helps differentiate the mechanisms of metabolic acidosis.

The anion gap is an expression of the excess unmeasurable anions in the body (the phosphate, sulfate, and other organic anions). To derive the value, add the bicarbonate and the chloride values to get a sum of the measured anions and subtract this sum from the measured cation, Na^+. The normal difference is 8–16 mEq/L. For example, if Na is 140, HCO_3^- 20, and chloride 100:

$$20 + 100 = 120$$
$$140 - 120 = 20 \text{ mEq of unmeasurable anions}$$

This value indicates there is an elevation of the unmeasurable anions in this patient.

The anion gap increases in metabolic acidosis resulting from an abnormal increase in organic acids. Examples are starvation, diabetic ketoacidosis, and lactic acidosis. The anion gap remains normal in metabolic acidosis owing to bicarbonate loss (for example, in diarrhea or lower gastrointestinal fistulas) or administration of chloride-containing acids, such as ammonium chloride.

Other Laboratory Data

Other laboratory data also may provide clues to causes of acid–base disturbances. For instance, an elevated blood urea nitrogen would suggest renal failure and possible metabolic acidosis, while abnormal pulmonary function tests would suggest potential respiratory acid–base imbalances.

NURSING DIAGNOSES

As is apparent from the earlier discussion of signs and symptoms, the most frequent nursing diagnoses for a patient with an acid–base imbalance are:

- Sensory-perceptual alteration
- Ineffective breathing pattern
- Altered tissue perfusion

Nursing measures for these diagnoses are discussed in detail in Chapters 3, 9, and 13.

Planning and Implementation of Care

Collaborate with the physician to relieve both the causes and the effects of acid–base disturbances.

Respiratory Acidosis

If the patient has a compensated respiratory acidosis from chronic pulmonary disease and is asymptomatic, no treatment is necessary. Should the acidosis be acute, uncompensated, and/or symptomatic, treatment is directed toward removing the cause. The nurse plays a major role in judicious use of a vigorous regimen of pulmonary hygiene to clear secretions and promote optimal ventilation. Mechanical ventilation may be necessary to lower the Pco_2 and maintain ventilation. If so, it must be provided cautiously. Excessive lowering of the Pco_2 can precipitate respiratory alkalosis. Also, if renal compensation is underway, a too-rapid lowering of the Pco_2 (before the elevated HCO_3^- level has time to decrease) can precipitate metabolic alkalosis.

Bicarbonate administration may be indicated if the acidosis is severe. Any electrolyte imbalances present also may require treatment. For example, significant hyperkalemia may necessitate insulin and dextrose infusions, ion exchange resins, or dialysis.

Metabolic Acidosis Treatment of metabolic acidosis involves both therapy of the underlying disorder and bicarbonate replacement. Treating the underlying disorder involves such activities as insulin and glucose administration in diabetic ketoacidosis, improvement of oxygenation in lactic acidosis so that aerobic metabolism can resume, and so on. Bicarbonate replacement is calculated using the American Heart Association's *Golden Rule 3* (Sladen 1981):

Sodium bicarbonate dose (mEq/L)

$$= \text{Base deficit (mEq/L)} \times \frac{\text{Patient weight (kg)}}{4}$$

For instance, for a 70-kg person with a base deficit of -10:

$$10 \times \frac{70}{4} = 10 \times 17.5$$

$$= 175 \text{ mEq bicarbonate dose}$$

Particular care must be taken to avoid rapid replacement of bicarbonate. As mentioned above, HCO_3^- ions do not equilibrate across the blood-brain barrier as rapidly as CO_2. This fact may be responsible for a lag of variable length between the rapid onset of metabolic acidosis and the maximal development of hyperventilation, and another lag between the rapid administration of bicarbonate and the cessation of hyperventilation. If the blood pH is returned rapidly to normal, the patient will continue to hyperventilate (because it takes several hours for the bicarbonate to alter the CSF pH), and the patient may develop a respiratory alkalosis. Usually, about half of the calculated dose is given initially, and the patient's response is checked before the physician decides whether further bicarbonate administration is necessary.

Respiratory Alkalosis

Respiratory alkalosis is treated by reducing the patient's need to hyperventilate. For example, correction of an underlying hypoxia often will restore the respiratory pattern and therefore the P_{CO_2} to normal. If the patient is being mechanically ventilated, decreasing the rate or tidal volume or adding extra tubing (to increase deadspace) will cause the P_{CO_2} to rise. Should the hyperventilation result from emotional excitement, having the person breathe into a paper bag is a convenient way to restore normal P_{CO_2} and eliminate the frightening symptoms of numbness, tingling, lightheadedness, and so on. This intervention must be followed by counseling to help the person become aware of the role he or she plays in inducing symptoms and to relieve emotional stress.

Metabolic Alkalosis

Metabolic alkalosis is treated by removing the underlying cause, promoting hydrogen retention, and by enhancing bicarbonate excretion. Examples of treating the underlying problem are relieving prolonged vomiting and replacing fluid and electrolytes lost through nasogastric suction. Depending on the patient's electrolyte status, hydrogen retention and bicarbonate excretion may be promoted by the administration of potassium chloride, acetazolamide, or ammonium chloride. If symptoms of calcium deficiency are present due to the decrease in ionized calcium, calcium gluconate may be given intravenously.

Mixed Disorders

Treatment of mixed disorders combines the principles governing the treatment of each individual disorder. For instance, to relieve a combined respiratory and metabolic acidosis due to severe hypoventilation, you must improve both ventilation (to relieve the respiratory acidosis) and oxygenation and circulation (to relieve the lactic acidosis). The combination of two acidoses or two alkaloses must be treated promptly and vigorously. They tend to block compensation for each other and therefore produce severe acid–base and electrolyte disturbances. The combination of an acidosis and an alkalosis is tolerated better by the body. They tend to have opposite effects on the bicarbonate/carbonic acid ratio and therefore produce a nearly normal pH.

General Nursing Care Measures

In addition to the measures specific to the acid–base disturbance(s), the nurse should provide the more general nursing care related to cerebral status changes; respiratory changes; and dysrhythmias, angina, or shock. For instance, for the confused patient, provide a safe environment, orient him or her to reality, and reassure him or her that the confusion probably will disappear as the condition is treated. Place the hyperventilating patient in a position that does not compromise diaphragmatic excursion. Decrease angina by assisting the person with activities of daily living to reduce myocardial workload. For more ideas on how to help these patients, review other chapters related to these symptoms.

Outcome Evaluation

Evaluate the patient's progress toward a healthy acid–base status. Outcome criteria by which you can judge the effectiveness of care are as follows:

- Level of consciousness restored to preimbalance state.
- Respiratory rate and tidal volume WNL for patient.
- Cardiac rate and rhythm WNL for patient.
- Extremities warm and dry (and pink if the patient is Caucasian).
- Serum electrolytes WNL for patient.
- Arterial blood gases WNL for patient.

REFERENCES

Burrell L, Burrell Z: *Critical care,* 4th ed. St Louis: Mosby, 1982.

Crabtree A, Jorgenson M: Exploring the practical knowledge in expert critical-care nursing practice. Unpublished master's thesis, University of Wisconsin, Madison, 1986.

Gilman et al.: *Goodman and Gilman's the pharmacological basis of therapeutics,* 7th ed. New York: Macmillan, 1985.

Guyton A: *Textbook of medical physiology,* 7th ed. Philadelphia: Saunders, 1986.

Laschinger HK: Demystifying arterial blood gases. *Canadian Nurse* (November) 1984; 45–47.

Littrell K: Arterial blood gas analysis. *Focus Crit Care* 1983; 10(4):49–51.

McFadden EA, Zaloga GP: Calcium regulation. *Crit Care Quart* 1983; 6(3):12–21.

Porth, CM: *Pathophysiology, concepts of altered health states,* 2d ed. Philadelphia: Lippincott, 1986.

Rice V: The role of potassium in health and disease. *Crit Care Nurse* (May/June) 1982; 54–73.

Rose BP: *Clinical physiology of acid–base and electrolyte disorders,* 2d ed. New York: McGraw-Hill, 1984.

Sladen A: Acid–base balance. In *Textbook of advanced life support,* McIntyre K, Lewis A (eds). Dallas: American Heart Association, 1981.

Stein, JM: Interpreting arterial blood gases. *Emerg Med* (January) 1986; 61–68.

Wodniak C, Szwed J: Fluid and electrolytes. Ch 5 in *Critical care nursing, A physiologic approach,* Abels L (ed). St Louis: Mosby, 1986.

Zaloga GP, Chernow B: Magnesium metabolism in critical illness. *Crit Care Quart* 1983; 6(3):22–27.

Zucker A, Chernow B: Diabetes Insipidus and the Syndrome of Inappropriate Anti-Diuretic Hormone Release. *Crit Care Quart* 1983; 6(3):63-74.

SUPPLEMENTAL READING

Baker WL: Hypophosphatemia. *Am J Nurs* 1985; 85(9):998–1003.

Jansen, C et al.: Hypophasphatemia. *Ann Emerg Med* 1983; 12:107–116.

Juan D: Clinical review: The clinical importance of hypomagnesemia. *Surgery* 1982; 91:510.

Kee J: *Fluids and electrolytes with clinical applications: A programmed approach,* 3d ed. New York: Wiley, 1982.

Price SA, Wilson LM: *Pathophysiology: Clinical concepts of disease processes,* 3d ed. New York: McGraw-Hill, 1986.

Reinhart RA, Desbiens NA: Hypomagnesemia in patients entering the ICU. *Crit Care Med* 1985; 13(6):506–507.

Sampson L et al.: *Methods in critical care.* Philadelphia: Saunders, 1980.

Shapiro B et al.: *Clinical application of blood gases,* 3d ed. Chicago: Year Book Medical Publishers, 1982.

17

Endocrine/Metabolic Disorders and Treatment

CLINICAL INSIGHT

Domain: Effective management of rapidly changing situations

Competency: Identifying and managing a patient crisis until physician assistance is available

Because of the swiftness with which crises occur and the physician's inability to be continually at the bedside, critical-care nurses often must manage patient crises until physician assistance is available. Functioning with aplomb in these situations requires an amalgam of nursing and medical knowledge, gleaned during on-the-job training and polished by practice. Because delay or misjudgments can have severe repercussions, the nurse who can function with poise in the face of an ongoing crisis is a special nurse, as this exemplar from Benner (1984, pp. 116-117) shows.

I came on duty at 3 P.M. and was assigned to a fresh postop open heart surgery. The patient had returned to the ICU around 11 A.M. that day and had all the usual paraphernalia for postops—IVs, respirator, chest tubes, foley catheters, etc. The patient had had a lot of IV fluid and blood replacement on days—this is the usual procedure for open heart surgery—give lots of fluid at first (usually have had mannitol), then

level off. Blood pressure will drop as the patient begins to warm up and dilate peripherally, but will usually level off soon. However, this patient continued to be hypovolemic—low blood pressure, low central venous pressure—and was diuresing in enormous amounts. We were pouring fluids in, in an attempt to catch up, but were managing, barely, to stay even with output. Clearly something was amiss here. I telephoned the surgeon's exchange but was not able to locate him. I tried also to contact the assistant, but he was off call to another doctor who was not terribly familiar with open heart surgery. Meanwhile, we were pouring in fluids, blood and packed cells, without orders, just to stay even, for the patient was continuing this diuresis. I began reviewing the possible causes for this and decided a likely one was hyperglycemia. I then ordered a blood glucose level and the results came back—more than 600 mg percent. About this time the assistant surgeon had come back on call and I was finally able to contact him. He prescribed on the basis of the blood glucose level and we were then able to stabilize the patient.

Metabolism refers to the cellular processes that support the functions of the human body. The *endocrine system* regulates the secretion of hormones that alter metabolic function. Endocrine and metabolic disorders are common in critical-care units and are often secondary to other disorders. The nurse must be intimately familiar with this system and ever alert to its possible dysfunction, as illustrated in the Clinical Insight. This chapter, while not all-inclusive, provides the critical-care nurse an understanding of four common endocrine/metabolic disorders and a common therapeutic technique affecting endocrine/metabolic function.

DIABETIC KETOACIDOSIS

Assessment

Pathophysiology

Diabetic ketoacidosis (DKA) is an emergency condition resulting from inadequate amounts of insulin. Insulin, secreted by the pancreatic islet cells, is an anabolic hormone that facilitates the transport of glucose into cells for metabolic processes and inhibits the breakdown of glycogen stores, fats, and proteins (Guthrie 1982).

It is important for the critical-care nurse to understand in detail the major pathophysiologic mechanisms that occur. Insulin lack causes complex physiologic derangements, the most important of which follow.

Hyperglycemia and Hyperosmolarity Decreased cellular uptake of glucose results in increased serum glucose concentration (hyperglycemia), which in turn increases overall serum concentration (hyperosmolarity).

Dehydration The increased osmolarity provokes a fluid shift from the intracellular to the extracellular space as a compensatory mechanism to dilute the excess glucose. This fluid shift, which causes intracellular dehydration, is ineffective because it is counteracted by another compensatory mechanism, increased renal excretion of glucose.

When glomerular filtration of glucose exceeds the transport maximum, glucose is spilled into the urine. This event usually occurs when the serum glucose level is greater than 180 mg/dl. The increased renal filtration of glucose is an important protective mechanism, but the glucose in the renal tubular filtrate increases osmotic pressure and provokes osmotic diuresis. The resulting extracellular volume depletion worsens dehydration.

Ketoacidosis Acidosis occurs as lipids used for metabolism yield ketoacids. Because no carbohydrates are being metabolized, lipolysis (breakdown of fats) occurs as an alternate source of energy. In addition, insulin normally inhibits lipase (an enzyme that stimulates lipolysis), so insulin lack accelerates lipolysis.

This breakdown results in free fatty acids, which are oxidized and cause accumulation of ketone bodies. Increased numbers of hydrogen ions (from the ketones) consume bicarbonate ions and result in metabolic acidosis (Price and Wilson 1986). In addition to the obvious effects of ketoacidosis, a decrease of extracellular sodium can occur. Keto acids have a low tubular reabsorption threshold in the kidneys. Thus, when the serum level of keto acids rises, a large amount is lost in the urine. The keto acids are mostly excreted along with extracellular sodium ions. The lost sodium ions are replaced in the extracellular fluid by hydrogen ions, which replacement worsens the acidosis (Guyton 1986). In addition, lactic acid accumulates secondary to the anaerobic metabolism of decreased cellular oxygenation, further worsening the metabolic acidosis.

Risk Conditions

Diabetic ketoacidosis can occur in undiagnosed insulin-dependent diabetics with inadequate secretion of endogenous insulin. It also can occur with known diabetics who reduce the amount of insulin per dose or miss an insulin dose entirely. Also at risk are people with an increased insulin need due to physical or emotional stress such as trauma, surgery, infection, or psychosocial stress disorders. The hormonal responses to stress responsible for the increased insulin need include release of glucagon from the liver, secretion of adrenal glucocorticoids, and adrenal secretion of catecholamines (Hudak 1986). Infection is the most common cause of DKA in these patients (Swearingen et al. 1986).

Signs and Symptoms

The client with DKA is acutely ill. Signs of dehydration from the osmotic diuresis include flushed dry skin, poor skin turgor, and dry mucous membranes. The client, if conscious, will complain of the "three Ps": thirst (polydipsia), hunger (polyphagia), and large amounts of urine (polyuria) due again to osmotic diuresis. However, these characteristic early signs of lack of insulin may not be associated with onset of DKA.

Respiratory symptoms include a tachypnea, Kussmaul's breathing (deep respiration), and acetone odor to the breath, all compensatory mechanisms for metabolic acidosis. Acetoacetic acid is converted to acetone, which is volatile and can be exhaled through breathing. Acetone normally has a "fruity" odor and acetone breath is characteristic of diabetes mellitus and DKA. The presence of Kussmaul's respiration indicates severe acidosis.

Neurologically, the client may demonstrate changes ranging from confusion to coma, related to dehydration and decreased cellular oxygenation. Deep tendon reflexes may be decreased or absent.

Cardiovascularly, the nurse will note tachycardia related to sympathetic nervous system discharge, hypotension related to dehydration, and flushed skin related to increasing amounts of carbonic acid. Other presenting symptoms may include nausea, vomiting, and abdominal pain.

Laboratory Tests

Laboratory assessment will reveal an elevated serum glucose level. Typically elevated to no more than 180-500 mg/dl because of the osmotic diuresis, serum glucose may soar to 1000 mg/dl or higher in the severely volume-depleted patient or one with impaired renal function. A widening anion gap ($Na - (Cl + HCO_3)$) reflects acid accumulation (normal is between 12 and 14 mEq/L). Also important are urine studies, to ascertain the presence of glucose and ketones. When the serum glucose level is above 300 mg, 100 grams of glucose may be lost in the urine in 24 hours. Additionally 100-200 grams of ketoacids may be lost in the urine in 24 hours. Arterial blood gases usually show a pH less than 7.3 and decreased bicarbonate levels. Increased plasma creatinine and blood urea nitrogen indicate decreased renal perfusion. Plasma osmolality will be above 300 mOsm/L. Electrolytes will demonstrate hyperkalemia due to displaced intracellular potassium (K^+) with acidosis, although a low total body potassium may be present with osmotic diuresis. Additionally, total serum sodium will be low because of urinary losses of sodium secondary to keto acid excretion; however, if the patient is severely dehydrated, serum sodium will reflect normal or high levels (see Chapter 16 for detailed discussion of sodium). Finally, to differentiate and confirm DKA it is important to rule out other disorders. To this end, EKG and cardiac enzymes rule out myocardial infarction; serum amylase rules out pancreatitis; and chest x-ray and urine and blood cultures are done to rule out possible infection.

NURSING DIAGNOSES

A variety of nursing diagnoses may apply to the patient with DKA.

- Fluid volume deficit
- Acid–base imbalance*
- Sensory perceptual alteration
- Chemical imbalance*
- Altered gas exchange
- Knowledge deficit

*Diagnosis developed by contributor.

Planning and Implementation of Care

DKA is an emergency, life-threatening condition. Early assessment, diagnosis, and intervention are vital to the patient's recovery.

Fluid Volume Deficit Related to Urinary Losses Secondary to Osmotic Diuresis

Rapid replacement of fluid is very important, because dehydration is the most immediate life-threatening aspect of the condition. As soon as intravenous access is established, administration of 0.9% sodium chloride ("normal" saline, NS) is usually initiated. The average fluid deficit in an adult is 3.5 liters, and the usual initial replacement is 1-2 liters in the first 2 hours (Foster and McGarry 1983). Serum osmolality often is used as a guide for fluid replacement.

Plasma expanders such as albumin and plasma concentrates may be necessary to forestall impending vascular collapse. However, their administration should follow NS, because the hypertonicity of these products can further cellular dehydration in a patient with a fluid deficit.

Although rapid fluid replacement is of utmost importance, the critical-care nurse should continue to assess carefully for complications. The rapid fluid replacement can cause hemodilution, hypotonicity, and subsequent interstitial edema, which may account for the pulmonary and cerebral edema that has been occasionally observed with DKA (Hillman 1983).

After the first few hours, the solution most likely will be changed to 0.45% normal saline or dextrose in water. There are three reasons for this. First, more water than sodium is lost during an osmotic diuresis, so free water (hypotonic) will need to be replaced. Second, reducing the amount of chloride in the solution will reduce the possibility of hyperchloremia. Finally, a 5% glucose solution should be given before hypoglycemia is likely to occur, which is discussed in more detail under the next nursing diagnosis (Foster and McGarry 1983).

During fluid replacement therapy it is important for the nurse to continually assess the patient. Assess for signs of circulatory overload, which may include the following:

- Neck vein distention
- Crackles in lungs
- Increasing CVP and pulmonary artery pressures
- Tachycardia
- Tachypnea

Also assess for signs of decreasing cardiac output:

- Decreasing urinary output related to decreasing renal perfusion secondary to dehydration. (*Note:* An indwelling catheter will be inserted to facilitate accurate hourly intake and output measurement.)
- Hypotension.
- Cool extremities related to sympathetic nervous system compensatory mechanisms.
- Additionally, see signs of circulatory overload above.

Chemical Imbalance Related to Electrolyte Losses and Lack of Insulin

As discussed previously, there are numerous chemical imbalances that occur with DKA.

Insulin   Insulin deficiency is the primary cause of all of the problems of DKA, so it follows that replacement is an important part of the therapy, although insulin alone will not correct all of the changes with DKA. Insulin has four main effects. First, insulin facilitates *transport of glucose across the cellular membrane*. It allows uptake and use of glucose by almost all cells and tissues of the body. Second, insulin facilitates *storage of glucose,* in the form of glycogen, in the liver. The glycogen is broken down to glucose at different periods during the day to maintain an adequate blood glucose level. Third, insulin promotes *fatty acid synthesis.* Fatty acids are then transported to adipose cells to be stored. Additionally, fatty acids are utilized by the liver to synthesize triglycerides. Insulin also inhibits the pancreatic enzyme lipase that causes breakdown of fatty acids into fat cells. Finally, insulin stimulates *active transport of amino acids into cells,* inhibits protein catabolism, and inhibits liver glyconeogenesis (Guyton 1986).

The most common methods (routes) of insulin administration are intravenous (IV) or subcutaneous (SQ). In DKA, the IV route is often preferred as it allows more reliable absorption. The amount administered should be guided by blood glucose levels assessed every hour. Usually, at approximately 250-300 mg/dl, the IV solution is changed to dextrose and water and/or the insulin dose is reduced. Generally, approximately 5-10 units per hour are given (Carroll and Matz 1983), and the blood glucose level decreases approximately 75-100 mg/dl per hour (Kriesberg 1983). Although some patients with DKA are insulin-resistant and require larger doses of insulin, most often low doses are effective (Barrett et al. 1982).

Electrolytes   Losses of electrolytes, including sodium, potassium, chloride, magnesium, phosphate, and calcium, are important considerations in patients with DKA. The electrolytes are usually replaced via the IV route and monitored by serum electrolyte levels.

Potassium (K^+) regulation is a bit more complex. Potassium is primarily an intracellular ion, with only a very small amount in the serum, so serum levels are not reflective of total body potassium (see Chapter 16 for detailed discussion of potassium). In acidosis, K^+ is shifted out of the cells (secondary to large amounts of hydrogen ions), so the serum level will be high. As acidosis is corrected, however, K^+ will move back into the cells and K^+ deficit may become evident due to K^+ loss during osmotic diuresis. If hypokalemia occurs, it probably will be 1–4 hours after treatment is begun (Kriesberg 1983). Potassium phosphate salts may be given, which also will correct phosphate depletion.

Acid–Base Imbalance Related to Abundance of Metabolic Acids Secondary to Insulin Deficiency

A significant number of patients with DKA do not require endogenous alkaline administration to correct acidosis. With prompt administration of fluid, electrolytes, and insulin, the kidney can begin to conserve bicarbonate and correct acidosis. However, the patient whose pH is less than 7.1, HCO_3 is less than 10 mEq/L, or Ca^{++} is less than 8 mEq/L may require bicarbonate (Swearingen et al. 1986; Hudak et al. 1986). The acidosis is corrected by administering either sodium bicarbonate or sodium lactate solution; correction should be guided by arterial blood gases.

The other important facet of acid–base imbalance for the critical-care nurse to remember is the K^+ shifts that occur with acidosis. As discussed previously, acidosis causes an efflux of K^+ out of cells. As acidosis is corrected and K^+ is driven back into cells, an actual K^+ deficit secondary to osmotic diuresis may appear. The critical-care nurse should monitor electrolytes carefully and report changes and/or abnormal levels.

There is another aspect of correction of acidosis that is important for the critical care nurse to understand. Remember that carbon dioxide (CO_2) diffuses into cerebrospinal fluid (CSF) much faster than bicarbonate. As bicarbonate (HCO_3) is administered, part of it dissociates into CO_2 and diffuses into the CSF, causing a transient but potentially serious further drop in CSF pH. In the patient whose pH is moving more toward normal range, this may manifest as a deepening coma.

Sensory-Perceptual Alteration Related to Changes in Level of Consciousness Secondary to Cellular Dehydration

The changes in sensation and perception that occur with DKA range from mental confusion to coma. The causes of the neurologic problems are multifactorial. First, the osmotic diuresis causes severe cellular dehydration and altered metabolism, which may precipitate sensory-perceptual alterations. Second, the anerobic metabolism that occurs as a result of hypoxemia and acidosis also will alter cerebral cellular metabolism and neuronal function. Finally, while insulin is being administered, there is risk of hypoglycemia, which will further impair cerebral and neuronal function.

Nursing care for the change in cerebral function should include decreasing the risk of vomiting and aspiration by positioning the patient on his or her side and having suction readily available. A nasogastric tube to low-intermittent suction may be ordered. If the patient is unconscious, it is important to have a cuffed endotracheal tube in place *prior* to gastric intubation, to reduce the risk of aspiration.

Altered Gas Exchange Related to Respiratory Pattern Changes Secondary to Acidosis and Decreased Level of Consciousness

The patient with DKA will demonstrate changes in breathing patterns related to the acidosis and also may demonstrate changes related to altered level of consciousness. The critical-care nurse should continually assess respiratory status for hyperpnea (Kussmaul's breathing) associated with acidosis and the potential for decreased respiratory movements, which may be associated with cerebral cell dehydration.

Assess arterial blood gases as ordered. Be alert for signs of inadequate gas exchange, which may include: decreased respiratory muscle excursion, tachycardia, dyspnea, and skin color changes (pallor or cyanosis). Report any changes in respiratory status, and administer oxygen as ordered. Be prepared for the possibility of endotracheal intubation.

Knowledge Deficit Related to Mechanisms of DKA

DKA is a largely preventable disorder. When the patient and family are ready, a teaching program should be instituted. An important function of the critical-care nurse is to initiate a program of self-care education, including signs and symptoms, appropriate interventions, and preventive measures.

Outcome Evaluation

Evaluation is based on the following outcome criteria:

- Plasma glucose less than 250 mg/dl.
- Electrolytes WNL.
- Serum osmolality WNL.
- Arterial blood gases WNL.
- Patient is alert and oriented.

- Urine output WNL.
- Vital signs WNL.
- Skin turgor is good.
- Mucous membranes are moist.

HYPERGLYCEMIC HYPEROSMOLAR NONKETOTIC COMA

Hyperglycemic hyperosmolar nonketotic coma (HHNK), a DKA-like syndrome with the absence of ketosis, is a medical and nursing emergency. It often is misdiagnosed because of clinical presentation similar to cerebral vascular accidents and DKA. However, it does not occur as frequently as DKA. If not treated promptly and correctly, it is fatal. It is a disorder of insulin deficiency that results in hyperglycemia and hyperosmolarity but no ketoacidosis. The hyperglycemia occurs because of decreased peripheral glucose uptake related to a relative insulin deficiency. An osmotic diuresis with glucosuria follows. This depletes electrolytes and precipitates extracellular and eventually intracellular dehydration; the dehydration and hyperglycemia increase serum osmolality. Cerebral impairment is the other major factor in HHNK, due in large part to dehydration of brain cells (Winters 1983).

What causes HHNK rather than DKA? One theory holds that, with HHNK, lipolysis from adipose tissue is inhibited. Patients with HHNK have lower levels of circulating fatty acids and lypolytic hormones, growth hormone, and cortisol. The limited cortisol and stress response may contribute to the lack of maximal response and lack of ketogenesis (Leske 1985).

Assessment

Risk Conditions

It is important to be able to identify the patient at risk. Certain patients with recent onset of Type II, non-insulin-dependent diabetes may be able to secrete enough insulin to prevent ketosis, but not enough to prevent high serum blood glucose levels, hyperosmolarity, and severe cellular dehydration. HHNK may also occur in previously stable patients whose insulin requirements increase, as with stress of surgery, trauma, or infection. HHNK also may be precipitated by pharmacologic therapy; for example, thiazide diuretics may decrease insulin release from the pancreas, as do diazoxide and phenytoin. Patients receiving high-calorie feedings, such as hyperalimentation and enteral feedings, also are at risk, because of increased glucose load. Last, although it may occur in patients with Type I or Type II diabetes, HHNK is much less common in Type I. Glucose processing dysfunction in Type I is more likely to be associated with ketone formation and precipitation of DKA.

Signs and Symptoms

The signs and symptoms of HHNK all result primarily from the effects of the high serum glucose level, which generally is greater than 600 mg/dl and may be as high as 1400–1600 mg/dl. Serum osmolality usually is greater than 350 mOsm/L, due to osmotic diuresis. Remember that serum ketones will be negative. Arterial blood gases usually are normal, because, without lipolysis, acidosis does not occur. It is important to note, however, that a slight acidosis may be present, related to either lactic acid production or decreased renal function, because of extracellular (intravenous) dehydration and decreased perfusion. Electrolyte levels will vary. Electrolytes are lost with the osmotic diuresis, however; depending on the state of hydration, sodium levels may be high, normal, or low. Similarly, potassium is drawn out of the cells with dehydration, so serum potassium may be initially high; then, when volume depletion is corrected, a total body K^+ deficit will be unmasked. Also contributing to the K^+ deficit is the dehydration-stimulated aldosterone response, which results in the renal tubular reabsorption of Na^+ and K^+ secretions.

Laboratory signs of decreasing kidney function may be present. An elevated blood urea nitrogen and serum creatinine indicate decreased glomerular filtration.

Examination of the urine reveals glycosuria, because the renal reabsorption transport maximum has been exceeded. Urine will be negative for ketones.

Early in this syndrome, the alert patient may complain of feeling drowsy and thirsty and may appear confused. Detection of accompanying physical changes is very important to early diagnosis and intervention.

Physical assessment will reveal clinical signs of dehydration. These may include dry mucous membranes, flushed dry skin, poor skin turgor, and postural hypotension. Sympathetic nervous system compensatory responses for the contracted intravascular volume include tachycardia, tachypnea, and constriction of peripheral blood vessels to shunt blood to more central organs. Of utmost importance and characteristic of this disorder are neurologic changes. These may be manifested by confusion, stupor or coma, or seizures. There is a direct relationship between plasma osmolality and degree of depressed cerebral functioning (Winters 1983). Because of the severe neurologic abnormalities, this disorder has the risk of being misdiagnosed as cerebrovascular accident. Finally, although Kussmaul's respiration is not present, the tachypnea and shallow respirations that do occur are related to a disturbance in respiratory-center functioning.

NURSING DIAGNOSES

The following nursing diagnoses may apply to the patient with HHNK:

- Fluid volume deficit
- Chemical imbalance*
- Sensory-perceptual alteration
- Alteration in tissue perfusion
- Altered respiratory function
- Knowledge deficit

*Diagnosis developed by contributor.

Planning and Implementation of Care

Fluid Volume Deficit Related to Decreased Volume Secondary to Osmotic Diuresis

---

The problem of extracellular and intracellular dehydration needs to be treated promptly. The type and volume of fluid replacement generally is determined by the physician, based on cardiovascular and renal status. The

following medical guidelines may be used when replacing fluids.

1. Isotonic saline (0.9% normal saline [NS]) if serum sodium is less than 130 mEq/L and plasma osmolality is less than 330 mOsm/L.

2. Hypotonic saline (0.45% NS) if hypernatremia is present (greater than 145 mEq/L).

3. Six to 8 liters may be replaced in the first 12 hours.

4. When blood glucose reaches approximately 250 mg/dl, switch to D5W to prevent hypoglycemia and/or switch from 0.9% NS to 0.45% NS to prevent lowering serum osmolality too rapidly, which can precipitate cerebral edema secondary to fluid shifts (Leske 1985).

Generally, patients with HHNK have a greater fluid deficit than patients with DKA because of a more prolonged and severe osmotic diuresis. Thus, they may require more fluid replacement. But remember, these patients often are elderly; may have renal, cardiac, or pulmonary disease; and are at risk for pulmonary edema and circulatory overload (Winters 1983). Therefore, it is important to assess for signs of circulatory overload, such as crackles in lung fields, distended neck veins, shortness of breath, dyspnea, bounding pulses, increased pulmonary artery pressures, increased pulmonary capillary wedge pressure, and tachycardia. During correction of the fluid volume deficit, it is important for the critical-care nurse continually to assess the patient for signs of decreasing cardiac output, which may accompany circulatory overload. These may include decreasing urinary output, tachycardia, and decreasing blood pressure.

Chemical Imbalance Related to Changes in Serum Levels Secondary to Relative Lack of Insulin

---

An important part of care is to reduce the blood glucose level below 300 mg/dl. The requirements for insulin usually are less than for patients with DKA, and some physicians treat HHNK with saline alone (Hudak 1986).

The goal of insulin therapy in HHNK is to gradually reduce the serum glucose level while preventing hypoglycemia and cerebral edema, as mentioned previously. Cerebral edema is a complication that occurs from reducing serum osmolality too rapidly. If osmolality is decreased rapidly, there is a substantial difference between brain cell osmolality and serum osmolality, causing a subsequent fluid shift to the intracellular space in the brain—hence, cerebral edema. Usually, short-acting regular insulin is administered. It is best to use the IV route, as subcutaneous administration does not provide adequate absorption secondary to dehydration.

Restoring electrolyte balance is the next intervention. As discussed previously, electrolyte levels often are low, and electrolytes need to be replaced. The critical-care nurse should assess for symptoms of electrolyte imbalances and administer repletion therapy, as ordered. (See Chapter 16 for a detailed discussion of electrolyte imbalances.)

Sensory-Perceptual Alteration Related to Decreased Level of Consciousness Secondary to Cellular Dehydration

The alterations in level of consciousness that occur are due to cellular dehydration in the central nervous system from the high plasma osmolality. It is important for the nurse to assess level of consciousness and neurologic status frequently and to report any seizure activity. Remember, phenytoin reduces endogenous release of insulin, so it probably would not be indicated for HHNK-induced seizures.

The neurologic changes also may be due to cerebral edema secondary to decreasing osmolality too quickly and/or impaired electrolyte balance and ideally will be reversed as the imbalance is corrected.

Alteration in Tissue Perfusion Related to Decreased Plasma Volume Secondary to Osmotic Diuresis

The critical-care nurse assesses for and assists in treating altered tissue perfusion. The decrease in tissue perfusion is mainly due to dehydration and hyperviscosity of the blood. These factors cause decreased renal perfusion and function, decreased cardiac output related to decreased preload, and decreased tissue perfusion and subsequent tissue hypoxia. Vascular thrombosis due to hemoconcentration can also occur (Winters 1983).

This problem will be relieved with fluid replacement. The nurse should assess for adequate renal output (1/2 cc/kg/hr), adequate tissue perfusion, and improving skin turgor. Additionally, observe for a decrease in sympa-

thetic compensatory responses as evidenced by a return to sinus rhythm (from tachycardia), normal blood pressure, palpable peripheral pulses, and increasing skin temperature.

Altered Respiratory Function Related to a Disturbance in Respiratory Center Functioning

The respiratory center in the brainstem may be affected by the severe cellular dehydration that occurs with HHNK. It is important to continually assess respiratory function and report any changes. Assess for respiratory excursion, air movement on auscultation, skin color, shortness of breath, dyspnea, and sympathetic compensatory responses for hypoxemia.

Administer oxygen as ordered, monitor blood gas values, and prepare for endotracheal intubation if alterations in respiratory function are observed.

Knowledge Deficit Related to Insufficient Information Regarding Mechanisms of HHNK and Prevention

Although critical-care patients sometimes are not ready for teaching programs, after the acute episode the nurse can assess the patient's readiness to learn and level of understanding and develop a teaching plan. This plan should include dietary restrictions and signs and symptoms of hyperglycemia and impending HHNK.

Outcome Evaluation

Evaluate the patient's progress according to these outcome criteria:

- Plasma glucose less than 300 mg/dl.
- Serum osmolality WNL.
- Patient is alert and oriented.
- Vital signs WNL.
- Skin turgor good.
- Serum electrolytes WNL.
- Urine output WNL.
- Serum creatinine and BUN WNL.

HYPOGLYCEMIA

Hypoglycemia is an emergency situation in which there is a decrease in plasma glucose levels to at or below 50 mg/dl.

Assessment

Risk Conditions

There are many potential causes of and contributing factors to hypoglycemia. The episode may be related to excessive insulin therapy or to change in absorption of insulin. It may be the result of insufficient nutritional intake or to decreased need for exogenous insulin (removal of stress, such as infection).

There are medications and drugs that also may precipitate this episode—for example, excessive oral hypoglycemic agents (sulfonylureas) and alcohol, which inhibits gluconeogenesis by the liver. Finally, other health problems, such as liver disease (depleted glycogen stores) and adrenal insufficiency (insufficient glucocorticoids), may be contributing factors.

Signs and Symptoms

Signs and symptoms usually are apparent when the blood glucose level is less than 50 mg/dl (Swearingen et al. 1986). The onset of symptoms usually is more rapid than with DKA. The physiologic symptoms patients demonstrate generally are related to nervous system function—more specifically, cerebral function. The cerebral changes result from insufficient supply of glucose to the brain cells (the brain does not utilize alternative energy sources as well as other tissues do).

Patients usually will first experience an inability to concentrate, apprehension, or light-headedness. Patients often are aware of these symptoms yet unable to verbalize their need for help. They often may present with slurred speech, trembling, and/or staggering gait, which may be mistaken for alcohol-induced signs. It is important to recognize these signs and be aware of the

possibility of hypoglycemia, because ignoring the signs may have a deleterious, even fatal, outcome.

The other signs involve the autonomic nervous system. The hypoglycemia stimulates release of catecholamines (epinephrine and norepinephrine). These hormones cause tachycardia, pallor, diaphoresis, cool skin, and tremors with potential seizure activity. This response is supported by glucocorticoid release from the adrenal glands, and liver glycogenolysis.

The central nervous system signs will progress to coma within minutes to an hour without treatment.

Diagnosis of hypoglycemia is based on low plasma glucose levels and on response when glucose is administered. Patients generally respond rapidly and dramatically to glucose administration.

NURSING DIAGNOSES

The following nursing diagnoses apply to the patient with a hypoglycemic episode:

- Chemical imbalance*
- Sensory-perceptual alteration
- Knowledge deficit

*Diagnosis developed by contributor.

Chemical Imbalance Related to Low Serum Glucose Level

The chemical disorder here is low blood sugar; administration of glucose is the treatment. The patient must be treated promptly to prevent cellular damage and infarction. If the patient is conscious, administer a fast-acting carbohydrate, such as 4 oz orange juice or apple juice or 2½ tablespoons of sugar. After this treatment, or if the patient is unconscious, start an intravenous line and be prepared to administer 50 ml of 50% dextrose IV push as ordered. When this is administered to an unconscious patient in the presence of uncomplicated hypoglycemia, consciousness will be promptly restored. An alternative therapy (but not as effective) is to administer exogenous glucagon IV to stimulate liver glycogenolysis. Be aware of the possibility of reoccurrence of the episode. Consult with the physician about continued nutrient/glucose support, and monitor blood glucose level.

If these measures do not reverse the symptoms, consider the following:

- The patient may not have uncomplicated hypoglycemia, *or*
- The patient needs more glucose.

Sensory-Perceptual Alteration Related to Decreased Cerebral Cellular Metabolism Secondary to Hypoglycemia

As discussed previously, the patient with hypoglycemia has central neurologic changes due to deficient glucose available to brain cells. These symptoms will promptly disappear with treatment. The key roles of the critical-care nurse in this situation are assessment and protection from injury. Monitor the level of consciousness and neurologic status frequently. Remember that this patient is at risk for seizures; therefore, pad the side rails, and have airways and suction equipment on hand.

Knowledge Deficit Related to Mechanisms of Hypoglycemia

Even though hypoglycemic episodes occur in stable, knowledgeable patients, they may be largely preventable. Patients need to know as much as possible about the causes and effects of hypoglycemic episodes. One factor that helps in the critical-care unit and at home is the use of capillary blood glucose monitoring devices rather than relying on urine glucose as a monitor of blood glucose (Miller 1986). Review diet and insulin doses with physician and patient. Finally, an episode of hypoglycemia usually is very frightening for the patient. Reassurance, explanations, and appropriate intervention by the nurse are vital.

Outcome Evaluation

Evaluation of the patient with a hypoglycemic episode can be based on the following criteria:

- Serum glucose level between 80 and 120 mg/dl.
- Patient is awake and alert.
- Vital signs WNL.

THYROID CRISIS

Assessment

Risk Conditions

Thyroid crisis, also known as *hyperthyroid crisis, thyroid storm,* and *thyrotoxicosis,* refers to the body's response to excessive amounts of circulating thyroid hormone. *Thyrotoxicosis* is simply a hyperthyroid state, whereas *thyroid crisis* and *thyroid storm* are emergency situations requiring critical care. The cause or precipitating factor in a crisis varies. It may be a stress situation that causes decompensation in a previously stable patient. Other possible causes include excessive exogenous thyroid hormone, withdrawal of antithyroid drugs, and palpation of the thyroid gland (D Johnson 1983).

One of the main effects of thyroid hormone is to maintain the body's cellular metabolism. In a thyroid crisis, one of the presenting signs is an increase in body temperature related to this mechanism. The increase in metabolic activity also uses a lot of body fluid, so the patient may be diaphoretic and dehydrated. Increased adrenergic activity causes tachycardia, increased blood pressure, and a hyperdynamic heart. Respiratory function eventually may deteriorate, and there may be skeletal muscle weakening because of muscle mass catabolism. Gastrointestinally, the patient with thyroid crisis usually has an increased appetite, because of metabolic needs, and may have increased GI motility. Skin is thin and friable. Red blood cell volume may be increased because of increased O_2 requirements; however, about 3% of patients have pernicious anemia (D Johnson 1983). Nervous system changes such as nervousness, emotional lability, delirium, and tremors are common.

Laboratory assessment of a thyroid crisis is based primarily on serum levels of triiodothyronine (T_3) and thyroxine (T_4), the thyroid hormones that regulate metabolic activity. The synthesis of these hormones depends on the presence of iodine in the gland. When T_3 and T_4 enter the bloodstream, they are bound by plasma proteins. In the periphery, thyroid hormone is free or unbound and then active and available to the tissues and cells. Levels of T_3 and T_4 will increase during a thyroid crisis. Radionuclear scanning may demonstrate an enlarged or nodular thyroid. Radioactive iodine uptake may be done to indicate the functional state of the thyroid gland. Radioimmunoassay studies demonstrate decreased plasma thyroid-stimulating hormone (TSH) concentrations in most patients (Guyton 1986). TSH is released by the anterior pituitary gland by a negative feedback mechanism stimulated by low circulating levels of thyroid hormone. Low TSH concentrations rule out inappropriate pituitary secretion as the cause of the thyroid crisis.

NURSING DIAGNOSES

The following nursing diagnoses may apply to the patient with thyroid crisis:

- Fluid volume deficit
- Potential alteration in body temperature
- Potential decrease in cardiac output
- Potential for impaired gas exchange
- Alteration in nutrition: less than body requirements
- Impaired tissue integrity
- Sensory-perceptual alteration

Planning and Implementation of Care

Fluid Volume Deficit Related to Increased Metabolic Activity Secondary to Increased Circulating Thyroid Hormone

As discussed previously, patients may become dehydrated because of increased metabolism and diaphoresis. Therefore, fluid replacement is an important part of therapy. Assess for signs of dehydration, such as decreased urine output, poor skin turgor, and dry mucous membranes, and consult with the physician. Use caution when replacing fluids, however, and observe for any signs of congestive heart failure, such as increasing dyspnea, crackles in the chest, and increasing pulmonary vascular pressures. The patient may require large amounts of fluid to replace metabolic losses and maintain a state of hydration. At the same time, however, the patient is in a very hyperdynamic cardiovascular state secondary to increased adrenergic activity, so the nurse must assess for heart failure related to increased cardiac workload.

Potential Alteration in Body Temperature Related to Increased Metabolic Activity Secondary to Increased Thyroid Hormone

Patients in thyroid crisis often present with hyperthermia related to the heat produced by exaggerated metabolic processes. Body temperature can increase to as much as 104°F. The nurse needs to assess rectal temperature, degree of peripheral vasodilatation, and diaphoresis. A hypothermia blanket may be used (see page 437 for discussion of therapeutic hypothermia). Also, institute general supportive measures that may help decrease metabolic rate, such as maintaining a quiet environment, reducing stimulation, and providing periods of undisturbed rest. It is important not to administer acetylsalicylic acid (ASA), because one of its actions is displacement of thyroxine from thyroid-binding hormones and making it available to tissues. Insulin may be required to prevent hyperglycemia from glycogenolysis.

Potential Decreased Cardiac Output Related to Increased Cardiac Workload Secondary to Increased Adrenergic Activity

The stress of thyroid crisis on the cardiovascular (CV) system is usually quite obvious as tachycardia, hypertension, and other signs of the hyperdynamic state. The increased inotropic state of the myocardium may be observed as bounding peripheral pulses, systolic murmur on auscultation, and a precordial heave palpated at the apex. It is important to assess for dysrhythmias, most commonly tachycardias. Assess for clinical indicators of adequate cardiac output, such as urine output, sensorium, vital signs, and tissue perfusion. Beta-adrenergic blocking drugs such as propranolol may be ordered to block the effect of catecholamines on the heart. Beta blockade also blocks the conversion of T_4 to T_3, the metabolically active form of thyroid hormone (D Johnson 1983). Vasodilators such as hydralazine and sodium nitroprusside may be used to reduce workload on the heart by decreasing afterload and systemic vascular resistance. An arterial line may be placed to facilitate accurate titration of the vasoactive drugs and measurement of systemic vascular resistance.

Potential for Impaired Gas Exchange Related to Decreased Muscle Strength Secondary to Protein and Muscle Catabolism

During thyroid storm, the amount of protein in muscles decreases. Since thyroid hormone inhibits synthesis of protein, protein catabolism exceeds anabolism. Therefore, respiratory muscles weaken. Second, if heart failure develops as a result of increased cardiac workload, pulmonary congestion will ensue. Assess respiratory function frequently, auscultate the lungs, and administer oxygen as ordered.

Alteration in Nutrition: Less Than Body Requirements Related to Increased Nutrient Requirements Secondary to Increased Metabolic Activity

The patient in thyroid crisis cannot keep up with nutrient requirements. Supplemental feeding and vitamins are an important part of care. The patient should be weighed daily; if a state of adequate nutrition cannot be maintained, hyperalimentation should be administered.

Finally, the critical-care nurse administers pharmacologic therapy to decrease the deleterious effects of thyroid crisis. This therapy may include the following.

- Propylthiouracil (PTU) blocks the synthesis of thyroid hormones by interfering with conversion of thyroxine (T_4) to triiodothyronine (T_3).

- Methimazole (Tapazole) also works to inhibit thyroid hormone synthesis.

- Iodide inhibits the release of thyroid hormone from the gland. It should be given approximately 1-2 hours after PTU. This is important, because with earlier administration, PTU may cause an accumulation of iodide in the gland, which would be used for further synthesis.

- Glucocorticoids may be given to replace the rapidly metabolized cortisol. Dexamethasone, if used, also suppresses the conversion of T_4 to T_3.

Outcome Evaluation

Evaluate the recovery of a patient from thyroid crisis by the following criteria:

- Vital signs WNL.
- Body temperature normal.
- Patient is awake and oriented.
- Skin is warm and dry.
- State of hydration normal.
- Lung sounds clear bilaterally.
- Weight stable.
- Patient is calm and steady.

THERAPEUTIC HYPOTHERMIA

Assessment

Candidates

Therapeutic hypothermia is the deliberate lowering of body temperature. Patients who may benefit from therapeutic hypothermia fall into two main categories. The first includes those who have a temperature above normal due to heat stroke, thyroid crisis, or infection, and who remain febrile in spite of antipyretics and conservative measures such as tepid baths, cooling fans, and ice packs. These patients are candidates for hypothermia because each degree centigrade of temperature elevation above normal raises metabolism approximately 7%; this increases physiologic stress in a patient whose resources may be nearing depletion due to the critical nature of the illness. The second group of patients includes those who are normothermic and who suffer an insult whose effects can be minimized by reducing the normal metabolic demand. Examples are patients undergoing cardiovascular surgery or neurosurgery, or those with acute cerebral ischemia or edema, severe gastrointestinal bleeding, or persistent coma following cardiac arrest. Both groups may be helped by moderate hypothermia, which can reduce the total metabolic demand by 50%. The effect on the function of individual organs varies, with some, such as the brain, being affected profoundly and others, such as the kidney, being affected minimally.

Signs and Symptoms

To comprehend the signs and symptoms seen in hypothermic patients, it is helpful to understand the major physiologic principles of thermoregulation. Body temperature is controlled by the *thermoregulatory center* in the anterior hypothalamus (Guyton 1986). Two types of sensory receptors supply information to the thermoregulatory center: the peripheral receptors, which sense surrounding or ambient temperature, and the central receptors, located near the center itself, which sense the temperature of blood (L Johnson 1981). The center uses a number of mechanisms to preserve body temperature, among which are shunting of blood and the potent heat-producing response of shivering.

The body's thermoregulatory zones can be conceptualized as three concentric rings. The outermost zone is the *shell,* which consists of the skin and subcutaneous adipose tissue. The skeletal muscles form the middle zone. The innermost zone, the *core,* consists of the viscera, which the body tries to protect at all costs, whether body temperature falls precipitously or gradually.

The physiologic effects and signs and symptoms of hypothermia can be roughly correlated with the degree of temperature drop. They are summarized in Tables 17–1 and 17–2.

NURSING DIAGNOSES

Nursing diagnoses applicable to the hypothermic patient include:

- Altered comfort
- Altered tissue perfusion
- Shivering*
- Altered level of consciousness*
- Impaired gas exchange
- Potential impairment of skin integrity
- Potential decreased cardiac output
- Potential for injury

*Diagnosis developed by author.

Planning and Implementation of Care

Introduction of Therapeutic Hypothermia

The range of therapeutic hypothermia associated with the greatest physiologic benefit and least hazard is the

---

TABLE 17-1 PHYSIOLOGIC EFFECTS OF HYPOTHERMIA

Mild	37°C
	Neurologic: autonomic stimulation
	Metabolic: BMR increased 3× normal
	32°C
Moderate	Neurologic: cerebral metabolism 66% of normal, cerebral blood flow 70% of normal, CSF pressure 64% of normal
	Metabolic: BMR 50% of normal, depressed hypothalamic thermoregulation
	Cardiac: HR 50% of normal, prolonged diastole
	Respiratory: decreased CO_2 production, leftward shift of O_2/hemoglobin dissociation curve, total O_2 demand 50% of normal
	Liver: depressed function
	Kidney: moderately decreased GFR
	28°C
Severe	Metabolic: BMR < 25% of normal, paralyzed thermoregulation, mixed metabolic and respiratory acidosis
	Cardiac: prolonged systole, prolonged conduction time, depressed pacemaker activity, hemoconcentration, hypovolemia
	20°C
Profound	Absent thermogenesis

TABLE 17-2 SIGNS AND SYMPTOMS OF HYPOTHERMIA

Mild 32-37°C	Level of consciousness: agitation→confusion→apathy Heart: HR increased→decreased; BP increased→decreased Peripheral vasoconstriction: intense→decreased Respiration: RR increased→decreased Musculoskeletal: shivering moderate→intense→decreased Muscular coordination: poor→staggering
Moderate 28-32°C	Level of consciousness: stupor→coma Heart: dysrhythmias Respiration: decreased RR, decreased gag and cough reflexes Musculoskeletal: shivering alternating with rigor
Severe 20-28°C	Respiration: severe depression, absent gag reflex Musculoskeletal: absent reflexes, rigor Heart: high risk of ventricular fibrillation
Profound below 20°C	Level of consciousness: coma→absent EEG Heart: ventricular fibrillation→asystole Respiration: apnea Musculoskeletal: rigidity

moderate range, 28–32°C. Since this is the range used most commonly at the bedside, this chapter will focus on effects of moderate hypothermia and *not* those of deep hypothermia (below 28°C).

To initiate hypothermia, place the blanket on the bed and precool it if possible. Place a bed pad at the top of the blanket where the head will rest and another at the bottom where the feet will be. Cover the bedpads and hypothermia blanket with a single layer of a bath blanket, which will absorb skin perspiration and provide a softer surface on which the patient can lie.

Place the patient on the blanket. Prepare the skin and extremities as explained later. Insert the rectal temperature probe at least 2 inches, making sure it is not embedded in feces. Tape the probe in position; if it falls out, it will register the cold blanket temperature and cause the machine to heat the patient. Set the blanket temperature several degrees centigrade lower than the body temperature. Adjust the machine to shut off automatically when the desired hypothermic level is detected by the probe. Because probes and machines may be inaccurate, it is a wise precaution to periodically check the patient's temperature with a rectal thermometer during hypothermia induction and maintenance. If desired, a second hypothermia blanket may be placed on top of the patient to enhance cooling.

During induction, monitor the patient closely for the phenomena of drift and after-fall.

Drift *Drift* is defined as a sudden change in body temperature greater than 1°C in 15 minutes. Many nurses have observed that drift precedes frank shivering, shock, and dysrhythmias.

After-Fall *After-fall* is the phenomenon of continuing drop in core temperature after the hypothermia machine is turned off. It may occur even though the machine is turned off because the chilled coolant in the blanket remains in contact with the patient's body. In addition, during hypothermia the periphery cools more than the core, so even after hypothermia is discontinued, the warmer core continues to lose heat to the superficial tissues; in addition, temperature may drop as chilled blood is returned from the periphery. Therefore, the cooling device should be reset and the top cooling blanket removed when the rectal temperature is a few degrees centigrade above the desired temperature. The patient usually shows an after-fall of 2–5°C. The more rapid the drift, the greater the after-fall. Drift and after-fall are intensified when the patient is obese. Muscle tone, thermoregulatory and vascular responses, and ambient temperature and humidity also affect drift and after-fall, so you cannot predict the extent to which these phenomena will develop in a given patient.

Expected and Potential Effects

Altered Comfort Related to Cold Hypothermia is an unpleasant experience for the patient, both physically and emotionally. When the patient complains of being cold, let the patient express the discomfort, and reinforce the value of the cooling. Help focus on the fact that it is temporary. Be patient if the patient becomes irritable from the continuing discomfort. Follow the measures listed in later sections to prevent shivering which worsens the discomfort.

Altered Tissue Perfusion Related to Normal Thermoregulatory Responses Monitor vital signs, neurostatus, and peripheral perfusion every 15 minutes until stable, and then every 1–2 hours. During the first 20 minutes of hypothermia, the pulse rate rises, blood pressure increases, and respiratory rate accelerates due to sympathetic and metabolic responses to the drop in temperature. The body initially responds to the cold stimulus by conserving body heat and increasing heat production. Peripheral vasoconstriction minimizes surface heat loss, and skin coldness and pallor occur. The increased venous return due to the vasoconstriction causes the blood pressure to rise. Increased heat production is achieved by the intense muscular activity known as shivering, which occurs in nearly all people exposed to intense cold.

After about 20 minutes, vasoconstriction ceases and superficial blood flow returns. Reactive hyperemia causes reddened skin. As body heat continues to be lost, all vital signs decrease. They stabilize at lower levels when the desired degree of hypothermia is maintained. At moderate hypothermia, the cardiac refractory period and ventricular relaxation are prolonged. The heart rate slows, coronary arterial filling is proportionally enhanced, and ventricular contractility improves.

Urinary output does not change significantly. Although a moderate decrease in glomerular filtration occurs, secretion of antidiuretic hormone is inhibited. Thus, the output will increase and the urine osmolality and specific gravity may decrease; however, electrolyte excretion by the kidney is unchanged.

It is crucial that you interpret the patient's vital signs and urinary output in light of the expected changes. For example, a pulse rate of 90 at 30°C is an abnormal finding that requires prompt investigation. Similarly, a progressive drop in urinary output may signal the onset of hypovolemia or renal failure.

Shivering Related to Normal Thermoregulatory Response Shivering is a normal physiologic response to cold. Shivering is produced by stimulation of the shivering center in the posterior hypothalamus. This center appears to respond to superficial temperature receptors in the skin, which detect changes in skin temperature, and deep thermoreceptors in or near the hypothalamus, which detect changes in the temperature of blood perfusing this area (DeLapp 1983).

It is important to prevent or minimize shivering in the hypothermic patient for several reasons. Shivering increases the patient's discomfort. It also accelerates the metabolic rate, pulse, arterial pressure, venous pressure, cerebrospinal fluid pressure, oxygen consumption, carbon dioxide production, depletion of glycogen stores, and production and accumulation of lactic acid. These effects occur at a time when perfusion to the core organs already is reduced. Since blood flow to the muscles is increased during shivering, the temperature gradient between the core and periphery steepens, and core heat loss worsens. Shivering therefore is only a short-term mechanism for coping with hypothermia, with numerous undesirable effects (Holtzclaw 1986).

To minimize shivering (without pharmacologic therapy) implement the following:

1. Prevent rapid cooling of the distal limbs. Because the hands and feet are most distal from the body, they lose heat very rapidly. Slowing their rate of heat loss appears to slow the change in core temperature. Wrap the upper extremities from fingertips to elbows and the lower extremities from toes to knees, until the patient has stabilized at the desired temperature.

2. During induction of hypothermia, initially set the blanket temperature to provide a steep gradient between it and the patient (15°C is a common initial setting). Monitor the rectal temperature. If it drops more than 1°C per 15 minutes, reduce the gradient between the patient and blanket by increasing the setting for the blanket temperature.

3. Observe the patient for shivering. Premonitory signs of frank shivering are muscle tremor artifact on the ECG, and tensing or clenching of the masseter muscles, which close the jaw (Figure 17–1). Actual shivering begins in the masseters as a twitch and moves to

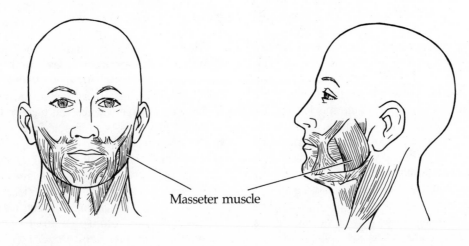

Masseter muscle

FIGURE 17-1

Location of masseter muscle.

the neck or pectoral areas. Frank shivering in the extremities and chattering teeth are later signs that usually necessitate pharmacologic intervention.

4. If shivering occurs, try reducing the rate of temperature decline by removing the top blanket or increasing the blanket temperature. If this action is contraindicated by the gravity of the patient's condition, the physician may prescribe chlorpromazine (Thorazine) in 10–25-mg doses. The effect of chlorpromazine on shivering is unpredictable. In addition, it causes vasodilatation, which produces hypotension, tachycardia, and increased core heat loss.

Altered Level of Conciousness Related to Decreased Cerebral Metabolism Cerebral metabolism drops more than the rest of the body, approximately 6.7% per degree centigrade. Cerebral blood flow decreases about a third, while cerebral metabolic demand diminishes about 54%. Since the decrease in cerebral metabolism is greater than the decrease in cerebral blood flow, cerebral perfusion is relatively improved. Cerebrospinal fluid pressure drops 5.5% per degree centigrade with moderate hypothermia.

At normal temperatures, the brain is slightly colder than the rest of the body. With surface cooling, it becomes 1–2°C warmer than the body core. Highly integrated centers are depressed first by hypothermia, providing a valuable cerebral protective mechanism even at moderately hypothermic levels. The sensorium, including hearing, fades at a body temperature of 33–34°C.

Nursing implications related to the decreased sensorium include applying artificial tears and taping the eyelids shut if blinking becomes infrequent. To evaluate changes in the level of consciousness, assess the more primitive responses, such as those elicited by painful stimuli, rather than higher integrative responses, such as response to a simple command.

Impaired Gas Exchange Related to Decreased Temperature and Decreased Tissue Perfusion The respiratory system undergoes several significant changes during hypothermia. Carbon dioxide production decreases, but ventilation decreases more rapidly. This imbalance between carbon dioxide production and excretion can lead to respiratory acidosis. Oxygen uptake increases, but cold shifts the oxyhemoglobin dissociation curve to the left, reducing the dissociation of O_2 from the red blood cells. This effect contributes to tissue hypoxia, which can precipitate ventricular irritability. If the hypoxic patient shivers, the cells must rely more heavily on anaerobic metabolism for energy production, which produces lactic acid and ketone bodies as by-products. Because circulation is reduced, these by-products accumulate and metabolic acidosis can occur.

Minimize the risk of acidosis by monitoring the blood gases closely. Prevent shivering. Once shivering occurs, consideration must be given to increased oxygen consumption, so administer oxygen as ordered. Promote ventilation through elevating the head of the bed, turning the patient frequently, and implementing a program of chest physiotherapy to enhance CO_2 elimination and removal of secretions. The physician may prescribe the addition of 2–5% CO_2 to the patient's ventilation. This treatment induces respiratory acidosis, which shifts the oxyhemoglobin dissociation curve back toward normal (the Bohr effect), thus promoting the release of oxygen to the tissues. It also dilates the cerebral vasculature, thus enhancing cerebral perfusion.

Potential Impairment of Skin Integrity Skin breakdown and frostbite can result from both diminished perfusion to the skin and the patient's decreased awareness of skin damage. Take the following steps to avoid these problems.

Keep the face, hands, and feet off the blanket. Place lamb's wool between the fingers and toes. Cover the hands and feet loosely with cotton and wrap them with stretch gauze. When bathing the patient, use tepid water and massage the skin gently to avoid producing heat. Turn the patient at least every 2 hours to relieve pressure points and massage the skin gently. To maintain the hypothermia, turn the blanket with the patient.

Potential Decreased CO Related to Dysrhythmias Be alert for dysrhythmias. Dysrhythmias (other than sinus bradycardia, which is an expected response) are unlikely to occur with moderate hypothermia if precautions are taken to ensure slow cooling and to avoid unintended deep hypothermia. During hypothermia, the total cardiac refractory period lengthens and and the vulnerable period is prolonged. The length of the vulnerable period is of concern, since an ectopic ventricular beat falling during the vulnerable period of the ventricles may initiate ventricular tachycardia or fibrillation. The likelihood of ectopic beats producing ventricular tachycardia or fibrillation does not increase dangerously during hypothermia until the temperature drops below 28°C. To minimize ventricular irritability, limit the temperature drop to 1°C per 15 minutes and preferably do not allow the core temperature to go below 28°C.

Hypothermia prolongs all intervals on the ECG. In addition, it often causes a slowly inscribed terminal portion of the QRS, called a J wave or Osborn wave. This wave, illustrated in Figure 17–2, does not signify any danger; it is an incidental finding. It is most pronounced in leads V_3–V_6.

Other electrocardiographic findings may include a

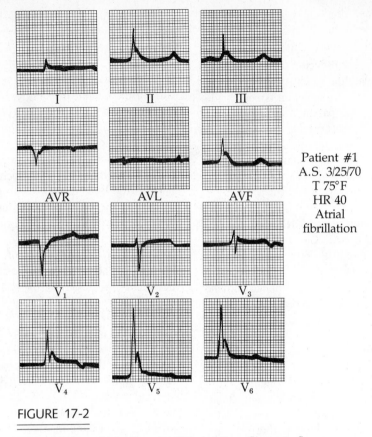

Patient #1
A.S. 3/25/70
T 75°F
HR 40
Atrial
fibrillation

FIGURE 17-2

ECG of accidental hypothermia. (Adapted from Clements S, Hurst J: Diagnostic value of electrocardiographic abnormalities observed in subjects accidentally exposed to cold. *Am J Cardio* 1972; 29:729. Used with permission of the author and publisher.)

fine muscle tremor and, at lower hypothermic levels, atrial fibrillation with a slow ventricular response.

Potential Decreased Tissue Perfusion Related to Thrombosis and Embolization During hypothermia, fluid shifts from the intravascular space into the intracellular and interstitial spaces. This shift leaves the blood more concentrated, and thrombosis and embolization may occur. Use support stockings, frequent turning, and range of motion exercises. See Chapter 8 for further suggestions on avoiding this complication.

Potential for Injury Related to Altered Drug Absorption Because of the altered absorption of drugs produced by decreased perfusion, avoid subcutaneous and intramuscular injections; give medications intravenously instead. If a medication must be given intramuscularly, use a deep injection technique.

Although few liver functions are decreased by moderate hypothermia, the ability to detoxify morphine and some barbiturates is reduced. The physician may prescribe reduced doses or substitutes for these drugs.

Rewarming

When hypothermia is no longer needed, rewarm the patient gradually. Although active (artificial) surface rewarming can be used, it carries the danger of warming the periphery before the core. The still-cold heart then may be unable to produce a CO adequate for the metabolic demands of the warmer areas. Dilatation of the surface vessels causes blood pooling, a diminished venous return, and a further decrease in cardiac output. These conditions may lead to "rewarming shock."

NURSING RESEARCH NOTE

Rafalowski M: Relationship of core temperature at time of blanket removal to subsequent core temperature in patients immediately after coronary artery bypass. *Heart Lung* 1987; 16:9–13.

One commonly used nursing measure to reverse hypothermia after cardiac surgery is the application of warmed blankets. Does the core temperature at which the nurse removes these blankets have any relationship to patients' subsequent temperatures?

Twenty-four stable male cardiac surgical patients were studied. Subjects met a number of criteria (such as no intraoperative myocardial infarction) designed to eliminate other factors that might affect body temperature regulation. Blankets were warmed for at least 20 minutes in a blanket warmer at a temperature equal to or less than 60°C (140°F).

The researcher applied three blankets on completion of the surgery. Patients were randomly assigned to one of two treatment groups: Group A had blankets removed when rectal temperatures reached 36.9°C (98.4°F); group B had them removed when temperatures reached 37.4°C (99.4°F). Temperatures were monitored every 15 minutes until blanket removal and every hour for 8 hours thereafter. Mean core temperatures were calculated from these readings. Demographic, preoperative, intraoperative, and postoperative data were recorded, including time of blanket removal and doses of antipyretics.

A one-way analysis of variance (ANOVA) revealed a significant difference between the time of blanket removal and mean core temperature (no significant difference was detected for peak temperatures). Using an analysis of covariance to control for antipyretic administration, the relationship between the groups' mean core temperature and time of blanket removal was statistically significant ($p = 0.0096$). Hourly temperature recordings following blanket removal were analyzed using an ANOVA of nested repeated measures. The thermal curves of the groups were significantly different ($p = 0.0001$): group B had a statistically significant sustained temperature elevation.

The researcher concluded that the simple nursing measure of promptly removing warming blankets when core temperature nears normal does affect postoperative temperature curves. She recommends further studies to substantiate the results and to identify the optimal temperature for warm blanket removal.

When therapeutic hypothermia has been used, natural rewarming is preferred. Simply remove the cooling blanket and place a bed blanket over the patient. The temperature should return to normal at the rate of approximately 1.0°C per hour.

Possible Complications

Shock and Acidosis During the rewarming period, which may take several hours, observe for shock and acidosis. Shock may result from too rapid warming, as explained above; this can occur even if the rewarming is achieved naturally. Acidosis may result from inadequate perfusion of the warmer areas or a release of the lactic acid that accumulated during shivering. During rewarming, the level of consciousness, pulse, blood pressure, and respiratory rate should increase proportionately to the core temperature. When any decrease or disproportionate increase occurs, alert the physician, who may want to investigate other possible causes (such as a bleeding ulcer), prescribe vasopressors, or initiate recooling.

Cumulative Drug Effects During the rewarming phase, remember to observe for the cumulative effects of previously administered drugs, particularly those given intramuscularly. Also, remember that hearing will return at about 34°C; you can use this knowledge to gradually reorient the patient to the surroundings.

Ulcers Another problem that may appear during rewarming is gastritis or peptic ulceration. During hypothermia, pepsin production continues, although the secretion of gastric juice diminishes. When rewarming occurs and gastric juice flow increases, it contains an increased concentration of pepsin. Notify the physician if signs of gastritis or ulceration appear.

Overhydration Rewarming causes fluid to shift from the intracellular and interstitial spaces back into the intravascular compartment. If fluids were not given cautiously during hypothermia, signs of overhydration may appear during rewarming. Recognition and management of fluid volume excess is discussed in detail in Chapter 16.

Outcome Evaluation

- Temperature WNL.
- BP and pulse WNL.
- ABGs WNL.
- Level of consciousness WNL.
- Urinary output 60–100 ml/hr.

REFERENCES

Baer C: Regulation and assessment of water and electrolyte balance. In *AACN's clinical reference for critical care nursing.* Kinney M et al. (eds). New York: McGraw-Hill, 1982.

Barrett EV et al.: Insulin resistance in diabetic ketoacidosis. *Diabetes* 1982; 31:923–938.

Benner P: From novice to expert. Menlo Park, CA: Addison-Wesley, 1984.

Carroll P, Matz R: Uncontrolled diabetes mellitus in adults: Experience in treating diabetic ketoacidosis and hyperosmolar nonketotic coma with low-dose insulin and a uniform treatment regime. *Diabetes Care* 1983; 6(6).

DeLapp T: Accidental hypothermia. *Am J Nurs* 1983; 83:63–67.

Foster DW, McGarry JD: The metabolic derangements and treatment of diabetic ketoacidosis. *N Engl J Med* 1983; 309:159–169.

Guthrie DW, Guthrie RA: *Nursing management of diabetes mellitus,* 2d ed. St Louis: Mosby, 1982.

Guyton A: *Textbook of medical physiology,* 7th ed. Philadelphia: Saunders, 1986.

Hillman DM: Resuscitation in diabetic ketoacidosis. *Crit Care Med* 1983; 11:53–54.

Holtzclaw BJ: Postoperative shivering after cardiac surgery: A review. *Heart Lung* 1986; 15:292–300.

Hudak CM et al.: *Critical care nursing: A holistic approach.* Philadelphia: Lippincott, 1986.

Johnson D: Pathophysiology of thyroid storm: Nursing implications. *Crit Care Nurse* 1983; 3:80–86.

Johnson L: Hypothermia and cold injury. *STAT* 1981; 2:108–116.

Kriesberg R: Diabetic ketoacidosis, alcoholic ketosis, lactic acidosis, and hyporeninemic hypoaldosteronism. In *Diabetes mellitus: Theory and practice,* 3d ed. Ellinberg M, Ritkin H (eds). New York: Medical Publishing Co., 1983.

Leske JS: Hyperglycemic hyperosmolar nonketotic coma: A nursing care plan. *Crit Care Nurse* 1985; 5:49–56.

Miller VG: Diabetes: Let's stop testing urine. *Am J Nurs* 1986; 86:54.

Price S, Wilson L: *Pathophysiology: Clinical concepts of disease processes,* 3d ed. New York: McGraw-Hill, 1986.

Sommers MS: Nonketotic hyperosmolar coma. *Crit Care Nurse* 1983; 3:58–61.

Swearingen PL et al.: *Manual of nursing therapeutics.* Menlo Park, CA: Addison-Wesley, 1986.

Winters B: Nursing implications of hyperosmolar coma. *Heart Lung* 1983; 12:439–446.

SUPPLEMENTAL READING

Alspach JG, Williams SM (eds): *Core curriculum for critical care nursing,* 3d ed. Philadelphia: Saunders, 1985.

Burman KD: Interpretation of thyroid function tests in systemically ill patients. *Crit Care Quart* 1983; 6:1–9.

Clochesy JM: Profound hypothermia. *Focus Crit Care* 1984; 11:19–21.

Cooke SS: Major thermal injury: The first 48 hours. *Crit Care Nurse* 1986; 6:55–62.

Fournier AM et al.: Blood pressure, insulin, and glycemia in non-diabetic patients. *Am J Med* 1986; 80:861–864.

Laakso M et al.: Prevalence of insulin deficiency among initially non-insulin-dependent middle-aged diabetic individuals. *Diabetes Care* 1986; 9:228–231.

McCarthy JA: The continuum of diabetic coma. *Am J Nurs* 1985; 85:878–880.

Nyberg G et al.: Time as a risk factor in diabetic nephropathy. *Diabetes Care* 1985; 8:590–593.

Hematologic/Immunologic Disorders

CLINICAL INSIGHT

Domain: The helping role

Competency: Being with a patient

Expert nurses know that there are times when words no longer comfort a patient, and they then provide solace through their very presence. The exquisite comfort provided by deeply felt, unspoken communication elegantly exemplifies the primacy of caring in expert nursing practice. In this extract, from Crabtree and Jorgenson (1986, p. 107), Kelly, the nurse, talks about Jon, an AIDS patient. Jon is struggling with whether to request resuscitative measures if he codes—knowing that he would thereby expose others to the disease. Kelly describes how Jon, surrounded by people who love him, wrestles with his poignant dilemma:

Then we decided that we needed to talk to him about what he wanted done . . . did he want to be a blue cart? We needed to explain to him totally what a blue cart was. His sister was in the room, and he had a very close friend, who was also a nurse—a public health nurse—and she had come in. We sat down with him and said, this is what a blue cart is. . . . You will have to be bagged; there will be a lot of peo-

ple in the room; more than likely you will have central lines placed because everything was peripheral at this time. Then I told him that blood will be everywhere, and there will be a lot of people exposed to it. And, there's probably not a whole lot we could do because of the cancer; your lungs are just not responding to treatment, and we're not oxygenating you, and I just flat out told him, somebody's going to be pushing on your chest; you may have to be shocked a couple times; I stressed the facts of everything.

Armed with this explicit information, Jon reaches the decision Kelly already knew he would—and she remains to comfort him with her very presence.

He was very aware of his disease and how it affected other people, and he said, no, I don't want to be coded because I don't want to expose people to that, to me, not knowing what's going to happen, getting blood all over, tracking blood everywhere, and I respected his opinion, and he seemed to deal real well with knowing that. But, after we were all done talking about it, he just, like, held on to my hand and just, you know. And then, afterwards, he wrote me a note saying, thank you for being so honest and thanks for being here, and he said he just wanted time, he said, just to be with me for a few minutes even

*though we were so busy in the unit; it's like I can't
just walk out on him, so I stayed in there with him
for awhile.*

The number of patients in critical-care units with hematologic and immunologic disorders has been increasing over the last few years. This chapter will focus on
the two major hematologic/immunologic disorders challenging the critical-care nurse: disseminated intravascular coagulation (DIC) and acquired immunodeficiency
syndrome (AIDS). Although both of these disorders are
quite complex and researchers are still learning more
about them at a rapid rate, this chapter provides the
nurse a knowledge of common laboratory tests used to
assess hematologic function, an understanding of the
critical care of a patient with disseminated intravascular
coagulation, and an understanding of current knowledge
and care of the patient with acquired immunodeficiency
syndrome. Even more challenging than these patients'
physical care is sensitivity to their emotional needs,
movingly illustrated in the Clinical Insight.

Laboratory Tests

Laboratory measures of hematopoiesis and coagulation
can provide helpful assessment clues when used as adjuncts to the patient's history and physical examination.

Complete Blood Count (CBC) and
Reticulocyte Count

The complete blood count (CBC) is a series of tests
that provides a fairly comprehensive evaluation of the
blood's formed elements. This common group of laboratory tests measures red blood cells *(erythrocytes),*
white blood cells *(leukocytes),* and platelets (Figure 18-
1). Red blood cells (RBCs) have three major functions:
oxygen transport, carbon dioxide transport, and acid–
base buffering. In the normal adult, RBC production occurs in the marrow of membranous bones, for example,
the vertebrae, sternum, ribs, and pelvis. Production is
stimulated by *erythropoietin,* a glycoprotein formed primarily in the kidneys in response to hypoxia. Normal
red blood cell formation requires the presence of amino
acids, iron, Vitamin B_{12}, folic acid, and other nutrients
(Porth 1986).
Red blood cell measures contained in the CBC are

the red cell count, hemoglobin level, and hematocrit.
The normal *red cell count* varies with sex, age, altitude,
and exercise. It usually falls within 4.5–6.0 million per
μl for males and 4.0–5.5 million per μl for females. *Hemoglobin* is an iron–protein complex, formed and carried
inside RBCs, that functions in O_2 and CO_2 transport and
in acid-base buffering. Males usually have a hemoglobin
level between 14 and 18 g per 100 ml and females between 12 and 16 g. The *hematocrit* expresses the volume percentage of red blood cells in whole blood, and
normally ranges between 40% and 54% for males and
37–47% for females. The red cell count, hemoglobin
level, and hematocrit usually follow the same trend. Elevated values, for instance, occur with hemoconcentration due to blood loss; dehydration; and polycythemia.
Decreased values are seen in fluid overload, recent
hemorrhage, and anemia.

Additional information on red cell production can be
obtained from a separately ordered reticulocyte count.
Reticulocytes are immature RBCs, which usually represent 0.5–2.0% of the RBC count. An increased reticulocyte count indicates an accelerated rate of RBC production, such as in hemolysis or hemorrhage. A
decreased count means depressed bone marrow production of red cells, as in aplastic anemia, or acute blood
loss.

White blood cells (WBCs), or leukocytes, are mobile
cells that function to protect the tissues from inflammatory agents, remove cellular debris, and participate in
the immune response. The CBC contains both a total
white cell count and a differential white cell count.

The *total white cell count* normally ranges between
5,000 and 10,000/dl. An increased count is a common,
nonspecific finding seen in various types of inflammation, tissue necrosis, and leukemia. A decreased count,
signifying bone marrow depression, occurs in viral infections, hepatitis, radiation therapy, and toxic reactions,
and certain immune disorders.

On the basis of their cytoplasmic, nuclear, and staining characteristics, WBCs are subdivided into five major
classes, which are reported in the *WBC differential
count.* Both the total WBC count and the differential
count are important in diagnosis. The white cell count
can indicate the presence of a general abnormality, such
as infection. The differential's detailed information on
white cell distribution, when interpreted in conjunction
with the total count, can provide information on the
stage and severity of specific disorders.

Those WBCs formed in the bone marrow are termed
granulocytes (because their cytoplasm contains numerous granules) or *polymorphonuclear leukocytes* (due to
the irregular shapes of their nuclei). Granulocytes are
divided further, on the basis of their staining characteristics, into neutrophils, eosinophils, and basophils. *Neu-*

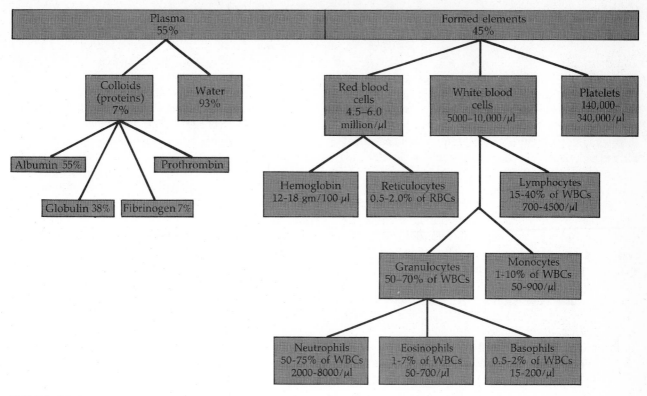

FIGURE 18-1

Blood constituents.

trophils are phagocytic cells that represent the body's first line of defense. Almost any process causing tissue damage, whether or not accompanied by inflammation, attracts neutrophils that phagocytize and digest foreign particles and damaged tissue. Among the conditions in which the neutrophil percentage rises are infection, surgical procedures, and myocardial infarction. A decreased neutrophil count occurs with hepatitis, aplastic anemia, some viral infections, and some medications, such as sulfonamides and antihistamines.

Eosinophils also are phagocytic cells. Although their exact function is unclear, they appear to detoxify foreign proteins and ingest antigen/antibody complexes. The eosinophil count rises in administration of foreign proteins, allergic reactions, and parasitic infections. It decreases with high levels of epinephrine and adrenocorticotropic hormone, as in severe stress reactions.

Basophils also have an unclear role. They are believed to carry histamine, appear to participate actively in allergic responses, and secrete heparin. The percentage increases with splenectomy, radiation therapy, and hemolytic anemia.

In addition to the WBCs formed in bone marrow, some are formed in the lymphoid tissues, which include the lymph glands, thymus, and spleen. These cells, which do not have granular cytoplasm but do have nuclei, are termed *lymphocytes* and *monocytes*. *Monocytes* are capable of transforming into *macrophages*, the highly powerful cells that ingest and digest foreign substances and cellular debris. *Lymphocytes* (also termed *immunocompetent cells*) have the capability of becoming sensitized against specific antigens and secreting antibodies. The lymphocyte count rises in inflammation, viral infections, hepatitis, and lymphocytic leukemia. It drops in radiation therapy and stress reactions. The monocyte count increases in inflammation and monocytic leukemia; decreases are rarely seen.

Platelets (thrombocytes) are another of the blood cell elements formed in the bone marrow. The normal platelet count is 140,000–340,000/μl. Platelets initiate blood clotting, as explained in detail in the next section (on blood coagulation). The platelet count is decreased in most leukemias and idiopathic thrombocytopenic purpura and elevated in some anemias, severe hemorrhage, and thrombocytosis (Porth 1986; Guyton 1986; Griffin 1986).

Blood Coagulation

Blood coagulation is an intricate sequence of chemical reactions that remains only partly understood despite years of investigation. The following simplified explanation is based on Guyton (1986).

When a blood vessel is ruptured, hemostasis occurs in several steps (Figure 18-2). First, vessel spasm limits the amount of blood loss. Second, a platelet plug forms because platelets adhere to the roughened endothelial surface and cause additional platelets to adhere to them. Third, a blood clot forms. Fourth, fibroblasts invade the clot and organize it into fibrous tissue within 8–10 days, or, less commonly, the clot dissolves.

Instrumental in clotting are prothrombin and fibrinogen, two plasma proteins formed by the liver. Coagulation occurs in three basic steps: the *formation of prothrombin activator* (Stage I), the *conversion of prothrombin to thrombin* (Stage II), and the *conversion of fibrinogen to fibrin* (Stage III).

Prothrombin can be activated by either of two systems. The systems are difficult to describe, as steps provoke others in a cascade and several steps occur si-multaneously (see Figure 18–2). Vascular injury itself initiates an intrinsic activator system, while damage to tissue initiates an extrinsic system. Although separated for purposes of analysis, these systems interact in the patient.

The factor that initiates the *intrinsic pathway* appears to be trauma to the blood itself or blood contact with subendothelial collagen. The initiating event causes platelets to release platelet phospholipids. It also activates Factor XII, which in turn activates Factor XI, which subsequently activates Factor IX. Activated Factor IX next activates Factor VIII, which in the presence of platelet phospholipids and calcium activates Factor X.

In the *extrinsic system,* damaged tissue releases thromboplastin and tissue phospholipids. Thromboplastin interacts with Factor VII in the presence of calcium and tissue phospholipids to activate Factor X.

From the activation of Factor X, clotting proceeds almost identically for both pathways. Activated Factor X interacts with Factor V, calcium, and platelet or tissue phospholipids to convert prothrombin to thrombin. Thrombin is a proteolytic enzyme that in turn converts fibrinogen to fibrin.

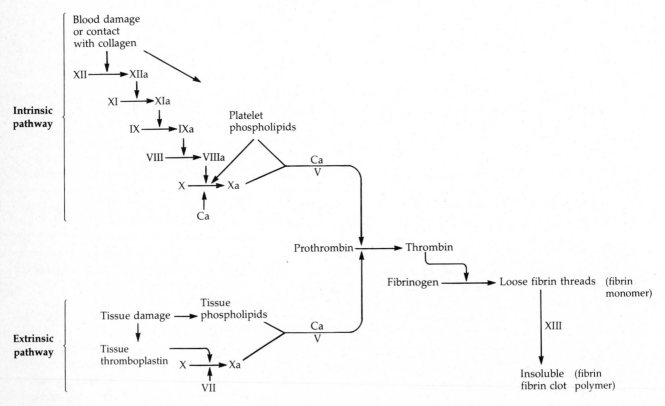

FIGURE 18-2

Coagulation process.

Loose fibrin threads adhere to the vessel wall, forming a network and trapping platelets, RBCs, and plasma. The loose threads are formed into an insoluble clot by Factor XIII. The clot then retracts, squeezing out the plasma and further binding the margins of the vessel rupture. Large numbers of platelets, which apparently bond the fibrin threads together, are needed for retraction.

The formation of fibrin activates a fibrinolytic system that serves to limit clotting to the area of injury. When a clot is formed, it incorporates a plasma protein called *plasminogen* (profibrinolysin). Although the mechanisms are unclear, plasminogen can be activated by several substances. Activated plasminogen becomes plasmin (fibrinolysin), a proteolytic enzyme that digests the fibrin threads and destroys the surrounding clotting factors.

Endogenous anticoagulants normally prevent both spontaneous blood clotting and clot extension. Among the most important anticoagulants are the smoothness of vascular endothelium and a negatively charged inner layer of endothelium that repels platelets and clotting factors. Also, the rapidity of blood flow tends to carry clotting factors away from a developing clot and thereby limit clot size. In addition, the clot's fibrin threads trap most of the thrombin. The remainder is inactivated by antithrombin-heparin cofactor, and by fibrin degradation products released during fibrinolysis.

Finally, the blood contains heparin. This strong anticoagulant is produced primarily by the mast cells located around the capillaries in the lungs and liver.

This brief explanation of the coagulation process helps to explain the various types of coagulation tests and the kinds of disorders that cause coagulation abnormalities.

A coagulation profile is used as a preoperative screening measure or an aid in diagnosis of a bleeding disorder. Although numerous tests may be ordered, the most common are the clotting time, activated partial thromboplastin time, prothrombin time, and fibrinogen level. (As with other laboratory tests, normal values vary among laboratories.)

The clotting or coagulation time is a general indicator of the blood's ability to clot and is used to evaluate the intrinsic pathway. It is determined on a venous sample by a number of methods, most commonly either the activated clotting time (ACT) or the Lee White. For the *Lee White* procedure, blood is mixed gently at 30-second intervals, and the time required for it to clot is noted. Since numerous factors participate in the clotting process, this test is nonspecific for clotting abnormalities. For the *ACT,* an activator that stimulates Factor XII is added to the blood. A prolonged clotting time may indicate anticoagulant therapy, liver disease, or a deficiency of any factor except VII. Results also are influenced by extraneous factors such as the size of test tubes and room temperature.

Because standardized results are so difficult to obtain for the clotting time, some physicians prefer the activated *partial thromboplastin time* (PTT). It too reflects the general clotting ability of the blood but is faster, more sensitive, and more easily standardized. It tests both the intrinsic and common pathways. The range of normal values is 30–40 seconds.

The clotting time and activated partial thromboplastin time are used primarily to monitor patients on heparin. They also are used to detect bleeding tendencies and evaluate hemorrhagic disorders.

Blood for the *prothrombin time* is a nonfasting, venous sample that is oxalated after drawing to prevent the conversion of prothrombin to thrombin. In the laboratory, calcium is added to neutralize the oxalate, and thromboplastin is added to provoke the conversion of prothrombin to thrombin. The time necessary for fibrin threads to appear then is noted. The test thus bypasses the intrinsic clotting process and evaluates the extrinsic system, as well as Stages II and III. A control value also is reported, based on the concurrent reactivity of reagents used in the test. The normal prothrombin time is 12-15 seconds. A prolonged prothrombin time may indicate coumarin therapy, liver disease, vitamin K deficiency, or obstructive jaundice (the deficiency of bile salts blocks intestinal absorption of vitamin K). The prothrombin time is the preferred test for monitoring oral anticoagulant therapy.

The *fibrinogen level* is determined on plasma extracted from a venous blood sample. The normal level is 200–400 mg/100 ml. The level is decreased in fibrinolytic disorders and in disseminated intravascular coagulation.

A test for the presence of *fibrin degradation products* (FDP) or *fibrin split products* (FSP) also may be done with hematologic disorders. Increased levels will be present when clot lysis is occurring, either endogenously or exogenously such as during intracoronary injection of streptokinase. The laboratory test method for measuring FDP is called the *red blood cell hemagglutination inhibition immune assay* (Hubner 1986).

When a platelet disorder is suspected, both the bleeding time and platelet count are evaluated. The platelet count determines the actual number of circulating platelets, and the bleeding time measures platelet function, the ability of the platelets to adhere and aggregate. Both are important in diagnosis. For example, a patient on large doses of aspirin may have adequate numbers of platelets; however, since aspirin prevents platelet aggregation and ability to adhere, bleeding time will increase.

DISSEMINATED INTRAVASCULAR COAGULATION (DIC)

Disseminated intravascular coagulation (DIC) is a complex disorder characterized, paradoxically, by simultaneous thrombosis and hemorrhage. It results from inappropriate, accelerated, systemic activation of the clotting system, which continues without its normal controls. To understand the pathophysiology of the disorder, you need to be familiar with the normal coagulation and fibrinolytic systems.

Assessment

Risk Conditions

There are numerous conditions that can place patients at risk for development of DIC. Among them are the following.

- *Tissue injury.* Trauma, burns, crush syndrome, snake bite
- *Antigen/antibody reactions.* Anaphylactic reactions, incompatible blood transfusions, transplant rejections
- *Obstetric emergencies.* Abruptio placentae, amniotic fluid embolism, incomplete abortion, retained dead fetus
- *Neoplasms.* Leukemia, solid tumors
- *Infections.* Septic shock
- *Prolonged hypotension*
- *Acidosis*

In DIC, the release of procoagulants initiates uncontrolled microcirculatory clotting. A number of procoagulants have been implicated, including bacterial toxins, free hemoglobin, and fragments of cancer or placental tissue. If the procoagulants cause endothelial wall damage, they can activate the intrinsic clotting pathway, the complement system, or the plasmin/kinin system. If they cause tissue injury, the procoagulants can activate the extrinsic clotting pathway. In many instances, of course, the triggering event activates more than one

pathway promoting coagulation (Kenner et al. 1986; Griffin 1986).

Whatever the triggering mechanism, explosive thrombin production occurs. The rapid thrombin formation causes three major problems: *diffuse fibrin deposition in the microcirculation, avid consumption of clotting factors, and provocation of the fibrinolytic system.*

Almost all patients with DIC have suffered an episode of prolonged hypotension. In arterial hypotension, arterial vasoconstriction combined with capillary dilatation and the opening of preferential arteriovenous shunts leads to stagnation of blood in many capillaries. The blood pooled in the capillaries rapidly becomes acidotic, which worsens the situation, as acidosis itself is another procoagulant. As the abnormal procoagulants accumulate in the acidotic blood, widespread clotting occurs in the microcirculation. This microcirculatory clotting in turn causes widespread organ ischemia and necrosis. As the capillaries of an average adult represent a total length of approximately 100,000 miles, clotting factors are consumed faster than they can be replaced (hence the term *consumption coagulopathy* sometimes used to describe DIC).

The presence of thrombin activates the fibrinolytic system, as a homeostatic mechanism to maintain patency of the microcirculation in compensation for the widespread obstruction to blood flow caused by the diffuse clotting (Rooney and Haviley 1985). The fibrinolytic system functions to limit clotting and in so doing produces FDPs (or FSPs). The FDPs also act as anticoagulants, interfering with the activity of thrombin, fibrin, and platelets.

Following the initial clotting and fibrinolysis, what is left in the microcirculation is a web of fibrin and FDPs. This web mechanically damages red blood cells trying to pass through it, causing the production of fragmented red blood cells, schistocytes, and hemolytic anemia (Kenner et al. 1986). As a result of the decreased availability of coagulation factors and the increased presence of anticoagulants, the patient's blood is unable to form stable clots in places where they are needed, and bleeding occurs into the skin, from body orifices, and at sites of catheters and incisions.

Although the clinical history is important in diagnosis, DIC is primarily a laboratory rather than clinical diagnosis. There is no specific test to diagnose DIC; instead, a panel of tests is evaluated to detect the presence and progress of DIC. The most common laboratory tests used to diagnose DIC are (a) prothrombin time, (b) partial thromboplastin time (PTT), (c) fibrinogen level, (d) platelet count, and (e) fibrin degradation products. In DIC, the prothrombin time and PTT are prolonged, due to the depletion of prothrombin and Factor V. The fibrinogen level is decreased, due to the depletion of fibrinogen. The platelet count is diminished, due to platelet consumption. In contrast to the decreased values of these two tests, fibrin degradation products are increased.

Signs and Symptoms

DIC can exist in chronic, subacute, and acute forms. The *chronic* form may be seen in patients with chronic DIC-provoking disorders, such as leukemia. The *subacute* form is present when the typical laboratory indications of DIC are present but the patient is not yet showing clinical signs. In the *acute* form, the earliest signs are blood oozing from multiple sites, such as IV line and blood sample puncture sites, or around nasotracheal or nasogastric tubes. The integumentary system shows petechiae, purpura, and ecchymotic areas. Signs of organ ischemia and necrosis, such as angina, may be present. Finally, significant, life-threatening bleeding episodes may occur.

NURSING DIAGNOSES

Because of the complexity of the disorder, multiple nursing diagnoses exist. They include:

- Fluid volume deficit
- Potential fluid volume excess
- Altered tissue perfusion
- Altered urinary elimination
- Impaired gas exchange
- Pain
- Altered level of consciousness
- Impaired skin integrity
- Altered oral mucous membrane
- Fear
- Disturbed self concept

Planning and Implementation of Care

Fluid Volume Deficit Related to Bleeding

1. *Note the presence and degree of bleeding.* Observe for the subtle signs that could signal the onset of DIC. In addition to observing for the persistent oozing and integumentary signs mentioned earlier, test GI drainage (nasogastric, emesis, and stool) and urinary drainage for the presence of occult blood. Also observe the degree of bleeding from wound sites, and, in women, check for the onset of vaginal bleeding.

2. *Monitor the blood pressure.* Try to prevent surges in blood pressure, which can disturb unstable clots and initiate new bleeding episodes. Also try to prevent hypotensive episodes, which, as mentioned earlier, contribute to the vicious cycle of clotting in DIC.

3. *Monitor laboratory values.* Evaluate the risk of bleeding episodes and the effectiveness of treatment measures.

4. *Administer medical and pharmacologic therapy as ordered.* Assist in the treatment of the underlying cause, as well as treatment of hypotension and acidosis when present. Meticulously administer and monitor the heparin therapy ordered. Heparin interrupts the cycle of clotting and bleeding, by inhibiting the action of thrombin (and therefore inhibiting platelet aggregation and the conversion of fibrinogen to fibrin), inhibiting the activation of Factor X (thereby blocking both the intrinsic and extrinsic pathways contributing to thrombin formation), and preventing further extension of already-developed clots (Rooney and Haviley 1985). Heparin usually is given as a continuous IV infusion of 1000 units per hour; lower doses are used in renal and liver failure. Use an infusion control device, and monitor it closely to ensure its accuracy. Also monitor the clotting time; the therapeutic level usually is 2–3 times normal. Finally, remember to double-check other drugs for compatibility with heparin, to avoid accidental over-anticoagulation. Heparin therapy is controversial in DIC; some experts argue that using heparin can cause thrombocytopenia and significant thromboses (Hewitt and Davies 1983; Griffin 1986).

After heparinization (if used) is underway, administer transfusion therapy as ordered. Administering transfusions prior to the establishment of heparinization is contraindicated, because administration of blood products with clotting factors will potentiate continuation of the process. Fresh whole blood, fresh frozen plasma, platelet concentrate, and factor concentrates are preferred for provision of coagulation factors and platelets (see Table 18-1).

Occasionally, antifibrinolytic drugs such as aminocaproic acid are administered with heparin. This drug retards the lysis of clots by inhibiting plasmin. It is given after heparin because there is the risk of further clot formation if given before.

TABLE 18-1 COMMONLY USED BLOOD PRODUCTS

PRODUCT	APPROXIMATE VOLUME	INDICATIONS	PRECAUTIONS/COMMENTS
Whole blood (WB)	500–510 ml (450 WB; 50–60 anticoagulants)	Acute, severe blood loss; hypovolemic shock. Increases both red cell mass and plasma	Must be ABO and Rh compatible. Do not mix with dextrose solutions; always prime tubing with normal saline. Observe for dyspnea, orthopnea, cyanosis, and anxiety as signs of circulatory overload; monitor VS. Hepatitis risk = 2*.
Packed red blood cells (RBCs)	250 ml	Increases RBC mass and oxygen-carrying capacity of the blood	Must be ABO and Rh compatible. Less immunologic risk than with WB because some donor antibodies are removed. Less volume, reducing risk of fluid overload. Hepatitis risk = 2*.
Fresh frozen plasma (FFP)	250 ml	Treatment of choice for combined coagulation factor deficiencies and Factor V and XI deficiencies; alternate treatment for Factor VII, VIII, IX, and X deficiencies when concentrates are not available	Must be ABO compatible. Supplies clotting factors. Usual dose is 10–15 ml/kg body weight. Hepatitis risk = 2**.
Platelet concentrate	25–50 ml (volumes may vary; usual adult dose is 5–6 U)	Treatment of choice for thrombocytopenia. Also used for leukemia and hypoplastic anemia	Usual dose is 0.1 U/kg body weight to increase platelet count to 25,000. Administer as rapidly as tolerated. ABO compatibility is preferable, but is expensive and usually not practical. Effectiveness is decreased by fever, sepsis, and splenomegaly. Febrile reactions are common. Use special "platelet" tubing and filter. Hepatitis risk = 2**.
Platelet concentrate by platelet pheresis	200 ml, but may vary	Treatment for thrombocytopenic patients who are refractory to random donor platelets	Involves removing donor's venous blood 200 ml at a time, removing the platelets by centrifuge, and returning the blood to patient. This is performed approximately six times to yield 200 ml platelets. Uses special donors, who usually are human leukocyte antigen (HLA) matched to the patient. Hepatitis risk = 2*.
Cryoprecipitate (Factor VIII)	10–25 ml	Routine treatment for hemophilia (Factor VIII deficiency) and fibrinogen deficiency (Factor XIII deficiency)	Made from FFP. Infuse immediately upon thawing. Hepatitis risk = 2*.
AHG (Factor VIII) concentrates	20 ml	Alternative treatment for hemophilia A	Allergic and febrile reactions occur frequently. Administer by syringe or component drip set. Can store at refrigerator temperature, making it convenient for hemophiliacs during travel. Hepatitis risk = 3**.
Factor II, VII, IX, X concentrate	20 ml	Treatment of choice for hemophilia B and Factor IX deficiencies	Can precipitate clotting. Allergic and febrile reactions occur occasionally. Contraindicated in liver disease. Hepatitis risk = 3**.

TABLE 18-1 COMMONLY USED BLOOD PRODUCTS (Continued)

PRODUCT	APPROXIMATE VOLUME	INDICATIONS	PRECAUTIONS/COMMENTS
Albumin	50 or 250 ml	Hypovolemic shock, hypoalbuminemia, plasma replacement for burn patients	Osmotically equal to 5X its volume of plasma. Used as a volume expander or in hypoalbuminemic states. Commercially available. Hepatitis risk = 0*.
Plasma protein fraction (PPF)	250 ml (83% albumin with some alpha and beta globulins)	Volume expansion	Commercially available; expensive. Certain lots reported to have caused hypotension, possibly related to vasoactive amines used in preparation. Hepatitis risk = 0*.
Granulocyte transfusion (collected from a single pheresis donor)	200 ml, but may vary	Leukemia with granulocytopenia related to treatment	Not a common treatment. Febrile and allergic symptoms are frequent. Must be ABO compatible. Hepatitis risk = 3*.

*Relative hepatitis risk: 0, no risk; 1 and 2, moderate to high risk; 3, maximum risk.
**Risk is greater when multiple donors are used.

Source: Tueller B: Hematologic disorders, in Swearingen P (ed): *Manual of nursing therapeutics* (Menlo Park, CA: Addison-Wesley, 1986), pp. 346–347.

Potential Fluid Volume Excess Related to Frequent Infusions

Monitor the intake and output closely. Observe for signs of fluid overload, particularly the development of crackles and of increased pulmonary capillary, pulmonary arterial, and right atrial pressures. Administer medical therapy, such as diuretics, to decrease fluid volume.

Pain Related to Tissue Ischemia

Frequently assess the patient's need for pain medications. Give pain medications intravenously whenever possible, to provide maximum effectiveness and to avoid creating another site for bleeding. Remove any tight straps that may restrict circulation.

Impaired Skin Integrity Related to Ischemia

Use a flotation mattress on the bed or an air-fluidized bed. Change the patient's position frequently and assess skin condition when doing so. Handle the patient very gently. Provide gentle skin care, being particularly careful to avoid scratching the skin or disturbing healing areas. Use such items as sheepskin and lamb's wool between toes to cushion the skin. Observe the skin frequently for areas of petechiae, purpura, ecchymoses, or redness.

Avoid needle sticks whenever possible. If unavoidable, use the smallest needle possible and apply pressure to the site for 10 minutes after giving the injection.

Altered Tissue Perfusion Related to Peripheral Microthrombi

Monitor peripheral perfusion by checking peripheral arterial pulses, skin temperature and color, and capillary filling time.

Altered Urinary Elimination Related to Renal Microthrombi

Monitor urinary output closely, as the patient is at particular risk for the development of acute tubular necrosis related to obstruction.

Impaired Gas Exchange Related to Pulmonary Microthrombi

Observe for early signs of hypoxemia, particularly tachycardia, increased respiratory rate, and restlessness. Monitor arterial blood gas values for the development of hypoxemia and hypercapnia.

Altered Level of Consciousness Related to Neurological Microthrombi

Frequently evaluate the patient's neurologic status. When assessing level of consciousness in patients who do not respond to verbal stimuli, avoid or minimize the use of painful stimuli such as pinching or pressure, which can result in ecchymoses.

Altered Oral Mucous Membrane Related to Ischemia

Observe the mucous membrane for petechiae and cyanosis. Provide very gentle mouth care with swabs rather than a toothbrush. If the patient is able to eat, provide a liquid or soft diet.

Fear Related to the Unknown and to Death

Provide emotional support; for example, consistently assign the same nurse to care for the patient to promote the development of rapport.

Relieve the patient's and family's anxiety; for example, provide brief explanations of procedures, and encourage short, frequent visits.

Use relaxation exercises or guided imagery to relieve patient stress. Use visualization exercises to help the patient capitalize on inner strengths in order to get well.

Support the coping mechanisms used by the patient and family, unless they are pathologic. If they are, encourage substitution of healthier coping mechanisms. See Chapter 3 for suggestions.

Disturbed Self-Concept Related to Loss of Ability to Care for Self and Unattractive Appearance

Whenever possible, allow the patient the opportunity to exercise control over decisions related to care. Explain that the oozing and bleeding is due to the disease process. Keep the patient and the environment clean and free of blood.

Outcome Evaluation

Evaluate the patient's progress according to these criteria:

- Cessation of overt and covert bleeding: no oozing or frank bleeding episodes, absence of petechiae and ecchymoses, secretions negative for occult blood.
- Relief of pain.
- Laboratory studies WNL.

ACQUIRED IMMUNE DEFICIENCY SYNDROME

Acquired immune deficiency syndrome (AIDS) has rapidly become a major health problem in this country and the world at large, reaching epidemic proportions. AIDS affects the body's ability to mount an immune response and therefore makes it vulnerable to opportunistic infections. Continuously growing knowledge about the disease enables the critical-care nurse to base care on a solid foundation of scientific data.

Assessment

Pathophysiology

Diagnosis of AIDS is based on clinical signs of opportunistic infection, malignancy, wasting syndrome, or dementia, and laboratory evidence of immunodeficiency not attributable to another cause. The virus associated with disruption of the immune response has been identified as the *human immunodeficiency virus* (HIV). This virus also is referred to as *human T-cell lympho-*

tropic retrovirus type III/lymphadenopathy associated virus (HTLV-III/LAV).

A brief, simplified description of the immune response follows to facilitate understanding of AIDS. The body's ability to mount an immune response is a complex, integrative process. Many types of cells are involved but most importantly the lymphocytes. Lymphocytes are the cells that provide antigen-specific response and "memory." The two classes of lymphocytes, B cell and T cell lymphocytes, each have distinct functional abilities. The *B cell lymphocytes,* when they encounter an antigen, either mature into plasma cells that secrete antibodies (immunoglobulins) or circulate as memory cells. The *T cell lymphocytes* have several "species" and functions. *Regulatory T cells,* also known as *helper T cells,* amplify responses of other T cells and also B cells. They do this by release of lymphokines (interleukin 2 and interferon). There also are *suppressor T cells,* which inhibit the immune response. The *cytotoxic T cells,* or *"killer" T cells,* provide cytotoxicity, by binding to the target cell and invading the cell membrane (Halliburton 1986).

The HIV belongs to the retrovirus group. It uses an enzyme called *reverse transcriptase* to convert viral RNA into DNA. It has a preference to locate in the helper T cells, where it destroys the cells and also breaks down the processes that depend on helper T cells, i.e., antibody-producing B cells. The virus also attacks cells in the brain, spinal cord, and peripheral nerves (Shaw et al. 1985).

AIDS, the final stage in the continuum of HIV infection, is characterized by the presence of an opportunistic disease. However, many people infected with HIV may be asymptomatic, have chronic lymphadenopathy, or have *AIDS-related complex* (ARC). ARC has been defined as the presence of two clinical conditions and two laboratory deviations associated with AIDS (*Abbott Diagnostics* 1986). An example would be a patient with lymphadenopathy in two or more noninguinal sites, fever greater than 100°F for 3 months, helper T cell count less than 400/mm^3, and thrombocytopenia.

In March 1985, the Food and Drug Administration (FDA) approved an HTLV-III antibody assay for screening donated blood and plasma. The test determines the presence of antibodies to the virus in the serum. The antibody test does not diagnose AIDS, and there is no certain clinical relevance of the presence of antibodies. One of the difficult aspects about infection with the HIV virus is that it does produce antibodies, but not in enough quantity to deactivate the virus. Additionally, the presence of antibodies in the serum indicates that exposure to the virus has occurred, but not necessarily that a person will present with an opportunistic infection associated with AIDS.

Risk Conditions

Transmission of the virus depends on several factors. The virus must be: (a) present in the fluid, (b) alive and stable in the fluid, (c) transmitted in a viable state, in a sufficient quantity to a susceptible host, and (d) able to penetrate the host and invade target cells. HIV is most commonly transmitted through sexual contact or direct injection into the bloodstream. Infection is dose related; for example, although small amounts of the virus have been identified in sweat and saliva, casual contact, sharing eating utensils, and hugging and kissing are not believed to transmit the virus (Friedland et al. 1986).

Epidemologic data have supported the identification of high risk groups. These include homosexual or bisexual men, intravenous substance abusers, hemophiliacs, and Haitian immigrants (LaCamera 1985). It is important to note, however, that AIDS increasingly is being reported in people not in these risk categories.

Signs and Symptoms

Disorders common in AIDS include Kaposi's sarcoma (KS) or one of the opportunistic infections. *Pneumocystis carinii* pneumonia (PCP), toxoplasmosis, cryptoccal meningitis, cytomegalovirus (CMV) of an organ other than the liver or lymph nodes, *Candida* esophagitis, or chronic herpes simplex (Bennett 1986).

AIDS-related complex usually manifests as persistent lymphadenopathy and T cell deficiency, mucous membrane disease or dermatologic disease, mild anemia, leukopenia, or thrombocytopenia.

Acute illness with AIDS may develop gradually or suddenly. Common complaints include fatigue, general malaise, night sweats, swollen lymph nodes, persistent diarrhea, cough, or shortness of breath (Carr and Gee 1986). The patient may present with weight loss, persistent fever, and frequent infection, or may have severe respiratory insufficiency or encephalitis. The spectrum is extremely variable and depends tremendously on the particular opportunistic infection. An outline of a hypothetical model of infection is as follows (*Abbott Diagnostics* 1986). Remember that this is only a possible course, which varies individually, and that not all persons who are antibody positive will develop AIDS.

- Infection
- Acute lymphproliferative syndrome
- Seroconversion
- Chronic lymphadenopathy
- Gradual depletion of helper T cells

- Gradual development of T cell deficiency:
  opportunistic mucous membrane disease
- Progressive defects in the immune system:
  severe T cell deficiency
  severe B cell failure
  defects in monocyte function
  defects in granulocyte function
- Recurrent opportunistic infections and/or neoplastic disorders
- Death

Laboratory studies demonstrate *cutaneous anergy* (unresponsiveness to injection of antigens subcutaneously); profound lymphopenia, especially T cell lymphocytes; diminished lymphocyte proliferation responses; thrombocytopenia; positive HIV antibody test; and T_4/T_8 ratio (ratio of helper T cells to suppressor T cells) less than 1.0.

NURSING DIAGNOSES

Because of the complexity of this disorder, multiple nursing diagnoses exist, and they vary with the opportunistic disorder present. They include but are not limited to:

- Altered gas exchange
- Sensory-perceptual alteration
- Potential for additional infection
- Altered nutrition: less than body requirements
- Impaired tissue integrity
- Altered comfort
- Self-care deficit
- Anxiety
- Fluid deficit

Planning and Implementation of Care

Altered Gas Exchange Related to Diffuse Consolidative Process

---

Frequently the person with AIDS seen in critical care has *Pneumocystis carinii* pneumonia (PCP). This person requires oxygen support and often mechanical ventilation. A serious problem occurs as the pneumocystis lodges in the interstitial space between the alveoli and the capillary and forms a hard cyst that replaces surfactant. Positive pressure breathing, including mechanical ventilation, can cause alveolar rupture because of the lack of surfactant. It is important for the critical-care nurse to assess for respiratory status frequently, including lung sounds, color, respiratory excursion, arterial blood gases, heart rate (which may increase as a compensatory mechanism for hypoxemia), and cough. With PCP, the lungs may sound clear or diffuse crackles may be present. PCP is a diffuse process, so no particular lobe of the lung is affected (Carr and Gee 1986). Administer medications as ordered to treat the pneumonia. These will most commonly be trimethoprim-sulfamethoxazole and pentamidine. These drugs are tolerated poorly, and side effects may include rash, neutropenia, and severe vomiting. Pentamidine can cause sterile abscesses when given IM (LaCamera 1985; Wollschlager et al. 1984).

Sensory-Perceptual Alteration Related to Viral Invasion of the CNS

Virtually every opportunistic infection associated with AIDS can and does affect the central nervous system, in the form of abscesses, meningitis, or encephalopathy. Headache may be the first symptom, which then progress to seizures, sensory or cognitive deficits, and coma (Bennett 1986). Initially, patients complain of decreased attention span, loss of memory, decreased mental acuity, or personality changes (Carr and Gee 1986).

If the problem is meningitis, pharmacologic therapy may include amphotericin B (IV) or 5-fluorocytosine (oral). Watch the patient carefully for side effects such as fever, chills, neutropenia, liver dysfunction, and anemia.

Toxoplasmosis encephalitis usually is treated with sulfadiazine or pyrimethamine. Both are given orally and may be associated with nephrotoxicity, gastrointestinal distress, and/or hypersensitivity.

Important nursing care includes the following:

- Monitor for neurologic signs such as headache and change in mentation or level of consciousness.
- Reorient the patient as necessary, and make frequent reference to the day's events.
- Protect the patient from injury.
- Explain to the patient and significant others about the behavioral and CNS changes.

• Provide emotional support, and assist the patient and family with coping with the effects of the disease.

Potential for Additional Infection Related to Decreased Immune Function

Septicemia can occur with any opportunistic infection, and AIDS patients are at high risk for nosocomial infections. Frequent and thorough handwashing probably is the most important part of care, and strict aseptic technique in care is vital. Reverse isolation will not prevent opportunistic infection from endogenous organisms, but the risk of additional infectious processes can be decreased.

Nursing care includes measures to help prevent infection:

• Maintain adequate fluid balance.
• Promote frequent handwashing.
• Maintain optimal nutritional status.
• Maintain aseptic technique during all invasive procedures.
• Turn and deep breathe every 2 hours.
• Monitor for cloudy urine, change in WBC count, visual disturbances, increased episodes of chills and diaphoresis, worsening dyspnea or redness or swelling at old IM or IV sites.

Altered Nutrition: Less Than Body Requirements, Related to Anxiety, Diarrhea, and Increased Metabolic Need

This problem has been referred to as the wasting syndrome associated with AIDS and has numerous etiologies (Schietinger 1986). First, there is an increased utilization of nutrients related to the disease process, and second, the patient may have anorexia related to fatigue, fear, anxiety, depression, or oral pain resulting from stomatitis. Enteral feedings or total parenteral nutrition (TPN) may be necessary to maintain adequate nutritional status. Enteral feedings are not adequate, and TPN is required if the absorption of nutrients is affected by diarrhea or GI involvement of KS.

The nurse can intervene with the following care measures:

• Consult with the patient to plan diet with adequate protein and calories.
• Offer soft foods and foods easily swallowed.
• Serve small portions.
• Encourage significant others to bring in favorite foods.
• Implement measures to reduce stomatitis (see impaired tissue integrity, next).
• Administer TPN or enteral feedings.

Note: If the patient is not tolerating oral feedings, consult the physician early, as malnutrition is more difficult to reverse once the process is severe.

Impaired Tissue Integrity Related to Bedrest and Deficient Immune System

Impairment of tissue integrity may occur as a complication of bedrest but often is seen specifically as stomatitis, pharyngitis, or esophagitis from *Candida* infection related to the incompetent immune system, altered nutritional status, and/or a side effect of chemotherapy. Pressure sores can be aggravated by chronic genital *Candida* infections or anal herpes lesions. Observe the patient for reddened or inflamed mucous membranes, ulcerations, and white opaque lesions on mucous membranes (Griffin 1986).

Nursing care includes the following:

• Assist with frequent oral hygiene.
• Encourage fluid intake of at least 2500 cc/day.
• Avoid offering spicy or hot foods.
• Maintain optimal nutritional status.
• Apply prescribed ointments.
• Wash and air the perineum and anal area frequently.

Altered Comfort: Pain Related to Damaged Nerves, Edema, and Immobility

Pain associated with AIDS may be related to immobility, neurologic involvement (peripheral neuropathy), dyspnea, swelling of KS lesions and herpes or Candida infections. Often it is difficult to relieve the pain completely; rather, the nurse seeks to decrease it to a tolerable level. Narcotics may be given, usually orally or IV. Decreasing muscle mass makes it difficult to give IM injections. Nursing care may involve positioning of comfort, meditation, imagery and relieving the pain pharmacologically before it becomes severe.

Self-Care Deficit Related to Progressive Weakness

AIDS often involves young, independent people. The nurse can encourage independence as much as possible and maintain optimal level of self-care. It is important to be sensitive to the patient's needs and desires for self-care and to promote as much independence as possible.

Anxiety Related to Life-threatening Illness

The diagnosis of AIDS and the subsequent implications most obviously will be a source of anxiety, fear, concern, anger, and depression. The patient and significant others often go through a grieving process when diagnosis is made. The nurse can have a positive effect by doing the following; also refer to Chapter 3.

- Encourage verbalization of fear.
- Encourage significant others to project a calm and concerned attitude.
- Include significant others in teaching.
- Explain all procedures.
- Respond to patient needs immediately.
- Use relaxation exercises or guided imagery to relieve patient stress.
- Use visualization exercises to utilize inner strength.
- Support the coping mechanisms used by the patient and significant others.

Fluid Deficit

Fluid deficit may be related to dehydration related to the infectious process or the severe unrelenting diarrhea that often occurs with AIDS. The critical-care nurse can administer prescribed antidiarrheal agents, encourage fluid intake, and monitor for signs of dehydration and electrolyte imbalance (see Chapter 16 for detailed discussion of fluid deficit and electrolyte imbalances).

Outcome Evaluation

Evaluate the patient's progress according to these criteria:

- Reduced fear and anxiety.
- Nutritional status is adequate.
- Mucous membranes are intact.
- Arterial blood gases WNL.
- Pain is relieved.
- Increased tolerance for activity.
- Patient is free of additional infections.
- Patient is alert and oriented.
- Skin turgor is good.
- Fluid status is adequate.

Current Investigational Areas

There are many areas of investigation regarding the treatment of AIDS. One area is the possibility of using drugs that help boost the defective immune system, that is, increase the number of T cells. Interleukin-2 has been shown to enhance T cell function in some studies (Lotze 1985). Interferons such as alpha interferon and gamma interferon have been tried, but with inconclusive results so far.

Antiviral agents to prevent HIV replication may be another way to boost the immune system. The antiviral agent must be able to cross the blood–brain barrier, since brain tissue and cells host the virus. Suramin, a drug used to treat parasitic infections, has been shown to stop the effects of HIV; however, the toxic effects of the drug limit its usefulness (Fischinger and Bolognesi 1985).

Other antiviral agents being investigated include azidothymidine (AZT), HPA-23, ribavirin, dideoxycytidine, ansamycin, and phosphonoformate (Bennett 1986). AZT is a promising drug that in a significant number of cases has stopped reproduction of the virus and allowed normal proliferation of T cells (*Abbott Diagnostics* 1986).

Many viral diseases can be controlled and prevented through vaccination, and this is another area of investigation. A problem with this approach is that HIV appears in several antigenic forms and is capable of altering its antigenic coating.

Current Guidelines for Preventing Transmission of HIV

Although HIV seroconversion in health care workers is very rare, there have been several reported cases. The following guidelines are recommended by the Centers for Disease Control to prevent transmission of agents between all patients and all health care workers (Centers for Disease Control 1986b).

1. All health care workers who perform or assist in invasive procedures must be educated regarding the epidemiology, modes of transmission, and prevention of HIV infection.

2. Wear gloves when touching mucous membranes or nonintact skin, and use other appropriate barrier precautions when indicated (e.g., masks, gowns, and eye coverings if aerosolization or splashes are likely to occur).

3. After delivery, use appropriate barrier precautions when handling the placenta or the infant until blood and amniotic fluid have been removed.

4. Use care to prevent injuries to hands caused by needles, scalpels, and other sharp instruments.

5. If the health care worker has exudative lesions or weeping dermatitis, that person should not assist in invasive procedures or other direct patient care activities.

6. Routine serologic testing for evidence of HIV infection is *not* necessary for health care workers who perform invasive procedures or for patients undergoing invasive procedures.

7. All health care workers with evidence of any illness that may compromise their ability to adequately and safely perform invasive procedures should be evaluated medically.

8. If an incident occurs that results in exposure of a patient to the blood of a health care worker, the patient should be informed and recommendations for management of such exposures should be followed.

REFERENCES

Abbott Diagnostics HTLV-III Education Series Monographs. Irving, TX: Abbott Laboratories, 1986.

Bennett J: What we know about AIDS. *Am J Nurs* 1986; 86:1016–1021.

Bennett J: HTLV-III AIDS link. *Am J Nurs* 1985; 85:1086–1089.

Carr GS, Gee C: AIDS and AIDS-related conditions: Screening for populations at risk. *Nurse Prac* 1986; 11:25–48.

Centers for Disease Control: Classification system for human T-lymphotropic virus type III/lymphadenopathy-associated virus infections. *Ann Intern Med* 1986a; 105:234–237.

Centers for Disease Control, Leads from morbidity and mortality weekly report: Recommendations for preventing transmission of infection with human T-lymphotropic virus type III/lymphadenopathy-associated virus during invasive procedures. *JAMA* 1986b; 256:1257–1258.

Crabtree A, Jorgenson M: Exploring the practical knowledge in expert critical-care nursing practice. Unpublished master's thesis, University of Wisconsin, Madison, 1986.

Darovic G: Disseminated intravascular coagulation. *Crit Care Nurse* 1982; 2:36–46.

Fischbach DF, Fogdall RP: *Coagulation: The essentials.* Baltimore, MD: Williams and Wilkins, 1981.

Fischinger PJ, Bolognesi DP: Prospects for diagnostic tests, intervention and vaccine development in AIDS. In *AIDS etiology, diagnosis, treatment and prevention,* Devita VT et al. (eds). Philadelphia: Lippincott, 1985.

Friedland GH et al.: Lack of transmission of HTLV III/LAV infection to household contacts of patients with AIDS or AIDS-related complex with oral candidiasis. *N Engl J Med* 1986; 314:344–349.

Griffin JP: Nursing care of the immunosuppressed patient in an intensive care unit. *Heart Lung* 1986; 15:179–187.

Guyton A: *Textbook of medical physiology,* 7th ed. Philadelphia: Saunders, 1986.

Halliburton P: Impaired immunocompetence. In *Pathophysiological phenomena in nursing.* Carrieri VK et al. (eds). Philadelphia: Saunders, 1986.

Hewitt PE, Davies SC: The current state of DIC. *Intens Care Med* 1983; 9:249–252.

Hubner C: Altered Clotting. In *Pathophysiological phenomena in nursing.* Carrieri et al. (eds). Philadelphia: Saunders, 1986.

Hudak et al.: *Critical care nursing,* 4th ed. Philadelphia: Lippincott, 1986.

Kenner C et al.: *Critical care nursing: Body–mind–spirit.* Boston: Little, Brown, 1986.

LaCamera et al.: The acquired immunodeficiency syndrome. *Nurs Clin North Am* 1985; 20:241–256.

Lotze MT: Treatment of immunologic disorders in AIDS. In *AIDS etiology, diagnosis, treatment, and prevention.* DeVita VT et al. (eds). Philadelphia: Lippincott, 1985.

Peabody B: Living with AIDS: A mother's perspective. *Am J Nurs* 1986; 86:45–46.

Porth CM: *Pathophysiology concepts of altered health states,* 2d ed. Philadelphia: Lippincott, 1986.

Rooney A, Haviley C: Nursing management of disseminated intravascular coagulation. *Oncol Nurs Forum* 1985; 12:15–22.

Schietinger H: A home care plan for AIDS. *Am J Nurs* 1986; 86:1021–1028.

Shaw GM et al.: HTLV-III infection in brains of children and adults with AIDS encephalopathy. *Science* 1985; 227:177–182.

Wollschlager CM et al.: Pulmonary manifestations of the acquired immunodeficiency syndrome. *Chest* 1984; 85:197–202.

SUPPLEMENTAL READING

Abrams DI: AIDS: Battling a retroviral enemy. *Calif Nurs Rev* 1986; 8:10–16, 36–38.

Au JP et al.: Kaposi's sarcoma presenting with endobronchial lesion. *Heart Lung* 1986; 15:411–413.

Brinkerhoff CE: DIC: Implications for clinical nursing in a pediatric burn population. *Crit Care Quart* 1984; 7:8–18.

Griffin JP: *Hematology and immunology concepts for nursing.* New York: Appleton-Century-Crofts, 1986.

Luce JM: The acquired immunodeficiency syndrome. *Am Rev Respir Dis* 1986; 134:859–861.

Swearingen P (ed): *Manual of nursing therapeutics.* Menlo Park, CA: Addison-Wesley, 1986.

Symposium: Therapy for immunocompromised patients. *Am J Med* (May 30) 1986; 80:(entire issue).

Turner JG, Williamson KM: AIDS, A challenge for contemporary nursing, Part I. *Focus Crit Care* 1986; 13:53–61.

Weiss SH et al.: HTLV III infection among health care workers. *JAMA* 1985; 254:2089–2092.

19

Nutrition

CLINICAL INSIGHT

Domain: The helping role

Competency: Maximizing the patient's participation and control in his or her own recovery

Expert nurses know how critically important it is that a patient be emotionally available to participate in recovery. Maximizing such participation requires the patient to have faith that he or she will get through the ordeal, and a recognition of his or her own power to influence recovery. A patient's making the commitment to engage in healing activities can be a hard-won step in recovery. It is a particularly difficult one if the patient is demoralized by prolonged illness and the feeling of being treated like an object. In the following exemplar, from Benner (1984, pp. 60-61), an expert nurse achieves a patient turnaround by challenging the patient to choose recovery.

*The patient was a 36-year-old man who had a history of multiple surgeries and complications. He had a history of ulcers and came as a transfer from another hospital after having surgery for hemorrhagic pancreatitis. He ended up with another surgery from which he emerged minus most of his pancreas and with multiple tubes, a huge abdominal wound, several IVs, etc. He was a person who had always been inde-*pendent and was having an extremely hard time coping with being ill and helpless. He finally reached a point where he was so angry and so depressed that he refused any further treatments, procedures, and blood work. He also refused to ambulate or do much of his self-care.

I went in to talk to him. He told me, "I'm so sick of being poked all the time, and not having any say in any of this. I'm so helpless. People are constantly doing things to me!" I told him that while the circumstances would be hard to change, he could shift his point of view. I told him that he did have a choice in all of this, and that instead of seeing himself as having things being done to him, he could view it as things being done for him to help him get better. I told him that while he felt helpless about what we were doing to him physically, he was the only one who could help himself mentally by keeping this whole thing in perspective . . . that he needed to remember that he was a person . . . that he was more than this sickness he was going through. I couldn't really tell if I was getting through.

The next morning when I came to work, I saw him sitting out in the hall by the window laughing and smiling. When I asked him what had changed for him, he said, "You were right! I'm just going to choose to be here and let all of you help me get well as fast as I can!"

I really felt like I made a difference in this man's life in helping him cope with circumstances he thought were beyond his control, just by helping him tap into inner strengths.

As illustrated in the Clinical Insight, the nurse can be instrumental in helping patients maintain both faith in their recovery and awareness of their power to influence it. Such nursing support is particularly important with patients whose illness requires prolonged hospitalization, often true of gastrointestinal disorders.

In the FANCAS system, *nutrition* is defined as the intake, digestion, and absorption of nutrients and the removal of solid waste products. To meet nutritional needs, a person requires a normally functioning GI system. This chapter therefore begins with a review of abdominal assessment and the most common GI abnormalities seen in the critically ill: upper GI bleeding, acute pancreatitis, hepatitis, and liver failure. The chapter then addresses the topic of nutrition in the critically ill.

GASTROINTESTINAL (GI) SYSTEM

GI Assessment

Gastrointestinal (GI) assessment can provide important data on the status of GI function. The assessment consists of two key areas: the history and the physical examination.

History

In eliciting the GI history, ask the patient about both general and specific signs and symptoms. *General symptoms* include changes in appetite or energy levels, and weight loss or weight gain. *Specific symptoms* about which to inquire include pain, nausea and vomiting, diarrhea or constipation, and heartburn or indigestion. The location of abdominal pain can be confusing, especially

in the beginning stages of a disorder, as pain may be referred along transmission pathways to a site distant from its source. The pain arising from an organ (*visceral pain*) often is dull, poorly localized, and hard for the patient to describe. In contrast, pain from the skin, peritoneum, or muscle wall (*somatic pain*) is sharp and easier to localize.

Physical Examination

The health assessment continues with a physical examination of the patient's general appearance, mouth, abdomen, anus, and rectum. A suggested format is shown in Table 19-1.

Mouth Examine the mouth for adequacy of dentition, tongue movement, and oral hygiene. Also note whether the gag and swallow reflexes are intact.

Abdomen Next, examine the patient's abdomen. As you do so, keep in mind the location of various abdominal organs (Figure 19-1). Instead of following the usual sequence of inspection, palpation, percussion, and auscultation, alter the order to inspection, auscultation, percussion, and palpation. Auscultation should precede percussion and palpation because the latter two can change the frequency of bowel sounds. Percussion should precede palpation because it usually is easier to identify the location of abdominal organs through percussion than through palpation. As you examine specific organs, you may find it helpful to alternate percussion and palpation. The following is a procedure for abdominal examination.

Be particularly careful when examining the person experiencing abdominal pain. Ask her/him to point to the area of pain, and examine that area last.

1. Inspect the abdomen, looking especially at its contour and symmetry. Also look for pulsations, scars, and distended superficial veins (seen in portal obstruction and venous thrombosis).

2. Auscultate the abdomen in all four quadrants. Apply the stethoscope diaphragm lightly to listen for *bowel sounds*. Normal bowel sounds are soft intermittent noises that occur about every 2-10 seconds and vary in frequency, intensity, and pitch. Sounds that are intensified, weak, or absent are abnormal. Loud gurgling sounds signify either increased intestinal motility, as in diarrhea or nervous tension, or early intestinal obstruction. Occasional weak sounds suggest poor peristalsis. Absent sounds occur after handling of the bowel during surgery, during severe electrolyte disturbances, in peritonitis, and in advanced intestinal obstruction.

TABLE 19-1 ABDOMINAL ASSESSMENT FORMAT

1. History _____
2. Physical
    Mouth: Dentition _____
        Tongue _____
        Oral hygiene/mucous membranes _____
        Gag reflex _____
        Swallow reflex _____
    Abdomen
        Inspection _____
        Auscultation _____
        _____

    Percussion and palpation:
        Liver _____
        _____
        Spleen _____
        _____

        Tenderness _____ Rigidity _____ Free fluid _____
    Anus and rectum _____
3. Laboratory tests and diagnostic procedures
    _____

4. Other _____

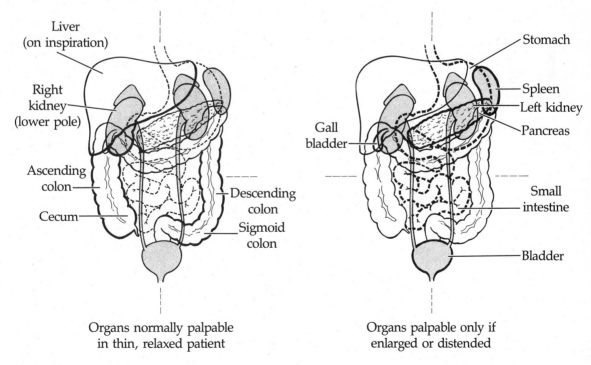

Organs normally palpable   Organs palpable only if
in thin, relaxed patient   enlarged or distended

Liver (on inspiration)
Right kidney (lower pole)
Ascending colon
Cecum
Descending colon
Sigmoid colon
Stomach
Spleen
Left kidney
Pancreas
Gall bladder
Small intestine
Bladder

FIGURE 19-1

Abdominal organs.

Listen for 5 minutes in each quadrant before deciding whether bowel sounds are absent.

The bell of the stethoscope is used to listen for vascular sounds and rubs. *Bruits* may be audible in patients with arteriosclerosis, hypertension, aortic aneurysms, masses compressing the aorta, or renal artery stenosis. Peritoneal *friction rubs* may be heard over the right lower costal margin, related to hepatic tumors or abscesses, or over the left lower costal area, related to splenic infarction.

3.   Percuss the abdomen lightly. Normally, you will hear tympany over the stomach and intestine (that is, over most of the abdomen). *Tympany* is a long, very hollow sound that indicates gas in an enclosed chamber. It resembles the sound you can hear by puffing out your cheek and percussing it. Over solid organs, a short, high-pitched sound (called *dullness*) will be heard. (If you wish to review percussion technique and the characteristics of percussion notes, see Chapter 7.)

Estimate the size of the *liver* by percussing in the right midclavicular line, down from lung resonance to dullness, and up from abdominal tympany to dullness. It is important to note both the location of the borders and the distance between them. The liver can normally be palpated 4 cm below the right costal margin (Bates 1987). A normal-sized liver may be displaced downward, as in emphysema, or upward, as in ascites or abdominal tumors. As a result, a liver edge below the costal margin does not necessarily indicate liver enlargement.

4.   Palpate the abdomen lightly. Use light touch to feel for tenderness and resistance. Resistance may be voluntary, due to patient discomfort, ticklishness, or apprehension, or involuntary, due to peritoneal irritation. If you encounter resistance, try to differentiate the type by ensuring that the patient is relaxed—make sure he or she is positioned comfortably and your hands are warm; try to distract the patient with conversation. You also can feel for the normal relaxation of the abdominal muscles on expiration. Rigidity that continues in spite of these maneuvers probably is involuntary.

Palpate areas of known tenderness last. If pain is present, check for rebound tenderness, a reliable sign of peritoneal inflammation. *Rebound tenderness* is pain that occurs after the release of pressure. To elicit this response, press firmly over a quadrant of abdomen other than the tender one and release the pressure suddenly. If the patient feels a sharp stab of pain over the suspected area (*not* over the site on which you pressed), rebound tenderness is present. This test can provoke severe pain and muscle spasm, which interfere with further examination. For this reason, it is wise to postpone it until the end of the examination.

5.   After light palpation to identify resistance and tenderness, palpate more deeply for masses and abdominal organs (refer back to Figure 19-1). Those which you normally may be able to feel in the thin, relaxed patient are the liver; the lower pole of the right kidney; ascending, descending, and sigmoid colon; cecum; and aorta. Unless they are enlarged or distended, you normally cannot feel the gallbladder, spleen, pancreas, stomach, small intestine, or bladder.

For deep palpation, ask the patient to breathe through the mouth. On each expiration, press slowly and firmly, each time increasing the depth of palpation until you have depressed the abdominal wall about 2-3 inches. During inspiration, maintain but do not increase the pressure. Instead, concentrate on feeling whether the organ is descending toward your fingers. Once you have located it, use your fingers to slide the abdominal wall back and forth over the organ to assess its shape, hardness, smoothness, and mobility.

To palpate the *liver,* stand on the patient's right side (Figure 19-2). Slide your left hand under and parallel to the eleventh and twelfth ribs. Place your right hand on the abdomen, below the lower border of liver dullness that you identified previously. Point your fingers toward the right costal border. Ask the patient to take a deep abdominal breath, blow it out, and take another deep breath. As the patient exhales, gently push your fingers inward and upward under the costal margin. You may be able to feel a firm ridge of pressure come down to meet your fingertips; this is the lower border of the liver. If you feel the edge, repeat the maneuver medially and laterally. An alternate technique is the *hooking* method: Stand at the patient's right shoulder. Hook the fingers of both hands over the right costal margin, and feel for the liver edge as the person inhales deeply. Note the smoothness of the edge and any tenderness. Since the liver normally is not palpable, *blunt percussion* over the liver is an alternate method of detecting tenderness. To perform blunt percussion, place your left hand on the lower right lateral rib cage. Make a fist with your right hand and lightly strike your left hand.

The *spleen* is not palpable unless it is enlarged about three times its normal size. To check for splenic enlargement, stand at the patient's right side (Figure 19-3). Reach over the patient and place your left hand under the left low back ribs. Place your right hand below the left costal margin on the anterior abdomen. Ask the patient to take a deep breath, lift with your left hand, and press inward with your right. As the normal spleen cannot be felt, be cautious if you do palpate the spleen. An enlarged spleen is friable and may rupture with aggressive palpation.

To palpate the *abdominal aorta,* press your thumb and fingers deep into the upper abdomen, slightly to the left of midline. Be very cautious in performing this ma-

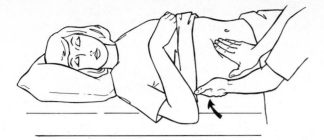

FIGURE 19-2

Palpation of liver.

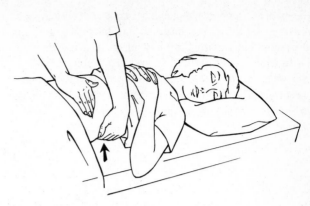

FIGURE 19-3

Palpation of spleen.

neuver on a patient with a suspected aortic aneurysm, as aggressive palpation can rupture the aneurysm.

Anus and Rectum Complete the physical examination of the gastrointestinal system by examining the anal area and rectum. Examine the anal area for hemorrhoids, fissures, rectal prolapse, or skin excoriation. If the date of the last bowel movement is not known, ask the physician whether it is safe to perform a digital examination of the rectum. Early detection of fecal matter in the rectum can avoid the development of a fecal impaction; but it may be necessary to delay this examination if the patient's condition is unstable or might be adversely affected by rectal stimulation.

Upper GI Hemorrhage

GI bleeds are classified as *upper GI bleeds,* which occur above the duodenojejunal junction, or *lower GI bleeds.* Because lower GI bleeds usually are not severe enough to warrant admission to a critical-care unit, this section focuses on assessment and management of the patient with an upper GI bleed.

Assessment

Patients at Risk Patients at risk of upper GI hemorrhage may include those with peptic ulceration (gastric or duodenal), stress ulceration (gastric or duodenal), venous ulcerations (esophageal or gastric), and Mallory-Weiss syndrome (Alspach and Williams 1985).

Mallory-Weiss syndrome is a linear, nonperforating tear of the gastric mucosa near the juncture between the esophagus and the stomach. It usually results from an episode of violent vomiting, most often in patients with a history of alcoholism, gastritis, or esophagitis.

About 75% of upper GI bleeds result from duodenal, gastric, or esophageal ulcers; 20% from erosive gastritis; and 5% from esophageal varices.

Signs and Symptoms The patient's clinical presentation will vary with the amount and speed of blood loss. Factors to include in assessment, in addition to the history and symptoms, are vital signs, peripheral perfusion, and hematemesis, hematochezia, or melena. Vital signs correlate roughly with the degree of blood loss. When blood loss is less than 500 ml, supine vital signs are likely to be normal due to compensatory mechanisms. Blood loss of 500-1000 ml causes sympathetic stimulation sufficient to cause tachycardia, and the patient may complain of being thirsty, dizzy, or nauseated. Blood loss in excess of 1000 ml will cause frank hypovolemic shock, with cool, clammy skin, rapid, thready pulse, and decreased level of consciousness.

An important clue in assessing the patient with a history of blood loss or suggestive symptoms but normal or equivocal vital signs is the response to *postural vital signs* (tilt test). Postural vital signs compare vital signs in the recumbent position with those in the sitting position. This test should not be performed if syncope, marked tachycardia, hypotension, or shock are present. To assess postural vital signs, work with a colleague to simultaneously measure the BP and pulse while the patient is recumbent. Then sit the patient up and immediately measure the BP and pulse again. (Be sure to observe the patient closely for fainting during the sitting up.) The comparison is considered *positive* for the presence of orthostatic hypotension if the systolic BP drops more than 10 mm Hg or if the pulse increases more than 20 beats per minute. Although nurses commonly are taught that positive postural vital signs means blood loss, this is not completely accurate. It is important to note that positive postural vital signs also can occur if the patient is on ganglionic-blocking agents for hypertension, receiving vasodilators, has taken alcohol, has peripheral neuropathy, or has adrenal insufficiency. A pulse increase of 20 beats or more per minute with no change in BP indicates a blood loss of 500 ml or less; a pulse increase of 30 beats per minute and a 10 mm Hg fall in BP correlate with a loss of approximately 1000 ml (Decker 1985).

Hematemesis (vomiting of blood) is common and usually indicates that the patient is bleeding from a source above the ligament of Treitz at the duodenojejunal junction. The blood may be bright red if bleeding is so profuse that there has been little time for gastric juices to act on it. Conversely, the blood may have a coffee-grounds appearance if bleeding has been slower and gastric juices have converted hemoglobin to a brown breakdown product.

Blood also may be present in stools, but its presence is of equivocal diagnostic value. The stool may appear black and sticky (tarry), bright red, or maroon. As little as 60 ml of blood in the gastrointestinal tract can cause *melena* (tarry stool). A black stool usually indicates an upper GI bleed, but also may be present in a lower GI bleed. *Hematochezia* (the presence of bright red blood) usually indicates massive upper GI bleeding with markedly increased GI motility, but it also can occur from a rapid lower GI bleed. The color of the stool also is affected by the intake of food; for example, beets can produce a red stool, whereas iron can produce a dark one. Stools should be hematested for occult bleeding if they appear normal.

NURSING DIAGNOSES

Nursing diagnoses that may apply to the patient with an upper GI bleed include:

- Fluid volume deficit
- Impaired tissue integrity
- Altered tissue perfusion
- Impaired gas exchange
- Sensory-perceptual alteration
- Anxiety

Planning and Implementation of Care

Planning and implementation of care can be divided into two phases: *emergency care,* to control shock; and *definitive care,* to control bleeding. Nearby is presented a nursing care plan for acute upper GI hemorrhage. The following section expands on selected aspects of care.

NURSING CARE PLAN

Acute Upper Gastrointestinal Bleeding

NURSING DIAGNOSIS	SIGNS AND SYMPTOMS	NURSING ACTIONS	DESIRED OUTCOMES

Fluid volume deficit related to bleeding/hemorrhage and loss of volume	Red blood or coffee-grounds material in nasogastric tube or emesis
	Sticky black or dark red stools
	If 30% or more of blood volume lost, shocklike symptoms:
	    increased heart rate
	    cold, clammy skin
	    shallow respirations
	    decreased blood pressure
	If less than 30% of blood volume lost:
	    pallor
	    weakness
	    positive orthostatic vital signs
	Decrease in urine output
	Increase in body temperature
		1. Maintain a large-caliber intravenous access.
		2. Prepare for possible insertion of pulmonary artery line and arterial line for assessment of hemodynamic status.
		3. Insert nasogastric tube
		4. Initiate intragastric lavage of iced saline as ordered.
		  a. Keep accurate records of amount used for irrigation.
		  b. Continue until return is clear.
		5. Add norepinephrine to irrigation if ordered to effect localized vasoconstriction.
			Normal circulating blood volume.
			Hemorrhage controlled.
			Hemodynamic stability.

NURSING CARE PLAN (Continued)

Acute Upper Gastrointestinal Bleeding (Continued)

NURSING DIAGNOSIS	SIGNS AND SYMPTOMS	NURSING ACTIONS	DESIRED OUTCOMES
		6. Administer colloids and crystalloids as ordered to replace volume. 　a. Maintain urine output of greater than 30 cc/hr. 　b. Assess hemodynamic parameters (CVP/RAP, PCWP, PAP, BP, HR, CO). 　c. Whole blood or packed cells may be given. 　d. After multiple transfusions, consider replacement of clotting factors, calcium and platelets. 7. Administer vitamin K as ordered. 8. Monitor BUN, electrolytes, hemoglobin, and hematocrit. 9. Administer vasopressin as ordered to control bleeding. Monitor for side effects such as hypertension, chest pain, abdominal pain, oliguria, water intoxication. 10. Administer topical thrombin through nasogastric tube as ordered to control bleeding. **CAUTION: Do not administer it IV, which would result in excessive clotting.** (Topical thrombin reacts with fibrinogen to cause clotting, and it must contact the capillary that is bleeding. Additionally, stomach acid must be buffered for thrombin to be effective.)	
* Impaired tissue integrity related to mucosal damage to GI tract and/or esophageal varices	Frank bloody emesis History of alcoholism Black, sticky, or dark red stools	1. Administer histamine H_2-receptor antagonists such as cimetidine, as ordered, to aid in healing of mucosa.	Absence or decreased bleeding from GI mucosa or esophageal varices

(Continues)

NURSING CARE PLAN (Continued)

Acute Upper Gastrointestinal Bleeding (Continued)

NURSING DIAGNOSIS	SIGNS AND SYMPTOMS	NURSING ACTIONS	DESIRED OUTCOMES
		2. Administer antacids as ordered.	
		3. Assist with insertion of a Sengstaken-Blackmore (SB) tube, as ordered.	
		a. Check patency of each lumen prior to insertion.	
		b. Explain procedure to patient.	
		c. Assess vital signs during procedure.	
		4. Once the tube is in place:	
		a. Ensure that x-ray is taken to confirm placement.	
		b. Inflate the gastric balloon with 200-500 cc of air.	
		c. Inflate the esophageal balloon with air to 20-40 mm Hg.	
		d. Secure tube using slight traction.	
		e. Keep scissors at bedside for emergency deflation of balloons in case of esophogeal rupture and tracheal occlusion by the balloon, as evidenced by sudden onset of respiratory distress and/or back pain.	
		f. Ensure patency of gastric aspiration port and oropharyngeal port.	
		g. Deflate esophageal balloon and reinflate as ordered.	
		h. Keep the head of the bed elevated to increase ventilation.	
		i. Check nostrils at least every 2 hours to prevent pressure sores.	
		j. Instruct patient to avoid coughing or straining.	
		k. Monitor for continued bleeding.	

NURSING CARE PLAN (Continued)

Acute Upper Gastrointestinal Bleeding (Continued)

NURSING DIAGNOSIS	SIGNS AND SYMPTOMS	NURSING ACTIONS	DESIRED OUTCOMES

		5. Assist with removal of tube
		  a. Usually removed after 24 hours of no bleeding.
		  b. Balloons usually are deflated for several hours prior to removal.
		6. Assist with injection sclerotherapy as a possible therapy for continued bleeding.
		7. Assist with bedside endoscopy for diagnosis of tissue damage.	

Altered tissue perfusion (decreased renal) related to decreased volume and compensatory vasoconstriction	Decreased urine output (30cc/hr or less) Serial increased potassium level Serial increases in BUN and creatinine High specific gravity of urine Presence of protein in urine	1. Assess hemodynamic parameters for indications of adequate vascular volume. 2. Assess urine output and specific gravity hourly. 3. Monitor serum levels of electrolytes, urea nitrogen, and creatinine. 4. Administer crystalloids and colloids as ordered to maintain vascular volume.	Urine output greater than 30 cc/hr. Serum electrolytes within normal limits BUN and creatinine normal Specific gravity normal

Potential for impaired gas exchange related to hemoglobin deficit or to pulmonary edema from fluid overload	Dyspnea
	Shortness of breath
	Crackles and/or wheezing heard on auscultation of chest
	Increased PCWP and RAP
	Increased HR, decreased BP
	Pink, frothy sputum
	Abnormal arterial blood gases
		1. Monitor ABGs.
		2. Administer supplemental oxygen, as ordered.
		3. Monitor hemodynamic status carefully during crystalloid and colloid replacement.
		4. Assess frequently for:
		  congestion in chest as evidenced by crackles and wheezes.
		  dyspnea, shortness of breath, orthopnea.
		  cough with pink, frothy sputum.
		5. If signs or symptoms occur, notify physician promptly and prepare to assist in treatment of pulmonary edema.
			ABGs within normal limits.
			Chest clear to auscultation.
			Hemodynamic stability.

Sensory-perceptual alteration related to increased blood ammonia levels (secondary to increased protein load from GI bleeding)	The following signs and symptoms may vary and/or appear in combination: Irritability	1. Administer antacids or histamine H$_2$-receptor antagonists as ordered to reduce bleeding.	Patient is alert and oriented. Absence of encephalopathy.

(Continues)

NURSING CARE PLAN (Continued)

Acute Upper Gastrointestinal Bleeding (Continued)

NURSING DIAGNOSIS	SIGNS AND SYMPTOMS	NURSING ACTIONS	DESIRED OUTCOMES

	Changes in level of consciousness
	Euphoria
	Increased drowsiness
	Confusion
	Slowed response
	Neuromuscular irritability
		2. Assess and monitor:
		BUN level, ammonia level.
		level of consciousness.
		neuromuscular function.
		response, alertness.
		3. Avoid therapies that may increase blood ammonia levels, such as:
		antacids with ammonium chloride.
		fluid volume deficit.
		excessive diuresis.
		4. Initiate actions to prevent encephalopathy as ordered:
		lactulose to promote excretion of ammonia.
		antibiotics to decrease formation of nitrogen-forming intestinal bacteria.
		volume replacement.
		5. If symptoms occur:
		  a. reorient patient frequently.
		  b. Provide a safe environment.
		  c. Administer sorbitol or magnesium citrate as ordered to decrease intestinal flora.
		  d. Administer low-protein nutritional support.
		  e. Administer lactulose as ordered to promote excretion of ammonia.	

Anxiety related to hospitalization, critical illness, or fear of death	Patient and family appear anxious, showing signs of fear: increased heart rate rapid, shallow breathing irritability asking numerous questions verbalizations of anxiety	1. Reassure patient. 2. Explain all procedures. 3. Maintain a calm, unhurried atmosphere. 4. Encourage verbalization of anxiety and fears. 5. Allow rest periods between treatments. 6. Keep patient warm and as comfortable as possible. 7. Demonstrate competency and efficiency.	Absence of anxiety, or tolerable level of anxiety

Fluid Volume Deficit Related to Hemorrhage

Among laboratory tests monitored is the BUN. The BUN rises because blood decomposes in the gastrointestinal tract and because liver metabolism slows due to decreased perfusion. If the creatinine level is normal (indicating normal kidney function), a markedly elevated BUN in a patient with an upper GI bleed indicates that a massive bleed has occurred.

Saline lavage is continued until the returns are clear. Traditionally, iced saline has been used to cause vasoconstriction; however, icing has become controversial because experimental data suggest that it may be no more effective than body-temperature saline in slowing bleeding and may cause adverse hemostatic effects (Dusek 1984). Levarterenol sometimes is added to the irrigating solution to increase vasoconstriction. Because Levarterenol is immediately metabolized by the liver, systemic vasoconstriction will not occur. When irrigating the stomach, be sure to keep meticulous records of intake and output to allow accurate determination of blood loss.

Blood transfusions are crucial. The patient should be monitored for a possible transfusion reaction, as well as for complications of massive transfusions, such as hypocalcemia. The hematocrit should rise 3% with each 500 ml of blood administered; if you do not observe this response, you should assume the patient is still bleeding actively. Immediate surgery is indicated if more than 6-8 units of blood must be administered, transfusions are ineffective in maintaining BP, or bleeding persists more than 24 hours (Alspach and Williams 1985).

Anxiety Related to Self-Soiling and Precarious Health Status

Patients often are acutely embarrassed about being unable to control their vomiting and diarrhea. The odors are unpleasant, and getting these excretions on one's body may activate memories of childhood struggles for mastery over one's body. It is helpful to reassure the patient that you understand it is impossible to control the vomiting and diarrhea. Keep the patient clean, and provide mouthwash to rinse blood out of the mouth after vomiting episodes. As the patient may feel humiliated if excretions get on you, wear an isolation gown over your uniform during acute bleeding episodes.

The patient with an upper GI bleed is anxious and frightened. The sight of one's own blood is very upsetting, and patients often fear that they are bleeding to death. A calm, professional attitude as you institute emergency procedures can convey a sense of safety to the patient. In addition, it is helpful to indicate that you understand the patient's fright and that everything is being done to stabilize the condition.

An upper GI hemorrhage often is acutely frightening to the family as well. For guidelines on nursing interventions with family members, please consult Chapter 3.

Definitive Care   The bleeding vessel often can be located with *fiberoptic endoscopy,* usually performed within 24 hours of admission. A local anesthetic is used, and the patient is sedated with diazepam. Electrocautery may be used to treat sites of bleeding. If the patient continues to bleed or is bleeding very rapidly (more than 0.5 ml per minute), *arteriography* is performed to visualize the arterial systems. Selective arteriography allows direct intra-arterial infusion of vasopressin to control bleeding.

Medical approaches to control bleeding include antacid administration, cimetidine or ranitidine administration, and tamponade of bleeding vessels. *Antacids* are used to promote healing and usually are titrated to achieve a gastric pH of 5 or more; therefore, the pH of the nasogastric aspirate is checked prior to administration. *Cimetidine* (Tagamet) is a specific histamine antagonist at a histamine$_2$ receptor site in gastric parietal cells (Pinilla et al. 1985). Although its use in prophylaxis of duodenal ulcers and treatment of hypersecretory disorders is accepted, its use in preventing and treating acute ulceration is controversial (Pinilla et al. 1985). Cimetidine can cause central nervous system side effects; hematologic disorders; slowed metabolism of warfarin-type anticoagulants, aminophyllin, and diazepam; and false-positive tests for occult blood. When both cimetidine and antacids are being used, they should be administered at separate times, as antacids decrease cimetidine absorption.

Ranitidine (Zantac), another histamine H_2-receptor antagonist, has fewer side effects. Side effects may include nausea, constipation, and GI pain; blood dyscrasias; and CNS effects.

When the patient has esophageal varices, tamponade of bleeding vessels is achieved most commonly with a triple-lumen *Sengstaken-Blakemore tube* (Figure 19-4). The three lumens lead to a gastric balloon, an esophageal balloon, and a drainage opening that may be used for gastric suction. (Also available on the market is a balloon compression tube with an additional port for esophageal suction.)

The nurse should assist the physician with insertion of the Sengstaken-Blakemore tube. The insertion procedure is similar to that for a nasogastric tube. Inflate both balloons prior to the start of the procedure and hold them under water to check for leaks. Insertion is frightening and uncomfortable for the patient because of the large diameter of the tube; so the patient usually is premedicated. Have suction readily available, because the patient often vomits during insertion, making aspiration a danger.

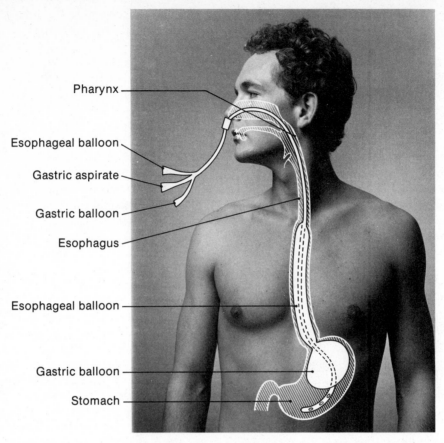

Pharynx

Esophageal balloon

Gastric aspirate

Gastric balloon

Esophagus

Esophageal balloon

Gastric balloon

Stomach

FIGURE 19-4

Triple-lumen esophageal-nasogastric (Sengstaken-Blakemore) tube. (Source: Swearingen PL: *The Addison-Wesley Photo-Atlas of Nursing Procedures.* Menlo Park, CA: Addison-Wesley, 1984, p. 228.)

Once the tube is positioned in the stomach, the *gastric balloon* is inflated with 50 ml air and the tube is clamped to prevent an air leak. The tube then is withdrawn until the balloon sits snugly up against the cardia of the stomach. Following an x-ray to verify correct placement, the balloon is inflated further to 200-250 ml. To prevent peristaltic movement of the tube, traction is placed on it by putting a football helmet on the patient and taping the tube to the chin guard. The gastric drainage lumen is irrigated as necessary to maintain patency.

If bleeding persists, the *esophageal balloon* also is inflated and clamped. Pressure of 25-40 mm Hg is maintained with the use of a sphygmomanometer for up to 24 hours; longer use could cause esophageal edema, ulceration, or perforation. When the esophageal balloon is inflated, the patient is unable to swallow, so you must suction the esophagus frequently. Alternatively, a na-

sogastric tube may be inserted above the esophageal balloon to provide continuous evacuation of secretions, or the four-lumen Minnesota tube, which has an additional lumen for esophageal aspiration, may be inserted (Amato 1983).

Potential complications with use of the Sengstaken-Blakemore tube include *airway obstruction* and *esophageal perforation.* If the gastric balloon ruptures, the whole tube will move upward and obstruct the airway. This is a true emergency, and you should promptly cut through all three lumens *(scissors always should be kept at the bedside)* and remove the tube. Notify the physician immediately if the patient experiences onset of back pain, upper abdominal pain, or shock, because these may herald esophageal perforation.

The Nachlas-Linton tube sometimes is used instead of the Sengstaken-Blakemore tube. It has one gastric balloon and two aspiration lumens, one that terminates in the stomach and one that terminates in the esophagus. It thus obviates the problem of accumulation of secretions in the esophagus that characterizes the Sengstaken-Blakemore tube. Because the Nachlas-Linton tube's gastric balloon has a much larger capacity than the Sengstaken-Blakemore's tube, it applies enough pressure to the intragastric veins that esophageal tamponade is unnecessary (White et al. 1985).

Surgery is indicated when the bleeding recurs, when shock is uncontrollable, or when esophageal bleeding persists.

Outcome Evaluation

Evaluate the patient's progress according to these desirable outcome criteria:

- Vital signs WNL.
- No complaints of dizziness, thirst, or syncope.
- Postural vital signs negative; that is, systolic BP change of less than 10 mm Hg and pulse change of less than 20 beats per minute.
- No hematemesis or hematochezia.
- Hemoglobin, hematocrit, and red blood cell count WNL.
- Arterial blood gas values WNL.
- Relaxed appearance.

Acute Pancreatitis

The pancreas has both endocrine (insulin-secretion) and exocrine (nonhormonal) functions. The exocrine function of the pancreas is to secrete enzymes that act to break down proteins, fats, and carbohydrates into simpler, absorbable forms. Pancreatic trypsin breaks down amino acid bonds in proteins, pancreatic amylase breaks down starches to disaccharides, and pancreatic lipase acts on triglycerides to produce fatty acids and glycerol. These powerful enzymes normally are stored in the pancreas in an inactive form and not activated until the secretion reaches the duodenum.

Under normal conditions, there are protective mechanisms to prevent premature activation and autodigestion. First, the enzymes are secreted and stored in an inactive form and are activated by trypsin. Second, trypsin inhibitor is present in the blood that supplies the pancreas.

Acute pancreatitis is a condition whose intensity varies from mild edema to hemorrhagic, necrotic inflammation. It is believed to be an autodigestive process. The enzyme responsible for initiating the process is trypsin, which activates elastase and phospholipase A. Elastase produces necrosis of blood vessel walls, and phospholipase destroys the cell membranes within the acinus. Trypsin causes edema and necrosis and further activates kallikrein. Kallikrein is a vasoactive substance that stimulates vasodilatation, increased vascular permeability, and edema (Geokas 1985; Alspach and Williams 1985; Toskes and Greenberger 1983). This facilitates leakage of the activated enzymes, blood, and fluid into the peripancreatic tissue.

Assessment

Risk Conditions The exact mechanism whereby pancreatic inflammation begins is unclear; however, many etiologic conditions are associated with pancreatitis, including alcohol abuse, biliary tract disease, hyperlipidemia, hypercalcemia, thiazide use, corticosteroid use, viral or bacterial infections, post traumatic injury, and vascular disorders (Geokas 1985). By far the most common such conditions are alcohol abuse and cholelithiasis. Presence of a gallstone in the common bile duct or ampulla of vater may precipitate reflux of bile and/or duodenal contents and subsequent activation of pancreatic enzymes (Price and Wilson 1986).

It is unclear exactly how alcohol abuse overcomes the natural safeguards of the pancreas and initiates premature pancreatic enzyme activation. Several mechanisms have been hypothesized (Geokas 1985); they are summarized as follows. First, alcohol stimulates and increases gastric and pancreatic secretions, which may induce duodenal inflammation and spasm of the ampulla of vater. Alcohol also decreases gastric pH, which is a stimulus for secretion of alkaline pancreatic fluid. In the presence of ampulla obstruction, stimulation of the pancreas can precipitate pancreatitis. Second, prolonged alcohol intake produces histologic changes in pancreatic tissue and the ducts, which may cause obstruction and cell membrane changes. It is important to note that not all people who abuse alcohol develop pancreatitis, indicating that other factors possibly are involved (Toskes and Greenberger 1983).

Signs and Symptoms

Physical Assessment The most common clinical feature of acute pancreatitis is severe abdominal pain. It may begin gradually or suddenly, but once present it persists and is unrelenting. It usually is located in the epigastrum, and often radiates to the back, chest, and flank areas. It is relieved by sitting forward. Nausea, vomiting, and abdominal distention, which may accompany the pain, usually are caused by hypomotility and peritonitis. Peritonitis occurs with cell and tissue destruction. If the condition is severe, shock may be present due to loss of large amounts of plasma into pancreatic and peripancreatic tissue. This hemorrhage may cause retroperitoneal bruising *(Grey-Turner's sign)* and discoloration around the umbilicus *(Cullen's sign)* (Toskes and Greenberger 1983). Rarely, pleural effusion may be present (Dewan et al. 1984). Additionally, low-grade fever and tachycardia are common.

Diagnostic Studies Traditionally, serum amylase concentration greater than 200 standard units is characteristic of pancreatitis. Serum amylase isoenzymes provide a more specific assessment. That is, elevation of *p*-isoamylase (greater than 40%) may indicate pancreatitis (Geokas 1985). A serum amylase level greater than 500 U/100 ml with positive isoenzymes confirms pancreatitis. Serum lipase levels rise later than amylase (usually at 5-7 days). Serum calcium is low because fat necrosis results in calcium precipitation. The resulting hypocalcemia may be severe enough to cause tetany. The white blood cell count is usually elevated, especially with peritonitis. Urinalysis reveals elevated urine amylase for 5-7 days and increased urine lipase for 5-7 days as well (Swearingen 1986).

Serum glucose and urine glucose may be elevated, as the inflammatory process affects endocrine (beta cell) function of the pancreas. Additionally, increased glucagon release and increased secretion of adrenal glucocorticoids may contribute to hyperglycemia.

Studies to assist in diagnosis of pancreatitis include ultrasound imaging, computerized tomography, angiography (rarely), and magnetic resonance imaging (Geokas 1985).

NURSING DIAGNOSES

The nursing diagnoses that may apply to the patient with acute pancreatitis include the following:

- Fluid volume deficit
- Alteration in comfort: pain
- Alteration in nutrition
- Potential for infection
- Chemical imbalance*

*Diagnosis developed by author.

Planning and Implementation of Care

Fluid Volume Deficit Related to Hemorrhage
Monitor the patient carefully for signs of hemorrhage and decreased fluid volume such as: decreased blood pressure, increased heart rate, peripheral vasoconstriction and decreased urine output (30-40 cc/hr). In addition, Grey-Turner's sign and Cullen's sign may indicate retroperitoneal and/or peripancreatic bleeding. Hemodynamic monitoring with a pulmonary artery line may be used to guide and evaluate fluid replacement. A right atrial pressure less than 2 mm Hg and a pulmonary capillary wedge pressure less than 6 mm Hg may indicate hypovolemia.

Administer fluid, blood replacement, and plasma expanders as ordered by the physician. Care must be taken when administering hyperosmotic solutions such as albumin because rapid fluid shifts may precipitate fluid overload.

Hypovolemia may contribute to renal failure with decreased renal perfusion, so monitor urine output hourly.

Alteration in Comfort: Pain Related to Inflammation Meperedine is the analgesic usually used for relief of the pain associated with pancreatitis. It is less likely to cause spasm of the sphincter of Oddi than an opiate such as morphine sulfate. Assist the patient to a position of comfort, usually Fowler's with knees flexed, as this relaxes abdominal muscles. Maintain bedrest to minimize pain and facilitate rest. Additionally, keep the patient NPO to decrease stimulation of pancreatic secretions.

The critical-care nurse may also intervene with nonpharmacologic techniques such as relaxation, massage, distraction, and guided imagery.

Alteration in Nutrition The patient with pancreatitis is at risk for nutritional deficiency for several reasons. First, the patient is NPO to decrease pancreatic secretions. Second, nasogastric suction is used to decrease abdominal distention and flow of acid into the small intestine, which stimulates pancreatic secretion. Finally, prior to hospitalization and implementation of suction, the patient has most likely been anorexic and nauseated and has experienced vomiting.

When nutritional support is needed, total parenteral nutrition often is administered and continued for approximately 2-3 weeks. The administration of lipids or amino acids intravenously does not stimulate the pancreas (Silverman et al. 1982; Fried et al. 1982).

When symptoms improve, start the patient on clear liquids very slowly as tolerated. Resumption of oral intake within the first 2 weeks has caused exacerbation, so caution should be exercised.

In addition to the above measures, make sure the patient avoids fat and alcohol intake.

Potential for Infection Related to Leakage of Enzymes The patient with pancreatitis is at risk for infection from peritonitis, pancreatic abscess, or pancreatic pseudocyst. These complications usually occur in the second or third week after the onset of pancreatitis (Price and Wilson 1986). Monitor the patient for signs of infection, such as increased WBC, increased polymorphonuclear cells (PMNs), increased temperature, and abdominal pain and rigidity.

Because of the toxicity of pancreatic secretions, peritoneal lavage may be done to remove the exudate and help prevent sepsis. However, lavage has not been shown to prevent pancreatic necrosis (Geokas 1985).

A treatment sometimes used for infected pseudocysts is aspiration by introducing a catheter into the cyst for drainage. If this is not possible, surgical removal is required (Geokas 1985). Another indication for surgery is necrotizing pancreatitis, as the necrotic tissue and abscess areas must be completely removed.

Chemical Imbalance Related to Changes in Metabolic Processes The patient with pancreatitis is at risk for numerous chemical imbalances. The critical-care nurse needs to know the possibilities and potential treatments.

- Hypocalcemia is treated with calcium substances.
- Albumin may be given to correct hypoalbuminemia that occurs with fat necrosis.
- Metabolic acidosis due to lack of insulin (ketoacidosis) and decreased renal function may be treated with glucagon and judicious use of insulin to promote glucose use.
- Cimetidine may be used to decrease gastric acid secretion.
- Hyperglycemia may occur due to decreased pancreatic function, and insulin may be required.

Additional Surgical Measures for Relief of Pancreatitis If more conservative treatment fails, further surgical options include:

- Total pancreatectomy, which will result in insulin-dependent diabetes.
- Pancreatectomy with islet cell autotransplantation. The patient's own healthy islet cells are injected into the portal vein and rest in the liver.
- Segmental pancreatic autotransplantation. Healthy segments of the pancreas are reimplanted and anastomosed to femoral vessels.

Outcome Evaluation

Evaluate the patient's progress according to the following outcome criteria:

- Fluid balance normal.
- Urine output 60 cc/hr or greater.
- Vital signs within normal limits.
- Relief of pain.
- No evidence of infection.
- No evidence of hemorrhage.

Hepatitis

Hepatitis is an inflammatory process of the liver. When hepatocytes are damaged due to the inflammatory process, cellular death occurs and liver function is impaired. Usually this process is reversible in hepatitis; however, hepatitis occasionally can lead to liver failure.

Hepatitis can be caused by drug toxicities or toxins such as alcohol. It can also be associated with infections such as salmonellosis, mononucleosis, and malaria (Porth 1986). The most common cause is viral, and four viruses have been identified: hepatitis A virus (HAV), hepatitis B virus (HBV), hepatitis Non-A Non-B (NANB), and, recently, hepatitis D virus (HDV). Table 19-2 compares the characteristics of Type A, Type B, and Non-A Non-B hepatitis.

Assessment

Risk Conditions

Hepatitis A This type of hepatitis formerly was known as infectious hepatitis. It usually has a mild clinical course. It is spread by oral ingestion of fecal contaminants (Gurevich 1983). Sources of the infection can include contaminated water, shellfish, oral–anal sex, and food handled by infected people. The highest incidence of HAV infections occurs in areas of poor sanitation and overcrowded living conditions. Small children often are sources of infection.

Hepatitis B This type of hepatitis formerly was known as serum hepatitis. The clinical course is more often serious than HAV and can result in a carrier and/or

TABLE 19-2 COMPARISON OF CHARACTERISTICS OF THREE TYPES OF VIRAL HEPATITIS

	TYPE A	TYPE B	NON-A NON-B
Mode of transmission	Fecal–oral route; large-scale outbreaks caused by contamination of food or water.	Percutaneous inoculation (needle stick); usually through blood, but may result from saliva or semen.	Usually blood; also semen and saliva.
Population affected	More common in children and in overcrowded areas with poor sanitation.	All ages. Drug addicts, male homosexuals, sexual partners of infected individuals. Patients and staff in hemodialysis units are at high risk.	All ages. Highest risk in recipients of blood transfusions. Also at risk are drug addicts, hemodialysis patients. Nosocomial spread possible.
Diagnosis of acute disease	Anti-hepatitis A virus (IgM) antibody in serum (anti-HAV IgM)	Hepatitis B surface antigen in serum (HBsAg)	When causes of type A and type B are ruled out
Incubation period	2–6 weeks	6 weeks–6 months	2 weeks–6 months
Carrier state	No	Yes	Yes
Chronicity	No	Yes	Yes
Measures for reducing exposure	Handwashing; stool precautions first 2–3 weeks	Handwashing; wearing gloves when handling body fluids and masks when fluids may splatter; using care when discarding needles and syringes; autoclaving all nondisposable items. Patient can never become a blood donor.	Same as for Type B
Prophylaxis	IG (immune globulin) before or within 1–2 weeks after exposure	HBIG (hepatitis B immune globulin) within 24 hours after exposure and 1 month later. Hepatitis B vaccine recommended for medical and laboratory personnel, male homosexuals, neonates of infected mothers, and sexual partners of chronic HBsAg carriers	Still controversial, but currently a single dose of IG is recommended
Common clinical features	Majority of symptoms are mild and flu-like. *3–12 days:* headache, nausea, fever, anorexia, epigastric pain, elevated SGOT, SGPT, LDH, and LDH3. *2 weeks:* jaundice, dark urine, clay-colored stools, elevated bilirubin abdominal tenderness	Often more severe; may require hospitalization	Same as Type A

Source: Adapted from Swearingen P: *Manual of nursing therapeutics* (Menlo Park, CA: Addison-Wesley, 1986), p. 326.

chronic state. HBV is not easily transmitted. The virus is present in serum and is transmitted by contact with contaminated serum. The virus can be transmitted by blood products, needles, sexual contact, and mothers to infants. Persons at risk are intravenous drug abusers, people with hemodialysis, health care workers, and male homosexuals.

Non-A Non-B Hepatitis This type of hepatitis is most commonly spread through blood transfusions, hemodialysis, or contaminated needles.

Hepatitis D The HDV is the smallest hepatitis virus known. It is an incomplete virus that relies on the presence of HBV to support its existence and replication

(Hansson 1985). The HDV is transmitted in the same manner as HBV.

Diagnosis

Hepatitis A Serum immune globulin M (IgM) type antibody to HAV appears approximately 4 weeks after initial infection and remains for 2-6 months after initial infection. It is diagnostic of acute infection, and the individual is considered contagious as long as it is detectable in the serum. After acute infection, IgG replaces

IgM, remaining for the life of the individual (Micozzi and London 1983).

Hepatitis B There are several serologic markers for HBV infection and three different antigen systems associated with the virus. Discussion of these follows.

Hepatitis B Surface Antigen (HBsAg) This antigen is present in the serum and is the first serologic manifestation of infection. It may appear as soon as 1 week after exposure. It persists throughout the period of clinical illness. The patient is contagious as long as HBsAg is present.

Antibody to Hepatitis B Surface Antigen (Anti-HBs) This antibody protects against future infection (that is, provides immunity). The presence of Anti-HBs usually means recovery has begun.

Hepatitis B Core Antigen (HBcAg) This antigen is found only on the hepatocyte; there is no serologic marker.

Antibody to HBc (Anti-HBc) This antibody is found in the serum in the late acute phase. It is the only serologic marker present when HBsAg has decreased and anti-HBs has not yet reached a detectable level.

Hepatitis B"e" Antigen (HBeAg) This antigen may be present in patients who are HBsAg positive. The patient usually is considered more infectious than if only HBsAg is present.

Antibody HB"e" (Anti HBe) Presence of this antibody usually is associated with resolution of infection (Micozzi and London 1983).

Antibody HDV (Anti-HDV) This antibody is the serologic marker for HDV and may be present with HBV infection.

Hepatitis Non-A Non-B There is no serologic marker for this type of hepatitis. Diagnosis is made by ruling out HAV and HBV.

Other Laboratory Tests Elevated SGOT, SGPT, and LDH isoenzymes 1 and 2 may occur. Additionally, elevated bilirubin (liver dysfunction), elevated urobilinogen, prolonged prothrombin time, and leukocytosis may occur.

Signs and Symptoms

Prodromal Period (Prior to Jaundice) Symptoms may include headache, nausea, vomiting, abdominal pain, mild elevation in temperature, and fatigue. Patients usually describe flu-like symptoms.

Icteral Period (Acute, Jaundice Phase) Symptoms include jaundice, dark urine, clay-colored feces, weight loss,

enlarged liver, and enlarged spleen. If severe, signs of hepatic failure may be present (see upcoming section).

NURSING DIAGNOSES

The approved nursing diagnoses that may apply to the patient with hepatitis include:

- Activity intolerance
- Altered nutrition: less than body requirements
- Potential for infection

Planning and Implementation of Care

Activity Intolerance Rest is the most important treatment for hepatitis patients. Patients usually pace their own activities, but the nurse needs to encourage rest and provide rest periods between activities and treatments. In the past, bedrest has been the treatment of choice; however, patients presently are encouraged to pace themselves.

Altered Nutrition: Less Than Body Requirements, Related to Decreased Vitamin Synthesis and Storage in the Liver and Decreased Appetite Food should be encouraged as tolerated, with a low-fat, high-carbohydrate diet usually being most desirable for anorexic patients. Assess nutritional intake and status and counsel the patient accordingly. Alcohol should be avoided for at least 6 months (Gurevich 1983). Pharmacologic therapy should be kept to a minimum because so many drugs are metabolized by the liver.

Potential for Infection Related to Decreased Resistance and Potential for Transmission of the Virus One of the best ways to prevent hepatitis is to prevent transmission of the virus. Isolate the patient from other patients; use aseptic technique for any invasive procedures, and handwashing when in contact with the patient. Maintain strict blood and enteric precautions.

Guidelines for Prophylaxis

Exposure to Acute HAV; anti-HAV, IgM positive

- Administer immune serum globulin (ISG).
- Order serologic tests.
- Administer additional dose of ISG if IgM positive.

Exposure to Non-A Non-B Hepatitis
- Controversial because no serologic marker is available.
- Usually, administer ISG.

Exposure to Acute HBV
- Order serologic profile.
- If HbsAg and anti-HBV negative, give HB immune globulin (HBIG) and repeat in 1 month. Follow-up serology is indicated.
- If anti-HBV positive, it indicates immunity and does not require HBIG administration.
- If HBsAg is positive, take hepatitis precautions.

Hepatitis B Vaccination   The HB vaccination uses noninfectious, inactivated virus. The purpose of the vaccine is to produce antibodies (anti-HBs) and subsequent immunity. People in high risk categories, such as nurses working in dialysis or blood banks, should consider taking the vaccine.

Outcome Evaluation

Evaluate the patient's progress based on the following outcome criteria:

- Serologic studies indicate recovery.
- Liver function tests indicate recovery.
- Patient is able to tolerate increasing levels of activity.

Liver Failure

Liver failure (hepatic failure) results when most liver functions have been altered. It may occur with a sudden onset or develop insidiously over a period of years.

The process of destruction of liver cells and decreasing liver function is called *cirrhosis*. Cirrhosis has three main etiologies, but eventually all lead to liver failure. *Postnecrotic cirrhosis* is characterized by formation of fibrous nodules and may follow hepatitis, or exposure to toxic chemicals or drugs. *Portal*, or *alcoholic (Laennec's)*, cirrhosis is characterized by fatty deposits and inflammation progressing to necrosis. *Biliary cirrhosis* begins in the bile ducts and is characterized by inflammation and scar formation in the ducts, eventually causing obstruction and destruction. The cause of biliary cir-

rhosis is often unknown but has been associated with gall stones (Porth 1986).

Liver Functions

The following summary of important liver functions is adapted from Keith (1985).

Vascular Functions
- Serves as a storage unit for blood volume and can release up to 400 cc as needed.
- Kupffer cells filter bacteria from the blood.

Secretory Functions
- Hepatocytes produce bile to aid in absorption of fats.
- Congugates bilirubin so it is water soluble.
- Removes unused cholesterol.

Metabolic Functions
- Stores sugar in the form of glycogen.
- Reconverts glycogen to glucose as needed for energy.
- Converts amino acids and fatty acids into new glucose (gluconeogenesis).
- Stores fat as triglycerides.
- Converts fatty acids to acetyl CoA (by a process called *beta oxidation*) for use in energy production.
- Converts excess acetyl CoA to ketones.
- Synthesizes serum proteins (albumin, globulins, and fibrinogen).
- Deaminates amino acids (removes an amino group so proteins can be used for energy production).
- Converts ammonia to urea.
- Produces vitamin-K-dependent clotting factors.
- Detoxifies hormones and drugs.

Storage Functions
- Stores large quantities of vitamins A, D, and B_{12} and iron.
- Stores vitamins E and K.

Assessment

Patients at Risk   There are three main precipitating conditions for hepatic failure: Laennec's (alcoholic) cirrhosis, postnecrotic cirrhosis, and biliary or obstructive processes. *Laennec's cirrhosis* occurs because of alcohol's direct toxic effect on the liver. The by-product of alcohol oxidation, acetaldehyde, causes mitochondrial membrane damage and necrosis of hepatocytes (Keith 1985). Alcohol also inhibits release of triglycerides from the liver (by increasing storage) and increases synthesis of fatty acids, thereby producing fatty infiltration and obstruction in the liver (Keith 1985). *Postnecrotic cirrhosis* and liver cellular destruction occurs with massive necrosis of liver cells, usually associated with viral hepatitis or hepatic destruction from toxic industrial chemicals (Swearingen 1986). *Obstructive processes* can occur with chronic biliary infections or ductal obstruction. In critically ill patients, liver failure also may be associated with circulatory failure and/or the shock state.

Signs and Symptoms The symptoms associated with the clinical presentation of liver failure vary with the severity and the extent of hepatic destruction. With early liver dysfunction, the patient may present with weakness, anorexia, weight loss, abdominal discomfort or pressure, and lack of energy. As the dysfunction progresses and the liver deteriorates, virtually every bodily system is affected.

Cardiovascular Symptoms Initially, the patient has a hyperdynamic cardiovascular system with flushed skin, hypertension, bounding pulses, and an enhanced precordial impulse. Blood pressure eventually decreases because of release of vasoactive substances from the damaged liver. Dysrhythmias may occur because of electrolyte changes (Alspach and Williams 1985).

Respiratory Symptoms Ascites may cause pressure on the diaphragm and prevent normal lung expansion. Additionally, pleural effusion may compress lung tissue as ascites fluid leaks into the pleural space. The patient usually is hypoxemic (Keith 1985).

Renal Symptoms Urine output decreases because of decreased renal perfusion.

Neurologic Symptoms Clinical manifestations range from minor personality changes to coma. Most neurologic changes result from accumulation of ammonia in the blood due to the liver's inability to convert it to urea. The excess ammonia then enters the central nervous system (Fraser and Arieff 1985). Additionally, the decreased storage of B vitamins may cause peripheral nerve degeneration and sensory alterations.

Hematologic Symptoms Coagulation problems occur because of deficient clotting factors. Bruising, nosebleeds, and gingival bleeding are common. The patient also may have petechiae associated with thrombocytopenia.

Fluid/Electrolyte Symptoms Electrolyte levels will vary with fluid balance. Initially, sodium and water retention

occur in the intravascular spaces due to decreased metabolism of ADH (prolonged half-life). As the liver becomes congested and portal vein pressure increases, fluid eventually seeps into the peritoneal cavity (ascites) and plasma volume decreases. This decrease results in compensatory mechanisms: release of ADH, release of aldosterone, and activation of the renin-angiotensin system. These mechanisms also result in sodium and water retention and eventually may cause dilutional hyponatremia (Keith 1985). Other electrolyte disturbances include:

- Hypokalemia due to diarrhea, aldosterone, or diuretics.
- Hypocalcemia due to decreased dietary intake and decreased absorption of vitamin D.
- Hypomagnesemia due to inability of the liver to store magnesium.

Gastrointestinal Symptoms Fetor hepaticus, a sweetish, almost fecal odor to the breath, is thought to be due to accumulation of methyl-mercaptan (Fraser and Arieff 1985). Because of the increased portal vein pressure, varices may develop, most frequently in rectal and esophageal vessels. These may be an additional source of gastrointestinal bleeding in hepatic failure.

Immunologic Symptoms Patients with hepatic failure have increased susceptibility to infection due to dysfunction of the filtering Kupffer cells.

Dermatologic Symptoms Jaundice occurs because of accumulation of bilirubin. Palmar erythema and erythema of the soles of the feet occur due to arteriovenous anastomoses (Keith 1985).

Diagnostic Tests The following summary is adapted from Swearingen (1986).

- Elevated SGOT and SGPT due to cellular destruction
- Elevated alkaline phosphatase due to inability to excrete
- Direct and total bilirubin elevated
- BUN may increase due to bleeding
- Plasma proteins decreased due to decreased synthesis in the liver
- Prolonged prothrombin time (PT) due to decreased synthesis of vitamin-K-dependent clotting factors
- Elevated urine bilirubin and urobilinogen
- Elevated ammonia
- RBCs may be decreased with hemorrhage
- Creatinine will be increased with decreased renal perfusion

---

NURSING DIAGNOSES

The approved nursing diagnoses that may apply to the patient with hepatic failure include:

- Potential fluid volume deficit
- Sensory-perceptual alteration
- Alteration in nutrition: less than body requirements
- Potential for infection
- Potential impaired gas exchange
- Impaired skin integrity

Planning and Implementation of Care

Potential Fluid Volume Deficit Related to Hemorrhage   The potential for hemorrhage is present for several reasons. First, there are decreased amounts of vitamin-K-dependent clotting factors. Second, thrombocytopenia related to splenomegaly usually is present. Finally, the increased portal venous pressure causes (a) development of collateral channels in systems with lower pressure, and (b) congestion in the venous systems, which results in engorged varicose veins. This can manifest as hemorrhoids and dilated abdominal veins *(caput medusae)*.

Another manifestation of collateral circulation is varices of esophageal submucosa and the upper stomach (Keith 1985). Bleeding varices are a life-threatening medical emergency. If bleeding occurs, the following care may be initiated:

- Oxygen therapy
- Hemodynamic monitoring and stabilization
  - volume replacement
  - fresh frozen plasma and vitamin K for clotting factors
- Gastric lavage with iced saline
- Emergency endoscopy
- Intravenous vasopressin to constrict the preportal arterioles, decrease blood flow to abdominal organs, and reduce portal pressure and portal blood flow (Quinless 1985). *Note:* Vasopressin may be given intraarterially, with placement of the arterial catheter by abdominal angiography (Bradford 1983). Vasopressin usually is given 0.4 U/min and gradually reduced as bleeding subsides. Side effects of vasopressin are due to its vasoconstrictor effects and increased afterload, so caution is exercised with patients with coronary artery disease.

- Esophagogastric tamponade via Sengstaken-Blakemore tube, which controls bleeding in 50-75% of patients (Quinless 1985). (See the care plan on Acute Upper Gastrointestinal Bleeding earlier in this chapter for related nursing care.) The esophageal and gastric balloons provide tamponade and hemostasis of the varices.

- Injection sclerotherapy involves the injection of a coagulating, sclerosing agent into the bleeding varices. The fiberoptic endoscope is most commonly used, and the procedure usually is done 12-24 hours after the initial bleeding episode, when the field is not obscured by blood (Bradford 1983). Vasopressin usually is continued postinjection, and the critical-care nurse observes for signs of rebleeding. Other possible complications of the procedure include fever due to inflammatory reaction, substernal chest pain due to sclerosing agent irritation of tissue, esophageal stenosis, aspiration, and allergic response to the sclerosing agent (Bradford 1983).

- Surgery may be done to divert blood flow from congested liver (see the discussion of ascites, next).

Potential Fluid Volume Alteration Related to Ascites   The ascites that occurs with liver failure is the result of several complicating factors. It can be understood by looking at Figure 19-5. Management of ascites may include the following (Dodd 1984):

- Dietary sodium limited to 200-500 mg/day
- Fluids restricted to approximately 1500 cc/day
- Daily calculation of weight, I & O, and abdominal girth
- Diuretics with an aldosterone antagonist such as spironolactone
- Intravenous albumin to increase plasma oncotic pressure
- Therapeutic paracentesis, using a small in-dwelling catheter for temporary relief, if respiratory function is impaired.

If ascites is refractory to medical management, peritoneovenous shunt procedures may be done. The collecting cannula lies in the peritoneal cavity and the outflow tubing is tunneled through subcutaneous tissue to the internal jugular vein. Important nursing actions for a patient with a shunt includes (Schumann 1983):

1. Maintain the patient in a supine position to facilitate flow.

2. Assist the patient with deep breathing to encourage flow.

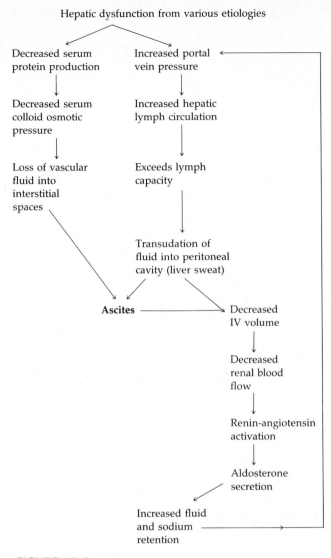

Hepatic dysfunction from various etiologies

Decreased serum protein production → Decreased serum colloid osmotic pressure → Loss of vascular fluid into interstitial spaces

Increased portal vein pressure → Increased hepatic lymph circulation → Exceeds lymph capacity → Transudation of fluid into peritoneal cavity (liver sweat)

→ **Ascites** → Decreased IV volume → Decreased renal blood flow → Renin-angiotensin activation → Aldosterone secretion → Increased fluid and sodium retention

FIGURE 19-5

Formation of ascites (Adapted from Dodd RP: Ascites: When the liver can't cope. *RN* (October) 1984; 26–30). Copyright (c) 1984 Medical Economics Company Inc., Oradell, N.J. Reprinted by permission.

3. Check patency of the shunt with a Doppler flow meter.

4. Observe for central fluid overload from drainage of fluid into the jugular vein.

5. If fluid overload occurs, treatment will include:
   a. Positioning the patient upright.
   b. Combination of digoxin and furosemide.
   c. Shunt ligation by the physician.

Sensory-Perceptual Alteration Related to Ammonia Retention Elevated plasma ammonia is a common occurrence in patients with hepatic failure. This problem is manifested as changes in neuromuscular and mental status. In early stages, patients show irritability, confusion, and clouding of sensorium. As it progresses, the patient may proceed into coma and demonstrate asterixis (characteristic "liver flapping").

Treatment is aimed at decreasing the amount of toxic protein metabolites that are absorbed into the blood. Initially, treatment includes excluding protein from the diet, since this diminishes the amount of bacterial breakdown of protein in the large intestine, which breakdown is the main source of ammonia. Another treatment involves introducing lactulose into the GI tract. Lactulose passes unchanged into the large intestine, where it is metabolized by bacteria, producing lactic acids and carbon dioxide. This decreases the pH to about 5.5, which favors conversion of ammonia to ammonium ions and subsequent excretion in the stool (Fraser and Arieff 1985).

Neomycin is used as a common treatment for hepatic encephalopathy. It is a nonabsorbable antibiotic that decreases the amount of urease-containing bacteria in the bowel, thereby decreasing ammonia production. For this purpose, it is given orally or by enema.

Alteration in Nutrition: Less Than Body Requirements, Related to Altered Hepatic Metabolism As discussed previously, liver dysfunction produces changes in carbohydrate, fat, and protein metabolism and alterations in storage and metabolism of vitamins and minerals. The dietary state of the patient in liver failure will improve when he or she stops drinking alcohol and receives nutritional support that includes vitamins, protein, fat, and usually increased carbohydrate.

The diseased liver needs protein to repair hepatocytes, but protein administration can result in ammonia retention and hepatic encephalopathy. The patient with symptoms of hepatic encephalopathy has lower protein requirements. Diets utilizing vegetable or dairy proteins have been suggested. Tube feeding preparations that provide up to half of the nitrogen content as branched-chain amino acids are appropriate (Guenter and Slocum 1983). Note that patients on these formulas will require supplements of vitamins, minerals, and trace elements. Additionally, since patients with ascites usually require restriction of fluids and sodium, it is important to note the sodium content of formulas. Calorie-rich formulas may be beneficial, and it is important to adjust electrolyte administration as needed (Guenter and Slocum 1983).

Potential for Infection Related to Decreased Detoxification of Bacteria by Liver With hepatic dysfunction, the liver Kupffer cells do not adequately filter and detoxify bacteria. Additionally, splenomegaly may contribute to leukopenia. These two conditions predispose the patient to infection. And increased circulating corticosteroids due to the stress response may decrease the immune response. This condition reemphasizes the importance of always using aseptic technique and frequent handwashing in patient care.

Potential Impaired Gas Exchange Related to Ascites, Possible Pleural Effusion As the patient with hepatic failure is predisposed to respiratory problems, frequently assess for adequate gas exchange. The patient is usually more comfortable and able to expand the chest in a semi-Fowler's position. Listen for adequate and clear lung sounds at least every 2 hours, and administer oxygen as prescribed.

Impaired Skin Integrity Related to Impaired Circulation and Nutritional Deficit Skin care is of utmost importance for the patient with hepatic dysfunction, because of jaundice, dry skin, and decreased peripheral circulation. Turn frequently, massage bony prominences, and keep the skin clean and dry.

Potential Alteration in Urinary Elimination Related to Decreased Renal Perfusion A serious complication of hepatic failure is decreased renal blood flow, decreased glomerular filtration, and subsequent renal failure. Renal failure in the presence of hepatic failure, termed *hepatorenal syndrome,* has a high mortality rate (Keith 1985). Treatment is directed toward improving hepatic function and supporting renal function. This includes:

- Fluid and electrolytes to maintain hemodynamic stability.
- Dextran or albumin to increase intravascular volume and increase glomerular filtration.
- Discontinuation of potentially nephrotoxic drugs such as neomycin.
- Monitoring of lab values indicative of renal function, such as BUN and creatinine.

Outcome Evaluation

Evaluate the patient's progress according to the following criteria:

- Patient is alert and oriented.
- Patient exhibits no signs of infection.
- Nutritional status is adequate.
- Gas exchange is adequate.
- No signs of hemorrhage.

- Abdominal girth is not increasing.
- Liver function tests within normal limits.
- Hemodynamics stable.

NOURISHMENT OF THE CRITICALLY ILL

Nutritional Assessment

As the key provider of care to the critically ill patient, it is essential that you be aware of common risk factors for and signs and symptoms of impending nutritional crisis so that you can promptly alert the appropriate member of the critical-care team. In most cases, a registered dietitian is available to assess thoroughly a patient's nutritional status.

The nutritional assessment can be divided conveniently into three major parts: diet history, physical examination, and laboratory data. A suggested screening assessment format is shown in Table 19-3.

History

Patterns of Eating and Elimination Include in your assessment the person's usual eating and elimination patterns. A knowledge of preferred foods, portion sizes, and meal frequency can be quite helpful in encouraging food intake in the anorexic patient. An awareness of normal bowel elimination patterns is essential in avoiding constipation, fecal impaction, or unnecessary use of laxatives, enemas, or suppositories.

Conditions That Limit Nutrient Intake or Absorption Patients may become malnourished through two general mechanisms: limited nutrient intake or absorption, and increased nutrient demand. Be alert for conditions that limit the patient's intake and absorption of nutrients.

High-risk conditions for malnourishment due to de-

TABLE 19-3 NUTRITIONAL ASSESSMENT

1. History
   Eating and elimination patterns _____

   Conditions limiting nutrient intake _____

   Conditions increasing needs _____

2. Physical examination
   General appearance _____
   Height _____
   Weight: Current _____ Usual _____ Ideal _____ Loss _____
   Triceps skinfold _____ Mid-upper arm circumference _____ Arm muscle circumference _____
3. Laboratory tests _____

creased nutrient intake and absorption include the following (Butterworth and Weinsier 1980):

- Pre-existing depletion
  - Alcoholism
  - Gross underweight
  - Gross overweight
  - Recent weight loss of 10% or more of usual body weight
- No oral intake for 10 days or more on simple IV solutions
- Drugs with catabolic or antinutrient properties: steroids, immunosuppressants, antitumor agents
- Prolonged nutrient losses: renal dialysis, draining abscesses or wounds, fistulas or short-gut syndromes, malabsorption syndromes

Conditions That Increase Needs A gross approximation of the minimum caloric needs of a healthy adult is 30 kcal/kg ideal body weight (Keithley 1983). Injury or stress can increase resting metabolic expenditure significantly. The Harris-Benedict equation and multiples by Long et al. (1979) provide the best means for estimating caloric needs. Although 2000-3000 calories will meet daily maintenance needs for most hospitalized adults, certain patients—such as those with acute head injury or burns—may require up to 4000 kcal/day. Protein intake for an average, healthy adult is 0.8 g/kg body weight per day based on the Recommended Dietary Allowances (1980).

Numerous conditions can increase protein/caloric needs. High-risk patients include those with the following conditions.

- Massive burns
- Severe infection
- Extensive trauma
- Prolonged fever

The most dramatic demand occurs in major burns, where requirements can increase up to four to six times normal.

Physical Examination

Physical examination can provide important indicators of malnourishment. The usual parameters evaluated by the nurse in a screening examination are general appearance, height, and weight.

General Appearance Many signs of nutritional deficiency are apparent on assessment of the general appearance of the patient. Among the signs of possible nutritional deficiencies are the following:

- Thin, frail appearance
- Hair loss
- Scaly skin
- Stomatitis
- Lethargy or confusion
- Easy fatiguability

The most important anthropometric parameter evaluated by the nurse is weight. Ideally, when evaluating weight, compare the current and usual weights to the ideal weight for the patient's height, using standardized height/weight tables. Also compare present weight to usual weight, noting particularly the approximate change in weight and the time period in which it has occurred. Finally, compare the amount and rapidity of recent weight loss with values indicating protein-calorie malnourishment: 1-2% of weight loss in last week, 5% in last month, or 10% in last 6 months (Williams 1981).

Another useful measure of nutritional deficiency is a recent absolute weight loss of 10 or more pounds. Although crude, this measure is statistically meaningful: Seltzer (1982) found that a recent loss of more than 10 pounds correlated with increased mortality. This measure has the advantage of immediate availability without need to resort to mathematical calculation or reference tables. It can alert you to the increased risk of mortality and the need for prompt initiation of nutritional repletion.

Anthropometric measures evaluated by the nutritional specialist are more detailed. An estimation of body fat reserves is obtained through measurement of both the triceps skinfold and the mid-upper-arm circumference. The *triceps skinfold* is measured at a reference point midway between the shoulder and elbow, on the back of the nondominant arm. The skinfold is lifted parallel to the arm's long axis. The thickness of the fold is measured with special calipers and compared to standard measurements. *Mid-upper-arm circumference* is measured at the same reference point as the triceps skinfold. This measurement also can be compared to a standard table.

Other measurements by the nutrition expert are meant to determine the status of protein in the body. Protein stores can be clustered in two categories: muscle protein and visceral protein (Keithley 1983). Muscle protein is assessed through anthropometric measures such as height, weight, muscle measurements (for example, mid-upper-arm muscle circumference), and the creatinine height index (Keithley 1983; Stotts and Friesen 1982). Visceral protein is evaluated through laboratory measurements (see next section).

Anthopometrics may be difficult to evaluate when the patient has edema or cannot sit. Weight trends may be hard to assess in patients with unstable volume status.

Laboratory Data

Among laboratory findings suggesting malnutrition are decreased hemoglobin and hematocrit levels. Measure-ment of serum albumin, total lymphocyte count, transferrin, and total iron-binding capacity are important because they reflect the status of visceral protein—that is, the most essential protein stores in plasma proteins, hemoglobin, clotting factors, hormones, enzymes, and antibodies (Keithley 1983). Additional findings include depressed serum glucose and insulin levels (Stotts and Friesen 1982). Urine studies can show increased volume and increased nitrogen levels in early starvation; late starvation is characterized by decreased nitrogen levels and increased urinary ketone bodies and ammonia levels (Stotts and Friesen 1982). In the critically ill patient who becomes stressed or septic and/or requires ventilatory support, the key assessment factors are weight, sodium, potassium, phosphorus, magnesium, and nitrogen balance. Serum albumin is only a nutritional value if the patient can be provided enteral nutrition.

In nutritionally depleted patients, potassium and phosphorus ions move out of the cells to maintain normal serum levels. With the provision of glucose, which stimulates endogenous insulin release, these ions are shifted back into the cells, producing symptoms related to hypokalemia and hypophosphatemia. Hypophosphatemia has a significant effect on respiratory function, and the respiratory-compromised patient may require ventilatory support.

Low serum albumin (less than 3.0 mg/dl) may affect the critically ill patient's tolerance of enteral feedings. Providing albumin is postulated to enhance feeding tolerance by decreasing bowel wall edema (Moss 1982).

Nitrogen balance is one of the most objective measurements for monitoring adequacy of nutritional therapy in the critically ill patient (Wilmore 1980). Negative nitrogen balance in patients receiving 0.8–1.5 g protein/kg/day suggests that the patient is receiving inadequate calories to spare protein and achieve an anabolic state. Measurement of urinary urea nitrogen losses requires a 24–hour urine collection. The urine is kept on ice to avoid excretion of nitrogen from bacteria, thus altering the measurement. Nitrogen (N) balance is calculated as follows:

$$N \text{ balance} = N \text{ intake} - N \text{ output}$$

1. Convert protein delivered to nitrogen. For example:

$$\frac{85g \text{ protein}}{6.4} = 13.2 \text{ g N/day}$$

2. Add 20% to urine urea nitrogen (UUN) value for non-urea nitrogen losses. For example:

$$UUN = 370 \text{ mg\%} \times 1.20\% = 444 \text{ mg\%}$$

3. Multiply the UUN value (mg/100 ml) by the urine volume (in liters per day). For example:

$$\text{Urine volume} = 2800 \text{ cc} = 2.8 \text{ L}$$

$$\frac{444\text{mg}/100 \text{ ml}/2.8 \text{ L/day}}{100} = 12.43\text{g}$$

4. Subtract "Nitrogen out" from "Nitrogen in":

$$
\begin{array}{rl}
13.20 \text{ g} & \text{N in} \\
-12.43 \text{ g} & \text{N out} \\
\hline
+ 0.77 \text{ g} & \text{N balance}
\end{array}
$$

5. Stool or fistula losses are accounted for by adding 2–4 g to total "Nitrogen out" before subtracting:

$$
\begin{array}{rl}
13.20 \text{ g} & \text{N in} \\
-14.43 \text{ g} & \text{N out} \\
\hline
- 1.23 \text{ g} & \text{N balance}
\end{array}
$$

These figures suggest that this hypothetical patient requires additional calories to achieve the optimum of +2–3 g positive nitrogen balance. During severe stress and sepsis, zero nitrogen balance may be the maximal response that can be achieved (Wilmore 1980).

Malnutrition

Physiology of Starvation

Stotts and Friesen (1982) have made a major contribution to the nursing literature on nutrition in the critically ill by delineating the metabolic characteristics of malnutrition. Early starvation begins within several hours of absent food intake; when the glucose from ingested food has been utilized, blood sugar decreases to 10–15% below its baseline value. This drop initiates two compensatory mechanisms: *alteration in insulin–glucagon balance* and *gluconeogenesis.*

Alteration in Insulin–Glucagon Balance When serum glucose falls, the level of circulating insulin decreases. This in turn stimulates *glycolysis,* the breakdown of liver glycogen stores. Unfortunately, the glycogen stores are exhausted within a few hours, so the rise in blood glucose is only temporary. The altered insulin-glucagon balance also initiates *lipolysis,* the breakdown of fat into free fatty acids and glycerol, both of which can be used by the heart and other body parts

for energy production. Finally, the insulin-glucagon change also initiates *proteolysis,* the breakdown of muscle tissue, which releases amino acids that the liver subsequently converts into glucose. Thus, proteolysis is an important energy source for glucose-dependent organs, especially the brain.

Gluconeogenesis The other compensatory mechanism initiated by a drop in serum glucose is *gluconeogenesis,* the formation of glucose from breakdown products of incomplete metabolism (lactate and pyruvate), amino acids, and glycerol. During this period of rapid catabolism, muscle mass decreases; urinary nitrogen loss accelerates; and rapid weight loss occurs, due to protein loss and an associated osmotic diuresis. This stage lasts up to 5 days if the patient ingests nutrients soon after injury (Moore and Brennan 1975) and up to 10 days if no nutrients are ingested (Saudek and Felig 1976).

Late Starvation If nutritional supplementation is not resumed, the patient enters the stage of late starvation after several days (Stotts and Friesen 1982). In this stage, the metabolic rate slows and the body's major energy source becomes fat, with the brain in particular adapting to the use of ketone bodies as its major energy source. The ketones also affect protein catabolism, so that muscle releases less of one amino acid, *alanine,* and more of another, *glutamine.* Alanine, the primary amino acid released during protein breakdown in the nonstarvation state, produces urea; thus in late starvation, when alanine release slows, urinary urea levels drop. Glutamine metabolism produces ammonia as a by-product, so urinary ammonia levels increase. Weight loss continues, but at a slower rate.

After several months, when fat stores are exhausted, the body turns to protein as its only remaining source of energy. Protein in muscles, organs, and cells is metabolized for energy, until death ensues.

The Injured or Infected Patient It is important to realize that fuel mobilization and utilization differ in patients with injury or infection as compared to patients who merely are nutritionally depleted. The nutritionally depleted patient follows the pattern of starvation and hypometabolism described above. In contrast, the injured or infected patient develops a hypermetabolic state and greater glucose mobilization in the immediate posttrauma period (Stotts and Friesen 1982). These differences are believed to be mediated by the release of catecholamines, epinephrine, and norepinephrine, triggered by sympathetic nervous system stimulation. The metabolic response of the injured or infected patient also is affected by the stress-provoked release of pituitary hormones, particularly ACTH. ACTH in turn stimulates the release of glucocorticoids, which promote glucose mobilization, and mineralocorticoids, which promote retention of sodium and water. The mineralocorticoid activity delays the onset of osmotic diuresis and rapid weight loss for up to 24–48 hours posttrauma.

NURSING DIAGNOSES

The nursing diagnoses appropriate for the malnourished person vary, depending on the cause and stage of starvation as well as on individual responses. Examples of individual or single diagnoses are:

- Fatigue
- Potential for infection
- Potential for fluid volume deficit
- Disturbed self-concept

A more global or general diagnosis is "altered nutrition: less than body requirements" or, more simply stated, "nutritional deficit."

Planning and Implementation of Care

Nutritional Supplementation Patients maintained solely on routine intravenous solutions receive highly inadequate nutrition. For example, a liter of 5% dextrose in water contains only approximately 170 calories of hydrated glucose. For the patient able to meet nutritional needs through *oral feeding,* ways to enhance the intake of adequate nutrients include such well-known nursing measures as small, frequent feedings, selection of foods the patient enjoys, provision of a pleasant eating environment, and social interaction during meals. Dietary supplements may be prescribed for patients whose calorie needs cannot be met with the usual oral diet.

For the patient unable to meet physiologic needs through oral intake, nutritional support via *enteral* or *parenteral* routes may be prescribed. If the patient has relatively normal GI function, *enteral feeding* is preferable. Tube feedings may be given via several routes, including nasogastric, gastrostomy, and jejunostomy tubes. Commercial formulas are available in three general categories: nutrient supplements, meal replacements, and defined-formula diets (Keithley 1983). Nutrient supplements are nutritionally incomplete and are intended to improve the intake of one or more nutrients. Meal replacement formulas are nutritionally complete, contain varying amounts of lactose, and re-

quire functioning digestion and absorption systems. Defined-formula diets are nutritionally complete clear liquid, and require minimal digestion. Formulas vary according to osmolality, caloric content, lactose content, electrolyte content, and nutrient sources. A clinical dietitian should be consulted in selection of a formula appropriate to patient needs.

Enteral feedings may be administered by intermittent or continuous infusion. Potential complications include diarrhea due, for example, to osmotic overload, bacterial contamination, or lactose intolerance; fluid and electrolyte disturbances; and aspiration.

Parenteral nutrition is prescribed for patients unable to meet nutritional needs through the GI system. Two routes are available: peripheral venous nutrition and central venous nutrition. *Peripheral venous nutrition* is appropriate for the patient with relatively lower caloric needs. Patients who need large amounts of calories and protein, however, usually require central venous nutrition, as the solutions used have greater caloric and protein density than do peripheral venous nutrition solutions.

The technique of *central venous nutrition* is referred to by several names, including *total parenteral nutrition* (TPN) and *hyperalimentation.* Among the patients who can benefit from this technique are those with gastrointestinal fistulas, bowel obstructions or resections, severe burns, or inflammatory bowel disorders. The nursing care of the person receiving total parenteral nutrition is complex. Because of the degree of nursing skill required, the remainder of this chapter is devoted to this nutritional technique.

Total Parenteral Nutrition (TPN) *Total parenteral nutrition* (TPN) is the delivery of total nutrition into the superior vena cava by means of a solution containing hypertonic glucose, crystalline amino acids, minerals, and vitamins, in amounts in excess of metabolic equilibrium needs. Indications for TPN are the following: hypermetabolism (for example, severe burns and septic shock), contraindications to eating (for example, acute pancreatitis, gastrointestinal fistula, inflammatory bowel disease, malabsorption syndromes, acute renal failure, hepatic failure), and pre-existing starvation (for example, due to cardiac surgical preoperative acute weight loss exceeding 10%, anorexia nervosa, cancer).

Initiating TPN Therapy If the physician orders TPN, assist him or her to initiate the therapy.

Baseline Laboratory Values Ensure that baseline laboratory values are obtained. Because of the complexity of TPN therapy, numerous baseline studies should be done. Authors differ somewhat on which studies to do and how frequently. The following studies usually are obtained before TPN is instituted: serum electrolytes, serum osmolality, fasting blood sugar, complete blood count, blood urea nitrogen, and serum protein and lipid levels. In addition, weigh the patient and obtain a chest x-ray, ECG, and urinalysis.

Adequate Hydration Assure adequate hydration. If the above studies or clinical evaluation indicate suboptimal hydration, consult with the physician and administer whatever fluids he or she recommends. Adequate hydration prior to the institution of TPN is essential. Not only is it technically difficult to insert the catheter in a constricted vein, but inadequate hydration also increases the risk of hyperosmolar nonketotic coma.

Catheter Insertion The catheter is inserted under local anesthesia, usually into the subclavian vein. This vein has a greater blood volume than other veins, so the hypertonic TPN solution is diluted more rapidly. This approach also allows the patient to move the neck and arms freely after insertion and simplifies the application of an occlusive dressing. The internal jugular vein may be used instead, but it is less desirable because it has a lesser volume, use of this site limits neck movement, and nearby hair makes it difficult to apply an occlusive dressing. The brachial and axillary veins are avoided. Their smallness limits blood flow between the catheter and the vessel wall. The concentrated solution and limited arm movement that occur with use of brachial or axillary veins both predispose to phlebitis.

Potential Complications There are numerous potential complications of catheter insertion, including injury to the vein, thrombosis, pneumothorax, arterial puncture, air embolism, dysrhythmias, and cardiac tamponade. Since these are the same as with any central venous catheter, see Chapter 11 if you wish to review signs, symptoms, and treatments. To help avoid these complications, maximize venous distention by positioning the patient as follows: Place a towel roll along the spine so the shoulders drop posteriorly, turn the head to the side opposite the insertion site, and place the patient in Trendelenburg position if tolerated.

Catheter Placement The physician will use a 2-inch 14-gauge needle and a 3-ml syringe to locate the vein by passing the needle through the skin, toward the suprasternal notch, and behind and below the clavicle. Once blood is obtained, the physician will have the patient hold breath and bear down *(Valsalva maneuver)* while the physician holds the needle hub, disconnects the syringe, and passes an 8-inch 16-gauge catheter its full length into the vein. When blood appears, attach the catheter hub to an isotonic intravenous solution. Tell the patient to breathe again, and flush the catheter. The physician will withdraw the needle and cover it with the needle guard to minimize the chance of shearing the catheter. The physician will place a single suture to keep the catheter in place and apply an antiseptic ointment. Finally, the physician will paint the skin with benzoin, apply a dressing, secure a loop of the tubing over the dressing to decrease traction on the catheter, and apply an occlusive dressing.

Starting the TPN Solution Obtain a stat chest x-ray to locate the catheter tip. It is important to verify catheter placement by x-ray because the catheter can curl up or travel up the internal jugular vein instead of going down the innominate vein into the superior vena cava. Once catheter placement is verified, discontinue the isotonic solution and begin the TPN solution.

Nutrients Supplied via TPN Table 19-4 shows how to calculate nutrient requirements for the TPN patient. As mentioned earlier, when protein undergoes proteolysis, tissue nitrogen is excreted. The negative nitrogen balance will continue even if exogenous nitrogen is supplied unless adequate calories also are supplied. When both adequate calories and nitrogen are provided, the calories will be used for energy and the nitrogen for protein synthesis.

Calories Theoretically, calories could be supplied as fat, alcohol, or carbohydrates. But use of alcohol and fat is limited by practical considerations. Alcohol causes sedation and possible liver toxicity. Although fat contains more calories per gram than carbohydrate or protein, fat emulsions cannot be used for total caloric intake because the rate of utilization of fat is limited and because the body requires the intake of some carbohydrate and amino acids as well as fat. Hypertonic glucose is used most frequently because it is inexpensive, available in several concentrations, and relatively safe.

Nitrogen Nitrogen (N) can be supplied as protein, protein hydrolysates, or amino acids. Although the body can use protein supplied in plasma, whole blood, or albumin, time and energy are required to convert it to forms suitable for protein synthesis. Although protein hydrolysates used to be the main source of N, synthetic crystalline amino acids now are preferred because they provide N in a form more easily and completely used by the body. Hydrolysates and amino acid solutions contain both essential and nonessential amino acids.

Ratio of Calories to Nitrogen As mentioned previously, calories must be supplied so that the nitrogen will be used for protein synthesis. The ratio of calories to nitrogen necessary for protein synthesis is approximately 150–250 cal to 1 g N. Usually, amino acids or the pro-

TABLE 19-4 CALCULATION OF NUTRIENT REQUIREMENTS FOR THE TPN PATIENT

For the depleted patient, use the ideal body weight to compute nutritional requirements. For the patient at or beyond ideal weight, use the current weight. Optimal
weight gain with nutritional support is 0.5-1.0 kg per week. This can be achieved by
giving 500 kcal per day *in addition to* calculated caloric requirements. Ideal body
weight for height can be calculated by the following formula:

Male: First 5 feet, 50 kg + 2.7 kg for every inch over 5 feet

Female: First 5 feet, 45.5 kg + 1.8 kg for every inch over 5 feet

Caloric Requirements

Consider the Harris-Benedict equation, with multiples developed by Long et al.
(1979), to calculate caloric requirements:

Men: $(66.47 + 13.75W + 5.0H) - (6.76A \times AF \times IF)$

Women: $(655.10 + 9.56W + 1.8H) - (4.68A \times AF \times IF)$

where W = weight (in kg), H = height (in cm), A = age (in years), AF = activity
factor, and IF = injury factor.

Activity Factor:		Injury Factor:	
Confined to bed	1.2	Minor operation	1.20
Out of bed	1.3	Skeletal trauma	1.35
		Major sepsis	1.60
		Severe thermal burn	2.10

Protein Requirements

The range is 0.8–2.0 g/kg body weight:

Normal	0 8–1.0 g/kg body weight
Moderate stress	1.0–1.5
Severe stress	1.5–2.0

Consider using 0.8 g protein/kg initially until nitrogen balance data can be obtained.
Protein calories should not be included in calculations of total caloric intake.

Fat Requirements

Approximately 30% of the nonprotein calories should be given via a fat emulsion. A
minimum of 4% of nonprotein calories must be given as fat to meet linoleic acid
requirements and to avoid essential fatty acid deficiency. Patients with increased CO_2
production may require 50% of their calories from the fat emulsion.

Trace Elements and Vitamin Requirements

Trace elements and vitamins are added to TPN solution in accordance with current
AMA group guidelines.

Trace Elements

Daily requirements (established by an AMA Council on Nutrition) are:

Zinc	5 mg	Manganese	0.5 mg
Copper	1 mg	Chromium	10 mcg

This requirement can be met by adding 5 ml per day of the trace element formula
(TEF) to the patient's TPN.

(Continues)

TABLE 19-4 CALCULATION OF NUTRIENT REQUIREMENTS FOR THE TPN PATIENT (Continued)

Vitamins

Daily requirements (established by an AMA Council on Nutrition) are:

Ascorbic acid	100 mg	Pyridoxine	4 mg
Vitamin A	3300 IU	Niacinamide	40 mg
Vitamin D	300 IU	Dexpanthenol	15 mg
Thiamine	3 mg	Vitamin E	10 IU
Riboflavin	3.6 mg	Biotin	60 mcg
Folic acid	400 mcg	Vitamin B_{12}	5 mcg

These requirements can be met by adding 10 ml *per day* of MVI-12® or its equivalent to the patient's TPN. Trace element formula and vitamins are ordered on a daily basis. The pharmacy staff should place the appropriate amount in each bottle to accumulate the daily dose.

tein hydrolysates are added to a 30–50% dextrose solution to obtain the proper cal/nitrogen ratio. Depending on its composition, the TPN solution's osmolality will be approximately 1200–2000 mOsm/kg. As normal serum osmolality is about 290 mOsm/kg, these solutions are extremely hypertonic.

Electrolytes A variety of electrolytes may be added to the solution. In the absence of definitive data on daily needs for some electrolytes, their supplementation must be determined empirically. In addition, supplementation is influenced by the multiplicity of factors affecting electrolyte needs in a given patient. Furthermore, minimal and optimal amounts of electrolyte intake may differ. For these reasons, the prescribed electrolyte supplementation may vary considerably from patient to patient and institution to institution. As electrolyte compositions of the different commercial solutions also vary, the physician should specify the desired total concentration of each electrolyte per liter. The pharmacist will add to the commercial solution the amounts necessary to provide the desired concentration.

Sodium chloride usually is added for maintenance and potassium for protein synthesis. Because potassium is excreted when muscle breaks down, patients in negative nitrogen balance often have a potassium deficit. If protein is supplied without potassium, these patients will be unable to synthesize protein. Calcium often must be provided; although intestinal loss ceases with hyperalimentation, urinary loss is exaggerated by immobilization. Magnesium deficit is common in starvation. Although magnesium is necessary for optimal functioning of enzyme systems, the amount that should be supplied has not been established definitely. Iron is supplied only if the patient is deficient; if so, it must be given intramuscularly rather than in the TPN solution.

Vitamins and Trace Elements Detailed discussion on the need for vitamins and trace elements (such as zinc and cobalt) is beyond the scope of this text. The patient usually is given 10 ml of fat- and water-soluble vitamins daily. Trace elements can be added to the solution or supplied in blood components. For a more complete discussion, consult Review Article (1980), cited in the reference list.

Prospects for the Future Although conventional parenteral nutrition is based on the delivery of hypercaloric solutions, recent investigations have called into question the usefulness of delivering more calories than the patient can use (Robin et al. 1981). Earlier, we mentioned that injured and infected patients have a different pattern of fuel mobilization and utilization than do patients who are just nutritionally depleted. Similarly, the former also have a different pattern of response to substrate administration (Elwyn 1980; Kinney and Felig 1979). Excessive glucose administration (when all nonprotein calories are provided as glucose) may result in increased CO_2 production, increased O_2 consumption, continued oxidation of fat, decreased capacity for lipogenesis, and excessive deposition of glycogen (Robin et al. 1981). The increased CO_2 production and O_2 consumption produce significant increases in ventilation, and may precipitate respiratory distress in the patient with poor pulmonary function (Askanazi et al. 1980). The excessive glycogen deposition may impose an additional stress on the liver and perhaps contribute to impaired liver function. Burke et al. (1979) have demonstrated that, in severely burned patients, there are maximal infusion rates beyond which there are no manifestations of additional increases in glucose oxidation or protein synthesis. Moreover, they noted large fat deposits in the livers of their patients who had received

TPN for 3 weeks or more preceding death from massive burns. They therefore suggest there may be a limit to the "physiological cost-effectiveness" of hypercaloric solutions. Robin et al. (1981) recommend that each patient requiring TPN be treated with an individualized approach that limits energy intake to approximate energy expenditure and utilizes fat as a significant energy source. Optimal nutritional support for the critically ill patient requires further research to define increased caloric needs through the use of indirect calorimetry, further assessment of optional amino acid profiles, and the actual utilization of fat emulsion, particularly in stressed or septic patients.

Importance of Physical Activity Promote optimal utilization of the calories and protein TPN provides by maintaining the patient's physical activity. If the patient can tolerate ambulation, encourage it. If not, provide activity through active or passive exercises. Exercise minimizes protein breakdown, helps to assure that weight is gained as lean muscle rather than adipose tissue, and lifts your patient's spirit as he or she sees bodily strength increasing. Explain the exercise's importance, and together set short-term goals by which the patient can judge improvement.

Potential Complications Prevent and/or respond promptly to complications of TPN. As you would expect with so complex a therapy, the potential problems are numerous. They include allergy, infection, hyper- or hypoglycemia, fluid overload, protein overload, bleeding, metabolic acidosis, fatty acid deficiency, and electrolyte imbalances.

Allergy Observe for allergy, a rare complication. Signs are fever or shaking chill within the first 15–30 minutes of administration or allergic signs such as wheals or hives. These reactions are seen only with the protein hydrolysates, not with the crystalline amino acids. If they occur, stop the TPN solution immediately and switch to 10% glucose temporarily while you notify the physician. The reactions usually disappear when the solution is discontinued.

Infection Guard against infection by following these guidelines:

1. Prevent infection through meticulous aseptic technique.

2. Use as few connections in the line as possible. Avoid "piggybacks" and stopcocks, and tape all connections securely. (These measures will prevent both infection and air embolism.) Some physicians advocate the use of filters in the line. Others avoid them, because they may clog, or release a bolus of bacteria if they

break; furthermore, they may stop bacteria but not their toxins.

3. Refrigerate solutions until 30 minutes before use, when you may allow them to warm naturally. Solutions usually are ordered daily from the pharmacy, which prepares them under a laminar-flow hood.

4. Do not hang solution that appears cloudy or has a precipitate. Do not save a discontinued bottle and rehang it later.

5. Minimize fibrin deposition along the catheter. Fibrin deposition is believed to provide a focus for infection and thrombosis. Do not administer blood through the line, or withdraw blood samples (unless checking for contamination of the catheter itself). Also, avoid using the line to measure central venous pressure.

6. Avoid administering drugs routinely via the line, as they may precipitate. (Most physicians do not add antibiotics routinely to the TPN solution, either. Routine use can promote superinfections, and some antibiotics may interact with chemicals in the fluid.)

7. Change the bottle, intravenous tubing, and filter (if you are using one) at least every 12–24 hours. Place the patient flat; if you do not, disconnecting the tubing may allow air to be sucked into the vein by negative thoracic pressure. Aseptically connect the new bottle to the new tubing and clear air from the line. Stop the flow in the old tubing. Then quickly and sterilely disconnect the old intravenous tubing from the extension tubing, which remains attached to the catheter hub underneath the dressing. Connect the new intravenous tubing to the extension tubing. Have the patient perform a Valsalva maneuver while you disconnect and reconnect the tubing to avoid a possible air embolism.

8. Change the dressing when soiled, and as specified by the physician (typically every other day). As you will change the extension tubing at the same time, again place the patient flat. Wear sterile mask and gloves. Remove the old dressing. Clean and examine the skin for erythema and any drainage. Examine the catheter to be sure it still is sutured in place, and make sure the needle guard still is closed. Apply antiseptic ointment if recommended at your institution. Change the extension tubing. (You may find it helpful to grasp the catheter *hub* with a hemostat while you do this. Do *not* clamp the catheter itself; although you may prevent an air embolus, you may produce a catheter embolus!) Redress the site occlusively. Write the date on the dressing so other staff can remember when the next change is due. Chart the procedure and your observations, and alert the physician to any troublesome signs, such as a loose suture.

9. Observe the patient closely for indications of bacterial or fungal infection. The most common bacterial contaminant is streptococcus. The catheter also may become contaminated with *Candida*. Because *Candida* sepsis may be asymptomatic in its early stages, routine weekly blood and urine cultures for both bacteria and fungi should be performed. Redness, swelling, heat, or tenderness at the insertion site or along the catheter course; fever; or chills are signs of infection. If you suspect infection, alert the physician. Change and culture the bottle, tubing, and filter. The physician will draw blood cultures from both the catheter and a peripheral vein and try to identify possible foci of infection other than the catheter itself, such as a urinary tract, respiratory, or wound infection. If one is identified, the physician will treat that infection and leave the catheter in place. If no other source can be located, the doctor will remove and culture the catheter. TPN may be resumed at another site. Note that only the development of a new infection warrants catheter removal. The patient with an established infection may be started on TPN precisely to reverse the nutritional depletion that contributed to that infection.

Hyperglycemia Be alert for hyperglycemia. The development of hyperglycemia is undesirable for a number of reasons. Excess glucose increases serum osmolality, causing a fluid shift from the intracellular to extracellular space. It also causes an osmotic diuresis, resulting in both extracellular and intracellular dehydration. The increased volume of plasma dilutes the serum sodium—producing hyponatremia—and also dilutes the serum bicarbonate—creating a hypertonic metabolic acidosis.

Hyperglycemia can result from an excessive total load of glucose, too rapid an infusion rate, or diminished glucose tolerance. Prevent hyperglycemia by incorporating these measures into the patient's care:

1. During the initial stabilization period (4–7 days), increase the TPN rate gradually according to the physician's orders and the patient's tolerance. TPN increases the glucose, protein, osmolar, and volume loads on the patient. Most patients can increase their ability to cope with these loads if they are introduced slowly. One example of administration follows. On the first day, the physician may order administration of 1000 ml of TPN solution over 24 hours and the rest of the patient's fluid requirements as routine intravenous fluid. Each day, one liter of TPN solution may be added and one liter of other fluid deleted, until the total desired TPN solution is being administered, typically 2–3 a day.

2. Maintain the flow rate ordered by the physician. Most physicians specify that a constant flow rate be maintained over 24 hours to prevent deleterious swings in blood glucose and serum osmolality. Use an infusion pump to maintain the flow of solution within 10% of the rate ordered by the physician. Check the accuracy of the flow rate periodically. (If no pump is available, use a volume control chamber to limit the volume that could be infused accidentally.) Time-tape the bottle to indicate how much solution should be infused over a given period. This will provide a double check on pump accuracy.

Do *not* increase flow rate to "catch up" an infusion that is behind schedule.

3. Monitor blood glucose levels daily during stabilization and one to three times weekly thereafter. Anticipate that the blood glucose will rise. It should stabilize under 200 mg%.

4. Check urine sugar and ketones every 6 hours, using a double-voided specimen. Urinary sugar and ketones should be negative. Due to variations in renal threshold for glucose, urine glucose determinations do not indicate accurately blood glucose levels. If you and the physician anticipate or experience difficulty in stabilizing the patient on TPN, do not rely on urine glucose determinations. Instead, use reagent indicator strips (BG chemstix) to test the patient's blood glucose level.

5. Expect that diabetic patients or those with relative pancreatic insufficiency will need exogenous insulin. Administer supplementary insulin as ordered.

6. Exogenous insulin often is needed due to the critically ill patient's altered glucose metabolism. Anticipate that patients who are on high-dose steroids or undergoing increased stress (such as during surgery, the early postoperative period, or sepsis) will have a relative glucose intolerance. These patients will need insulin coverage when TPN is used.

7. Anticipate that patients with cardiac, renal, or hepatic disease will require adjustments in TPN volume or composition.

8. Monitor the patient for signs of hyperglycemia. Signs of hyperglycemia are: an increased urinary output, a urinary glucose level of 3–4$^+$, and/or ketone level greater than small; confusion, headache, lethargy, convulsions, or coma; nausea, vomiting, or diarrhea; dehydration; and a blood glucose level over 200 mg%. Notify the physician, who will order the infusion rate slowed or supplemental insulin administered.

Hyperglycemic Hyperosmolar Nonketotic State (HHNK) If a decreased level of consciousness is accompanied by profound dehydration, a blood sugar over 600 mg%, and a serum osmolality over 350 mOsm/L, the patient has developed a *hyperglycemic hyperosmolar nonketotic state* (HHNK). In this condition, an inadequate supply of insulin, probably due to pancreatic exhaustion, allows glucose to accumulate in the blood. Enough insulin is produced to prevent the use of fatty acids as an energy source, so ketones are *not* released. The syndrome thus differs from diabetic acidosis, in which diminished glucose utilization *does* provoke ketone production. Urinary glucose and ketone levels reflect this distinction. In diabetic acidosis, both glucose and ketone levels are high. In HHNK, marked glycosuria occurs without ketonuria.

In addition to hyperalimentation, HHNK may occur in other conditions, such as pancreatitis, severe infection, stress, and dialysis. (For a detailed discussion, see Chapter 17.) The mortality of the syndrome is high.

A hyperglycemic hyperosmolar nonketotic state is best prevented by vigilant attention to the measures outlined above to prevent hyperglycemia. If HHNK does occur, collaborate with the physician to treat it aggressively. The following procedure is recommended.

1. Stop the TPN infusion.

2. Rapidly replace the fluid deficit with hypotonic fluids, as ordered by the physician. One-half the needed volume should be replaced in the first 24 hours. If the patient is hypotensive or hyponatremic, normal saline is used; otherwise 0.45% sodium chloride solution usually is used. When the blood sugar reaches 250 mg%, glucose solutions may be resumed.

3. Administer insulin as ordered by the physician. Doses depend on hourly blood glucose and serum osmolality levels. Give the insulin intravenously, and watch the patient closely because she or he may be more sensitive to insulin than the ketoacidotic patient.

4. Administer potassium according to the physician's orders. Patients with diabetic ketoacidosis develop a systemic acidosis that causes hyperkalemia. Those with HHNK do not and may require earlier potassium replacement due to urinary losses. Doses depend on serum potassium determinations.

Hypoglycemia Hypoglycemia also is a constant threat to patients on TPN. Signs and symptoms of hypoglycemia include profuse sweating, palpitations, convulsions, and/or coma, accompanied by a normal urine volume and negative urinary glucose level. Hypoglycemia can occur as a rebound phenomenon if the TPN solution is stopped suddenly, especially in patients receiving exogenous insulin. In this situation, the pancreas continues to produce high levels of insulin, causing blood glucose to drop precipitously. Prevent rebound hypoglycemia with these measures:

1. Use an infusion pump to maintain a constant flow rate.

2. Prevent kinking, clotting, and displacement of the catheter. If the flow slows, check for these causes.

If they are absent, try changing the filter, if one is in use.

3. Avoid giving blood or other solutions through the catheter, because you will interrupt the flow of TPN solution and increase risk of infectious complications.

4. If the patient is receiving insulin, give it intravenously rather than subcutaneously. By doing so, any accidental interruption in solution flow will be accompanied by an appropriate interruption in insulin administration.

5. If the patient is receiving exogenous insulin, keep urine glucose at 0, to prevent chronic water loss. Monitor BG chemstix to prevent hypoglycemia.

6. If you are unable to use an infusion pump and there is an unplanned interruption in administration, restart the infusion promptly; this may avoid a hypoglycemic reaction.

7. If abrupt changes in flow occur, notify the physician promptly so he or she can order appropriate changes in therapy.

8. When the physician orders the solution discontinued, taper it off gradually. Guidelines are presented later in this chapter.

Fluid Overload Observe for fluid overload. Weigh the patient daily under the same conditions, and maintain strict intake and output records. Also consult with the physician about the expected rate of weight gain from tissue synthesis; the goal usually ranges up to 2½ pounds per week. More may be desirable, especially if the patient's hydration is very poor or fat stores are depleted severely. A gain in excess of the amount for a specific patient may represent fluid overload rather than increased lean body mass. Patients without cardiac, renal, or hepatic disease usually can tolerate 3000–4000 ml fluid per day.

Protein Overload Watch for signs of protein overload. Monitor the BUN and creatinine daily until stable and then weekly. If signs of prerenal azotemia appear, the physician may change from the previous TPN solution to solutions containing only essential amino acids to lower the protein load on the kidneys.

Bleeding Be alert for bleeding. Monitor CBC, prothrombin time, and platelet count weekly. Malnourished patients often have anemia and/or hypoproteinemia. Alert the physician if you suspect either condition, as administration of whole blood, plasma, or albumin may be needed.

Metabolic Acidosis Be alert for the signs of metabolic acidosis. They include restlessness, disorientation, coma, hyperventilation, hyperkalemia, arterial pH below 7.35, and serum bicarbonate below 23 mEq/L. Possible causes of metabolic acidosis in TPN patients include hyperglycemia, excessive additions of sodium chloride or potassium chloride to TPN solutions, or administration of crystalline amino acid solutions that contain cationic amino acids or that are derived from chloride or hydrochloride salts. If the problem results from excessive sodium or potassium chloride administration, the physician can substitute sodium or potassium bicarbonate, acetate, or phosphate for electrolyte replacement.

Fatty Acid Deficiency Watch for fatty acid deficiency. Scaly skin, skin eruptions around the nose and mouth, mouth or tongue tenderness, hair loss, poor skin turgor, poor wound healing, and decreased resistance to infections result from fatty acid deficiency. Such deficiency occurs because hypertonic dextrose provokes hyperinsulinemia, which in turn inhibits lipolysis, and because the TPN solution does not contain fatty acids. Alert the physician if you note these signs, and administer fat emulsions as ordered.

Commercially available fat emulsions contain safflower or soybean oil, egg yolk phospholipids, and glycerin in water (Gever 1981). Two to three 500-ml bottles are administered weekly through a Y-site or piggyback into a peripheral venous line. If a filter is used in the peripheral line, the fatty acid (lipid) emulsion should be connected below it because the fat particles can be trapped in the filter. Inspect the bottle before administration to detect separation of the emulsion. Avoid shaking the bottle, because shaking can cause aggregation of fat particles and separation of the emulsion. You may give fat emulsion safely via a peripheral vein because it is isotonic. Do not add any drugs, electrolytes, or other nutrients to the bottle because you may disturb the emulsion's stability. For the first 30 minutes, give the solution at the rate of 1 ml/min while you observe for dyspnea, allergic reactions, vomiting, or chest pain. If no untoward reactions occur, you may increase the rate to the limit specified by the physician, typically 500 ml over a 6–12 hour period.

Electrolyte Imbalances Maintain electrolyte balance. Monitor serum electrolytes daily until stabilized and weekly thereafter. Watch for signs and symptoms of developing imbalances. Potential electrolyte imbalances during TPN include hypo/hypernatremia, hypokalemia, and hypophosphatemia.

Changes in weight, blood pressure, pulse volume, skin turgor, level of consciousness, and respiratory rate may indicate sodium imbalances, which are discussed in detail in Chapter 16. Hyponatremia is fairly common and may be due to true sodium loss or dilution of serum sodium by fluid shift from the intracellular to extracellular compartment. As mentioned above, sodium is added routinely to the solution to meet maintenance needs.

Hypernatremia may occur secondary to excessive osmotic diuresis. If the elevation in serum sodium is accompanied by lethargy, hyperventilation, or coma, suspect the occurrence of hyperglycemic hyperosmolar nonketotic state, discussed earlier.

Weakness, cramps, nausea or vomiting, paresthesias, and ECG changes suggest hypokalemia, also discussed in Chapter 16. Potassium needs are increased during TPN, due to stress, osmotic diuresis, and increased protein synthesis.

Weakness, confusion, paresthesias, seizures, coma, and dysarthria may be signs of hypophosphatemia. This condition can develop from the increased demand for phosphate for production of proteins, membrane phospholipids, deoxyribonucleic acid, and adenosine triphosphate (ATP), and from the increased need for buffering of acidic wastes produced by the accelerated metabolic rate. A diminished phosphate level can cause decreased levels of ATP and 2,3 diphosphoglycerate in red cells (Janson et al. 1983). Since these compounds bind to hemoglobin, their deficiencies are associated with a leftward shift of the oxyhemoglobin dissociation curve; that is, the red cells' affinity for oxygen is increased, so less oxygen is available to the tissues. Hypophosphatemia also may produce a decreased ATP level in leukocytes, leading to a theoretical decrease in ability to combat infection (Janson et al. 1983). To prevent these problems, the physician often will order 10–15 mEq/L of phosphate added to the TPN solution. Since supplemental phosphate can cause a drop in serum calcium, calcium must be provided also. Add the calcium and phosphate to separate bottles, because they precipitate when mixed together.

Vitamin–Mineral Abnormalities Be alert for signs of vitamin and mineral deficiencies. For example, monitor the patient for signs and symptoms of poor wound healing, impaired immunity, and mental abnormality (Review Article 1980).

Discontinuation of TPN The physician will discontinue TPN when the condition necessitating its use is alleviated and the patient shows progress toward adequate nutrition. The rate of solution usually is tapered to avoid insulin rebound and hypoglycemia.

While returning to oral intake, the patient may have little appetite because of all the glucose being supplied intravenously. Slowing the infusion rate and providing appetizing meals, perhaps with some pleasant social interaction, will help to stimulate appetite.

Outcome Evaluation

Evaluate the patient's progress toward adequate nutrition according to these outcome criteria:

- Weight gain within limits specified for the patient, usually 2½ pounds per week.

- Increased muscle mass.

- Improved wound healing.

- Absent or diminishing signs of infection.

- Hemoglobin, serum albumin, and lymphocyte levels WNL for patient.

- Water balance WNL for patient.

- Serum electrolytes WNL for patient.

REFERENCES

GI Disorders

Alspach JG, Williams SM: *Core curriculum for critical care nursing.* Philadelphia: Saunders, 1985.

Amato E: A nursing reference: Gastrointestinal tubes and drains. *Crit Care Nurse* Part I, (Nov/Dec) 1982; 50–57. Part II (Jan/Feb) 1983; 46–48.

Bates B: *A guide to physical examination,* 4th ed. Philadelphia: Lippincott, 1987.

Benner P: *From novice to expert.* Menlo Park, CA: Addison-Wesley, 1984.

Bradford KS: Injection sclerotherapy in the management of bleeding esophageal varices. *Crit Care Nurse* 1983; 3:36–40.

Brunner LS, Suddarth DS: *Textbook of medical-surgical nursing,* 5th ed. Philadelphia: Lippincott, 1984.

Decker SI: The life-threatening consequences of a GI bleed. *RN* (October) 1985; 18–25.

Dewan et al.: Chronic massive pancreatic pleural effusion. *Chest* 1984; 85:497–501.

Dodd RP: Ascites: when the liver can't cope. *RN* (October) 1984; 26–30.

Dusek J: Nursing rules—Fact or myth?: Iced gastric lavage slows bleeding in gastric hemorrhage. *Crit Care Nurse* (July/Aug) 1984; 8.

Fraser CL, Arieff AI: Hepatic encephalopathy. *N Engl J Med* 1985; 313:865–873.

Fried GM et al.: Pancreatic protein secretion and gastrointestinal hormone release in response to parenteral amino acids and lipid in dogs. *Surgery* 1982; 92:902–905.

Geokas MC: Acute pancreatitis. *Ann Intern Med* 1985; 103:86–100.

Guenter P, Slocum B: Hepatic disease: Nutritional implications. *Nurs Clin North Am* 1983; 18:71–80.

Gurevich I: Viral hepatitis. *Am J Nurs* 1983; 83:571–586.

Hansson BG: Virology and clinical significance of delta agent infection. *J Virol Meth* 1985; 10:295–298.

Keith JS: Hepatic failure: Etiologies, manifestations, and management. *Crit Care Nurse* 1985; 5:60–86.

Micozzi MS, London WT: The clinical laboratory diagnosis of viral hepatitis. *Lab Manag* (January) 1983; 18–27.

Mushahwar LK et al.: Interpretation of hepatitis B virus and hepatitis delta virus serological profiles. *Pathologist* 1984; 38:648–650.

Pinilla JC et al.: Does antacid prophylaxis prevent upper gastrointestinal bleeding in critically ill patients? *Crit Care Med* 1985; 13:646–650.

Porth CM: *Pathophysiology concepts of altered health states,* 2d ed. Philadelphia: Lippincott, 1986.

Price SA, Wilson LM: *Pathophysiology, clinical concepts of disease processes,* 3d ed. New York: McGraw-Hill, 1986.

Quinless FW: Severe liver dysfunction, client problems and nursing actions. *Focus Crit Care* 1985; 12:24–32.

Schumann D: Correction of ascites with peritoneovenous shunting, a study of clinical management. *Heart Lung* 1983; 12:248–257.

Silverman et al.: The safety and efficacy of a lipid-based system of parenteral nutrition in acute pancreatitis. *Am J Gastroent* 1982; 77:494–497.

Swearingen P (ed): *Manual of nursing therapeutics.* Menlo Park, CA: Addison-Wesley, 1986.

Toskes PP, Greenberger NJ: Acute and chronic pancreatitis. *Disease-a-Month* 1983; 29:5–81.

White et al.: Management of massive hemorrhage from esophageal varices. *Crit Care Quart* 1985; 8:69–79.

Nutrition

Askanazi J et al.: Respiratory distress secondary to a high carbohydrate load: A case report. *Surgery* 1980; 87:596.

Burke J et al.: Glucose requirements following burn injury. *Ann Surg* 1979; 190:274–278.

Butterworth C, Weinsier R: Malnutrition in hospital patients: Assessment and treatment. Pages 660–720 in *Modern nutrition in health and disease,* Goodhart R, Shils M (eds). Philadelphia: Lea and Febiger, 1980.

Elwyn D: Nutritional requirements of adult surgical patients. *Crit Care Med* 1980; 8:10–36.

Gever L: Intravenous lipids. *Nurs 81* (Nov) 1981; 160–161.

Janson C et al.: Hypophosphatemia. *Ann Emerg Med* 1982; 12:107–116.

Keithley J: Infection and the malnourished patient. *Heart Lung* 1983; 12:23–27.

Kinney J, Felig P: The metabolic response to injury and infection. *Endocrinology* 1979; 3:1963–1968.

Long CL et al.: Metabolic response to injury and illness: Estimation of energy and protein needs from indirect calorimetry and nitrogen balance. *J Enteral Parenteral Nutrition* 1979; 3:452–456.

Moore F, Brennan M: Surgical injury: Body composition, protein metabolism, and neuroendocrinology. Pages 169–224 in *Manual of surgical nutrition,* Ballinger W (ed). Philadelphia: Saunders, 1975.

Moss G: Malabsorption associated with extreme malnutrition: Importance of replacing plasma albumin. *J Am Coll Nutr* 1982; 1:89–92.

Recommended dietary allowances, revised 1980. Washington, DC: Food and Nutrition Board, National Academy of Sciences-National Research Council.

Review Article: Trace metal abnormalities in adults during hyperalimentation. *J Enteral Parenteral Nutrition* 1980; 5:424–429.

Robin A et al.: Influence of hypercaloric glucose infusions on fuel economy in surgical patients: A review. *Crit Care Med* 1981; 9:680–686.

Saudek C, Felig P: The metabolic events of starvation. *Am J Med* 1976; 60:118–125.

Seltzer MH: Instant nutrition assessment: Absolute weight loss and surgical mortality. *J Enteral Parenteral Nutrition* 1982; 6:218–221.

Stotts N, Friesen J: Understanding starvation in the critically ill patient. *Heart Lung* 1982; 11:469–478.

Weinsier R, Butterworth C: *Handbook of clinical nutrition.* St Louis: Mosby, 1981.

Williams S: *Nutrition and diet therapy,* 4th ed. St Louis: Mosby, 1981.

Wilmore DW: *The metabolic management of the critically ill.* New York: Plenum, 1980.

SUPPLEMENTAL READING

GI Disorders

Hussey KP: Vasopressin therapy for upper gastrointestinal tract hemorrhage. *Arch Int Med* (1985); 145: 1263–1267.

Johanson BC et al.: *Standards for critical care,* 2d ed. St Louis: Mosby, 1985.

Malangoni MA et al.: Factors contributing to fatal outcome after treatment of pancreatic abscess. *Ann Surg* (1986); 203:605–613.

Rubin W: The spectrum of cirrhosis. *Emerg Med* 1983; 15:29–58.

Smith SL: Liver transplantation: Implications for critical care nursing. *Heart Lung* 1985; 14:617–628.

Traiger GL, Bohachick P: Liver transplantation: Care of the patient in the post-operative period. *Crit Care Nurse* 1983; 3:96–103.

Tuckerman M, Turco S: *Human nutrition.* Philadelphia: Lea and Febiger, 1983.

Nutrition

Bernard et al.: *Nutritional and metabolic support of hospitalized patients.* Philadelphia: Saunders, 1986.

Keithley J: Nutritional assessment of the patient undergoing surgery. *Heart Lung* 1985; 14:449–455.

Morgan J: Nutritional assessment of critically ill patients. *Focus Crit Care* (Jun) 1984; 28–34.

Palys C: Patients receiving total parenteral nutrition can be weaned from mechanical ventilation without difficulty. *Crit Care Nurs* (Nov/Dec) 1984; 28–29.

20

Activity

CLINICAL INSIGHT

Domain: Monitoring and insuring the quality of health care practices

Compentency: Assessing what can safely be omitted from or added to medical orders

Nurses must exercise judgment when carrying out medical orders. They are expected, for example, to spot an unsafe dose of medication and withhold its administration, or to recognize when a change in a patient's condition makes an order no longer apppropriate and to seek updated orders. A more sophisticated application of nursing judgment involves weighing conflicting orders and deciding which one is more appropriate at a given time. Conflicting orders occur so frequently and over so many gradations of significance that the nurse soon learns that he or she cannot apply to every situation the textbook solution (i.e., turn to a physician to resolve the dilemma); the nurse must learn to differentiate which conflicting orders are important enough to warrant physician consultation (for example, those clearly within the realm of medicine and with major repercussions if an error is made) and which should be resolved independently.

Learning to make such differentiations requires an intimate awareness of medical therapies, ongoing dialogue with physicians, and an ability to analyze what's most appropriate for a particular patient at a particular time. The ability to act confidently on one's decision thus depends on an abundant fund of clinical experience, as well as trust between physician and nurse, a trust built on a foundation of established credibility. Discretion often is called for in relation to orders regarding vital signs or those that affect patients' rest and sleep, since sleep deprivation is a major problem in the critical-care unit. In this paradigm, from Benner (1984, pp. 140–141), a nurse discusses the uncertainties involved resolving conflicting orders.

I took care of a patient . . . who had an open–and–close exploratory laparotomy for pancreatic cancer. He had been febrile. For three nights I woke him every four hours and helped him do all his breathing exercises and lung physical therapy. He was really depressed and wasn't talking about anything that had to do with his diagnosis. . . . The fourth night his temperature had come down some, and by now he was exhausted from lack of sleep. I figured that he was going to have a lot better chance to focus on things that he needed and wanted to focus on if he could just get some uninterrupted sleep. His temperature remained the same in the morning. His lungs probably would have been clearer had I awakened him at 3 A.M., but I elected not to, given his extreme fatigue and depression. It's not clear what is the right *thing to do. There are studies done about the effectiveness of chest physical therapy and then there are other studies done about the effectiveness of sleep. But there is never anything that proves that X is better than Y, especially in a particular situation, so that I know that chest physical therapy every four hours is really going to help or that sleep is going to help. It is expected that I will use my best judgment under the circumstances.*

In the FANCAS model, *activity* is defined as the *expenditure of physical or emotional energy.* The physical inactivity suffered by critically ill patients can have far–reaching consequences. As demonstrated in the Clinical Insight, your efforts can influence not only your patients' survival but also their convalescence and eventual resumption of a satisfying lifestyle.

Assessment

Any patient can suffer the detrimental effects of decreased activity. However, some patients need only minimal teaching and supervision, while others need extensive assistance to avoid complications from decreased mobility. To assess the type and amount of assistance your patient needs, you should obtain an activity history and perform a physical assessment of the patient. A recommended format for activity assessment is shown in Table 20-1.

History

Begin your assessment by soliciting an activity history. Ask the person to describe his or her activities of daily living both before and after the illness. Include such activities as sleep, hygiene, physical exercise, and recreation. Often, asking the person to describe a typical day will elicit revealing information about self-imposed activity restrictions. If the patient is too ill to answer these questions early in the hospitalization, defer them or seek the assistance of family or significant others.

Determine both the current activity level prescribed by the physician and the patient's actual activity level. Evaluating both aspects of current activity can help you identify the patient who is physically or emotionally unable to cope with the degree of activity the physician approves. Under the prescribed activity level, it is helpful to include a projection of the expected length of ac-

TABLE 20-1 ACTIVITY ASSESSMENT FORMAT

1. History

   Past activity level _____

   Current activity

     Prescribed (include estimated duration) _____

   _____

   _____

     Actual _____

   Risk factors for complications: ☐ age over 40 ☐ lengthy bedrest ☐ vascular disease ☐ abdominal or pelvic surgery ☐ fractures ☐ paralysis ☐ paresthesias ☐ decreased level of consciousness ☐ weakness ☐ decreased activity tolerance ☐ dehydration ☐ other (specify) _____

2. Physical

   Skin: color _____ moisture _____ ☐ reddened areas
   ☐ broken skin ☐ blisters ☐ swelling ☐ bruises
   ☐ other (specify) _____

   Activity impediments: ☐ cast ☐ traction ☐ other (specify) _____

   Assistive devices: ☐ cane ☐ walker ☐ crutches ☐ wheelchair
   ☐ other (specify) _____

3. Diagnostic procedures and laboratory tests _____

   _____

4. Other relevant data _____

   _____

tivity restriction. While obtaining the history, be alert for the presence of the risk factors identified in Table 20-1.

Physical Examination

Examine the patient physically to evaluate skin integrity and possible impediments to activity. Determine whether the skin, especially that over bony prominences, appears intact and healthy. Note the presence of casts, precarious intravenous lines, or other impediments. Also note the presence of assistive devices such as a cane.

Diagnostic Procedures and Laboratory Tests

Under the category of diagnostic procedures and laboratory tests, make a note of formal range of motion evaluation by a physical therapist, electromyography, or other diagnostic data related to activity, if any have been obtained.

NURSING DIAGNOSES

Activity–related NANDA diagnoses are:

- Activity intolerance
- Impaired physical mobility
- Self-care deficit

Planning and Implementation of Care

The activity assessment described above will help you plan and implement ways to prevent or combat the effects of restricted activity. These effects are numerous and can be grouped conveniently according to the six FANCAS categories: fluid balance, aeration, nutrition, communication, activity, and stimulation.

Fluid Balance

Fluid balance is controlled by the cardiac, vascular, and renal systems, each of which suffers when activity is restricted.

Altered CO and/or Altered Tissue Perfusion

The cardiovascular system deteriorates rapidly on complete bedrest. The detrimental effects of bedrest, well-known to most nurses, in the past have been attributed to physical inactivity. Recent studies, however, have shown that body fluid shifts are a major determinant of many of bedrest's undesirable cardiovascular effects (Winslow 1985). The critical-care nurse can use both the information derived from classic studies and this new information to anticipate and counteract the negative consequences of bedrest.

Fluid Shift When a person changes from supine to standing, gravity causes about 500 cc of blood to shift from the upper to the lower half of the body (Gauer and Thron 1965). This shift from the thorax to the periphery decreases venous return, stroke volume, cardiac output, and arterial pressure. It also triggers multiple compensatory responses (mediated by the carotid, aortic, and cardiopulmonary baroreceptors) to maintain arterial pressure. Conversely, when a person lies down, a central fluid shift increases venous return, stroke volume, and cardiac output and activates depressor responses that include a compensatory decrease in heart rate (Winslow 1985).

Blomqvist et al. (1980) studied 10 healthy young men on 24 hours bedrest with a 5-degree head-down tilt (a maneuver that produces effects similar to prolonged bedrest but in a shorter period). The central fluid shift changes were transient, returning to normal supine levels after 6 hours and reflecting normal upright levels after 24 hours. The subjects demonstrated orthostatic hypotension, tachycardia, decreased stroke volume, and decreased exercise tolerance—all effects commonly observed with prolonged bedrest.

Other investigators have documented a decrease in stroke volume with prolonged bedrest. Saltin et al. (1968) studied five healthy young men on 20 days' bedrest. They noted a decrease in stroke volume of 17% during supine rest and 24% during upright rest.

A classic study by Taylor et al. (1949) revealed that healthy young men developed tachycardia at work, and tachycardia at rest after 21 days of bedrest. Tachycardia at rest increased at the rate of one beat per minute every 2 days. Convertino et al. (1982) also documented increased heart rates during quiet sitting and exercise after 10 days bedrest in healthy middle-aged men.

The strain on the heart is intensified during *Valsalva maneuvers,* which bedfast patients do frequently while moving in bed or straining to move their bowels. Valsalva maneuvers increase intrathoracic pressure and decrease venous return; when intrathoracic pressure drops again, it is followed by a rebound increase in venous return.

The increased myocardial work provoked by bedrest increases myocardial oxygen consumption. This increased oxygen demand can be deleterious when superimposed on potentially ischemic myocardium.

Orthostatic Hypotension Normally, neurovascular reflexes cause automatic blood pressure adjustment to changes in body position. Arteriolar and venous constriction, tachycardia, decreased intrathoracic pressure, the pumping action of leg muscles, and venous valves all help to compensate for assumption of an upright posture. With prolonged bedrest, venous pooling results from loss of muscle tone. The nervous system also appears to habituate to the decreased pressure, lessened resistance, increased flow, and dilated vessels that characterize the supine position (Browse 1965). Because the person no longer can compensate quickly for position changes, sudden upright posture causes blood to pool in the muscles and abdomen, and the person faints. The abrupt drop in blood pressure due to the change of position is called *orthostatic hypotension.*

Orthostatic intolerance may begin after only 6 hours of bedrest (McCally et al. 1966). After 21 days of bedrest, it may take up to 7 weeks of reconditioning to reverse (Taylor et al. 1949). Orthostatic intolerance is the most important determinant of bedrest-induced exercise intolerance, and 3.5 hours a day of gravitational stress can prevent much of the cardiovascular deterioration that occurs with bedrest (Convertino et al. 1982). This level can be provided by getting the patient out of bed for meals and toileting (Winslow et al. 1984). In one study, acute MI patients treated with modified bedrest (active leg exercises, sitting on the edge of the bed, and commode use from the day of admission) did not develop orthostatic intolerance (Fareeduddin and Abelmann 1969).

Decreased Cardiovascular Reserve Cardiovascular deconditioning occurs rapidly on bedrest. The tachycardia present at rest becomes more pronounced with exercise, particularly upright exercise (Winslow 1985). Taylor et al. (1949) reported that in their normal subjects after 3 weeks' bedrest, moderate work provoked tachycardia of 40 beats per minute over baseline values, and the ability to walk a 10% incline at 3.5 miles per hour decreased by 75%. The diminished cardiac reserve significantly interferes with the patient's ability to perform

muscular work. These healthy men needed 5–10 weeks of physical conditioning before their cardiovascular functions returned to normal.

Most of the research on the effects of bedrest has been done with healthy young subjects. Although these studies are valuable, the physiologic findings may not be generalizable to older adults.

To provide more clinically applicable data, Convertino et al. (1982) studied 12 normal males, 46–54 years old, to determine the impact of bedrest on people in the common age range for MI. Bedrest was maintained for 10 days, a duration similar to that for patients recovering from acute MI. The investigators detected a significant decrease (15%) in maximal oxygen uptake during upright exercise following the period of bedrest. (*Maximal oxygen uptake* represents the maximum rate of oxygen delivery to the tissues and as such is an important measure of cardiovascular reserve (Winslow 1985). It equals maximal cardiac output times maximal arteriovenous difference.) This decrease occurred in spite of great increases in exercise heart rates and was attributable to orthostatic factors: decreased left ventricular volume and filling pressure due to venous pooling in the legs.

Similar effects were noted in an earlier study by Saltin et al. (1968). Their subjects, five healthy young men, showed a 28% fall in oxygen uptake after 20 days of bedrest. Oxygen uptake returned to baseline after 8–12 days in previously sedentary subjects, but took as long as 43 days to return to normal in previously active subjects. Saltin et al. also documented a 23–35% decrease in stroke volume during exercise following the bedrest period. Despite pronounced tachycardia, this significant reduction in stroke volume kept cardiac output lower than before bedrest.

Plasma Volume Most studies have found a plasma volume loss with bedrest. These losses, which occur early and level off at a reduced volume, are variable and may range up to 15% (Winslow 1985). Plasma volume is an important (but not the only) determinant of orthostatic tolerance and exercise capacity (Winslow 1985). Blood volume also decreases, though not as much as plasma volume; Wenger (1983) reports a 700–800-cc loss of circulating blood volume after 7–10 days of bedrest.

Nursing Interventions To minimize cardiovascular deterioration, recall that the central fluid shift is more important than physical inactivity in producing cardiovascular dysfunction. Nursing measures should aim to counteract this fluid shift (Winslow 1985):

1. Get the person out of bed for meals, chairsitting, and ambulation, unless specifically contraindicated.

2. Teach the patient to change position slowly to allow time for the neurovascular system to accommodate.

3. Monitor and help the patient when he or she first gets out of bed. Have the patient lie down if any sign of orthostatic intolerance appears, such as dizziness or marked tachycardia.

4. Avoid or counteract conditions that increase venous pooling, such as hot baths and varicosities.

5. Question orders for bedrest and activity levels you consider inappropriate to the patient's condition. Physicians may not review and revise these orders as often as appropriate.

6. For patients unable to get out of bed, consider using a chair-bed, oscillating bed, or other devices.

7. Encourage the patient who tolerates an upright position to get out of bed to bathe. Winslow et al. (1985), comparing the physiologic responses associated with basin, tub, and shower bathing, found that the three types of baths have similar physiologic costs. Patients rated all three as light exertion and strongly disliked the basin bath (performed sitting on the edge of the bed). Additional recommendations from these authors are:

a. Carefully assess orthostatic tolerance before allowing a standing shower or tub bath.

b. Before the first tub bath, evaluate the patient for possible difficulty getting out of the tub. If the patient is weak or obese or has had difficulty getting out of tubs before, use a tub chair or hand rails or have other personnel help the patient. This is important because the isometric activity involved in getting out of the tub can increase myocardial workload and cause blood pressure to soar.

c. Adjust water temperature to 95°–98°F, because the vasodilatation caused by hot water accentuates orthostatic intolerance.

Altered Urinary Elimination Pattern The major renal problems associated with bedrest are diuresis, stasis, infection, and stone formation. When a person moves from the erect to the supine position, renal blood flow increases 54% and renal plasma flow increases 71% (Underhill et al. 1982). The effects are mediated by decreased ADH release resulting from stimulation of baroreceptors by increased thoracic blood volume. The resulting diuresis is greatest during the first 4 days of bedrest.

Although the supine position does not significantly affect nephron function per se, the kidney must excrete a greater solute load than normal because of tissue breakdown and bone demineralization. Urinary stasis develops because the supine position inhibits both the flow of urine into the ureter and the expulsion of urine from the bladder. In the upright position, gravity helps urine to empty from the renal pelvis into the ureter. In the supine position, the beneficial effect of gravity is lost, and renal stones may develop because of urinary stasis in the renal pelvis.

Bedrest also can lead to bladder distention and stasis. Urination normally requires coordinated interaction among the detrusor muscle of the bladder and the internal and external urethral sphincters. An emptying reflex is triggered when the volume of the adult bladder approaches 400–500 ml, although a person can inhibit it for a while because the external sphincter is under voluntary control. In the upright position, when a person responds to the urge to empty the bladder, he or she relaxes the external sphincter. The detrusor muscle contracts reflexly, increasing bladder pressure and opening the internal sphincter so urine is released. In the supine position, however, it is harder to relax the external sphincter, so reflex emptying is more difficult to achieve. Sometimes the person can compensate with an increase in abdominal pressure. If the urge to void is ignored or not perceived, however, the bladder distends and urine eventually spills out due to the pressure of the excessive volume. Urinary incontinence contributes to skin breakdown and to patients' discouragement and anxiety. With repeated bladder distention, the urge to urinate becomes weaker, and back pressure may damage the kidneys. The stagnant urine also becomes more alkaline than normal, making the bladder more prone to infection and stone precipitation.

Several factors contribute to precipitation of urinary stones. The excretion of calcium, phosphates, and other minerals is increased due to protein breakdown and bone demineralization, so their concentration in urine is increased. Deitrick et al. (1948) discovered that urinary calcium loss increased by the third day of bedrest and peaked by the fourth–fifth weeks. Urine becomes alkaline because of infection and decreased production of acid metabolites owing to lessened muscular activity. Stones precipitate more easily in an alkaline solution.

Nursing Interventions To discourage stasis, infection, and stone precipitation, include these measures in your nursing care:

1. Encourage getting out of bed to void. Winslow et al. (1984) compared two toileting methods: urination in bed (using a bedpan or urinal) and out of bed (using a commode for females and standing urinal for males). They studied 95 normal subjects, cardiac outpatients, medical inpatients, and MI patients (2–28 days postinfarction). Data were collected on oxygen consumption, peak heart rate, peak rate pressure product, the patient's rating of perceived exertion, and preference. The results showed that both in-bed and out-of-bed methods required slight energy cost. Patients clearly preferred getting out of bed to toilet, stating it was easier and more comfortable than in-bed use of the urinal or bedpan.

Getting the patient out of bed for toileting helps provide the gravitational stress necessary to minimize the orthostatic intolerance provoked by bedrest. The upright posture also contributes to improved kidney drainage, and the weight-bearing activity lessens nitrogen and mineral loss. Reserve in-bed toileting for patients with specific contraindications to getting out of bed.

2. Diminish protein breakdown and bone demineralization with position changes, range of motion exercises and, if possible, weight bearing (by getting the patient up in a chair, standing at the bedside, or walking).

3. Encourage production of dilute, acid urine. Place the patient on intake and output monitoring. If not contraindicated, give about 3000–4000 ml fluid daily to maintain a dilute urine. Maintain physical activity and avoid urinary tract infections.

4. Facilitate bladder emptying. If the patient's condition precludes voluntary urination, provide for urinary drainage by using intermittent catheterization, a condom catheter (for males), or an indwelling catheter. Catheterization is at best a mixed blessing because of its potential as an infection route. Employ a closed urinary drainage system, and use a needle and syringe to withdraw urine specimens from the tubing without breaking the system.

For the person who can urinate voluntarily, try to encourage relaxation of the external sphincter by providing privacy when the person needs to void, using a commode chair, or letting the male patient stand. If the patient must remain in bed, promote urination by elevating the head of the bed, pouring warm water over the perineum, running water in a sink, or teaching the patient to empty the bladder manually if necessary. Periodically check for bladder distention.

5. In addition to these general nursing measures, specific interventions are determined by the characteristics of renal stones present or for which the patient is at risk (Metheny 1982).

Measures may include decreased intake of precursors, acidification or alkalinization of urine, and administration of medications to inhibit stone formation. If not passed spontaneously, stones are removed by irrigation or surgery.

Aeration

Bedrest compromises a number of factors affecting aeration. The slumped posture patients on bedrest often assume interferes with both diaphragmatic and costal movement (Browse 1965). Ventilation decreases due to diminished tidal volume and minute volume. Muscle weakness and loss of reserve muscle power alter the mechanics of ventilation, so patients have to work harder to match pre-bedrest maximum ventilatory capacity. Incisions that restrict diaphragmatic or costal movement, and obesity may further restrict respiratory excursion.

Secretion clearance also is decreased on bedrest. Normally, position changes and coughing aid gravity drainage from the smaller bronchi and bronchioles. Bedrest reduces position changes that help clear secretions and stimulate coughing. Ciliary action may diminish, because bedrest interferes with the usual distribution of mucus into an even film around the bronchioles (Browse 1965). As a result, drainage and expulsion of respiratory secretions is more difficult. This problem is exacerbated by dehydration or medications that depress respiration or the cough reflex. In addition, because the patient is not engaging in activity, he or she takes fewer deep breaths, which normally reexpand collapsed alveoli. Atelectasis may develop and predispose the person to respiratory infections.

Regional ventilation/perfusion ($\dot{V}/\dot{Q}$) relationships also are affected by body position. The dependent portion of the lung receives greater ventilation and perfusion than the nondependent portion (Kaneko et al. 1966).

The greatest aeration risk posed by bedrest is the increased danger of thromboembolism. According to West (1987), blood pooling occurs with bedrest because of lack of leg skeletal muscle contraction, loss of vasomotor tone, and sacculated vessels (common in the elderly). Risk factors include the following (West 1987).

Physiologic—dehydration, weakness, increased blood viscosity (due to greater plasma volume loss than blood volume loss)

Physical—flaccidity, positioning (such as gatching bed at knees, restricting popliteal flow), prolonged bedrest, lack or improper use of support wraps or hose

Pharmacologic—birth control pills producing hypercoagulability

Pathologic—cancer, stroke, varicosities, sacculations, lower abdominal and pelvic surgery, limb paresthesia, trauma, blood dyscrasia

Psychologic—altered mental status

Nursing Interventions   Common measures to prevent pulmonary complications of bedrest include turning and deep-breathing, in-bed leg exercises, careful positioning, elastic compression devices, early ambulation, and anticoagulants for high-risk patient subgroups. Please see the detailed sections in Chapter 8 on pulmonary embolism, atelectasis, and respiratory failure for further information about interventions to prevent pulmonary complications of bedrest.

Nutrition

Both the intake and elimination of food suffer in the bedridden patient. During the acute phase of illness, the patient often receives only parenteral fluids, which are notoriously inadequate as a source of nutrition (see Chapter 19). Even when an oral diet is resumed, intake may suffer because of fasting for laboratory tests, poor appetite, nausea, and diminished interest in self-care. Compounding the problem is accelerated catabolism leading to protein breakdown and negative nitrogen balance. Measures to promote nutrition are discussed in Chapter 19.

Normal elimination of bowel contents depends on involuntary visceral reflexes assisted by voluntary breath holding and contraction of abdominal muscles. The bedridden patient may be less aware of the defecation reflex, be too weak to use the abdominal muscles, or try to inhibit the reflex because of embarrassment over lack of privacy. Then, too, with a diminished or absent food intake the gastrocolic reflex may be provoked only infrequently or weakly.

Nursing Interventions   To prevent constipation and impactions, follow these guidelines.

1. If admission to the critical-care unit was sudden and unexpected, the patient may develop constipation due to material present in the intestines at the time of falling ill. Check on the date of the last bowel movement, and determine the patient's normal frequency of bowel movements. If one does not occur in the normal pattern, consult the physician about digitally examining the rectum for stool and about measures to promote bowel evacuation.

2. Maintain an adequate fluid intake. According to Hirschberg et al. (1976), if the patient is producing 1500 ml of urine daily, he or she probably also is getting enough fluid for normal bowel activity.

3. Discuss the patient's usual bowel pattern with the patient or family, and try to duplicate it as closely as possible. If the patient is allowed to eat, high roughage foods and naturally laxative foods can be quite helpful, as can simple exercises to strengthen abdominal muscles, such as contracting them several times an hour (while exhaling).

4. Straining with bowel movements should be avoided because it is a Valsalva maneuver that in susceptible patients can provoke hemorrhoids, rectal prolapse, bradycardia, heart block, MI, or stroke. If the person is straining, teach how to exhale while tightening the abdominal muscles. Also ask the physician to order a stool softener.

5. Occasional use of suppositories, laxatives, or enemas may be necessary; but avoid relying on them, because they disrupt the normal bowel pattern.

6. Bedridden patients often view the bedpan as an invention of the devil, finding it uncomfortable, embarrassing, and tiring to use. Check with the physician about use of a commode instead; it requires less energy to use and more closely duplicates the American culture's usual position for bowel movements.

7. Try to provide as much privacy as possible. For example, your patient will appreciate your thoughtfulness in supplying a call bell to signal when done rather than having you inquire brightly every few minutes, "Are you done yet?" Another aid is to attach a sign to the curtain or door saying "Please don't interrupt for a few minutes" to avoid intrusion—by doctors on rounds, x-ray or laboratory technicians, dietary or housekeeping personnel, and visitors. It is amazing how many people unwittingly can troop in during the "private, relaxed, unhurried" time the patient needs to move the bowels! Because patients may inhibit bowel activity due to embarrassment over expulsive smells and noises, it is helpful to provide air freshener and sound from a radio or television.

Communication

The patient on bedrest may be less motivated to communicate with others because of fatigue, anxiety, depression, or poor self-esteem; or less able to communicate because of coma, lethargy, confusion, or actual impediments such as an endotracheal tube. Deitrick et al. (1948) reported dramatic emotional changes during 6 weeks' immobilization: each of their four healthy male subjects manifested signs of increased stress, anxiety, hostility, increased sexual tension, and violent emotional reactions whenever their positive personal relationships with physicians and nurses were threatened.

Nursing Interventions   Please see Chapter 3 for ways to assist patients with communication of their needs, wishes, hopes, and fears.

Activity

Normal musculoskeletal function depends on both tonic activity and periodic increases in stress. Immobilization contributes to four undesirable musculoskeletal consequences. The first three—muscle weakening, restricted range of joint motion, and pressure ulcers—can develop rapidly. The fourth, osteoporosis, is a long-term complication of chronic bedrest.

Muscle Weakening   When maintained at full rest, a muscle loses 10–15% of strength per week (Kottke 1971). After a few weeks of bedrest, even a healthy person develops disuse atrophy (West 1987). An unused muscle may atrophy to one-half its normal size within one month (Guyton 1986). In addition to causing generalized weakness and poor stamina, muscle disuse also can contribute to limitations of joint movement.

Restricted Range of Motion Sometimes when you try to move a joint passively through its full range of motion, you will encounter resistance, with or without pain. Such resistance can result from a variety of causes, such as spasticity, scars, edema, arthritis, and disuse. Kottke (1965) states that gross evidence of restricted motion begins within a few days and develops progressively. When soft tissue structures around a joint shorten and the joint cannot be moved even when the person is anesthetized, a *contracture* exists. Contractures are extremely difficult to treat, often requiring prolonged physiotherapy or surgery.

Limitations of joint movement often reflect a patient's position in bed. Prolonged plantar flexion may lead to contractures of the gastrocnemius and soleus muscles and Achilles tendon (*footdrop*). These contractures seriously interfere with a person's ability to walk. Limited movement of the hip and knee joints makes walking difficult because balance is precarious when joints are out of alignment. Hip adductor tightness can make perineal care difficult and cause a scissors gait. Shoulder or hand contractures limit many activities of daily living and job skills. Restricted range of motion also may harm joints further by placing unusual stresses on them.

Pressure Ulcers Pressure ulcers are necrotic areas that develop from excessive pressure sustained over prolonged periods. Approximately 1.1–1.8 million patients per year develop pressure ulcers in American hospitals (Maklebust et al. 1986). These ulcers commonly involve the skin and soft tissue but over time can extend through muscle and fascia into bone. There may be a significant amount of tissue necrosis before the overlying skin breaks down.

One of the major contributors to ulcer development is the application of pressure to the skin that exceeds pressure at the arteriolar end of capillaries (Narsete et al. 1983). This is approximately 32 mm Hg (Romm et al. 1982). Pressures higher than this impede nutritional capillary flow, producing ischemia and eventual necrosis. Hirschberg et al. (1976) assert that a pressure ulcer can be caused by as little as one hour of pressure and immobility, and frequently results from one episode of continuous pressure. Pressure of 70 mm Hg for 2 hours will cause irreversible damage to healthy tissue (Elliott 1982).

Pressure ulcers develop first as tender, reddened areas. As pressure continues, the skin becomes edematous and then necrotic. In the necrotic stage, the tissue becomes blue and then becomes black and sloughs off.

The cause of pressure ulcers is multifactorial. Certain factors can help you predict whether a patient is at increased risk for pressure ulcer development. Risk factors include decreased sensation, impaired circulation, poor nutrition, infection, decreased activity, damaged skin, incontinence, altered level of consciousness, and old age.

Prevention of pressure ulcers includes frequent position changes, proper positioning techniques, correction of nutritional deficits, and patient/family education. Among the pressure-relieving devices that may be used are sheepskin, egg-crate mattresses, air mattresses, flotation mattresses, air-fluidized bead systems, and the low-air-loss bed system.

Treatment of pressure ulcers is difficult. A variety of methods is used, mostly on an empirical basis. Among the treatment methods that have been advocated are applying granulated sugar, absorption beads or gels, or various ointments to the ulcer; exposing it to ultraviolet light; and applying an elastic polyurethane film.

Osteoporosis Osteoporosis results from progressive depletion of bone due to an imbalance between the rates of bone formation and destruction. *Osteoblasts* lay down the matrix in which bone salts precipitate. *Osteoclasts* are believed to secrete enzymes that absorb the matrix and bone salts. During immobilization, osteoclastic destruction exceeds osteoblastic deposition, and the bone becomes depleted of matrix, calcium, phosphorus, and nitrogen. The result is porous bone that is readily

NURSING RESEARCH NOTE

Maklebust J et al.: Pressure—relief characteristics of various support surfaces used in prevention and treatment of pressure ulcers. *J Enterostom Ther* 1986; 13:85–89.

Preventing pressure ulcers is a major concern of nurses caring for bedridden patients. Many pressure-relieving devices are marketed. Just how effective are they? This study objectively evaluated various support surfaces marketed to reduce pressure on bony prominences, thereby preventing or treating pressure ulcers. The researchers hypothesized there would be no significant difference between conventional hospital mattresses and several "pressure—relieving" support surfaces. The products tested were a conventional hospital mattress, a 2-inch convoluted foam pad, the Biogard critical-care flotation unit, and the Sof-Care bed cushion. A pressure transducer connected to an inflation system and aneroid gauge was used to measure pressure at the contact between the support surface and the tissue. Pressures under the sacrum, heel, and greater trochanter were measured in 13 healthy subjects, who ranged in height, weight, and age. Three consecutive measurements, with the sensor repositioned each time, were recorded for each combination of site and support surface. The means and standard deviations of the contact pressures were determined for each of the subjects and analyzed with the Wilcoxon signed rank test, a parametric equivalent to a paired t test. The alpha level was set at Wα/2 = 0.01.

The level of pressure against which the surfaces were evaluated was 32 mm Hg, considered to be the pressure at which capillary closure occurs. All support surfaces, including the hospital mattress, reduced sacral pressure below 32 mm Hg. Only the Sof-Care bed cushion reduced trochanteric pressure below 32 mm Hg. None of the surfaces reduced heel pressure below this level, although all the support surfaces had pressures significantly lower than the mattress. These findings were consistent with other studies reporting heel pressures above 32 mm Hg even with air-fluidized beds.

The authors concluded that trochanteric pressure was more reliable than sacral for comparing pressure relief in this group of patients, and that even when a surface reduces pressure adequately for the trochanter, the heels still may be at risk (necessitating the use of other techniques or products to protect them).

---

compressed or fractured. Osteoporosis takes weeks to develop and therefore is a problem more of the chronically ill person than of the acutely ill one. Most studies show that in-bed exercise is effective in maintaining muscle mass, strength, and exercise capacity, but ineffective in preventing orthostatic intolerance and calcium loss (Winslow 1985). Passive range of motion exercises or vigorous supine or sitting exercises cannot prevent osteoporosis, but standing for 3 hours a day can (Winslow 1985).

Nursing Interventions To minimize muscle weakening, restricted ranges of motion, pressure ulcers, and osteoporosis, utilize these measures:

1. The bed should have a firm mattress. Place a footboard at its end, preferably leaving space between it and the mattress for the patient's heels or toes.

2. Avoid excessive, prolonged pressure on soft tissue over bony prominences (such as the sacrum, ischium, heels, greater trochanters of the femur, and malleolus) through frequent turning, judicious positioning, and use of pressure-relieving devices.

If the person has diminished sensation or motor activity, turn him or her at least every 2 hours. If the patient is completely unable to sense pressure or shift body weight, turn him or her at least hourly. Each time you turn the person, leave him or her in a position that maintains functional alignment and minimizes pressure on bony prominences.

The supine position encourages hip and knee flexion contractures, especially if the head or foot of the bed is elevated. To avoid these contractures, if the patient can tolerate it, place him or her prone at least twice a day for 30 minutes. The prone position also is helpful in draining posterior lung segments and relieving pressure on the back of the head, sacrum, and heels. Because this position is difficult to achieve or contraindicated when patients have anterior incisions, chest tubes, or artificial ventilators, critically ill patients often are turned only three-quarters prone.

With every position change, inspect the skin on which the patient was resting. Look for blanching, reactive hyperemia lasting more than 5 minutes, edema, tenderness, or blisters. These are early signs of skin breakdown. It is imperative that the site be relieved of further pressure. Among the common ways to relieve pressure are foam pads, sheepskins, or an alternating-pressure mattress. More elaborate methods include flotation mattresses, air-fluidized bead systems, and a low-air-loss bed system. An alternate method of relieving pressure depends on pillows placed to suspend bony prominences above the bed.

Patients who are completely alert usually can change positions at will, though they often need encouragement to turn and assistance so they do not entangle themselves in the various cables and tubes attached to them. Remind them to avoid Valsalva maneuvers.

3. Implement a graded exercise and activity program as described in the following section.

Exercise and Activity Recommendations Other than for cardiac rehabilitation, little has been written specifically about exercise suitable for patients in critical-care units. The following section presents concepts culled from physical therapy and nursing sources that are adaptable to the critical-care setting. The recommendations are offered to conserve the patient's energy, maintain muscle strength and joint mobility, and prevent disabilities secondary to prolonged bedrest. (They are not intended as therapeutic measures for patients who already have musculoskeletal disabilities; consult a physical therapist for guidance in those circumstances.)

To implement a safe and effective exercise program, you should know the patient's estimated capacity for activity, the energy cost of various activities, and signs that the patient should decrease or discontinue an activity. Guidelines for implementing an exercise program follow. As there are based on myocardial rehabilitation literature, you may need to adapt them to other types of patients. Furthermore, since guidelines by their very nature are general, a physician should evaluate any exercise program for a specific individual.

The New York Heart Association has identified four functional classes of cardiac patients, based on symptomatology with activity. This classification may be useful in judging appropriateness of activities. Class I patients have no limitation of physical activity; they do not have any unusual tiredness, dyspnea, angina, or palpitations with ordinary physical activity. Class II patients have slight limitation of physical activity; they are comfortable at rest but develop symptoms with ordinary physical activity. Class III patients have markedly limited physical activity; they are comfortable at rest but develop symptoms with less than ordinary activity. Class IV patients are unable to perform any physical activity comfortably; they may have symptoms even at rest, and these symptoms increase in severity with any physical activity. Most cardiac patients in critical-care units are in functional class III or IV.

Numerous studies of energy metabolism have identified the metabolic cost of various activities. One metabolic equivalent unit (MET) is the amount of energy the body requires while at rest, or approximately 3.5 ml O_2 per kg body weight per minute. The energy cost of activities is expressed as multiples of this basic requirement.

Table 20-2 shows the clinical correlation among the Heart Association functional classification, workload capacities, and sample energy expenditures for self-care activities for a 70-kg person

During the initial postadmission period, the patient's symptoms may worsen with any physical activity and may be present even at rest. Complete chair rest or bedrest is indicated. You should feed and completely bathe the patient. When the physician determines that the patient is stable and progressing satisfactorily, a graded exercise and activity program may be started. However, no such program should be started if any contraindications to activity are present (Table 20-3).

Initially, only low-level, 1–2 MET energy expenditures are permissible. Provide passive range of motion exercise to all extremities, five times each, several times a day. These exercises can be integrated pleasantly with daily patient care activities such as bathing, position changes, postural drainage, and chest physiotherapy. Remember to stabilize the body part proximal to the joint as you move the body part distal to it. (Also consider teaching family members to do some of these exercises. Performing the exercises may help them feel they are contributing to their loved one's well-being and reduce some of their anxiety and the boredom of long periods of inactivity in waiting rooms.)

As soon as feasible, teach the alert patient active exercises. There are many variations of active exercises. Whichever you prefer, be sure to give your patient specific directions, and instruct on how to avoid Valsalva maneuvers on exertion. Demonstrate the exercises, and have the patient return the demonstration.

Observe the patient closely as he or she performs physical activities, to detect untoward reactions. Signs that activity should be decreased or discontinued can be grouped into five categories (O'Brien 1982; Fardy et al. 1980):

Cardiovascular alerting signs
Heart rate or BP increase greater than 25%
Any drop in heart rate or BP
Development or increased frequency of dysrhythmias
ST segment displacement
Respiratory signs
Dyspnea
Irregular breathing
Decreased respiratory rate
Shallow breathing
Nervous system signs
Any decrease in level of consciousness

TABLE 20-2 WORKLOAD CAPACITIES FOR N.Y. HEART ASSOC. FUNCTIONAL CLASSIFICATIONS

CLASS	LIMITATION OF PHYSICAL ACTIVITY	COMFORTABLE AT REST?	RESPONSES TO PHYSICAL ACTIVITY	WORKLOAD CAPACITY (METS)*	EXAMPLES OF SELF-CARE ENERGY EXPENDITURES**
I	None	Yes	No undue responses to ordinary activity	6–10	Bowel movement—bedpan
II	Slight	Yes	Fatigue, dyspnea, angina, palpitations with ordinary activity	4–6	Walking 4 mph Bedside commode Showering
III	Marked	Yes	Fatigue, dyspnea, angina, palpitations with less than ordinary activity	2–3	Combing hair Washing hands, face Shaving—sitting Dressing, undressing Getting out of and into bed Walking 2 mph
IV	Severe	Yes or no	Worsening of symptoms with any activity	1	Eating—sitting Standing, relaxed Sitting in chair Conversation Rest—supine

* Data from Chung E: *Quick reference to cardiovascular diseases*, 2d ed. Philadelphia: Lippincott, 1983.
** Data from Chung and from Trombly C, and Scott A: *Occupational therapy for physical dysfunction*. Baltimore: Williams and Wilkins, 1977.

TABLE 20-3 CONTRAINDICATIONS TO EXERCISE

1. New or progressive angina pectoris
2. Impending or very recent myocardial infarction
3. Uncontrolled congestive heart failure
4. Uncontrolled hypertension
5. Arrhythmias
   a. Second- and third-degree A-V block
   b. Fixed rate pacemakers
   c. Ventricular tachycardia
   d. Uncontrolled atrial fibrillation
   e. Frequent premature ventricular contractions at rest that increase with exercise
6. Gross cardiac enlargement
7. Valvular disease—moderate to severe
8. Outflow tract obstructive disease
9. Recent pulmonary embolism
10. Uncontrolled diabetes mellitus
    Note: Use caution with certain drugs:
    Reserpine
    Propranolol
    Guanethidine
    Procainamide
    Ganglionic blocking agents

From Wenger N: *Rehabilitation after myocardial infarction*. Dallas: American Heart Association. Copyright © 1973. Reprinted with permission, American Heart Association.

Loss of coordination
Skin vital signs
Coolness
Paleness
Cyanosis

Other signs
Pain, especially chest pain (angina) or leg pain (intermittent claudication)
Frequent stopping or leaning
Severe anxiety
Unanticipated fatigue or weakness

One detailed model of a graded activity program is that used by the Cardiac Rehabilitation Program at Grady Memorial Hospital and the Emory University School of Medicine in Atlanta, Georgia (Wenger 1982). The inpatient phase of this program is subdivided into seven steps, progression through which is specified by the patient's primary physician. The exercises should be directly supervised by the nurse or physical therapist. The activities for each step are delineated in Table 20-4.

By completion of step 2, the patient usually is ready for transfer out of the coronary care unit. During the remainder of hospitalization, the person undertakes more difficult exercises and increasing self-care activi-

TABLE 20–4   INPATIENT REHABILITATION: SEVEN-STEP MYOCARDIAL INFARCTION PROGRAM (REVISED 1980): GRADY MEMORIAL HOSPITAL AND THE EMORY UNIVERSITY SCHOOL OF MEDICINE

STEP	SUPERVISED EXERCISE	CCU/WARD ACTIVITY	EDUCATIONAL-RECREATIONAL ACTIVITY
CCU			
1	Active and passive ROM all extremities, in bed Teach patient ankle plantar and dorsiflexion—repeat hourly when patient is awake	Partial self-care Feed self Dangle legs on side of bed Use bedside commode Sit in chair 15 min 1–2 times/day	Orientation to CCU Personal emergencies, social service aid as needed
2	Active ROM all extremities, sitting on side of bed	Sit in chair 15–30 min 2–3 times/day Complete self-care in bed	Orientation to rehabilitation team, program Smoking cessation Educational literature if requested Planning transfer from CCU
Ward			

3	Warm-up exercises, 2 METs:
	    Stretching
	    Calisthenics
	Walk 50 ft and back at slow pace
		Sit in chair ad lib
		To ward class in wheelchair
		Walk in room
			Normal cardiac anatomy and function
			Development of atherosclerosis
			What happens with myocardial infarction
			1–2 METs craft activity

4	ROM and calisthenics, 2.5 METs Walk length of hall (75 ft) and back, average pace Teach pulse counting	OOB as tolerated Walk to bathroom Walk to ward class, with supervision	Coronary risk factors and their control
5	ROM and calisthenics, 3 METs Check pulse counting Practice walking a few stairsteps Walk 300 ft bid	Walk to waiting room or telephone Walk in ward corridor prn	Diet Energy conservation Work simplification techniques (as needed) 2–3 METs craft activity

6	Continue above activities
	Walk down flight of steps (return by elevator)
	Walk 500 ft bid
	Instruct on home exercise
		Tepid shower or tub bath, with supervision
		To OT, cardiac clinic teaching room, with supervision
			Heart attack management:
			    Medications
			    Exercise
			    Surgery
			    Response to symptoms
			    Family, community adjustments
			    on return home
			Craft activity prn

7	Continue above activities
	Walk up flight of steps
	Walk 500 ft bid
	Continue home exercise instruction; present information regarding outpatient exercise program
		Continue all previous ward activities	Discharge planning:
			    Medications, diet, activity
			    Return appointments
			    Scheduled tests
			    Return to work
			    Community resources
			    Educational literature
			    Medication cards
			    Craft activity prn

ROM = range of motion, MET = metabolic equivalent unit, OOB = out of bed, OT = occupational therapy

From: Wenger N: Rehabilitation of the patient with symptomatic atherosclerotic coronary heart disease. Page 1151 in *The heart, arteries and veins*, 5th ed. Hurst J et al. (eds). New York: McGraw-Hill, 1982. Reproduced with permission.

ties. Following hospital discharge, the patient may perform exercises at home or ideally enter a long-term conditioning program.

The exercise and activity program is integrated with a predetermined educational program. The educational program is designed to facilitate adaptation to a healthier lifestyle and covers such topics as the anatomy and physiology of the heart, myocardial infarction, diet, discharge medications, activity after discharge, follow-up care, and community resources. Schedules such as those in Tables 20-5 and 20-6 may be used in educating patients and families about the energy cost of various activities.

A progressive activity program can promote venous flow, muscle strength, endurance, joint mobility, skin integrity, and other indices of physiologic health. Equally important is its impact on the person's psyche. It counteracts the feelings of helplessness, hopelessness, and powerlessness that accompany critical illness, and, as the person sees concrete evidence of returning strength, confidence and optimism for the future are promoted.

Stimulation

A frequent accompaniment to decreased mobility is impaired ability to perceive and respond to one's environment. Among the most common changes are sleep pattern disturbance, disturbed self-concept, and potential sexual dysfunction.

Sleep Pattern Disturbance   Disturbances of normal sleep patterns are inevitable in the critical-care environment. Among the factors responsible are interrupted sleep cycles, unfamiliar sleeping environment, alterations in normal sleep/activity cycles, pre-existing sleep deficits, and medications.

Stages of Sleep   To understand the effects of disturbed sleep patterns, you first need to be familiar with normal sleep structure. There are two distinct types of normal sleep: rapid eye movement (REM) sleep and non-REM sleep. Sympathetic stimulation is predominant during REM sleep, whereas parasympathetic stimulation is predominant during non-REM sleep (Hemenway 1980). REM sleep is characterized not only by rapid eye movements but also by marked physiologic activity. The REM electroencephalogram (EEG) is similar to that seen during waking. The REM electromyogram (EMG), which measures muscle tone, shows a low amplitude; although the brain is very active, impulse transmission to the muscles is blocked (Sanford 1981). Breathing, heart rate, and temperature fluctate (Walsleben 1982). According to Sanford, cardiovascular measurements are at or above waking levels and the incidence of ectopic beats increases; the respiratory pattern is like that of Cheyne-Stokes and oxygen consumption increases; and cerebral blood flow and metabolic rate accelerate. REM mentation is what we think of as dreams; it tends to be vivid, colorful, dramatic, very emotional, and implausible.

Non-REM sleep, in which parasympathetic activity predominates, occurs in four stages. Stage 1 is a tran-

sitional stage in which the person is just dropping off to sleep. The patient has fleeting thoughts and awakens at the slightest stimulus, remembering this period just as one of drowsiness. Slow rolling eye movements are present. The EEG shows low voltage waves of varying frequency. This stage usually lasts from 30 seconds to 7 minutes (Walsleben 1982). In stage 2, the person becomes more relaxed, eye movements cease, and thoughts become vaguer. Although clearly asleep, the person can be awakened readily. About 45% of total sleep time normally is spent in this stage (Walsleben 1982).

Stages 3 and 4, or "delta" sleep, are marked by deeper sleep during which the EEG shows slow, high amplitude delta waves. In stage 3, muscle relaxation deepens; pulse, respiratory rate, and temperature decrease; and the person sleeps through occasional, moderately loud stimuli. In stage 4, the person appears very relaxed and rarely moves. Vigorous stimulation is necessary to awaken him or her.

Mentation during non-REM sleep tends to be more realistic and logical, and often reflects recent activity. Non-REM dreams are rarely in color (Walsleben 1982); they also are harder to recall (Sanford 1981).

Sleep Cycles   Sleep cycles normally are synchronized with the person's circadian ("about a day") rhythm, in such a way that the greatest amount of sleep occurs during the low point of the circadian cycle. Superimposed on this basic sleep cycle is a continuation of the basic rest/activity cycles that operate during waking periods. These basic rest/activity cycles are cycles of central nervous system activity that peak an average of every 90 minutes. Once the person has completed stage 1 (falling asleep), the common, most effective progression is stages 2, 3, 4, 3, 2, REM, 2, 3, 4, and so on (Sanford 1982).

The length of time devoted to each stage of sleep varies during the night, with delta sleep most common during the first third of the night, and REM sleep periods increasing in duration during the night from 1–2 minutes at the start to 20–30 minutes by early morning (Wotring 1982). The percentage of total sleep time spent in REM sleep varies with age, from about 30% in adolescence to 15% at age 65 (Kogeorgos and Scott 1980).

Sleep Disturbances   There are numerous sleep disturbances that may affect critically ill patients. Among the most common are desynchronized sleep, sleep deprivation, and REM rebound. Rarer medical disorders include nocturnal cardiovascular symptoms, sleep apnea, and narcolepsy.

Desynchronized Sleep   Desynchronized sleep occurs when a person is unable to obtain the majority of sleep

TABLE 20-5 ENERGY COST (IN METS) OF ACTIVITY AND EXERCISE

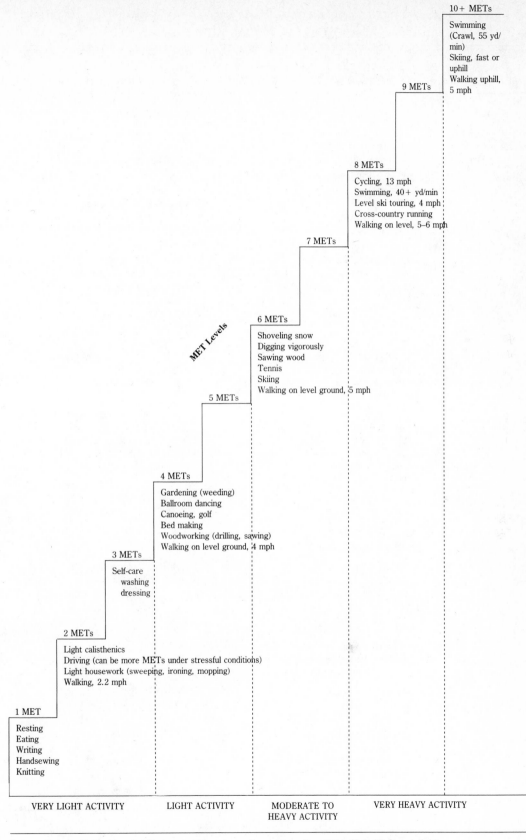

MET Levels

10+ METs
Swimming (Crawl, 55 yd/min)
Skiing, fast or uphill
Walking uphill, 5 mph

9 METs

8 METs
Cycling, 13 mph
Swimming, 40+ yd/min
Level ski touring, 4 mph
Cross-country running
Walking on level, 5–6 mph

7 METs

6 METs
Shoveling snow
Digging vigorously
Sawing wood
Tennis
Skiing
Walking on level ground, 5 mph

5 METs

4 METs
Gardening (weeding)
Ballroom dancing
Canoeing, golf
Bed making
Woodworking (drilling, sawing)
Walking on level ground, 4 mph

3 METs
Self-care
washing
dressing

2 METs
Light calisthenics
Driving (can be more METs under stressful conditions)
Light housework (sweeping, ironing, mopping)
Walking, 2.2 mph

1 MET
Resting
Eating
Writing
Handsewing
Knitting

VERY LIGHT ACTIVITY   LIGHT ACTIVITY   MODERATE TO HEAVY ACTIVITY   VERY HEAVY ACTIVITY

Source: Sivarajan E: Cardiac rehabilitation: Activity and exercise program. Page 555 in Underhill S et al. (eds), *Cardiac nursing*. Philadelphia: Lippincott/Harper & Row, 1982.

TABLE 20-6 MET LEVEL FOR RECREATIONAL, SELF-CARE, HOME MAINTENANCE, AND OCCUPATIONAL ACTIVITIES

MET LEVEL	RECREATIONAL, SELF-CARE, HOME MAINTENANCE	OCCUPATIONAL
1.5 or less	Watching TV Painting Sewing Conversation	
1.8–2.2	Walking 1.2 mph Driving Playing piano Self-care activities Playing cards	Typing Desk work Operating electrical office machinery
2–3	Walking 2 mph Level cycling 5 mph Golf with power cart	Manual typing Light janitorial work Shoesmith, tailor, locksmith Auto, radio, TV repair Bartending Hand dusting, dusting floor, vacuum cleaning Scrubbing floors
3–4	Walking 3 mph Cycling 6 mph Golf, pulling bag cart Gardening (raking, hoeing, weeding) Pushing power mower	Cleaning windows Making beds Machine assembly Trailor-truck in traffic
4–5	Walking 3.5 mph Cycling 8 mph Swimming 20 yards/min Light carpentry Golf, carrying clubs Table tennis	Painting, paperhanging, masonry Light carpentry Carrying (carpets, food, bags) Washing floors Stripping beds
5–6	Walking 4 mph Cycling 10 mph Stream fishing Digging garden Ice or roller skating 9 mph	Stair climbing, slowly Walking fast (4 mph) Scrubbing
6–7	Walking 5 mph Cycling 11 mph Ski touring 2½ mph Downhill skiing Splitting wood Singles tennis Snow shoveling Folk and square dancing Mowing lawn with push mower	Shoveling 10/min of 10 pounds Digging ditches
7–8	Jogging 5 mph Cycling 12 mph Vigorous downhill skiing	Pushing wheelbarrow Carrying heavy load >80 pounds Planing wood
8–9	Running 5½ mph Cycling 13 mph Ski touring 4 mph Squash and handball	Shoveling 10/min of 14 pounds
>9		Shoveling 10/min of 16 pounds

Source: Sivarajan E: Cardiac rehabilitation: Activity and exercise program. Page 558 in Underhill S et al. (eds),
Cardiac nursing. Philadelphia: Lippincott/Harper & Row, 1982.

during normal sleeping hours. When the period of the greatest amount of sleep shifts more than 1½ to 2 hours from the normal sleep period, the person experiences a decreased sense of well-being, irritability, anorexia, decreased stress tolerance, and numerous altered metabolic processes (Sanford 1981). If the person is in an environment in which all cues are consistent with a different bedtime (for instance, meals, lighting, and noise levels), he or she will need at least 3–5 days to resynchronize sleeping. A familiar example of this sleep disturbance is "jet lag."

Sleep Deprivation In the critical-care unit, sleep deprivation commonly occurs because patients are interrupted before completing their 90-minute sleep cycle. Each time they are interrupted, they must restart the cycle. As a result, they spend more time in transition and light sleep and less time in deep sleep than is normal. Sleep deprivation causes a loss of both non-REM and REM sleep time, with the loss of REM time disproportionately greater (Sanford 1981). Non-REM sleep loss is experienced as physical fatigue, whereas the effects of REM sleep loss are psychologic (Adams 1980). Signs of REM deprivation include irritability, confusion, anxiety, and short-term memory loss, which can progress to paranoia and hallucinations (Adams 1980; Helton et al. 1980). It is fascinating to note that the hallucinations may represent the breakthrough of REM sleep into waking periods, especially given that hallucinations are a hallmark of "ICU psychosis," which often occurs in sleep-deprived patients. In experimental studies, the signs of REM deprivation occurred after 2–5 nights of sleep deprivation, and they disappeared when the subjects were allowed one night of recovery sleep (Helton et al. 1980).

REM Rebound A compensatory increase in REM time that occurs when the person resumes sleep after REM sleep loss is called *REM rebound*. REM rebound can happen after sleep deprivation due to interruptions by staff, preadmission sleep loss, alcohol withdrawal, or discontinuation of the use of hypnotics (both alcohol and hypnotics suppress REM). REM rebound can impose increased physiologic stress on the patient, as REM sleep is marked by increased cardiovascular workload and irritability as well as increased cerebral blood flow, which can elevate intracranial pressure in those with central nervous system dysfunction (Sanford 1981).

Nocturnal Cardiovascular Disturbances These may include increased dysrhythmias and nocturnal angina. While there is conflicting evidence as to whether sleep increases or decreases dysrhythmogenesis, there is stronger evidence correlating the occurrence of angina at night with REM sleep patterns (Hemenway 1980). For people sleeping from 11 P.M. to 7 A.M., the longest

NURSING RESEARCH NOTE

Richards K: A description of sleep patterns in the intensive care unit. *Heart Lung* 1986; 15:306.

In recent years, nursing literature has documented nurses' increasing concern about the impact of sleep on recovery and psychologic well-being. Sleep disruption is a given in intensive care units; but before nurses can develop effective interventions, they need to know specifically how sleep differs in the ICU and have a valid, reliable tool for assessing sleep disruption in the ICU.

This study was designed to describe sleep patterns in an ICU and evaluate the validity of a visual analog scale developed to measure subjective sleep quality in the ICU. Ten male patients (ages 50–69 years) were studied for 15 nights in an open ward of a medical ICU. Polysomnographic data about these subjects were compared to tables of age- and sex-matched normal values. The ICU subjects' polysomnographic data also were correlated with the results of 14 visual analog scales describing the patient's subjective quality of ICU sleep, using Pearson correlation coefficients. Unpaired two-tailed *t* tests were used to examine the relationships between ICU sleep and selected medications, ICU night, previous ICU experience, and habitual at-home day sleep patterns.

Study subjects demonstrated dramatic changes in sleep patterns. They spent significantly more time awake and in stage 1 and less time in stage 2 and REM sleep. The analog scale showed beginning construct validity, but still needs reliability testing before it can be used as a basis for patient care management decisions.

This study adds to the fund of knowledge about sleep in the ICU by identifying specific disruptions observed in patients. The researcher emphasizes the need for additional studies on other types of ICU patients, as well as for research designed to examine the impact of disrupted sleep on recovery and the effect of nursing interventions on sleep.

REM period occurs between 4 A.M. and 5 A.M. (Walsle-ben 1982). This is also the time of peak incidence of nocturnal angina attacks and nonviolent deaths (Hemenway 1980; Walsleben 1982).

Sleep Apnea Sleep apnea is a disorder in which the patient stops breathing for up to 90 seconds. It is subdivided into obstructive, central, and mixed types. *Obstructive apnea* is caused by obstruction of the upper pharyngeal airway. The breathing pattern consists of very quiet or absent breaths followed by loud snoring and thrashing movements as the person attempts to clear the airway (Parkosewich 1986). *Central apnea,* the rarer form, is marked by absence of diaphragmatic movement; there appears to be no effort to breathe (Williams and Jackson 1982). *Mixed apnea* is a combination of the two types; central apnea may occur first, followed by obstructive apnea. The symptoms of sleep apnea include heavy snoring, snorting, extreme restlessness, falling out of bed, sleepwalking, bedwetting, and personality changes; the heart rate may decrease to 30 beats/minute and then increase up to 120 beats/minute, increased ectopic beats may occur, and oxygen saturation may fall as low as 20% (Walsleben 1982) during apneic episodes. Sleep apnea also can cause sudden death. Treatment of obstructive sleep apnea involves improving airway patency by means of a tracheostomy used at night, removal of obstructions such as enlarged tonsils, and weight loss in obese patients. Central apnea is difficult to treat and may include mechanical ventilation at night or insertion of a phrenic pacemaker.

Nursing Interventions The critical-care nurse can play a crucial role in safeguarding patients' sleep. Following are recommendations to minimize sleep disruptions and promote as near normal sleep as possible in the critical-care environment.

1. Obtain a sleep history as part of your nursing assessment. Include questions about when the patient normally sleeps, bedtime rituals, factors that promote sleep, and frequency and reasons for waking. When feasible, ask the sleeping partner about snoring and nighttime restlessness.

2. Whenever possible, duplicate the person's normal bedtime rituals.

3. Adjust the lighting, noise level, and temperature to make the room conducive to sleep. Close the door, dim the lights, and turn off any unneeded machinery.

4. If the patient's condition allows, encourage daytime exercise periods.

5. Group nighttime treatments and observations that require touching the patient so as to allow uninterrupted periods of 90 minutes, if at all possible.

6. Encourage staff to muffle conversations at nighttime.

7. Avoid the use of hypnotics whenever possible by inducing sleep with backrubs, warm milk, or relaxation exercises.

8. If hypnotics must be used, encourage the physician to prescribe ones that minimize sleep disruption. These include flurazepam (Dalmane), chloral hydrate, and diazepam (Valium).

9. If patients have been using hypnotics prior to admission, it would be wise to taper use during hospitalization rather than abruptly discontinuing the drug. It has been estimated that up to 20% of the population uses hypnotics regularly (Kogeorgos and Scott 1980).

10. When patients have a history of chronic alcoholism, anticipate that REM rebound will occur and be especially alert for signs of cardiovascular instability or increased intracranial pressure.

11. Observe patients while they sleep to evaluate the quality of their sleep. Monitor cardiac rhythm and pulmonary pressures. If patients are extremely restless and snoring heavily, consider the possibility of sleep apnea. Dysrhythmias and elevated pulmonary pressures may indicate episodes of REM-related hypoxemia (Parkosewich 1986).

12. Be extremely cautious about giving narcotics or sedatives to patients suspected of having sleep apnea. Because these agents impair respiratory drive, sudden death may be precipitated.

Disturbed Self-Concept Related to Physical Alterations or Awareness of Internal Disorders

Decreased mobility often provokes an altered body image. Pitorak (1975) describes body image as "the picture of one's own body developed in his mind. Yet it isn't just a picture of the body, of course; it's a whole personal range of activity and possibility, an outstanding impression, the sum of one's life experiences and future hopes. It may not even be accurate, but it's real to the holder." Body image may include objects the person uses frequently (such as eyeglasses, dentures, or canes). It is shaped by powerful cultural norms and may have irrational aspects. Particularly in the American culture, those who are not young, slim, strong, and whole may view their bodies and themselves negatively.

In the critically ill, changes in body image may result from actual external physical alterations (such as scars or amputations) or awareness of internal disorders (such as chronic renal failure). Decreased mobility can affect body image through sensory deprivation or the increased dependency and changes in status and power that accompany immobility.

Body image changes create a distortion of self that

can be extremely anxiety-provoking. Among the factors influencing how the patient adapts to the change in body image are its visibility; changes it imposes on lifestyle and favorite activities; self-strengths; sources of support; and reactions of those around, whether loved ones, strangers, or professional staff.

Nursing Interventions Ways you can help the patient adapt to an altered body image are these:

1. Find out how the patient perceives the body image change. Asking the patient how he or she viewed his or her body before illness and how he or she feels now may unleash a torrent of feelings and give you clues to ways you can assist.

2. Listen supportively as the patient talks about and tries to work through feelings. Also be alert for nonverbal cues such as a panicky or disgusted expression when viewing a surgical wound.

3. Comment favorably upon those aspects of body image the patient values and still possesses.

4. Help the patient stay clean. A patient unable or too tired to care for self can become very embarrassed and depressed about dirty hair, poor oral hygiene, or unpleasant body odors.

5. As soon as possible, encourage the person to resume self-care. If the person seems reluctant to care for an altered part, ask him or her to assist you (by holding tape, for instance) and demonstrate a matter-of-fact acceptance as you care for that area, emphasizing positive aspects (for example, "The skin around your stoma's looking better—pink and healthy"). Nurses are in a unique position to help patients this way. Benner (1984) points out that expert nurses make "culturally avoided aspects of an illness approachable and understandable . . . and often the ways of . . . coping are transmitted without words but by demonstration, attitudes, and reactions."

6. Consider asking the patient whether he or she would like someone who has coped with the same life experience to visit him or her and family. Such a person can provide sensitivity, practical tips, and hope that surpass even those offered by well-intentioned, knowledgeable staff.

Potential Sexual Dysfunction Related to Fear, Physical Limitations, or Knowledge Deficit

Sexuality is an integral part of body image and is affected profoundly by decreased mobility. During the stage of fighting for survival, sexuality is low on the list of concerns of the patient, partner, and staff. After this initial period, however, it can become a primary (though often unexpressed) concern of the patient and/or partner. Because of their own discomfort with the topic,

staff may assume with relief that if the person does not bring it up, he or she is not thinking about it. In fact, the person may be waiting for a cue from you that it is a permissible topic of discussion.

Counseling about resumption of sexual activity after hospital discharge can be started while the patient is still in the critical-care unit. The critical-care nurse is in an excellent position to initiate this counseling because of the intimacy and trust that can characterize the nurse–patient relationship. Such early counseling can contribute to a smoother, more rapid recovery by forestalling or alleviating concerns that plague the patient and partner. Among these concerns may be the possibility of harming the patient, changes in sexual interest, and worry about their ability to satisfy each other or have children. The partner in particular may feel resentful and guilty about finding the patient less attractive sexually, discovering the patient's sexual interest has waned, or having to assume a more active sexual role in their relationship.

Several studies have reported the sexual concerns and effects of sexual counseling (or its lack) on MI patients and their spouses. As recently as 1980, more than one-half of the 100 wives of MI patients interviewed by Papadopoulos (1980) had received *no* sexual counseling prior to their husbands' hospital discharge. Nearly a quarter of the couples never resumed sexual activity, because of either impotence or lack of trying. The other three-quarters reported lessened frequency and quality in their sexual relationships. Interestingly, the majority of couples had made no changes in foreplay patterns or sexual positioning, in spite of any instructions they may have been given. The two primary fears of 92% of the spouses were that their mate would have chest pain or another MI during sexual activity.

Mann et al. (1981) reported a one-year post-MI survey of 88 patients who had attended a rehabilitation program that included discussion of sexuality. Of the 68 subjects who had been sexually active prior to infarction, 13 had not resumed sexual activity. Thiry-three others reported decreased frequency of intercourse due to impotence, loss of interest, or cardiac symptoms. The group discussion in the course had not prevented an overall decrease in sexual activity.

The major sexual dysfunctions reported after MI are impotence and premature ejaculation in male patients, temporary inability to reach orgasm in female patients, and loss of libido in both sexes (Scalzi 1982a). Secondary impotence and premature ejaculation (that is, problems not previously present) appear to be quite common.

Another group that often develops sexual dysfunction is chronic obstructive pulmonary disease (COPD) patients (Cooper 1986). Loss of libido, the most common complaint, may result from fear of shortness of breath or from coughing, sputum production, and the unpleasant mouth odor that characterize COPD.

Nursing Interventions Ways you can help the patient and/or partner include the following.

1. Develop an awareness of your own feelings and values about sex.

2. Examine your current nursing practice. Do you ask about sexuality when taking a patient's history? Zalar (1982) found that 60% of nurses polled never did. If you don't, examine the reasons why.

3. Assess readiness to discuss sexual concerns by being attentive to nonverbal as well as verbal cues about sexual concerns.

4. Maintain a nonjudgmental attitude. If you feel you would be too uncomfortable exploring the topic, refer the patient to other staff more comfortable with sexual counseling or to community groups such as a post-MI rehabilitation program or ostomy club for support in developing a satisfying sexual identity.

5. If you do feel comfortable responding, provide an appropriate environment for assessment and counseling.

6. Indicate your willingness to discuss the topic, perhaps by asking whether the patient has thought about how his or her disability might temporarily or permanently affect his or her sexual relationships.

7. Assess the patient and partner for baseline information (Table 20-7).

8. Consider the patient's physical status, psychologic status, and the physiologic cost of sexual activity (Table 20-8). MI patients usually are physically capable of resuming intercourse 6–8 weeks after infarction. The energy expenditure during orgasm is 4–6 METs, while the other stages of sexual response require 3–4 METs (Cohen 1986). If the patient can walk vigorously or climb stairs rapidly without abnormalities of pulse, blood pressure, or ECG, sexual activity usually can be resumed safely. The actual amount of physical energy that middle-aged, long-married couples require during sexual activity is approximately equal to that required for climbing two flights of stairs, scrubbing a floor, arguing with a spouse, or driving to work (Hellerstein and Friedman 1970).

9. Keep the issue of sexuality in perspective. Meet more immediate patient needs and concerns first. Present sexual activity as one of several types of physical activity that can be reincorporated into the person's life according to the level of recovery.

10. Learn about specific techniques that may apply to your patients; they vary with the disability. Couples may need to experiment with different times or positions for intercourse or alternative forms of pleasuring each other. The acceptability of these alternatives may vary with the person's age and religious, cultural, and ethnic background. You do not need to become an expert in order to share some basic knowledge that may help your patients. For instance, you can alert the male patient being discharged on antihypertensive medications that impotence may occur and point out that recent studies of female sexuality have shown that most women gain more pleasure from clitoral stimulation than from intercourse itself.

11. Discuss with the physician prophylactic measures to reduce the physiologic cost of sexual activity. Measures that may be used prophylactically include nitroglycerin, bronchodilators, and increased oxygen flow rates if the person is on continuous oxygen at home.

12. Cardiac patients should be advised to avoid intercourse after a heavy meal or heavy alcohol intake, when very tired or pressed for time, or with unfamiliar partners (Scalzi 1982a, 1982b). They also should be advised to contact their physician if rapid heart rate or breathing persists longer than 5 minutes after orgasm, chest pain develops, extreme fatigue is experienced the next day, or sexual difficulties occur.

13. If you detect long-standing sexual problems, offer a referral to a counselor with special expertise.

14. Above all, appreciate the importance of sexual expression. Cooper (1986) writes: "It is time for the nurse to acknowledge that people are sexual beings. Although disease, disability, and age may alter how they express their sexuality, patients rarely stop needing the feelings of love, comfort, and belonging that are normally associated with sexual expression."

Outcome Evaluation

Evaluate the effectiveness of your nursing care. This chapter has stressed nursing measures to prevent the hazards of decreased mobility. It is important also that you be able to spot developing problems early, call them to the physician's attention, and implement appropriate nursing care activities. Table 20-9 presents the signs and symptoms that should alert you to the possible ineffectiveness of preventive measures.

·TABLE 20-7 ASSESSMENT AND PLANNING FOR SEXUAL COUNSELING

ASSESSMENT	RATIONALE	EXPECTED OUTCOMES	INTERVENTIONS

1. Previous patterns of sexual activity
  a. Availability of sexual partner
  b. Frequency of activity
  c. Duration of coitus
  d. Usual time of day
  e. Favored positions of intercourse.
	Data collected identifies need for sexual counseling, previous stressful patterns, and provides a base of information to individualize the counseling.	Patient will return to the same level of sexual activity as prior to infarction.	1. Instruct patient to:
			  a. Adopt positions of intercourse that require less energy and strain.
			  b. Avoid intercourse after a large meal or excessive alcohol intake (3-hour wait is advised), when tired, under time pressure, or with unfamiliar partners.

2. Experience with chest pain during sexual stimulation, activity	Experience can increase fear or anxiety in patient or spouse.	Patient will identify how to use nitroglycerin prophylactically (before activity) to avoid chest pain.	2. Instruct patient:
			  a. To take nitroglycerin prior to any activity that might precipitate chest pain.
			  b. About purpose, side effects, method of taking nitroglycerin, and the need to replace outdated medications (6 months or more).

3. Sexual difficulty prior to myocardial infarction (1–3 months)
  a. Type of difficulty:
    Men—premature ejaculation, inability to maintain erection
    Women—inability to achieve orgasm
  b. Frequency of difficulty
  c. Surrounding stressful circumstances
  d. Medications taken pre- and postinfarction
  e. Pre-existing disease that may interfere with sexual function
	Previous sexual difficulty is not uncommon and for sporadic periods postinfarction. It may be related to fatigue, stress, or effects of medications. Memories of sexual difficulty prior to MI may increase fear or permanent sexual difficulties.	Patient will identify the effect of stress and medications on sexual performance.	3. a. Instruct patient about cardiac drugs that can lead to sexual difficulty:
			    Reserpine—decreased libido and impotence
			    Methyldopa—impotence, lack of sexual desire, disorders of ejaculation
			    Propranolol—increased fatigue, decreased sexual desire
			  b. Emphasize the relationship between stressful conditions (fatigue, long working hours, anxiety) and sexual difficulty.

4. Patient's and partner's understanding of when they can resume sexual activity	Data collected identifies expectations, fears, what information has been acquired and retained, and any further myths or misconceptions.	Patient and spouse will identify when they can safely resume sexual activity.	4. a. Instruct patient and partner that resumption of sexual activity postinfarction is safe after 6–8 weeks, and depends on physical condition, extent of damage from infarction, and, of course, hospitalization.
			  b. Instruct patient on learning signals of intolerance for sexual activity:
			    Rapid heart rate and breathing rate that persists 4–5 min after orgasm
			    Chest pain during or after intercourse
			    Extreme fatigue the day after intercourse
			    Sleeplessness after sexual experience

Source: Cohen J: Sexual counseling of the patient following myocardial infarction. *Crit Care Nurse* 1986; 6(6): 18–28.

TABLE 20-8　CONSIDERATIONS IN SEXUAL COUNSELING

1. *Patient's physical status*
   General health preinfarction
   Physical activity tolerance preinfarction
   Frequency and severity of angina
   Ability to tolerate progressive activity postinfarction

2. *Patient's psychologic status*
   Fear/anxiety
   Depression/grief response
   Changing roles within the family/disruption of sexual roles
   Medications

3. *Physiologic requirements during four stages of sexual response*
   Excitement: 3–4 METs*
   Plateau: 3–4 METs
   Orgasm: 4–6 METs
   Resolution: 3–4 METs

*One MET is the amount of energy used to consume 3.5 ml/kg/min of oxygen when the body is at rest.

Source: Cohen J: Sexual counseling of the patient following myocardial infarction. *Crit Care Nurse* 1986; 6(6):18–28.

At the time of the patient's discharge from the critical-care unit, the desirable outcome criteria following ideally should be met:

- Maintenance of consciousness, warm dry skin, and normal blood pressure when head is elevated suddenly.
- Resting heart rate not exceeding admission heart rate plus 0.5 beat per minute per day of bedrest.
- No redness, tenderness, or swelling over veins.

- Urine at least 1500 ml/day, clear, acidic, with no stones and no foul odor.
- Breath sounds clear bilaterally.
- Arterial blood gas values WNL for patient.
- Weight WNL for patient.
- Bowel movement of normal color and soft consistency at least twice a week.
- No erythema, edema, tenderness, or pressure ulcers (over bony prominences, in particular).
- Joints freely movable within range normal for patient.
- If alert and physically able, patient correctly demonstrates appropriate exercises and states their purpose and frequency.
- Patient has verbalized satisfaction with amount and quality of sleep.
- Patient may verbalize beginning awareness of changes in body image and sexuality and beginning ability to cope with them.

REFERENCES

Adams R: Sleep and its abnormalities. Pages 1015–1020 in *Harrison's principles of internal medicine.* Isselbacher K (ed). New York: McGraw-Hill, 1980.

Asher R: The dangers of going to bed. *Brit Med J* (Dec) 1947; 967–968.

Benner P: *From novice to expert.* Menlo Park, CA: Addison-Wesley, 1984.

Blomqvist CG et al.: Early cardiovascular adaptation to zero gravity simulated by head-down tilt. *Acta Astronautica* 1980; 7:543.

TABLE 20-9　KEY SIGNS AND SYMPTOMS OF PHYSIOLOGIC COMPLICATIONS OF IMMOBILITY

SIGNS AND SYMPTOMS	POSSIBLE CAUSE
When head or upper body elevated suddenly: pallor, fainting, weakness, clammy skin, tachycardia, hypotension	Orthostatic hypotension
Tender, inflamed veins	Venous thrombosis
Dyspnea, chest pain	Pulmonary embolus
Cold, painful, white, blue or mottled extremities, diminished pulses	Arterial embolus
Bone pain, easy fracturing	Osteoporosis
Resistance (with or without pain) to joint movement	Restricted range of joint motion
Abdominal distention, decreased appetite, headache, malaise, sacral pain, hard infrequent stools, straining, liquid stools	Constipation
Urinary frequency, urgency, burning; small amounts of cloudy, foul-smelling, alkaline urine; flank pain	Urinary tract infection
Flank pain, colicky abdominal pain, nausea and vomiting, hematuria, stones in urine	Kidney stone
Altered breath sounds, fever, productive cough	Respiratory infection
Skin blanching, erythema, edema, tenderness, or blisters, particularly over a bony prominence	Pressure ulcer

Browse N: *Physiology and pathology of bedrest.* Springfield, IL: Charles C Thomas, 1965.

Cohen JA: Sexual couseling of the patient following myocardial infarction. *Crit Care Nurse* (Nov/Dec) 1986; 6(6): 18–28.

Convertino V et al.: Cardiovascular responses to exercise in middle-aged men after 10 days of bedrest. *Circ* 1982; 65:134–140.

Cooper D: Sexual counseling of the patient with chronic lung disease. *Focus Crit Care* (Jun) 1986; 13:3:18–20.

Deitrick JE et al.: Effects of immobilization upon various metabolic and physiologic functions of normal man. *Am J Med* 1948; 4:3.

Downs F: Bed rest and sensory disturbances. *Am J Nurs* 1974; 74:434–436.

Elliott RM: Pressure ulcerations. *Am Fam Physician* 1982; 25:171–180.

Fardy P et al.: *Cardiac rehabilitation.* St Louis: Mosby, 1980.

Fareeduddin K, Abelmann WH: Impaired orthostatic tolerance after bed rest in patients with myocardial infarction. *N Engl J Med* 1969; 280:345–350.

Garber S: Trochanteric pressure in spinal cord injury. *Arch Phys Med Rehabil* 1973; 63:549–552.

Gauer OH, Thron HL: Postural changes in the circulation. Pages 2409–2439 in *Handbook of physiology.* Hamilton WF (ed). Section 2: Circulation. Washington, DC: American Physiological Soc., Vol III, 1965.

Guyton A: *Textbook of medical physiology,* 7th ed. Philadelphia: Saunders, 1986.

Hellerstein HG, Friedman EG: Sexual activity and the post coronary patient. *Arch Int Med* 1970; 125:987–999.

Helton M et al.: The correlation between sleep deprivation and the intensive care unit syndrome. *Heart Lung* 1980; 9:464–468.

Hemenway J: Sleep and the cardiac patient. *Heart Lung* 1980; 9:453–463.

Hirschberg G et al. (eds): *Rehabilitation: A manual for care of the disabled and elderly,* 2d ed. Philadelphia: Lippincott, 1976.

Kaneko K et al.: Regional distribution of ventilation and perfusion as a function of body position. *J Appl Physiol* 1966; 21:767.

Kogeorgos J, Scott D: Sleep and sleep disorders. *Practitioner* 1980; 224:717–721.

Kottke F: Deterioration of the bedfast patient: Causes and effects. *Public Health Reports* 1965; 80:437–447.

Kottke F: Therapeutic exercise. Pages 365–406 in *Handbook of physical medicine and rehabilitation,* eds. F. Krusen et al. Philadelphia: Lippincott, 1971.

Maklebust J et al.: Pressure relief characteristics of various support surfaces used in prevention and treatment of pressure ulcers. *J Enterostom Ther* 1986; 13:85–89.

Mann S et al.: The effects of myocardial infarction on sexual activity. *J Cardiac Rehab* 1981; 1:187–190.

McCally M et al.: Tilt table responses of human subjects following application of lower body negative pressure. *Aerospace Med* 1966; 37:1247–1249.

Meissner J: Which patient on your unit might get a pressure sore? *Nurs 80* (June) 1980; 64–65.

Metheny N: Renal stones and urinary pH. *Am J Nurs* (Sep) 1982; 137–1375.

Narsete TA et al.: Pressure sores. *Am Fam Physician* 1983; 28:135–139.

Norton LC, Conforti CG: The effects of body position on oxygenation. *Heart Lung* (Jan) 1985; 14:45–52.

O'Brien M: Assessing activity tolerance in critical care settings. *Focus* (Dec/Jan) 1982; 11–12.

Papadopoulos C et al.: Sexual concerns and needs of the post coronary patient's wife. *Arch Int Med* 1980; 140:38–41.

Parkosewich JA: Sleep-disordered breathing: A common problem in chronic obstructive pulmonary disease. *Crit Care Nurse* (Nov/Dec) 1986; 6:60–64.

Pitorak E: Rheumatoid arthritis: living with it more comfortably. *Nurs* 1975; 5:33–35.

Roberts S: *Behavioral concepts and the critically ill patient.* Englewood Cliffs, NJ: Prentice-Hall, 1976.

Romm S et al.: Pressure sores: State of the art. *Tex Med* 1982; 78:52.

Saltin B et al.: Response to exercise after bedrest and after training. *Circ* 1968; 38(VII):1–55.

Sanford S: Sleep I: Dynamics; Sleep II: Nursing implications. Pages 175–178 in *Proceedings of the eighth annual 1981 NTI.* Newport Beach, CA: American Assn. of Critical Care Nurses, 1981.

Scalzi C: Sexual counseling. Pages 592–600 in *Cardiac nursing.* Underhill S et al. (eds). Philadelphia: Lippincott, 1982a.

Scalzi C: Sexual counseling and sexual therapy for patients after myocardial infarction. *Cardiovasc Nurs* 1982b; 18:13–17.

Sivarajan E: Cardiac rehabilitation: Activity and exercise program. Pages 551–561 in *Cardiac nursing.* Underhill S et al. (eds). Philadelphia: Lippincott, 1982.

Taylor H et al.: Effects of bedrest on cardiovascular function and work performance. *J Appl Physiol* 1949; 2:223–239.

Trombly C, Scott A: *Occupational therapy for physical dysfunction.* Baltimore: Williams and Wilkins, 1977.

Underhill S et al. (eds): *Cardiac care nursing.* Philadelphia: Lippincott, 1982.

Walsleben J: Sleep disorders. *Am J Nurs* (Jun) 1982; 936–940.

Wenger N: Exercise prescription for patients with coronary disease and for healthy individuals. Pages 30–42 in *Quick reference to cardiovascular diseases,* 2d ed. Chung E (ed). Philadelphia: Lippincott, 1983.

Wenger N: Rehabilitation of the patient with symptomatic atherosclerotic coronary heart disease. In *The heart arteries and veins,* 5th ed. Hurst J et al. (eds). New York: McGraw-Hill, 1982.

Wenger N: Rehabilitation after myocardial infarction. Dallas, TX: American Heart Association, 1972.

West J: Evolution of concepts: Movement, posture and compression for stasis-prone bedfast patients. Unpublished paper, 1987.

Williams R, Jackson D: Problems with sleep. *Heart Lung* 1982; 11:262–267.

Winslow EH: Cardiovascular consequences of bed rest. *Heart Lung* (May) 1985; 14:236–246.

Winslow EH et al.: Oxygen uptake and cardiovascular responses in control adults and acute myocardial infarction patients during bathing. *Nurs Res* (May/Jun) 1985; 34:164–169.

Winslow EH et al.: Oxygen uptake and cardiovascular response in patients and normal adults during in-bed and out-of-bed toileting. *J Cardiac Rehab* 1984; 4:348–354.

Wotring K: Using research in practice. *Focus* (Oct/Nov) 1982; 34–35.

Zalar M: Role preparation for nurses in human sexual functioning. *Nurs Clin North Am* 1982; 3:331–361.

SUPPLEMENTAL READING

Beaver MJ: Mediscus low-air-loss beds and the prevention of decubitus ulcers. *Crit Care Nurse* 1986; 6:5:32–39.

Berliner H: Aging skin, part one. *Am J Nurs* (Oct) 1986a; 1138–1141.

Berliner H: Aging skin, part two. *Am J Nurs* (Nov) 1986b; 1259–1261.

Birdsall C: How do you use the continuous passive motion device? *Am J Nurs* (Jun) 1986; 657–658.

Bramwell L: Wives' experiences in the support role after husbands' first myocardial infarction. *Heart Lung* (Nov) 1986; 15:578–584.

Burke LJ, Fischer LE: Nursing diagnoses, indicators, and interventions is an outpatient cardiac rehabilitation program. *Heart Lung* (Jan) 1986; 15:1:70–86.

Dunbar S, Redick E: Should patients with acute myocardial infarctions receive back massage? *Focus Crit Care* (Jun) 1986; 13:42–45.

Fisch R: Preventing minor sexual difficulties from becoming sexual problems. *Human Sexuality* 1981; 15:67–71.

Melville S: Relaxation techniques in acute myocardial infarction: The theoretic rationale. *Focus Crit Care Nurs* (February) 1987; 7:9–12.

Mickens D: Activities of daily living in women after myocardial infarction. *Heart Lung* (July) 1986; 15:376–381.

Mickus D: Activities of daily living in women after myocardial infarction. *Heart Lung* (Jul) 1986; 15:376–382.

Nicklin WM: Postdischarge concerns of cardiac patients as presented via a telephone callback system. *Heart Lung* (May) 1986; 15:268–272.

Shenkman B: Factors contributing to attrition rates in a pulmonary rehabilitation program. *Heart Lung* (Jan) 1985; 14:53–58.

Simmons K: Sexuality and the female ostomate: patient-to-patient advice. *Am J Nurs* 1983; 83:409–411.

21

Trauma

CLINICAL INSIGHT

Domain: The teaching-coaching function

Competency: Timing—capturing a patient's readiness to learn

In the hectic environment of the intensive care unit, nurses rarely have the luxury of waiting for an optimal time to teach. Instruction, often hurried, occurs under the most extreme circumstances. Teaching in this environment requires a special sensitivity to patients: an awareness of when someone is ready to learn, the flexibility to capitalize on this readiness, and an ability to stay in tune with how the patient is responding to the information.

In the following paradigm, from Crabtree and Jorgenson (1986, pp. 124–125), Robin is caring for a head-injured patient who is scheduled to undergo surgery as soon as he is stabilized. As his disorientation from subdural hematoma clears, he becomes increasingly apprehensive. Robin recognizes that she may be able to alleviate some of his fear, as well as ready him for crucial participation in his postoperative recovery:

I started slowly. I started with the most important thing, the intubation. Because I knew he was going to be tubed, and I knew if I couldn't go any farther,

it was at least important for him to know about that. . . . I was aware that he would probably be intubated 24 hours post-op, just as a maintenance type thing, because of his cardiac problems. Tom also had some pulmonary problems, some COPD or emphysema. But, I started there, in that, if I didn't get any farther, he would know that he wouldn't be able to talk. He would know what the tube was like. He would know what we were doing when we were bagging him and/or suctioning.

And I figured, if he couldn't handle it, I think I, maybe even subconsciously, knew that I could stop there. Because, when it comes right down to it, I think that was my priority; that is, if he didn't know about the Swan, you know, the placement, or what I was using it for, at least he would understand the most important thing. And I also went through the fact that his hands would be tied down, because coming out of the anesthesia, you might pull on your tubes, you might pull them out—those kinds of things. And, he handled that real well, and I think just as a natural flow . . . we went through everything. And, a lot of it, I think, you do subconsciously. You know, I would have stopped if he got too apprehensive, but once we started, I think he was more curious and wanted to know more. . . .

Well, Tom came back the next day post-op, and of course, intubated, with a Swan and an art-line and

*the whole nine yards that we talked about. They ex-
pected to have just tons of problems with him: heart-
wise, cardiac output, pulmonary-wise, apprehension.
They figured they'd have to sedate him.*

Robin's teaching and coaching, however, have a major
impact on the patient's recovery:

*He did beautifully. He was extubated the next day.
He had his Swan out the next day. And, he went to
the floor the third day post-op. He did just wonder-
fully. He was so relaxed. He knew what was going
on. He knew when it was going to happen and how
things were going to happen. You know, he didn't
need any of the Valium they thought he was going to
need to relax him; he had some pain meds, but nothing like we had expected. He was like a different person, considering pre-op he was so nervous; he was so
teary-eyed initially. He wasn't sure if this was really
worth being 71 years old and all.*

Introduction

By its very nature, trauma is thrust upon an individual suddenly and dramatically; there is no time for psychologic preparation or anticipatory teaching. As illustrated in the Clinical Insight, the nurse plays a pivotal
role not only in caring for the patient physically after a
traumatic experience but also in helping the person cope
psychologically with the aftermath of trauma.

Trauma is defined as injury resulting from an external force. It may be accidental, self-inflicted, or an act
of violent aggression. The neglected disease of modern
society, trauma is the leading cause of death for individuals between ages of 1 and 44 years; and for all ages it
ranks third behind cancer and cardiovascular disease.
Affecting primarily males, its peak incidence is in the
15–24 age group. Each year in this country, over
140,000 individuals die as a result of trauma; and for
every death, another two to four individuals are permanently disabled. Trauma is of epidemic proportions
and is a major health issue facing today's society. The
costs associated with trauma in this country exceed $83
billion annually. This amounts to $228 million each day,
which is greater than the costs associated with cardiovascular disease and trails only the amount spent for
individuals with cancer or other terminal illness.

Trauma may be classified as blunt, penetrating, or a
combination of both. *Penetrating trauma* (gunshot
wounds and stabbings) frequently occurs in urban inner-

city areas; *blunt trauma*, often associated with motor
vehicle accidents, falls, assaults and other similar mechanisms of injury, is seen more frequently in rural and
suburban areas. Burns resulting from thermal, chemical
and electrical causes are often referred to as traumatic
events.

Trauma may be further categorized into minor or
major injuries. A *minor trauma* is a single-system injury
that does not pose a threat to life or limb. Appropriate
treatment for such minor injuries can be provided in
hospital emergency departments. On the other hand,
victims of *major trauma*—serious, multiple-system injuries—require immediate and specialized intervention
to prevent loss of life or limb. Table 21–1 lists types of
injuries and physiologic states that require trauma-center care. Regionalization of trauma care and the designation of trauma centers helps to provide optimum care
for victims of major trauma. Recent studies indicate
that, since the advent of trauma care systems, there
has been a significant decrease in mortality and morbidity related to traumatic injury (West et al. 1983; San
Diego County 1987).

A systems approach to trauma care involves not only
the designation of trauma centers (that is, hospitals
making a special commitment to the care of trauma patients), but also the development and maintenance of a
community trauma system. Regionalized trauma care
requires organization of activities from time of injury
through discharge from the hospital, rehabilitation, and

TABLE 21–1 TYPES OF INJURIES AND PHYSIOLOGIC STATES THAT POTENTIALLY BENEFIT FROM TRAUMA-CENTER CARE

- Systolic blood pressure < 90 (adult)
- Systolic blood pressure < 60 (child)
- Delayed capillary refill
- No spontaneous eye opening
- Penetrating cranial injury
- Penetrating thoracic injury between the midclavicular lines
- Gunshot wound to abdomen or thorax
- Unstable chest wall (flail chest)
- Penetrating injury to neck
- Falls from heights greater than 15 feet
- Survivors of vehicular accidents in which fatalities occurred
- Pedestrians struck by automobiles
- Patients ejected from open or closed vehicles
- Patients requiring extended extrication from accident vehicle, etc.
- Very young and very old patients and those with precarious medi-
  cal histories

TABLE 21–2 ESSENTIAL COMPONENTS OF A TRAUMA CARE SYSTEM

- Triage and in-field treatment
- Communications network
- Transportation: air and ground
- Patient management within hospital (trauma-team concept)
- Education of medical and paramedical professionals and public about trauma care and prevention
- Evaluation of care

return to society. Essential components of a trauma system are presented in Table 21–2.

Prevention is the ultimate goal of a trauma care system. Unlike physiologic changes due to medical disease processes, the occurrence of trauma is entirely preventable. Community education and awareness programs are successful in decreasing the mortality and morbidity associated with traumatic injury. Such effort should be aimed toward the 15–24 age group, where peak incidence occurs. Additional efforts should be directed at alcohol and drug use, since that is frequently a factor in major accidents and injuries.

Nursing Roles

An organized approach to trauma care requires the delineation of specific roles and responsibilities for trauma team members. The trauma team responsible for the initial resuscitation and stabilization of critically injured

TABLE 21–3 TYPICAL MAKEUP OF A HOSPITAL TRAUMA TEAM

- Trauma surgeon—team captain
- Emergency physician
- Anesthesiologist
- Trauma nurse team leader (TNTL)—emergency nurse
- Trauma resuscitation nurse—critical-care nurse
- Trauma scribe—emergency nurse
- Trauma surgical nurse
- Radiology technologist
- Laboratory technologist
- Respiratory technologist
- Social worker
- Nursing supervisor

individuals usually includes the health care providers listed in Table 21–3. The typical trauma team includes 3–5 professional nurses, usually from the emergency department, critical-care unit, and surgical suite. Each individual has specifically delineated roles and responsibilities meant to provide the trauma patient with optimal care.

The critical-care nurse in the trauma resuscitation areas assists with the initial resuscitation and provides continuity of care by remaining with the patient throughout resuscitation and definitive care. Table 21–4 shows a typical trauma team protocol for the critical-care nurse functioning as a member of the trauma team.

Once the resuscitation and diagnostic studies are completed, the major trauma victim will be transferred to either the operating room (for necessary surgical intervention) or the intensive care unit (for continued assessment and intervention).

The critical-care nurse must be knowledgeable about the physiologic responses to injury and potential injuries

TABLE 21–4 TRAUMA RESUSCITATION TEAM PROTOCOL FOR THE CRITICAL-CARE NURSE

Title: critical-care trauma nurse, who is a registered nurse with specialized training in caring for the critically ill and traumatized patient, who is preassigned to the trauma team by the critical-care charge nurse, and who functions as trauma support nurse

How notified: by trauma beeper and voice page

Who responds: the designated critical-care nurse

Responds to: trauma resuscitation area

Reports to: trauma nurse team leader (TNTL)

Functions performed:

1. Obtains report on patient status from TNTL.
2. Assists with removal of clothing.
3. Assists with trays and procedures as directed by TNTL.
4. Monitors intravenous fluids and blood therapy (rates, patency, infectious control techniques, proper taping), replaces solutions, and obtains flow rates from trauma surgeon. Informs trauma scribe of fluid intake and replacements for documentation.
5. Obtains central venous pressure readings and reports to trauma surgeon and trauma scribe for documentation.
6. Inserts foley catheter, dips urine for blood, sends specimen to lab, reports output to trauma scribe for documentation.
7. Communicates with critical-care unit as to bed availability and estimated time of patient transfer.
8. Assists with taking the vital signs every 5 minutes.
9. Assists with airway management as indicated.
10. Provides continuity of care by accompanying patient through diagnostic studies and definitive care.
11. Assumes primary care in critical-care unit.

related to patterns of trauma and mechanisms of injury. For example, a trauma patient admitted to the intensive care unit after involvement as a driver in a high-speed motor vehicle accident has potential for injuries that include:

- Increased intracranial pressure (IICP)
- Cervical spine injury
- Major vessel disruption
- Cardiac tamponade
- Pneumothorax
- Tension pneumothorax
- Pulmonary contusions
- Thoracoabdominal injuries
- Orthopedic traumas

These injuries may not be apparent initially; therefore, the knowledgeable critical-care nurse maintains a high index of suspicion in assessing the trauma patient, determining appropriate diagnoses, and implementing specialized nursing care. The critical-care nurse frequently has more interaction and longer direct care responsibility for the major trauma victim than any other health care professional. Therefore, it is essential that the critical-care nurse acquire and maintain an advanced knowledge base and skills specific to the needs of critically injured patients.

The registered nurse, as a member of the multidisciplinary trauma team, is expected to function in interdependent and independent roles. Through utilization of the nursing process, the nurse determines the priorities for the nursing care of the major trauma victim and identifies the presence of one or more nursing diagnoses.

An essential component of nursing care throughout the resuscitation, definitive care, and rehabilitation phases of care is the anticipation of needs prior to their actual occurrence. An important example of this anticipatory role includes the ability to determine the needs for special equipment and supplies prior to the arrival of the patient, utilizing information reported by paramedics or other prehospital care personnel. This anticipation of needs requires a thorough knowledge and understanding of the pathophysiology of major traumatic injury and appropriate interventions.

During the initial resuscitation, stabilization, and critical care of the trauma victim, the nurse may utilize advanced assessment skills to identify injuries that require immediate intervention to prevent loss of life or limb. For example, a nurse may identify decreased breath sounds and a deviated trachea in the patient who has experienced major chest trauma. This information alone

will immediately alert the trauma team to life-threatening injuries (especially tension penumothorax) and the need for immediate intervention. Inherent in the trauma team concept is the fact that the trauma team members are competent, through advanced education and training, to respond to the specialized needs of the critically injured patient.

Documentation of care modalities, diagnostic procedures, therapeutic interventions, and patient response is a responsibility of the critical-care and trauma resuscitation nurse. During the initial resuscitation, a nurse scribe frequently is used to assure accurate documentation of the specific individuals involved and the chronology of events. In the critical-care unit, an extensive nursing flow sheet is ideal for documenting appropriate and necessary information.

MULTIPLE TRAUMA

To combat the disheartening mortality and morbidity from trauma, critical-care nurses should make sound clinical decisions based on current scientific principles of therapy. This section focuses on the assessment and implementation of care in managing the multiple trauma patient. Key concepts pertaining to the etiology and mechanisms of traumatic injury also are presented.

Key Concepts

The Body's Response to Injury

Injury occurs when an energy load applied to the body exceeds the body's ability to withstand that energy. This energy load, defined as kinetic energy or energy of motion, can be represented by the following equation:

$$\text{Kinetic energy} = \frac{\text{Mass} \times \text{Velocity}^2}{2}$$

Kinetic energy applied to the body causes either blunt or penetrating trauma. The extent of the injury depends on the amount of energy absorbed by the body tissues at the time of impact.

Principles of Injury in Blunt Trauma

Not all kinetic energy produced in a collision is applied to the body tissues. For example, in blunt trauma from motor vehicle accidents, kinetic energy is dissipated in two impacts. The *primary* impact occurs as the car hits an immovable object; the kinetic energy expended at this point is evidenced by damage to the exterior of the vehicle. The *secondary* impact occurs as the body set in motion by the primary impact collides with immovable objects such as the steering wheel, the dashboard, and the windshield. The extent or severity of injury following the secondary impact is determined by the amount of energy remaining after the primary impact; that is, the secondary impact energy. This also may be influenced by *stopping distance*. The importance of the relationship between stopping distance and the extent of injury was first identified in 1942, when it was discovered that the greater the stopping distance, the more kinetic energy is dissipated and the smaller the extent of bodily injury (May 1984).

The term *force* is used to describe the amount of energy that is directed at body tissues, taking into account any factors influencing stopping distance. Force can be represented by the following equation:

$$\text{Force} = \frac{\text{Kinetic energy}}{\text{Stopping distance}}$$

There have been reported cases of survivals from free falls varying from 55–146 feet. In each case survival was possible because the victims landed in a prone or supine position onto a yielding structure, such as a roof or soft earth, that allowed time for deceleration (May 1984). Airbags and sturdy automobile frames increase stopping distance and decrease the force applied to body tissues, respectively, thereby increasing survivability following major motor vehicle accidents.

There are three basic types of force as characterized by their effects on a given mass: tension, compression and shear. A *tensile* force tends to pull apart; a *compressive* force tends to push together; and a *shearing* force tends to make part of a tissue slide over an immediately adjacent part (May 1984). These forces can act alone or in combination; the result is always deformity. The extent to which this deformity causes injury is determined by the characteristics of the tissues. In response to an applied force, highly elastic tissue such as colon and bowel can stretch tremendously without damage. Even

normal bone possesses a small amount of elasticity. However, if the force exceeds the tissue's ability to withstand that force, injury will result.

Blunt forces of great magnitude cause multiple injuries. This is because the force is distributed over larger body areas. A major study analyzing data from 57,597 victims of rural automobile accidents found that only 30% of the injuries were limited to one body area; 70% involved at least two body areas; and 38% involved more than two. The victims that were critically injured had injuries to the head, neck, thorax, and abdomen in some combination (Gurdjian et al. 1970).

Factors that influence the severity of the body's response to an injuring force include (May 1984):

1. *Area over which the force is concentrated.* The wider the area, the greater the body's chance of absorbing the force and avoiding severe organ injury.

2. *Location of the impact.* Vital structures such as the heart and lungs may be spared, since the rib cage and sternum may absorb much of the applied force. The abdominal organs are more prone to injury, since they lack the protective bony structures of the chest wall.

3. *Safety equipment and protective clothing.* These can often prevent or greatly reduce morbidity and mortality following severe impacts. Following primary collision, seat belts keep the victim in the automobile and help avoid the secondary collision of body parts against such structures as the steering wheel, windshield, and dashboard, which can be fatal. Airbags increase the stopping distance of body parts and also prevent their impact with the previously mentioned unyielding automobile structures. Protective leather clothing and helmets can absorb much of the tearing and shearing forces following motorcycle accidents.

Falls, motor vehicle accidents (including motorcycle accidents), and pedestrian trauma account for the majority of injuries from blunt trauma. The forces responsible for producing injury via these particular mechanisms can be either direct or indirect. A *direct* force causes injury by direct impact or forced compression. An *indirect* force causes injury during rapid acceleration or deceleration as body tissues and vessels are stretched, rotated, and torn from points of attachment. Ordinarily, a combination of these forces is involved in producing blunt injuries.

Often, blunt injuries are difficult to diagnose, since surface trauma may or may not be present. Due to this fact, blunt trauma presents a major challenge to the critical-care team. A high index of suspicion is needed when assessing these injuries, to avoid missing occult internal injuries that, if undetected, can lead to preventable deaths.

Principles of Injury in Penetrating Trauma

The theory of kinetic energy is used to illustrate the importance of mass and velocity as they relate to the extent of injury in penetrating trauma. The most common types of penetrating trauma are stab and gunshot wounds. Weapons that inflict these wounds can be classified according to their velocity at impact. *Knives* or other sharp instruments are low-velocity-impact weapons. As these instruments enter the body, tissues are pushed aside and the damage inflicted is limited to a small area surrounding the center of the wounding track. Morbidity and mortality depend only on the structures that have been penetrated; however, these wounds can be rapidly lethal if a vital structure such as the heart, the brain, or a large vessel has been injured. *Firearms* can be classified as low-, medium-, or high-velocity-impact weapons. The extent of injury inflicted by these weapons is directly related to the amount of kinetic energy the bullet expends in the tissue. Factors that determine the amount of energy delivered to the tissue in gunshot wounds are:

- Caliber of the weapon
- Construction of the bullet
- Velocity of the weapon
- Firing distance

To understand the relationship of these factors to energy release, certain terms need to be clarified. Table 20–5 defines common terms used in the assessment of gunshot wounds.

The velocity of a missile contributes more to its kinetic energy and wounding capability than the mass of the bullet. The following principle is a good rule of thumb in estimating kinetic energy of firearms:

TABLE 21–5 BALLISTICS TERMINOLOGY

TERM	DEFINITION
Ballistics	Science of the motion of traveling projectiles: barrel of firearm → trajectory through air → final complicated motion after projectile strikes target
Caliber	Approximate diameter of the bullet, in inches
Gauge	Diameter of the shotgun barrel
Velocity	Speed of the projectile, in ft/sec
Magnum	Addition of extra gunpowder to a bullet to increase its weight and destructiveness

Doubling the *size* of a bullet *doubles* its energy.

Doubling the *speed* of a bullet *quadruples* its energy.

Another important factor in estimating kinetic energy of firearms and their wounding capability is *firing distance*. The velocity of all bullets falls off with increasing distance. This is especially true of handguns, since they ordinarily are effective only at short ranges (less than 50 yards).

A bullet that merely passes through, only severing structures as it goes, transmits very little energy to the tissue. To be able to transmit its energy and thus inflict greater damage, the missile must slow down dramatically or stop in the tissue. Various bullets have been designed to do just that. Bullets that are hollow-point or soft-nosed tend to mushroom after perforating the target, expanding to several times their original caliber (diameter). This flattening out of the bullet gives up greater amounts of kinetic energy to the tissue. Other bullets are designed to disintegrate or to tumble once they have penetrated the target. Any of these actions increases their wounding power.

The density of the tissue penetrated by bullets also influences the amount of kinetic energy released. The greater the density of the tissue the bullet passes through, the more the bullet is slowed down and the more kinetic energy is expended in the tissue. For example, lung tissue, because of its low density, is minimally damaged by bullets, whereas the high-density liver tissue is severely damaged, as greater energy is expended.

A temporary cavity may be formed in the tissue by the transmission of kinetic energy from the bullet to the surrounding tissue. The energy shock waves develop after penetration with high-velocity weapons as the tissue is accelerated forward and laterally away from the bullet. This millisecond acceleration generates a transient, water-vapor-filled cavity around the bullet and its track. The cavity may be up to 30 times the diameter of the bullet. The subatmospheric conditions inside the cavity can cause further damage by drawing contaminants such as clothing and soil into the wound. The cavity alternately stretches and compresses until energy is dissipated, so extensive damage can occur to tissues even though they are not in the direct path of the bullet. This phenomenon of cavity formation is illustrated in Figure 21–1 (Barach et al. 1986).

Critical-care nurses who understand these concepts of kinetic energy and the body's response to blunt and penetrating forces will be better equipped to assess and manage these challenging trauma patients.

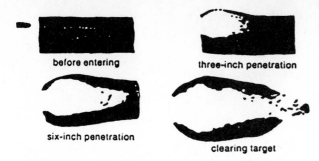

FIGURE 21–1

A high-velocity bullet fired into a block of gelatin demonstrates the formation of a temporary cavity. The cavity is formed by the transmission of kinetic energy from the bullet to the surrounding tissue. Cavitation lasts only 5–10 milliseconds, but pressure on the walls can be 100 times atmospheric, causing damage to the surrounding tissues. (Reprinted from: Swan KG, Swan RC: *Gunshot wounds: Pathophysiology and management.* Littleton, MA: PSG Publishing, 1980.)

Assessment

Risk Factors

Epidemiologic studies have identifed specific factors that predispose individuals to increased risk of becoming a victim of traumatic injury. Injury no longer is viewed as a result of chance, but rather as "an event that is caused by the interaction of specific factors which are amenable to preventive interventions" (Thompson 1986). These risk factors follow.

Alcohol use: Greater than 50% of all trauma is reported to occur in the presence of elevated blood alcohol concentrations.

Sex: Males are at 50% greater risk for fatal injury than females.

Age: The highest rates of both fatal and nonfatal injuries occurs in the 15–24-year-old age group, with the highest incidence of fatal injury occurring in the elderly population (60 years and older).

Though education regarding injury prevention is not a priority in the initial care of these multiple trauma victims, patient and family education regarding preventable measures is still a responsibility of trauma nurses in the critical-care setting.

A prioritized, systematic approach to the assessment of the multiple trauma patient is the key to planning and implementing effective care. This is more difficult than it sounds, since the bloody, disfiguring injuries that accompany trauma, though often not fatal, can be distracting and prevent the early identification of life-threatening conditions.

There are two components to a complete assessment of the multiple trauma patient:

The history—This involves the identification of the mechanism of injury and the past medical history of the patient.

The physical examination—This is divided into the primary and secondary surveys.

History

Mechanism of Injury and Past Medical History

Identification of the mechanism of injury (MOI) involves defining the who, what, where, when, and why of the injuring event. The prehospital report sheet or the emergency resuscitation record can help identify these factors. If the patient is alert and oriented, he or she may be able to provide some of these details. Table 21–6 lists some factors that may be used to ascertain such details. The key point to remember in identifying the mechanism of injury is to make it specific to each individual patient, i.e., to determine the amount of force that was directed at *that* patient's body tissue at the moment of impact.

The complete history of the mechanism of injury may reveal information that will heighten your index of suspicion regarding actual and potential injuries. Subsequently, the physical examination will become more individualized as areas of the body are preidentified for being at risk and requiring in-depth assessment. This focus leads to earlier identification and treatment of all injuries and greatly affects mortality and morbidity following multiple trauma.

The past medical history of the patient always has been an important component in the assessment of critically ill or injured individuals. In trauma care the pneumonic "AMPLE" has been used to elicit crucial data points:

A Allergies

M Medications

P Present illnesses

L Last meal

E Events preceding injury (chest pain, seizure before the accident, etc.)

TABLE 21–6 FACTORS TO ASSESS TO DETERMINE TRAUMATIC FORCE AND BODY AREAS MOST SUSCEPTIBLE TO INJURY

MOTOR VEHICLE ACCIDENTS	FALLS	PENETRATING TRAUMA

Estimated speed of accident:
  Freeway vs surface street
Direction of vehicle impact:
  Frontal
  Lateral
  Rear
Damage to vehicle:
  Front end
  Rear end
  Side doors caved into passenger space
  Steering wheel bent
  Windshield broken
Position of victim in vehicle:
  Front seat—driver/passenger
  Back seat
  Victim ejected from vehicle
Seat belt/no seat belt
Extrication of victim required
Another passenger (in same or other vehicle) dead at scene
Motorcycle:
  Helmet/no helmet
  Protective clothing
  Distance victim found from motorcycle
Pedestrian:
  Type of vehicle that struck victim
  Traveling speed of vehicle
  Estimated distance victim was thrown and body points of impact
	Height of fall
	Any evidence of stopping distance
	Surface onto which victim fell
	Position which victim was found after fall
	Evidence of any other injury prior to fall (gunshot wounds, stab wounds, physical assault)
		Gunshot Wounds
		
		Location of wounds
		Caliber/velocity of weapon
		Distance from which patient was shot:
		  Close range
		  Long range
		Character of wounds:
		  Size
		  Extent of external tissue destruction
		  Powder burns surrounding wounds (indicates victim was shot at close range)
		  Number of "shots" heard by bystanders or victim
		
		Stab Wounds
		
		Location of wounds
		Type of weapon
		Length of blade
		Depth of penetration

Physical Examination

Primary Survey The primary survey is a rapid (60–90 seconds) evaluation of the airway, breathing, circulatory, and disability or neurologic (ABCD) status of the trauma patient. It involves look–listen–feel techniques to identify life-threatening injuries in order of ABCD priority. The necessity for speed in managing these critically injured patients often dictates that assessment and resuscitative interventions become simultaneous functions. If a problem is encountered in the ABCD primary survey, it is dealt with at that time. Interventions are discussed in the planning and implementation phases of care. Table 21–7 summarizes the steps of the primary survey.

Secondary Survey The secondary survey is the head-to-toe, front-to-back physical examination of the patient. The steps of physical assessment are done in their correct order (inspection, percussion, palpation, auscultation) and according to the body region involved. An example of some signs and symptoms to look for in the secondary survey of a multiple trauma patient are outlined in Table 21–8. This assessment format should

TABLE 21–7 THE PRIMARY ASSESSMENT SURVEY

Airway	Assess patency while ensuring cervical spine immobilization.
Breathing	Assess for presence or absence of breathing; if present, assess effectiveness.
Circulation	Assess for presence or absence of a major pulse. Assess overall peripheral perfusion. Look for major external signs of hemorrhage.
Disability (neurologic status)	Assess level of consciousness. Assess pupillary response to light. Assess gross motor and sensory function.

TABLE 21–8 THE SECONDARY ASSESSMENT SURVEY (ANTERIOR AND POSTERIOR)

Head/Face	Inspect/palpate bones and skin for bony deformities, malocclusion, edema, and surface trauma. Inspect eyes for extraocular movements; assess for visual changes. Inspect ears for otorrhea; assess hearing. Inspect nose for rhinorrhea or nasal flaring.
Neck	Inspect/palpate for tracheal deviation, neck vein distention, cervical spine tenderness, edema, subcutaneous emphysema, surface trauma. Assess for hoarseness or dysphagia.
Chest	Inspect chest wall for wounds, ecchymoses, abrasions, or other surface trauma. Inspect/palpate thoracic cage for unequal chest excursion, paradoxical movement, crepitus, retractions. Auscultate for diminished or absent breath sounds or muffled heart sounds.
Abdomen	Inspect abdominal wall for wounds, ecchymoses, other surface trauma, distention. Auscultate for abnormal bowel sounds. Palpate for rigidity, guarding, pain, rebound tenderness.
Pelvis/Genitalia	Palpate pelvis for instability. Inspect perineum and genitalia for lacerations, hematomas, edema. Inspect urinary meatus and anus for blood. Palpate vagina for masses and lacerations; palpate rectum for masses, sphincter tone, prostatic displacement.
Extremities	Inspect for bony deformities, edema, hematomas, surface trauma. Palpate bones for tenderness, crepitus, instability. Palpate peripheral pulses for absent or unequal pulses.

be used regardless of when the nurse encounters the trauma patient. It is a prioritized approach that identifies life-threatening problems first and organizes a head-to-toe physical examination in order of priority body regions.

A full set of vital signs (temperature, pulse, respiratory rate, blood pressure) is obtained at this time. And all clothing is removed, to enable thorough assessment (which may entail cutting off the clothing if the patient needs to remain in full spinal immobilization throughout the assessment phase). After the patient is completely exposed, measures to prevent hypothermia are used, such as warm blankets or heat lamps. Diagnostic tests are completed at this time, and specialty consultants, such as neurosurgery and orthopedics, are notified as needed.

In the presence of life-threatening or potentially life-threatening ABCD injuries, physical examination begins immediately, and the full details of the subjective history are obtained as the patient stabilizes.

Cardinal Rules in Major Multiple Trauma

With these assessment data, a plan of care can be developed and interventions carried out in their order of priority. There are a few axioms or cardinal rules in the assessment of the multiple trauma patient that, if adhered to, can guide the critical-care team in organizing and prioritizing the plan of care to avoid delays in diagnosis and treatment. Table 21–9 lists these cardinal rules.

Planning and Implementation of Care, Emergent Period

In the emergent phase, the goal of therapy is the immediate institution of organized life-saving therapeutic interventions to reverse respiratory and cardiovascular compromise and manage elevated intracranial pressure.

NURSING DIAGNOSES (ACTUAL OR POTENTIAL)

Most of the approved nursing diagnoses can be used at one point or another in the care of multiple trauma patients. The major actual or potential nursing diagnoses that may be encountered during the emergent and acute phases of care include:

EMERGENT PERIOD

Airway

- Ineffective airway clearance

Breathing

- Ineffective breathing patterns
- Impaired gas exchange

Circulation

- Alteration in cardiac output: decreased
- Alteration in tissue perfusion: cardiopulmonary and peripheral
- Fluid volume deficit, actual or potential

Disability (Neurological)

- Alteration in tissue perfusion: cerebral
- Impaired physical mobility: spinal cord injury

ACUTE PERIOD

Physical

- Potential for infection
- Impaired tissue integrity
- Alteration in comfort: pain
- Activity intolerance
- Hypothermia
- Alteration in urinary elimination
- Alteration in bowel elimination
- Alteration in nutrition: less than body requirements

Psychosocial

- Impaired verbal communication
- Anxiety
- Fear
- Powerlessness
- Posttrauma response
- Ineffective individual family coping related to traumatic experience

TABLE 21–9 CARDINAL RULES IN MULTIPLE TRAUMA

Until proven otherwise:

1. All patients with head and facial trauma have a cervical spine injury.
2. All patients with an altered level of consciousness have a head injury.
3. All young, healthy patients lacking a palpable radial pulse are in shock.
4. Hypotension, tachycardia, and pallor indicate bleeding into the chest, abdomen, or pelvis if no obvious external injuries are present.
5. All patients with chest trauma are presumed critical.
6. All patients with distended neck veins have a pericardial tamponade or tension pneumothorax.
7. Penetrating wounds at or below the nipple line involve the chest and abdomen.
8. Systolic blood pressure is estimated to be:
   Palpable radial pulse = 80–100 mm Hg.
   Palpable femoral pulse = 70 mm Hg.
   Palpable carotid pulse = 60 mm Hg.

Ineffective Airway Clearance Related to Obstructed Airway

Airway obstruction in the multiple trauma patient may be due to the following

- The tongue
- Blood or vomitus
- Soft tissue facial or neck trauma
- Instability of maxillary or mandibular structures

Complete airway obstruction will present with no evidence of breathing. *Partial* obstruction will present with noisy, stridorous breathing and deep intercostal and substernal retractions. The presence of an airway obstruction necessitates the following interventions:

1. Perform a jaw thrust or a chin lift to open the airway. (Hyperextension of the head and neck is avoided at all costs due to suspected cervical spine injury.)
2. Remove debris from the oral cavity—suction as needed.
3. Insert an oral or nasal pharyngeal airway.
4. Ventilate the patient with 100% oxygen via bag-valve mask device as needed.
5. Prepare to assist with oral or nasal tracheal intubation.

6. If intubation is unsuccessful (two attempts), prepare to assist with initiation of a surgical airway—either cricothyroidostomy or tracheostomy (selection will be based on physician preference and skill level).

7. If patient does not require intubation, monitor patency and be prepared to intervene as needed.

8. If patient is not intubated, consider insertion of a naso/orogastric tube as a second-line airway protection to prevent respiratory compromise from aspiration of blood or vomitus.

Ineffective Breathing Patterns

Ineffective breathing patterns in the multiple trauma victim may be related to the following:

- Decreased level of consciousness (head injury, drugs, alcohol)
- Tension pneumothorax
- Flail chest
- Pulmonary vessel injury with large hemothorax
- Penetrating chest trauma
- Pulmonary contusion
- Tracheal-bronchial tear
- Spinal cord injury
- Pain from any combination of injuries

In the presence of any of the above identified injuries, the critical-care nurse should observe for the following signs and symptoms:

- Dyspnea, tachypnea
- Tachycardia, hypotension
- Asymmetric chest wall expansion
- Use of accessory or abdominal muscles for breathing
- Distended neck veins
- Tracheal shift
- Paradoxical chest wall movement
- Decreased lung sounds
- Bloody secretions from the airway
- Sucking chest wounds
- Reduced arterial P_{O_2}

Measures to alleviate the ineffective breathing patterns are directed toward the specific cause and include the following interventions.

1. Establish and maintain airway patency.

2 Oxygenate and ventilate according to specific patient needs.

3. Obtain ABGs and chest x-ray as needed.

4. Prepare for interventions specific to cause—for example:

- Needle thoracostomy followed by chest tube insertion for tension pneumothorax
- Chest tube insertion for hemo/pneumothorax
- Occlusive dressing to sucking chest wound
- Intubation, high-flow oxygen, aggressive pulmonary toilet for pulmonary contusion
- Bronchoscopy and surgical repair for tracheal-bronchial tear

Impaired Gas Exchange

This may result from injury to the central nervous system, the chest, or the abdomen, with alteration in oxygenation and ventilation, or major hemorrhage.

Monitor the patient's respiratory and cardiovascular status continuously. Administer humidified high-flow oxygen (6–8 liters) to all multiple trauma patients. Monitor arterial blood gas values and ventilation as measured by tidal volume, vital capacity, and FEV_1, etc. Suction the patient as needed. Be prepared to assist with intubation or a surgical airway procedure as needed.

Alteration in Cardiac Output: Decreased

Signs and symptoms depend on the cause. Common causes of decreased cardiac output in the multiple trauma patient are:

- Cardiac tamponade
- Tension pneumothorax
- Acute major loss of circulating blood volume

Treatment is directed at relieving the cause.

Cardiac Tamponade   A pericardiocentesis is done to relieve cardiac tamponade. (Keep in mind that, if the cause of the tamponade is a penetrating injury to the heart, an emergency thoracotomy will need to be done as definitive therapy.) A pericardiocentesis is a short-term, emergency measure to allow for some return of function of the left ventricle. If cardiac tamponade occurs as a result of blunt trauma to the chest, the blood in the pericardial sac most likely will not be clotted blood, and aspiration—even with a large-bore (19-gauge) spinal needle—will be inadequate to remove the obstruction. A surgical procedure ("pericardial window") will have to be performed in the operating room.

Tension Pneumothorax   In the critical-care unit, tension pneumothorax may be seen as a result of mechanical ventilation. The classic signs and symptoms are:

- Decreased systolic blood pressure
- Increased central venous pressure as manifested by elevated CVP readings (15–20 cm H_2O) or distended neck veins
- Tracheal deviation away from the affected side
- Absent lung sounds on affected side
- Severe dyspnea

The immediate measure to relieve the tension pneumothorax is decompressive thoracostomy with a large-bore (12–16-gauge) needle in the second intercostal space, midclavicular line, followed by chest tube insertion. See the section on chest trauma for further details.

Acute Major Loss of Circulating Blood Volume
Decreased cardiac output as a result of major blood loss is treated with crystalloid and blood replacement.

Decreased Tissue Perfusion Related to Acute Loss of Circulating Blood Volume

Fluid Volume Deficit Related to Acute Loss of Circulating Blood Volume

Interventions directed at correcting these two nursing diagnoses in the multiple trauma patient are very similar. The section on shock in Chapter 13 covers the general interventions. Specifics for the multiple trauma patient include:

- High-flow oxygen administration or intubation with mechanical ventilation to maintain Po_2 at more than 80 mm Hg
- Control of major external hemorrhage with direct pressure
- Major venous access and establishment of a minimum of two large-bore (14–16 gauge) peripheral

intravenous lines closest to the central circulation (antecubital lines are the best)

- If unable to access peripheral lines, be prepared to assist the physician with a saphenous vein cutdown, femoral, internal jugular, or subclavian vein cannulation

Hemorrhage in trauma is classified according to the physiologic response to percent of acute blood volume lost. Fluid resuscitation proceeds according to the class of hemorrhage (Table 21–10). In Class I and II hemorrhage the "3:1" rule of fluid replacement applies: 3 ml of crystalloid solution is given for every 1 ml blood lost. This amounts to a fluid challenge of 1–3 liters of fluid. The patient's response is observed during the fluid administration; if there is not a satisfactory response ($\uparrow$BP, $\downarrow$HR, $\downarrow$RR, improvement in peripheral skin signs), the patient is assumed to be in Class III to Class IV hemorrhage. Blood products are begun on a 1:1 ratio of replacement: for every milliliter of blood lost a milliliter of blood is replaced.

The pneumatic antishock garment (PASG) (Figure 21–2) may be used along with fluid resuscitation to raise the systolic blood pressure to an acceptable level (100 mm Hg). The use of this device is clouded in controversy, but some trauma centers still use it in the period immediately following acute blood loss (1–2 hours).

If the patient does not respond to fluid replacement and the use of the PASG, operative intervention must be considered to definitively control major chest or abdominal cavity hemorrhage.

Hemodynamic monitoring in the critically injured volume-depleted patient usually includes measurements of arterial pressure, CVP, PAP, PCWP, and cardiac output. Pulmonary artery catheters are particularly useful in assessing the response of an impaired left ventricle to fluids and blood products (e.g., elderly patients with underlying cardiac disease).

Altered Tissue Perfusion, Cerebral

All interventions are aimed at maximizing cerebral perfusion with well-oxygenated blood. The goal of therapy is to prevent or minimize elevations in increased intracranial pressure following head trauma. Chapter 5 presents the specific interventions aimed at decreasing increased intracranial pressure.

Remember that an adult with multiple trauma cannot be hypotensive due to blood loss from a closed head injury. If the unconscious multiple trauma patient is hypotensive from acute blood loss, you must assess the chest or abdomen to determine the source of bleeding. Major long-bone fractures (femur) and displaced pelvic fractures also can cause major blood loss.

TABLE 21–10 ESTIMATED FLUID AND BLOOD REQUIREMENTS* (BASED ON PATIENT'S INITIAL PRESENTATION)

	CLASS I	CLASS II	CLASS III	CLASS IV
Blood loss (ml)	up to 750	750–1500	1500–2000	2000 or more
Blood loss (%BV)	up to 15%	15–30%	30–40%	40% or more
Pulse rate	<100	>100	>120	140 or higher
Blood pressure	Normal	Normal	Decreased	Decreased
Pulse pressure (mm Hg)	Normal or increased	Decreased	Decreased	Decreased
Capillary blanch test	Normal	Positive	Positive	Positive
Respiratory rate	14–20	20–30	30–40	>35
Urine output (ml/hr)	30 or more	20–30	5–15	Negligible
CNS-mental status	Slightly anxious	Mildly anxious	Anxious and confused	Confused-lethargic
Fluid replacement (3:1 rule)	Crystalloid	Crystalloid	Crystalloid and blood	Crystalloid and blood

*For a 70-kg male.

Reprinted from American College of Surgeons, Committee on Trauma: *Advanced trauma life support course for physicians*. Chicago, IL: American College of Surgeons, 1984.

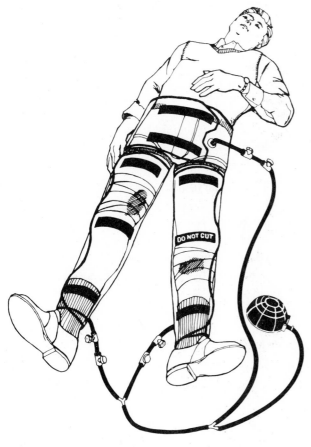

FIGURE 21–2

Pneumatic antishock garment (PASG). (Reprinted from Hammond BB, Lee G: *Emergency nursing*, 1984. By permission of David Clark Co., Inc., Worcester, Ma.

Impaired Physical Mobility Related to Spinal Cord Injury: Actual or Potential

The multiple trauma patient will be brought to the hospital by the prehospital providers in "full spinal immobilization." This means the patient is immobilized on a long backboard with a hard cervical collar, sandbags to the neck, and adhesive tape or body straps across the forehead, shoulders, and pelvis. The patient must remain immobilized until the spinal cord injury is ruled out (usually by radiographic determination) or definitive stabilization is achieved, e.g., application of cervical traction tongs, a halo device, or open-reduction, internal fixation of thoracic and lumbar vertebral fractures.

Outcome Evaluation, Emergent Period

Evaluate the patient's progress according to these outcome criteria:

• Patent airway is maintained.

• Adequate oxygenation and ventilation within patient's normal limits.

• Adequate signs of resuscitation, as evidenced by: ↑ BP and ↓ HR to within normal range; improved peripheral perfusion; preload increased to CVP 3–8 cm H_2O, PCWP 4–12 mm Hg.

- Improved cardiac output (>3.5 L/min).
- Urine output $\geq$ 0.5 ml/kg/hr.
- Increased pH.
- Patient is oriented to person, place, and time.
- Neurologic signs WNL.
- Absence or resolution of increased ICP.
- Stabilization of spinal fracture.
- Degree of sensation and movement of extremities remains stable or improved.

Planning and Implementation of Care, Acute Period

Once the emergent phase has passed and the condition of the patient stabilizes, the critical-care nurse should determine which aspects of care have priority. Infection, sepsis, and multiple organ failure are the major physical complications that are commonly seen in the multiple trauma patient. The psychosocial problems seen in multiple trauma are numerous. This section discusses two physical nursing diagnoses and one psychosocial nursing diagnosis frequently encountered in this period of care. The other diagnoses listed earlier are discussed in detail in other sections of this text, and the interventions identified there are applicable to the multiple trauma patient.

Impaired Tissue Integrity

Traumatic events resulting in open wounds are considered dirty injuries. Often the accident occurs in an unclean environment, or wounding instruments were impaled through dirty clothing. The resulting wound is considered dirty and frequently contains foreign debris. Because of these factors, the risk of infection and sepsis is significant.

Treatment is specific to the type and location of the wound. The following are guidelines for the management of wounds in multiple trauma patients.

1. Handle the wound carefully to prevent further contamination. Initially, cover all open wounds with normal-saline–soaked dressings.
2. If possible, elevate the area to promote venous and lymphatic drainage and decrease edema.
3. Observe wounds for signs of inflammation, purulent drainage, and ischemia.

4. Change dressings using meticulous sterile technique.
5. With multiple wounds, take extra care to prevent cross-contamination.
6. Establish proper nutrition and caloric intake, which are vital to wound healing.
7. Provide tetanus immunization as indicated (tetanus toxoid 0.5 ml IM if previous immunization is current; human immune globulin 250 units IM if immunization status is unknown or there is no previous immunization).
8. Pay special attention to extremity wounds occluded by plaster, to assess systemic and local extremity temperatures, capillary refill, edema, and sensory and motor capability of affected limb.

Potential for Infection

Following injury, the body instantly begins to mobilize a highly organized series of neurohumoral and cellular responses in its effort to prolong survival. The sequelae resulting from any major ABCD complications place the patient at increased risk for infection and sepsis. Prolonged periods of hypoxia and inadequate tissue perfusion are the major factors leading to alterations in cellular activity that increase the potential for infection and sepsis.

To minimize the potential for infection and sepsis in the multiple trauma patient, the critical-care nurse should do the following.

1. Monitor the patient for any signs of infection.
2. If signs or symptoms of infection or sepsis are identified, assist in rapid identification of the source.
3. Obtain cultures of any suspected sources.
4. Initiate antibiotic therapy (as ordered by the physician) as soon as possible.
5. Monitor culture and sensitivity results, and notify the physician for any needed changes in therapy.
6. Improve host defense through improved nutrition and initiation of isolation as indicated.

Ineffective Individual/Family Coping Related to Traumatic Experience

A traumatic event is sudden, unplanned, and disrupting to an individual and the significant support group. The psychologic and sociologic results can be devastating if not recognized and included in the treatment regimen. One of the most challenging aspects of nursing care for the trauma patient is the provision of psychosocial support for the patient, family, and friends as they attempt to cope with the traumatic injury.

The trauma patient will be assessed by a interdisciplinary team of experts, a team usually consisting of ten or more individuals. Invasive and often life-saving procedures will be completed simultaneously, sometimes without prior explanation. The procedures, in combination with memories of the incident resulting in injury, are often overwhelming to the trauma patient. Nursing interventions should be aimed at allowing the patient an opportunity to verbalize and to participate in the care. Chapter 3 provides specific interventions related to communication and psychosocial aspects of injury.

Outcome Evaluation, Acute Period

The overall goal for the acute period is to transfer the patient from the critical-care unit with intact and functional respiratory, cardiovascular, neurologic, genitourinary, and gastrointestinal systems. The following outcome evaluation criteria are related specifically to the nursing diagnoses discussed in this section.

- Vital signs WNL.
- Wounds free of signs of infection.
- Patient and significant others are utilizing appropriate coping mechanisms.
- Patient is physically and psychologically ready for any needed rehabilitation.

Summary

In the care of multiple trauma patients, critical-care nurses can make a difference. Trauma must be considered as a disease that has its own natural history and specialized problems. In order to deliver effective nursing care, the critical-care nurse should be able to understand and integrate the variety of data representing multiple organ systems. Based on these data, the critical-care nurse then should develop a plan of care that addresses life-threatening problems in order of priority and prevents delays in intervention and treatment. This approach enables the critical-care nurse to have the

greatest impact on traumatic injury by decreasing morbidity.

The care of multiple trauma patients is often multidisciplinary, involving all hospital departments. The critical-care nurse, in conjunction with the primary surgeon, should coordinate these efforts in order to provide optimal care and to minimize the physiologic and psychologic impacts of the injury.

HEAD INJURY

In the United States, over 400,000 people require hospitalization each year for head injury (Henkle 1986). For people under the age of 35, trauma is the number-one cause of death and neurologic disability (Lillehei and Hoff 1985). Substance abuse and noncompliance with speed limits or seat belt laws contribute to a vast majority of vehicular accidents, with two-thirds of the victims sustaining head injury. Other causes of head injury include falls, violence, and sports-related accidents. Men are victims 2–3 times more frequently than women, with the majority being between 15–24 years old. The impact of this devastating injury is not only the death toll but also the disabilities sustained, which affect patient, family, and society.

Assessment

Mechanism of Injury

Several mechanisms operating individually or simultaneously produce the injuries associated with craniocerebral trauma. When the head is struck by a moving object, such as a lead pipe, an *acceleration* injury occurs. A *deceleration* injury results when the head hits a stationary object, such as a cement sidewalk. When the head hits a stationary object while in motion, an *acceleration-deceleration* injury occurs. The *coup-contrecoup* phenomenon causes injury to the brain at the point of impact *(coup)* and on the side opposite *(contrecoup)* due to rebound from the force of the injury. Twisting of the brain is associated with rotation of the head. With these mechanisms in mind, let us review the anatomic relationship of the bony skull and the semisolid brain to bring into perspective the range of injuries encountered.

The base of the skull has bony prominences, such as the wing of the sphenoid bone and the petrous part of the temporal bone. The intracranial contents are further compartmentalized by the falx cerebri and the tentorium cerebelli (see Figure 21–3). Essentially, the skull is a closed box, with the foramen magnum being the major opening. The semisolid brain is suspended within the cranial vault and anchored by the union of the brainstem to the spinal cord.

According to Hickey (1986), acceleration-deceleration and rotation result in intracranial stresses to the brain, which take the following form: (1) compression or pushing of tissue together, (2) tension or pulling apart of tissue, and (3) shearing or sliding of portions of tissue over other portions.

Types of Injuries

Head injury occurs either primarily at the moment of impact or secondarily as a delayed event (Shpritz 1983; Ward 1984).

Primary Injury   *Primary injury* is damage to brain tissue produced at the time of impact; it includes frac-

ture, concussion, contusion, and laceration (Shpritz 1983).

Skull Fractures   Skull fractures are classified as linear, comminuted, depressed, compound, or basal skull fractures. The majority of skull fractures are *linear,* which involves a single crack in the skull. Fragmentation of the bone is referred to as a *comminuted* fracture; if bone is displaced inward into the brain, it is called a *depressed* fracture. If a linear, comminuted, or depressed fracture occurs with an external opening, it is referred to as a *compound* fracture. Compound fractures communicate directly with intracranial contents, providing a direct route for bacterial invasion.

Basal skull fractures warrant special attention because of the potential for more serious sequelae. The base of the skull is divided into the anterior, middle, and posterior fossae. A fracture of the anterior fossa may traverse the paranasal air sinuses, while a fracture of the middle fossa involves the temporal petrous bone. The dura closely adheres to the bone, resulting in a dural tear and leakage of cerebrospinal fluid when a fracture occurs. *Rhinorrhea* is the drainage of cerebrospinal fluid and blood from the nose; leakage of the same components from the ear is called *otorrhea*. The danger to the patient is an intracranial infection, since organisms can enter via the dural tear.

Diagnosis of a skull fracture commonly is based on

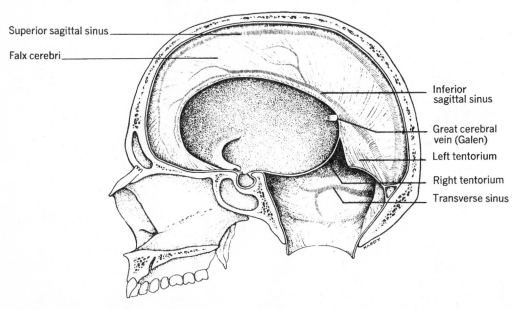

FIGURE 21–3

Cranial dura mater. The skull opened to show the falx cerebri and the right and left portions of the tentorium cerebelli, as well as some of the cranial venous sinuses. (From Chaffee EE, Lytle IM: *Basic physiology and anatomy.* Published by Lippincott/ Harper & Row, 1980. Reprinted by permission of EE Chaffee.

skull films. Basal fractures are difficult to visualize on x-ray, so physical findings play a major role in making the diagnosis. Rhinorrhea, subconjunctival hemorrhage, and periorbital ecchymosis (racoon's eyes) are clinical indicators of an anterior fossa fracture. Fracture of the middle fossa, involving the middle ear, causes otorrhea, ecchymosis over the mastoid bone (Battle's sign), hemotympanum, and possibly facial nerve palsy.

Concussion Concussion is a clinical term describing temporary, diffuse neuronal dysfunction due to head injury, often described as "jarring" the brain. Signs and symptoms last from minutes to hours and include altered consciousness, confusion, headache, visual disturbances, dizziness, and irritability. Amnesia is a frequent sequela and may involve the inability to recall events that occur after the injury (posttraumatic amnesia) or events that occurred before the injury (retrograde amnesia) (Manifold 1986).

Contusions and Lacerations According to Hickey (1986), *contusion* is a bruising of part of the brain without interruption of the pial covering, although the underlying cortical tissue and white matter may be hemorrhagic. A traumatic break in the continuity of the brain tissue describes a *laceration*. Contusions and lacerations may be found with open head injuries (depressed fracture or penetrating objects) or closed (blunt) head injuries.

Common sites for contusions and lacerations include the anterior surfaces of the frontal and temporal lobes, the inferior and lateral surfaces of the temporal lobes, and the orbital areas. (The structure of the base of the skull, with its irregular surfaces, causes contusions or lacerations on impact.)

The clinical presentation of the patient with a cerebral contusion or laceration depends on the exact area of involvement and the extent of the damage. Consciousness generally is lost at the time of impact, with depth and length of unconsciousness correlating with morbidity and mortality of the patient. Other symptoms include motor, sensory, or speech disturbances.

Diagnosis and Treatment of Primary Injuries History, physical exam, skull films, and CT scanning when indicated are used to differentiate concussion from cerebral contusion and/or laceration. Patients diagnosed with a cerebral concussion may be sent home if they have a responsible party to observe them for any significant change in neurologic status. Contusions and lacerations are more serious injuries and require hospitalization. Depending on the severity, therapeutic measures might include hypertonic agents, assisted ventilation with hyperventilation, and corticosteroids.

Secondary Injury Secondary processes that may follow the primary injury include hematomas and cerebral edema (Shpritz 1983). Hematomas and edema may lead to increased intracranial pressure (IICP) and brain herniation.

Hematomas Intracranial hemorrhage may result from an open or closed head injury. When a single vessel or many small bridging vessels are torn, the blood collects and forms an expanding mass lesion. Hematomas are classified as: (1) epidural, (2) subdural, or (3) intracerebral. Intracranial hemorrhage in an adult does not produce hypovolemic shock.

Epidural Hematoma An epidural hematoma is a neurosurgical emergency associated with arterial bleeding in the potential space between the skull and the dura mater. Because the bleeding is under great pressure, it quickly can become life-threatening. Since the bleeding has to strip the dura away from the inner table of the skull, it is a more confined bleed and lenticular in shape. Fracture of the temporal bone and tearing of the middle meningeal artery lead to an epidural hematoma. Hickey (1986) reports that epidural hematomas account for about 2% of all types of head injury.

Signs and Symptoms of Epidural Hematoma The classical presentation of epidural hematoma is one of temporary loss of consciousness at the scene of the accident, followed by a lucid interval and then progressive deterioration in neurologic function. Since epidural hematomas more commonly occur unilaterally, the patient should be observed for the signs and symptoms of uncal herniation. (Refer to Chapter 5 for a detailed discussion of uncal herniation.)

Diagnosis and Treatment of Epidural Hematoma The diagnosis of epidural hematoma is made by CT scanning. Early surgical intervention optimizes the patient's chance for a more favorable outcome. Burr holes are made in the skull, allowing for clot evacuation and ligation of bleeding vessels.

Subdural Hematoma Subdural bleeding occurs in the potential space between the dura and the arachnoid layers of the meninges. Subsequent to tearing of small cerebral arteries or bridging veins, the bleeding can spread over the hemispheres in this space and put direct pressure on the brain. Hickey (1986) reports that 10–15% of head injury patients develop subdural hematomas.

Signs and Symptoms of Subdural Hematoma Categories of subdural hematomas have been formulated based on time between injury and appearance of signs and symptoms. *Acute* subdural bleeding is often associated with significant primary impact damage, such as contusions and lacerations. Within 24–48 hours, signs and symptoms of neuronal dysfunction and IICP will present. *Subacute* subdural hematomas lead to symptoms within 2 days to 2 weeks. Clinical presentation relates to the area of the brain involved, which may give localizing signs such as a dilated pupil and abnormal motor response or generalized signs of IICP.

Chronic subdurals may not cause symptoms for over 2 weeks or until months later. Due to the time lag and the seeming insignificance of the blow to the head, many patients may not remember the initial injury. Headache, mental confusion, drowsiness, and/or seizure activity cause the patient to seek medical care.

Diagnosis and Treatment of Subdural Hematoma Diagnosis of subdural hematoma is based on the CT scan. Acute, subacute, and chronic subdurals that are large enough to produce significant symptoms require surgical evacuation. Small subdurals may be followed medically if symptoms are receding.

Intracerebral Hematoma Intracerebral hemorrhage frequently accompanies contusions or lacerations, especially if there has been a penetrating head injury. According to Hickey (1986), bleeding into the cerebral substance is seen in about 2–3% of head injury patients.

Signs and Symptoms of Intracerebral Hematoma Clinical presentation of intracerebral hematoma is a combined picture of neuronal dysfunction due to cerebral contusion or laceration and the intracerebral bleeding. The patient generally is rendered unconscious from the time of the injury. Localizing signs include hemiplegia on the contralateral side, and a dilated pupil on the side of the clot. As intracranial pressure increases, signs of transtentorial herniation with accompanying changes in respirations, pupils, and motor response occur.

Diagnosis and Treatment of Intracerebral Hematoma CT scan verifies the extent of intracerebral bleeding. Due to parenchymal involvement, neurologic deficit generally is permanent, regardless of whether medical or surgical management is used.

Cerebral Edema Cerebral edema is an increase in the amount of water in the intracellular and/or extracellular space of the brain (Rudy 1984). Cerebral edema results directly from primary head injury and occurs secondarily from cerebral ischemia, anoxia, and hypercapnia. *Vasogenic edema* results from breakdown of the normal capillary membrane integrity. The altered membrane permeability allows proteins to leak into the extracellular space. This affects white matter most commonly. *Cytotoxic edema* involves increased fluid within the intracellular space. The accumulation of metabolic waste products related to anaerobic metabolism interferes

with normal cellular function. Dysfunction of the sodium pump results in an increased number of intracellular sodium ions. This displaced sodium draws water with it, leading to cellular swelling.

Cerebral edema may be localized or generalized. The extent of its development relates directly to the severity of the injury and reaches its maximum level in 24–72 hours. Cerebral edema increases brain mass, leading to IICP. Signs and symptoms depend on the primary injury and are exacerbated by the presence of cerebral edema. The CT scan is used to diagnose cerebral edema. Pharmacologic intervention for cerebral edema includes: (1) osmotic diuretics, (2) furosemide, and (3) corticosteroids.

NURSING DIAGNOSIS

The main nursing diagnosis for head injuries is:

- Altered tissue perfusion (cerebral) related to head injury

Planning and Implementation of Care

Managing the head-injured patient is a real nursing challenge. The main goals when planning and implementing care are:

1. Maintain a patent airway with adequate respiratory exchange.
2. Monitor and assess neurologic status.
3. Prevent or control IICP.
4. Maintain normal body functions.
5. Prevent or control infection and seizure activity.

Maintaining a Patent Airway with Adequate Respiratory Exchange

Assuring adequate respiratory exchange will minimize the detrimental, cerebral vasodilating effects of a low Po_2 and a high Pco_2. You can appreciate the danger hypoxia or hypercapnia presents to the patient with a contused, swollen brain or the one with an expanding hematoma. The increase in intracranial volume may ex-

NURSING RESEARCH NOTE

McQuillan K: The effects of Trendelenburg position for postural drainage on cerebrovascular status in head-injured patients. *Heart Lung* 1987; 16:327.

Nurses often wonder how to reconcile two seemingly conflicting goals in caring for head-injured patients: clearing pulmonary secretions and maintaining normal intracranial pressure (ICP). If a nurse puts a head-injured patient in Trendelenburg position to perform chest physiotherapy (CPT), won't the resulting increased ICP harm the patient? This study, conducted at the Institute for Emergency Medical Services System (MIEMSS), Baltimore, Md., was designed to answer that question by determining the acute cerebrovascular physiologic changes that occur in head-injured patients during CPT in the Trendelenburg position.

Using a convenience sampling technique, 20 head-injured patients were studied. All were hemodynamically stable, mechanically ventilated, and without severe pulmonary complications. They were monitored with a Richmond screw or intraventricular catheter, arterial line, intravascular P_aO_2 monitoring system, and capnometer. Using a repeated-measures pretest–posttest experimental design, two consecutive CPT treatments were administered to each subject, in a randomly assigned order, 2–6 hours apart. One CPT treatment utilized a horizontal position; the other utilized the Trendelenburg position. Each subject served as his or her own control. Data (recorded every minute for 10 minutes before, during, and after each treatment) included heart rate, mean arterial BP (MABP), ICP, cerebral perfusion

pressure (CPP), and P_aO_2, and, in 10 patients, end-tidal CO_2 values.

Data were analyzed using repeated-measures analysis of variance, *t* tests, and Pearson's correlations. With both treatments, MABP and CPP remained adequate. Changes in heart rate, P_aO_2, and end-tidal CO_2 did not significantly affect cerebrovascular status. Although ICP was higher ($p < 0.05$) with the Trendelenburg position, it returned to baseline level more rapidly than with the horizontal position. With both treatments, MABP and CPP remained adequate. P_aO_2 improved only with Trendelenburg CPT. The researcher concluded that Trendelenburg CPT was safe for the head-injured patients in this sample, providing cerebrovascular status was closely monitored.

ceed the brain's compensatory mechanisms, leading to increased intracranial pressure. Refer to Chapters 5 and 9 for ways to maintain airway patency and to prevent hypoxemia and hypercapnia.

Monitoring and Assessing Neurologic Status

In the setting of head injury, the neurologic exam focuses on changes indicative of increasing intracranial pressure and compromise to vital brainstem areas. Astute assessment and documentation of level of consciousness, pupil size and reactivity, eye movements, motor response, and respiratory patterns aid in the prompt recognition of changes in neurologic status. Significant changes, such as decreasing level of consciousness, development of unequal pupils, abnormal flexion or extension, and a change from normal breathing to Cheyne-Stokes, need to be reported to the physician immediately. Early institution of measures to decrease intracranial pressure and surgical intervention when indicated provide the best chance for preventing permanent neurologic dysfunction.

Preventing/Controlling IICP

The reader is referred to Chapter 5, where IICP is discussed thoroughly.

Maintaining Normal Body Functions

Nursing the head-injured patient requires vigilance in monitoring all body systems. One significant pulmonary complication is the development of *central neurogenic pulmonary edema*. Muwaswes (1985) reports that, with this disorder, there is a centrally mediated, massive sympathetic discharge that produces systemic vasoconstriction. This forces blood into the low-resistance pulmonary circuit. Pulmonary hypertension and altered capillary permeability lead to extravasation of protein-rich fluid into the alveoli and interstitium. Pulmonary artery pressure monitoring reveals normal pulmonary capillary wedge pressure with elevated pulmonary artery systolic and diastolic pressures. This rules out cardiac failure as a cause for the pulmonary edema. The nurse should monitor lung sounds for the early detection of crackles and report elevated pulmonary pressures to the physician.

Zegeer (1984) explains that *cardiac disturbances* are caused by overactivity or depression in either the parasympathetic or sympathetic nervous system related to intracranial disorders. Electrocardiogram changes include ST-segment elevation or depression, T-wave inversion, large U waves, and QT prolongation. Dysrhythmias encountered include sinus bradycardia, ectopic beats, junctional rhythm, and atrial and ventricular tachycardia. Nursing measures instituted are continuous EKG monitoring and patient assessment whenever there is a significant change in rhythm.

Fluid and electrolyte balance is assessed by accurately recording intake and output and following the lab data. Urine output that exceeds 200 cc/hour for 2 hours when no diuretic has been given may be indicative of *diabetes insipidus*. Dehydration and hypernatremia can occur if the condition isn't recognized and fluid replacement and vasopressin administration initiated. On the opposite extreme, urine output less than 30 cc/hour and hyponatremia are suggestive of the syndrome of *inappropriate antidiuretic hormone* (SIADH). SIADH is treated with water restriction. If the hyponatremia is severe, sodium chloride administration may be necessary.

The gastrointestinal system should be monitored for signs of bleeding. Nasogastric aspirant and stool should be tested for blood. *Stress ulcers* may be directly related to the head injury or may be a complication of steroids. Cimitedine (Tagamet) or ranitidine (Zantac) are used to prevent stress ulcers. Nutritional requirements are met early with parenteral or enteral feeding.

Preventing/Controlling Seizure Activity

Since seizures occur in approximately 10% of head-injured patients in the acute phase, must be instituted measures to protect the patient (Rudy 1984). This includes keeping side rails up at all times, and a padded tongue blade and an airway at the head of the bed. When seizure activity occurs, the nurse should note: time of onset and duration, generalized or localized motor involvement, pupillary reaction or eye deviation (if possible), and incontinence. Anticonvulsant medications may be ordered prophylactically or started once the patient exhibits seizure activity. The nurse should ensure that anticonvulsants are administered as ordered. For a more thorough discussion of seizures, the reader is referred to Chapter 5.

Preventing/Controlling Infection

Nurses play a major role in preventing infections. The development of an infection prolongs the patient's hospital stay and, if severe enough, may threaten the patient's life. Key areas of concern after head injury are invasive lines (especially ICP), basal skull fractures with leakage of cerebrospinal fluid, scalp wounds, and the lungs. If invasive lines are in place, be sure to maintain a closed system, and swab ports or connections with betadine and then alcohol before entering or changing tubing.

Since cerebrospinal fluid has a high glucose content, the existence of rhinorrhea or otorrhea contribute to the potential for an infection. The nose or ear should not be packed with gauze or probed with a cotton swab. A loose dressing should be placed under or over the orifice and changed when wet with drainage.

Scalp wounds, whether from head injury or after craniotomy, should be kept clean, dry, and covered. Venous drainage from the scalp empties into venous sinuses inside the skull. Good handwashing prior to changing head dressings and keeping the patient's hands away from the scalp wound will aid in preventing infection.

Good pulmonary hygiene is critical in preventing atelectasis and pneumonia. Specifics have been covered in Chapters 8 and 9 and are not reiterated here.

Outcome Evaluation

Evaluate the patient's progress according to these outcome criteria:

- Patient returns to premorbid level of consciousness.
- Cranial nerves are functioning appropriately.
- Patient responds appropriately to stimuli.
- Normal motor responses (no posturing, absent Babinski reflex).
- Absence of infection.
- Vital signs WNL for the patient.

SPINAL CORD TRAUMA

Approximately 10,000 people sustain a permanent spinal cord injury each year in the United States, 57% resulting in quadriplegia (Richmond 1985). The etiology parallels that of head injury. Richmond (1985) reports that 50% of spinal cord injuries affect individuals below the age of 25, most commonly males.

This section deals mainly with the cervical-cord-injured patient, the quadriplegic. This person suddenly finds the world turned upside down and inside out: a frightened mind held captive by a body that won't move. Complete independence is abruptly replaced with total dependence on others for all activities of daily living.

Key Concepts

Mechanisms of Injury

Traumatic injury more commonly affects the cervical area and is related to flexion, extension, rotation, and/or compression forces. These forces cause vertebral fractures and dislocations, disruption of longitudinal ligaments, and spinal cord damage.

According to Cerullo (1985), maximum mobility and force of movement make C_6 the most common site of cervical fractures. The next areas that are frequently involved include C_5 and C_7.

Classification of Spinal Cord Injury

The degree of functional impairment of the spinal cord may be divided into complete versus incomplete lesions.

Complete Cord Lesion A *complete* cord lesion involves the total loss of sensory and motor function below the level of the lesion. When this occurs in the cervical region, the person becomes a *quadriplegic*. *Paraplegia* is paralysis of both legs. See Table 21–11 for the classification of neurologic deficits according to the level of spinal cord injury.

Incomplete Cord Lesion An *incomplete* cord lesion involves a varying degree of loss of sensory and motor function below the level of the lesion. Intact function reflects sparing of certain tracts.

Central cord syndrome consists of motor weakness that is more marked in the upper extremities than in the lower extremities. It is also characterized by variable sensory impairment and bladder dysfunction. Hyperextension injuries are more likely to cause this injury. Pathophysiology is related to compression of the

TABLE 21–11 CLASSIFICATION OF NEUROLOGIC DEFICITS ACCORDING TO THE LEVEL OF SPINAL CORD INJURY

LEVEL OF INJURY	NEUROLOGIC DEFICIT
Cervical	
C_1 to C_2	Quadriplegia: no respiratory function, with an immediate respiratory arrest if untreated
C_3 to C_4	Quadriplegia: loss of phrenic nerve innervation to the diaphragm, causing absence of respirations
C_4 to C_5	Quadriplegia: no motor power in the arms
C_5 to C_6	Quadriplegia: gross motor function in the arms only
C_6 to C_7	Quadriplegia: no triceps function; biceps spared
C_7 to C_8	Quadriplegia: no intrinsic muscle function in the hands; triceps spared
Thoracic and lumbar	
T_1 to T_{12} and L_1 to L_2	Paraplegia: arm function preserved; some loss of intercostals; loss of bladder, bowel, and sexual function
L_2 and below	Cauda equina damage: a combination of loss of sensory, motor, bowel, bladder, and sexual function; degree of injury depends on which nerve roots are involved
Sacral	Loss of bowel, bladder, and sexual function

Source: Adapted from Kneisl CR, Ames SW: *Adult health nursing—A biopsychosocial approach.* Menlo Park, MA: Addison-Wesley, 1986, p. 1200.

central portion of the spinal cord and/or interruption of blood flow via the anterior spinal arteries (Dudas 1984).

Anterior cord syndrome usually results from flexion injuries. There is complete paralysis with hypesthesia (decreased sensibility to touch) and hypalgesia (decreased sensitivity to pain) below the level of the lesion. Since the dorsal columns are intact, the sensations of touch, motion, positions, and vibration are preserved. Pathophysiology of this lesion is related to compression or interruption of the anterior spinal artery, which supplies blood to the anterior two-thirds of the spinal cord (Hickey 1986).

The *Brown–Séquard syndrome* results from a penetrating injury that causes a transverse hemisection of the spinal cord. Clinically, the patient presents with ipsilateral (same-side) paresis or paralysis; ipsilateral loss of pressure, touch, vibration, and position senses; and contralateral (opposite-side) loss of pain and temperature. This clinical picture may seem odd but is easily understood if you recall how the tracts are carried in the spinal cord (refer to Figures 4–10 and 4–11). The motor (corticospinal) tract travels on the same side that its fibers exit the cord. The dorsal columns that carry the sensations of pressure, touch, vibration, and position transmit these impulses on the same side and do not cross until they reach the brain. In contrast, pain or temperature impulses cross almost immediately to the opposite side of the spinal cord and ascend in the lateral spinothalamic tract. The patient with hemisection of the right half of the cord will present with right-sided motor loss; right-sided loss of pressure, touch, vibration, and position senses; and left-sided loss of pain and temperature senses.

Spinal Cord Shock   *Spinal cord shock* is the loss of all reflex activity below the level of the lesion. It is due to the abrupt cessation of descending impulses as a direct result of the spinal cord injury. This inability of the spinal cord to respond occurs immediately after injury and lasts from days to months.

Flaccid paralysis is a hallmark of spinal cord shock. Other signs and symptoms include hypotension, bradycardia, loss of bowel and bladder function, and impaired temperature regulation.

The appearance of involuntary reflexes signifies that spinal cord shock is abating. The anal reflex may be tested, as it frequently is one of the earliest to return. Other indications include return of the ankle and knee jerk. With the return of reflex activity, the development of spasticity poses a problem for the quadriplegic.

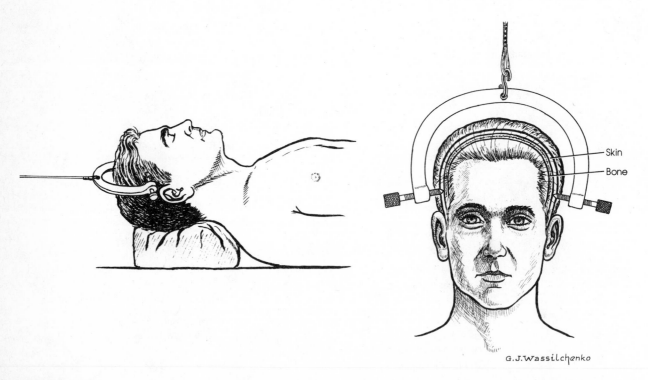

G.J.Wassilchenko

FIGURE 21–4

Gardner-Wells tongs. (From: Rudy EB: *Advanced neurological and neurosurgical nursing.* St Louis: Mosby, 1984, Figure 12–7, p. 404.)

Diagnosis and Treatment of Spinal Cord Injuries

All patients suspected of head and neck injuries should have cervical spine films taken. Anteroposterior films assess alignment, while the lateral view helps to assess stability. CT scan, tomography, or myelography may be employed to visualize the problem if plain films are not conclusive. Throughout the diagnostic workup, extreme care should be exercised to keep the head and neck immobilized so as to prevent further injury.

Early management of the patient with injured spinal cord is aimed at decompression and stabilization. Indications for surgical intervention include open, penetrating injuries, an unstable spine, and progressive neurologic deficit.

Nonsurgical reduction and stabilization of the cervical spine is accomplished using skeletal traction. There are various types of skull tongs available, such as Vinke, Gardner-Wells, Trippi-Wells, and Crutchfield. Figure 21–4 illustrates the Gardner-Wells tongs. The Gardner-Wells tongs have two spring-loaded pins that are seated into the temporal bone just above and in front of the ears. Once the tongs are inserted, weights are applied in an effort to restore the normal alignment of the spinal column. The physician determines the amount of weights to be used. The nurse should assure that weights hang freely at all times, so traction is not interrupted. X-rays may be taken after weights are applied and with each increase, to assess alignment. The patient with tongs may have to remain in traction, flat in bed, for up to 8 weeks. The patient may be cared for on a regular bed or placed on a turning frame.

Assessment in the Emergency Department

All multiple trauma victims should have cervical spine precautions instituted and maintained until ruled out by x-rays. This is accomplished with the use of a hard cervical collar, sandbags, and tape.

The ABCs should be attended to, as with all acutely ill patients. The airway is checked for patency. The jaw thrust or chin lift without hyperextension of the neck may be used to open the airway. Respiratory effort is evaluated by examining the chest for bilateral, symmetric movement and assessing skin color, nailbeds, and earlobes. If intubation is required, the nasotracheal route is preferred, to prevent neck extension.

Pulse, capillary refill, and blood pressure are evaluated for evidence of circulatory embarrassment. Signs of hypovolemic shock include hypotension and tachycardia; whereas signs of spinal cord shock include hypotension and bradycardia. The nurse should ensure adequate intravenous access for infusion of volume and/or vasopressors as indicated.

A quick neurologic exam should be performed to establish a baseline for future comparison. To evaluate for potential head injury, level of consciousness and pupillary response should be assessed. The extremities are observed for any spontaneous movement. If none, then response to stimulus and reflexes are checked. Sensation is tested using pinprick, starting at the toes and quickly moving up to the torso to determine the sensory level. Documentation should reflect frequent assessment of respiratory effort and the baseline neurologic exam.

NURSING DIAGNOSES

Nursing diagnoses for the cervical-cord-injured patient encompass physical and emotional needs in the acute stage as well as in the long-term rehabilitative stage. The following nursing diagnoses should be utilized to guide patient care.

- Potential ineffective breathing pattern
- Potential altered tissue perfusion
- Potential ineffective thermoregulation
- Impaired physical mobility
- Altered urinary elimination pattern
- Altered bowel elimination
- Alteration in comfort: pain
- Potential infection
- Disturbance in self-concept: body image, self-esteem, role performance, personal identity

---

Planning and Implementation of Care

In the acute phase, management of the patient is geared toward monitoring for effective ventilation, ensuring an adequate blood pressure, maintaining neck immobilization, providing for urinary and bowel elimination, and alleviating pain.

Potential Ineffective Breathing Pattern Related to Spinal Cord Injury

Injury to the spinal cord above C_4 interrupts the phrenic nerve to the diaphragm and often is fatal due to respiratory arrest. Cervical cord injury below C_4 spares the phrenic nerve, but it may become compromised as cord edema develops. Astute monitoring of the patient's vital capacity and ABGs will alert you to diminished ventilatory reserve. If the vital capacity drops below 1,000 cc, you should be prepared to assist with nasotracheal intubation and assisted ventilation.

Potential Altered Tissue Perfusion Related to Spinal Cord Shock

The loss of sympathetic activity due to spinal cord shock causes arterial vasodilation and venous pooling, leading to a hypotensive state. Since the parasympathetic nervous system is unopposed, marked bradycardia can occur. Management of these two acute complications consists of administering fluids, a vasopressor, and/or atropine. If the bradycardia does not respond to atropine, a temporary transvenous pacer needs to be placed to maintain good perfusion. Frequent monitoring of vital signs and the ECG for cardiac dysrhythmias is imperative.

Potential Ineffective Thermoregulation Related to Spinal Cord Shock

An additional problem related to the loss of sympathetic tone is difficulty maintaining a normal body temperature. The combination of vasodilation and the inability to shiver causes heat loss. Patients should have their temperatures taken every 4 hours and body exposure to the environment minimized. Additional warming methods may be necessary to maintain normal body temperature.

Impaired Physical Mobility Related to Spinal Cord Injury

In the critical-care unit the patient who is in skull tongs is on complete bedrest on a Stryker frame or a regular hospital bed. Each shift, the nurse needs to check the tongs to be sure they are secure and the traction weights are hanging freely. The weights should never rest against the bed or on the floor or be released, because cord injury may be extended. If the patient is in a regular hospital bed, turning should be accomplished using a log-rolling technique. At all times, the head and neck should be at 90° to the body, with the nose in line with the navel.

Altered Urinary Elimination Pattern Related to Spinal Cord Injury

In the acute phase of spinal cord shock, the patient has an atonic bladder because impulses from the brain are unable to reach it. A urinary catheter must be inserted to prevent overdistention of the bladder. An indwelling catheter may be used for a few days to monitor output closely in the acutely unstable patient. Intermittent catheterization is then employed to maintain bladder capacity. When spinal shock wears off, the bladder becomes spastic and reflex emptying may occur.

Altered Bowel Elimination Related to Spinal Cord Injury

The abdomen should be assessed for the presence of bowel sounds. The stomach may need to be decompressed with a nasogastric tube. Depending on associated gastrointestinal injuries and bowel function, nutritional requirements are met via parenteral or enteral feeding.

Bowel evacuation should be undertaken as soon as the patient is over the critical period. Bowel control can be regained in most cord-injured patients with an appropriate bowel training program. Constipation should be prevented, as it may trigger autonomic dysreflexia or aggravate spasticity. A high-roughage diet, plenty of fluids, and the use of stool softeners, mild cathartics, suppositories, or digital stimulation are all part of a bowel retraining program.

Alteration in Comfort: Pain Related to Injury or Surgical Intervention

The patient may experience pain at the site of injury or related to surgical intervention. Paresthesias (burning, tingling) or hyperesthesias (increased sensitivity) may occur and be a source of discomfort to the patient. Pain should be alleviated with analgesics and other comfort measures. (See the section on pain in Chapter 6 for specifics.)

Potential for Infection

Infection is a threat to the patient acutely and for the rest of his or her life. Potential sources of infection are the lungs, bladder, and skin.

The loss of intercostal and abdominal muscles to assist in effectively clearing the airway makes the quadriplegic prone to atelectasis and pneumonia. Good pulmonary hygiene along with early mobilization may help to decrease pulmonary infections.

According to Hickey (1986), urinary tract infections can lead to renal disease, which is one of the chief causes of death in the long-term management of these patients. An overdistended bladder can cause ischemia, which predisposes tissue to bacterial invasion and infection. Strict aseptic technique should be used when catheterizing patients. Antiseptic bladder irrigations may be ordered. Vitamin C, cranberry juice, and apple juice are taken to acidify the urine, which discourages bacterial growth and bladder stone formation. Dairy products should also be limited, to control urinary stone formation.

Another potential site for infection is the skin. The insertion sites of the skull tongs should be inspected daily for signs of redness or excess drainage. Pin care should include cleansing with hydrogen peroxide and then with betadine, followed with a sterile split 2×2 dressing.

The development of a decubitus ulcer not only poses a risk of infection but delays the rehabilitation process and can aggravate spasticity or precipitate an episode of autonomic dysreflexia. The key is prevention. Establish a turning schedule. Be sure to scrutinize the skin for reddened areas, and straighten the linen so there are no bumps or wrinkles to put pressure on the patient. Pay special attention to pressure points. Utilize pressure-relieving devices (see Chapter 20).

Altered Tissue Perfusion Related to Autonomic Dysreflexia

Autonomic dysreflexia is a potentially life-threatening situation seen in patients with cord lesions above the T_6 level. Autonomic dysreflexia does not occur until spinal cord shock is over. It is a massive sympathetic discharge stimulated by sensory input that cannot traverse the spinal cord to communicate with the brain (Richmond 1985). Signs and symptoms include throbbing headache, flushing of the face and neck, nasal congestion, sweating above the lesion, hypertension, and bradycardia. A distended bladder, full rectum, decubitus ulcer, ingrown toenail, and bladder spasm are a few examples of stimuli that may trigger this response. (See Figure 21–5.)

The danger to the patient is that uncontrolled blood pressure will precipitate a stroke. Therefore, management is aimed at eliminating the cause. But if that cannot readily be ascertained, then blood pressure control is instituted.

Patients at risk of developing autonomic dysreflexia should be identified by tagging their chart so hospital personnel are alerted to the condition. Indepth patient/family education is vital, since this will be a problem for the patient for the rest of life.

Disturbance in Self-Concept: Body Image, Self-Esteem, Role Performance, Personal Identity Related to Spinal Cord Injury

Of all the problems we have talked about, probably none will require the time and patience needed to deal with the emotional care of the patient and significant others. Chapter 3 discusses the grieving process, coping mechanisms, and communication with the patient and family. Following are humanistic principles particularly important in caring for spinal-cord-injured patients.

- Know what the physician has told the patient and family so you can reinforce what they are told.
- Deal openly and honestly with the patient and family.
- Provide reassurance by touching. (Be sure to touch where the patient can feel.)
- Be in the patient's visual field so the patient knows to whom he or she is talking.
- Avoid talking "about," "over," or "for" the patient.
- Always explain what is being done and why.
- Allow the patient some control over daily activities.
- Provide for privacy.
- Pay special attention to personal care, to maintain the person's sexual self-image (e.g., the use of after-shave cologne, make-up, nail polish).
- Acknowledge the family's feelings, and include them in daily care activities as soon as possible.

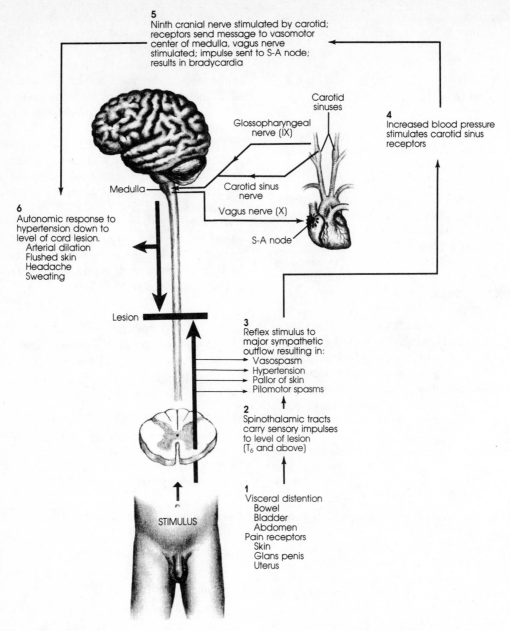

5
Ninth cranial nerve stimulated by carotid; receptors send message to vasomotor center of medulla, vagus nerve stimulated; impulse sent to S-A node; results in bradycardia

Carotid sinuses

Glossopharyngeal nerve (IX)

4
Increased blood pressure stimulates carotid sinus receptors

Medulla

Carotid sinus nerve

Vagus nerve (X)

6
Autonomic response to hypertension down to level of cord lesion.
  Arterial dilation
  Flushed skin
  Headache
  Sweating

S-A node

Lesion

3
Reflex stimulus to major sympathetic outflow resulting in:
  → Vasospasm
  → Hypertension
  → Pallor of skin
  → Pilomotor spasms

2
Spinothalamic tracts carry sensory impulses to level of lesion (T_6 and above)

1
Visceral distention
  Bowel
  Bladder
  Abdomen
Pain receptors
  Skin
  Glans penis
  Uterus

STIMULUS

FIGURE 21–5

Autonomic dysreflexia pathway. (From Rudy EB: *Advanced neurological and neurosurgical nursing.* St Louis: Mosby, 1984, p. 413.)

Outcome Evaluation

The patient's progress should be evaluated according to these outcome criteria:

- Motor strength remains the same or improves.

- Adequate ventilation.
- ABGs WNL for patient.
- Absence of signs of infection.
- Absence of pain.
- Absence of bladder and bowel incontinence.
- Patient can direct own care.

- Patient utilizes adaptive aides to assist with ADLs within limits of injury.
- Patient verbalizes signs and symptoms of autonomic dysreflexia and relief measures.

CHEST TRAUMA

Chest injuries are the second leading cause of death for all victims of trauma, resulting in 25% of all sudden trauma deaths in the United States. Head trauma is the only fatal injury surpassing chest trauma in incidence. Trauma to the chest comprises life-threatening traumatic injuries and requires accurate diagnosis and immediate intervention. Less than 15% of all thoracic injuries require surgical intervention, with the remaining 85% successfully managed with simple procedures during the initial assessment and resuscitation.

Key Concepts

Etiology

Trauma to the thorax may be blunt or penetrating. *Blunt* chest trauma tends to occur in suburban and rural areas, most often results from motor vehicle accidents, and frequently involves injuries sustained from steering wheel impact. In a pediatric population, bicycle handlebars are a frequent cause of blunt chest trauma. The majority of penetrating injuries result from stabbing or gunshot wounds, many of which occur in urban inner-city areas.

Mechanism of Injury

A significant force is required to cause major chest trauma and often results in associated injuries of other vital organs and systems. A high index of suspicion must be maintained for injury to the head, cervical spine, and abdominal contents when chest injuries are evident. Associated abdominal trauma most often involves liver and spleen injuries.

Blunt Trauma Three types of mechanical forces contribute to the pathology of blunt trauma (Jurkovich and Moore 1984):

1. Direct blows to the chest (disruption of the bony thorax)
2. Deceleration (aortic disruption, cardiac contusion, pulmonary contusion, tracheobronchial rupture)
3. Compression (aortic disruption, cardiac rupture, diaphragmatic rupture, tracheal disruption)

Ordinarily, a combination of these forces is involved in producing a chest injury. Figure 21–6 illustrates those forces and their relationship in injury production.

Penetrating Trauma The pathology depends on the type of weapon, missile pathway, and velocity at impact. All penetrating injuries that enter or traverse the mediastinum must be evaluated for potential cardiac tamponade, cardiac injury, or injury to a great vessel (aorta or innominate or subclavian arteries). More than 80% of penetrating chest wounds cause a hemothorax; virtually all cause a pneumothorax (Jurkovich and Moore 1984).

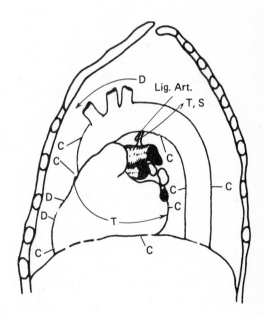

FIGURE 21–6

Some of the forces involved in injury to the chest. D = deceleration, T = torsion, S = shearing, C = compression, D = direct impact. (Reprinted from May HL: The critically injured patient. In *Emergency medicine.* New York: John Wiley & Sons Medical Publications, 1984, p. 241.)

Pathophysiology

Chest trauma often leads to tissue hypoxia. Three pathologic consequences of thoracic injury, alone or in combination, are responsible for inadequate oxygen delivery. These consequences and their possible causes are as follows (Jurkovich and Moore 1984):

- *Hypoxemia* (possibly due to airway obstruction, pneumothorax, flail chest, pulmonary contusion, tracheobronchial injury, or diaphragmatic rupture)
- *Hypovolemia* (possibly caused by hemothorax, great vessel disruption, or cardiac rupture)
- *Myocardial failure* (possibly due to pericardial tamponade, cardiac contusion, myocardial ischemia, or coronary air embolus)

Assessment

Signs and Symptoms

Signs and symptoms associated with chest trauma are varied and depend largely on the specific injury. As previously stated, chest trauma may result in injury, and subsequent alteration or disruption, to the respiratory and cardiovascular systems. Anatomic and physiologic signs and symptoms associated with chest trauma are identified in Table 21–12. Signs and symptoms specific to certain chest injuries are presented in Table 21–13 along with pathophysiology and interventions.

Diagnostic Considerations

Diagnostic studies can provide valuable data in diagnosing specific chest injuries. However, many situations that result from chest trauma require immediate intervention based on the patient's signs and symptoms, and a delay for diagnostic studies, e.g., chest x-ray, will prove detrimental to patient outcome. Laboratory data, radiographic examination, electrocardiography, oximeter monitoring, and angiography play important roles in the management of major chest trauma. Diagnostic studies commonly used to assess chest trauma are presented in Table 21–14.

TABLE 21–12 ANATOMIC AND PHYSIOLOGIC SIGNS AND SYMPTOMS ASSOCIATED WITH CHEST TRAUMA

ANATOMIC

Paradoxical chest wall movement
Chest wall abrasions, contusions, ecchymosis
Open wounds (penetrating and perforating)
Tracheal deviation
Distended neck veins
Chest wall crepitus

PHYSIOLOGIC

Dyspnea, shortness of breath
Tachypnea
Respiratory distress, mild to severe
Cyanosis
Decreased or absent breath sounds
Hyperresonance or dullness to percussion
Signs of hypovolemic shock
Chest pain, especially on inspiration
Muffled heart sounds
Pulsus paradoxus
Widened mediastinum
Cardiac dysrhythmias

NURSING DIAGNOSES

Chest trauma may result in many applicable nursing diagnoses, including:

- Impaired gas exchange
- Ineffective breathing pattern
- Alterations in tissue perfusion
- Fluid volume deficit
- Alterations in cardiac output
- Alteration in comfort: pain
- Potential ineffective family coping

Numerous additional nursing diagnoses may apply to the chest trauma patient at various stages of hospitalization.

INJURY	PATHOPHYSIOLOGY	SIGNS AND SYMPTOMS	NURSING/MEDICAL INTERVENTIONS
Tension pneumothorax	Air enters the pleural space on inspiration without any mechanism for release. Intrathoracic pressure increases on affected side, resulting in complete collapse of the lung. Occurs more frequently than cardiac tamponade.	Severe shortness of breath Respiratory distress Tracheal deviation to unaffected side Distended neck veins (may be flat if severe hypovolemia) Decreased or absent breath sounds, affected side Hyperresonance on percussion, affected side	1. Prepare for insertion of 14–16-gauge needle into 2nd intercostal space in midclavicular line of affected side. 2. Prepare for insertion of chest tube into 5th/6th intercostal space, anterior to midaxillary line.
Open pneumothorax (sucking chest wound)	Defect in chest wall allows passage of air from atmosphere into pleural space and out of the plurae.	Respiratory distress Tachypnea, grunting Penetrating chest wound Sucking sound as air enters pleural space Unilateral decrease or absence of breath sounds, affected side	1. Cover wound with sterile, occlusive dressing. 2. Monitor for development of tension pneumothorax. 3. Remove dressing if tension pneumothorax develops. 4. Prepare for insertion of chest tube into 5th/6th intercostal space, anterior to midaxillary line. 5. Definitive care usually is surgical closure of chest wall defect.
Massive Hemothorax	Accumulation of 1500 ml or more of blood in pleural space. May cause severe hemodynamic compromise due to major blood loss, mediastinal shift and compression of unaffected lung.	Signs of shock Dyspnea Unilateral decrease/absence of breath sounds, affected side Dullness to percussion, affected side Distended or flat neck veins	1. Restore blood volume with crystalloid, blood, and/or colloids before chest tube insertion. 2. Consider PASG. 3. Consider autotransfusion. 4. Prepare for insertion of large bore chest tube 5th/6th intercostal space, anterior to midaxillary line. 5. Continuous monitoring of chest tube drainage. 6. Emergency thoracotomy if severe hypovolemia or unable to control blood loss.
Flail Chest	Usually occurs in relation to blunt trauma with the flail segment resulting in paradoxical movement of the chest wall. Occurs when two or more ribs are fractured in at least two sites, when the sternum is separated from the rib cage due to multiple fractures. Results in impaired ventilation and gas exchange due to pain and associated lung injury.	Shortness of breath, [respiratory distress] Flail segment, paradoxical chest wall movement Severe chest pain, affected side Crepitus and abnormal chest wall movement may be palpable	1. Stabilize flail segment with manual pressure or position on affected side if not contraindicated. 2. Control of pain with intercostal nerve blocks and/or systemic intravenous analgesics. 3. Aggressive respiratory care. 4. If severe respiratory distress, endotracheal intubation and ventilatory support.
Cardiac tamponade	Most often occurs from a penetrating injury to the myocardium which results in an acute accumulation of blood in the pericardial sac. May less frequently result from blunt cardiac trauma. Results in alterations in diastolic filling of ventricles and mechanical function of the heart. Venous hypertension often occurs due to the backup of blood resulting from the decreased diastolic filling.	Signs of shock Beck's triad (venous pressure with JVD-may be absent in severe hypovolemia; B/P; muffled heart sounds) Pulsus paradoxus (fall in systolic B/P 15 mmHg during inspiration) Possible inability to palpate apical pulse Dyspnea, possibly Kussmaul's respirations	1. Pericardiocentesis by the subxyphoid route (pericardial blood has Hct lower than venous blood and will not clot). 2. Placement of central line to assess central venous pressure. 3. Emergency thoracotomy if unable to aspirate pericardial blood. 4. Definitive care requires thoracotomy for surgical repair of cardiac injuries.

TABLE 21–14 DIAGNOSTIC STUDIES COMMONLY USED TO ASSESS CHEST TRAUMA

STUDY	DIAGNOSTICALLY SIGNIFICANT DATA
Laboratory:	
Complete blood count (CBC)	Hemoglobin/hematocrit
Electrolytes	Baseline data
Arterial blood gas	$\uparrow P_{CO_2}$; $\downarrow P_{O_2}$; $\downarrow pH$
Urinalysis	Positive for blood
Radiography: chest x-ray	Collapsed lung; widened mediastinum
Electrocardiogram	Elevated ST segment; dysrhythmias
Transconjunctival oximetry	$P_{cj}O_2 < 50$ torr

Planning and Implementation of Care

Resuscitation and Stabilization

Immediately following chest trauma, acute resuscitation and stabilization must occur. Basics of this resuscitation effort include attention to airway, breathing, circulation, and cervical spine stabilization.

Airway Insure patient airway.

Breathing

1. Provide high-flow oxygen.
2. Provide ventilatory assistance, as indicated.
3. Prepare for aggressive ventilatory support, as indicated.

Circulation

1. Provide hemorrhage control, as indicated.
2. Initiate/provide volume replacement.
3. Initiate pneumatic antishock garment (PASG), as indicated.
4. Initiate autotransfusion, as indicated.

Cervical spine stabilization Initiate/maintain cervical spine stabilization, as indicated.

Additional interventions and strategies in relation to nursing diagnoses and specific chest injuries follow.

Impaired Gas Exchange

Impaired gas exchange can result from anatomic or physiologic dysfunction as a result of injury. To minimize the effects of impaired gas exchange in chest trauma victims, monitor for signs and symptoms of increasing respiratory distress, administer high-flow humidified oxygen, and prepare to assist with intubation or surgical airway and mechanical ventilation as needed. Monitor the patient's progress by frequent measurements of arterial blood gases (ABGs). Therapeutic interventions are directed at relieving the specific cause of impaired gas exchange.

Ineffective Breathing Patterns

The loss of integrity of the bony thorax or underlying pulmonary parenchymal injury may cause ineffective breathing patterns. Observe the patient for the effectiveness of breathing, i.e., rate and depth of respirations, cyanosis, use of accessory muscles, tracheal deviation, paradoxical chest wall movement, and lung sounds. Measures to alleviate the ineffective breathing pattern are aimed at the specific cause. See Table 21–13 for detailed discussion of nursing and medical interventions.

Fluid Volume Deficit Related to Blood Loss

Blood loss from chest trauma may be the result of a hemothorax occurring from a major pulmonary tear, aortic disruption, or a penetrating heart wound. Initiation of volume replacement is the first priority. Consider use of the pulmonary antishock garment (PSAG) and autotransfusion to support circulation, as ordered. Carefully monitor the patient's hemodynamic response. Assist with treatment of cardiac tamponade, if present (see Chapter 13 for details). Assist with insertion of central venous or pulmonary artery lines. Prepare the patient for arteriography and/or surgery as needed.

Alteration in Comfort: Pain Related to Disruption of Nerves and Tissues

The patient with trauma to the chest, either blunt or penetrating, usually will experience chest pain. The pain itself, if untreated, will result in impaired gas exchange and ineffective breathing patterns due to guarding and splinting to decrease the chest pain. As soon as life-saving interventions have been initiated, the critical-care nurse should assess the level of pain and the patient's response to pain. Administration of various forms of pain medication is appropriate in chest trauma. Systemic analgesics and intercostal nerve blocks frequently are utilized to alleviate pain in relation to chest trauma.

Outcome Evaluation

The patient's response to nursing and medical intervention should be evaluated through the assessment of physiologic function. Criteria for outcome evaluation should therefore include:

- Vital signs WNL.
- Capillary refill < 3 seconds.
- Skin vitals (color, moisture, turgor, mucous membranes) WNL.
- Patient is alert and oriented.
- Urine output $\geq$ 30–50 ml/hour.
- Arterial blood gas WNL, normally: pH 7.35–7.45, P_{CO_2} 35–45 mm Hg, P_{O_2} $\geq$ 80 mm Hg/room air.
- Cardiac rhythm normal.
- Peripheral pulses strong and equal bilaterally.
- Patient expresses relief from pain.

ABDOMINAL TRAUMA

Abdominal trauma occurs as a result of either blunt or penetrating forces. Trauma resulting from blunt impact is the most common abdominal injury, frequently from motor vehicle accidents and physical assault. Penetrating abdominal trauma, occurring less frequently and resulting from stabbing and gunshot wounds, tends to occur in inner-city urban areas. Victims of multiple trauma often experience abdominal injury as a life-threatening component. In addition, 75% of patients with blunt injury to the abdomen have concomitant injury to the head, chest, or extremities. Abdominal trauma may result in massive blood loss with subsequent hemorrhagic

shock or peritonitis and later septic shock. Abdominal injuries therefore may lead to fluid volume deficit, alteration in tissue perfusion, potential for infection, alteration in comfort, and alteration in bowel and urinary elimination.

The severity of blunt injury is directly related to the force of impact, the amount of time the force is applied, and the anatomic area where the force is directed. The abdominal wall offers minimal support and protection from injury in relation to protection provided by the skull and bony thorax. Abdominal viscera consists of both hollow and solid organs, with solid organs frequently injured by blunt force and hollow organs injured by penetrating trauma. The hollow organs include the stomach, intestines, and bladder and a portion of the esophagus. The liver, spleen, pancreas, kidneys, and uterus comprise the solid organs, with the liver and spleen being the most frequently injured abdominal organs. When the stomach, bladder or intestines are filled with fluid, they act as solid organs in response to severe impact or force.

Assessment

Signs and Symptoms

The initial signs and symptoms exhibited by the abdominal trauma patient may be as severe as those indicative of profound hypovolemia or as subtle as no signs of injury or complaint of pain.

Assessment findings may include:

- Signs and symptoms of shock
- Ecchymosis of abdominal wall
- Decreased or absent bowel sounds
- Pain, rebound tenderness, muscle guarding
- Left shoulder pain

This last phenomenon, referred to as *Kehr's sign*, is a classic finding in patients with splenic rupture and is caused by blood below the diaphragm irritating the phrenic nerve. This pain radiates to the left shoulder.

The major life-threatening concern in abdominal injuries is severe blood loss and the resulting hemorrhagic shock (see section on shock in Chapter 13). Peritonitis and sepsis are life-threatening concerns that cause increased mortality and morbidity in the later stages of care.

Diagnostic Considerations

Specific information regarding the mechanism of injury, events preceding the incident, location of the patient at the time of injury, and the force of impact provides significant data for diagnosis of abdominal injury. Diagnostic studies must occur as life-saving intervention is initiated. As with chest trauma, initial diagnostic efforts should address airway, breathing, and circulatory status.

The most important diagnosis in abdominal trauma or suspected abdominal trauma is whether or not the patient will require immediate surgical intervention to prevent death or disability. During the early resuscitation and stabilization phases of care, the diagnosis of specific intraabdominal injuries is unimportant; of great importance, however, is the decision, in a timely manner, to move the patient to the surgical suite.

Laboratory Studies The patient with abdominal trauma requires laboratory studies similar to those for the chest trauma victim. Early determination of hemoglobin and hematocrit, electrolytes, urinalysis, and arterial blood gases is essential to direct resuscitative measures as well as to establish baseline data for ongoing assessment and comparison. Actual or potential abdominal injury may require transfusion of blood products; therefore, a type and screen or type and crossmatch should occur as a part of the initial laboratory studies.

Additional laboratory studies specific to abdominal trauma may include determination of amylase, BUN, and creatinine. Although often obtained, controversy exists as to their actual value in identifying significant injury. Guaiac of stool and gastric contents may indicate injury and bleeding. Analysis of peritoneal lavage fluid is completed to determine the presence of blood cells, bile, amylase, or feces—all indicative of intraabdominal injury.

Radiographic Studies Radiographic studies vary with the severity of injury and institutional and community practices. Prior to the widespread use of computerized axial tomography (CAT) to assess abdominal trauma, abdominal films were obtained routinely. With increasing use of the CAT scan to determine significant injury, a decrease in the use of abdominal films is evident.

Radiographic studies that may be indicated include the following:

- *Upright abdominal film* may reveal air below the diaphragm, indicating disruption of a hollow organ, or abnormal densities associated with bleeding from solid organs (less than 800 ml of blood may not be visualized on x-ray).
- *Lateral decubitus film* may reveal disruption of hollow organs through air along the lateral aspects of the abdomen.
- *Intravenous pyelogram* (IVP) may be used to determine extravasation of contrast media, indicating injury to the kidney, ureters, or bladder.
- *Computerized axial tomography* may be used to determine actual sites of bleeding and quantify bleeding in the abdominal cavity.

Peritoneal Lavage The *peritoneal lavage* is used to determine nonspecific intraabdominal injury and subsequent bleeding. It is most useful in the assessment of blunt abdominal trauma and is considered to be 95% accurate in identifying the need for surgical intervention. Controversy exists regarding the effectiveness and accuracy of peritoneal lavage versus computerized axial tomography. Current modalities indicate a rise in popularity of the CAT scan determination of abdominal injuries.

Prior to initiation of the peritoneal lavage, a nasogastric or orogastric tube and urinary catheter should be inserted. The nasogastric tube is both diagnostic and therapeutic, since it decompresses the stomach, prevents aspiration, and minimizes gastric content contamination of the abdominal cavity. The urinary catheter is inserted to empty the bladder, thereby decreasing the risk of puncturing the bladder during the procedure. It further allows monitoring of urine output and analysis of urine for gross or occult blood.

Warmed saline solution or Ringer's lactate should be infused into the peritoneal cavity to prevent the risk of hypothermia induced by the infusion of cold or room-temperature fluids. If frank blood is not initially aspirated, 1000 ml of fluid should be infused over 10–15 minutes. The fluid then drains via gravity, and analysis of peritoneal lavage fluid is completed to determine the presence of blood cells, bile, amylase, or feces, all indicative of intraabdominal injury.

Positive peritoneal lavage findings include:

- Frank, non-clotting blood
- 100,000 red cells/mm^3 (blunt trauma)
- 1,000–100,000 red cells/mm^3 (penetrating trauma)
- Hematocrit greater than 2%
- More than 500 white cells/mm^3
- Amylase greater than 200 Somogyi units
- Presence of bile
- Presence of fecal material or bacteria

Frequently a quick method is used to determine the need for immediate surgical intervention when evaluating peritoneal lavage fluid. The rule of thumb is that, if newsprint can be read through the lavage return, the peritoneal lavage is negative. This rule may not always be accurate, and immediate laboratory analysis of lavage fluid is necessary to ensure appropriate treatment (American College of Surgeons 1984).

NURSING DIAGNOSES

Nursing diagnoses that may apply to the abdominal trauma patient are multiple. The major important diagnoses include:

- Fluid volume deficit
- Potential for infection

Planning and Implementation of Care

Critical life-saving interventions are instituted immediately and include activities to support or reestablish vital physiologic functions. Immediate intervention must be directed toward ensuring a patent airway, providing high-flow oxygen, and supporting effective ventilation. Airway patency requires ongoing assessment, optimal positioning with cervical spine consideration, and suctioning as indicated. Fluid resuscitation should begin immediately, since the major concern in abdominal trauma is massive blood loss and subsequent hypovolemia.

As diagnostic procedures and stabilization continue, the critical-care nurse should provide ongoing assessment and prepare for immediate transport to surgery if indicated. Insertion of a nasogastric/orogastric tube and urinary catheter, although not life-saving, should occur during stabilization of the patient.

Interventions related specifically to the patient with abdominal trauma may include stabilization of foreign or impaled objects. Such objects should not be removed prior to surgery due to the risk of massive bleeding once the tamponading agent is removed. To minimize complications, all open wounds or eviscerations should be covered with sterile, saline-moistened dressings.

Tetanus immunization status and the need for antibiotics should be determined during the resuscitation and stabilization of the trauma victim. Antibiotics are indicated if intraabdominal organs have been perforated and leakage of contents has occurred. The risk of peritonitis and sepsis is great in this event.

Major concerns for the abdominal trauma patient during the critical-care phase are hemodynamic stability, recognition and identification of occult injuries, risk of sepsis, nutritional support, and psychosocial support for the patient and significant others. The psychologic aspects of care are specifically addressed in Chapter 3. Through an understanding and appreciation of patterns of trauma or mechanisms of injury and the various associated injuries, the critical-care nurse can suspect certain injuries. This enables the prioritization of specific assessment parameters and guides the establishment of plans for patient care.

One current trend is to take a conservative approach in the treatment of abdominal trauma. In essence, this means that surgical intervention is not necessarily viewed as an immediate treatment modality except in life-threatening situations. This patient should be closely monitored through ongoing assessment and frequent computerized axial tomographic studies of the abdomen. The critical-care nurse should observe for subtle changes in level of consciousness, respiratory and circulatory status, and pain response to determine alterations indicating a need for immediate surgery.

Fluid Volume Deficit Related to Blood Loss

Initial circulating volume replacement should be provided through large-bore (14–16-gauge) peripheral intravenous catheters. Warmed crystalloids, such as normal saline or Ringer's lactate, should be infused as indicated by patient status and estimation of blood loss. Blood products should be available for immediate use as indicated. The pulmonary antishock garment (PASG) may be considered to provide circulatory support. Autotransfusion is not indicated in abdominal trauma, due to the risks associated with infusion of contaminated blood. The critical-care nurse should prepare to assist with insertion of central venous lines, Swan-Ganz catheter, and other invasive modalities that may be used to monitor hemodynamic status.

Potential for Infection Related to Ruptured Hollow Viscus

Sepsis is a major concern in the trauma patient and is of particular importance when injury results in perforation of the bowel. The perforation is liable to cause leakage of virulent bacterial bowel contents into the peritoneum, with subsequent peritonitis and septic shock. The critical-care nurse should be ready to administer prophylactic antibiotics as ordered and to prepare the patient for surgery to repair the perforated bowel. Carefully monitor the patient's hemodynamic status and observe for signs of sepsis, including elevated temperature.

Outcome Evaluation

Effective treatment of abdominal trauma requires immediate attention to airway, breathing, and circulatory status and a high index of suspicion for severe injury. Criteria for outcome evaluation should include:

- Vital signs WNL.
- Systolic blood pressure ≥ 90 mm Hg.
- Capillary refill < 3 seconds.
- Skin vitals (color, moisture, turgor, mucous membranes) WNL.
- Patient is alert and oriented.
- Urine output ≥ 30–50 ml/hour.
- Patient expresses relief from pain.
- Signs of returned gastrointestinal functioning (ileus disappears, bowel sounds become active).
- Diet is consumed and tolerated without problems.

ORTHOPEDIC TRAUMA

Orthopedic trauma, often the most visibly dramatic injury, must be managed only after life-threatening situations have been assessed and appropriately treated. Airway, breathing, and circulation require immediate attention to ensure a patent airway, effective ventilation, and adequate tissue perfusion. Several orthopedic injuries do constitute life- or limb-threatening emergencies and require intervention during the initial resuscitation and primary survey phases of care. These injuries include uncontrolled hemorrhage, neurovascular compromise (absence of pulse or sensation), and amputations.

Once life-threatening situations have been corrected and an initial head-to-toe assessment has been completed, definitive care is initiated. At this time actual or potential orthopedic injuries are managed, including splinting and immobilization of injured parts. Assessment and management of orthopedic trauma requires an understanding of mechanisms of injury and injuries that frequently are associated with specific traumatic incidence. It is not unusual for injuries to bones to be missed because of the patient's inability to verbalize complaints of pain and the lack of obvious deformity.

Assessment

Risk Conditions

Incidence of orthopedic trauma correlates to the incidence of major traumatic injury. The peak incidence is in the 15–24-year-old age group and affects predominately males. Risk groups and conditions therefore include teenagers and young adults, especially those involved in contact sports, vehicular accidents, falls, assaults and other sports-related events, such as skiing, hang-gliding, and jogging. Additionally, the use of alcohol and drugs, emotional problems, underlying illnesses, and previous injuries to the same extremity are conditions that potentially result in an increased incidence of orthopedic trauma. The extremely young and elderly populations also are at risk due to developmental phases of bone growth or events related to the aging process, respectively.

Prevention As with other traumatic events, orthopedic injuries frequently are associated with the use of alcohol and drugs. Community education regarding drinking and driving, safe sports activities, and industrial safety will play a major role in preventing orthopedic trauma. Additionally, the use of seat belts when riding in motor vehicles will result in less severe injury and possibly prevent loss of life or limb.

Pathophysiologic Changes

Orthopedic injuries may result in fractures, sprains, strains, ligament tears, tendon lacerations, arterial disruption, and joint dislocations. Such injuries may involve interruption of skin integrity. A *sprain* is a ligament in-

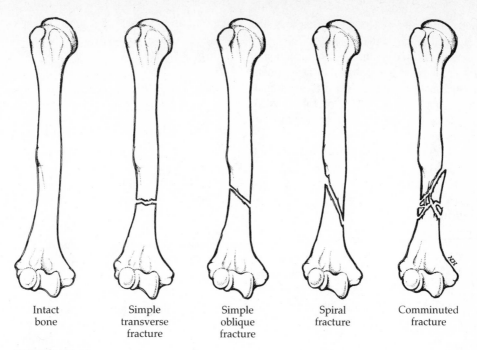

Intact bone   Simple transverse fracture   Simple oblique fracture   Spiral fracture   Comminuted fracture

FIGURE 21–7

Types of fractures. (Adapted from Cosgriff JH, Anderson DL: *The practice of emergency care,* 2d ed. Published by Lippincott/Harper & Row. Reprinted by permission of JH Cosgriff.

jury that occurs when a joint exceeds its normal range of motion. The most common sprains occur in the ankles, knees, and shoulders. A weakening or overstretching of a muscle where it attaches to the tendon is a *strain*. Any type of abnormal movement may result in a strain, with frequent occurrence related to sports injuries.

Fractures are classified as closed or open. In a *closed* or *simple, fracture,* the bone is fractured but the skin remains intact. *Open,* or *compound, fractures* involve both fractures of the bone and disruption of the skin. Any disruption near the site of an actual or potential fracture is categorized as an open fracture. Figure 21–7 depicts types of fractures. Fractures, whether open or closed, result in a significant blood loss. A closed femur fracture may cause a blood loss of up to 2–3 units, and pelvic fractures result in one unit of blood lost with each fracture.

Dislocations frequently are limb-threatening because of subsequent neurovascular compromise. Therefore, dislocations of major joints require immediate intervention to prevent further harm and prevent disability. Dislocations result when joints exceed the normal range of motion and the joint surfaces are no longer intact.

Crush injuries and amputations may cause life-threatening situations due to massive blood loss associated with such events. Crush injuries often occur when heavy objects fall on extremities. Amputations result from either penetrating trauma, shearing forces, or dismemberment by extreme force.

Signs and Symptoms

Orthopedic injuries may be evident through observation of an obvious deformity or may be missed due to no complaint of pain and no visual signs of injury. As with other forms of trauma, a history of the accident and information about the mechanism of injury provide data to guide the assessment process. Typical signs of orthopedic injury include obvious deformity of the injured extremity, pain, swelling, muscle spasm, crepitus, limited movement, and possible neurovascular compromise. Signs of shock may appear due to a substantial blood loss from either external hemorrhage or internal bleeding resulting from disruption of tissue and vessels. External wounds and protruding bone are obvious indicators of major orthopedic trauma.

The "five Ps" (pain, pallor, pulselessness, paresthesias, and paralysis) often are utilized to assess potential or actual orthopedic injuries. Additional assessment must include comparison of the injured extremity with the uninjured extremity. Assessment of blood loss should take into consideration actual external loss and an estimation of blood lost into the closed space.

Special attention to occult injuries or frequently missed injuries is important during the assessment phase of care. Such injuries include cervical spine injuries, especially C_6 and C_7; fractures of the clavicle, scapula, and humerus; nondisplaced forearm, pelvic, or femoral neck fractures; and fractures of the malleoli, metacarpals, metatarsals, or phalanges (American College of Surgeons 1984).

Diagnostic Considerations

Laboratory Data The patient with orthopedic injuries must be assumed a major trauma victim until that is ruled out. To provide appropriate treatment, including resuscitation and stabilization, initial laboratory studies should include:

- Complete blood count (CBC)
- Type and cross-match or type and screen for blood products
- Urinalysis
- Arterial blood gas determination

Additional laboratory studies are based on patient status. See assessment of multiple trauma, earlier in this chapter.

Radiologic Studies Initial x-rays should be completed for obvious or suspected injury. Radiographic studies should also be used to identify or rule out associated or concurrent injuries. As indicated, x-ray studies should include the joint above and below the site of injury.

Computerized axial tomography may be utilized to diagnose orthopedic trauma in situations where x-ray does not completely rule out an injury. This is particularly useful in questionable cervical spine x-rays.

NURSING DIAGNOSES

Nursing diagnoses related to orthopedic trauma are:

- Alterated tissue perfusion
- Alteration in comfort:pain
- Impaired physical mobility
- Impaired skin integrity

Other possible radiologic studies include arteriograms to identify specific vessel injury associated with orthopedic trauma.

Planning and Implementation of Care

Nursing intervention initially should address airway with cervical spine immobilization, breathing, and circulation with hemorrhage control. All clothing must be removed to allow thorough assessment of actual and potential injuries. See shock (Chapter 13) or chest trauma (this chapter) for specific interventions related to hypovolemia and hemorrhagic shock.

High-flow oxygen via nasal cannula, mask, or endotracheal tube should be given. Two large-bore (14- or 16-gauge) intravenous lines should be initiated with warmed, normal saline or Ringer's lactate infusing as indicated. Hemorrhage should be controlled with manual pressure.

Once life-threatening and limb-threatening situations are controlled, assessment and intervention related to other orthopedic trauma is appropriate. All injured extremities, whether actual or potential, should be immobilized, with the joint distal to and proximal to the injury included in the splint. Neurovascular status distal to the site of injury must be assessed and documented prior to and after splinting. Various devices may be utilized for immobilization to maintain stability and prevent further injury, including cardboard splints, molded splints, and backboards.

Extremities should be immobilized as they lie, except in situations where a neurovascular compromise is evident. *Neurovascular compromise* is delayed capillary refill, absence of pulse, and/or loss of movement or sensation. In such an event, the extremity should be aligned prior to splinting, with reassessment of neurovascular status after immobilization. The pneumatic antishock garment (PSAG) is ideal for immobilizing pelvic fractures, preventing associated pain, and slowing blood loss.

Closed fractures of the femur should be managed with a traction splint, such as the Hare traction or Sager splint. Lower-extremity traction devices, when properly applied, decrease pain, slow blood loss, and prevent further injury. Again, neurovascular status must be assessed and documented both prior to and after application of the traction splint. Once traction is applied, it must remain intact until an orthopedic surgeon is available or a neurovascular compromise exists.

Any orthopedic injury potentially will result in swelling and pain. To decrease the severity and extent of such results of trauma, ice should be applied at the site of injury or suspected injury. Additionally, the extremity should be elevated above the level of the heart to further reduce swelling and associated pain.

Alteration in Comfort: Pain

Severe pain frequently is experienced in orthopedic trauma. Although the patient complains of pain, intervention must be aimed toward assessment and identification of life- and /or limb-threatening injuries and appropriate treatment. Once other injury is managed or ruled out, intervention related to pain can be initiated. Pain relief is best obtained through intravenous infusion of analgesics such as morphine in small, frequent doses. The use of Nitronox also is useful in alleviation of pain. This is a self-administered analgesic consisting of 50% oxygen and 50% nitrogen. Pain relief additionally is obtained through limiting movement of the injured extremity and immobilization.

Impaired Skin Integrity

In the event of an open or compound fracture, special attention must be given the disruption of skin integrity. An extremity with an open fracture always is splinted as it lies in an effort to prevent further contamination of the site. The wound should be covered with a saline-moistened sterile dressing. Prophylactic antibiotics via the intravenous route should be initiated during the stabilization and definitive care phase.

Remember that traumatic injuries are prone to infection and tetanus. Tetanus and tetanus immune globulin should be administered as indicated. If you are unable to accurately determine the patient's tetanus status, both active and passive immunization must be attained.

Selected Orthopedic Injuries

Amputations Amputations present a challenge to prehospital care and trauma personnel. An amputation may be partial or complete, usually involving digits, the lower leg, the hand, or the forearm. In the event of a complete amputation, bleeding may be less than with a partial amputation. Complete severance of a vessel allows constriction, with the ends clamping down onto each other, whereas the partially severed vessel will remain open, since pressure results from the proximal and distal ends.

Signs and symptoms of amputations include visual evidence, pain, and bleeding. X-ray of both the stump and amputated part will determine the presence of foreign bodies. Microsurgery techniques have advanced the replantation of amputated parts, with resulting use of the extremity.

After life-saving intervention, priorities in care are directed toward preservation of the amputated part and the stump, to enhance chances for replantation. The amputated part always should be transferred to the hospital with the trauma victim. Care of the amputated part should include the following:

1. Do not attempt to clean the part.
2. Wrap in a saline-moistened gauze dressing.
3. Place in an airtight container.
4. Maintain in a hypothermic state, but do not freeze or place directly on ice.

Without proper preservation, the amputated part is viable for only 4–6 hours; with preservation, this may be extended to 18 hours.

Stump care includes the control of active bleeding, ideally using manual pressure, pressure dressings, and elevation of the extremity. Tourniquets and hemostats are not indicated for hemorrhage control unless all other interventions are unsuccessful. Remove gross debris from the stump, and cover with a saline-moistened dressing once bleeding is controlled.

Crush Injuries Crush injuries frequently occur as industrial-related accidents and often involve heavy machinery. Loss of limb and possibly loss of life are realistic concerns with massive crush injuries. Such injury results in severe damage and destruction of tissues, vessels, nerves, and bones. Pathophysiologically, there is major blood loss and hypovolemia; myoglobinuria damages the kidneys and may result in renal failure.

Signs and symptoms associated with crush injury are:

- Signs of shock
- Severe pain
- Massively crushed extremity

Intervention in the emergency department and critical-care unit are supportive, as indicated by patient status. Life-saving intervention must be implemented immediately. Active bleeding is best controlled with direct pressure and pressure dressings. Elevation of the affected extremity will decrease pain and swelling. The injured area should be gently cleansed while taking care not to increase surface trauma.

Pelvic Fractures Fractures of the pelvis result from vehicular and motorcycle accidents, falls from heights, and crush injuries. Each fracture of the pelvis may cause a blood loss of 1–2 units; therefore, hypovolemia is a major concern. Death related to pelvic fractures usually occurs because of uncontrollable hemorrhage. Later consequences often are related to massive blood transfusions and their sequelae.

Signs and symptoms include pain, signs of shock, instability of the pelvic ring, pelvic ecchymosis, and hematuria. A high index of suspicion for associated abdominal, chest, head, and spine trauma must be maintained.

Intervention includes immobilization with a backboard and application of pneumatic antishock garment (PASG) to tamponade bleeding and promote stabilization of bony structure. Treatment of pelvic fractures may include external fixation, internal fixation, arterial embolization, and supportive care.

Selected Complications

Complications frequently associated with orthopedic injuries are compartment syndrome and fat embolization.

Compartment Syndrome Compartment syndrome occurs as pressure increases inside the fascial compartment enveloping the injury site. The increasing pressure may result from internal bleeding and swelling or from external sources such as a cast or pneumatic antishock garments. Compartment syndrome predominately occurs in relation to injuries involving the lower leg and forearm. This condition causes compression of nerves, vessels, and muscle and must be identified immediately to prevent permanent damage.

Signs and symptoms associated with compartment syndrome include:

- Progressive severe pain, frequently described as pain not relieved by narcotic analgesics
- Absent or decreasing distal pulse
- Cyanosis or pallor of distal extremity
- Delayed capillary refill
- Loss of motor function
- Paresthesia (loss of sensation, numbness)

An increased compartment pressure becomes evident with measurement. Normal compartment pressure is 20 mm Hg or less, with 21–40 mm Hg indicating decreased tissue perfusion and 41 mm Hg or above signalling ischemia.

Immediate intervention is based on early recognition of signs and symptoms. Elevation of the affected extremity only to the level of the heart will help prevent further swelling. The critical-care nurse should prepare for a fasciotomy if compartment pressure is greater than 40 mm Hg, indicating tissue ischemia. The fasciotomy will immediately relieve elevated compartment pressure and may prevent permanent neurovascular damage and possible loss of limb.

Fat Embolism Fat embolism frequently is associated with long-bone fractures and immobility. Although the pathophysiology of fat embolism syndrome is not agreed upon, two theories have been proposed to explain the occurrence of fat embolization: the mechanical theory and the biochemical theory. Originally it was thought that neutral fat droplets escaping from the site of the fracture entered the circulation and lodged in the lung and the brain, causing local ischemic areas (the *mechanical* theory).

The *biochemical* theory places importance on the stress caused by trauma and the activation of the sympathetic nervous system. A subsequent release of catecholamines, epinephrine, and norepinephrine triggers the release of free fatty acids and neutral fats from the fracture site. Fat globules then form and become coated with platelets that have aggregated at the site of injury. The coated globules enter the circulation through the severed vessels and lodge in the lung and brain, again causing local ischemic areas.

The typical signs and symptoms of fat embolism tend to occur between 24 and 72 hours after injury, with some appearing as early as 12 hours. Patients at risk usually are young and have experienced multiple trauma or a single lower-extremity long-bone fracture. The initial signs and symptoms associated with fat embolism are tachypnea (with a decreased arterial oxygen tension), tachycardia, fever, and central nervous system changes (altered level of consciousness and behavior changes). Later clinical findings include petechiae (especially pronounced in the axillary creases, the chest, and the conjunctivae), retinal changes, fat globules in the urine, decreasing hemoglobin, thrombocytopenia, and increased erythrocyte sedimentation rate.

Interventions to prevent and treat fat embolization related to long-bone trauma are controversial. Immobilization of fractures may minimize embolism from the site of fracture. The administration of supplemental high-flow oxygen is indicated for all trauma patients, with aggressive ventilatory support needed for patients with progressive signs and symptoms of fat embolism syndrome. Positive end-expiratory pressure (PEEP) may be required in some situations. The inflammatory process in the lung may be diminished by the use of corticosteroid therapy; therefore, the administration of methylprednisolone succinate (Solu-Medrol) is recommended. Care should be taken to prevent overhydration. Diuretic administration may be indicated in the patient who has received crystalloid resuscitation resulting in fluid overload.

Other, less conventional, modes of therapy may include the administration of alcohol, heparin, and low-molecular-weight dextran. Although these treatment modalities are not widely accepted, some authorities utilize one or all because of beneficial results reported in various studies.

Definitive Care

Definitive care for orthopedic injuries includes accurate diagnosis, reduction of dislocations, and application of pins, casts, or traction to promote healing. Open reduction and internal fixation (ORIF) may be required in certain situations, with a closed reduction and casting appropriate at other times. Nursing care should involve frequent assessment of the affected extremity to include assessment of the five Ps and early recognition of neurovascular compromise and associated complications.

Outcome Evaluation

Evaluate the patient's progress and the effects of your nursing interventions according to these outcome criteria:

- Signs of shock are absent.
- Tissue perfusion is maintained, as evidenced by normal skin temperature, normal skin color, capillary refill less than 3 seconds.
- Pain relief is attained, as evidenced by patient verbalization.
- Mobility is restored to maximum potential, as evidenced by appropriate fracture care.
- Skin integrity is maintained, as evidenced by absence of infection and/or tissue breakdown.

BURNS

A major thermal insult is one of the most devastating traumas that can befall the critically ill. The patient not only has to cope with the complex physiologic sequelae of the insult but also with its psychologic effects and long-term implications for the quality of life. No wonder that nursing the burned patient is one of the most demanding—and yet most satisfying—challenges to face the critical-care nurse.

Key Concepts

The skin is composed of three layers: the epidermis, the dermis, and the hypodermis, or subcutaneous fat (Figure 21–8). The *epidermis,* the outermost layer, is thin and nonvascular. It consists primarily of epithelial cells, which form a protective coating and are being shed constantly. The epidermis contains *keratin,* which limits fluid loss, and *melanin,* which contributes to the basic color of the skin. The *dermis,* the middle layer, has a complex structure, consisting of blood vessels, sensory receptors for temperature, pain, touch, and pressure, portions of hair follicles, sebaceous glands, and ducts of sweat glands. The deepest layer is the *hypodermis,* the subcutaneous fat (containing the roots of sweat glands and hair follicles), under which lies the fascia, muscles, and organs.

The skin is such an accepted part of our being that we sometimes forget its important physiologic functions. It protects the body and plays major roles in perception, temperature regulation, and fluid and electrolyte balance. In addition, because of its cosmetic features, it forms an essential defining feature of a person's self-identity and self-concept.

Assessment

Patients can be burned through several different mechanisms, usually classified as *thermal, electrical, chemical,* and *radiation agents.* Thermal causes, the most common, include flame, scald, and tar.

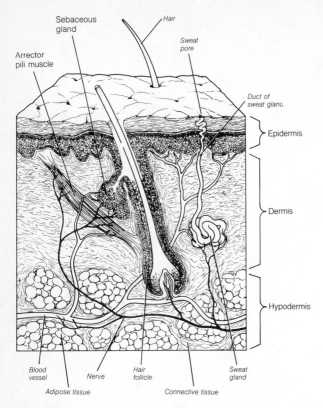

Arrector pili muscle

Sebaceous gland

Hair

Sweat pore

Duct of sweat gland

Epidermis

Dermis

Hypodermis

Blood vessel

Nerve

Hair follicle

Sweat gland

Adipose tissue

Connective tissue

FIGURE 21–8

Structure of the epidermis, dermis, and hypodermis layers. (From Spence A, Mason E: *Human anatomy and physiology,* 3d ed. Menlo Park, CA: Benjamin/Cummings, 1987, Fig. 5.2a.)

TABLE 21–15 CLASSIFICATION OF BURNS

BURN TYPE	AREA DAMAGED	CHARACTERISTICS
Partial Thickness		

Superficial	Epidermis	Epidermal inflammation:
		   Erythema
		   Pain
		   Little or no edema
		   Dry, intact skin

Deep	Epidermis Dermis	Erythema Blanching on pressure Hair still present Blisters that increase in size Intense pain Minimal to moderate edema Oozing/weeping
Full Thickness	Epidermis Dermis Hypodermis (subcuta-neous fat)	Dry Blisters absent or do not increase in size Red, white, black charred Leathery texture No pain No blanching on pressure Blood vessels may be visible
All Tissues	Skin Muscle Bone	Charred tissue Very deep wounds Pronounced edema

Signs and Symptoms

The signs and symptoms of a burn vary with the extent of skin damage (Table 21–15).

Burn Depth

Superficial Partial-Thickness Burns (First-Degree Burns)
These burns involve only the epidermis; common examples are sunburn and scald burns. The signs and symptoms are those of epidermal inflammation: redness and pain, with little edema. The skin remains dry and intact at the time of the burn. It desquamates within 3–7 days, and spontaneous healing occurs within a few days.

Deep Partial-Thickness Burns (Second-Degree Burns)
These involve both the epidermis and dermis. They often are the result of exposure to flames, scalding substances, or hot tar. Because the epidermis is involved, the sensory receptors, the capillaries, the hair follicles, and the sebaceous and sweat glands are damaged. The burn is characterized by a red or mottled appearance, blanching on pressure, intense pain, and moderate edema. The skin has blisters or vesicles that increase in size, and oozing and weeping of fluid is apparent. Hair is still present. Healing usually occurs spontaneously within about 3–5 weeks but sometimes requires grafting.

Full-Thickness Burns (Third-Degree Burns) Such burns result from flame, scald, tar, chemical agents, or electrical agents. They involve all three layers of the skin. Because all the structures in the dermal layer are destroyed, the burn, which may appear red, white, or charred, does not blanch on pressure, and the area of full-thickness burn is painless. It may have a dry, leathery texture; either no hair is present or the hair pulls out easily. Blisters are absent or, if present, do not increase in size. Blood vessels may be visible in the exposed tissue. A small burn (less than 4 cm diameter) may heal from granulation and migration of healthy epithelium from the wound edges (Wooldridge-King 1982). A more extensive burn cannot heal spontaneously and instead requires skin grafting.

Fourth-Degree Burns A fourth-degree burn is an extremely deep burn commonly seen with charring. It involves all the skin layers plus muscle and bone.

It is important to realize that the degree of burn varies with the intensity and duration of exposure to the burning agent. In addition, it is common for areas with different degrees of burn to be interspersed, and for areas of severe burn to be surrounded by areas of lesser burn. The full extent of a burn may not be apparent for several hours or days. A lesser-degree burn can convert to greater degree if the burning process continues or if blood supply to the area is impaired due to edema, hypotension, infection, or simple pressure.

Burn Area The burned area can be determined in several ways. A quick, convenient method in the prehospital or emergency department setting is the *rule of nines,* which assigns percentages to various areas of the body (Figure 21–9). For small or peculiarly shaped burns, a useful method is to compare the size of the burn to the size of the patient's palm. The palmar surface approximates 1% of the total body surface area (TBSA). The *rule of nines* is relatively inaccurate for determining specific therapies, as it does not account for differences in body proportions among age groups. The most precise determination of burn extent is achieved with the Lund and Browder chart, which correlates body surface area percentages with age (Figure 21–10).

Burn Severity The severity of a burn can be categorized as *minor, moderate,* or *major* according to the guidelines developed by the American Burn Association

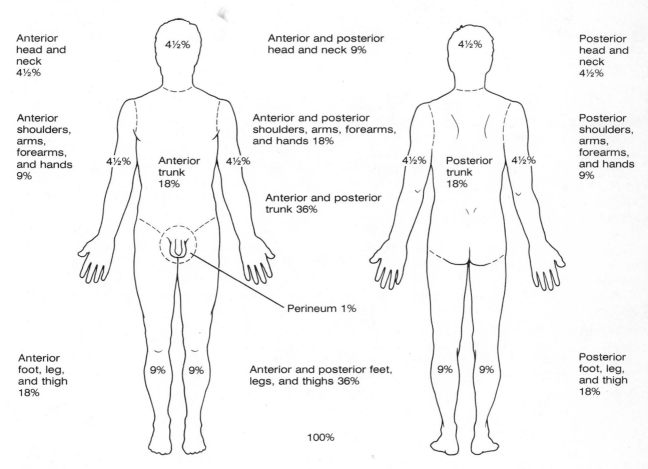

FIGURE 21–9

Estimating the extent of burns on the body surface area using the rule of nines. (From Spence A, Mason E: *Human anatomy and physiology,* 3d ed. Menlo Park, CA: Benjamin/Cummings, 1987, Fig. 5.7.)

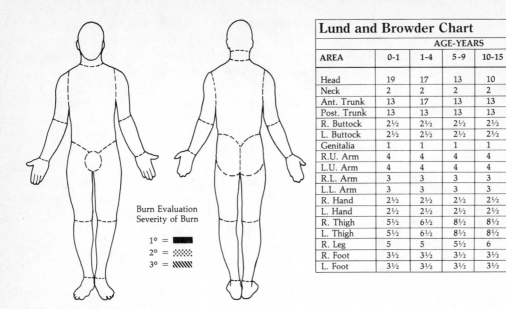

Lund and Browder Chart								
	AGE-YEARS					**%**	**%**	**%**
AREA	**0-1**	**1-4**	**5-9**	**10-15**	**ADULT**	**2°**	**3°**	**TOTAL**
Head	19	17	13	10	7			
Neck	2	2	2	2	2			
Ant. Trunk	13	17	13	13	13			
Post. Trunk	13	13	13	13	13			
R. Buttock	2½	2½	2½	2½	2½			
L. Buttock	2½	2½	2½	2½	2½			
Genitalia	1	1	1	1	1			
R.U. Arm	4	4	4	4	4			
L.U. Arm	4	4	4	4	4			
R.L. Arm	3	3	3	3	3			
L.L. Arm	3	3	3	3	3			
R. Hand	2½	2½	2½	2½	2½			
L. Hand	2½	2½	2½	2½	2½			
R. Thigh	5½	6½	8½	8½	9½			
L. Thigh	5½	6½	8½	8½	9½			
R. Leg	5	5	5½	6	7			
R. Foot	3½	3½	3½	3½	3½			
L. Foot	3½	3½	3½	3½	3½			
					Total			

Burn Evaluation
Severity of Burn

1° =
2° =
3° =

FIGURE 21–10

Lund and Browder chart for precise determination of burn extent. (Adapted from Lund C, Browder N: The estimation of areas of burns. *Surg Gynecol Obstet* 1944; 79:352–358.)

(1976). The categories are determined by the *depth* of burn, *area* of burn, and *high-risk factors*. The remainder of this discussion focuses on the care of the patient who has suffered a major thermal insult.

According to the ABA guidelines, patients with major burns should be cared for in a regional burn center. A major burn presents with any of the following characteristics: (a) a full-thickness burn greater than 10% TBSA; (b) a partial-thickness burn greater than 25% TBSA; (c) a burn in a *critical area:* the face, eyes, ears, hands, perineum/genitalia, or feet; or (d) a high-risk burn. A high-risk burn is one complicated by inhalation injuries, electrical burning, fractures or other major trauma, pre-existing serious medical disease (such as diabetes or heart failure), or age below 2 years or above 60 years. Another type of high-risk situation is social circumstances indicating abuse (such as child abuse or spouse abuse) or indicating that follow-up care may not be attended to.

Nursing Diagnoses

Burn care can be conceptualized as a continuum with three overlapping periods: emergent (resuscitation) phase, acute period, and rehabilitative period. According to Archambeault-Jones and Feller (1981), the *emergent period* lasts from the onset of injury to 2 days–2 weeks posttrauma, depending on the severity of injury. The *acute period* lasts from the end of the emergent period until all the full-thickness burns are covered with autografts. The *rehabilitation period* may last up to 5 years except in the case of a severely burned infant or small child, in which case the social and physical rehabilitation may last until the child is fully grown.

These periods are distinguished by the emphasis placed on different aspects of the burn patient's recovery. In the emergent phase, major concerns are maintenance of pulmonary function and cardiovascular integrity. In the acute phase, primary concerns are protection against infection and enhancement of wound healing. In the rehabilitation phase, the chief concern is restoration of the patient to useful participation in society.

This section focuses on nursing care during the emergent and acute periods. For further information on rehabilitation, the reader is referred to the burn literature, particularly Archambeault-Jones and Feller (1981).

NURSING DIAGNOSES

EMERGENT PERIOD

- Pain
- Impaired gas exchange
- Decreased cardiac output
- Decreased tissue perfusion
- Altered urinary elimination pattern
- Altered bowel elimination
- Potential altered level of consciousness

ACUTE PERIOD

- Potential for injury
- Ineffective thermoregulation
- Altered nutrition: less than body requirements
- Potential for infection
- Potential impaired gas exchange
- Potential activity intolerance
- Potential poor wound healing
- Potential ineffective individual coping
- Potential ineffective family coping

Planning and Implementation of Care

Pain Related to Continued Burning or Exposure of Sensory Receptors

It is critical that the first person who aids a burned patient stop the burning process. Everyone should be taught to *stop, drop, and roll* to put out flames on the body. If the victim is too disoriented to have done that, the rescuer should establish eye contact, if possible, and drop and roll the victim or use a blanket or any other method at hand to smother the flames. Clothing and jewelry should be removed, because they retain heat. In the emergency department, small burns can be soaked in cool saline to further halt the burning process and relieve pain.

The patient with a full-thickness burn may not need as much immediate pain control as you would initially expect; because the skin's pain receptors have been destroyed, the full-thickness burn area is anesthetized.

Deep partial-thickness burns, however, are ex-

tremely painful. Patients rarely have only full-thickness burns, so they will experience pain from other burn sites. Analgesia can be provided with intravenous morphine titrated to achieve pain control.

Impaired Gas Exchange Related to Upper or Lower Airway Injury

Burned patients can develop upper airway obstruction, manifested by laryngeal edema, laryngospasm, or profuse airway secretions due to mucosal trauma in the naso- and oropharynx. This damage can occur with or without actual smoke inhalation. Observe for the signs of stridor, dyspnea, and intense hoarseness; if these signs are present, the patient requires intubation for airway protection until the swelling subsides in a few days.

Ineffective gas exchange also can result from lower airway damage related to inhalation injury. The lower airway usually is not directly burned, as heat is dispersed on inhalation; steam burns of the airway are an exception. Usually, lower airway damage is related to inhalation of the toxic products of combustion, which cause a chemical pneumonitis.

Be alert for dyspnea, tachypnea, cough, crackles, and rhonchi, as well as decreasing PO_2. On admission, the patient should receive a chest x-ray (which usually is normal), have a set of baseline arterial blood gases drawn, and have a sputum specimen sent for culture and sensitivity. The critical-care nurse should be especially wary of lower airway damage with smoke inhalation. Clues to smoke inhalation include a history of being burned within an enclosed space, singed nasal hairs, burns around the nose and mouth, and carbonaceous particles in the sputum. If smoke inhalation is suspected, the physician may elect to perform a laryngoscopy or bronchoscopy on admission to the critical-care unit or order Xenon lung scans. Positive findings include carbon particles, and mucosal erythema, swelling, blistering, and sloughing.

Poor gas exchange also may result from carbon monoxide poisoning. Because carbon monoxide has a much greater affinity for hemoglobin than does oxygen, oxygen saturation is significantly impaired. A carboxyhemoglobin level should be drawn on any patient with a history suggesting smoke inhalation. The normal value is less than 5%. Symptoms associated with increased levels of carbon monoxide are confusion, headache, dyspnea, nausea, vomiting, hallucinations, ataxia, coma, and, finally, cardiopulmonary arrest (Vermeer 1982).

The final factor that can cause impaired gas exchange in the initial postburn period is a circumferential burn of the chest, which limits thoracic expansion necessary for respiration and commonly leads to alveolar hypoventilation. A circumferential chest burn is relieved via escharotomy.

Initial airway care should include intubation if upper airway damage is present; administration of humidified oxygen; frequent auscultation of breath sounds; monitoring of arterial blood gases; measurements of tidal volume, vital capacity, and inspiratory force every 4 hours; suctioning as necessary; and encouragement of the patient to turn, cough, and breathe deeply every hour. Carbon monoxide poisoning is treated with 100% oxygen, or, if available, hyperbaric oxygenation.

Decreased Cardiac Output Related to Burn Shock and Other Factors

Burn shock is the term used to describe the hypovolemic shock suffered by patients with major thermal insults. In the first 24–36 hours postburn, capillary permeability increases significantly. This increase is most marked at the site of injury, but also occurs throughout the rest of the body. The leaky capillaries allow translocation of fluid, electrolytes, and proteins into a nonfunctional interstitial space, nicknamed "the third space." This fluid movement and the accumulation of cellular debris exceed the ability of the venous ends of the capillaries and of the lymphatics to absorb the excess fluid. The degree of fluid shift can be hard to comprehend; a patient with a 40% TBSA burn can third-space up to 75% of his plasma volume (Davies 1982). In addition, of course, fluid is lost via the exposed surface of the burn. Other factors that contribute to decreased cardiac output include hypothermia, acidosis, decreased coronary artery perfusion, and, in extensive burns, the possible release of a myocardial depressant factor.

Nursing measures to combat burn shock include the prompt establishment of large-bore IV lines (through the burned skin itself if necessary) and management of the fluid replacement prescribed by the physician. Fluid resuscitation must be aggressive to combat the deleterious effects of burn shock.

The content of the fluid used in the initial 24-hour resuscitation period is controversial. Some experts argue that it should be partially crystalloids and partially colloids, as both crystalloids and colloids are lost in burn shock. Others believe that colloids are contraindicated, because they can leak out into the interstitial spaces pulling fluid along with them, increasing the likelihood of early development of pulmonary edema and causing further risk of pulmonary edema when the capillary leak seals over and the colloid particles are trapped outside

the vascular system. According to Demling (1987), the most popular resuscitation fluid in the United States is crystalloid, particularly lactated Ringer's solution. The point to remember here is that fluid resuscitation in the burn patient is dynamic. No one formula can be considered correct all the time. The key is understanding the pathophysiology of burn shock in order to make the best choice for the individual patient.

A number of different formulas may be used to guide fluid resuscitation (Table 21–16). When replacement of both crystalloids and colloids is preferred, the most universally known formula is the Brooke formula. It calls for 1.5 ml crystalloid and 0.5 ml colloid per kg body weight per percent TBSA burned, plus 2000 ml electrolyte-free solution (glucose in water).

If only crystalloid therapy is preferred initially, the most commonly used formula is the Baxter (Parkland) formula. This formula states that the amount of fluid to be replaced in the first 24 hours postburn equals 4 ml lactated Ringer's solution per kg body weight per percent TBSA burned. (If the percent of TBSA burned exceeds 50%, the maximal figure used still is 50%.) Using this formula, for example, a 70-kg patient with a 60% burn would receive 14 L of fluid in the first 24 hours (4 $\times$ 70 $\times$ 50 = 14,000 ml = 14 L). One-half the fluid is given in the first 8 hours postburn (not postadmission), when the capillary leak is greatest; one-quarter in the next 8 hours; and the final quarter in the next 8 hours. This calculation is only a guideline, of course. The least amount of fluid necessary to produce adequate tissue perfusion should be used.

The adequacy of fluid resuscitation must be carefully monitored by the physician and nurse according to vital signs, peripheral perfusion, urinary output, and hemodynamic parameters. Hematocrit values also are used to monitor fluid resuscitation. In the immediate postinjury period, the hematocrit rises due to hemoconcentration. As fluid volume is restored, the hematocrit drops, reflecting adequate fluid resuscitation.

Given the massive amounts of fluid that are administered, meticulous monitoring of infusions and precise intake and output records are essential. If the burn exceeds 25% TBSA, a central venous line and PA line are inserted to guide fluid resuscitation. Fluid replacement after the initial 24 hours involves colloids, crystalloids, and electrolyte-free solutions in varying amounts according to the patient's needs.

The end of burn shock is signalled by the onset of spontaneous diuresis about 48 hours postburn, due to the mobilization of burn edema and reestablishment of normal capillary permeability. The patient should be monitored carefully for signs of excess fluid volume, CHF, and pulmonary edema. During this diuretic phase, fluid infusion rates can be diminished, provided that sat-

TABLE 21–16 FLUID RESUSCITATION FORMULAS, FIRST 24 HOURS*

FORMULA	URINE OUTPUT	RATE OF INFUSION	BASIS FOR CALCULATED VOLUME
Brooke			
Colloid: 0.5 ml/kg/% burn (plasma protein solutions, e.g., albumin) Crystalloid: 1.5 ml/kg/% burn (lactated Ringer's) 5% DW: 2000 ml/meter²	Adult: 0.5–1.0 ml/kg/hr Child: 1.0 ml/kg/hr	One-half the total in the first 8 hours; one-quarter the total in the next 8 hours; one-quarter the total in the next 8 hours	Burn surface area to a maximum of 50% TBSA. Burns greater than 50% are calculated the same as 50% TBSA
Parkland			
Crystalloid: 4 ml/kg/% burn (lactated Ringer's)	Same as for Brooke	Same as for Brooke	Total burn area for all sizes of burns
Monafo			
Hypertonic saline (Na 250 mEq/L, lactate 150 mEq/L, Cl 100 mEq/L)	Same as for Brooke	Rate and volume titrated to urine production	

*It must be remembered that the "first 24 hours" means from the time of the burn injury, not from the beginning of treatment.

Sources: Demling R: Fluid replacement in burned patients. *Surg Clin North Am* (Feb) 1987; 67(2):15–30; Dingeldein GP: Fluid and electrolyte therapy in the burned patient. *Manual of burn therapeutics,* Boston: Little, Brown 1983, p. 11.

isfactory tissue perfusion and urinary output are maintained.

The patient should be weighed on a metabolic scale soon after admission, to gain a baseline weight prior to the peak of edema, and weighed daily thereafter. Edema development gradually increases over the first 3 days, and the patient can be expected to gain approximately 15% of baseline weight during the initial few days (Wooldridge-King 1982). Burn edema has a gel-like consistency due to its high protein content. It is slowly mobilized over a period of about 2 weeks.

Potential Decreased Cardiac Output Related to Potassium Imbalances

During the first 24–36 hours, cellular destruction and impairment of the sodium-potassium pump cause hyperkalemia to develop. During this period, the nurse should not add potassium to intravenous solutions and should monitor the patient for ECG signs necessitating treatment of the hyperkalemia. After 72 hours, during burn diuresis, hypokalemia may develop. During this time, add potassium to intravenous solutions to replace urinary losses, as ordered.

Decreased Tissue Perfusion Related to Progressive Thrombosis

Major burn trauma causes a progressive ischemia due to several interrelated factors. Aggregation of platelets and leukocytes and intravascular hemolysis causes sludging of cellular debris in the microcirculation. In conjunction with decreased perfusion due to decreased CO, this sludging causes thrombosis of both the micro- and macrocirculation. Peripheral pulses, skin temperature, and capillary filling should be monitored closely. If pulses are not palpable, flow should be checked with an ultrasonic flowmeter. Perfusion of the fingers should be watched especially closely, because fingers have poor peripheral perfusion. Elevating the extremities helps to reduce edema formation, thereby improving capillary flow. Due to the unreliability of tissue perfusion, medications must be given intravenously.

Perfusion is particularly likely to become compromised if there is a circumferential burn of an extremity; the constriction of the eschar combined with the tissue pressure from edema formation can severely impair blood flow. Escharotomy (surgical incision of the eschar) is indicated if distal pulses become weak or absent, distal unburned skin becomes cyanotic, capillary filling weakens, or progressive paresthesias or motor impairment develop (Wooldridge-King 1982). Less frequently, a fasciotomy (surgical incision through the fascia to expose underlying tissue) may be needed. A fasciotomy may be particularly helpful in an electrical burn, to release the pressure caused by major edema and to assess tissue viability.

Altered Urinary Elimination Pattern Related to Volume Changes

A Foley catheter should be inserted if the burn exceeds 20% TBSA, and the urinary output monitored hourly. Normal urinary output is 1 ml/kg per minute, or 60 ml per hour. A minimally acceptable urinary output is 0.5 ml/kg per minute, or 30 ml per hour. A urinary specimen should be sent to the laboratory for routine examination and culture and sensitivity on admission. Dark, concentrated urine may be present due to sludging of hemoglobin or myoglobin from damaged cells, indicating massive hemolysis or tissue destruction and possible renal damage. The abnormal concentration usually clears with adequate fluid administration, although mannitol may be indicated if it is pronounced.

Altered Bowel Elimination Related to Paralytic Ileus and Gastric Hemorrhage

Development of gastric dilatation and paralytic ileus is a normal response to the stress of a major burn. The patient should not be allowed oral food or fluids until bowel sounds return. A nasogastric tube usually is placed because of the real danger of vomiting and aspiration. The intense thirst present for the first 2 days, which is a compensatory mechanism for the fluid volume deficit, can be relieved with ice chips and mouth swabs.

GI bleeds can occur due to hemorrhagic gastritis, which develops secondary to capillary congestion and rupture, or to Curling's ulcer. Nursing measures to prevent GI bleeding include checks of nasogastric fluid aspirate pH and occult blood every 2 hours, administration of antacids down the nasogastric tube every 2 hours, and administration of ranitidine or cimetidine, as ordered.

Potential Altered Level of Consciousness

The patient with a major burn normally is alert and oriented, although intensely anxious, on admission. There-

fore, if a decreased level of consciousness is present, alternative causes should be investigated—for example, associated head trauma, decreased cardiac output (shock), inhalation of toxic materials, carbon monoxide poisoning, and drug or alcohol overdose.

Potential for Injury Related to Anemia

Patients with massive burns develop a profound anemia, characterized by abnormal RBC morphology and decreased RBC half-life. Hemolysis begins when some red blood cells are destroyed by heat as they pass through the burned areas or get trapped in swollen capillaries. Hemolysis contributes to capillary thrombosis, and the resulting anemia may significantly reduce oxygen-carrying capacity.

The initial injury may destroy up to 10–15% of the red blood cell mass. It is followed by a progressive anemia whose exact cause is unknown but appears to be an extrinsic mechanism unrelated to initial heat or mechanical damage (Davies 1982). In addition, the patient loses blood during debridement. Most patients require transfusions of packed red cells to maintain acceptable serum hematocrits.

Ineffective Thermoregulation Related to Heat Loss

A significant amount of body heat is lost through a major burn. Beginning in the emergent period, the patient should be kept warm by using a heat cradle and warm environmental temperature in the unit.

Altered Nutrition: Less Than Body Requirements, Related to Stress Response

As part of the normal physiologic response to an overwhelming stress, the burned patient becomes hypermetabolic, developing increased catecholamine release, increased glucose production from the breakdown of glycogen (glycogenolysis) and formation of glucose from fats and proteins (gluconeogenesis), and protein catabolism leading to negative nitrogen balance. The increased metabolic rate peaks at about 1 week postburn. Because of these factors, the patient needs to be protected from additional stressors in his environment, provided with as much uninterrupted rest as possible, and given a high-calorie diet of approximately 5,000–6,000 calories per day. Once bowel sounds have returned, oral feedings are preferred. If nutritional needs cannot be met through oral feedings, then enteral feedings, peripheral venous fat emulsions, or hyperalimentation may be necessary. Patients should be weighed daily to monitor the effectiveness of the program.

Potential for Infection Related to Broken Skin, Traumatized Tissue, and Suppressed Inflammatory Response

Infection presents a major problem for seriously burned patients, sepsis being a leading cause of death in these patients. The burn wound itself is a frequent source of infection. The skin is the body's first line of defense against infection, so loss of the skin barrier is a significant risk condition. In addition, the injured tissue is a superb culture medium. Finally, inflammatory response is impaired. In full-thickness burns, blood vessels undergo coagulation necrosis, so white blood cells cannot reach burned tissue. Areas without complete arterial occlusion still suffer impaired defense; although phagocytic cells may be able to reach them, the neutrophils' ability to kill ingested bacteria is depressed (Davies 1982).

Because of these factors, burn patients are seriously jeopardized by infection, both from themselves and their environment. Burn wounds often are colonized by the patient's endogenous GI, respiratory, and skin flora *(autocontamination)*. Exogenous sources of infection include invasive procedures, such as IV catheterization, hemodynamic monitoring lines, Foley catheterization, hyperalimentation, endotracheal intubation, and so on. Manipulation of the burn wound during tubbing, debridement, and surgery can seed the bloodstream with infectious organisms.

Wound infections occur with a variety of organisms, especially *Staphylococcus aureus, Pseudomonas aeruginosa,* beta-hemolytic *Streptococcus,* and *Candida albicans* (Pruitt 1984). Tetanus prophylaxis is provided on admission. The patient is treated on sterile sheets, by personnel in sterile attire, and, when possible, in special units that reduce the flow of airborne contaminants. Meticulous attention to aseptic care of invasive devices is critical. Other measures to reduce infection include conscientious handwashing and decontamination of equipment such as hydrotherapy tanks. Surface cultures, blood cultures, and full-thickness biopsies (the most reliable indicators of infection) are obtained every

few days. Infections are particularly prone to develop at the juncture of eschar and living tissue. The subeschar tissue is left without a blood supply initially, due to coagulation of blood vessels in the burned layers. For this reason, systemic antibiotics cannot be delivered to subeschar tissues in therapeutic levels. Because of the vascular dynamics, many units no longer give systemic antibiotics prophylactically. Instead, subeschar infections must be fought with eschar removal, drugs that penetrate the eschar, and subeschar antimicrobial infusions. Granulation tissue starts developing about 2 weeks postburn and matures by about 4 weeks, at which time capillary supply is firmly reestablished and phagocytic cells can reach the subeschar layer.

If wound infection is not controlled, bacteria will seed the bloodstream, resulting in bacteremia that may lead to septicemia. *Bacteremia* is defined as colonization of microorganisms greater than 10^5 per gram of viable tissue (Salisbury et al. 1983). In major burns, bacteremia is a constant threat to the patient until the burn wound is completely covered by autografts. It is not uncommon to have recurrent episodes of bacteremia following hydrotherapy treatment and/or major debridement procedures. The nurse should be alert for such signs of impending septicemia as fever, chills, malaise, elevated WBC, increased pulse or respiratory rate, gradual hypotension, and altered mental status. Treatment includes aggressive wound cleansing, daily wound and blood cultures, administration of appropriate antimicrobials and antipyretics as ordered by the physician, and promotion of adequate rest and nutrition.

Overwhelming septicemia can provoke the development of septic shock. Septic shock carries a high mortality, and its development in the burn patient is an ominous prognostic sign. Recognition and management of septic shock is covered in Chapter 13.

Potential Impaired Gas Exchange Related to Shock, Trauma, and Infection

The importance of pulmonary care continues during the acute phase, but emphasis shifts from management of early complications, such as airway obstruction, to later complications, primarily ARDS and pneumonia. For principles of care related to these, please consult Chapter 8. Bronchopneumonia is a grave danger. Airborne sources are most common, but pneumonia also may occur via blood-borne bacterial seeding from another site, most commonly the burn wound itself.

Potential Activity Intolerance Related to Contractures

Hypertrophic scarring and contractures of scar tissue can cause severe functional impairment of burned areas. Because contractures tend to form in positions of comfort, it is important to begin splinting burned areas in positions of function early, and to explain to the patient why you are doing so. The patient should be turned at least every 2 hours, and a physical therapist should be consulted to design a program of range of motion exercises and appropriate splints. The patient should be encouraged to exercise in bed and to ambulate as soon as possible.

Potential Poor Wound Healing Related to Inadequate Wound Care

Wound healing can be conceptualized as a triad of interrelated factors: *wound damage, endogenous host defense mechanisms,* and *exogenous support for healing.* As the

TABLE 21–17 TOPICAL PREPARATIONS USED IN BURN CARE

PREPARATION	ADVANTAGES	DISADVANTAGES	NURSING ACTIONS
Silver sulfadiazine (Silvadene)	Wide-spectrum antimicrobial Antifungal Nonstaining Relatively painless Usable without dressings No systemic metabolic abnormalities	Less eschar penetration than Sulfamylon Decreased granulocyte formation	Check for allergy to sulfa; sometimes causes rash.
Mafenide acetate (Sulfamylon)	Eschar penetration Effective with *Pseudomonas* Topical of choice for electrical burns Suitable for open method of treatment Used for gram-negative organisms	Severe pain and burning sensation (lasts 30 min) Acidic breakdown product Carbonic anhydrase inhibitor Ineffective against fungi May cause hypersensitivity rash	Administer pretreatment analgesic. Monitor for metabolic acidosis and hyperventilation. Check for allergy to sulfa; observe for rash.
Povidone-iodine (Betadine)	Antifungal Wide-spectrum microbicidal	Iodine absorption Staining of clothing Dressing necessary Metabolic acidosis	Assess for allergy to iodine. Check serum iodine levels.
Bismuth tribromphenate (Xeroform)	On Vaseline gauze, so conforms to wound	Painful removal	Alert patient to discomfort before removing.
Silver nitrate	Low cost	Continuous wet soaks Superficial penetration Black staining Stinging Electrolyte imbalances (low sodium, low chloride, low calcium), alkalosis	Keep dressings wet. Perform active debridement. Check serum electrolytes daily.
Enzymatic Debriding Agents			
Fibrinolysin and deoxy-ribonuclease (Elase)	Digestion of necrotic material	Burning sensation	Remove dry eschar before applying.
Sutilains (Travase)	Digestion of necrotic material	Refrigeration necessary Irritation of wound and skin Can cause some bleeding Can cause fluid loss Painful on partial-thickness burn	Limit use to 10–15% of burn surface at one time. Observe for infection. Cross-hatch eschar if necessary to allow optimal penetration. Monitor fluid balance. Assess need for analgesic.

manager of the healing support mechanisms prescribed by the physician, the critical-care nurse plays a crucial role in the healing process.

Therapeutic approaches can be broadly subdivided into conventional and aggressive therapies. *Conventional* therapy consists of hydrotherapy with debridement of necrotic tissue, application of topical antimicrobials and dressings, and skin grafting. Hydrotherapy is used to soften eschar, wash away topical agents, and aid in debridement. Unfortunately, hydrotherapy may increase the risk of wound contamination, is very painful, and causes heat loss. Debridement, a procedure dreaded by burn patients because of the severe pain involved, involves either removal of eschar with forceps and scissors or scalpel, or wet-to-dry dressings that are then peeled away from the burn wound surface. A variety of methods of wound care may be used. In the *open* (exposure) method, wounds are left exposed to air. This method allows easy visibility of the site as well as increased dryness, but may require reverse isolation and a warm room to minimize heat loss. *Dry occlusive dressings,* consisting of thick bandages, are used less frequently, because they limit observation and mobility and may promote infection. They are used primarily to stabilize grafts. The method most commonly used is *partial exposure.* A thin layer of antimicrobial cream is applied, and this then may be covered by a thin layer of gauze. A variety of antimicrobial agents also is available. Advantages and disadvantages of different agents and dressings are summarized in Tables 21–17 and 21–18.

Aggressive therapies consist of tangential or staged removal of eschar down to a bleeding base (granulating tissue), followed with dressings and grafting. Compared to conventional therapy, early aggressive surgical therapy shortens hospitalization, reduces the development of sepsis, and decreases scar formation; however, it increases blood loss. Excisions can be started during the first week postburn. In the past, they have been limited to removal of no more than 15% TBSA at one procedure, although some centers are experimenting with more liberal guidelines.

Skin grafts can be obtained from animals such as pigs *(heterografts),* cadavers *(homografts),* or the patient *(autografts).* Synthetic grafts also are available. Heterografts, homografts, and synthetic grafts are used as temporary biological dressings to minimize infection, prevent fluid and heat loss, and protect nerve endings. Homografts and heterografts also are used to prepare the granulating wound bed for autografting.

Autografts are used to provide permanent coverage for full-thickness burns. Full-thickness grafts, which

TABLE 21–18 TYPES OF BURN DRESSINGS

PREPARATION	ADVANTAGES	DISADVANTAGES
Poly-2-hydroxyethylmethacrylate (Hydron)	Spray powder Flexible Conforms to wound	Fluid loss via oozing
Pigskin	Relief of pain Reduction of water and heat loss Available in several forms Can be meshed	Costly Can provoke rejection
Cadaver skin	Relief of pain Reduction of water and heat loss Can be meshed	Expensive Scarce and not always available
Amniotic membrane	Biologic dressing Relief of pain Reduction of water and heat loss	Difficult to apply at times
Op-site (polyurethane)*	Permeable to air Not permeable to fluid or bacteria—promotes wound healing in moist environment No scab formation No debridement necessary Immediate pain reduction Painless removal Transparent Significantly shortens healing time	Time-consuming application Self-adhesive—can be difficult to apply Not suitable for full-thickness burns

*From Conkle W: Op-site dressing: New approach to burn care. *J Emer Nurs* (January/February) 1981; 9–16.

contain both the epidermis and all the dermis, are less commonly used than split-thickness grafts because they "take" less easily and require a longer time to heal. Split-thickness skin grafts, which include the epidermis and part of the dermis, can be taken from anywhere there is intact skin; preferred donor sites are those that match the skin texture of the area to be grafted and will be covered by clothing, such as the thigh. Skin layers are removed with a dermatome. *Sheet grafts,* which are used to cover the face, hands, fingers, and jointed areas, are left exposed or open to the air and are carefully rolled with sterile cotton-tipped applicators to remove trapped fluid or air that accumulates (Salisbury et al. 1983). *Mesh grafts* are skin grafts that are put through the Tanner dermatome, which meshes them and allows expansion to three or more times their original size. Mesh grafts, which are used to cover large surface areas such as the chest, back, arms, and legs, are dressed and kept moist for the first 48–72 hours postgrafting (Salisbury et al. 1983). The graft sites are immobilized by splints to insure the grafts will "take." Although mesh grafts have the advantage of numerous openings through which fluid can drain, they have the disadvantages of additional portals for infection and an unattractive appearance, which cosmetically limits their use to areas that will be covered by clothing.

In order for a graft to take, it must be placed on a healthy recipient bed that can generate granulation tissue and a capillary network. The graft must be immobilized for up to 10 days until a fibrin network and granulation tissue are firmly established (Fisher and Helm 1984). Blood flow usually is established by the third day. Nursing responsibilities during the early postgraft period include: (a) prevention of shearing between the graft and site by appropriate positioning, dressings, and sedation; (b) removal of serous accumulations or hematomas under the graft, if approved by the surgeon; and (c) observation of the graft site for infection. More conservatively, dressings may be left in place for up to 10 days. When they are removed, range of motion exercises may be resumed. Donor sites also must be cared for. They usually are covered with a light gauze dressing and left exposed to air, with drying encouraged by use of a heat lamp. Analgesics may be necessary for the first day or two. Donor sites also should be observed carefully for infection.

Advance in Burn Wound Coverage Gallico et al. (1984) have reported that human epidermal cells from a small skin biopsy about the size of a postage stamp (2 cm^2) can be cultured to produce an epitheal sheet suffi-

cient to cover the entire body surface. Culture time is about 3–4 weeks. This development has been cited by experts as the most significant advance in burn wound coverage since skin grafting was developed in the early 1900s.

Potential Ineffective Individual and/or Family Coping Related to Psychotraumatic Experience

Among the most challenging aspects of caring for the burned patient is the provision of psychologic support for the patient, family, and friends as they try to cope with the devastating impact of the burn. Psychologic reactions may include: (a) anxiety or fear about prognosis and treatment; (b) anger at self or others for contributing to the burn accident; (c) guilt for not being "more careful" to avoid dangerous circumstances; (d) resentment if the person views the burn as undeserved punishment; and (e) increased awareness of vulnerability, especially if the burn is perceived as resulting from an act of senseless violence. Patients often go through a grieving process for loss of their body image; loved ones may undergo a parallel grief process for loss of the patient's appearance or other valued characteristics.

Depending on the individual, applicable nursing diagnoses may include anxiety, altered family dynamics, fear, grieving, rational anger state, social isolation, disturbed self-concept, and spiritual distress.

Chapter 3 on communication and Chapter 20 on activity detail ways to assist the patient with the adaptation process and also contain specific suggestions on meeting the needs of critically ill patients' families. Among the nursing measures most effective in helping burned patients and families are: (a) projecting a calm, confident attitude as procedures are performed; (b) being honest and as hopeful as reality allows; (c) giving "bad news" in small doses appropriate to current coping levels; (d) focusing on small goals and their achievement; (e) willingly repeating explanations, which often are not heard initially through the screen of fear, pain, and anxiety; (f) preparing family and friends for bedside visits; (g) seeking assistance and consultation with psychologists and other burn team members skilled at dealing with psychotrauma; and, after the initial life threat has passed, (h) having the patient and loved ones put in contact with successfully rehabilitated burn survivors.

Outcome Evaluation

During the emergent and acute periods, the burned patient's progress can be judged according to these criteria:

- Vital signs WNL.
- CVP and PA readings normal.
- Alert and oriented level of consciousness.
- Urinary output 30–50 ml per hour during resuscitation phase.
- Bowel sounds present.
- Ventilation and oxygenation adequate as manifested by lung sounds and arterial blood gases WNL.
- Wounds free of "soupy" appearance or other signs of infection.

REFERENCES

Introduction

Cales RH, Heilig RW (ed): *Trauma care systems: A guide to planning, implementation, operation, and evaluation.* Rockville, MD: Aspen Publishers, 1986.

Committee on Trauma Research, Commission on Life Sciences, National Research Council and the Institute of Medicine: *Injury in America.* Washington, DC: National Academy Press, 1985.

Crabtree A, Jorgenson M: Exploring the practical knowledge in expert critical-care nursing practice. Unpublished master's thesis, University of Wisconsin, Madison, 1986.

San Diego County Department of Health Services, Division of Emergency Medical Services: *Trauma system annual report,* January 1987.

Trunkey D: Trauma. *Scientific American* 1983; 249:28–35.

Trunkey D: The value of trauma centers. *ACS Bulletin* 1982; 67; 5–7.

West JG et al.: Impact of regionalization: The Orange County experience. *Arch Surg* 1983; 118:740–744.

Multiple Trauma

Barach E et al.: Ballistics: A pathophysiologic examination of the wounding mechanism of firearms: Part I. *J Trauma* 1986; 26(3):114–124.

DeMuth WE: The mechanisms of shotgun wounds. *J Trauma* 1971; 11:219.

Gurdjian ES et al. (eds): *Impact injury and crash protection.* Springfield, IL: Charles C Thomas, 1970, p. 14.

Johanson BC et al. (eds): *Standards for critical care,* 2d ed. St Louis: Mosby, 1985, pp. 543–560.

Kenner CV et al.: *Critical care nursing: Body-mind-spirit,* 2d ed. Boston: Little, Brown, 1985.

May HL: The critically injured patient. Pages 231–245 in *Emergency medicine.* New York: John Wiley & Sons Medical Publications, 1984.

Swan KG, Swan RC: *Gunshot wounds: Pathophysiology and management.* Littleton, MA: PSG Publishing Co., 1980, p. 75.

Thompson JM et al.: *Clinical nursing.* St Louis: Mosby, 1986.

Head Injury

Hickey JV: *The clinical practice of neurological and neurosurgical nursing.* Philadelphia: Lippincott, 1986.

Hinkle J: Treating traumatic coma. *Am J Nurs* (May) 1986; 551–556.

Kneisl CR, Ames SW: *Adult health nursing—A biopsychosocial approach.* Menlo Park, CA: Addison-Wesley, 1986.

Lillehei KO, Hoff JT: Advances in the management of closed head injury. *Ann Emerg Med* (Aug) 1985; 789–795.

Manifold SL: Craniocerebral trauma. *Focus Crit Care* (Apr) 1986; 22–35.

McGuffin JF: Basic cerebral trauma care. *J Neuro Nurs* 1983; 15:189–193.

Muwaswes M: Increased intracranial pressure and its systemic effects. *J Neuro Nurs* 1985; 17:238–243.

Nikas DL (ed): *The critically ill neurosurgical patient.* New York: Churchill Livingstone, 1982.

Rudy EB: *Advanced neurological and neurosurgical nursing.* St Louis: Mosby, 1984.

Shpritz DW: Craniocerebral trauma. *Crit Care Nurse* (Mar/Apr) 1983; 49–61.

Ward JD: Axioms on head injury. *Hosp Med* (Nov) 1984; 115–134.

Webster M: Trends and controversies in head-trauma care. *Nurs Life* (Nov/Dec) 1984; 46–51.

Weiss MH, Stern M: Step-by-step management of head injury. *Crit Care Monitor* (Mar/Apr) 1985.

Zegeer LJ: Systemic cardiovascular effects of intracranial disorders: Implications for nursing care. *J Neuro Nurs* 1984; 16:161–167.

Spinal Cord Trauma

Anderson DK et al.: Spinal cord injury and protection. *Ann Emerg Med* 1985; 14:816–821.

Bell J, Hannon K: Pathophysiology involved in autonomic dysreflexia. *J Neuro Nurs* 1986; 18:86–88.

Brackett TO et al.: The emotional care of a person with a spinal cord injury. *JAMA* 1984; 252:793–795.

Cerullo LJ, Quigley MR: Management of cervical spinal cord injury. *J Emerg Nurs* 1985; 11:182–187.

Dudas S, Stevens KA: Central cord injury: Implications for nursing. *J Neuro Nurs* 1984; 16:84–88.

Egerton J et al.: ABC of spinal cord injury: Nursing. *Brit Med J* 1986; 292:325–329.

Grundy D, Russell J: ABC of spinal cord injury: Medical management in the spinal injuries unit. *Brit Med J* 1986; 292:183–187.

Grundy D et al.: ABC of spinal cord injury: Early management and complications—I. *Brit Med J* 1986a; 292:44–47.

Grundy D et al.: ABC of spinal cord injury: Early management and complications—II. *Brit Med J* 1986b; 292:123–125.

Hickey JV: *The clinical practice of neurological and neurosurgical nursing.* Philadelphia: Lippincott, 1986.

The injured patient's injured neck. *Emerg Med* (Apr) 1984; 16:24–58.

In the aftermath of head injury. *Emerg Med* (Jan) 1985; 17:88–116.

Kneisl CR, Ames SW: *Adult health nursing—A biopsychosocial approach.* Menlo Park, CA: Addison-Wesley, 1986.

Persaud DH: Assessing sexual functions of the adult with traumatic quadriplegia. *J Neuro Nurs* 1986; 18:11–12.

Ricci MM (ed): *Core curriculum for neuroscience nursing,* 2d ed. Oak Park, IL: American Association of Neuroscience Nurses, 1984.

Richmond TS: The patient with a cervical spinal cord injury. *Focus AACN* 1985; 12:23–33.

Rudy EB: *Advanced neurological and neurosurgical nursing.* St Louis: Mosby, 1984.

Stewart T: A threat to the spine-injured. *Emerg Med* (Mar) 1985; 107–110.

Szymanski D et al.: Central cord syndrome. *Ann Emerg Med* 1983; 12:45–47.

Trafton PG: Spinal cord injuries. *Surg Clin North Am* 1982; 62:61–72.

Chest Trauma

American College of Surgeons, Committee on Trauma: *Advanced trauma life support course: Instructor manual.* Chicago: American College of Surgeons, 1984, pp. 205–222.

Cosgriff J, Anderson D: *The practice of emergency care,* 2d ed. Philadelphia: Lippincott, 1984, pp. 354–381.

Hammond B, Lee G: *Emergency nursing: A quick reference.* Philadelphia: Lippincott, 1984, pp. 36–58.

Hoyt K: Chest trauma assessment. *Trauma Quart* 1986; 2(2):1–7.

Hoyt K: Chest trauma. *Nurs 83* 1983; 13(5):34–41.

Jurkovich E, Moore E: Thoracic trauma. *Trauma Quart* 1984; 1(1):37–51.

Rhodes M: Update on chest trauma. *Crit Care Quart* 1983; 6(2):306–319.

Sheehy S, Barber J: *Emergency nursing: Principles and practice.* St Louis: Mosby, 1985, pp. 306–319.

Trunkey D, Lewis F: *Current therapy of trauma—2.* Philadelphia: Decker, 1986, pp. 235–265.

Abdominal Trauma

American College of Surgeons, Committee on Trauma: *Advanced trauma life support course: Instructor Manual.* Chicago: American College of Surgeons, 1984, pp. 223–233.

Cosgriff J, Anderson D: *The practice of emergency care,* 2d ed. Philadelphia: Lippincott, 1984, pp. 367–381.

Grant HD et al.: *Emergency care,* 2d ed. Bowie, MD: Robert S. Brady Co., 1982, p. 243.

Rea R et al. (eds): *Trauma nursing core course: Instructors manual.* Chicago: Award Printing Corp., 1987.

Thal ER et al.: Abdominal trauma. Pages 291–344 in Shires TA (ed): *Principles of trauma care,* 3d ed. New York: McGraw-Hill, 1985.

Turnkey D, Lewis F: *Current therapy of trauma—2.* Philadelphia: Decker, 1986, pp. 266–306.

Wiener SL, Barrett J: Penetrating and nonpenetrating abdominal injuries. Pages 212–250 in Wiener SL, Barrett J (eds): *Trauma management for civilian and military physicians.* Philadelphia: Saunders, 1986.

Orthopedic Trauma

American College of Surgeons, Committee on Trauma: *Advanced trauma life support course: Instructor manual.* Chicago: American College of Surgeons, 1984. pp. 269–278.

Cosgriff J, Anderson D: *The practice of emergency care.* Philadelphia: Lippincott, 1984, pp. 570–594.

Epps CH (ed): *Complications in orthopaedic surgery,* 2d ed. Philadelphia: Lippincott, 1986.

Rea R et al. (eds): *Trauma nursing core course: Instructors manual.* Chicago, Award Printing Corp., 1987.

Stevenson CK: Take no chances with fat embolism. *Nurs 85* 1985; 15(6):58–63.

Wiener SL, Barrett J (eds): *Trauma management for civilian and military physicians.* Philadelphia: Saunders, 1986.

Burns

American Burn Association: Specific Optimal Criteria for Hospital Resources for Care of Patients with Burn Injury. The Association, April 1976.

Archambeault-Jones C, Feller I: Burn Care. Pages 741–794 in Kenney M et al. (eds): *AACN's clinical reference for critical care nursing.* New York: McGraw Hill, 1981.

Davies J: *Physiological responses to burning injury.* London: New Academic Press, 1982, pp. 45–91, 108, 246, 396, 558–612.

Demling R: Fluid replacement in burned patients. *Surg Clin North Am* 1987; 67(2):15–70.

DiMola M et al.: Burn Care Protocols. *J Burn Care and Rehab* (Jan/Feb) 1986; 60–65.

Dyer C: Burn care in the emergent period. *J Emerg Nurs* (Jan/Feb) 1980; 9–16.

Fisher S, Helm P: *Comprehensive rehabilitation of burns.* Baltimore, MD: Williams and Wilkins, 1984, pp. 19–20.

Gallico G et al.: Permanent coverage of large burn wounds with autologous cultured human epithelium. *N Engl J Med* 1984; 3(11):448–451.

Johnson C, Cain V: Burn care: The rehab guide. *Am J Nurs* (Jan) 1985; 48–50.

Pruitt B: The diagnosis and treatment of infection in the burn patient. *Burns* 1984; 11:79–91.

Robertson K et al.: Burn care: The crucial first days. *Am J Nurs* (Jan) 1985; 30–45.

Rosequist C, Shepp P: Burn care: The nutrition factor. *Am J Nurs* (Jan) 1985; 45–48.

Ruberg R: Advances in burn care. *Clin Plastic Surg* 1986; 13:3–159.

Salisbury et al. (eds): *Manual of burn therapeutics: An interdisciplinary approach,* 1st ed. Boston/Toronto: Little, Brown, 1983, pp. 23–59.

Vermeer C: Carbon monoxide poisoning. *J Emerg Nurs* 1982; 8:217–220.

Wooldridge-King M: Nursing considerations of the burned patient during the emergent period. *Heart Lung* 1982; 11:353–363.

SUPPLEMENTAL READING

Head Injury

Cooper KR et al.: Safe use of PEEP in patients with severe head injury. *J Neurosurg* 1985; 63:552–555.

Heiden JS et al.: Severe head injury. *Phys Ther* 1983; 63:1946–1951.

Heise T: Management of the multiple trauma patient with increased ICP. *J Neuro Nurs* 1983; 15:201–204.

Hockberger RS et al.: Blunt head injury: A spectrum of disease. *Ann Emerg Med* 1986; 15:202–207.

Montgomery J: Overview of head injuries. *Phys Ther* 1983; 63:1945.

Scherer P: Assessment: The logic of coma. *Am J Nurs* (May) 1986; 542–550.

Warren JB: Pulmonary complications associated with severe head injury. *J Neuro Nurs* 1983; 15:194–200.

Yanke J: Head injuries. *J Neuro Nurs* 1984; 16:173–180.

Spinal Cord Trauma

Agee BL, Herman C: Cervical logrolling on a standard hospital bed. *Am J Nurs* (Mar) 1984; 315–318.

Friedman-Campbell M, Hart CA: Theoretical strategies and nursing interventions to promote psychosocial adaptation to spinal cord injuries and disability. *J Neuro Nurs* 1984; 16:335–342.

Ingersoll GL: Abdominal pathology in spinal cord injured persons. *J Neuro Nurs* 1985; 17:343–348.

Mackechnie J, Wade PA: Case report: Electrophrenic respiration and discharge planning with a C_1 quadriplegic. *J Neuro Nurs* 1984; 16:347–352.

Stanton GM: A needs assessment of significant others following the patient's spinal cord injury. *J Neuro Nurs* 1984; 16:253–256.

Chest Trauma

Hart LH: Hidden chest trauma in the head-injured patient. *Crit Care Nurse* (July/August) 1986; 51–57.

Sommers MS: Cardiac tamponade after non-penetrating cardiac trauma. *Dimen Crit Care Nurs* (July/August) 1986; 206–215.

Orthopedic Trauma

Larson M et al.: Detecting compartmental syndrome using continuous pressure monitoring. *Focus Crit Care* (October) 1986; 51–56.

Martin SL: Fat embolism syndrome. *Dimen Crit Care Nurs* (May/June) 1983; 158–161.

Burns

Bernstein N: *Emotional care of the facially burned and disfigured.* Boston: Little, Brown, 1976.

Cooke S: Major thermal injury—the first 48 hours. *Crit Care Nurse* 1986; 6(1):55–63.

Heck E et al.: Composite skin graft: Frozen dermal allografts support the engraftment and expansion of autologous epidermis. *J Trauma* 1985; 25:106–112.

Hudak C et al.: *Critical care nursing: A holistic approach,* 4th ed. Philadelphia: Lippincott, 1986, pp. 642–658.

Hyperbaric oxygenation therapy now making careful comeback. Medical News, in *JAMA* (September 4) 1981; 1057–1066.

Kenner CV: Burn injury. Pages 1101–1146 in Kenner CV et al. (eds): *Critical care nursing: Body-mind-spirit.* Boston: Little, Brown, 1985.

Klein DG, O'Malley P: Topical injury from chemical agents: initial treatment. *Heart Lung* 1987; 16(1):49–54.

Ross M: Healing under pressure. *Am J Nurs* 1986; 10:1118–1120.

Winkler J (issue ed): Burn care update. *Crit Care Quart* 1984; 7(3):1–84.

Yoshitsugu K, Inoue H: Ultrastructural study of regenerated skin after deep dermal and third degree burns. *Annals Plastic Surg* 1985; 15(5):386–393.

Appendix 1

FANCAS

This book utilizes a conceptual approach that is based on a teaching tool developed by a nurse, Dr. June C. Abbey (1976). Dr. Abbey identified six areas of universal concern to nurses interested in promoting the goal of a living, interacting, pain-free person: fluid balance, aeration, nutrition, communication, activity, and pain. The teaching tool she developed to help nurses remember these concerns carries the mnemonic FANCAP. FANCAP is compatible with most nursing models based on a framework of problem solving, basic needs, general systems, or adaptation (Abbey 1980). The approach used in this book is an adaptation of FANCAP called FANCAS (Swendsen 1975), in which the "P" for "pain" is replaced by an "S" for the broader area of "stimulation."

FANCAS serves as a memory aid to help you diagnose a patient's problems and project solutions to them. The categories deliberately are broad to allow maximum flexibility of the tool in various clinical settings. The definitions and subcategories shown in Table A–1 are derived from Abbey and Swendsen. Any categorization of a given problem is correct provided it can be supported logically. The order of the letters is unimportant. In fact, this edition has rearranged the letters to emphasize the significance of particular areas. The order used is:

C Communication
S Stimulation
A Aeration
F Fluid balance
N Nutrition
A Activity

Throughout this book, the components of FANCAS are isolated for analysis and description. A patient, of course, cannot be compartmentalized so neatly. The very nature of a patient mandates a holistic approach to care, one that interweaves consideration of physiologic, psychologic, social, and spiritual attributes.

Previous chapters discuss in detail not only the *what* of patient care but also the *how to* and *why*. Such detail is appropriate for educational purposes. In the setting of a busy critical-care service, however, such detail is inappropriate if not impossible to include on a patient's care plan. This appendix presents one feasible method of care planning in a critical-care setting and illustrates its application with a clinical example.

An in-depth discussion of nursing care planning theory is beyond the scope of this appendix. The reader who wishes to know more about that theory is referred to the many excellent references on care planning in the nursing literature. Instead, the intent here is to demonstrate the transformation of data obtained with a FANCAS assessment tool into a clinically useful plan of care. To that end, the major components of a nursing care planning system are discussed briefly.

TABLE A–1 FANCAS AND SELECTED CORE CONCEPTS AND SKILLS IN CRITICAL-CARE NURSING

LETTER	CATEGORY	DEFINITION	CORE CONCEPTS	CORE SKILLS

C	Communication	Verbal and nonverbal interchange between person and environment	Anatomy and physiology of vision, hearing, and speech
			Stages of adaptation
			Nursing care in:
			  Impaired verbal communication
			  Sensory-perceptual alteration
			  Ineffective individual coping
			  Ineffective family coping
			  Death and dying
				Assessment of communication process and content
				Crisis intervention

S	Stimulation	Perception, interpretation, and integration of stimuli	Anatomy and physiology of nervous system
			Nursing care in:
			  Increased intracranial pressure
			  Herniation syndromes
			  Status epilepticus
			  Pain
			  Guillain-Barré syndrome
			  Myasthenia gravis
			  Vascular disorders
			  Craniotomy
			  Ventricular shunting
				Stimulation physical assessment
				Interpretation of reports of neurodiagnostic procedures
				Intracranial pressure monitoring
				Pain relief measures

A	Aeration	Movement of gases to provide energy and eliminate volatile waste products	Respiratory anatomy and physiology
			Nursing care in:
			  Pulmonary edema
			  Adult respiratory distress syndrome
			  Atelectasis
			  Pulmonary embolus
			  Respiratory failure
			  Status asthmaticus
			  Pneumothorax
			  Pneumonia
			  Thoracotomy
				Aeration physical assessment
				Interpretation of bedside pulmonary function test reports
				Interpretation of arterial blood gases
				Interpretation of reports of chest x-rays and other diagnostic procedures
				Nursing skills related to oxygen therapy, chest physiotherapy, artificial airways, tracheal suctioning, mechanical ventilation, chest drainage, and thoracotomy

F	Fluid balance	Movement of fluids and electrolytes among body compartments	Cardiovascular anatomy and physiology
			Nursing care in:
			  Dysrhythmias and conduction defects
			  Acute chest pain
			  Acute myocardial infarction
				Cardiovascular physical assessment
				Interpretation of reports of cardiovascular laboratory tests
				Interpretation of reports of cardiac diagnostic procedures

(Continues)

TABLE A–1 FANCAS & SELECTED CORE CONCEPTS & SKILLS IN CRITICAL-CARE NURSING (Continued)

LETTER	CATEGORY	DEFINITION	CORE CONCEPTS	CORE SKILLS
			Altered cardiac output (cardiac failure)	Hemodynamic pressure monitoring
			Acute cardiac tamponade	ECG interpretation
			Decreased tissue perfusion (shock)	Advanced cardiac life support
			Intraaortic balloon counterpulsation	Nursing skills related to pacemakers, drug therapy, and intraaortic balloon counter pulsation
			Cardiac surgery	
			Renal anatomy and physiology	Renal physical assessment
			Nursing care in:	Interpretation of urinalysis, BUN, creatinine, and related laboratory tests
			Acute renal failure	
			Dialysis	Nursing skills related to hemofiltration, peritoneal dialysis, protection of hemodialysis; Vascular access
			Fluid and electrolyte physiology	Fluid and elctrolyte physical assessment
			Nursing care in fluid and electrolyte imbalances:	Interpretation of serum osmolality, serum electrolytes, and related laboratory tests
			Fluid excess	
			Fluid deficit	
			Hypo/hypernatremia	
			Hypo/hyperkalemia	
			Hypo/hypercalcemia	
			Hypo/hypermagnesemia	
			Acid–base physiology	Interpretation of arterial blood gases
			Nursing care in acid–base imbalances:	
			Respiratory acidosis	
			Respiratory alkalosis	
			Metabolic acidosis	
			Metabolic alkalosis	
			Nursing care in therapeutic hypothermia	Use of hypothermia blanket
			Endocrine/metabolic physiology	Endocrine/metabolic assessment
			Nursing care in:	Interpretation of serum glucose and thyroid tests
			Diabetic ketoacidosis	
			HHNK	
			Hypoglycemia	
			Thyroid crisis	
			Hematologic/immunologic physiology	Hematologic/immunologic assessment
			Nursing care in:	Interpretation of CBC and coagulation profile
			Disseminated intravascular coagulation	
			AIDS	

TABLE A–1 FANCAS & SELECTED CORE CONCEPTS & SKILLS IN CRITICAL-CARE NURSING (Continued)

LETTER	CATEGORY	DEFINITION	CORE CONCEPTS	CORE SKILLS
N	Nutrition	Intake, digestion, and absorption of nutrients; removal of solid waste products	Abdominal anatomy and physiology Nursing care in: Gastrointestinal bleeding Hepatitis Hepatic failure Pancreatitis	Abdominal assessment Assessment of nutritional status Nursing skills related to hyperalimentation
A	Activity	Expenditure of physical or psychologic energy	Physiological effects of bedrest Sleep Sexuality Nursing care in: Sleep pattern disturbance Disturbed self-concept Potential sexual dysfunction	Assessment of activity Prevention of detrimental effects of bedrest: range-of-motion exercises, positioning procedures Environmental control
All	Trauma	Injury	Trauma physiology Mechanisms of injury Trauma resuscitation roles Nursing care in: Head trauma Spinal cord trauma Chest trauma Abdominal trauma Orthopedic trauma Multiple trauma Burn physiology Nursing care in emergent and acute burn phases	Trauma assessment Trauma priority-setting Nursing skills related to cervical spine stabilization, chest tube insertion, peritoneal lavage, orthopedic stabilization Assessment of burn severity Calculation of burn fluid requirements Burn wound care

Nursing Care Plan

The nursing care plan contains nursing diagnoses, signs and symptoms, nursing actions, and desired outcomes. Nursing problems are written as diagnostic statements: a *nursing diagnosis* joined (by the words "related to") to an etiology, the most probable cause of the problem. Table A–2 presents nursing diagnoses grouped according to FANCAS.

Problems may be actual or potential. An *actual* problem is one the patient definitely will experience. A *potential* problem is one for which the patient is at high risk. For instance, for patients with chest tubes, pain is an actual problem, whereas infection is a potential problem.

Signs and symptoms are the subjective and objective data on which the diagnoses are based, that is, its common manifestations.

Nursing actions are activities designed to facilitate the patient's achievement of the outcomes desired. They specify what is to be done, under what circumstances, and how frequently. An example might be "Perform passive range of motion exercises for the paralyzed extremity five times every 4 hours while patient is awake."

Desired outcomes are short-term objectives that must be achieved before the overall discharge criteria can be met. They should be specific, measurable patient behaviors, that is, statements of what you can observe with your senses. For instance, suppose you were writing a standard care plan for congestive heart failure (CHF) and had identified as a nursing diagnosis "potential knowledge deficit related to post-discharge medications." A statement such as "understands medications" would not be acceptable as a desired outcome. Because it does not specify what you would observe the patient doing, it is too subject to varying interpretations by different members of the nursing staff. An acceptable desired outcome might be "Correctly states name, purpose, and dosage schedule for each discharge medication."

Nursing diagnoses, signs and symptoms, nursing actions, and desired outcomes can be derived from clinical experience, a review of patient charts, and/or a review of nursing literature. Nursing care for many critical-care disorders is presented in this book. For disorders not specifically addressed in this book, the core concepts can be used as building blocks in the construction of a care plan.

Purpose of the Standard Care Plan

Standard care plans delineate the *usual* problems that can be predicted from a patient's condition and those nursing actions likely to lead to successful resolution of the problems. They are written *in advance* and should

TABLE A-2 NURSING DIAGNOSES GROUPED ACCORDING TO FANCAS

COMMUNICATION

Anxiety
Fear
Grieving, anticipatory
Grieving, dysfunctional
Hopelessness
Powerlessness
Posttrauma response
Rape-trauma syndrome

Coping, ineffective individual
Coping, ineffective family: compromised
Coping, ineffective family: disabling
Coping, family: potential for growth

Communication, impaired verbal
Family processes, alteration in
Social interaction, impaired
Parenting, alteration in
Social isolation
Violence, potential for

Spiritual distress

STIMULATION

Comfort, altered: chronic pain
Comfort, alteration in: pain

Knowledge deficit (specify)
Thought processes, alteration in

Sensory-perceptual alteration: visual, auditory, kinesthetic, gustatory, tactile, olfactory
Unilateral neglect

AERATION

Airway clearance, ineffective
Breathing pattern, ineffective
Gas exchange, impaired

FLUID BALANCE

Cardiac output, alteration in: decreased
Tissue perfusion, alteration in

Tissue integrity, impaired

Fluid volume deficit
Fluid volume, alteration in: excess

Body temperature, potential alteration in
Hypothermia
Hyperthermia
Thermoregulation, ineffective

FLUID BALANCE (Continued)

Functional incontinence
Reflex incontinence
Stress incontinence
Urge incontinence
Total incontinence
Urinary elimination, alteration in patterns
Urinary retention

NUTRITION

Oral mucous membrane, alteration in
Nutrition, alteration in: less than body requirements
Nutrition, alteration in: more than body requirements
Swallowing, impaired

Bowel elimination, alteration in: constipation
Bowel elimination, alteration in: diarrhea
Bowel elimination, alteration in: incontinence

ACTIVITY

Activity intolerance
Diversional activity, deficit
Home maintenance management, impaired
Mobility, impaired physical
Self-care deficit (specify level): feeding, bathing/hygiene, dressing/grooming, toileting
Self-concept, disturbance in: body image, self-esteem, role performance, personal identity

Sleep pattern disturbance

Injury, potential for: poisoning, suffocation, trauma
Infection, potential for
Skin integrity, impairment of

Adjustment, impaired
Growth and development, altered
Health maintenance alteration
Noncompliance (specify)

Sexuality patterns, altered
Sexual dysfunction

Within FANCAS categories, related diagnoses have been grouped. The distinction in the official NANDA list between actual and potential diagnoses (for: activity intolerance; fluid volume deficit; nutrition, alteration in: more than body requirements; parenting, alteration in; and skin integrity, alteration in) has been dropped to simplify the list and because most diagnoses can be used in either form.

These nursing diagnoses are from McLane A (ed): *Classification of nursing diagnoses: Proceedings of the seventh conference.* St Louis: Mosby, 1987.

be readily accessible to the nursing staff. Standard care plans are appropriate for patients whose problems and progress fall within expected norms.

Standard care plans can be written for diagnoses, situations, or general physiologic states. An intensive care unit, for example, might have standard care plans on pulmonary edema, knowledge deficit, and sleep deprivation.

Individual Care Plan

When a standard care plan is available to cover predictable care, an individual care plan needs to be handwritten only for *unusual problems,* that is, those that are unique or require special attention. They may be unanticipated problems or anticipated ones with which the patient is not coping satisfactorily. Frequently, you may determine from your assessment that the patient does not have any unusual problems. In that case, you would use only the standard care plan. If you did identify unu-

sual problems, you would state for each one: its probable etiology, signs and symptoms, nursing actions, and expected outcomes.

This care planning system is efficient, flexible, and promotes individualized care. Writing a new comprehensive care plan "from scratch" on every patient is unrealistic in today's busy critical-care environment. With this system, the nurse writes only the unusual problems, if any.

Care Planning Application: Karen J.

Table A–3 presents data obtained during a critical-care nurse's assessment of Karen J. on the day before her cardiac surgery. The nurse used a FANCAS assessment format, which leads logically into identification of patient problems.

TABLE A–3 CRITICAL-CARE NURSING ASSESSMENT GUIDE

Name *Karen J.*   Hospital # *000000*

Date *9/24*   Assessor *Nancy Holloway, RN*

Chief complaint *"short of breath, very tired, weight loss × 1½ yrs"*

Medical diagnosis *severe mitral regurgitation, significant mitral stenosis;*
for valve replacement 9/25

Allergies *penicillin*

VITAL SIGNS

Temperature ___*98.6°*___ Pulse ___*72*___ Respirations ___*16*___ BP ___*120/70*___

GENERAL APPEARANCE

Age ___*48*___ Sex ___*F*___ Race ___*W*___ Height ___*5'2"*___ Weight ___*46.5 kg*___

General: development ___*frail*___ nourishment ___*appears poor*___

degree of distress *no acute distress*

COMMUNICATION

Process

1. History *congenital deafness and slurred speech*
2. Physical
   Vision *nl*

TABLE A–3   CRITICAL-CARE NURSING ASSESSMENT GUIDE *(Continued)*

COMMUNICATION (Continued)

Reading ability *college level*

Hearing *deafness—greater in R ear*

Tactile perception *nl*

Speech *slurred, hesitant*

Writing ability *nl*

Gesturing ability *nl*

3. Diagnostic procedures and laboratory tests
   none

4. Other relevant data *none*

Content

1. History
   Ethnic background *Caucasian*
   Religion *Baptist "but not strong faith"*
   Education *2 yr RN—did not complete*
   Occupation *homemaker*
   Usual coping methods
   Pain *withdraws physically and emotionally; has tears in eyes; doesn't like to ask for pain medication because of seeming weak and babyish*
   Anger *withdraws until cooled off*
   Substance abuse *none*
   Emotional problems *neg except for "hard time adjusting" when illness caused her to lose scholarship and drop out of school 2 years ago*

2. Current information
   Expressed concerns *will be embarrassed without dentures; husband will be shocked and upset when sees her post-op; won't know when daughter's baby born*

   Expectations of hospitalization *expects dangerous surgery, painful, unpleasant post-op period; worried about competence of staff, esp. supervision of students and new nurses; anticipates difficulty making needs understood*

   Significant others *husband Raymond and daughter Melissa. Raymond works in construction 8 AM–6 PM; off only on day of surgery. Melissa expecting baby any day. Neither present for any teaching–home is 3-hr drive from hospital*

   Apparent stage of adaptation to illness *disorganization—anxiety*

3. Diagnostic procedures *none*
4. Other relevant data *none*

STIMULATION

1. History *neg*
2. Physical
   LOC *alert and oriented*
   Skull *intact*   Neck *flexible*
   Eyes: Corneal reflex *nl*
   Pupil size *3 mm, equal*
   Reaction to light *brisk and equal*
   Extremities:
   Sensation *nl*

(Continues)

TABLE A–3 CRITICAL-CARE NURSING ASSESSMENT GUIDE *(Continued)*

STIMULATION (Continued)

Voluntary movement *moves all extremities freely*

Reflex movement *DTRs 2⁺ and equal bilaterally*

Babinski *nl bilaterally*

Posturing *absent*

Smoothness and coordination of movement *nl*

3. Diagnostic procedures and laboratory tests
none

4. Other relevant data *none*

AERATION

1. History *DOE, PND, orthopnea × 1½ years; smoking history neg*

2. Physical

   A. Inspection

      Thoracic shape *symmetrical, AP < lateral diameter*

      Respirations: Rate _____ *16* _____ Rhythm _____ *eupnea* _____

      Chest expansion *equal bilaterally*

   B. Palpation

      Trachea *midline*

      Tactile fremitus *nl*

   C. Percussion *nl*

   D. Auscultation

      Breath sounds *nl*

      Adventitious sounds: *few rales at bases; clear with coughing*

      Voice and whispered sounds *nl*

   E. Extrathoracic signs

      Cyanosis _____ *neg* _____ Clubbing _____ *neg* _____

      Use of accessory muscles _____ *neg* _____

   F. Other _____

3. Diagnostic procedures and laboratory tests

   A. Chest x-ray *results not available*

   B. Pulmonary function tests *not done*

      Inspiratory force _____ Compliance _____

      FEV_1 _____ TV _____ RV _____

      FRC _____ TLC _____ VC _____

      V_D/V_T ratio _____

      Other _____

   C. Other *NA*

(Continues)

TABLE A–3 CRITICAL-CARE NURSING ASSESSMENT GUIDE *(Continued)*

FLUID BALANCE

Cardiovascular system

1. History *Rheumatic fever, age 12*

    P.A.T. after catheterization 3 weeks ago—converted p̄ treatment

    c̄ Quinidine. Has been on Lanoxin, Hydrodiuril, KCl—last doses 9/23

2. Physical

    A. Inspection/palpation—vasculature

    Skin color _____ *pale* _____ temperature _____ *warm* _____

    trophic changes _____ *neg* _____

    vascular lesions _____ *neg* _____

    tenderness _____ *neg* _____ Homan's sign _____ *neg* _____

    edema _____ *neg* _____

    Arterial pulses

    carotid _____ $2^+ =$ _____ brachial _____ $2^+ =$ _____ radial _____ $2^+ =$ _____

    femoral _____ $2^+ =$ _____ popliteal _____ $2^+ =$ _____

    dorsalis pedis _____ $2^+ =$ _____ posterior tibial _____ $2^+ =$ _____

    B. Auscultation—vasculature

    BP *120/70—bilateral brachial*

    Bruits *neg*

    C. Neck veins *distended at 90°* HJR *neg*

    PTT *47 (control 45.5)*

    D. Inspection/palpation—heart

    PMI *5th ICS at anterior axillary line*

    Precordial movements *apical thrill*

    E. Auscultation—heart

    Heart sounds

    S₁ _____ *nl* _____ S₂ _____ *opening snap* _____

    S₃ _____ *none* _____ S₄ _____ *none* _____

    Murmurs *holosystolic III/VI apex → axilla*

    diastolic IV/VI axilla → apex

    rubs *none*

3. Diagnostic procedures and laboratory tests

    A. CBC RBC _____ *4,200,000* _____ Hgb _____ *14.5* _____ Hct _____ *38%* _____

    Reticulocytes _____ *NA* _____ WBC _____ *8600* _____

    Differential _____ *nl* _____

    B. Clotting time _____ *NA* _____ PT _____ *12.9 (control 13.0)* _____

    C. Enzymes *SGOT 23, LDH 212, CPK 8*

    D. ECG *NSR at 72*

    E. Chest x-ray *results not yet reported*

    F. Cardiac cath *3 weeks ago. Cardiac output and index nl; LV function good. Mitral valve gradient 16, area 0.9 cm²*

    G. Cardiac pressures RA _____ *2* _____ RV _____ *40/4* _____ LA _____ *19* _____

    LV _____ *120/8* _____ PA _____ *40/16* _____ Aorta _____ *120/70* _____ PCWP _____ *22* _____

    CVP _____ *16* _____

(Continues)

TABLE A–3 CRITICAL-CARE NURSING ASSESSMENT GUIDE *(Continued)*

FLUID BALANCE *(Continued)*

H.   Other _____

4.   Other relevant data *none* _____

Renal system

1.   History *neg* _____

2.   Physical *neg* _____

3.   Diagnostic procedures and laboratory tests
     Urine volume *24 hour unknown. Urinalysis sample 200 ml; voids* _____
          7–8 x/day s̄ difficulty

     spg __*1.020*__   osmolality __*NA*__
     urinalysis: color __*straw*__   clarity __*clear*__
     pH __*6*__   cells __*few white*__
     crystals __*0*__   casts __*0*__
     bacteria __*0*__

FLUID BALANCE

BUN __*7*__ Creatinine __*0.8*__
Creatinine clearance __*NA*__ Hgb __*see above*__
Hct __*see above*__

Other _____

4.   Other relevant data *none* _____

Fluid and electrolyte balance

1.   History *anorexia × 1½ yrs, diuretics × 1 yr* _____

2.   Physical *skin turgor nl; mucous membranes hydrated; BP, pulse rate, pulse volume normal* ___

3.   Diagnostic procedures and laboratory tests
     Intake and output (24 hr) *no definite data; pt describes as "average"* _____
     Blood sugar __*100 mg%*__
     Osmolality: serum __*NA*__ urine __*NA*__
     Electrolytes: serum Na^+ __*136*__ K^+ __*3.6*__
          Cl^- __*98*__ Ca^+ __*NA*__ Mg^{2+} __*NA*__
          urine: Na^+ __*NA*__ K^+ __*NA*__ Cl^- __*NA*__

Other _____

4.   Other relevant data *none* _____

Acid–base balance

     Arterial blood gases *not done* _____
     F_1O_2_____ Po_2_____
     A-a gradient_____ Shunt_____
     pH _____ Pco_2 _____ HCO_3 _____ BE _____
     anion gap _____

(Continues)

TABLE A–3　CRITICAL-CARE NURSING ASSESSMENT GUIDE *(Continued)*

NUTRITION

1.　History *anorexia, fatigue × 1½ years. Usual elimination pattern 1/day—nl color and consistency*

2.　Physical

　　General appearance *thin, frail, pale*

　　Weight ____*46.5 kg*____ Change? _____*loss of 13 kg in last 1½ yr*_____

Mouth: Dentition *upper and lower dentures*

　　　　Tongue *nl appearance and movement*

　　　　Gag reflex *intact*

　　　　Swallow reflex *intact*

　　Abdomen

　　　　Inspection *nl appearance*

　　　　Auscultation *nl bowel sounds in all 4 quadrants; no bruits or rubs*

　　　　Percussion and palpation

　　　　　　Tenderness ____*neg*____ Rigidity ____*neg*____

　　　　　　Liver *upper border 6th ICS, lower at costal margin; not tender*

　　　　　　Spleen *5 cm oval 9th–11th ribs at MAL; not palpable*

　　　　Rectum and anus *Ō hemorrhoids*

3.　Diagnostic procedures and laboratory tests

4.　Other relevant data *none*

ACTIVITY

1.　History

　　Past activity level *sedentary × 1½ yrs due to fatigue and dyspnea; played tennis and other active sports before that. Sleeps 8 hrs a night (10 PM–6 AM) plus 3 naps per day; bathes in evening; likes to read and sew.*

　　Current activity level

　　　　Prescribed (include estimated duration)

　　　　complete bedrest; probably up in chair on 2nd p.o. day and ambulating with assistance on 5th p.o. day

　　　　Actual *bedrest, moving about freely*

2.　Physical

　　Perception of pressure ____√____ normal _____ absent _____ diminished _____

　　　　If absent or diminished, specify how _____

　　Skin integrity *no signs of breakdown*

　　Activity impediments _____ cast _____ diminished joint mobility _____

　　　　　　____√____ low tolerance for physical exertion

　　　　　　_____ other (specify) _____

3.　Diagnostic procedures and laboratory tests
　　NA

4.　Other relevant data *none*

Abbreviations: nl = normal, neg = negative, NA = not available, LOC = level of consciousness.

After assessing the patient and recording the data, the nurse's next step is to analyze the data in order to identify the nursing diagnoses. The following paragraphs describe the nurse's thinking as the nurse reviews and analyzes the data under each FANCAS section.

Communication

There are a lot of problem signals here.

Worry About Cost of Hospitalization She says their insurance won't cover the bill. The Social Service Department might be able to help with this.

Worry About Her Husband and Daughter She's really upset about not being with her daughter during labor. She also seems concerned her husband will lose his job if he takes time off, yet angry that he's not here when she needs him. She also said she's afraid he'll be shocked and upset when he first sees her after the operation. This amount of anxiety about her family is unusual.

Communication Barriers She has trouble both hearing and speaking, and is worried that staff will ignore her or not understand what she needs. Also, she'll be intubated for several hours postoperatively. She may have unusual trouble getting adequate pain relief and emotional support because of her tendency to withdraw, too. These difficulties make communication an unusual problem for her.

Anxiety About Staff Competence She is knowledgeable about technical details of care and apprehensive about a painful, unpleasant postoperative period. She's also concerned about poor care from inexperienced staff. This degree of anxiety about staff competence is unusual.

Stimulation

Everything looks good here except her speech difficulty, which has already been considered.

Aeration

Her dyspnea on exertion and paroxysmal nocturnal dyspnea are signs of her mitral valve disease and should be relieved by her surgery. Her lungs are clear now, and she'll need the usual postop chest care to keep them that way. No unusual problems here.

Fluid Balance

Cardiac Her left atrial, pulmonary capillary wedge, and right-sided pressures are elevated; but these elevations are typical for her disorders. The apical thrill, murmurs, increased mitral valve gradient, and decreased valve area are all typical, too. Potential atrial dysrhythmias are usual problems with mitral stenosis and regurgitation, due to volume overload of the atria or hypoxia secondary to pulmonary congestion. Her cardiac strengths are her normal rhythm, left ventricular and aortic pressures, left ventricular function, cardiac output, cardiac index, and serum enzymes. Our standard care plan on mitral valve replacement is appropriate for her.

Vascular Her vascular status doesn't pose any problems. The only pathologic finding is the jugular venous distention; but that's just another sign of her right-sided failure.

Renal Everything's normal here.

Fluid and Electrolytes Everything's normal here, too.

Nutrition

She says she's not been hungry for a long time and often is too tired to fix nourishing meals; this is borne out by her chronic weight loss. She'll be N.P.O. during the operative period; as she's already depleted of nutrients, poor wound healing and resistance to infection are possibilities. This is an unusual problem.

Activity

She is sedentary because of her fatigue and is on bed-rest. She really sleeps a lot now. Although she'll be sedated from the anesthetic and analgesics, her decreased mobility will probably not be much of a problem, as she is moving about in bed freely now and the surgeon anticipates getting her out of bed within 3 days after the surgery. This decrease in mobility represents a usual problem.

After identifying the patient's problems and differentiating the usual and unusual problems, the nurse develops a care plan. The nurse begins with the standard care plan for mitral valve replacement developed by the nursing staff of the intensive care unit. Table A–4 lists the usual problems included in the standard care plan for a patient undergoing mitral valve replacement.

After identifying actual and potential usual problems, the staff had written possible causes, signs and symptoms, nursing actions, and desired outcomes. Table A–5 illustrates the development of four problems selected from this standard care plan for patients undergoing mitral valve replacement: anxiety, potential sensory-perceptual alterations, potential decreased cardiac output, and potential for infection.

TABLE A-4 NURSING DIAGNOSES FOR STANDARD CARE PLAN ON MITRAL VALVE REPLACEMENT—INTENSIVE CARE UNIT PHASE

Communication

Anxiety
Potential sensory-perceptual alterations

Stimulation

Pain

Aeration

Potential ineffective airway clearance
Potential ineffective breathing pattern
Potential impaired gas exchange

Fluid balance

Potential decreased cardiac output
Potential alteration in tissue perfusion
Potential excess fluid volume
Potential alteration in urinary elimination pattern

Nutrition

Potential decreased nutrition

Activity

Impaired physical mobility
Potential for infection
Potential sensory-perceptual alterations

TABLE A-5   STANDARD CARE PLAN*

Nursing discharge criteria

1. *Vital signs within normal limits (WNL) for patient*
2. *Urinary output above 30 ml/hr with specific gravity WNL for patient*
3. *Arterial blood gas values WNL for patient after extubation*
4. *Arterial line discontinued*
5. *Peripheral pulses, limb temperature, and limb color WNL for patient*
6. *Level of consciousness WNL for patient*
7. *Medical/surgical problems (for example, dysrhythmias) controlled by medical therapeutic plan*
8. *Patient and/or family demonstrate awareness of therapeutic plan and ability to cooperate with it*

NURSING DIAGNOSIS	SIGNS AND SYMPTOMS	NURSING ACTIONS	DESIRED OUTCOMES
Communication			
Anxiety related to pain and separation from loved ones; unfamiliar environment; dependency	Tense expression or posture Restless Withdrawn Hypertension Tachycardia Tachypnea	1. Implement preoperative cardiac surgery teaching program in conjunction with nursing staff on preoperative unit. 2. Nurse who will receive patient postoperatively: Visit patient on day be-	Relaxed facial expression. Relaxed body posture. Discusses questions and worries with staff. BP, pulse, and respirations WNL for patient.

(Continues)

TABLE A-5   STANDARD CARE PLAN* *(Continued)*

NURSING DIAGNOSIS	SIGNS AND SYMPTOMS	NURSING ACTIONS	DESIRED OUTCOMES
		fore surgery, assess understanding of preop teaching program and appropriateness of taking patient and family to visit ICU.	
		3. Assess need for analgesics by noting groaning, frowning, unexplained restlessness, unwillingness to move. Control pain by giving analgesics before patient requests.	
		4. When stripping chest tubes, turning patient, or performing other painful procedures, alert patient to likelihood of pain, premedicate if necessary, and provide reassurance and encouragement.	
		5. Splint incision with pillow or sheet during movement, coughing, and chest physiotherapy.	
		6. Assist patient to cope with fears of dependency and loss of control by acknowledging their presence, involving patient in individualizing plan of care as necessary, emphasizing ways patient can contribute to recovery, allowing patient to make choices about timing of care, and encouraging patient to perform self-care when appropriate to physical status.	
		7. Assign same staff to care for patient whenever feasible.	
		8. Explain bedside activities and likely patient sensations, even if patient appears unconscious.	
		9. Encourage visits and phone calls from loved ones.	
		10. If severe anxiety persists despite nursing measures, consult MD re sedation.	

TABLE A-5 STANDARD CARE PLAN* *(Continued)*

NURSING DIAGNOSIS	SIGNS AND SYMPTOMS	NURSING ACTIONS	DESIRED OUTCOMES
Stimulation Potential sensory perceptual alterations related to sleep deprivation; medications; post-cardiotomy or ICU psychosis; cerebral hypoxia or emboli	Confused Disoriented Tired appearance	1. As soon as patient returns to unit, begin orienting to reality. 2. Assess level of consciousness every hr until stable. 3. Make environment meaningful by explaining objects and noises; remind patient if discussed during preop teaching. 4. Schedule care to allow as much undisturbed sleep as possible.	Patient is alert and oriented to person, place, time, recent and remote memory. Patient appears rested.
Fluid balance Potential decreased cardiac output related to altered cardiac rhythm or chemical imbalance	Hypotension Decreased level of consciousness Urinary output < 60 cc/hr Cool, clammy skin Decreased peripheral pulses Dysrhythmias Electrolyte imbalances Acid–base imbalance	1. Check BP and peripheral perfusion every 15 minutes until stable and then every 1–4 hours. 2. Place on continuous ECG monitor on admission to ICU. 3. Run rhythm strip and mount it in chart with analysis every 4 hrs and prn for serious dysrhythmia. 4. Obtain 12-lead ECG daily and prn for serious dysrhythmia. 5. Reduce catecholamine stimulation by minimizing patient anxiety and pain and treating hypotensive episodes promptly. 6. Reduce Valsalva maneuvers (after extubation) by: reminding patient to exhale when moving about in bed; controlling pain; administering stool softeners when ordered by MD. 7. Keep informed of serum electrolyte and blood gas values. 8. Check chart for medical orders re treatment of: dysrhythmias, electrolyte imbalances, acid–base imbalances, hypo- or hypertension.	BP ± 20 mm Hg of patient's normal BP. Adequate peripheral perfusion as manifested by: mental state WNL for patient; urinary output WNL for patient; warm, dry skin; peripheral pulse volume WNL for patient. Normal sinus rhythm (ideal) or spontaneous or artificial rhythm with regular ventricular rate between 60 and 100 beats per minute. If premature beats present: 10 or fewer APBs or JPBs per minute; 4 or fewer VPBs per minute; no VPBs that are multifocal, more than 3 consecutive, or encroaching on T waves. Serum electrolytes and acid–base values WNL.

(Continues)

TABLE A-5   STANDARD CARE PLAN* *(Continued)*

NURSING DIAGNOSIS	SIGNS AND SYMPTOMS	NURSING ACTIONS	DESIRED OUTCOMES
Potential for infection related to contamination of indwelling arterial, venous, and urinary catheters; surgical incisions; artificial airway; atelectasis	Fever Purulent drainage Erythema, edema, tenderness at sites Nonhealing incision Purulent respiratory secretions	1. Check termperature every 4 hours. 2. Check indwelling catheter and incision sites every shift. 3. Use meticulous sterile technique with catheter care, wound care, and suctioning. 4. Discontinue catheters per MD orders as soon as BP stable, patient taking fluids orally, and patient alert enough to use urinal or bedpan. 5. Inform MD of temperature spikes; obtain blood cultures and catheter cultures as ordered. 6. Check chart for orders for antipyretics and/or antibiotics.	Temperature WNL for patient. No purulent drainage, erythema, edema, or unusual tenderness at sites of indwelling catheters. Incisions healing without purulent drainage, skin breakdown, or wound dehiscence. No purulent respiratory secretions.

Abbreviations: WNL = within normal limits, APB = atrial premature beat, JPB = junctional premature beat, VPB = ventricular premature beat, MD = doctor of medicine, po = postoperative, BP = blood pressure; ICU = intensive care unit, re = regarding, ECG = electrocardiogram, prn = as necessary, q = every.
*This table presents an expansion of four selected diagnoses from Table A–4.

(For teaching purposes, only selected, representative problems are fully illustrated here, with possible causes, signs and symptoms, nursing actions, and desired outcomes. The remaining problems are discussed in the text, and the reader can easily derive causes, signs and symptoms, nursing actions, and outcomes for these problems if desired.)

This standard care plan represents a consensus of the staff's judgments about nursing care and is supported by documentation in the nursing and medical literature. Because this plan had been developed prior to Karen's expected ICU admission, the nurse does not need to rewrite an extensive care plan. Instead, the nurse need only review the SCP and individualize the patient's care plan if any unusual problems are present.

Because Karen J. does have unusual problems, the nurse writes the personalized care plan in Table A–6.

This plan of care clearly indicates much of the care anticipated for Karen the next day. It will, of course, be updated when her postoperative orders arrive in the unit and as changes in her condition necessitate. Left in the cardiac surgical unit the evening before surgery, it can alert the nurses to Karen's unusual problems in advance of her actual admission. It thus can reduce the staff's anxiety about their unknown patient and ensure that attention is paid early to her unusual problems. Because it will accompany her upon discharge from the critical-care unit, it also can facilitate continuity of care. It shows which of Karen's unusual problems received early care-planning attention, which ones are receiving continued nursing intervention, and which ones still need to be explored. A care plan such as this is invaluable in facilitating personalized nursing care, both during the crucial early postoperative days and beyond the critical-care experience.

INDIVIDUAL NURSING CARE PLAN

Name: _Karen J._   Age: _48_   Sex: _female_

Physician: _Dr. Sabatier_   Primary nurse: _Nancy Holloway, RN_

Medical diagnosis: _Severe mitral regurgitation, significant mitral stenosis. For mitral valve replacement 9/25_

Nursing discharge criteria _____

As specified in mitral valve replacement SCP

Home care coordination activities _Referral to Social Service 9/24_

Significant others: _husband Raymond, grown daughter Melissa_

Activities of daily living

Activity   ☑ bedrest
         ☐ OOB to bathroom ⎱ Assistance needed?
         ☐ up ad lib   ⎰ ☐ yes   ☐ no

Bathing   ☑ bed bath   ☐ complete   ☑ partial   ☐ self
         ☐ shower
         ☐ tub

Meals   ☑ NPO   ☐ diet _____
         ☐ feeds self   ☐ assistance needed

Toileting   ☐ bedpan/urinal   ☐ commode   ☐ bathroom

DATE	NURSING DIAGNOSIS	SIGNS AND SYMPTOMS	NURSING ACTIONS	DESIRED OUTCOMES
9/24	Anxiety related to: a. Worry over husband and daughter b. Expectation of painful and unpleasant postoperative period c. Fears about staff competence d. Also see mitral valve replacement SCP, problem: anxiety	Verbalizes anxiety Appears tense Worried facial expression	1. See SCP. 2. Allow husband to visit whenever able to come. 3. Before husband's first visit, explain wife's and unit's appearance. 4. Accompany husband on first visit. 5. Encourage husband to verbalize reactions after visit and clarify misconceptions. 6. Notify patient promptly of baby's birth when daughter or husband calls. 7. If possible, do not assign students or new nurses to care for her. If unavoidable, provide supervision and discuss their uncertanties re: knowledge or skill away from bedside.	See SCP.

(Continues)

INDIVIDUAL NURSING CARE PLAN *(Continued)*

DATE	NURSING DIAGNOSIS	SIGNS AND SYMPTOMS	NURSING ACTIONS	DESIRED OUTCOMES
9/24	Impaired verbal communication related to: a. Congenital deafness R > L b. Slurred speech c. Tendency to withdraw emotionally when upset or in pain. d. Postoperative intubation	Congenital deafness Slurred speech When upset or in pain, has tears in eyes but does not volunteer information or answer questions	1. Look directly at her. 2. Enunciate clearly and slowly. 3. Direct speech more toward her left ear. 4. Use gestures to supplement speech. 5. While she is intubated, use personalized communication cards on ring (already prepared for her at unit secretary's desk). 6. After her extubation, listen to speech patiently and attentively; watch gestures. 7. After her extubation, use Magic Slate if speech unintelligible. 8. Watch for withdrawn expression or tears in eyes. 9. Offer pain medication according to your judgment in addition to her requests. 10. If she is withdrawn, gently ask why. If no reply, allow short period of withdrawal (her usual pattern) and ask again.	1. Able to indicate needs. 2. No tense expression, frowning, or other signs of frustration. 3. No periods of emotional withdrawal longer than 30 minutes.
9/24	Potential poor wound healing or wound infection related to inadequate nutrition (also see mitral valve replacement SCP, potential for injury)	Anorexia Weight loss	1. See SCP. 2. Replace dentures after extubation. 3. As soon as bowel sounds return, check with MD about high calorie diet and desired rate of weight gain. 4. Send consult to dietitian to plan hospital meals around favorite foods, and (before hospital discharge) to help her plan nutritious meals needing minimal preparation at home. 5. During meals, encourage eating; help her if she is too tired. 6. Save uneaten meal items (if appetizing) and offer as snacks. 7. Weigh q.o.d.	1. See SCP. 2. Eats all food on tray. 3. Gains weight at rate specified by MD.

REFERENCES

Abbey J: FANCAP: A descriptive study of a useful tool for teaching clinical nursing. Unpublished doctoral dissertation. University of California, San Francisco, 1976.

Abbey J: FANCAP: What is it? Pages 107–118 in *Conceptual models for nursing practice,* 2d ed. Riehl J, Roy C Sr (ed). New York: Appleton-Century-Crofts, 1980.

Swendsen L: FANCAS: A framework for nursing assessment. University of California School of Nursing, San Francisco, 1975.

SUPPLEMENTAL READING

Gordon, Marjory (1987): *Nursing Diagnosis, Process and Application,* 2nd ed. New York: McGraw-Hill, 1987.

Grady, Rita: Comprehensive management of nursing care delivery, *Nursing Management* 16(5):47-49.

Iyer, Patricia, Taptich, Barbara, and Bernocchi-Losey, Donna (1986): *Nursing Process and Nursing Diagnosis.* Philadelphia: W.B. Saunders.

McLane, Audrey (ed.) (1987): *Classification of Nursing Diagnoses: Proceedings of the Seventh Conference of the North American Nursing Diagnosis Association.* St Louis: Mosby, 1987.

Appendix 2

Pharmacology*

Designed for easy reference or review, this section offers vital information on drugs commonly used in critical care that are not specifically discussed in the text. Each drug table lists the *Common use, Mechanism of action, Dosage, Administration, Anticipated response, Side effects, Interactions,* and *Other pertinent information.* Specific nursing implications are italicized. Such nursing implications as "Obtain a thorough drug history to check for interaction" and "Teach patient about side effects of the drug" have not been listed in the tables. These implications apply in *every* situation where drugs are being administered and competent nursing care is being practiced. Since nurses are held legally responsible for safe and effective drug administration, the nurse should consult other sources as well as this reference section for pharmacologic management.

Certain drugs have been described as groups rather than individually due to their similarities other than dosages. This format eliminates unnecessary duplication and, more importantly, emphasizes the interrelationships of these drugs.

The author and the publisher have exerted every effort to ensure that drug selections and dosages set forth in this text are in accord with current recommendations and practice at the time of publication. (Note that pediatric doses are *not* included.) In view of ongoing research, changes in government regulations, and the constant flow of information relating to drug therapy and drug reactions, the reader is urged to check the package insert for each drug for any change in indications or dosage and for added warnings and precautions. This is particularly important where the recommended agent is a new and/or infrequently employed drug.

The appendix tables are arranged alphabetically by generic drug name or group heading. The index that precedes the appendix tables, however, lists alphabetically not only the drugs' generic names but also their trade names (in italics) and (when appropriate) group names.

*Adapted from Saxton D et al.: *The Addison-Wesley manual of nursing practice.* Menlo Park, CA: Addison-Wesley, 1983.

Index to Critical Care Drugs

Abbokinase; see Thrombolytic agents

Acebutolol; *see* Beta-adrenergic blocking agents

Acetylcysteine, 595, Table 8-2

Adrenal corticosteroids, inhalation, 595, Table 8-2
systemic, 596

Albuterol, 597, Table 8–2

Alevaire, *see* Tyloxapol

Alprazolam; *see* Benzodiazepines

Alupent; see Metaproterenol sulfate

Amicar; see Aminocaproic acid

Aminocaproic acid, 597

Aminophyl; see Aminophylline

Aminophylline, 598

Amiodarone, 599

Amrinone, 330

Aramine; see Metaraminol

Atenolol; *see* Beta-adrenergic blocking agents

Ativan; see Benzodiazepines

Atropine, 348, Table 14–1, Table 8–2

Beclomethasone; *see* Adrenal corticosteroids, inhalation

Beclovent; see Adrenal corticosteroids, inhalation, also Table 8–2

Benzodiazepines, 599

Beta-adrenergic blocking agents, 600

Betamethasone; *see* Adrenal corticosteroids, systemic

Blocadren; see Beta-adrenergic blocking agents

Brethine; see Terbutaline

Bretylium, 348, Table 14–1

Bretylol, *see* bretylium

Brevibloc, see Beta-adrenergic blocking agents

Bricanyl; see Terbutaline

Bronkometer; see Isoetharine

Bronkosol; see Isoetharine

bumetanide; *see* Loop diuretics

Bumex; see Loop diuretics

Calan; see Calcium channel blocking agents

Calcium channel blocking agents, 601

Calcium chloride, 601, 348, Table 14–1

Capoten, see Captopril

Captopril, *see* 330

Cardilate; see Nitrates

Cardioquin; see Quinidine

Cardizem; see Calcium channel blocking agents

Chlordiazepoxide; *see* Benzodiazepines

Cimetidine, 602

Cin-Quin; see Quinidine

Cordarone; see Amiodarone

Corgard; see Beta-adrenergic blocking agents

Corticotropin; *see* Adrenal corticosteroids, systemic

Cortisone; *see* Adrenal corticosteroids, systemic

Coumadin; see Warfarin

Cromolyn sodium, 602, Table 8–2

Crystodigin; see Digitalis glycosides

Dalmane; see Benzodiazepines

Decadron; see Adrenal corticosteroids, systemic

Decadron Respihaler; see Adrenal corticosteroids, inhalation

Dexamethasone; *see* Adrenal corticosteroids, inhalation and systemic

Diazepam; *see* Benzodiazepines
Diazoxide, 603
Digitalis glycosides, 603
Digitoxin; *see* Digitalis glycosides
Digoxin; *see* Digitalis glycosides
Dilantin; see Hydantoin anticonvulsants
Diltiazem; *see* Calcium channel blocking agents
Disopyramide, 604
Dobutrex, see dobutamine
Dobutamine, 329
Dopamine, 329, 330

Edecrin; see Loop diuretics
Edrophonium chloride, 604
Epinephrine, 346, Table 8–2, Table 14–1
Erythrityl tetranitrate; *see* Nitrates
Esmolol, see Beta-adrenergic blocking agents
Ethacrynic acid; *see* Loop diuretics
Ethotoin; *see* Hydantoin anticonvulsants

Flurazepam; *see* Benzodiazepines
Furosemide; *see* Loop diuretics

Halcion; see Benzodiazepines
Heparin, 605
Hydantoin anticonvulsants, 605
Hydrocortisone; *see* Adrenal corticosteroids, systemic
Hyperstat; see Diazoxide

Inderal; see Beta-adrenergic blocking agents
Inocor, see Amrinone
Intropin, see Dopamine
Intal; see Cromolyn sodium
Isoetharine, 606
Isoproterenol, 348, Table 8–2, Table 13–1
Isoptin; see Calcium channel blocking agents
Isordil; see Nitrates
Isosorbide dinitrate; *see* Nitrates
Isuprel, see Isoproterenol

Kayexalate; see Sodium polystyrene sulfonate

Labetolol; *see* Beta-adrenergic blocking agents
Lanoxicaps; see Digitalis glycosides
Lanoxin; see Digitalis glycosides
Lasix; see Loop diuretics
Levophed; see Norepinephrine
Librium; see Benzodiazepines
Lidocaine, 348, Table 14–1
Lixaminol; see Aminophylline
Loop diuretics, 607
Lopressor; see Beta-adrenergic blocking agents
Lorazepam; *see* Benzodiazepines

Mannitol, 607
Mephenytoin; *see* Hydantoin anticonvulsants
Mesantoin; see Hydantoin anticonvulsants
Metaproterenol sulfate, 608, Table 8–2
Metaraminol, 608
Methylprednisolone; *see* Adrenal corticosteroids, systemic
Metoprolol; *see* Beta-adrenergic blocking agents
Midazolam, see Benzodiazepines
Morphine sulfate, 609
Mucomyst; see Acetylcysteine

Nadolol; *see* Beta-adrenergic blocking agents
Naloxone, 610
Narcan; see Naloxone
Nifedipine; *see* Calcium channel blocking agents
Nipride, see Nitroprusside
Nitrates, 610
Nitro-Bid; see Nitrates
Nitrodisc; see Nitrates
Nitro-Dur; see Nitrates
Nitroglycerin; *see* Nitrates
   intravenous, 330
   ointment; *see* Nitrates
Nitrol; see Nitrates
Nitroprusside, 330
Nitrospan; see Nitrates
Nitrostat; see Nitrates
Norepinephrine, 611
Normodyne; see Beta-adrenergic blocking agents
Norpace; see Disopyramide

Osmitrol; see Mannitol
Oxazepam; *see* Benzodiazepines

Pancuronium bromide, 611
Panwarfin; see Warfarin
Pavulon; see Pancuronium bromide
Peganone; see Hydantoin anticonvulsants
Pentaerythritol tetranitrate; *see* Nitrates
Peritrate; see Nitrates
Phenytoin; *see* Hydantoin anticonvulsants
Pindolol; *see* Beta-adrenergic blocking agents
Prednisolone; *see* Adrenal corticosteroids, systemic
Prednisone; *see* Adrenal corticosteroids, systemic
Procainamide, 612, 349, Table 14–1
Procardia; see Calcium channel blocking agents
Pronestyl; see Procainamide
Propranolol; *see* Beta-adrenergic blocking agents
Proventil; see Albuterol

Quinaglute; see Quinidine
Quinidine, 612
   gluconate, 612
   polygalacturonate, 612
   sulfate, 612

Ranitidine, 613
Restoril; see Benzodiazepines

Sectral; see Beta-adrenergic blocking agents
Serax; see Benzodiazepines
Sodium bicarbonate, 346, Table 14–1
Sodium polystyrene sulfonate, 613
Somophyllin; see Aminophylline
Sorbitrate; see Nitrates
Steroids; *see* Adrenal corticosteroids
Streptase; see Thrombolytic agents
Streptokinase; *see* Thrombolytic agents
Sustachron; see Nitrates

Tagament; see Cimetidine
Temazepam; *see* Benzodiazepines
Tenormin; see Beta-adrenergic
    blocking agents
Tensilon; see Edrophonium chloride
Terbutaline, 614
Thrombolytic agents, 614
Timolol; *see* Beta-adrenergic
    blocking agents
Trandate; see Beta-adrenergic
    blocking agents
Transderm-Nitro; see Nitrates

Triamcinolone; *see* Adrenal corti-
    costeroids, systemic
Triazolam; *see* Benzodiazepines
Tridil; see Nitrates
Tyloxapol, *see* Table 8-2

Urokinase; *see* Thrombolytic
    agents

Valium; see Benzodiazepines
Vanceril; see Adrenal corticoste-
    roids, inhalation, also Table 8-2
Ventolin; see Albuterol

Verapamil, 349; *also see* Calcium
    channel blocking agents
Versed, see Benzodiazepines
Visken; see Beta-adrenergic block-
    ing agents

Warfarin, 615

Xanax; see Benzodiazepines

Zantac; see Ranitidine

Acetylcysteine (Mucomyst)

Common use   to assist patient in clearing mucous secretions in acute and chronic lung disease.
Mechanism of action   mucolytic agent; lowers the viscosity of mucous secretions.

Dosage   **1.** 1–10 ml of 20% or 2–20 ml of 10% solution 3–4 times daily. **2.** For direct instillation, 1–2 ml of 10–20% solution every 1–4 hours.
Administration   via inhalation, or direct instillation into trachea.

---

1. *Refrigerate opened bottles; use within 96 hours.* **2.** *Wash patient's face after inhalation treatment, because area may be sticky.* **3.** *Dried particles of medication may occlude respiratory therapy equipment; clean equipment after each treatment.*

Anticipated response   expectoration of loosened secretions.

---

1. *Encourage coughing; provide ample tissues and basin for discarding secretions.* **2.** *Suction secretions if the patient is unable to cough and expectorate.*

Side effects   **1.** *GI:* nausea, stomatitis, sulfur taste. **2.** *Respiratory:* May increase airway obstruction in asthmatic or elderly patients with severe respiratory insufficiency.

Auscultation of the patient's lung sounds before and during treatment is advised; if wheezing and increased bronchial congestion occur, bronchodilators may be necessary.

Interactions   physically incompatible with many inhalation antibiotics.

Administer drug separately.

Other   **1.** Medication hardens rubber and discolors certain metals on contact. **2.** Acetylcysteine administered orally is also used to prevent liver damage following acetaminophen overdose.

Use only glass, plastic, aluminum, or stainless steel with this drug.

Adrenal Corticosteroids (inhalation): beclomethasone (Beclovent, Vanceril), dexamethasone (Decadron Respihaler)

Common use   treatment of bronchial asthma that does not respond to nonsteroid medications.
Mechanism of action   mechanism of local action is not clear; it may involve the systemic antiinflammatory and immunosuppressant actions of these drugs.

Dosage   **1.** *beclomethasone:* (inhalation aerosol) 2 metered sprays 3 or 4 times a day, increased if necessary up to a total daily dose of 20 metered sprays. **2.** *dexamethasone:* (inhalation aerosol) 2–3 metered sprays 2, 3, or 4 times a day, increased if necessary up to a total daily dose of 12 metered sprays.
Administration   inhalation.

1. When transferring patients from systemic to inhalation adrenal corticosteroids, the systemic drug should be continued at full dose for at least 1 week after beginning inhalation therapy, and decreased very gradually after that. Monitor patient for signs of adrenal insufficiency. 2. Instruct patient not to puncture or burn aerosol container.

Anticipated response   improved pulmonary function.

1. These drugs are unsuitable for acute asthmatic episodes. 2. Significant improvement may not be evident for 1–4 weeks after the start of therapy.

Side effects   **1.** *GI:* irritation, dry mouth and nose, oral candidiasis. **2.** *Dermatologic:* skin rash (allergy). **3.** *Respiratory:* paradoxical bronchospasm, hoarseness.

1. Rinse patient's mouth after each dose to prevent throat irritation and candidiasis. 2. At high doses or in sensitive individuals, systemic adrenocorticosteroid effects are possible with these aerosols. See Adrenal corticosteroids, systemic, for a complete discussion.

Interactions   **1.** Inhalation aerosol forms of bronchodilators contain fluorocarbon propellants, as do adrenal corticosteroid aerosols. The use of both drugs close together can cause fluorocarbon toxicity. **2.** These aerosols may increase or decrease the effects of oral anticoagulants. **3.** Dexamethasone may increase the risk of GI side effects when used with nonsteroid antiinflammatory agents or alcohol. **4.** Dexamethasone may increase the risk of GI hemorrhage when administered concurrently with any anticoagulant or thrombolytic agent. **5.** Dexamethasone may increase blood glucose and therefore antagonize the effects of antidiabetic drugs.

1. Allow at least 15 minutes to elapse between bronchodilator and adrenal corticosteroid aerosols. 2. Monitor prothrombin time carefully in the patient receiving oral anticoagulants and these drugs.

Adrenal Corticosteroids (systemic): betamethasone, corticotropin, cortisone, dexamethasone, hydrocortisone, methylprednisolone, prednisolone, prednisone, triamcinolone (There are many brand names for each drug.)

Common use   in adrenal insufficiency, and as antiinflammatory or immunosupressant agents in a wide variety of disorders.

Mechanism of action   exact mechanisms are unknown; these drugs interfere with inflammatory processes and suppress cell-mediated immune reactions; increase sodium and water retention and potassium excretion through actions on the renal distal tubules; decrease calcium absorption and increase calcium excretion; decrease bone formation and increase bone resorption; stimulate protein catabolism; mobilize fatty acids; and induce gluconeogenesis.

Dosage   **1.** *betamethasone:* (oral) 0.6–7.2 mg daily in single or divided doses; (intra-articular) up to 12 mg; (IM, IV) up to 12 mg daily. **2.** *corticotropin:* (IM) 40–80 USP units daily; (IV diagnostic aid) 10–25 USP units in 500 cc D_5W run over 8 hours. **3.** *cortisone:* (oral) 25–300 mg/day in single or divided doses; (IM) 20–300 mg/day. **4.** *dexamethasone:* (oral) 0.5–9 mg daily in single or divided doses; (intra-articular) 4–16 mg of the acetate suspension, or 0.2–6 mg of the phosphate; (IM) 8–16 mg of the acetate suspension, or 0.5–9 mg of the phosphate; (IV) 0.5–9 mg of the phosphate daily. **5.** *hydrocortisone:* (oral) 20–240 mg daily in single or divided doses; (IM) 15–240 mg of the suspension daily; (intra-articular) 5–75 mg; (IM, IV, SC) 100–500 mg of the phosphate or sodium succinate, repeated every 2–6 hours; (rectal) 90–100 mg retention enema. **6.** *methylprednisolone:* (oral) 4–48 mg daily as single or divided doses; (intra-articular) 40–80 mg; (IM) 4–12 mg of the acetate suspension; (IM, IV) 10–40 mg of the sodium succinate; (rectal) 40 mg 3–7 times a week. **7.** *prednisolone:* (oral) 5–60 mg daily as single or divided doses; (intra-articular) 4–100 mg of suspension; (IM) 2–60 mg. **8.** *prednisone:* (oral) 5–60 mg daily in single or divided doses. **9.** *triamcinolone:* (oral) 4–48 mg daily in single or divided doses; (intra-articular) 2.5–15 mg; (IM) 40–80 mg.

Administration   oral, intramuscular, intravenous, intra-articular, rectal.

1. Administer IM injections deep into gluteal muscle to avoid local tissue atrophy. Rotate sites if repeated doses are necessary. 2. Rest patient's weight-bearing joints for 24–48 hours after intra-articular injection. 3. Rapid IV injection can cause life-threatening cardiac dysrhythmias. Keep resuscitation equipment and medications on hand.

Anticipated response   See Common use, Mechanism of action, and Side effects. Adrenal corticosteroids are used for a wide variety of disorders.

Corticotropin should not be used in emergencies or when an immediate effect is needed.

Side effects   **1.** *GI:* nausea, peptic ulceration, pancreatitis. **2.** *CV:* hypertension, edema. **3.** *Metabolic:* poor wound healing, increased blood glucose, abnormal fatty deposits, adrenal suppression. **4.** *Musculoskeletal:* muscle weakness, osteoporosis, growth suppression. **5.** *CNS:* depression, euphoria, insomnia, confusion, disorientation. **6.** *Ophthalmic:* increased intraocular pressure, cataracts, blurred vision. **7.** *Dermatologic:* hirsutism, acne, subcutaneous tissue atrophy. **8.** *Other:* increased susceptibility to infection; carcinogenic with long-term use.

1. *Administer oral doses with food to decrease GI irritation. The administration of antacids has not been shown to prevent severe GI problems in adrenal corticosteroid therapy.* **2.** *Adrenal recovery may occur within a week after very-short-term therapy; recovery may take a year or more after long-term administration, and some patients never fully recover their adrenal function. Adrenal function monitoring may be needed to assess patient's continued ability to respond to stress.* **3.** *A low-calorie, low-carbohydrate, low-fat, high-protein, or sodium-restricted diet may be necessary during long-term therapy. Potassium and/ or calcium supplementation also may be needed.*

Interactions **1.** With alcohol or nonsteroid antiinflammatory drugs, increased risk of GI ulceration and hemorrhage. **2.** With anticoagulants or thrombolytic agents, increased risk of GI hemorrhage. **3.** May increase or decrease the effects of oral anticoagulants. **4.** These drugs may antagonize the effects of antidiabetic drugs. **5.** Estrogen-containing medications may increase both the therapeutic and the toxic effects of adrenal corticosteroids. **6.** Adrenal corticosteroids increase the potential for digitalis toxicity. **7.** These drugs antagonize the diuretic effects of diuretics and enhance the hypokalemia of potassium-depleting diuretics. **8.** With other immunosuppressive agents, increased risk of infection and lymphomas. **9.** These drugs may antagonize the effects of potassium supplements. **10.** The administration of live virus vaccines may result in viral infection rather than immunization. With other immunizations, possible decreased or absent antibody response and increased risk of neurologic complications.

Many of the potential drug interactions involving the adrenal-corticosteroids have serious consequences. Multiple drug therapy must be monitored very closely, and the benefits and risks of these combinations weighed carefully.

Albuterol (Proventil, Ventolin)

Common use relief of bronchospasm in patients with reversible obstructive airway disease, such as asthma.
Mechanism of action sympathomimetic agent, beta-adrenergic agonist, bronchodilator; directly relaxes bronchial smooth muscle.
Dosage (inhalation) 1 or 2 inhalations repeated every 4–6 hours; (oral) 2–8 mg 3 or 4 times a day.
Administration inhalation, oral.

1. *Advise patient to take amount prescribed—excessive dosage may result in paradoxical bronchospasm.* **2.** *Store away from heat and light.* **3.** *Do not puncture or burn container.* **4.** *Avoid*

contact with eyes. **5.** *Advise patient to notify physician if he or she becomes nonresponsive to usual dose or if condition worsens.* **6.** *Use lower doses with the elderly.*

Anticipated response relief of bronchospasm and wheezing.

Onset of action within 5–15 minutes by inhalation, within 30 minutes orally. Maximum effect within 60–90 minutes, and duration of action 3–6 hours after inhalation; orally, 2–3 hours to maximum effect, and 6 hours or more duration.

Side effects **1.** *CV:* tachycardia, hypertension, palpitations, angina, dysrhythmias, headache, chest pain. **2.** *CNS:* tremor, nervousness, dizziness, insomnia. **3.** *GI:* heartburn, nausea, vomiting, unusual taste. **4.** *Respiratory:* paradoxical bronchospasm, drying or irritation of oropharynx. **5.** *GU:* difficult urination.

1. *Monitor blood pressure and apical pulse.* **2.** *Rinse mouth with water after each inhaled dose to relieve dry mouth.*

Interactions **1.** Beta blockers inhibit drug's effect. **2.** Additive effect when given with other sympathomimetic drugs. **3.** With monoamine oxidase inhibitors or tricyclic antidepressants, excessive and potentially dangerous hemodynamic responses. **4.** With digitalis glycosides, increased risk of dysrhythmias.

1. *Beta-blockers generally should not be administered to people with obstructive lung disease.* **2.** *Avoid concurrent use of albuterol and MAO inhibitors or tricyclic antidepressants.* **3.** *Monitor the digitalized patient closely.*

Other **1.** Patients who are hypersensitive to other sympathomimetics, or to fluorocarbon propellents, may be hypersensitive to albuterol. **2.** Use with caution in patients with cardiovascular disorders, diabetes mellitus, hyperthyroidism, or enlarged prostate. **3.** Used experimentally to delay preterm labor.

Aminocaproic Acid (Amicar)

Common use to control excessive bleeding.
Mechanism of action antihemorrhagic; inhibits plasminogen activator substances and inhibits fibrinolysin activity.
Dosage oral or IV, initially, 4–5 g over 1 hour followed by 1–1.5 g/hour until bleeding is controlled (up to 30 g within 24 hours).
Administration oral and intravenous

1. Do not administer unless there is laboratory documentation of hyperfibrinolysis. 2. Never administer IV form undiluted. 3. Dilute solution for IV use with sterile water for injection, 5% dextrose and water, normal saline, or Ringer's solution. 4. To avoid thrombophlebitis, use care inserting IV needle, fixing its position, and maintaining the site.

Anticipated response   control of bleeding.

1. Keep careful intake and output records to determine fluid loss. 2. Monitor coagulation studies carefully.

Side effects   1. *CNS:* headache, tinnitus, dizziness, fatigue. 2. *GI:* nausea, vomiting, cramps, diarrhea. 3. *CV:* slow or irregular heartbeat, hypotension. 4. *GU:* difficult or painful urination, oliguria.

1. Change in pulse rate usually indicates too-rapid IV administration; slow the rate. 2. Urinary problems may indicate renal failure.

Interactions   increased potential for blood clotting when used with oral contraceptives or other estrogens.

Other   Use with caution in cardiac, hepatic, or renal disease or in patients predisposed to thrombosis.

Aminophylline (Aminophyl, Lixaminol, Somophyllin)

Common use   treatment of bronchial asthma, bronchospasm, COPD.
Mechanism of action   bronchodilator; relaxes bronchial smooth muscle.

Dosage   maintenance dosages (initial loading doses may be higher):

EQUIVALENT OF ANHYDROUS THEOPHYLLINE

	ORAL/RECTAL	IV
Smoker	4 mg/kg every 6 hours	0.7 mg/kg/hour
Nonsmoker	3 mg/kg every 8 hours	0.43 mg/kg/hour
Elderly	2 mg/kg every 8 hours	0.26 mg/kg/hour
CHF, liver failure	2 mg/kg every 12 hours	0.2 mg/kg/hour

Administration   oral, intravenous, rectal.

1. Before administering loading dose, ascertain if patient has recently been on theophylline therapy. 2. Rectal absorption is erratic. Administer after evacuation, if possible. 3. Do not use if solution is crystallized. 4. Oral form is absorbed best on an empty stomach but can be given with meals if GI irritation develops. 5. Give IV form at a rate no faster than 25 mg per minute. 6. IM use is possible but not recommended. 7. Dose must be individualized, due to narrow therapeutic range and wide patient variation. 8. When changing from IV to oral dosing, the first oral dose should be given 4–6 hours after the IV infusion is completed. When using an extended-release oral form, the initial dose should be given at the time the IV infusion is discontinued. 9. Enteric-coated or extended-release dosage forms should never be crushed or broken. If the patient cannot tolerate the whole pill, obtain an order for liquid or rectal aminophylline.

Anticipated response   1. Increased ease of respiration. 2. Decreased rate of respiration.

Observe patient for improved ventilation: improved color, decreased pulse and respiratory rates, decreased use of accessory muscles for respiration, decreased anxiety.

Side effects   1. *CNS:* anxiety, headache, seizures. 2. *CV:* flushing, palpitations, hypotension, dysrhythmias, tachycardia, precordial pain. 3. *GI:* bitter aftertaste, nausea, vomiting, anorexia, dyspepsia, feeling of gastric fullness, epigastric pain, bleeding; rectal irritation (rectal dosage forms only). 4. *GU:* diuresis.

1. Monitor blood pressure and pulse and respiratory rates while patient is on therapy. 2. GI side effects may diminish if taken with food. 3. IV form should be diluted, and infused slowly to avoid severe hypotension.

Interactions   1. When used with ephedrine or other sympathomimetics, excessive CNS stimulation may occur. 2. Mutual antagonism in effects on bronchial smooth muscle exists between aminophylline and beta-blocking drugs. 3. Phenytoin, tobacco, or marijuana may increase aminophylline metabolism, necessitating dosage increases. 4. Cimetidine or erythromycin may decrease aminophylline clearance, resulting in possible toxicity.

Instruct patient not to use over-the-counter preparations without consulting a physician.

Other   1. Aminophylline therapy may exacerbate cardiac disease or peptic ulcer; use with caution. 2. Hepatic disease, severe hypoxemia, or prolonged fever may decrease aminophylline clearance and result in toxic plasma concentrations. 3. Monitoring of serum levels is highly recommended, due to wide variation in therapeutic dose and relatively narrow therapeutic serum level range.

Amiodarone (Cordarone)

Common use prevention and treatment of ventricular dysrhythmias.

Mechanism of action antidysrhythmic; prolongs refractory period, slows AV conduction, suppresses automaticity in the Purkinje network.

Dosage (oral) 800–1600 mg/day initially, in divided doses if necessary, until satisfactory patient response or side effects occur; decrease gradually over 1 month to a maintenance dose of 200–400 mg/day.

Administration oral.

Because of its delayed onset of action and complicated dosing, amiodarone is not recommended as a first-line antidysrhythmic drug.

Anticipated response control of dysrhythmia.

Side effects **1.** *Respiratory:* cough, dyspnea, SOB; potentially fatal pulmonary fibrosis. **2.** *CV:* tachycardia, bradycardia, other dysrhythmias. **3.** *Neurologic:* peripheral neuropathy, tremors, ataxia. **4.** *Ophthalmic:* blurred vision, dry eyes, photophobia. **5.** *Dermatologic:* photosensitivity, blue-gray coloration of skin, rash. **6.** *Metabolic:* hypothyroidism, hyperthroidism. **7.** *GI:* constipation, anorexia, nausea. **8.** *CNS:* headache, dizziness (without hypotension). **9.** *GU:* impotence, decreased libido.

1. Side effects may not be evident until therapy has continued for several days or weeks, and they may persist for several months after amiodarone withdrawal. 2. The elderly may experience more ataxia than younger adults. 3. Auscultate chest regularly; employ x-ray, pulmonary function studies, or bronchoscopy as needed if pulmonary toxicity is evident. 4. Protect skin from excess sunlight during therapy, and for several months afterwards. 5. Ophthalmoscopic exam is recommended prior to therapy and as a follow-up to ophthalmic signs and symptoms.

Interactions **1.** With other antidysrhythmic drugs, including beta blockers and calcium channel blockers, possible additive cardiac effects and increased tachydysrhythmias. **2.** Amiodarone potentiates coumarin anticoagulants, and this effect can persist for weeks or months after amiodarone is discontinued. **3.** Amiodarone increases serum digitalis levels and may cause digitalis toxicity. **4.** Amiodarone increases serum phenytoin levels and may cause phenytoin toxicity. **5.** Potassium-depleting diuretics may increase risk of hypokalemia-related dysrhythmias.

1. Use with extreme caution with other antidysrhythmic drugs.

2. Decrease anticoagulant dose by one-third to one-half and monitor prothrombin time closely when amiodarone is given with anticoagulants. 3. When amiodarone is given to a digitalized patient, discontinue the digitalis, or decrease the dose by 50%, and carefully monitor cardiac function.

Other Do not use if severe bradycardia is present, unless controlled by a pacemaker.

Benzodiazepines: alprazolam (Xanax), chlordiazepoxide (Librium), diazepam (Valium), flurazepam (Dalmane), lorazepam (Ativan), midazolam (Versed), oxazepam (Serax), temazepam (Restoril), triazolam (Halcion)

Common use treatment of anxiety, insomnia, and alcohol withdrawal; skeletal muscle relaxant; anticonvulsant; anesthesia adjunct.

Mechanism of action central nervous system depressants whose specific mechanisms of action are not completely established.

Dosage **1.** *alprazolam:* (oral) 0.25–0.5 mg 3 times a day, increased gradually as needed. **2.** *chlordiazepoxide:* (oral) 5–25 mg 3 or 4 times a day; (IM, IV) 50–100 mg initially, followed by 25–50 mg 3 times a day if needed. **3.** *diazepam:* (oral) 2–10 mg 3 or 4 times a day; (IM, IV) 2–10 mg, repeated in 3 or 4 hours as needed. **4.** *flurazepam;* (oral) 15–30 mg at bedtime. **5.** *lorazepam:* (oral) 1–4 mg 2 or 3 times a day, or once at bedtime; (IM) 50 mcg/kg; (IV) 44 mcg/kg or a total of 2 mg, whichever is less. **6.** *midazolam:* (IM) 70–80 mcg/kg 30–60 min. before surgery; (IV) 75–200 mcg/kg, administered slowly; (IV anesthesia adjunct) 150–600 mcg/kg **7.** *oxazepam:* (oral) 10–30 mg 3 or 4 times a day. **8.** *temazepam:* (oral) 15–30 mg at bedtime. **9.** *triazolam:* (oral) 0.25–0.5 mg at bedtime.

Administration oral, intramuscular, intravenous.

*1. Begin with lower doses in elderly, debilitated, or very young patients or in those with impaired renal or hepatic function. 2. Parenteral administration, especially rapid IV administration, may cause apnea, hypotension, bradycardia, or cardiac arrest. Keep **emergency** equipment and medications on hand. 3. In general, the IM route is avoided because of possible erratic absorption. 4. For IM chlordiazepoxide, prepare solution with the manufacturer's diluent only. 5. An IV solution of diazepam may precipitate; give as IV bolus only.*

Anticipated response   relief of anxiety; shortened time to fall asleep; prevention of most physical manifestations of alcohol withdrawal; relief of muscle spasm and pain; suppression of seizure activity; facilitated anesthesia.

Physical dependence will develop with regular use. Depending on the specific benzodiazepine, withdrawal symptoms may occur 2–20 days after abrupt discontinuance of the drug; therefore, gradual dosage reduction is necessary.

Side effects   **1.** *CNS:* confusion, paradoxical excitement, mental depression, drowsiness, headache. **2.** *Ophthalmic:* blurred vision. **3.** *Musculoskeletal:* weakness, ataxia, clumsiness. **4.** *GI:* constipation, diarrhea, nausea, dry mouth. **5.** *CV:* hypotension, dizziness. **6.** *Overdose:* confusion, drowsiness, shakiness, slurred speech, bradycardia, dyspnea, severe weakness.

Elderly and debilitated patients are more sensitive to the CNS effects of these drugs; use with caution.

Interactions   **1.** Increased CNS depression when used with other CNS depressants. **2.** Possible additive hypotension with antihypertensives, diuretics, or other medications that lower blood pressure. **3.** Cimetidine may increase plasma level of benzodiazepines, thereby increasing their effects. **4.** With the anticonvulsants primidone, valproic acid, or carbamazepine, possible increased seizure activity or other change in seizure pattern.

Use cautiously with interacting drugs, monitor carefully, and adjust doses as needed.

Other   **1.** Avoid use during pregnancy; several benzodiazepines have been implicated in congenital malformations. **2.** These drugs may exacerbate mental depression, myasthenia gravis, narrow-angle glaucoma, or respiratory distress.

Beta-Adrenergic Blocking Agents: acebutolol (Sectral), atenolol (Tenormin), esmolol (Brevibloc), labetolol (Normodyne, Trandate), metoprolol (Lopressor), nadolol (Corgard), pindolol (Visken), propranolol (Inderal), timolol (Blocadren)

Common use   control of angina, dysrhythmias, hypertension; postmyocardial infarction cardiac preservation.
Mechanism of action   selectively block beta-receptors in sympathetic nervous system without causing general inhibition of adrenergic activity.

Dosage   **1.** *acebutolol:* 200 mg twice a day. **2.** *atenolol:* initially, 12.5–25 mg once a day, increased as needed to 50–100 mg once a day. **3.** *esmolol:* (IV) 500 mcg/kg over 1 min, followed by 50 mcg/kg/min. **4.** *labetolol:* (oral) 100–400 mg twice a day; (IV) 20 mg bolus over 2 minutes, followed by 40–80 mg every 10 minutes, titrated to BP response; or 2 mg/min up to a total dose of 50–300 mg. **5.** *metoprolol:* (oral) 100–450 mg once daily or divided into 2 doses; (IV) 5 mg every 2 minutes for 3 doses, then change to oral. **6.** *nadolol:* 40–320 mg daily. **7.** *pindolol:* 10–60 mg daily, divided into 2–4 doses. **8.** *propranolol:* (oral) 30–640 mg divided into 3 or 4 doses; extended-release tablets, 80, 120, or 160 mg daily; (IV) 1–3 mg bolus, administered at 1 mg/min, repeated in 2 minutes and again in 4 hours as needed. **9.** *timolol:* 20–60 mg/day, divided into 2 doses.

Atenolol and nadolol have longer half-lives: give only once a day.

Administration   oral; *labetolol, metoprolol, and propranolol may also be given intravenously. Older people may be sensitive to the effects of beta-blocker drugs; adjust doses carefully.*

Anticipated response   **1.** Slowed heart rate. **2.** Decreased blood pressure. **3.** Less frequent dysrhythmias. **4.** Possible decrease in rate of postmyocardial infarction mortality.

1. Patients should be advised not to discontinue drug abruptly, because rebound angina or even myocardial infarction can occur; withdraw drug over at least 3 days, preferably 1–2 weeks. 2. Some practitioners recommend gradual beta-blocker withdrawal 48 hours prior to surgery. 3. Labetolol may cause pronounced hypotensive effects, because it blocks both alpha and beta receptors. Monitor closely.

Side effects   **1.** *CNS:* weakness, fatigue, drowsiness, depression, insomnia, nightmares, confusion. **2.** *Respiratory:* bronchospasm. **3.** *GI:* nausea, dry mouth, vomiting. **4.** *Metabolic:* hypoglycemia. **5.** *CV:* congestive heart failure, bradycardia, AV blocks, peripheral ischemia, fluid retention (high doses).

1. Beta-blockers generally are contraindicated in patients with a history of COPD or asthma. 2. Atenolol and metoprolol are most "cardioselective" and are least likely to cause blood sugar or respiratory problems. 3. Contraindicated in overt congestive heart failure. 4. Contraindicated in patients with a history of mental depression.

Interactions   **1.** With other antihypertensive drugs, including diuretics, increased hypotension. **2.** Possible excessive bradycardia or heart block when given with digitalis.

3. Mutual inhibition of effects when given with sympathomimetic drugs such as aminophylline and isoproterenol. 4. May potentiate antidiabetic drugs.

When giving a beta-blocker and digitalis, check pulse at least daily, especially during initial therapy or after dosage revisions of either drug.

Calcium Channel Blocking Agents: diltiazem (Cardizem), nifedipine (Procardia), verapamil (Calan, Isoptin)

Common use   control of angina; (verapamil) treatment of supraventricular tachycardia; used experimentally in the treatment of hypertension.
Mechanism of action   inhibit flow of calcium ions into cardiac and vascular smooth muscle cells, resulting in decreased muscle tone.

Dosage   1. *diltiazem:* (oral) 30 mg 3–4 times a day, increased gradually as needed up to 240 mg daily. 2. *nifedipine:* (oral) 10 mg 3 times a day, increased gradually as needed up to 180 mg daily. 3. *verapamil:* (oral) 80 mg 3–4 times a day, increased gradually as needed up to 480 mg daily; (IV) initially, 5–10 mg over 2 minutes, with a 10-mg dose 30 minutes later if needed.
Administration   oral, (verapamil) IV

1. *Advise patient not to discontinue these drugs abruptly.* 2. *In elderly patients, administer IV dose over at least 3 minutes.*

Anticipated response   decrease in frequency of angina episodes or dysrhythmias; improved coronary artery perfusion and decreased coronary artery spasm; peripheral vasodilation (especially nifedipine); depressed SA and AV nodal conduction (diltiazem and verapamil).

1. *Observe patient for reduction of anginal pain.* 2. *Monitor blood pressure, especially during initial dose titration.* 3. *Emphasize the benefits of weight loss, proper diet, exercise, and eliminating smoking in control of angina and hypertension.*

Side effects   1. *CNS:* dizziness, light-headedness, syncope, headache, nervousness. 2. *CV:* hypotension, flushing, peripheral edema, palpitations, tachycardia, bradycardia. 3. *GI:* nausea, constipation. 4. *Musculoskeletal:* weakness. 5. *Respiratory:* dyspnea, cough, nasal congestion. 6. *Metabolic:* hypoglycemia. 7. *Dermatologic:* urticaria, pruritus.

1. *Monitor BP, especially during initial therapy or when the dose is changed. Instruct patient to change position slowly to avoid orthostatic hypotension.* 2. *Observe for peripheral edema.* 3. *Monitor frequency, duration, and severity of anginal attacks.* 4. *Have vasopressors available during initial therapy in case of severe hypotension.*

Interactions   1. With beta-adrenergic blockers, possible dangerously prolonged AV conduction or severe hypotension. 2. With other drugs that lower BP, additive hypotensive effect. 3. With nitrates, possible additive antianginal effect. 4. With digitalis, increased serum digitalis and possible toxicity. 5. Disopyramide with verapamil or diltiazem may have a dangerous negative inotropic effect on the heart. 6. With other highly protein-bound medications, such as the nonsteroid antiinflammatory drugs, salicylates, coumarin anticoagulants, phenytoin, or quinidine, possible erratic effects of either drug.

1. *Monitor digitalis serum levels if both drugs are given concurrently, and closely monitor cardiac status. Reduction of digitalis dose may be necessary.* 2. *Do not give disopyramide within 48 hours before or 24 hours after verapamil administration.*

Calcium Chloride

Common use   treatment of hypocalcemia and hyperkalemia; an adjunct drug in cardiac resuscitation efforts.
Mechanism of action   electrolyte replenisher; the exact mechanism of action of calcium ions in such physiologic processes as muscle contraction, nerve impulse transmission, and blood clotting is not understood.

Dosage   200–1000 mg administered at no greater than 100 mg/min. Repeat in 1–3 days as needed.
Administration   intravenous.

1. *Warm solution to body temperature before administering.* 2. *Infuse at a rate no greater than 100 mg/min.*

Anticipated response   correction of electrolyte imbalance.

Side effects   1. *GI:* bitter taste, nausea. 2. *CV:* flushing, warmth. 3. *Neurologic:* tingling sensations. 4. *Overdose or intolerance:* bradycardia, cardiac arrest, hypotension, diarrhea, vomiting, mental depression, high urine output. 5. *Other:* sweating, burning sensation at injection site, necrosis at injection site.

1. Infuse slowly to decrease incidence of side effects. 2. Use a small-gauge needle and a large vein to minimize local irritation, and infuse slowly. 3. A serum calcium greater than 10.5 mg/100 ml is considered hypercalcemic. Initial treatment is conservative—withhold calcium. In serious hypercalcemia, employ hydration, loop diuretics, chelating agents, calcitonin, and corticosteroids as needed.

Interactions   **1.** Calcitonin will antagonize the effects of calcium chloride in hypercalcemia. **2.** With vitamin D, other calcium-containing medications, or thiazide diuretics, possible hypercalcemia. **3.** Calcium chloride may cause serious dysrhythmias in digitalized patients. **4.** May antagonize parenteral magnesium sulfate.

When calcium chloride is given to digitalized patients, carefully monitor cardiac function.

Other   **1.** Do not use in digitalis toxicity or ventricular fibrillation. **2.** Use with caution if renal function is impaired, because of the danger of hypercalcemia.

Cimetidine (Tagamet)

Common use   treatment and prevention of gastric or duodenal ulcer and hypersecretory states.
Mechanism of action   histamine H_2 receptor antagonist; inhibits gastric acid secretion.

Dosage   (oral) 300 mg 4 times daily; for prevention of recurrent duodenal ulcer, 400 mg at bedtime; (IM, IV) 300 mg every 6 hours.
Administration   oral, intramuscular, intravenous.

1. Maximum daily dosage is 2400 mg. 2. Give with meals and at bedtime. 3. When administering IV push, inject over a 2-minute period. 4. For piggyback administration, use 100 ml of dextrose or saline; infuse over 15–20 minutes. 5. Do not use for minor digestive complaints.

Anticipated response   relief of pain, healing of ulcers, prevention of recurrence.

In most cases, limit dosage to period of 8 weeks (pathologic hypersecretory states may need indefinite course of therapy).

Side effects   **1.** *GI:* transient diarrhea. **2.** *GU:* gynecomastia, impotence, possible decrease in sperm count (apparently returns to normal after discontinuing drug therapy). **3.** *Hematologic:* blood dyscrasias. **4.** *CNS:* dizziness, head-

ache, confusion. **5.** *CV:* hypotension, cardiac rate or rhythm changes may occur after too-rapid IV injection.

1. Check for melena. 2. Assess pain relief. 3. Older patients are more susceptible to CNS side effects.

Interactions   **1.** May potentiate oral anticoagulants. **2.** Antacids may decrease cimetidine absorption. **3.** May increase blood levels of phenytoin, propranolol, theophylline, and tricyclic antidepressants, possibly resulting in toxicity.

1. Monitor patient for adjustment of anticoagulant drug dosage. 2. Give antacid at least 1 hour before or after cimetidine dose. 3. Monitor interacting drugs closely for toxic effects, and adjust doses as needed.

Cromolyn Sodium (Intal)

Common use   prophylactic treatment of asthma.
Mechanism of action   mast cell stabilizer; inhibits bronchoconstriction by preventing release of substances that mediate allergic response.

Dosage   20 mg (in capsule or solution) 4 times daily.
Administration   inhalation.

1. If a bronchodilator inhaler is also prescribed, use it 20–30 minutes prior to cromolyn. 2. Protect capsules from moisture, and store at room temperature. 3. Teach patient correct use of inhaler: exhale before placing mouthpiece between lips, then inhale deeply with even breath. Hold breath and exhale. Repeat until powder is gone. 4. Rinse mouth after each dose to prevent throat irritation. 5. Full benefit of the drug may not be evident for 3–4 weeks.

Anticipated response   reduction in frequency of asthmatic attacks.

Not effective in relieving acute attack. Cromolyn is not a bronchodilator or anti-inflammatory drug.

Side effects   **1.** *CNS:* dizziness, headache. **2.** *Respiratory:* bronchospasm, cough, stuffy nose, throat irritation. **3.** *Dermatologic:* skin rash, itching, swelling of lips or eyes. **4.** *GI:* nausea, dry mouth. **5.** *GU:* frequent or difficult urination.

Interactions   none reported.

Other The inhalation-capsule form contains lactose. Patients who are lactose-intolerant may not tolerate this form.

Diazoxide (Hyperstat)

Common use lowers blood pressure in hypertensive crisis.
Mechanism of action antihypertensive; vasodilator.

Dosage 1–3 mg/kg, up to 150 mg, repeated as needed in 5–15 minutes.
Administration intravenous.

---

1. Administer IV bolus over 30 seconds, with patient lying down. Maintain patient in supine position for 15–30 minutes after adinistration. 2. Patient should be maintained on oral medication after blood pressure is under control.

Anticipated response rapid fall in blood pressure.

Monitor vital signs frequently. Peak effect in 2–5 minutes, duration of action 2–12 hours.

Side effects 1. *CNS:* dizziness, light-headedness, flushing, drowsiness, confusion. 2. *CV:* hypotension, angina, sodium and water retention, tachycardia. 3. *Metabolic:* hyperglycemia, hyperuricemia. 4. *GI:* constipation, nausea, vomiting, anorexia.

1. Weigh patient daily. 2. Instruct patient to rise slowly to avoid orthostatic hypotension. 3. Check blood sugar regularly. 4. Keep norepinephrine on hand, and notify physician to treat severe hypotension. 5. Often administered with a diuretic (given IV 30–60 minutes prior to diazoxide) to potentiate antihypertensive effect and to prevent congestive heart failure from salt and water retention.

Interactions 1. May increase the effect of oral anticoagulants. 2. Hypotension will be potentiated if given with other drugs that lower blood pressure. 3. Thiazide or loop diuretics may increase the hyperglycemic, hyperuricemic, and antihypertensive effects of this drug. 4. Antagonizes effects of antidiabetic drugs.

Other Use with extreme caution in patients with poor cardiac reserve or coronary or cerebral insufficiency.

Digitalis Glycosides: digitoxin (Crystodigin), digoxin (Lanoxin, Lanoxicaps)

Common use treatment of congestive heart failure, atrial fibrillation, and atrial flutter.
Mechanism of action cardiotonic, antidysrhythmic; increases strength and force of heart contraction, causing increased cardiac output; decreases heart rate and lengthens atrioventricular and sinoatrial conduction time.

Dosage 1. digitoxin: (oral, IM, IV) 0.05–0.3 mg every day. 2. digoxin (oral, capsules) 0.05–0.35 mg daily; (oral, tablets or elixer) 0.125–0.5 mg daily; (IV, IM) 0.1–0.5 mg daily.
Administration oral, intramuscular, intravenous.

1. Higher doses may be needed initially as loading doses. 2. Do not substitute digoxin for digitoxin or vice versa; these drugs cannot be interchanged without dosage revisions. 3. Do not change brands of either digoxin or digitoxin without consulting physician; there are differences in bioavailability that can result in different therapeutic effects. 4. IM routes are usually avoided because of pain of injection and erratic rate of absorption. If absolutely necessary, administer deep IM and massage the site well afterwards.

Anticipated response slowed heart rate, decreased edema, increased urine output, resolution of CHF symptoms, control of dysrhythmias.

1. Digoxin acts faster than digitoxin. 2. Digoxin is safer than digitoxin in presence of liver disease. 3. Digitoxin is safer than digoxin in presence of renal disease. 4. Instruct patient about importance of weight control, regular exercise, and low-salt diet in controlling heart disease. 5. Note: Digitalized patients are more sensitive than others to electrical countershock, and they are more likely to respond with ventricular dysrhythmias. If electrical intervention is necessary, begin with minimal energy levels and increase carefully. 6. Elderly or debilitated patients, those with impaired renal function, or those using electronic pacemakers may develop digitalis toxicity at lower doses than other patients. Monitor carefully.

Side effects 1. *GI:* discomfort, anorexia, nausea, vomiting. 2. *CV:* unusually slow pulse. 3. *CNS:* mental depression, confusion. 4. *Other:* gynecomastia. 5. Signs of toxicity include anorexia, nausea and vomiting, diarrhea, drowsiness, lethargy, fatigue, headache, confusion, personality changes, blurred vision, blue/green vision, photophobia, and dysrhythmias.

1. Take apical-radial pulse for 1 minute before administering drug; do not give if patient's pulse is too low (minimum safe pulse rate varies: know the patient's usual pulse range and check with prescriber for guidelines). 2. Low serum potassium and high serum calcium predispose patient to digitalis toxicity. 3. Therapeutic serum digitalis levels vary greatly from person to person, and digitalis toxicity is better diagnosed on the basis of signs and symptoms than on blood levels.

Interactions **1.** Quinidine, propranolol, and calcium channel blockers may increase effect of digitalis, possibly resulting in digitalis toxicity. **2.** Cholestyramine or bran may decrease oral digitalis absorption. **3.** Phenobarbital increases digitalis metabolism, leading to decreased serum digitalis levels. **4.** Adrenocorticosteroids and potassium-depleting diuretics increase the possibility of digitalis toxicity because of their tendency to cause hypokalemia. **5.** Parenteral calcium salts, parenteral magnesium sulfate, other antidysrhythmic drugs, or sympathomimetics may increase the risk of cardiac dysrhythmias.

1. Adjust doses of digitalis or other drugs as needed. 2. Allow at least 2 hours to elapse from time of digitalis dose before administering cholestyramine or bran. 3. Monitor serum potassium levels.

Disopyramide (Norpace)

Common use suppression or prevention of recurrent ventricular dysrhythmias, such as premature ventricular contractions or ventricular tachycardia.
Mechanism of action antidysrhythmic agent; depresses myocardial responsiveness; normalizes regional cardiac electrical impulse conduction.

Dosage **1.** 150 mg every 6 hours, or 300 mg extended-release capsules every 12 hours; average daily doses range from 400 to 800 mg in divided doses. **2.** A 300-mg loading dose may be given for rapid control of dysrhythmias.
Administration oral.

1. Small patients and patients with moderate renal or hepatic insufficiency, cardiomyopathy, or possible cardiac decompensation usually require reduced doses. 2. Hypokalemia should be corrected before therapy is begun. 3. Monitor vital signs for potential hypotension and bradycardia during initial therapy; alert physician if significant (approximately 25%) widening of QRS complex is observed on EKG. 4. Contraindications: cardiogenic shock and second or third-degree AV block.

Anticipated response maintenance of normal sinus rhythm; reduced frequency or duration of recurrent ventricular dysrhythmias.

Onset of effects takes 30 minutes to 3 hours.

Side effects **1.** *GU:* urinary retention. **2.** *CV:* hypotension, heart failure, conduction disturbances, dizziness. **3.** *GI:* constipation, dry mouth, hepatotoxicity. **4.** *CNS:* blurred vision, confusion. **5.** *GU:* impotence. **6.** *Other:* increased intraocular pressure.

1. Observe for possible urinary retention, particularly among older males. 2. Caution patient to rise slowly from sitting or recumbent position to avoid orthostatic hypotension. 3. Patients with glaucoma may react with increased intraocular pressure; instruct them to report immediately any visual changes or eye pain. 4. Observe for signs of hepatotoxicity—for example, jaundice. 5. Caution patient against driving or operating machinery if dizziness or blurred vision occurs.

Interactions **1.** May produce profound heart failure or conduction delays (or block) when given with other antidysrhythmic drugs. **2.** With alcohol, possible hypoglycemia and/or hypotension. **3.** With oral anticoagulants, possible erratic anticoagulant effect.

1. Give cautiously with similar antidysrhythmic drugs. Do not administer within 48 hours before or 24 hours after verapamil. 2. Do not use with alcohol. 3. Use caution in giving oral anticoagulants with disopyramide.

Other worsening of heart failure may occur in patients with compromised ventricular function.

Edrophonium Chloride (Tensilon)

Common use to diagnose myasthenia gravis; as curare antagonist; experimentally, in the treatment of supraventricular tachycardias.
Mechanism of action cholinergic; inhibits destruction of acetylcholine, facilitating parasympathetic nerve impulse transmission across the neuromuscular junction.

Dosage *to diagnose myasthenia gravis:* 10 mg IM, or 2–10 mg IV; *as curare antidote:* 10 mg IV; *as antidysrhythmic:* 5–10 mg IV.
Administration intramuscular, intravenous

Accurately record each dose given and patient's response.

Anticipated response **1.** Increase in muscle strength in patients with myasthenia gravis. **2.** Reversal of curare-induced neuromuscular blockade. **3.** Termination of dysrhythmia.

Side effects   **1.** *CNS:* weakness, blurred vision, watery eyes. **2.** *CV:* hypotension, bradycardia. **3.** *Respiratory:* increased secretions, apnea, wheezing. **4.** *Musculoskeletal:* muscle weakness, cramps, twitching. **5.** *GI:* diarrhea, nausea, salivation. **6.** *GU:* frequent urination.

Keep atropine available to reverse edrophonium effects in sensitive individuals.

Interactions   **1.** With other cholinergic drugs in patient with myasthenic weakness, may cause cholinergic crisis and worsening of patient's condition. **2.** With digitalis, may cause excessive bradycardia.

Other   Do not use in patients with bronchial asthma, GI obstruction, or urinary tract obstruction.

Heparin

Common use   treatment of pulmonary embolism; prevention and treatment of vein thrombosis; disseminated intravascular coagulation.
Mechanism of action   anticoagulant; prevents formation of fibrin and thrombin.

Dosage   (SC) 10,000–20,000 units initially, then 8,000–10,000 units every 8 hours; (IV) 10,000 units initially, then 5,000–10,000 units every 4–6 hours; (continuous IV infusion) 20,000–40,000 units in 1000 ml sodium chloride solution, infused over 24 hours.
Administration   intravenous, subcutaneous.

1. *Obtain report of partial thromboplastin time before administering (½ hour before administration time); partial thromboplastin time values are usually maintained at 1½–2 times the control value.* **2.** *When administration is SC, inject above iliac crest or in lower abdomen deep into fat; do not aspirate prior to injection, or massage area.* **3.** *Avoid IM route because of irregular absorption of drug, increased incidence of hematoma, and pain.* **4.** *IV pump is recommended for continuous IV infusion.* **5.** *When taking blood samples from patient, apply continuous pressure for 3–5 minutes.* **6.** *Intermittent IV infusion may be given diluted and piggybacked into main IV line, or IV push.* **7.** *Do not use solution if discolored or if precipitate is present.* **8.** *Heparin is strongly acidic and incompatible with many IV medications. Use separate infusion sites, or flush tubing carefully before and after each dose.*

Anticipated response   anticoagulation and prevention of embolism formation.

Have protamine sulfate available as antidote for frank bleeding; because heparin is short-acting, treatment of overdose is conservative unless frank bleeding occurs.

Side effects   **1.** *Hematologic:* hemorrhage, prolonged clotting time, thrombocytopenia. **2.** *Dermatologic:* urticaria (allergy). **3.** *CV:* vasospastic hypersensitivity, with pain and cyanosis of limbs (not reversed by protamine sulfate). **4.** *Other:* with long-term therapy, possible hair loss or osteoporosis.

1. *Check patient's urine and feces for overt signs of bleeding; watch for easy bruising, unexplained nosebleeds, prolonged menses, dizziness, severe headache.* **2.** *People over 60, especially women, are more susceptible to hemorrhage during heparin therapy.*

Interactions   **1.** Aspirin, ibuprofen, indomethacin, oxyphenbutazone, phenylbutazone, and other antiplatelet drugs may increase risk of hemorrhage. **2.** Blood transfusions should be undertaken cautiously: heparin activity lasts up to 22 days after refrigeration of ACD-converted blood, and there is a possible risk of hemorrhage when such blood is given to a patient receiving heparin. **3.** With steroids and nonsteroid anti-inflammatory agents, increased risk of GI hemorrhage because of these drugs' potential to cause GI ulceration.

Warn patient not to take OTC preparations that contain aspirin or ibuprofen.

Other   Contraindicated in bleeding disorders (except disseminated intravascular coagulation), when an aneurysm is present, and in severe uncontrolled hypertension.

Hydantoin Anticonvulsants: ethotoin (Peganone), mephenytoin (Mesantoin), phenytoin (Dilantin)

Common use   management of grand mal and psychomotor seizures, and status epilepticus; treatment of dysrhythmias.

Mechanism of action   anticonvulsants, exact mechanism unknown; believed to alter the movement of sodium ions across cell membranes, thereby stabilizing neuronal membranes and inhibiting seizure activity.

Dosage   1. *ethotoin:* (oral) initially, 500–1000 mg, increased gradually up to 5 grams per day, divided into 4–6 doses. **2.** *mephenytoin:* (oral) 50–100 mg daily, increased as needed up to 800 mg. **3.** *phenytoin:* (oral) 100 mg 3 times a day, increased as needed to 600 mg daily; (IV) (in status epilepticus) 150–200 mg, followed by 100–150 mg after 30 minutes if needed; (as antidysrhythmic) 50–100 mg every 10–15 minutes as needed and tolerated.

Administration   oral, intravenous.

1. IV phenytoin should be administered at a rate no greater than 50 mg/min. Clear tubing with normal saline before and after each dose. 2. IV phenytoin precipitates easily in solution. If intermittent infusion, rather than bolus injections, are necessary, use normal saline solution, mix immediately before infusing for a concentration of 10 mg/ml, infuse within 4 hours, and use an in-line filter. 3. Avoid extravasation of phenytoin, as it is very caustic to tissues. 4. Mephenytoin is the least safe of the hydantoins and generally is used only after safer anticonvulsants have failed to control seizures. 5. When discontinuing an anticonvulsant, gradual dosage reduction is necessary. 6. Oral absorption differs greatly among different brands of phenytoin. The prescribing physician should be informed of any brand change.

Anticipated response   decreased frequency of seizures, control of status epilepticus, or decreased dysrhythmias.

Side effects   1. *GI:* constipation, nausea, gingival hyperplasia. **2.** *CNS:* drowsiness, fatigue, insomnia, dizziness, headache, diplopia. **3.** *Hematologic:* agranulocytosis, thrombocytopenia. **4.** *Musculoskeletal:* muscle twitching, bone fractures or slowed growth. **5.** *Dermatologic:* excessive growth of body and facial hair. **6.** *Toxicity:* continuous rolling or back-and-forth movements of eyes, blurred vision, confusion, behavioral changes, hallucinations, slurred speech, ataxia, increased frequency of convulsions.

1. Administer oral forms with food or milk to decrease GI side effects. 2. Until drug's sedative effects are known, instruct patient to be careful in tasks requiring alertness. 3. Teach proper mouth and dental care, including regular teeth cleaning by a professional. The use of ethotoin may decrease gum hyperplasia.

Interactions   1. Hydantoins increase the rate of metabolism of many other drugs, including adrenocorticoids, oral contraceptives and other estrogens, digitalis, disopyramide, quinidine, and levodopa, and may decrease the therapeutic effects of these drugs. **2.** Oral anticoagulants, cimetidine, disulfiram, phenylbutazone, and sulfonamides may increase the effects of hydantoins, resulting in hydantoin toxicity. **3.** Aluminum, magnesium, or calcium antacids may decrease the bioavailability of phenytoin. **4.** Hydantoins may increase blood sugar and thereby antagonize the effects of antidiabetic drugs. **5.** Barbiturates have variable effects on hydantoin metabolism. **6.** Hydantoins deplete folic acid; folic acid supplements may lower serum hydantoin levels and cause loss of seizure con-

trol. **7.** Additive cardiac depression when IV phenytoin is used with lidocaine or beta-blocker drugs. **8.** Phenytoin may increase methadone metabolism and precipitate withdrawal symptoms. **9.** Hydantoins may decrease serum theophylline levels. **10.** Chronic alcohol use may decrease hydantoin effects, while high-dose acute use may increase serum hydantoins.

1. Separate the doses of antacids and phenytoin by at least 2 hours. 2. Adjust antidiabetic therapy as needed to control blood sugar. 3. Carefully monitor hydantoin blood levels when phenobarbital or another barbiturate is part of the regimen.

Other   Hydantoins administered before delivery increase the risk of life-threatening hemorrhage in the neonate.

Isoetharine (Bronkosol, Bronkometer)

Common use   treatment of chronic bronchitis, asthma, and emphysema.
Mechanism of action   sympathomimetic bronchodilator; relaxes bronchial smooth muscle.

Dosage   1. mesylate: 1 inhalation, repeated after 1–2 minutes, every 4 hours. **2.** hydrochloride salt: *hand nebulizer—* 3–7 inhalations of 1% solution every 4 hours; *IPPB or oxygen aerosolization—*0.5–4 ml of 0.125–0.25% solution every 4 hours.
Administration   inhalation.

1. Avoid contact with eyes. 2. Instruct patient to use inhaler correctly (Exhale; deeply inhale on mouthpiece while squeezing bulb of inhaler; hold breath for several seconds; exhale slowly into the air.) 3. When drug is administered with oxygen, flow of oxygen should be adjusted to 4–6 L/min for 15–20 minutes. Do not administer if solution is discolored or contains a precipitate.

Anticipated response   relief of bronchospasm, increased vital capacity, and decreased airway resistance.

1. Observe patient's respirations for rate and depth. 2. Vital capacity monitoring may be ordered to confirm effectiveness of drug. 3. May decrease in effectiveness with continued use, necessitating a switch to another drug.

Side effects   1. *CNS:* insomnia, tremor, headache, anxiety, dizziness. **2.** *CV:* palpitation, tachycardia, chest pain. **3.** *GI:* nausea. **4.** *Other:* sulfite preservative used in some brands can cause allergic reactions and worsen bronchospasm.

Elderly patients are more sensitive than younger adults to sympathomimetic effects.

Interactions 1. Beta-blocking drugs will antagonize bronchodilating effect of this drug. 2. With other sympathomimetic drugs, increased sympathomimetic effects and possible increase in uncomfortable side effects and/or toxicity. 3. Inhalation-aerosol forms of adrenocorticoids contain fluorocarbon propellants, as does isoetharine, and the use of both drugs close together can cause fluorocarbon toxicity. 4. May antagonize antihypertensive medications. 5. With digitalis, increased risk of dysrhythmias.

1. *Allow at least 15 minutes to elapse between isoetharine and adrenocorticoid aerosols.* 2. *Monitor cardiac status when isoetharine is used in digitalized patient.*

Loop Diuretics: bumetanide (Bumex), ethacrynic acid (Edecrin), furosemide (Lasix)

Common use treatment of congestive heart failure, essential hypertension, and edema, including acute pulmonary edema.

Mechanism of action inhibits reabsorption of electrolytes and thereby increases excretion of water in renal tubules.

Dosage 1. *bumetanide:* (oral) 0.5–2 mg daily; (IV, IM) 0.5–1 mg, repeated every 2–3 hours as needed. 2. *ethacrynic acid:* (oral) 50–200 mg daily; (IV) 50 mg, repeated in 2–6 hours as needed. 3. *furosemide:* (oral) 20–80 mg daily; (IV) 20–40 mg, repeated or increased at 2-hour intervals as needed.

Administration oral, intravenous, intramuscular.

1. *When administering IV, dilute with 5% dextrose or sodium chloride.* 2. *If solution is hazy (due to diluents with a pH below 5), discard.* 3. *Discard reconstituted drug after 24 hours.* 4. *IV solution is physically incompatible with whole blood or whole-blood derivatives.* 5. *Do not add drug to IV solution; inject through Y-tube or 3-way stopcock.* 6. *Avoid IM or SC administration, because these routes will cause local irritation.*

Anticipated response diuresis.

1. *Onset of action after IV administration is within minutes; after oral administration, 30–60 minutes. Keep bedpan or urinal available, or Foley tubing patent.* 2. *Explain to patient importance of low-sodium diet.* 3. *Check patient's weight; keep accurate intake and output records, and monitor electrolyte lev-*

els. 4. *These drugs generally are prescribed for people who don't respond to thiazides, or for rapid mobilization of extreme edema.*

Side effects 1. *CNS;* tinnitus, deafness, mood changes, headache, confusion, drowsiness, muscle cramps, lethargy. 2. *GI:* abdominal cramps, dry mouth, thirst, diarrhea, nausea. 3. *CV:* orthostatic hypotension, dizziness, circulatory collapse. 4. *Metabolic:* hypokalemia, hyponatremia, hyperglycemia, hyperuricemia, hypocalcemia.

1. *Encourage intake of foods and fluids high in potassium.* 2. *Potassium salts or potassium-sparing diuretic may be prescribed in lieu of dietary potassium supplementation.* 3. *Check patient for signs of electrolyte depletion.* 4. *Elderly patients are more sensitive than younger adults to hypotensive and electrolyte effects, and at greater risk of circulatory collapse.* 5. *Monitor the patient's hearing during therapy, using audiometric testing if necessary.*

Interactions 1. When taken with other nephrotoxic or ototoxic drugs, increased potential for toxicity. 2. May potentiate antihypertensives and muscle relaxants. 3. May cause cardiac dysrhythmias with digitalis. 4. With corticosteroids, increased potassium loss. 5. With lithium, increased serum lithium levels. 6. With alcohol, barbiturates, or narcotics, possible increased orthostatic hypotension. 7. Antagonizes antigout drugs. 8. May increase or decrease the effects of anticoagulants or thrombolytic agents. 9. May antagonize hypoglycemic medications. 10. For furosemide only (in addition to above): with chloral hydrate, possible diaphoresis, hot flashes, and hypertension. With clofibrate, may increase the effects of both medications and cause uncomfortable side effects.

Other 1. Contraindicated in cases of anuria or severe renal disease. 2. Furosemide usually is the first choice over ethacrynic acid, because it is easier to give IV and because it has a lower risk of ototoxicity. 3. Diuretics do not prevent toxemia of pregnancy, and there is no evidence that they are useful in the treatment of toxemia. Contraindicated during pregnancy. 4. These drugs may exacerbate lupus erythematosus.

Mannitol (Osmitrol)

Common use treatment of acute renal failure and cerebral edema; reduction of intraocular and intracranial pressure; in overdose, to promote urinary excretion of toxic substances and to prevent renal damage.

Mechanism of action osmotic diuretic; increases osmotic pressure of glomerular filtrate, thereby decreasing renal tubular reabsorption of water; elevates blood plasma osmolality.

Dosage   usual dose is 50–200 g as a 5–25% solution; adjust rate of administration to maintain urine flow of at least 30–50 ml/hour.

Administration   intravenous.

1. Begin with a test dose if inadequate renal function is suspected. 2. Dissolve all crystals by warming ampules in hot water; cool to body temperature before administering. 3. Use IV filter when administering a 15% or greater solution of mannitol.

Anticipated response   diuresis; decreased intraocular and intracranial pressure.

1. Monitor urine output and specific gravity hourly throughout course of therapy. 2. Monitor electrolytes.

Side effects   1. *GI:* thirst, nausea, vomiting, dry mouth. 2. *CNS:* headache, dizziness, blurred vision. 3. *Metabolic:* fluid and electrolyte imbalance. 4. *CV:* circulatory overload with congestive heart failure, pulmonary edema, tachycardia, hypotension.

1. Observe patient for signs of electrolyte imbalance. 2. Monitor intake and output. 3. Weigh patient daily. 4. Monitor vital signs frequently. 5. Monitor renal function.

Interactions   1. With digitalis, enhances the possibility of digitalis toxicity associated with hypokalemia. 2. Mannitol solution may cause pseudoagglutination of blood during transfusion.

If blood and mannitol must be administered together, add at least 20 mEq of sodium chloride to each liter of mannitol solution.

Other   Do not use mannitol if acute tubular necrosis, severe pulmonary congestion, or intracranial bleeding are present.

Metaproterenol Sulfate (Alupent)

Common use   symptomatic treatment of bronchial asthma, bronchitis, emphysema.

Mechanism of action   sympathomimetic bronchodilator; enhances beta-adrenergic receptor activity, resulting in bronchodilation, decreased airway resistance, and relief of bronchospasm.

Dosage   acute episodes: 1. (inhalation aerosol) 2–3 inhalations no more often than every 3–4 hours. (Do not exceed 12 inhalations in 24 hours.) 2. (inhalation, solution, via hand nebulizer) 5–15 inhalations no more often than every 4 hours. 3. (inhalation, solution, via IPPB) 0.2–0.3 ml no more often than every 4 hours. 4. (oral) 20 mg 3–4 times a day.

Administration   oral, via inhalation.

1. Teach patient how to administer inhalation dose. (Exhale through nose; shake container; deeply inhale on mouthpiece; hold breath for several seconds; exhale slowly. Repeat in 2 minutes.) 2. Store drug in light-resistant container.

Anticipated response   increased vital capacity.

Observe patient carefully for response to drug. If no response is apparent, or if respiratory distress worsens, discontinue drug immediately and contact physician.

Side effects   1. *CNS:* nervousness, restlessness, dizziness, weakness, headache, drowsiness. 2. *CV:* tachycardia, hypertension, angina, dysrhythmia. 3. *GI:* nausea, vomiting. 4. *Other:* sulfite preservative used in some brands can cause allergic reactions and worsen bronchospasm.

1. Explain the importance of not overusing this drug. 2. Elderly patients are more sensitive than younger adults to sympathomimetic effects.

Interactions   1. With beta-blocker drugs, mutual antagonism of effects. 2. With other sympathomimetic drugs, possible increased effects (or side effects) of metaproterenol. 3. Inhalation aerosol forms of adrenocorticoids contain fluorocarbon propellants, as does metaproterenol, and the use of both drugs close together can cause fluorocarbon toxicity. 4. May antagonize the effects of antihypertensive or antianginal drugs. 5. With digitalis, may increase the risk of dysrhythmias.

1. Allow at least 15 minutes to elapse between metaproterenol and adrenocorticoid aerosols. 2. Monitor cardiac status when metaproterenol is used in digitalized patients.

Other   Use with caution in individuals with hypertension, coronary disease, diabetes, or thyroid disease.

Metaraminol (Aramine)

Common use   prevention and treatment of acute hypotension resulting from hemorrhage, shock, surgery, drug reactions, etc.

Mechanism of action sympathomimetic vasopressor; stimulates alpha-adrenergic receptors, increasing systolic and diastolic blood pressures.

Dosage (IM, SC) 2–10 mg; (IV bolus) 0.5–5 mg, followed by IV infusion; (IV infusion) 15–100 mg in 500 ml sodium chloride or D_5W, adjusting rate to BP response.
Administration Intravenous, intramuscular, subcutaneous.

1. IV route is preferred; use large veins. 2. Administer IV infusion with an infusion control device. 3. Too-rapid administration may cause pulmonary edema, dysrhythmias, and cardiac arrest. 4. Correct blood volume depletion immediately or concurrently. 5. Discard solution after 24 hours. 6. Physically incompatible with barbiturates, penicillins, and phenytoin—administer via separate IV line, or flush tubing carefully.

Anticipated response increased blood pressure and improved circulation.

Withdraw drug gradually to avoid recurrent hypotension.

Side effects 1. *CV:* dysrhythmias; sloughing of tissue at injection site (in extravasation); hypotension with prolonged use. 2. *Overdose:* convulsions, severe hypertension, severe dysrhythmias. 3. *Other:* sulfite preservative used in some brands can cause allergic reactions.

1. In case of extravasation, infiltrate site with phentolamine. 2. IV phentolamine can be used to counteract excessive hypertension.

Interactions 1. Alpha-adrenergic blockers such as phentolamine and prazosin will decrease the pressor effect of metaraminol. 2. With a hydrocarbon inhalation anesthetic such as cyclopropane or halothane, increased risk of severe ventricular dysrhythmias. 3. With beta-blockers, possible mutual inhibition, or hypertension, bradycardia, and heart block. 4. With digitalis or levodopa, increased risk of dysrhythmias. 5. With ergotamine, possible increased vasoconstriction, followed by ischemia and gangrene. 6. With guanadrel or guanethidine, possible enhanced pressor effect and hypertension. 7. With tricyclic antidepressants or MAO inhibitors, possible dysrhythmias, tachycardia, hypertension, and hyperpyrexia.

1. Decrease metaraminol dose in patients who are receiving hydrocarbon anesthetics, and closely monitor cardiac function. 2. Carefully monitor cardiac function in the digitalized patient receiving metaraminol.

Morphine Sulfate

Common use treatment of moderate to severe pain; as preoperative medication; in acute pulmonary edema secondary to left ventricular failure.
Mechanism of action narcotic analgesic; exact mechanism of action is unknown; believed to alter perception of and emotional response to pain.

Dosage (oral) 10–30 mg every 3–4 hours. (oral, extended release) 30 mg every 8–12 hours. (IM, SC) 5–20 mg every 3–4 hours. (IV bolus) 4–10 mg, diluted in 4–5 ml of water for injection. (IV infusion) 4–12 mg/hour. (rectal) 10–20 mg every 3–4 hours.
Administration oral, subcutaneous, intramuscular, intravenous, rectal.

1. For analgesic effect, administer before pain peaks; inform patient that he or she may request medication. 2. In chronic pain, around-the-clock dosing is more effective than p.r.n. administration. 3. This drug is a controlled substance, Schedule II. 4. Rapid IV injection can cause anaphylaxis, circulatory collapse, or cardiac arrest. IV morphine should be injected slowly over a period of several minutes. 5. Administer extended-release tablets whole, never crushed. 6. Dosages are highly individualized, depending on the severity of pain, patient response, and degree of tolerance. Dosages listed above are initial ranges only.

Anticipated response relief of pain; vasodilatation

1. Use nondrug measures to increase patient's comfort: proper positioning, environmental temperature, and so on. 2. Physical dependence will develop with regular use. Taper dosage when drug is discontinued, to avoid withdrawal symptoms.

Side effects 1. *CNS:* euphoria, mood changes, dysphoria, depressed cough reflex, sedation. 2. *CV:* bradycardia, orthostatic hypotension. 3. *GI:* nausea, vomiting, dry mouth, constipation. 4. *GU:* urinary tention, urgency, impotence. 5. *Respiratory:* decreased respiratory rate and depth. 6. *Other:* tolerance.

1. Observe patient for onset of side effects. 2. Keep narcotic antagonist and resuscitative equipment on hand when administering drug. 3. Warn patient not to undertake tasks requiring alertness until drug's sedative effect has been assessed. 4. Begin a bowel regimen (usually, a stimulant laxative) at the time of initiation of around-the-clock dosing. 5. Elderly patients may be more sensitive to respiratory depressant effects. 6. Tolerance develops much more rapidly with parenteral dosage forms than with other forms. 7. If hypotension, dizziness, or nausea make the patient particularly uncomfortable, keep the patient recumbent during periods of the drug's peak effect.

Interactions   1. With other CNS depressants, increased CNS depression. 2. Additive hypotension when used with other drugs that decrease blood pressure. 3. With anticholinergics or other constipating drugs, increased risk of severe constipation, impaction, or paralytic ileus. 4. With hydroxyzine, possible increased analgesia, hypotension, and CNS depressant effects. 5. With MAO inhibitors, possible severe and even fatal reaction involving excitation, rigidity, hyper/hypotension, respiratory depression, hyperpyrexia, and cardiovascular collapse.

Use a small test dose (1/4 dose) on patients who are already taking MAO inhibitor drugs.

Other   Contraindicated in patients with increased intracranial pressure; use with caution in COPD, supraventricular tachycardia, liver disease, Addison's disease, prostatic hypertrophy, pregnancy, acute abdomen, drug abuse history or emotional instability, severe inflammatory bowel disease.

Naloxone (Narcan)

Common use   antidote for narcotic-induced respiratory depression.
Mechanism of action   narcotic antagonist; exact mechanism of action is unknown; believed to work by competitive inhibition of narcotics at tissue receptor sites.

Dosage   0.1–0.4 mg, repeated as needed.
Administration   intravenous, subcutaneous, intramuscular.

1. IV route is preferred for better dose titration. Initial IV bolus may be followed by repeat boluses, IV infusion, or IM injection. 2. Because narcotic duration of action may exceed that of naloxone, respiratory depression may recur; observe respiratory pattern before and after administration.

Anticipated response   reversal of narcotic effects.

1. Will precipitate withdrawal symptoms in narcotic-dependent patients. 2. Prepare for agitation and combativeness as naloxone takes effect. 3. Naloxone will reverse analgesia as well as respiratory effects; if applicable, reinstitute pain control as soon as possible. 4. Use other resuscitative measures as needed.

Side effects   1. *GI:* nausea and vomiting (rare). 2. *CV:* tachycardia, hypertension. 3. *CNS:* nervousness, restlessness. *Nausea and vomiting only with high doses.*

Nitrates: erythrityl tetranitrate (Cardilate); isosorbide dinitrate (Isordil, Sorbitrate); nitroglycerin—buccal (Sustachron), oral (Nitro-Bid, Nitrospan), parenteral (Nitrol, Tridil), sublingual (Nitrostat), transdermal (Nitro-Bid, Nitrodisc, Nitro-Dur, Transderm-Nitro); pentaerythritol tetranitrate (Peritrate)

Common use   treatment and prevention of angina pectoris.
Mechanism of action   generalized peripheral vasodilation results in decreased peripheral resistance and increased venous pooling, thus decreasing cardiac workload.

Dosage   1. *erythrityl tetranitrate:* (oral, sublingual, buccal) 5–10 mg 3–4 times a day. 2. *isosorbide dinitrate:* (oral) 5–10 mg every 6 hours; (chewable form) 5 mg every 2–3 hours; (extended-release) 40 mg every 8–12 hours; (sublingual or buccal) 2.5–5 mg every 2–3 hours. 3. *nitroglycerin:* (oral extended-release) 1–9 mg every 12 hours; (buccal extended-release) 1 mg 3 times a day; (sublingual) 150–600 mcg, repeated at 5-minute intervals as needed for angina relief; (ointment) 15–30 mg (2.5–5 cm) every 8 hours; (transdermal system) 1 dosage system every 24 hours; (intravenous) initially 5 mcg/min, increased at 3–5-minute intervals until desired effect is achieved or rate reaches 20 mcg/min. 4. *pentaerythritol tetranitrate:* (oral) 10–20 mg 4 times a day; (oral extended-release) 30–80 mg 2 times a day.
Administration   oral, sublingual, buccal, transdermal, intravous.

1. Ointment: spread evenly over skin, but do not rub in; cover with plastic wrap if increased absorption is desired. 2. Transdermal ointment or patches are best applied to skin that is not hairy and that is free of scars or lesions. Avoid the distal extremities and thick adipose tissue. 3. Transdermal patches should never be trimmed in an attempt to modify dosage. 4. Although newer forms of sublingual nitroglycerin have improved stability, the sublingual form generally should be replaced every 6 months to ensure continued effectiveness. 5. Many people cannot digest extended-release dosage forms. A partially dissolved tablet or capsule may be found in the patient's stool. The patient's response to nitrate therapy should be determined through the use of regular dosage forms before an extended-release form is tried. 6. IV nitroglycerin should be administered with an infusion monitoring device. 7. Standard IV infusion sets are made of polyvinyl chloride plastic and unpredictably absorb up to 80% of nitroglycerin from solution. Use non-PVC plastic for tubing and connections. Be aware that non-PVC plastic may be incompatible with consistent operation of the infusion monitoring device.

Anticipated response   decreased frequency (or, with nitroglycerin sublingual, prompt relief) of anginal pain.

1. Long-acting forms will not provide relief during acute attack. 2. Tolerance may develop with prolonged use. Discontinuing nitrate therapy briefly and then restarting may restore its effectiveness.

Side effects   1. *CV:* orthostatic hypotension, headache, flushing, dizziness. 2. *GI:* nausea. 3. *Dermatologic:* skin irritation.

1. Treat occasional headache with aspirin or acetaminophen. 2. Frequent headaches warrant decrease in level or frequency of dose, or change to nonnitrate antianginal medication. 3. Advise patient to rise slowly to avoid orthostatic hypotension. 4. Rotate transdermal sites to avoid skin irritation. 5. Nurses or others administering topical nitroglycerin should avoid contact with the ointment or patch surface, and wash hands thoroughly after preparing the dose, to avoid transdermal absorption of the drug.

Interactions   1. With other drugs that lower blood pressure, possible aggravated hypotension. 2. Sympathomimetic drugs may antagonize effects of nitrates.

Other   1. Use cautiously with cerebral hemorrhage or recent head trauma (nitrates may raise cerebrospinal fluid pressure). 2. Use cautiously with recent MI; hypotension and tachycardia may aggravate ischemia.

Norepinephrine (Levophed)

Common use   treatment of severe hypotension, as in shock, cardiac arrest, and drug reactions.
Mechanism of action   vasopressor, sympathetic stimulant; raises blood pressure, improves myocardial contractility, and increases coronary artery blood flow.

Dosage   adults: initially, 8–12 µg/min; then adjust flow rate to maintain low-normal blood pressure; maintenance dose is usually about 2–4 µg/min.
Administration   intravenous infusion.

1. If possible, give into a large vein to avoid accidental extravasation. 2. Mix with IV fluids that contain dextrose—for example, D₅W or D₅NS. (Dextrose protects against loss of the drug's potency in solution.) 3. Individual response to this drug varies greatly, so flow rate must be adjusted according to patient's response. 4. Reduce infusion gradually when discontinuing drug.

Anticipated response   increase in blood pressure; improved tissue perfusion.

1. Blood flow to all areas except heart and brain may be reduced. Renal vasoconstriction occurs. Monitor accordingly. 2. Treat underlying cause of shock as soon as possible.

Side effects   1. *CV:* hypertension, bradycardia, other dysrhythmias. 2. *CNS:* headache, restlessness. 3. *Dermatologic:* skin necrosis (from severe vasoconstriction) if drug extravasates. 4. *Other:* sulfite preservative used in preparing norepinephrine injection can cause allergic reactions.

1. Monitor blood pressure, pulse, and ECG continuously during therapy. 2. Monitor intake and output. 3. In case of extravasation, inject solution of saline and phentolamine locally to try to prevent skin necrosis and sloughing.

Interactions   1. Hydrocarbon anesthetics such as halothane and cyclopropane sensitize the heart to the action of norepinephrine and may result in severe ventricular dysrhythmias. 2. With beta-blocker drugs, mutual inhibition, or hypertension, excessive bradycardia, and possible heart block. 3. With other CNS stimulants, additive CNS stimulation, possibly resulting in convulsions or dysrhythmias. 4. With digitalis, increased risk of cardiac dysrhythmias. 5. With ergotamine, possible peripheral vascular ischemia and gangrene. 6. With oxytocin or tricyclic antidepressants, possible prolonged and severe hypertension.

1. Avoid use with interacting drugs. If norepinephrine is essential in these patients, begin with a reduced dosage. 2. Carefully monitor cardiac function when norepinephrine is given to digitalized patients.

Other   Norepinephrine crosses the placenta and can cause fetal hypoxia.

Pancuronium Bromide (Pavulon)

Common use   to facilitate mechanical ventilation; to aid in intubation; as adjunct to anesthesia.
Mechanism of action   neuromuscular blocking agent blocks nerve impulse transmission at myoneural junction, resulting in skeletal muscle paralysis.

Dosage   0.04–0.1 mg/kg; then increments of 0.01 mg/kg.

Administration   intravenous.

1. *Do not administer unless under* direct *supervision of physician experienced in the use of this drug.* **2.** *Do not store in plastic containers.* **3.** *Store in refrigerator.* **4.** *Ventilatory assistance must be available.* **5.** *Patient needs to be sedated during administration.*

Anticipated response   rapidly induced skeletal-muscle paralysis.

1. *Monitor vital signs closely.* **2.** *Anticholinesterase agents usually are used for reversal of paralysis. Observe patient closely after administration of antagonist for possible return of muscle relaxation.*

Side effects   **1.** *CV:* tachycardia. **2.** *Dermatologic:* transient rash. **3.** *GI:* salivation. **4.** *Neurologic:* prolonged neuromuscular blockade. **5.** *Respiratory:* depression, apnea. **6.** *Overdose:* deep respiratory depression, cardiovascular collapse.

Interactions   **1.** Possible intensified neuromuscular blockade when given with beta-blockers, procainamide, quinidine, aminoglycoside or polymixin antibiotics, lithium, inhalation anesthetics, or massive blood transfusions. **2.** Additive respiratory depression with opiates or other drugs that depress respiration. **3.** Calcium salts usually reverse pancuronium effects. **4.** Possible increased cardiac dysrhythmias in digitalized patients. **5.** Hypokalemia may potentiate pancuronium effects.

1. *When drugs that may enhance neuromuscular blackade are given concurrently or sequentially, the primary potential danger is incomplete reversal of neuromuscular blockade postoperatively. Monitor patient carefully.* **2.** *Check serum potassium prior to administration. Use caution if potassium-depleting drugs, such as thiazide diuretics, loop diuretics, or corticosteroids, are administered.*

Other   Hyperthermia may intensify and prolong pancuronium's effect.

Procainamide (Pronestyl)

Common use   treatment of premature ventricular contractions, ventricular tachycardia, paroxysmal atrial tachycardia, and atrial fibrillation.
Mechanism of action   antidysrhythmic; depresses automaticity of heart muscle fibers; slows rate of atrioventricular conduction; increases refractory period.

Dosage   **1.** (oral) 250–500 mg every 3 hours. **2.** (IM) 500–1000 mg 4 times a day. **3.** (IV) 100–1000 mg, diluted and infused at 20–50 mg/min, then 2–6 mg/min as maintenance.
Administration   oral, intramuscular, intravenous.

1. *Patient should be placed on cardiac monitor during parenteral therapy.* **2.** *Observe for indications of heart block or prolonged Q-T interval.* **3.** *Constantly observe patient receiving drug IV drip.* **4.** *Patient should be in supine position when drug is administered IV.* **5.** *IV rate should not exceed 50 mg/min.*

Anticipated response   control of irregular cardiac activity.

Instruct patient to take this drug exactly as prescribed.

Side effects   **1.** *CNS:* confusion, depression, hallucinations, dizziness. **2.** *CV:* hypotension (especially with IV form). **3.** *GI:* nausea, vomiting, anorexia, diarrhea. **4.** *Musculoskeletal:* lupus. **5.** *Hematologic:* agranulocytosis, leukopenia, thrombocytopenia.

1. *Elderly patients are more sensitive to the drug's hypotensive effects.* **2.** *Discontinue drug if lupus occurs.* **3.** *Do routine CBCs and cardiac function monitoring during long-term therapy.*

Interactions   **1.** With other antidysrhythmics, possible additive effects. **2.** With antihypertensives, additive hypotension. **3.** Procainamide may inhibit the effects of antimyasthenic drugs on skeletal muscle. **4.** May enhance the effects of neuromuscular blocking drugs.

Other   Use with caution in patients with congestive heart failure or renal disease.

Quinidine: quinidine gluconate (Quinaglute), quinidine polygalacturonate (Cardioquin), quinidine sulfate (Cin-Quin)

Common use   treatment of atrial dysrhythmias, premature ventricular contractions.
Mechanism of action   antidysrhythmic agent; increases cardiac refractory period; slows A-V conduction; depresses automaticity.

Dosage   **1.** *sulfate:* (oral) 200–400 mg every 2–3 hours initially, followed by 100–300 mg 3–6 times a day; (IV) 600 mg in 40 ml of D_5W, administered at 1 ml/min. **2.** *gluconate:* (IV) diluted inD_5W to 800 mg/40 ml, infuse at 1 ml/min. (IM) initially 600 mg, then 400 mg up to 12 times a day. **3.** *polygalacturonate:* (oral) 275–825 mg every 3–4 hours initially, then gradually increase dose as needed.

Administration　oral, intravenous, intramuscular.

1. Do not use discolored solutions. 2. Check apical rate and blood pressure before administration. 3. Utilize continuous ECG and BP monitoring during IV administration.

Anticipated response　control of dysrhythmia.

Monitor EKG when initiating therapy.

Side effects　**1.** *Hematologic:* blood dyscrasias. **2.** *CNS:* restlessness, vertigo, confusion. **3.** *CV:* hypotension, pallor. **4.** *GI:* nausea, vomiting, diarrhea, hypersalivation. **5.** *Other:* signs of toxicity include nausea, vomiting, tinnitus, dizziness, headache, fever, tremor, visual changes, widening QRS interval, ventricular ectopic beats, AV block.

1. Administer drug with food, to lessen GI irritation. 2. Notify physician if you suspect toxicity. Check blood levels of quinidine (normal levels are 2–6 μg/ml).

Interactions　**1.** With anticoagulants, possible increased anticoagulant effect. **2.** With digitalis, possible increased serum digitalis, resulting in toxicity. **3.** With urinary alkalizers such as sodium bicarbonate, other antacids, or large amounts of citrus fruit juices, increased serum quinidine and possible toxicity. **4.** With other antidysrhythmics, additive cardiac effects. **5.** Quinidine may antagonize the inotropic effect of bretylium and potentiate hypotension. **6.** Cimetidine prolongs quinidine half-life. **7.** Quinidine may potentiate the effects of neuromuscular blocking agents. **8.** Potassium-containing medications may enhance quinidine effects, while hypokalemia tends to decrease quinidine effect. **9.** Phenytoin and phenobarbital decrease serum quinidine levels.

1. Use caution when giving quinidine with anticoagulants. 2. Monitor patient closely if quinidine must be given with cardiac glycosides; decrease digoxin dose as needed. 3. Adjust drug doses as needed when quinidine is given with other interacting drugs.

Other　Do not give quinidine for digitalis-induced dysrhythmias.

Ranitidine (Zantac)

Common use　treatment and prevention of gastric or duodenal ulcer and hypersecretory states.

Mechanism of action　histamine H_2-receptor antagonist; inhibits gastric acid secretion.

Dosage　(oral) 150 mg 2 times daily; for prevention of recurrent duodenal ulcer, 150 mg at bedtime. (IM, IV) 50 mg every 6–8 hours.

Administration　oral, intramuscular, intravenous.

1. Administer IV ranitidine over not less than 5 minutes. 2. Do not use for minor digestive complaints. 3. Instruct patient to avoid food, drinks, or other medications that cause GI distress.

Anticipated response　relief of pain, ulcer healing, prevention of recurrence.

In most cases, limit dosage to a period of 8 weeks. Pathologic hypersecretory states may need an indefinite course of therapy.

Side effects　**1.** *GI:* nausea, constipation, pain. **2.** *Hematologic:* blood dyscrasias. **3.** *CNS:* dizziness, headache, confusion.

1. Check for melena. 2. Assess pain relief. 3. Older patients are more susceptible to CNS effects.

Interactions　**1.** Ranitidine may decrease absorption of the antifungal agent ketoconazole. **2.** May create false negative results when testing skin for allergies.

1. Give ranitidine at least 2 hours after ketoconazole. 2. Discontinue ranitidine use before testing skin for allergies.

Sodium Polystyrene Sulfonate (Kayexalate)

Common use　treatment of hyperkalemia.

Mechanism of action　antihyperkalemic; sodium in the resin is partially replaced by potassium and excreted.

Dosage　**1.** (oral) 15 g up to 4 times daily diluted in water or sorbitol. **2.** (rectal) 25–100 g as needed.

Administration　oral, rectal.

1. Chill solution for oral administration. 2. For rectal administration, prepare medication at room temperature. 3. Administer cleansing enema before and after Kayexalate enema; explain procedure to patient, and advise that minimum retention time is 30–60 minutes. Post-Kayexalate enema should be nonsodium and be administered via Y-tubing for continuous drain-

age. **4.** *A mild laxative given concurrently will help prevent constipation.*

Anticipated response reduction of excessively high serum potassium level when resin is eliminated through bowel movement.

1. *Not useful in emergency treatment because of slow action.* **2.** *Monitor patient for signs and symptoms of electrolyte depletion.* **3.** *Monitor serum potassium levels daily, and run periodic ECGs.*

Side effects **1.** *GI:* anorexia, nausea, vomiting, constipation, fecal impaction. **2.** *Metabolic:* hypokalemia, sodium retention, and other electrolyte disturbances. **3.** *CNS:* confusion, irritability.

Sorbitol may be given with both forms to combat constipation.

Interactions **1.** With antacids and laxatives, possible reduction in sodium/potassium exchange and possible systemic alkalosis. **2.** Other drugs that affect potassium levels, such as intravenous sodium bicarbonate and insulin, should be used with caution.

Do not use this drug with antacids or laxatives that contain calcium or magnesium.

Terbutaline (Brethine, Bricanyl)

Common use management of bronchial asthma, bronchitis, emphysema.
Mechanism of action sympathomimetic action relaxes bronchial smooth muscle.

Dosage (oral) 2.5–5 mg 3 times a day, with a maximum of 15 mg daily; (SC) 0.25 mg repeated once after 15–30 minutes if necessary; (inhalation) 2 inhalations 60 seconds apart every 4–6 hours.
Administration oral, subcutaneous, inhalation.

1. *Space 3 daily doses 6 hours apart.* **2.** *Administer subcutaneously in deltoid region.*

Anticipated response decreased airway resistance; relief of bronchospasm.

Side effects **1.** *CNS:* tremors, dizziness, nervousness, drowsiness, anxiety, headache. **2.** *CV:* tachycardia, palpitations. **3.** *GI:* nausea, vomiting.

1. *Careful observation is essential when administered to patients with elevated blood pressure, dysrhythmias, or hyperthyroidism.* **2.** *Elderly patients are more sensitive than younger adults to sympathomimetic effects.*

Interactions **1.** Beta-blockers may antagonize this drug's bronchodilatory effect. **2.** With other sympathomimetic drugs, potentiation of effects and increased side effects. **3.** Inhalation aerosol forms of adrenocorticoids and terbutaline contain fluorocarbon propellants; concurrent use can lead to fluorocarbon toxicity. **4.** With hydrocarbon inhalation anesthetics such as halothane or cyclopropane, increased risk of severe ventricular dysrhythmias. **5.** May antagonize the effects of antihypertensive or antianginal medications. **6.** Increased risk of dysrhythmias in the digitalized patient.

1. *Separate corticosteroid and terbutaline aerosols by at least 15 minutes.* **2.** *Monitor cardiac function as needed when terbutaline is given with interacting drugs.*

Other Use with caution in patients with a history of dysrhythmias, high blood pressure, convulsions, diabetes, or hyperthyroidism.

Thrombolytic Agents: streptokinase (Streptase), urokinase (Abbokinase)

Common use dissolution of acute pulmonary emboli, coronary artery thrombi, and deep venous thromboses, and clearance of intravenous catheter obstruction.
Mechanism of action activate plasmin, which in turn breaks down fibrin clots.

Dosage **1.** *streptokinase:* (coronary artery thrombi) intracoronary infusion of 20,000 IU bolus followed by infusion of 2,000 IU/min for 1 hour; (other) IV loading dose of 250,000 IU over 30 minutes, then maintenance dose of 100,000 IU/hour for up to 24–72 hours. (catheter obstruction) 100,000–250,000 IV, administered slowly. **2.** *urokinase:* (coronary artery thrombi) 6000 IU/min, up to a usual total dose of 500,000 IU; (other) 4,400 IU/kg over 10 minutes, then 4,400 IU/kg/hour; (catheter obstruction) fill catheter with a solution of 5,000 IU/ml urokinase.

Administration   intravenous.

1. *For best results after coronary artery thrombus, streptokinase should be administered within 6–8 hours of myocardial infarct.* 2. *These drugs are not used for superficial thrombophlebitis.* 3. *Reconstitute immediately before use. Do not shake.*

Anticipated response   dissolution of thrombi and emboli, with improved circulation to previously occluded vascular beds.

1. *Monitor coagulation panels.* 2. *Action is almost immediate and persists up to 12 hours after infusion is discontinued.* 3. *The patient usually is kept on bedrest during therapy.*

Side effects   1. *Hematologic:* bleeding. 2. *Metabolic:* fever. 3. *Other:* allergic reactions, including anaphylaxis, in sensitive patients; streptokinase is antigenic and induces antibody formation, and resistance to subsequent streptokinase therapy may persist for 3–6 months.

1. *Keep antifibrinolysin aminocaproic acid (Amicar) on hand to reverse severe bleeding.* 2. *Blood should be available for transfusion in case of severe bleeding.* 3. *Keep epinephrine 1:1000 units on hand in case of anaphylaxis.* 4. *Check for blood in urine and stools, as well as at any traumatized areas, including IV sites; and for reperfusion dysrythmias.* 5. *The risk of hemorrhage is greater with these drugs than with heparin or the oral anticoagulants.* 6. *Elderly patients may have an increased risk of cerebral hemorrhage when these drugs are administered.*

Interactions   1. With other anticoagulants, possible uncontrolled, excessive bleeding. 2. With other drugs that alter platelet function (aspirin, indomethacin, and so on), increased potential for bleeding.

1. *Do not give with other anticoagulants.* 2. *Do not give with other drugs that alter platelet function (including OTC drugs containing aspirin).*

Other   Use these drugs with extreme caution in patients with recent bleeding disorders or active hemorrhage; suspected aneurysm; recent childbirth; bacteial endocarditis, recent invasive procedure or biopsy; recent trauma or surgery.

Warfarin (Coumadin, Panwarfin)

Common use   treatment of pulmonary emboli; prevention or treatment of venous thrombosis and atrial fibrillation with embolization.

Mechanism of action   interferes with activity of vitamin K, which in turn interferes with the formation of active procoagulation factors.

Dosage   2–10 mg daily (maintenance dose).
Administration   oral.

1. *Prothrombin times are done daily at the start of therapy and then weekly; prothrombin times should not exceed 2½ times normal. (Best to maintain patient at 1½–2 times normal.)* 2. *Administer drug at same time daily.* 3. *Elderly and debilitated patients are extrasensitive to this drug's effects.*

Anticipated response   decreased blood clotting, as evidenced by laboratory tests; prevention of thrombus formation and/or uneventful resolution of existing clots.

1. *Inform patient of importance of complying with medication regimen and laboratory tests.* 2. *Onset of action may take up to 3 days.*

Side effects   1. *GI:* cramps, nausea, vomiting, diarrhea. 2. *Hematologic:* hemorrhage, leukopenia. 3. *Other:* unusual hair loss.

1. *Watch for signs of bleeding.* 2. *Instruct patient to shave with electric razor.* 3. *Instruct patient to carry card identifying ongoing anticoagulant therapy.* 4. *Avoid IM injections and repeated blood drawing.* 5. *Anticoagulant effect may increase during prolonged fever or diarrhea. Monitor patient closely for altered response to anticoagulants.*

Interactions   Because warfarin is highly but weakly protein bound, there is potential for numerous drug interactions. In addition, any drugs that can affect platelets or vitamin K or that are ulcerogenic contribute to risk of bleeding. Therefore, prothrombin time should *always* be checked when anything is added to or subtracted from the regimen of the patient on warfarin.

Encourage patient to avoid self-medication and alcohol.

Other   1. Contraindicated during pregnancy; congenital malformations have been documented. 2. Warfarin therapy is contraindicated when any of the following conditions exist: cerebral or aortic aneurysm, suspected cerebrovascular hemorrhage, any active bleeding, recent neurosurgery or ophthalmic surgery, known blood dyscrasias, uncontrolled hypertension. 3. Use with caution in renal or hepatic function impairment, visceral carcinomas, severe diabetes, recent childbirth, or vitamin C or K deficiencies.

REFERENCES

Clark JF et al.: *Pharmacological basis of nursing practice.* St Louis: Mosby, 1982.

Gahart BL: *Intravenous medications: A handbook for nurses and other allied health personnel,* 4th ed. St Louis: Mosby, 1981.

Hahn AB et al.: *Pharmacology in nursing,* 15th ed. St Louis: Mosby, 1982.

Rodman MJ, Smith DW: *Pharmacology and drug therapy in nursing,* 3rd ed. Philadelphia: Lippincott, 1985.

Sheridan EH et al.: *Falconer's the drug, the nurse, the patient,* 7th ed. Philadelphia: Saunders, 1982.

Shlafer M, Marieb EN: *Pharmacology for nurses.* Menlo Park, CA: Addison-Wesley, in press.

U.S. Pharmacopeial Convention, Inc. (Ed.): *USP DI: Drug information for the health care provider* (Vol. I) and *Advice for the patient* (Vol. II), 7th ed. Rockville, MD: USPC, Inc, 1987.

SUPPLEMENTAL READING

For drug information updates

The Medical Letter, published every two weeks by The Medical Letter, Inc., 56 Harrison Street, New Rochelle, NY 10801.

USP DI Updates, published bimonthly by USPC, Inc, 12601 Twinbrook Pky, Rockville, MD 20852.

INDEX

A small "f" following a page number refers to a figure; a "t" refers to a table.

Abbokinase, 614
Abdomen, physical examination of, 462–465
Abdominal aorta, palpation of, 465
Abdominal assessment format, 463t
Abdominal organs, location of, 463f
Abdominal trauma, 549–552
  assessment of, 549–551
  nursing diagnoses and, 551
  outcome evaluation in, 552
  planning and implementation of care in, 551–552
Aberration, cardiac conduction, 292
Absolute refractory period, 266
Absorption atelectasis, oxygen therapy and, 188
Abstract thinking, assessment of, 56
Accelerated junctional rhythm, ECG tracing of, 283t
Accelerated ventricular rhythm, ECG tracing of, 284t
Acebutolol, 600–601
Acetazolamide, 405
Acetylcysteine, 595
Acid-base imbalances, 413–424
  assessment of, 413–423
  diabetic ketoacidosis and, 430
  outcome evaluation in, 424
  planning and implementation of care in, 423–424
  signs and symptoms of, 417–418
  See also specific type

Acidemia, 414
Acidosis
  definition of, 414
  DIC and, 450
  hypothermia and, 443
  mixed, 417, 418t
  See also specific type
Acids, definition of, 413
Acquired immune deficiency syndrome (AIDS), 454–459
  assessment in, 454–456
  current investigational areas in, 458
  nursing diagnoses and, 456
  outcome evaluation in, 458
  pathophysiology of, 454–455
  planning and implementation of care in, 456–458
  prevention of transmission, 459
  risk factors in, 455
  signs and symptoms of, 455–456
Actin, 323
Action potential, cardiac, 264, 265f, 268–269
Activity, 496–516
  assessment of, 497–498
    format for, 497t
  energy cost of, 509t
  outcome evaluation in, 514–516
  planning and implementation of care in, 498–514
  restricted, minimizing complications of, 503–508
  total parenteral nutrition and, 490

Activity intolerance
  accepted nursing diagnosis, 498
  acute myocardial infarction and, 313, 316t
  burns and, 566
  hepatitis and, 477
  renal failure and, 381
  status asthmaticus and, 182
Acute Physiology and Chronic Health Evaluation (APACHE), 18
Adaptation to crisis, stages of, 37, 41–43
Adenosine triphosphate, 323, 334–335
ADH. *See* Antidiuretic hormone
Adrenal corticosteroids
  for cerebral edema, 88
  pharmacology of, 595–597
Adrenocorticotropic hormone, eosinophil count and, 447
Adult hyaline membrane disease, 163
Adult respiratory distress syndrome (ARDS), 163–166
  assessment of, 163–165
  etiologies of, 163t
  nursing care plan for, 167–168t
  nursing diagnoses and, 165
  outcome evaluation in, 166
  pathophysiology of, 163–164f
  planning and implementation of care in, 165–166
  risk factors in, 163
  septic shock and, 336
  signs and symptoms of, 164–165
Aeration, restricted activity and, 501–502

Aeration assessment, 135–159
  bedside pulmonary function tests in 142–146
  blood gas values in, 146–154
  diagnostic procedures in 154–159
  format for, 136t
  history and physical examination in, 136–142
Aeration disorders. *See specific disorders*
Aeration treatment techniques, 185–211
  artificial airways, 192–197
  chest drainage, 207–210
  chest physiotherapy, 189–192
  mechanical ventilation, 201–207
  oxygen therapy, 186–189
  tracheal suctioning, 197–200
  thoracic surgery, 210–211
Afferent arteriole, 370, 372
After-fall, hypothermia and, 439
Afterload, 323, 362
  cardiac failure and, 328
  cardiac failure risk and, 324
  cardiac output and, 256
  central venous pressure and, 251
AIDS. *See* Acquired immune deficiency syndrome
AIDS-related complex (ARC), 455
Air bronchogram sign, 155
Air emboli
  causes of, 174
  preventive measures for, 175
  pulmonary artery catheterization and, 257
  signs and symptoms of, 175
Airway, artificial. *See* Artificial airways
Airway clearance, ineffective acute respiratory failure and, 178
  ARDS and, 166
  myasthenia gravis and, 111
  status asthmaticus and, 180, 181f
  status epilepticus and, 95
  trauma and, 528–529
Airway damage, to and from artificial airway, 195–196
Airway obstruction
  artificial airways and, 195, 196–197
  drug treatment for, benefits of, 181f
  Sengstaken-Blakemore intubation and, 472
Airway resistance
  ARDS and, 166
  measurement of, 145
Alanine, malnutrition and, 485
Albuterol, 597
Alcoholism, REM rebound and, 512
Aldosterone
  sodium concentration and, 401
  sodium reabsorption and, 374
  water output control and, 397
Alkalemia, 414
Alkalosis
  definition of, 414
  mixed, 417, 418t
  See also specific type
Allergic reactions, eosinophil count and, 447
Allergy, total parenteral nutrition and, 490
Alpha receptors, 329

Alprazolam, 599–600
Alupent, 608
Alveolar-arterial gradient, 153
Alveolar ventilation, calculation of, 146
Amicar, 597–598
Aminocaproic acid, 597–598
Aminophyl. *See* Aminophylline
Aminophylline
  pharmacology of, 598
  status asthmaticus and, 182
  upper GI bleeding and, 471
Amiodarone, 302, 599
Ammonia buffer system, 414, 415f
Amphotericin B, 456
Amputations, 555
Amrinone, for cardiac failure, 330
Analgesics, for PTCA 357t
Anaphylactic shock, 334
Anatomic shunt, 153, 154
Anemia
  acute renal failure and, 381
  burns and, 564
  See also specific type
Aneurysm, cerebral, 98–99, 102t
Angina pectoris
  chest pain profile in, 305t
  pre-infarction, IABP and, 362
Angiography, 100, 158, 246
Angioplasty. *See* Percutaneous transluminal coronary angioplasty
Angiotensin, arteriolar
  vasoconstriction and, 225
Angiotensin II, formation and effects of, 372–373
Angle of Louis, 227
Anion gap, 422–423
Anions, definition of, 398
Ankylosis, chest drainage and, 209–210
Ansamycin, 458
Antacids, for upper GI bleeding, 471
Anterior cord syndrome, 540
Antianginal agents, 601
Antiasthmatic agents
  pharmacology of, 602–603
  for status asthmaticus, 182t
Antibiotics, for pneumothorax, 171
Anticoagulant agents
  pharmacology of, 605, 615
  for upper GI bleeding, 471
Anticonvulsants, 605–606
Antidiuretic hormone (ADH)
  sodium concentration and, 397, 401
  tubular reabsorption and, 373
  water output control and, 397
Antidysrhythmic (antiarrhythmic) agents, 604, 605
Antiemetic agents, for pneumothorax, 171
Antigen/antibody reactions, DIC and, 450
Antihistamines, neutrophil count and, 447
Antihypertensive agents, 603
Antishock garment, 340, 343, 531f, 554
Antithrombin-heparin cofactor, blood coagulation and, 449
Anus, physical examination of, 465

Anxiety
  acute myocardial infarction and, 313,
  AIDS and, 456, 458
  ARDS and, 166
  pulmonary edema and, 162
  upper GI bleeding and, 470, 471
Aorta
  function of, 229
  IAB catheter in, 363f
Aortic aneurysm
  dissecting, chest pain profile in, 306t
  sudden death and, 346
Aortic area, location of, 229–230
Aortic pressure, normal, 249
Aortic valve, location of, 229
Aortography, 246
Aphasia, 35, 39
Aplastic anemia, neutrophil count and, 447
Apnea, status epilepticus and, 95
Apneustic breathing, 73
Apneustic center, inspiration and, 139
Apprehension, artificial airways and, 194
Arachnoid, 56
Aramine, 608–609
Aristocort. *See* Adrenal corticosteroids
Arterial blood gases, 418–421 in shock, 339t
Arterial lines, blood pressure monitoring and, 257–258
Arterial pressures
  mean
    determination of, 222
    regulation of, 225–226
  normal tracing of, 257f
Arterial pressure waveform, balloon pressure waveform and, 364f
Arterial pulses
  abnormal, 221f
  peripheral, evaluation of, 220
Arterial-steal syndrome, hemodialysis and, 385
Arteriography, 76–77, 247
  upper gastrointestinal hemorrhage and, 471
Arterioles, control of, 224
Artificial airways, 192–197
  complications of
    prevention of, 194–196
    treatment of, 196–197
  outcome evaluation in, 197
  removal of, 197
  types of, 192, 193t, 194
Ascites, 480–481
Aspirin, for PTCA, 357t
Assessment
  communication and, 32–38
  critical-care assessment guide, 579–584t
  in nursing process, 6–8
Assessment guides, critical care, 579–584t
Asthma. *See* Status asthmaticus
Asystole, management of 347t
Ataxic breathing, 73–74
Atelectasis, 166–169
  assessment of, 168–169
  mechanical ventilation and, 205

nursing diagnoses and, 169
outcome evaluation in, 169
oxygen therapy and, 188
planning and implementation of care in, 169
restricted activity and, 501, 502
risk conditions in, 168–169
signs and symptoms of, 169
tracheal deviation and, 140
Atenolol, 600–601
Atherosclerosis
bruits and, 222
coronary, sudden death and, 346
Ativan, 599–600
ATP, 323, 334–335
Atria, location of, 228–229
Atrial depolarization, P wave and, 268
Atrial fibrillation, ECG tracing of, 282t
Atrial flutter, ECG tracing of, 281t
Atrial gallop, 234
Atrial premature beat, ECG tracing of, 296–297t
Atrial rhythms, ECG tracings of, 281–282t
Atrial tachycardia with block, ECG tracing of, 281t
Atrioventricular blocks, 276
ECG tracings of, 287–289t
Atrioventricular dissociation, 276–292
Atropine
actions of, 348
for cardiac arrest, 347t, 348
Attention, assessment of, 56
Auditory input, communication and, 34
Auscultation
aeration assessment and, 141–142
heart examination and, 230–236
See also Blood pressure auscultation
Auscultation sites, 230f
mnemonics for, 231ft
Auscultatory gap, 222
Autocontamination, 565
Autografts, for burns, 567
Autoimmune disorders, 102–114
Guillain-Barré syndrome, 103–107
myasthenia gravis, 108–114
Automaticity, 267
Automobile accidents, force in, 523, 526t
Autonomic dysreflexia, 543, 544f
Autonomic nervous system, 71f
assessment of, 70–72
kidney autoregulation and, 373
Autonomy principle, 20, 21, 25–26
Autoregulation
kidney and, 371–372
pressure, 82
AV fistula, 385, 386f
AV graft, 385
AV shunt
hemodialysis and, 384–385
standard, 384f
straight, 384f
Azidothymidine (AZT), 458

Babinski sign, 67, 69f
Bacteremia, 565

Balloon rupture, pulmonary artery catheterization and, 257
Barbiturate coma, for cerebral edema, 89
Barometric pressure, definition of, 149
Baroreceptor reflexes, mean arterial pressure regulation and, 225
Baroreceptors, water output control and, 397
Basal ganglia, 52, 69
Basal skull facture, 534, 535
Bases, definition of, 413
Basophils, 447
Battle's sign, 535
Beclomethasone, 595–596
Beclovent, 595–596
Beneficence principle, 20, 26
Benzodiazepines, 599–600
Berry aneurysm, 98
Beta-adrenergic blocking agents
pharmacology of, 600–601
thyroid crisis and, 436
Betadine, for burns, 566t
Betamethasone, 596–597
Beta receptors, 329
Bicarbonate, reabsorption and creation of, renal mechanisms for, 415f
Biliary cirrhosis, 478
Bismuth tribromphenate, for burns, 566t
Blindness, communication and, 32
Blocadren, 600–601
Blood chemistries, in shock, 338–339t
Blood coagulation, 448–449
calcium and, 408
process of, 448f
Blood constituents, 447f
Blood flow, physics of, 222–224
Blood gas values, 146–154
mixed venous, 152–153
Blood pressure. See Arterial pressures
Blood pressure auscultation, 220–226
abnormal findings in, 222
interpretation of, 222–226
technique of, 220–222
Blood pressure changes, assessment of, 72
Blood products, commonly used, 452–453t
Blood supply, to brain, 57
Blood transfusions, upper gastrointestinal hemorrhage and, 471
Blood urea nitrogen (BUN)
in acute renal failure, 377
renal function and, 375
Blood vessel expansion, 358f
Blunt trauma, 520, 523, 545
Body fluids
compartments of, 396–397
intake and output of, 397–398
osmolality of, 398
requirements with trauma, 531t
Bone disease, acute renal failure and, 382
Botterel scale, for grading ruptured cerebral aneurysms, 99t
Bowel elimination
acute myocardial infarction and, 313, 316–317t
alterations in burns and, 564

peritoneal dialysis, 390
spinal cord injury and, 542
Bowel sounds, 462, 464
Bowman's capsule, 371
Bradycardia
cardiac failure risk and, 323
cardiac output and, 302
definition of, 275
hyperkalemia and, 407
Bradykinin, capillary permeability and, 335
Brain
blood supply to, 57
lateral view of, 54f
structures of, 52, 534f
functions of, 55t
Brainstem, 52
Brainstem depression, status epilepticus and, 95
Breathing pattern, ineffective acid-base imbalances and, 418, 423
chest trauma and, 548
chronic respiratory failure and, 179
hyperglycemic hyperosmolar nonketotic coma and, 433
pneumothorax and, 172
spinal cord injury and, 542
status epilepticus and, 94
trauma and, 529
Breath sounds, aeration assessment and, 141–142
Brethine, 614–615
Bretylium
actions of, 348
for cardiac arrest, 347t, 348–349
for ventricular tachycardia, 302
Brevibloc, 600–601
Bricanyl, 614–615
Bronchitis, 177–179
assessment of, 177–178
nursing diagnoses and, 178
outcome evaluation in, 179
planning and implementation of care in, 178–179
pneumothorax and, 171
risk factors in, 177–178
signs and symptoms in, 178
Bronchodilators
pharmacology of, 597, 598, 606–607, 608
for pneumothorax risk reduction, 171
for status asthmaticus, 182t
Bronchopneumonia, burns and, 565
Bronchoscopy, 157–158
Bronchospasm, status asthmaticus and, 180–181
Bronkometer, 606–607
Bronkosol, 606–607
Brown-Séquard syndrome, 540
Bruits, 222, 464
Bumetanide, 607
Bumex, 607
BUN. See Blood urea nitrogen Bundle branch blocks, 276, 289–290t, 291–292
Burkitt's lymphoma, 454

Burns, 557–569
  assessment of, 557–560
  classification of, 558t
  Lund and Browder chart for, 560f
  nursing diagnoses and, 560–561
  outcome evaluation in, 569
  planning and implementation of care in,
      561–568
  rule of nines and, 559f
  signs and symptoms of, 558–560
  topical preparations for, 566t
  types of dressings for, 567t
Burn shock, 562–563
Burr hole, 118

Calan, 349, 601
Calcium, roles of, 408–409
Calcium channel blockers, 601
Calcium chloride
  actions of, 348
  for cardiac arrest, 347t, 348
  for hyperkalemia, 407
  for hypocalcemia, 410
  pharmacology of, 601–602
Calcium imbalances, 408–411, 409t
Calcium ion imbalance, 422
Calcium stones, precipitation of restricted
      activity and, 500
Calipers, 273, 275f
Calories, total parenteral nutrition and, 487
Candida albicans, wound infections and,
      565
CAPD, 388
Capillary beds, local blood flow control and,
      224
Capillary dynamics
  altered, cardiovascular system assessment
      and, 219–220
  edema formation and, 219–220
Capillary permeability, bradykinin and, 335
Capillary shunt, 153, 154
Captopril, 330
Capture beat, 276
Carbonic acid/bicarbonate buffer system,
      414
Cardiac arrest, drugs used in, 346–349,
      347t
Cardiac blood pool imaging, 243
Cardiac catheterization, 244–247
  complications of, 247
  data recorded in, 246–247
  patient preparation for, 244–246
  procedures of, 246
  ventricular tachycardia and, 302
Cardiac conduction defects
  diagnosis of, 276–292
  See also specific defect
Cardiac conduction system,
      266–268, 266f
  re-entry mechanism and, 267f
Cardiac cycle
  auscultation of, 230–231
  hemodynamics of, 232f
Cardiac depolarization
  normal patterns of, 272f

related vectors and, 270–273
  sequence of, 271f
Cardiac disturbances, and trauma, 538
Cardiac failure, 322–331
  assessment of, 323–325
  chest trauma and, 546
  nursing diagnoses and, 325
  outcome evaluation in, 331
  planning and implementation of care in,
      325–331
  risk conditions in, 323–324
  signs and symptoms of, 324–325
Cardiac index, 256
Cardiac interventions, 340–366
  cardiopulmonary bypass, 359–361
  emergency cardiac drug therapy, 346–350
  intra-aortic balloon counterpulsation,
      361–366
  outcome evaluation, 365–366
  pacemakers, 350–356
  percutaneous transluminal coronary angio-
      plasty, 356–359
Cardiac output, 322
  calculation of, 346
  determinations, 256
  measurement of, 256
  normal, 256
Cardiac output decrease
  activity intolerance and, 498–500
  acute chest pain and, 307
  acute myocardial infarction and, 313, 316t
  burns and, 562–563
  cardiac failure and 322–323
  cardiac tamponade, 332
  continuous ultrafiltration and, 392
  dysrhythmias and, 302
  hemodialysis, 387
  mechanical ventilation and, 205
  pneumothorax and, 172, 173
  pulmonary embolus and, 175, 176–177
  status asthmaticus, 183
  status epilepticus and, 95–96
  thyroid crisis and, 436–437
  trauma and, 529–530
Cardiac pressures
  measurement of, 247–249
  normal, 248f
Cardiac reserve, restricted activity and, 499
Cardiac shunts. See specific type
Cardiac structures, 227–230
  blood flow in, 229f
  position of, 228f
Cardiac sympathectomy, ventricular tachy-
      cardia and, 302
Cardiac tamponade
  acute, 331–333
    nursing diagnosis and, 332
    outcome evaluation in, 333
    planning and implementation of care in,
      332–333
    risk conditions in, 331–332
    signs and symptoms of, 332
  central venous pressure and, 251
  chest trauma and, 547t
  etiologies of, 332

pulmonary artery pressures and, 254
  pulsus paradoxus and, 222, 332
  trauma and, 529–530
Cardiac trauma, cardiac tamponade and, 331
Cardiac valves, functions of, 229
Cardilate, 610–611
Cardiogenic shock
  acute renal failure and, 376
  causes of, 333
  post-infarction, IABP and, 362
  signs and symptoms of, 337
Cardiomyopathy, cardiac failure risk and,
      324
Cardiopulmonary bypass, 359–361
  postoperative implications of, 360–361
  principles of, 359–360
Cardioquin, 612–613
Cardiovascular diagnostic procedures,
      237–258
  diagnostic procedures, 239–247
  hemodynamic monitoring, 247–258
  laboratory tests, 238–239
  See also specific procedure
Cardiovascular physical assessment,
      215–236
  blood pressure auscultation in, 220–226
  format for, 216–217t
  general inspection in, 218–219
  heart examination in, 227–236
  history in, 216–218
  neck vein examination in, 226–227
  peripheral arterial pulse evaluation in, 220
  PQRST mnemonic for, 218t
  skin examination in, 219–220
Cardioversion, 349–350
Cardizem, 601
Carotid endarterectomy, 100
Carpal spasm, 410
Catecholamine stimulation, dysrhythmias
      and, 301
Catheter emboli
  causes of, 174
  preventive measures for, 175
Catheter fling, 255
Cation exchange resins, for hyperkalemia,
      407
Cations, definition of, 398
CBC, 446–447
Cellular hypoxia, energy availability and,
      335
Central cord syndrome, 539–540
Central cyanosis, respiratory distress and,
      140
Central nervous system ischemic response,
      mean arterial pressure regulation and,
      225
Central neurogenic pulmonary edema,
      537–538
Central venous nutrition, 486
Central venous pressure
  measurement of, 249
  monitoring with transducer, 250f
Central venous pressure lines, 249–252
  insertion of, 249–250
  measurements with, 250–251

Cerebellar peduncles, 52
Cerebellum, 52, 69
Cerebral aneurysm, 98–99, 102t
Cerebral arteries, areas of distribution of, 58f
Cerebral arteriography, 76–77
Cerebral cortex, subdivisions of, 52
Cerebral dysfunction, motor responses to noxious stimulation in, 68f
Cerebral edema, 536
Cerebral metabolism, hypothermia and, 441
Cerebral perfusion pressure (CPP), 82
Cerebral tracts, 52
Cerebrospinal fluid, 57
    leaks, 57
    sampling of, 74–75
Cerebrospinal fluid drainage, for cerebral edema, 88–89
Cerebrum, 52
Chemical buffers, 413
Chemical imbalance, acute pancreatitis and, 475
Chemoreceptor reflexes, mean arterial pressure regulation and, 225
Chest drainage, 207–210
    chest tube removal and, 210
    complication prevention and, 209–210
    maintenance of, 208–209
    outcome evaluation in, 210
    Pleurevac system of, 208f
    techniques of, 207–208
Chest expansion, 139–140
Chest landmarks, external, 227–230
Chest pain
    acute, 305–307
        nursing diagnoses and, 307
        profiles of, 305–307t
    cardiovascular assessment and, 216
    pneumothorax and, 172
    precordial, cardiac tamponade and, 332
    pulmonary embolus and, 176
    thromboembolism and, 175
    ventricular fibrillation and, 346
Chest percussion, 189, 191f
Chest physiotherapy, 189–192
    chest percussion and, 189, 191f
    outcome evaluation in, 191
    postural drainage positions and, 190f
    techniques of, 189–191
Chest roentgenology, 240
    See also Chest X-ray
Chest trauma, 545–549
    assessment of, 546–548
    blunt, 545
    diagnostic studies and, 548t
    nursing diagnoses and, 546
    outcome evaluation in, 549
    penetrating, 545
    planning and implementation of care in, 548–549
    pneumothorax and, 171
    signs and symptoms of, 546t, 547t
Chest X-ray, 154–157, 156f
    abnormal signs in, 155–157
    normal characteristics of, 155

Cheyne-Stokes respiration, 73, 90, 537
CHF. See Congestive heart failure
Chloral hydrate, for sleep disturbances, 512
Chlordiazepoxide, 599–600
Chloride ion imbalance, 422
Chlorpromazine, for shivering, 441
Cholinergic agents, 604–605
Chronic obstructive pulmonary disease (COPD), 161
    breathing patterns in, 138–139
    central venous pressure and, 251
    sexual dysfunction and, 513–514
Chronic respiratory failure, 177–183
    bronchitis, 177–179
    emphysema, 177–179
    status asthmaticus, 179–183
Chvostek's sign, positive, 410
Cimetidine
    pharmacology of, 602
    stress ulcers and, 538
    upper gastrointestinal hemorrhage and, 471
CinQuin, 612–613
Circulation
    factors affecting, 223f
    humoral control of, 225
    local, intrinsic control of, 224
    nervous control of, 224–225
Cirrhosis, 478–479
Cisternal puncture, 75
Cisterna magna, 57
Clicks, 234
Closed fracture, 553
Clotting time, 449
Clubbing, respiratory distress and, 140
Cluster breathing, 73
Collapse, lung, 155–157
Colloid osmotic pressure, definition of, 219
Coma
    barbiturate, 89
    definition of, 55
    Glasgow coma scale and, 55–56
    hyperglycemic hyperosmolar non-ketotic, 431–433
    pupils during, 61
Comminuted fracture, 534, 553f
Communication, 31–47
    assessment of, 32–38
        format for, 33t
        content of, 35–38
        nursing diagnoses and, 37, 38t
        outcome evaluation in, 47
    planning and implementation of care and, 38–47
    restricted activity and, 502–503
Compartment syndrome, 556
Complete blood count, 446–447
Compliance, measurement of, 145–146
Compound fracture, 534, 553
Computerized tomography, 75–76, 243, 550
Concentration, mental, assessment of, 56
Concentration, solution, definition of, 398
Concussion, 535
Confusion, definition of, 55
Congestive atelectasis, 163

Congestive heart failure
    fluid volume excess and, 500
    nursing care plan for, 326–328
    nursing diagnoses and, 325
    shortness of breath and, 216, 218
Conjugate eye movement, 60
Consciousness
    assessment of level of, 52–56
    reticular activating system and, 54
Consciousness, altered level of acid-base imbalances and, 417–418, 423
    burns and, 564
    diabetic ketoacidosis and, 430
    DIC and, 454
    hemodialysis and, 387
    hyperglycemic hyperosmolar non-ketotic coma and, 433
    hypoglycemia and, 435
    hypothermia and, 438, 441
    peritoneal dialysis and, 390
    upper GI bleeding and, 470
Consensual light reflex, 60
Consolidation, chest X-ray and, 157
Continuous ambulatory peritoneal dialysis, 388
Contusion, 535
Coping, ineffective
    acute myocardial infarction and, 313, 317t
    burns and, 568
    family, 43–47, 107
    Guillain-Barré syndrome and, 107
    individual, 39–43, 113
    myasthenia gravis and, 113
    trauma and, 532–533
Cordarone, 599
Corgard, 600–601
Corneal reflex, cranial nerve assessment and, 61
Coronary arteriography, 246–247
Coronary artery perfusion time
    decreased, myocardial ischemia/infarction and, 324
Coronary artery thrombosis, acute myocardial infarction and, 308
Coronary blood supply, 309
Coronary blood vessels, 310f
Coronary cardiogenic shock, 333
Corticosteroids, for cerebral edema, 88
Corticotropin, 596–597
Cortisone, 596–597
Coumadin. See Warfarin
Coumarin therapy, prothrombin time and, 449
Coup-countrecoup phenomenon, 533
CPK. See Creatinine phosphokinase
Cranial nerves, 59f
    assessment of, 57–62
    screening test for function of, 57t
Craniectomy, 118
Craniotomy, 100, 118–121
Creatinine
    in acute renal failure, 377
    renal function and, 375
Creatinine clearance, determination of, 375–376

Creatinine phosphokinase, evaluation in cardiac disease, 238–239
Crepitus, 141
Crisis
  ineffective family coping and, 43–47
  ineffective individual coping and, 39–43
  stages of adaptation to, 37
Critical-care environment, 5t
Critical-care nursing
  assessment guide in, 579–584t
  changes in, 17–19
  core concepts and skills in, 13, 573–575t
  ethics in, 20–22, 25–26
  legal issues in, 22–25
  satisfactions of, 17
  scope of practice of, 5t
  stresses of, 17–19
  technological advances and, 17
Critical-care planning and implementation, 11–13
Cromolyn sodium, 602–603
Crush injuries, 555
Crush syndrome, acute renal failure and, 376
Crystalloid solutions, parenteral fluid replacement with, 342t
Crystodigin. See Digitalis glycosides
Cullen's sign, 474
Cutaneous anergy, 456
CVP. See Central venous pressure
Cyanosis, respiratory distress and, 140, 178
Cystine stones, precipitation of restricted activity and, 500
Cytotoxic edema, 536

Dalmane. See Flurazepam
Damping, 255
Deadspace, calculation of, 146
Debridement, for burns, 567
Decadron. See Dexamethasone
Decerebrate posturing, 66
Decorticate posturing, 66
Decortication, 211
Deep partial-thickness burns, 558
Defibrillation, 349
Delirium, definition of, 55
Deontological ethical method, 21
Depressant drugs, cardiac failure risk and, 324
Depressed fracture, 534
Dermatomes, 64f
Dermis, structure of, 557, 558f
Dexamethasone
  for cerebral edema, 88
  pharmacology of, 595–596
  thyroid crisis and, 437
Diabetes insipidus, 538
Diabetes mellitus
  glycosuria in, 375
  sudden cardiac death and, 346
Diabetic ketoacidosis, 427–431
  assessment of, 427–428
  ketonuria in, 375
  nursing diagnoses and, 428
  outcome evaluation in, 430–431

  pathophysiology of, 427
  planning and implementation of care in, 428–430
  risk factors in, 427
  signs and symptoms of, 428
Diagnosis. See Nursing diagnoses
Dialysis, 382–392
  for hyperkalemia, 407
  See also Hemodialysis; Peritoneal dialysis
Dialysis disequilibrium syndrome, 387
Dialyzers, 383
Diaphoresis, status asthmaticus and, 180
Diastolic augmentation, 362
Diastolic murmurs, 235
Diazepam
  pharmacology of, 599–600
  for sleep disturbances, 512
  for status epilepticus, 96
  for upper GI bleeding, 471
Diazoxide, 603
DIC. See Disseminated intravascular coagulation
Dideooxycytidine, 458
Diencephalon, 52
Diffusion
  definition of, 219
  tubular reabsorption and, 373
Diffusion coefficient, gas exchange in lungs and, 150
Digitalis glysosides
  for cardiac failure, 329
  pharmacology of, 603–604
Digitalis toxicity
  hypercalcemia and, 410
  hypokalemia and, 404
Digitoxin. See Digitalis glycosides
Digoxin. See Digitalis glycosides
Dihycon. See Phenytoin
Dilantin. See Phenytoin
Diltiazem, 601
Dilutional hyponatremia, 401
Dipridamole, for PTCA, 357t
Disopyramide, 604
Dislocations, 553
Disseminated intravascular coagulation (DIC), 450–454
  assessment of, 450–451
  nursing diagnoses and, 451
  outcome evaluation in, 454
  planning and implementation of care in, 451–454
  risk conditions in, 450–451
  septic shock and, 336
  shock and, 450
  signs and symptoms of, 451
Distributive shock, causes of, 333–334
Diuretics
  for ARDS, 165
  for hyperkalemia, 407
  pharmacology of, 607
  for renal failure in shock, 343
Dobutamine, for cardiac failure, 329–330
Dobutrex, 329–330
Doll's eyes phenomenon, 61, 62f

Dopamine
  for cardiac failure, 329, 330, 331
  for shock, 343
Dopaminergic receptors, 329
Doppler ultrasonography, arterial flow evaluation and, 241–242
Drift, hypothermia and, 439
Drug absorption, hypothermia and, 442
Drug therapy
  for cardiac failure, 328–331
  as cardiovascular intervention, 346–349, 347t
Dura mater, 56
Dysarthria, 101
Dysconjugate eye movement, 60
Dysphasia, 101
Dyspnea, pneumothorax and, 172
Dysrhythmias, 260–303
  assessment of, 294–295
  cardiac output and, 302
  diagnosis of, 260–294
  hypothermia and, 441–442
  intervention, 302–303
  outcome evaluation in, 303
  prevention of, 301–302
  risk conditions and, 295, 301
  See also specific type

Echocardiography, 240–241, 241f
Ectopic beats, 292
  hypokalemia and, 404
  premature beats, 292–294
    ECG, tracings of, 296–299t
Ectopy, ventricular aberration vs., 294f
Edecrin, 607
Edema, mechanisms causing, 219–220
Edrophonium chloride, 604–605
Efferent arteriole, 372
Egophony, 142
Einthoven's triangle, 260, 260f
Elase, 566t
Electrocardiogram artifacts, 263f
Electrocardiographic patterns, causes of, 301t
Electrocardiograph tracing
  of accidental hypothermia, 442f
  balloon pressure waveform and, 364f
  potassium levels and, 406f
Electrocardiography, 260–275
  acute myocardial infarction and, 309–311
  analysis in, 264–275
  atrial rhythms and, 281–282t
  atrioventricular blocks and, 287–289t
  bedside monitoring and, 261–264
  bundle branch blocks and, 289–290t
  deflections in, 269f, 270f
    labeling, 268, 270f
  junctional rhythms and, 282–283t
  leads in, 260–261
    placement of, 260f, 261f, 263f
  membrane potentials and, 264–266
  noncompensatory vs. compensatory pauses and, 293f
  premature beats and, 296–299t
  problems in recording, 262–264

refractory periods and, 266
sinus rhythms and, 277–279t
supra ventricular rhythms and, 280t
12-lead technique of, 260–261
vectors in, 268–273
    depolarization and, 270–273, 271f, 272f
    interpretation of mean, 270
    plotting of, 269–270
    ventricular aberration vs. ectopy and, 294f
    ventricular rhythms and, 284–286t
Electrocautery, upper gastrointestinal hemorrhage and, 471
Electroencephalography, 75
Electrolyte imbalances, 421–423
    cardiac failure risk and, 324
    diabetic ketoacidosis and, 429
    dysrhythmias and, 295
    head trauma and, 538
    liver failure and, 479
    total parenteral nutrition and, 493
Electrolytes, 387, 398–399
    total parenteral nutrition and, 489
Electrophysiologic studies, 244
Embolization, hypothermia and, 442
Emphysema, 177–179
    assessment of, 177–178
    nursing diagnoses and, 178
    outcome evaluation in, 179
    planning and implementation of care in, 178–179
    pneumothorax and, 171
    risk factors in, 177–178
    signs and symptoms in, 178
Endocardial pacing, 351
Endocrine system, definition of, 426
Endotracheal tube, 192, 194
End-plate, 108
Energy production, cellular aerobic and anaerobic, 334f
Enteral feeding, 486
Enterobacter, septic shock and, 335
Eosinophils, 447
Epicardial pacing, 351
Epidermis, structure of, 557, 558f
Epidural hematoma, 535
Epileptic seizures. See Status epilepticus
Epinephrine
    actions of, 346
    blood vessel constriction/dilation and, 224–225
    for cardiac arrest, 346, 347t
    eosinophil count and, 447
    for ventricular fibrillation, 346
Equivalent weight, definition of, 398
Erb's point, 230
Erythrityl tetranitrate, 610–611
Erythrocytes, 446
Erythropoietin
    kidney disease and, 376
    red blood cell production and, 446
Escape beats, 292
Escape rhythms, hyperkalemia and, 407
Escherichia coli, septic shock and, 335
Esmolol, 600–601

Esophageal balloon, esophageal varices and, 472
Esophageal perforation, Sengstaken-Blakemore intubation and, 472
Esophageal varices, Sengstaken-Blakemore tube and, 471–472, 472f
Ethacrynic acid, 607
Ethics, 20–22, 25–26
Ethotoin, 605–606
Exercise
    contraindications to, 506t
    energy cost of, 509t
Extrapyramidal system, assessment of, 69
Eye position and movement, cranial nerve assessment and, 57–62
Eye response, consciousness and, 56

Falls, force in, 523, 526t
Falx cerebri, 56, 89
Family
    ineffective coping related to crisis, 43–47, 107, 532–533, 568
    role of, 36
FANCAS, 4, 572
    core concepts and skills in, 573–575t
    nursing diagnosis classification and, 577t
Fascicular blocks, 291
Fat embolism
    causes of, 174
    orthopedic trauma and, 556–557
    signs and symptoms of, 170
Fatique, malnourishment and, 486
Fatty acid deficiency, total parenteral nutrition and, 493
Fear
    acute chest pain and, 307
    acute myocardial infarction and, 313, 314–315t
    AIDS and, 456, 458
    cardiac tamponade and, 332
    DIC and, 454
    renal failure and, 389
    sexual dysfunction and, 513–514
    status asthmaticus, 180, 183
    upper gastrointestinal hemorrhage and, 471
Fiberoptic bronchoscope, 157
Fiberoptic endoscopy, upper gastrointestinal hemorrhage and, 471
Fibrillation, definition of, 276
Fibrin, blood coagulation and, 448–449
Fibrin degradation products, 449
    DIC and, 450
Fibrinogen, blood coagulation and, 448
Fibrinogen level, 449
    DIC and, 450
Fibrinolysin and desoxyribonuclease, for burns, 566t
Fibrin split products, 449
    DIC and, 450
Fick method, cardiac output calculation and, 246
Filtration, definition of, 219
Flail chest, 139–140, 547t

Fluid and electrolyte imbalances
    assessment of, 396–399
        format for, 396t
    See also specific type
Fluid balance, restricted activity and, 498–501
Fluid exchange, mechanics of, 219
Fluid imbalances, 399–401
    outcome evaluation in, 400–401
    serial body weight monitoring in, 396–397
Fluid overload
    cardiac failure risk and, 324
    CVP line insertion and, 252
    pulmonary artery pressures and, 254
    total parenteral nutrition and, 492
Fluid resuscitation formulas, 563t
Fluid volume deficit, 399t
    abdominal trauma and, 551
    acute cardiac failure and, 324
    acute pancreatitis and, 474
    AIDS and, 456
    chest trauma and, 548
    continuous ultrafiltration and, 391–392
    diabetic ketoacidosis and, 428–429
    DIC and, 451
    hemodialysis and, 387
    hyperglycemic hyperosmolar nonketotic coma and, 432
    liver failure and, 480
    malnutrition and, 486
    nursing diagnoses and, 399
    renal failure and, 382
    renal transplantation and, 392
    signs and symptoms of, 399–400
    status asthmaticus and, 182
    thyroid crisis and, 436
    trauma and, 530
    treatment of, 400
    upper gastrointestinal hemorrhage and, 466, 471
    See also Hypovolemia
Fluid volume excess, 400t
    DIC and, 453
    hemodialysis and, 387
    nursing diagnoses and, 400
    peritoneal dialysis and, 389
    renal failure and, 380
    signs and symptoms of, 400
    treatment for, 400
Flurazepam
    pharmacology of, 599–600
    for sleep disturbances, 512
Flutter, definition of, 276
Foramen magnum, 56
Fractures
    bone, 553, 553f
    pelvic, 556
    skull, 534–535
Frank-Starling mechanism, 256, 322
Friction rubs, 464
Full-thickness burns, 558–559
Functional residual capacity, measurement of, 144
Furosemide
    for ARDS, 165

pharmacology of, 607
for renal failure in shock, 343
Fusion beat, ECG tracing of, 299t

Gallop rhythms, 232, 234
Gardner-Wells tongs, 540f
Gas exchange, impaired
  acid-base imbalances and, 418
  acute myocardial infarction and, 313, 316t
  AIDS and, 456
  ARDS and, 165–166
  atelectasis and, 169
  burns and, 561–562, 565
  cardiac failure and, 325
  chest trauma and, 548
  chronic respiratory failure and, 179
  diabetic ketoacidosis and, 430
  DIC and, 454
  hypothermia and, 438, 441
  liver failure and, 482
  peritoneal dialysis and, 390
  plural effusion and, 173
  pulmonary edema and, 162
  pulmonary embolus and, 176
  status asthmaticus and, 180
  status epilepticus and, 95
  thyroid crisis and, 437
  trauma and, 529
  upper gastrointestinal hemorrhage and, 469
Gastric balloon, esophageal varices and, 472
Gastric hemorrhage, burns and, 564
Gastrointestinal hemorrhage. See Upper gastrointestinal hemorrhage
Gastrointestinal system, assessment of, 462–465
  format for, 463t
Gated cardiac blood pool imaging, 243
GFR. See Glomerular filtration rate
Glasgow coma scale, 55–56
Glomerular filtration, 371
Glomerular filtration rate, autoregulation of, 371–372
Glomerulonephritis, acute renal failure and, 376
Glomerulus, 370
Gluceptate, for hypocalcemia, 410
Glucocorticoids, thyroid crisis and, 437
Gluconate, for hypocalcemia, 410
Gluconeogenesis, 485, 564
Glucose level, hypoglycemia and, 434–435
Glutamine, malnutrition and, 485
Glycogenolysis, 564
Glycolysis, 334
  malnutrition and, 485
Glycosuria, diabetes mellitus and, 375
Granulocytes, 446
Grey-Turner's sign, 474
Guillain-Barré syndrome, 103–107
  assessment of, 103–105
  diagnosis of, 104–105
  nursing diagnoses and, 105
  outcome evaluation in, 107
  planning and implementation of care in, 105–107

signs and symptoms of, 104
  variants of, 104t
Gunshot wounds, 524, 525f, 526t

Halcion, 599–600
Hare traction, 554
Head, examination of, 56–57
Head injury, 533–538
  assessment of, 533–536
  nursing diagnoses and, 536
  outcome evaluation in, 538
  planning and implementation of care in, 536–538
  types of, 534–536
Health potential, depleted
  atelectasis and, 169
  DIC and, 451–454
Hearing deficit, impaired verbal communication and, 38–39
Heart, ECG views of, 262f
Heart block, hyperkalemia and, 407
Heart disease, sudden cardiac death and, 346
Heart examination, 227–236
  auscultation and, 230–236
  external chest landmarks and, 227–230
  percussion and, 230
  precordial pulsation palpation and, 230
Heart murmurs
  auscultation of, 234–235
  characteristics of, 235t
Heart rate, cardiac output and, 222, 224
Heart sounds
  abnormal, 233t
  acute myocardial infarction and, 308
  auscultation of, 230–234
Hematemesis, 466
Hematochezia, 466
Hematocrit, normal, 446
Hematology, in shock, 338–339t
Hematomas, 535–536
Hemianopia, 32
Hemiblocks, 291–292
Hemodialysis, 382–392
  circulatory access in, 384–385
  dialyzers and dialysate solutions in, 383
  discontinuing, 388
  fistulas and grafts in, 385
  monitoring, 387–388
  peritoneal dialysis compared to, 383t
  preparation for, 385–387
  problems between sessions in, 388
Hemodynamic lines, uses of, 247
Hemodynamic monitoring, 247–258
  arterial lines and, 257–258
  cardiac cycle and pressure waves and, 247
  central venous pressure lines and, 249–252
  hemodynamic lines and, 247
  pressure measurements and, 247–249
  pulmonary arterial lines and, 252–257
Hemofiltration, 390–392, 390f
Hemoglobin, function of, 446
Hemorrhage
  AV shunts and, 385

thoracic surgery and, 211
  total parenteral nutrition and, 492
  upper GI, 465–473
Hemorrhagic shock, emergency measures for, 339
Hemostatic agents, 597–598
Henle's loop, 371
Heparin, 449
  for DIC, 451
  pharmacology of, 605
  for PTCA, 357
  for pulmonary embolus, 175
  for thromboembolism, 176
Heparinization, 386
Hepatitis, 475–478
  assessment of, 475–476
  characteristics of types of, 476t
  diagnosis of, 476–477
  guidelines for prophylaxis, 477–478
  lymphocyte count and, 447
  neutrophil count and, 447
  nursing diagnoses and, 477
  outcome evaluation in, 478
  planning and implementation of care in, 477
  risk conditions in, 475–476
  signs and symptoms of, 477
Hepatojugular reflux test, 227
Hering-Breuer reflex, inspiration and, 139
Herniation syndromes, 89–93
  assessment of, 89–93
  care planning and implementation in, 93
  nursing diagnoses and, 93
  outcome evaluation in, 93
  risk factors in, 89
  signs and symptoms of, 89–93, 90–91f, 92f
Heterografts, for burns, 567
Hexaxial reference system, 270, 271f
HIV. See Human immunodeficiency virus
Holosystolic murmurs, 234, 235
Homografts, for burns, 567
Human immunodeficiency virus (HIV), 454–455
  in current investigations, 458
  preventing transmission of, 459
Hyaline membranes, ARDS and, 163
Hydantoin anticonvulsants, 605–606
Hydrocephalus
  communicating, 99
  high-pressure, 121
  noncommunicating, 121
  normal-pressure, 121–122
Hydrocortisone, 596–597
Hydrometer, urine specific gravity and, 374
Hydrostatic pressure, definition of, 219
Hydrotherapy, for burns, 567
Hyperaldosteronism, fluid volume excess and, 400
Hyperalimentation, 486
Hypercalcemia, 410–411
  nursing diagnoses and, 411
  signs and symptoms of, 410
  treatment for, 411

Hypercapnia
  cerebral blood vessel dilation and, 86–87
  pulmonary artery pressures and, 254
Hyperglycemia
  diabetic ketoacidosis and, 427
  peritoneal dialysis and, 390
  total parenteral nutrition and, 491
Hyperglycemic hyperosomolar nonketotic
      coma, 431–433
  assessment of, 431–432
  nursing diagnoses and, 432
  outcome evaluation in, 433
  planning and implementation of care in,
      432–433
  risk factors in, 431
  signs and symptoms of, 431–432
Hyperkalemia, 407
  acute renal failure and, 381
  emergency treatment for, 408t
  nursing diagnoses and, 407
  signs and symptoms of, 407
  treatment for, 407
Hypermagnesemia, 411–412
  signs and symptoms of, 412
  treatment for, 412
Hypernatremia, 402–403, 403t
  nursing diagnoses and, 403
  signs and symptoms of, 403
  total parenteral nutrition and, 493
  treatment for, 403
Hyperosmolar hyperglycemic nonketotic
      state, 491–492
Hyperosmolarity, diabetic ketoacidosis and,
      427
Hyperpolarization, 404
Hyperstat, 603
Hypertension
  auscultatory gap and, 222
  sudden cardiac death and, 346
Hypertonic agents, for cerebral edema, 88
Hypertonicity, definition of, 398
Hypertrophic myocardiopathy, sudden death
      and, 346
Hyperventilation, for cerebral edema, 88,
      118
Hypocalcemia, 409–410
  liver failure and, 479
  nursing diagnoses and, 410
  signs and symptoms of, 410
  treatment for, 410
Hypodermis, structure of, 557, 558f
Hypoglycemia, 434–435
  assessment of, 434–435
  nursing diagnoses and, 434
  outcome evaluation in, 435
  total parenteral nutrition and, 492
Hypokalemia, 404–406
  acute renal failure and, 382
  liver failure and, 479
  nursing diagnoses and, 404
  signs and symptoms of, 404–405
  total parenteral nutrition and, 493
  treatment for, 405–406
Hypomagnesemia, 411–412
  liver failure and, 479

signs and symptoms of, 412
  treatment for, 412
Hyponatremia, 401–402, 402t
  nursing diagnoses and, 402
  signs and symptoms of, 402
  total parenteral nutrition and, 493
  treatment for, 402
Hypophosphatemia, total parenteral nutri-
      tion and, 493
Hypopolarization, 407
Hypotension
  DIC and, 450
  intracranial lesions and, 118
Hypothalamus, 52
Hypothermia
  ECG of, 442f
  intracranial lesions and, 119
  physiologic effects of, 438t
  signs and symptoms of, 438, 439t
  See also Therapeutic hypothermia
Hypotonicity, definition of, 398
Hypotonic solutions, parenteral fluid re-
      placement with, 342t
Hypoventilation
  oxygen therapy and, 188
  thoracic surgery and, 211
Hypovolemia, 399
  acute renal failure and, 376
  chest trauma and, 546
  pulmonary artery pressures and, 254
  See also Fluid volume deficit
Hypovolemic shock
  causes of, 333
  emergency measures for, 340
  pathophysiologic changes in, 334–335
  signs and symptoms of, 336–337
Hypoxemia
  cerebral blood vessel dilation and, 86–87
  chest trauma and, 546
  chronic respiratory failure and, 178
  pulmonary artery pressures and, 254
  status asthmaticus and, 182
  tracheal suctioning and, 199
Hypoxia
  pneumothorax and, 172
  thromboembolism and, 175

IABP. See Intra-aortic balloon counterpulsa-
      tion
Ice water calorics, 61, 62
Idiopathic thrombocytopenic purpura, plate-
      let count and, 447
Immobility, physiologic complications of,
      signs and symptoms of, 516t
Immunocompetent cells, 447
Incor, 330
Inderal, 600–601
Individual nursing care plan, 589–590t
Infection
  abdominal trauma and, 551–552
  acute pancreatitis and, 475
  acute renal failure and, 381
  AIDS and, 455, 456, 457
  artificial airways and, 195, 197
  atelectasis and, 169

AV shunts and, 385
  burns and, 565
  CVP line insertion and, 252
  DIC and, 450
  eosinophil count and, 447
  Guillain-Barré syndrome and, 106
  head injuries and, 538
  hepatitis and, 477
  IABP and, 365
  intracranial pressure monitoring and, 86
  liver failure and, 481–482
  lymphocyte count and, 447
  malnutrition and, 485–486
  mechanical ventilation and, 205
  neutrophil count and, 447
  renal transplantation and, 393
  spinal cord injury and, 490–491
  total parenteral nutrition and, 490–491
  trauma and, 532
  ventricular shunt and, 124, 125
Inflammation, lymphocyte count and, 447
Injury, potential for
  abdominal, 549–552
  in blunt trauma, 523
  body's response to, 522–523
  chest, 545–459
  head, 533–538
  hypothermia and, 438, 442
  mechanism of, 525
  orthopedic, 552–557
  in penetrating trauma, 524, 525f
  renal failure and, 378
  spinal cord, 531, 539–545
  status epilepticus and, 96
  See also Trauma
Inotropes
  for cardiac failure, 329–330, 331
  for shock, 341
Insight, assessment of, 56
Inspiratory area, 138
Inspiratory force, maximum, 145
Inspired gas, composition of, 149t
Insulin deficiency
  diabetic ketoacidosis and, 429
  hyperglycemia hyperosomolar nonketotic
      coma and, 432–433
Insulin-glucagon balance, malnutrition and,
      485
Intal, 602–603
Intercostal spaces, location of, 228f
Intermittent claudication, cardiovascular
      system assessment and, 218
Intermittent mandatory ventilation, 201–202
Internal capsule, 52
Intra-aortic balloon catheter, position in
      aorta, 363f
Intra-aortic balloon counterpulsation,
      361–366
  complications in, 364–365
  equipment in, 362
  indications for, 362
  insertion of, 362–363
  nursing care and, 363–364
  physiologic effects of, 362
  timing of, 363–364

weaning from, 364–365
Intra-aortic balloon waveform, 264f
Intracardiac shunts
  cardiac failure risk and, 323
  pulmonary artery pressures and, 254
Intracerebral hematoma, 536
Intracerebral hemorrhage, sudden death
  and, 346
Intracranial dynamics, 82
Intracranial lesions, treatment of,
  118–121
Intracranial pressure
  increased, 81–89
    assessment of, 81–86
    nursing diagnoses and, 86
    outcome evaluation in, 89
    planning and implementation of care in,
      86–89
    risk conditions in, 81
    signs and symptoms of, 82
  monitoring of, 82–86
    methods of, 83f
    set-up procedure for, 83–86
    subarachnoid screw and, 83, 84f
Intracranial pressure waves, 85f
Intracranial volume, 81
Intrarenal pressure theory, 371–372
Intrathoracic pressure, preventing increases
  in, 87–88
Intravenous pyelogram (IVP), 55
Intropin. See Dopamine
Involuntary motor activity, cranial nerve as-
  sessment and, 66–69
Iodide, thyroid crisis and, 437
Ions, definition of, 398
Ischemia, AV shunts and, 385
Isoetharine, 606–607
Isoproterenol
  actions of, 348
  for cardiac arrest, 348
  for shock, 343
Isoptin, 601
Isordil, 610–611
Isosorbide dinitrate, 610–611
Isuprel. See Isoproterenol

Judgment, assessment of, 56
Junctional escape rhythm, ECG tracing of,
  282t
Junctional premature beat, ECG tracing of,
  297–298t
Junctional rhythms, ECG tracings of,
  282–283t
Junctional tachycardia, ECG tracing of, 283t
Juxtaglomerular complex, 372
  structure of, 372f

Kaposi's sarcoma, 454
kayexalate. See Sodium polystyrene sulfo-
  nate Kehr's sign, 549
Keratin, 557
Kerley's B lines, 155
Ketoacidosis, 427–431
Ketonuria, diabetic ketoacidosis and, 375

Kidneys
  anatomy of, 369f, 370–371
  See also Renal assessment
Klebsiella, septic shock and, 335
Knife wounds, 524, 526t
Korotkoff sounds, cause of, 220–221
Krebs cycle, 335, 413
Kussmaul's sign, 227

Labetalol, 600–601
Laceration, 535
Lactic acidemia, cerebral blood vessel dila-
  tion and, 86
Laenec's cirrhosis, 478–479
Lanoxicaps. See Digitalis glycosides
Lasix. See Furosemide
Lateral decubitus film, 550
Lee-White test, 449
Left atrial pressure, 248
  normal, 249
Left-to-right cardiac shunts, central venous
  pressure and, 251
Left ventricular failure
  left ventricular compliance and, 248
  pulmonary artery pressures and, 255
  signs and symptoms of, 325
Left ventricular pressure, normal, 249
Legal issues, 22–25, 26–27
Leukemias, platelet count and, 447
Leukocytes, 446–447
Levarterenol, for upper GI bleeding, 471
Levophed. See Norepinephrine
Librium, 599–600
Lidocaine
  actions of, 348
  for cardiac arrest, 347t, 348
  for PTCA, 357t
  for ventricular tachycardia, 302
Linear fracture, 534
Lipolysis, malnutrition and, 485
Liver, palpation of, 464, 464f
Liver failure, 478–482
  assessment of, 478–479
  nursing diagnoses and, 480
  outcome evaluation in, 482
  planning and implementation of care in,
    480–482
  signs and symptoms of, 479
Liver functions, 478
Living wills, 22
Lixaminol. See Aminophylline
Lobectomy, 211
Loop diuretics, 607
Lopressor, 600–601
Lorazepam, 599–600
Lower airway injury, burns and, 561–562
Lumbar puncture, 75
Lund and Browder chart, burn evaluation
  and, 560f
Lung biopsy, 159
Lungs
  boundaries of, 137f
  examination of, 137–138
Lung scans, 157
Lung volumes and capacities, 142–145, 144f

Lymphocytes, 447
Lymphocytic leukemia, lymphocyte count
  and, 447

Macrophages, 447
Macula densa, 372
Mafenide acetate, for burns, 566t
Magnesium, roles of, 411
Magnesium imbalances, 411–413, 412t
  outcome evaluation in, 412–413
Magnetic resonance imaging (MRI), 77–79,
  243
Mallory-Weiss syndrome, 465
Malnutrition, 485–494
  nursing diagnoses and, 486
  outcome evaluation in, 494
  physiology of, 485–486
  planning and implementation of care in,
    486–493
Malpractice, definition of, 23
Mannitol
  for cerebral edema, 88
  pharmacology of, 607–608
  for renal failure in shock, 343
Massive hemothorax, chest trauma and,
  547t
Mechanical ventilation, 201–207
  complications of
    prevention of, 203–205
    treatment of, 205–206
  discontinuation of, 206–207
  outcome evaluation in, 207
  procedure for, 201–203
Mechanism of injury (MOI), 525
  with chest trauma, 545
  with head injury, 533–534
  with spinal cord injury, 539
Mediastinal shift, pneumothorax and, 172,
  173
Medical Anti-Shock Trousers, 340, 343,
  531f, 554
Medical diagnosis, nursing diagnosis vs.,
  9–10
Medications
  myasthenia gravis and, 111t
  nebulized, guide to, 182t
Medulla oblongata, 52
Melena, 466
Membrane potentials, electrocardiography
  and, 264–266
Memory, assessment of, 56
Meninges, 56–57
Meningitis, 81, 456
Mentation, assessment of, 56
Mephenytoin, 605–606
Mesantoin, 605–606
Mesh grafts, 568
Metabolic acidosis, 414, 416t
  acute myocardial infarction and, 308
  planning and implementation of care in,
    423
  shock and, 335–336
  total parenteral nutrition and, 492–493
Metabolic acids, definition of, 413

Metabolic alkalosis, 414, 417t
  planning and implementation of care in, 424
  septic shock and, 335
Metabolism, definition of, 426
Metaproterenol sulfate, 608
Metaraminol, 608–609
Metarterioles, control of, 224
Methimazole, thyroid crisis and, 437
Methylprednisolone
  for cerebral edema, 88
  pharmacology of, 596–597
Methylprednisolone succinate, 557
Metoprolol, 600–601
Midazolam, 599–600
Midbrain, 52
Minute ventilation, calculation of, 146
Mitral area, location of, 229, 230f
Mitral stenosis, central venous pressure and, 251
Mitral valve, location of, 229
Mitral valve disease, pulmonary artery pressures and, 254
Mitral valve prolapse, sudden death and, 346
Monocytes, 447
Morphine sulfate, 609–610
Motor activity
  reflex, 66–70
  voluntary, 66
Motor neuron lesions, 69, 70t
Motor response, consciousness and, 56
Motor tracts, left side, 67f
Mouth, physical examination of, 462
Mucolytic agents
  pharmacology of, 595
  for status asthmaticus, 182t
Mucomyst, 595
Multiple-gated acquisition scanning, 243
Mucous membrane, altered oral DIC and, 454
Murmurs. See Heart murmurs
Muscle contractility, calcium and, 408
Muscle metabolism, creatinine and, 375
Muscle weakening, restricted activity and, 503
Musculoskeletal disorders, 161
Myasthenia gravis, 108–114
  assessment of, 108–111
  classifications of, 110t
  diagnosis of, 110–111
  drugs and, 111t
  nursing diagnoses and, 111
  outcome evaluation in, 114
  planning and implementation of care in, 111–114
  risk factors in, 108
  signs and symptoms of, 108–110
Myocardial contractility, 323
  cardiac failure risk and, 323–324
Myocardial depressant factor, septic shock and, 335
Myocardial hypoxia, dysrhythmias and, 295
Myocardial infarction
  acute, 307–322

  assessment of, 308–314
  chest pain profile in, 306t
  diagnostic procedures in, 308–314
  nursing diagnoses in, 313
  risk conditions in, 308
  signs and symptoms of, 308
  causes of, 308–309
  coronary blood supply and, 309
  ECG indicators of, 309–311
  inpatient rehabilitation program, 507t
  left ventricular compliance and, 248
  location and evolution of, 311–313
  nursing care plan for, 314–322
  nursing diagnoses and, 313
  outcome evaluation in, 314
  serum enzymes and, 238f, 313–314
  sexual dysfunction and, 513
  SGOT levels and, 239
  shock and, 344
  shortness of breath and, 216, 218
  sudden death and, 346
  type of, 309
Myocardial infarction imaging, 242
Myocardial infarcts
  evolutionary changes in, 313f
  localization of, 312f
Myocardial ischemia
  cardiac failure risk and, 324
  ECG patterns of, 309, 311f
Myocardial perfusion imaging, 242–243
Myocardial revascularization, ventrilcular tachycardia and, 302
Myocarditis, cardiac failure risk and, 324
Myofibrils, 323
Myoglobinuria, 555
Myosin, 323

Nachlas-Linton tube, 472–473
Nadolol, 600–601
Naloxone, 610
Narcan, 610
Narcotic analgesics, 600–601
Nasopharyngeal airway, 192
Nebulized medications, guide to, 182t
Neck, examination of, 56–57
Neck vein examination, 226–227
Negligence, definition of, 23
Neoplasms
  DIC and, 450
  LDH elevations and, 239
Nephron, 370–371
  structures of, 371f
Neurogenic shock, signs and symptoms of, 337
Neurologic assessment, 74–79
  observation chart, 53t
Neurologic status, monitoring and assessing, 537
Neuromuscular blocking agents, 611–612
Neuromuscular transmission, schema of, 109f
Neurovascular compromise, 554
Neutrophils, 447
Nifedipine, 601
Nipride. See Sodium nitroprusside

Nitrates, 610–611
Nitro-Bid, 610–611
Nitrodisc, 610–611
Nitro-Dur, 610–611
Nitrogen, total parenteral nutrition and, 487
Nitroglycerin
  for cardiac failure, 330
  pharmacology of, 610–611
  for PTCA, 357t
  for shock, 343
Nitrol, 610–611
Nitroprusside, for cardiac failure, 330–331
Nitrospan, 610–611
Nitrostat, 610–611
Nocturnal cardiovascular disturbances, 511–512
Nodes of Ranvier, 103
Noncardiogenic pulmonary edema, 163
Noncoronary cardiogenic shock, 333
Nonmalefescence principle, 20
Norepinephrine
  for cardiac failure, 329
  pharmacology of, 611
  for shock, 343
  vasoconstriction and, 224
Normal-pressure hydrocephalus (NPH), 121–122
Normodyne, 600–601
Norpace, 604
Nuchal rigidity, 57
Nuclear magnetic resonance (NMR), 243
Nuclear scans, myocardial infarction and, 313–314
Nursing care plan, 576–590
  for acute renal failure, 379–380t
  for ARDS, 167–168t
  for congestive heart failure, 326–328
  for ruptured cerebral aneurysm, 102t
  standard care plan, 585–588t
  for uncomplicated myocardial infarction, 314–322
  for upper GI bleeding, 466–470
Nursing diagnoses, 8–11
  for abdominal trauma, 551
  for activity intolerance, 498
  for acute chest pain, 307
  for acute myocardial infarction, 313
  for acute pancreatitis, 474
  for acute renal failure, 378
  for adult respiratory distress syndrome, 165
  for AIDS, 456
  for atelectasis, 169
  benefits of, 9
  for bronchitis, 178
  for burns, 560–561
  for cardiac failure, 325
  for cardiac tamponade, 332
  for chest injuries, 546
  for communication, 37, 38t
  for craniotomy, 119
  critical care and, 8–9
  for diabetic ketoacidosis, 428
  for DIC, 451
  for dysrhythmia, 301

for emphysema, 178
FANCAS classification of, 577t
for fluid volume deficity, 399
for fluid volume excess, 400
for Guillain-Barré syndrome, 105
for head injuries, 536
for hepatitis, 477
for herniation syndromes, 93
historical background of, 8
for hypercalcemia, 411
for hyperglycemic hyperosmolar nonke-
    totic coma, 432
for hyperkalemia, 407
for hypernatremia, 403
for hypocalcemia, 410
for hypoglycemia, 434
for hypokalemia, 404
for hyponatremia, 402
for hypothermic patient, 438
for increased intracranial pressure, 86
for liver failure, 480
for malnutrition, 486
medical diagnosis vs., 9–10
for myasthenia gravis, 111
North American Nursing Diagnosis Asso-
    ciation and, 8, 10
for orthopedic trauma, 554
for pain, 128
for pleural effusion, 173
for pneumonia, 170
for pneumothorax, 172
process of, 10–11
for pulmonary edema, 162
for pulmonary embolus, 176
for shock, 339
for spinal cord injury, 541
for status asthmaticus, 180
for status epilepticus, 95
for stroke, 101
for thyroid crisis, 436
for trauma, 528
for upper GI hemorrhage, 466
for ventricular shunts, 125
Nursing model, 4
Nursing process, 4–13
    assessment in, 6–8
    diagnosis in, 8–11
    evaluation in, 13
    flow chart of, 7f
    planning and implementation in, 11–13
Nursing skills, 11–13
Nursing stress, 17–19
    mechanisms for reducing, 19–20
Nutrient demand theory, 224
Nutrient requirements, calculation of,
    488–489t
Nutrition, altered
    acute pancreatitis and, 474
    AIDS and, 456, 457
    burns and, 564–565
    hepatitis and, 477
    liver failure and, 481
    peritoneal dialysis and, 390
    renal failure and, 381
    shock and, 339, 343
    thyroid crisis and, 437

Nutrition, restricted activity and, 502
Nutritional assessment, 482–485
    format for, 483t
Nutritional supplementation, 486

Obstetric emergencies, DIC and, 450
Obstructive disorders, definition of, 161
Obstructive hydrocephalus, 81
Obstructive jaundice, prothrombin time and,
    449
Obtundation, definition of, 55
Oculocephalic reflex, cranial nerve assess-
    ment and, 61–62
Oculovestibular reflex, cranial nerve assess-
    ment and, 62
Oliguria, differential diagnosis of, 378t
Open fracture, 553
Open pneumothorax, chest trauma and,
    547t
Oral feeding, 486
Organ donation
    kidneys, 392
    legal issues in, 26–27
Orientation, assessment of, 56
Orthopedic trauma, 552–557
    assessment of, 552–554
    complications with, 556–557
    nursing diagnoses and, 554
    outcome evaluation in, 557
    planning and implementation of care in,
        554–557
    risk conditions in, 552
    signs and symptoms of, 553–554
Orthostatic hypotension, restricted activity
    and, 499
Orthostatic intolerance, 499
Osmitrol. See Mannitol
Osmol, definition of, 398
Osmolality
    definition of, 398
    of urine, 374
Osmolarity, definition of, 398
Osmoreceptors, water output control and,
    397
Osmosis, definition of, 398
Osmotic diuretics, 607–608
Osteoporosis, restricted activity and,
    503–504
Otorrhea, 534, 535
Oxazepam, 599–600
Oxygenation, indices of, 151
Oxygen therapy, 186–189
    complications of, 188–189
    guidelines for initial selection, 186
    methods of, 186–188
    options in, 187t
    outcome evaluation in, 189
Oxygen toxicity
    mechanical ventilation and, 205
    prevention of, 189
Oxyhemoglobin dissociation curve, 151–152
    shifts in, 152f

Pacemaker cells, cardiac, 267
Pacemaker rhythms, 355f

Pacemakers, 350–356
    external, 353f
    indications for, 350, 351t
    modes of pacing and, 351–352
    pacing catheters and, bedside insertion,
        352–353
    postinsertion nursing care and, 354–356
Pain, 126–130
    acute chest pain and, 305
    acute myocardial infarction and, 308
    acute pancreatitis and, 474
    AIDS and, 456, 457–458
    assessment of, 126–128
    burns and, 561
    cardiac tamponade and, 332
    chest trauma and, 548–549
    DIC and, 453
    gastrointestinal assessment and, 462
    nursing diagnoses and, 128
    orthopedic trauma and, 555
    outcome evaluation in, 130
    peritoneal dialysis and, 389–390
    planning and implementation of care in,
        128–130
    pneumothorax and, 172
    pulmonary embolus and, 175
    renal failure and, 381, 382
    risk conditions in, 126–128
    signs and symptoms of, 128
    somatic, 462
    spinal cord injury and, 542–543
    visceral, 462
Palpation
    aeration assessment and, 140–141
    gastrointestinal assessment and, 462–465
    renal assessment and, 370
Palpitations, cardiovascular system assess-
    ment and, 218
Pancreatectomy, 475
Pancreatitis, acute, 473–475
    assessment of, 473–474
    nursing diagnoses and, 474
    outcome evaluation in, 475
    planning and implementation of care in,
        474–475
    risk conditions in, 473
    signs and symptoms of, 473–474
Pancuronium bromide, 611–612
Panwarfin. See Warfarin
Paralytic ileus, burns and, 564
Paraplegia, 539, 539t
Parenteral fluid replacement, for shock,
    341–342t
Parenteral nutrition, 486
    See also Total parenteral nutrition
Paroxysmal atrial tachycardia (PAT), ECG
    tracing of, 279t
Partial pressure, definition of, 149
Partial thromboplastin time, 449
    DIC and, 450
Paternalism, 20–21
Patient
    adaptation stages of, 37, 41–43
    concerns of, 36
    death of, 18, 46–47

expectations of, 36
medical history of, 35–36
sensory-perceptual alterations in, 39–41
terminal, 22, 46–47
See also Coping, ineffective
Pavulon, 611–612
PEEP. *See* Positive-end expiratory pressure
Peganone, 605–606
Pelvic fractures, 556
Penetrating trauma, 520, 524, 545
Pentaerythritol tetranitrate, 610–611
Pentamidine, 456
Percussion
    aeration assessment and, 141
    blunt, 464
    gastrointestinal assessment and, 462–464
    renal assessment and, 370
Percutaneous transluminal coronary angio-
        plasty (PTCA), 356–359
    candidates for, 356
    care following, 358–359
    medications used for, 357t
    patient preparation for, 357
    procedure, 357–358
Perfusion, skin, cardiovascular system as-
        sessment and, 219
Perfusion scans, lung, 157
Pericardial tap, pneumothorax and, 171
Pericardiocentesis, for cardiac tamponade,
        333
Pericarditis
    cardiac tamponade and, 331
    chest pain profile in, 306t
    pulmonary artery pressures and, 254
    pulsus paradoxus and, 222
Peripheral arterial pulses, evaluation of, 220
Peripheral cyanosis, respiratory distress
        and, 140
Peripheral resistance, determination of, 224
Peripheral venous nutrition, 486
Peritoneal dialysis, 388–390
    access in, 388
    hemodialysis compared, 383
    monitoring, 389–390
    preparation for, 389
    systems of, 388
Peritoneal lavage, 550–551
Peritonitis, peritoneal dialysis and, 389–390
Peritrate, 610–611
Peritubular system, 370
pH, definition of, 413
Pharmacologic therapy. *See* Drug therapy
Pharyngeal airways, 192
Phenobarbital, for status epilepticus, 96–97
Phenytoin
    pharmacology of, 605–606
    for status epilepticus, 96
Phosphate buffer system, 414, 415f
Phosphonoformate, 458
Physical activity. *See* Activity
Physical examination, cardiovascular,
        218–236
    blood pressure auscultation in, 220–226
    general inspection in, 218–219
    heart examination in, 227–236

neck vein examination in, 226–227
peripheral arterial pulse evaluation in, 220
skin examination in, 219–220
Physical mobility, and spinal cord trauma,
        531, 542
Physiologic shunt, 153–154
Pia mater, 56
Pindolol, 600–601
Plasma expanders, parenteral fluid replace-
        ment with, 341t
Plasmin, blood coagulation and, 449
Plasminogen, blood coagulation and, 449
Platelet aggregation, IABP and, 365
Platelet count, DIC and, 450
Platelets, 446, 447
    blood coagulation and, 448
Pleural effusion, 173–174
    assessment of, 173–174
    chest X-ray and, 157
    nursing diagnoses and, 173
    outcome evaluation in, 174
    risk conditions in, 173
    signs and symptoms in, 173
Pleurevac disposable chest drainage sys-
        tem, 207, 208f
Pneumatic antishock garment (PASG), 340,
        343, 531f, 554
Pneumocystis carinii pneumonia, 455, 456
Pneumonectomy, 211
Pneumonia, 170–171
    assessment of, 170–171
    chest pain profile in, 306t
    nursing diagnoses and, 170
    outcome evaluation in, 171
    planning and implementation of care in,
        171
    risk factors in, 170
    signs and symptoms of, 170–171
Pneumotaxic area, inspiration and, 138
Pneumothorax, 171–173
    assessment of, 171–172
    chest drainage and, 209
    chest X-ray and, 157
    CVP line insertion and, 252
    mechanical ventilation and, 205
    nursing diagnoses and, 172
    outcome evaluation in, 173
    planning and implementation of care in,
        172–173
    risk conditions in, 171
    signs and symptoms of, 171–172
    spontaneous, chest pain profile in, 306t
    thoracic surgery and, 211
    tracheal deviation and, 140
Polymorphonuclear leukocytes, 446
Pons, 52
Positive end-expiratory pressure (PEEP),
        202
    airway pressure curves of, 202f
    ARDS and, 164
    discontinuation of, 206
    fat embolism and, 556
    intrathoracic/intracranial pressure and, 87
Positive pressure ventilation, pneumothorax
        and, 171

Positron-emitted tomography (PET), 243
Postnecrotic cirrhoses, 478, 479
Postural drainage positions, 190f
Postural vital signs, assessment of,
        465–466
Posturing, 66
Potassium, roles of, 404
Potassium imbalances, 404–408, 405t
    in acute renal failure, 378
    burns and, 563
    outcome evaluation in, 407
Potassium ion imbalance, 421–422
Potassium-removing resins, 613–614
Povidone-iodine, for burns, 566t
PQ interval, 273
PQRST mnemonic, cardiovascular system
        assessment and, 218t
Precapillary sphincters, control of, 224
Precordium, 227
Prednisolone, 596–597
Prednisone, 596–597
Preload, 322–323, 362
    cardiac failure and, 328
    cardiac failure risk and, 323
    cardiac output and, 256
    central venous pressure and, 251
Premature beats, 292–294
    ECG tracings of, 296–299t
Premature ventricular beats, sudden cardiac
        death and, 346
Pressure autoregulation, 82
Pressure gradients, O2 and CO2, gas ex-
        change and, 149–150
Pressure ulcers, restricted activity and, 503
Presystolic gallop, 234
PR interval, 273
Procainamide
    for cardiac arrest, 347t, 349
    pharmacology of, 612
    for ventricular tachycardia, 302
Procardia, 601
Pronestyl. *See* Procainamide
Propranolol, 600–601
Propylthiouracil (PTU), thyroid crisis and,
        437
Protein overload, total parenteral nutrition
        and, 492
Proteinuria, renal disease, and, 375
Proteolysis, malnutrition and, 485
Proteus, septic shock and, 335
Prothrombin, blood coagulation and, 449
Prothrombin time, 449
    DIC and, 450
Protodiastolic gallop, 234
Proventil, 597
Pseudomonas aeruginosa
    septic shock and, 235
    wound infections and, 565
Pulmonary angiography, 158
Pulmonary artery, function of, 229
Pulmonary artery catheters, 252–257
    complications of, 256–257
    insertion of, 252–253
Pulmonary artery end-diastolic pressure,
        248

Pulmonary artery pressures
  monitoring of, 253–254
  normal, 248f
  waveform of, 254f
Pulmonary blood volume, pulmonary artery
    pressures and, 254
Pulmonary capillary (artery) wedge pres-
    sure
  measurement of, 248
  monitoring of, 254–255
  normal, 248f
  waveform of, 254f
Pulmonary edema, 161–162
  assessment of, 161–162
  nursing diagnoses and, 162
  outcome evaluation in, 162
  planning and implementation of care in,
    162
  signs and symptoms of, 162
  trauma and, 537–538
Pulmonary embolus, 174–177
  assessment of, 174–176
  cardiac failure risk and, 324
  central venous pressure and, 251
  chest pain profile in, 306t
  nursing diagnoses and, 176
  outcome evaluation in, 177
  planning and implementation of care in,
    176–177
  pulmonary artery pressures and, 239
  restricted activity and, 502
  risk conditions in, 174–175
  signs and symptoms of, 175–176
Pulmonary function, symbols related to,
    147–149f
Pulmonary function tests, 142–146
Pulmonary hypertension
  cardiac failure risk and, 324
  pulmonary artery pressures and, 254
Pulmonary infarction
  pulmonary artery catheterization and, 256
  signs and symptoms of, 175–176
Pulmonary thromboembolism, sudden death
    and, 346
Pulmonary vascular resistance, pulmonary
    artery pressures and, 254
Pulmonary veins, function of, 229
Pulmonic area, location of, 229, 230f
Pulmonic stenosis, central venous pressure
    and, 251
Pulmonic valve, location of, 229
Pulse. See specific type
Pulse pressure, definition of, 221
Pulse rate, changes in, assessment of, 72
Pulsus paradoxus, 222, 332
Pump lung, 163
Pupillary responses, cranial nerve assess-
    ment and, 60
Pupils
  abnormal, cranial nerve assessment and,
    60
  in comatose patients, 61f
Pupil size and shape, cranial nerve assess-
    ment and, 60

P wave, 270–273
  atrial depolarization and, 268
Pyrimethamine, 456

Q RS complex, 268–270, 273
QRST complex, 268
QT interval, 273
Quadriplegia, 539, 539t
Quinaglute, 612–613
Quinidine, 612–613
Q wave, 273

R adiation therapy, basophil count and, 447
Radiographic studies, abdominal trauma and,
    550
Radionuclide studies, 242–244, 313–314
Rales, 141
Ramirez shunt, hemodialysis and, 384
Range of motion, restricted activity and,
    503
Ranitidine
  pharmacology of, 613
  for stress ulcers, 538
  for upper GI bleeding, 471
RBCs, 446
Rebound tenderness, peritoneal inflamma-
    tion and, 464
Rectum, physical examination of, 465
Red blood cell hemaglutination inhibition im-
    mune assay, 449
Red blood cells, functions of, 446
Red cell count, normal, 446–447
Refractometer, urine specific gravity and,
    374
Refractory periods, 266
Relative refractory period, 266
REM rebound, 511
  alcoholism and, 512
REM sleep, 508
Renal arterial thrombosis, acute renal failure
    and, 376
Renal assessment, 369–376
  format for, 369t
  history and physical examination in, 370
  laboratory tests in, 370–376
Renal blood flow, autoregulation of,
    371–372
Renal buffer system, 414
Renal disease, proteinuria in, 375
Renal failure
  acute, 376–392
    assessment of, 376–392
    care planning and implementation in,
      380–382
    dialysis and, 382–392
    nursing care plan for, 379–380t
    nursing diagnoses and, 378
    phases of, 378, 380
    prevention of, 377
    risk conditions in, 376–377
    shock and, 343
    signs and symptoms of, 377–378
  fluid volume excess and, 400
Renal function, tests of, 374–376
Renal infarction, LDH elevations in, 239

Renal transplantation, 392–393
Renal tubule, 371
Renin, angiotensin II formation and, 372
Residual volume, measurement of, 143–144
Respiratory acidosis, 414, 416t
  planning and implementation of care in,
    423
Respiratory acids, definition of, 413
Respiratory failure
  chronic, 177–183
  definition of, 161
  restricted activity and, 502
Respiratory alkalosis, 414, 417t
  acute myocardial infarction and, 308
  planning and implementation of care in,
    424
Respiratory buffer system, 414
Respiratory center, 138–139
Respiratory changes, assessment of, 72–74
Respiratory patterns, abnormal, 73f
Respiratory rate and rhythm, aeration as-
    sessment and, 138–139
Respondeat superior, 23
Resting membrane potential, cardiac, 264
Restoril, 599–600
Restrictive disorders, definition of, 161
Reticular activating system, 54f
  consciousness and, 54
Reticulocyte count, 446–447
Reverse transcriptase, 455
Rhinorrhea, 534, 535
Rhonchi, 141–142
Rhythmicity, 267
Ribavirin, 458
Right atrial pressure
  normal, 253
  waveform of, 252f
Right heart failure, status asthmaticus and,
    183
Right ventricular failure signs and symptoms
    of, 324–325
  thromboembolism and, 175
Right ventricular infarction, central venous
    pressure and, 251
Right ventricular pressure
  monitoring of, 253
  normal, 249, 253f
Rigid bronchoscope, 157
Rule of nines, burn evaluation and, 559,
    559f

S ager splint, 554
Sarcomere, 323
Sarcoplasmic reticulum, 323
Scribner shunt, hemodialysis and, 384
Sectral, 600–601
Sedation, for cerebral edema, 89
Seizures, head trauma and, 538
  See also Status epilepticus
Self-concept, disturbed
  acute chest pain and, 307
  altered body image and, 512–513
  DIC and, 454
  malnutrition and, 486
  spinal cord injury and, 543

Sengstaken-Blakemore tube, esophageal varices and, 471–472, 472f
Sensation, assessment of, 62–66
Sensorimotor function, assessment of, 62–70
Sensory-perceptual alterations, 39–41
    AIDS and, 456–457
    liver failure and, 481
    upper GI bleeding and, 469–470
Sensory tracts, right side, 65f
Septicemia, 457
Septic shock
    acute renal failure and, 376
    pathophysiologic changes in, 335–336
    signs and symptoms of, 337
Serax, 599–600
Serial body weights, monitoring of, 396–397
Serratia spp., septic shock and, 335
Serum amylase concentration, acute pancreatitis and, 474
Serum enzymes
    evaluation of, 238–239
    myocardial infarction and, 238t, 313–314
    shock and, 338t
Serum glutamic oxaloacetic transaminase (SGOT), 239, 479
Sexual counseling, 513, 515t, 516t
Sexual dysfunction, restricted activity and, 513–514
SGOT, 239, 479
Shaldon catheter, hemodialysis and, 384
Sheet grafts, 568
Shivering, normal thermoregulatory responses and, 440–441
Shock, 333–344
    assessment of, 333–339
    hemodynamic responses in, 336t
    hypothermia and, 443
    laboratory data in, 337, 338–339t
    nursing diagnoses and, 339
    outcome evaluation in, 344
    parenteral fluid replacement in, 341–342t
    pathophysiologic changes in, 334–336
    planning and implementation of care in, 339–344
    prevention of, 337
    risk conditions in, 333–334
    signs and symptoms of, 336–337
    spinal cord, 540
Shock lung, 163, 344
Shortness of breath, cardiovascular assessment and, 216, 218
SIADH, 401, 538
Silhouette sign, 155
Silvadene, 566t
Silver nitrate, for burns, 566t
Silver sulfadiazine, for burns, 566t
Simple fracture, 553, 553f
Sinoatrial node action potential location, 266
    ventricular action potential vs., 267f
Sinus arrest
    ECG tracing of, 279t
    hyperkalemia and, 407
Sinus arrhythmia, ECG tracing of, 278t

Sinus blocks, 276
Sinus bradycardia, ECG tracing of, 276, 277t
Sinus rhythms, 277–279t
Sinus tachycardia, ECG tracing of, 278t
Skin, structure of, 557, 558f
Skin examination, cardiovascular system assessment and, 219–220
Skin grafts, for burns, 567–568
Skin integrity, impaired
    DIC and, 453
    Guillain-Barré syndrome and, 106
    hypothermia and, 438, 441
    liver failure and, 482
    orthopedic trauma and, 555
Skull bones, 56
Skull fractures, 534–535
Sleep
    cycles of, 508
    desynchronized, 508
    pattern disturbance, 508, 511–512
    stages of, 508
Sleep apnea, 512
Sleep deprivation, 511
Sleep pattern disturbances, restricted activity and, 508, 511–512
Smoking
    bronchitis and, 177–178
    emphysema and, 177–178
    sudden cardiac death and, 346
Snaps, 234
Sodium, roles of, 401
Sodium bicarbonate
    for acidosis in shock, 343
    actions of, 346–348
    for cardiac arrest, 346–348, 347t
Sodium concentration, control of, 397
Sodium edecrin, 607
Sodium imbalances, 401–404
    outcome evaluation in, 403–404
Sodium ion imbalance, 421
Sodium nitroprusside
    for cardiac failure, 330–331
    for shock, 343
Sodium polystyrene sulfonate
    for hyperkalemia, 407
    pharmacology of, 613–614
Solu-medrol. *See* Methylprednisolone
Somatic pain, 462
Somophyllin. *See* Aminophylline
Sorbitrate, 610–611
Sound transmission, aeration assessment and, 140
Specific gravity, of urine, 374
Speech loss, impaired verbal communication and, 34–35, 38–39
Spinal cord, cross section of, 64f
Spinal cord shock, 540
Spinal cord trauma, 539–545
    assessment in emergency department, 541
    classification of, 539–540, 539t
    diagnosis and treatment of, 541
    impaired physical mobility with, 531, 542
    nursing diagnoses and, 541

outcome evaluation in, 544–545
    planning and implementation of care in, 541–543
Spinal nerve plexuses, peripheral nerves arising from, 63f
Spinal reflexes, cranial nerve assessment and, 66–69
Spleen, palpation of, 464–465, 465f
Splenectomy, basophil count and, 447
Sprain, 552–553
Stab wounds, 524, 526t
Standard care plans, 585–588t
    for mitral valve replacement, 585t
    purpose of, 576–578
Staphylococcus aureus, wound infections and, 565
Starling's law of capillaries, 219
Starvation
    ketonuria in, 375
    physiology of, 485–486
    See also Malnutrition
Status asthmaticus, 179–183
    assessment of, 180
    nursing diagnoses and, 180
    outcome evaluation in, 183
    planning and implementation of care in, 180–183
    risk conditions in, 180
    signs and symptoms of, 180
Status epilepticus, 93–97
    assessment of, 94–95
    causes of, 94t
    classification of seizures, 93t
    nursing diagnoses and, 95
    outcome evaluation in, 97
    planning and implementation of care in, 95–97
    risk factors in, 94
    signs and symptoms of, 94–95
Sternal angle, 227
Steroids
    for ARDS, 165–166
    for cerebral edema, 88
    fluid volume excess and, 400
    for pneumothorax, 171
    for status asthmaticus, 182t
Stiff lung, 163
Stimulation, restricted activity and, 508–514
Stimulation assessment, 51–79
    diagnostic procedures in, 74–79
    history in, 52
    physical examination in, 52–74
Stimulation disorders, 80–114
    See also specific disorder
Stimulation treatment techniques, 117–130
    craniotomy, 118–121
    pain management, 128–130
    ventricular shunts, 121–126
Strain, 553
Streptase, 614
Streptococci, beta-hemolytic, wound infections and, 565
Streptokinase, 614

Stress
    in critical-care nursing, 17–19
    fluid volume excess and, 400
    of organ donation, 25
Stress response, burns and, 564–565
Stroke, 97–103
    body locus of, 98t
    diagnosis of, 99–100
    embolic, 98
    hemorrhagic, 98–99
    management of, 100
    nursing diagnoses and, 101
    occlusive, 97–98
    outcome evaluation in, 103
    planning and implementation of care in,
        101–103
    thrombotic, 97–98
Stroke volume
    cardiac failure and, 322
    cardiac output and, 222, 224
    restricted activity and, 499
ST segment, 273
Stupor, definition of, 55
Subarachnoid hemorrhage, 81
Subarachnoid screw, intracranial pressure
    monitoring and, 83, 84f
Subdural hematoma, 535–536
Sudden death, 346
Sulfadizine, 456
Sulfamylon, 566t
Sulfonamides, neutrophil count and, 447
Summation gallop, 234
Superficial partial-thickness burns, 558
Supraventricular rhythms, ECG tracings of,
    279–280t
Supraventricular tachycardia, ECG tracing
    of, 280t
Supraventricular tachycardia with aberra-
    tion, ECG tracing of, 280t
Surgical decompression, for cerebral
    edema, 89
Sustachron, 610–611
Sutilains, for burns, 566t
Swan-Ganz pulmonary artery catheter, 252
Sympathomimetic agents, 597, 611
Syncope, cardiovascular system assessment
    and, 218
Syndrome of inappropriate antidiuretic hor-
    mone, 401, 538
Systemic vascular resistance, determination
    of, 224
Systemic venous congestion, cardiac tam-
    ponade and, 332
Systolic ejection murmurs, 235
Systolic murmurs, 234, 235

Tachycardia
    cardiac output and, 302
    definition of, 275–276
    hypokalemia and, 404
    restricted activity and, 498
Tactile fremitus, 140–141
Tactile perception, communication and, 34
Tagamet. See Cimetidine
Tapazole, 437

T cells, 455, 456, 458
Technological advances, 17
Temazepam, 599–600
Temperature changes
    assessment of, 72
    thyroid crisis and, 436
Tenormin, 600–601
Tension pneumothorax
    chest trauma and, 547t
    trauma and, 530
Tensilon, 604–605
Tentorium cerebelli, 56
Terbutaline, 614–615
Terminal care, 22, 46–47
Tetany, 410
Thalamus, 52
Therapeutic hypothermia, 437–444
    assessment in, 437–438
    outcome evaluation in, 444
    planning and implementation of care in,
        438–442
    rewarming and, 442–443
Thermoregulation
    burns and, 564
    spinal cord shock and, 542
Thermoregulatory center, 438
Thermoregulatory response, normal
    altered tissue perfusion and, 439–440
    shivering and, 440–441
Third-spacing, fluid volume deficit and, 400
Thirst, sodium concentration and, 397
Thoracentesis, pneumothorax and, 158–159
Thoracic shape, aeration assessment and,
    138
Thoracic surgery, 210–211
Thorax, examination of, 137–138
Thorazine, 441
Thought, assessment of, 56
Thrombocytes. See Platelets
Thromboembolism
    causes of, 174
    IABP and, 365
    preventive measures for, 174–175
    pulmonary artery catheterization and, 257
    signs and symptoms of, 175
    See also Pulmonary embolus
Thrombolytic agents, 614
Thrombosis
    AV shunts and, 385
    hypothermia and, 442
Thyroid crisis, 435–437
    assessment of, 435–436
    nursing diagnoses and, 436
    outcome evaluation in, 437
    planning and implementation of care in,
        436–437
Thyroid storm, 435
Thyrotoxicosis, 435
Tidal volume, measurement of, 143
Timolol, 600–601
Tissue injury, DIC and, 450
Tissue integrity, impaired
    AIDS and, 456, 457
    trauma and, 532

Tissue perfusion, altered
    acid-base imbalances and, 418, 423
    activity intolerance and, 498–500
    acute chest pain and, 307
    burns and, 563–564
    cardiac tamponade and, 332
    continuous ultrafiltration and, 392
    DIC and, 453
    hyperglycemic hyperosmolar nonketotic
        coma and, 433
    hypothermia and, 438, 439–440, 442
    normal thermoregulatory responses and,
        439–440
    renal transplantation and, 392–393
    shock and, 339
    spinal cord injury and, 542, 543
    trauma and, 530
    upper GI bleeding and, 469
Tonicity, definition of, 398
Topical preparations, for burn care, 566t
Torsâde de pointes, 286t
Tort law, 23
Total lung capacity, measurement of, 144
Total parenteral nutrition, 486–493
    catheter insertion and, 487
    discontinuation of, 493
    initiation of, 486–487
    nutrients supplied via, 487–490
    physical activity and, 490
    potential complications of, 490–493
Total solids meter, urine specific gravity
    and, 374
Toxoplasmosis encephalitis, 456
Trace elements, total parenteral nutrition
    and, 489
Tracheal stimulation, dysrhythmias and, 301
Tracheal suctioning, 197–200
    complications of
        prevention of, 198–199
        treatment of, 200
    outcome evaluation in, 200
Tracheostomy tube, 194
Traction splint, 555
Trandate, 600–601
Transderm-Nitro, 610–611
Transducer, central venous pressure moni-
    toring with, 250f
Transient ischemic attack (TIA), 97
Transplants. See Organ donation
Transport maximum, tubular reabsorption
    and, 373
Transtentorial herniation, signs and symp-
    toms of, 90–91f
Trauma, 519–569
    abdominal, 549–552
    acute period
        outcome evaluation in, 533
        planning and implementation of care in,
            532–533
    assessment and, 525–527, 526t, 527t
    blunt, 520, 523, 545
    burns, 557–569
    chest injuries, 545–549
    definition of, 520

emergent period
  outcome evaluation in, 531–532
  planning and implementation of care in, 527–531
estimated fluid and blood requirements with, 531t
head injury, 533–538
major, 520
minor, 520
multiple, 522, 527, 528t
nursing diagnoses and, 528
orthopedic, 552–557
penetrating, 520, 524,545
physical examination with, 526–527
risk factors with, 525
spinal cord, 531, 539–545
Trauma care system, essential components of, 521t
Trauma-center care, injuries and physiologic states benefitting from, 520t
Trauma team
  makeup of, 521t
  protocol for critical-care nurse, 521–522, 521t
Travase, 566t
Trendelenburg position, 537
Triamcinolone, 596–597
Triazolam, 599–600
Tricuspid area, location of, 229, 230f
Tridil, 610–611
Trimethoprim-sulfamethoxazole, 456
Troponin, 323
Trousseau's sign, positive, 410
Tubular reabsorption, 373
  countercurrent mechanism and, 373
T wave, 273
  ventricular depolarization and, 268
Tympany, 464

Ulcers
  hypothermia and, 443
  pressure, 503
  stress, 538
Ultrafiltration, hemodialysis and, 383t, 387, 390–392
Uncal herniation, signs and symptoms of, 89, 91–93, 92f
Upper airway injury
  artificial airways and, 195–196
  burns and, 561–562
Upper gastrointestinal hemorrhage, 465–473
  assessment of, 465
  nursing diagnoses and, 466
  outcome evaluation in, 473
  planning and implementation of care in, 466–473
  signs and symptoms of, 465–466
Upright abdominal film, 550
Uremic pericarditis, acute renal failure and, 381–382
Ureteral colic, 370
Urinalysis, routine, 374–375
Urinary elimination pattern, alteration in activity intolerance and, 500–501

burns and, 564
DIC and, 453
liver failure and, 482
peritoneal dialysis and, 390
spinal cord injury and, 542
Urinary stones, precipitation of, restricted activity and, 500
Urinary tract obstruction, acute renal failure and, 376
Urine, dilute or concentrated, excretion of, 373–374
Urine concentration, countercurrent mechanism for, 374f
Urine formation, 370–374
Urine measurements
  in acute renal failure, 378t
  in shock, 339t
Urine osmalality/specific gravity, 374
  in acute renal failure, 377
Urine sodium levels, in acute renal failure, 377
Urine volume, 374
  in acute renal failure, 377
Urokinase, 614
Utilitarian ethical method, 21
U wave, 273

Vagal stimulation, dysrhythmias and, 301–302
Validation, nursing diagnosis and, 10
Valium. See Diazepam
Valsalva maneuver
  dysrhythmias and, 301
  restricted activity and, 499
Valvular insufficiency, central venous pressure and, 251
Valvular regurgitation, cardiac failure risk and, 323
Vanceril, 595–596
Vasa recta, 370
Vascular disorders, 97–103, 161
Vasoconstrictors
  for cardiac failure, 329
  for shock, 343
Vasodilators
  for cardiac failure, 330–331
  for shock, 343
Vasodilator theory, local blood flow control and, 224
Vasogenic edema, 536
Vasogenic shock, causes of, 334
Vasomotion, 224
Venous admixture, 154
Venous pressure, assessment of, 226–227
Venous pulse waves, 227f
  assessment of, 227
Ventilation-perfusion imbalance, impaired gas exchange and, 343
Ventilation/perfusion relationships, 150–151
Ventilation scans, lung, 157
Ventilators
  settings of, 203
  types of, 201
Ventolin, 597

Ventricles, heart, location of, 228–229
Ventricular aberration, ectopy vs., 294f
Ventricular action potential
  ionic movements and, 265f
  SA nodal action potential vs., 267f
Ventricular asystole
  ECG tracing of, 286t
  hyperkalemia and, 407
  hypokalemia and, 404
Ventricular catheter, intracranial pressure monitoring and, 83
Ventricular contractility
  cardiac output and, 256
  central venous pressure and, 251
Ventricular depolarization, QRS complex and, 268
Ventricular dysrhythmias
  pulmonary artery catheterization and, 256
  supraventricular aberration vs., 295t
Ventricular failure, acute renal failure and, 376
Ventricular fibrillation
  ECG tracing of, 285t
  hyperkalemia and, 407
  hypokalemia and, 404
Ventricular filling time, decreased, myocardial ischemia/infarction and, 324
Ventricular gallop, 234
Ventricular premature beats
  ECG tracing of, 298t
  subcategories of, ECG tracings of, 299–300t
Ventricular puncture, 75
Ventricular rhythms, ECG tracings of, 284–286t
Ventricular septal defect, central venous pressure and, 251
Ventricular shunts, 121–126, 123f
  complications of, 124
  function of, 123
  insertion procedure, 123
  planning and implementation of care with, 125–126
  rationale for insertion, 122
Ventricular tachycardia, ECG tracing of, 285t, 286t
Ventriculography, 246
Veracity principle, 20
Verapamil, 349, 601
Verbal response, consciousness and, 56
Versed, 599–600
Visceral pain, 462
Vision deficit, impaired verbal communication and, 38–39
Visken, 600–601
Visual input, communication and, 32
Visual pathways, 34f
Vital capacity, measurement of, 144–145
Vital signs, examination of, 70–74
Vitamin-mineral abnormalities, total parenteral nutrition and, 493
Vitamins, total parenteral nutrition and, 489
Voluntary motor activity, 66–70
Vulnerable period, 266

W andering baseline, 263f, 264
Warfarin
    pharmacology of, 615
    for PTCA, 357t
Water imbalances, mechanical ventilation
        and, 205
Water intoxication, 401
Water output, control of, 397–398

WBCs, 446–447
Wet lung, 163
Wheezes, 141
Whispered pectoriloquy, 142
White blood cells, functions of, 446–447
White cell count, normal, 446
White cell differential count, 446
Whole blood, parenteral fluid replacement
        with, 341t

Work load capacities, restricted activity
        and, 506t

X anax, 599–600
Xeroform, 566t
Xylocaine. *See* Lidocaine

Z antac. *See* Ranitidine